# Anesthesiologist's Manual of Surgical Procedures

# Anesthesiologist's Manual of Surgical Procedures

Editors

**Richard A. Jaffe, M.D., Ph.D.**
Assistant Professor of Anesthesia

and

**Stanley I. Samuels, M.B., B.Ch.**
Professor of Anesthesia

Stanford University School of Medicine
Stanford, California

Raven Press New York

**Raven Press, Ltd., 1185 Avenue of the Americas, New York, New York 10036**



Made in the United States of America

**Library of Congress Cataloging-in-Publication Data**

Anesthesiologist's manual of surgical procedures / edited by Richard A. Jaffe and Stanley I. Samuels.
p. cm.
Includes bibliographical references and index.
ISBN 0-7817-0012-4
1. Anesthesiology. 2. Surgery, Operative. 3. Operations, Surgical.
I. Jaffe, Richard A. II. Samuels, Stanley I.
[DNLM: 1. Anesthesia--methods. 2. Anesthesiology. 3. Surgery, Operative.
WO 235 A5795 1994]
RD81.A545 1994
617.9'6--dc20
DNLM/DLC
for Library of Congress 93-50933

---

The material contained in this volume was submitted as previously unpublished material, except in the instances in which credit has been given to the source from which some of the illustrative material was derived.

Great care has been taken to maintain the accuracy of the information contained in the volume. However, neither Raven Press nor the authors can be held responsible for errors or for any consequences arising from the use of the information contained herein.

9 8 7 6 5 4 3 2 1

This book is respectfully dedicated to
our friend, mentor, and teacher

*C. Philip Larson, Jr., M.D., M.S.*

# TABLE OF CONTENTS

# CONTRIBUTORS

**John Adler, MD**
Assistant Professor of Neurosurgery
Stanford University School of Medicine
Stanford, California 94305
(*Stereotactic Neurosurgery*)

**Edward J. Alfrey, MD**
Assistant Professor
Department of Surgery
Stanford University School of Medicine
Stanford, California 94305
(*Liver and Kidney Transplantation*)

**Sandra Leigh Bardas, RPh, BS**
Operating Room Pharmacist
Stanford University Medical Center
Stanford, California 94305
(*Drug Interactions*)

**John G. Brock-Utne, MA, MD, PhD, FFA**
Professor of Anesthesia
Stanford University School of Medicine
Stanford, California 94305
(*Otolaryngology*)

**Jay B. Brodsky, MD**
Professor of Anesthesia
Stanford University School of Medicine
Stanford, California 94305
(*Thoracic Surgery*)

**Gordon A. Brody, MD**
Clinical Assistant Professor of Orthopedics
Stanford University School of Medicine
Stanford, California 94305
Hand Surgeon
Stanford University Medical Center
Stanford, California 94305
Sports, Orthopedics and Rehabilitation Medicine Associates
Menlo Park, California 94025
(*Hand Surgery*)

**Sally Byrd, MD**
Clinical Instructor of Ophthalmic Surgery
Stanford University School of Medicine
Stanford, California 94305
Staff Surgeon
Department of Ophthalmology
Veterans Affairs Medical Center
Palo Alto, California 94304
(*Ophthalmic Surgery*)

**Eugene J. Carragee, MD**
Assistant Professor in Orthopedic Surgery
Director, Orthopedic Spine Service
Stanford University School of Medicine
Stanford, California 94305
(*Spine Surgery*)

**Carter Cherry, MD**
Staff Anesthesiologist
Santa Clara Valley Medical Center
San Jose, California 95128
(*Gynecology/Infertility, Obstetric Surgery*)

**Sheila E. Cohen, MB, ChB, FRCA**
Professor of Anesthesia
Director, Obstetrical Anesthesia
Stanford University School of Medicine
Stanford, California 94305
(*Gynecology/Infertility, Obstetric Surgery*)

**John J. Csongradi, MD**
Associate Chief
Department of Orthopedic Surgery
Santa Clara Valley Medical Center
San Jose, California 95128
Clinical Associate Professor
Stanford University School of Medicine
Stanford, California 94305
(*Orthopedic Surgery for Lower Extremities*)

**Donald C. Dafoe, MD**
Associate Professor, Department of Surgery
Chief, Division of Transplantation
Director, Multi-Organ Transplant Center
Stanford University School of Medicine
Stanford, California 94305
(*Liver and Kidney Transplantation*)

**Steven Deem, MD**
Assistant Professor of Anesthesia
University of Washington
Seattle, Washington 98195
(*Urology*)

**Jayshree Desai, MD**
Clinical Assistant Professor of Anesthesia
Stanford University School of Medicine
Stanford, California 94305
(*Ophthalmic Surgery*)

**Sarah S. Donaldson, MD, FACR**
Professor of Radiation Oncology
Stanford University School of Medicine

Director of Radiation Oncology
Lucile Salter Packard Children's Hospital at Stanford
Stanford, California 94305
(*Pediatric Radiation Therapy*)

**John A. Duncan III, MD, PhD**
Assistant Professor of Neurosurgery
Georgetown University Medical Center
Washington DC 20007
(*Pediatric Neurosurgery*)

**Babak Edraki, MD**
Staff Physician and Clinical Research Associate
Director
Stanford Women's Group Dysplasia Clinic
Department of Gynecology and Obstetrics
Stanford University School of Medicine
Stanford, California 94305
Instructor, Stanford Endoscopy Center for Training and Technology
Stanford University Medical Center
Stanford, California 94305
(*Gynecological Oncology, Obstetric Surgery*)

**Talmage D. Egan, MD**
Assistant Professor of Anesthesia
University Hospital
Salt Lake City, Utah 84112
(*Hand, Shoulder Surgery*)

**Peter R. Egbert, MD**
Professor and Chairman
Department of Ophthalmology
Stanford University School of Medicine
Stanford, California 94305
(*Ophthalmic Surgery*)

**Yasser El-Sayed, MD**
Chief Resident, Obstetrics and Gynecology
Stanford University Hospital
Stanford, California 94305
(*Obstetric Surgery*)

**James I. Lin Fann, MD**
Cardiovascular Surgery Fellow
Stanford University School of Medicine
Stanford, California 94305
(*Vascular Surgery*)

**Willard E. Fee, Jr, MD**
Professor and Chairman
Department of Otolaryngology
Stanford University School of Medicine
Stanford, California 94305
(*Otolaryngology Surgery*)

**Linda Foppiano, MD**
Clinical Assistant Professor of Anesthesia
Stanford University School of Medicine
Stanford, California 94305
(*Trauma Surgery*)

**Fuad S. Freiha, MD, FACS**
Chief, Urologic Oncology
Professor of Urology
Stanford University School of Medicine
Stanford, California 94305
(*Urology*)

**Raymond R. Gaeta, MD**
Assistant Professor of Anesthesia
Stanford University School of Medicine
Stanford, California 94305
(*Otolaryngology*)

**Michael W. Gaynon, MD**
Clinical Associate Professor of Ophthalmology
Stanford University School of Medicine
Stanford, California 94305
(*Retinal Surgery*)

**Ronald N. Gibson, MD**
Chief Resident
Department of Gynecology and Obstetrics
Stanford University School of Medicine
Stanford, California 94305
(*Obstetric Surgery*)

**Rona G. Giffard, MD, PhD**
Assistant Professor of Anesthesia
Stanford University School of Medicine
Stanford, California 94305
(*Aesthetic Surgery, Burn Surgery*)

**Stuart B. Goodman, MD, MSC, FRCS(C), FACS**
Associate Professor of Orthopedic Surgery
Stanford University School of Medicine
Stanford, California 94305
(*Orthopedic Surgery for Lower Extremities*)

**Alvin Hackel, MD**
Professor of Anesthesia and Pediatrics
Stanford University School of Medicine
Acting Head, Department of Anesthesia
Lucille Packard Childrens Hospital at Stanford
Stanford, California 94305
(*Pediatric General Surgery*)

**Gordon R. Haddow, MB, ChB, FFA(SA)**
Assistant Professor of Anesthesia
Stanford University School of Medicine
Stanford, California 94305

(*Cardiac, Vascular Surgery, Liver/Kidney Transplantation*)

**Gary E. Hartman, MD**
Associate Professor of Surgery and Pediatrics
Children's National Medical Center
Washington DC 20010
(*Pediatric General Surgery*)

**W. Leroy Heinrichs, MD, PhD**
Director, Section of Gynecology
Medical Director
Gynecology and Obstetrics Clinic
Stanford University School of Medicine
Stanford, California 94305
(*Gynecology/Infertility Surgery*)

**R. Harold Holbrook, Jr, MD**
Associate Professor, Maternal-Fetal Medicine
Stanford University School of Medicine
Stanford, California 94305
(*Obstetric Surgery*)

**Steven K. Howard, MD**
Assistant Professor of Anesthesia
Stanford University School of Medicine
Stanford, California 94305
Staff Anesthesiologist
Veterans Affairs Medical Center
Palo Alto, California 94304
(*General Surgery*)

**Richard A. Jaffe, MD, PhD**
Assistant Professor of Anesthesia
Stanford University School of Medicine
Stanford, California 94305
(*Dental, Ophthalmic, Restorative Surgery*)

**Stefanie S. Jeffrey, MD, FACS**
Clinical Associate Professor of Surgery
Stanford University School of Medicine
Stanford, California 94305
(*Breast Surgery*)

**Daniel S. Kapp, MD, PhD**
Professor of Radiation Oncology
Stanford University School of Medicine
Stanford, California 94305
Director, Clinical Hyperthermia
Department of Radiation Oncology
Stanford University Medical Center
Stanford, California 94305
(*Gynecological Oncology Surgery*)

**Amar Kaur, MD**
Senior Registrar
Singapore General Hospital
(*Otolaryngology*)

**Peter S. Kosek, MD**
Clinical Assistant Professor of Anesthesia
Stanford University School of Medicine
Stanford, California 94305
(*Orthopedic Surgery for Lower Extremities*)

**Amy L. Ladd, MD**
Assistant Professor
Department of Functional Restoration
Stanford University School of Medicine
Stanford, California 94305
Chief, Hand Clinic
Veterans Affairs Medical Center
Palo Alto, California 94304
Chief, Hand Clinic
Lucile Salter Packard Children's Hospital at Stanford
Stanford, California 94305
(*Shoulder Surgery*)

**C. Philip Larson, Jr, MD, MS**
Professor of Anesthesia and Neurosurgery
Stanford University School of Medicine
Stanford, California 94305
(*Adult and Pediatric Neurosurgery*)

**George Lederhaas, MD**
Staff Anesthesiologist
Nemour's Children's Clinic
Jacksonville, Florida 32209
(*Pediatric General Surgery*)

**Yuan-Chi Lin, MD**, MPH
Assistant Professor of Anesthesia and Pediatrics
Stanford University School of Medicine
Stanford, California 94305
(*Congenital Repair, Pediatric Orthopedic Surgery*)

**Padma Malipedi, MD**
Research Assistant
Department of Gynecology and Obstetrics
Stanford University School of Medicine
Stanford, California 94305
(*Gynecological Oncology Surgery*)

**James B.D. Mark, MD**
Johnson and Johnson Professor
Department of Cardiothoracic Surgery
Head, Division of Thoracic Surgery
Stanford University School of Medicine
Stanford, California 94305
(*Thoracic Surgery*)

**Frederick G. Mihm, MD**
Professor of Anesthesia
Stanford University School of Medicine
Stanford, California 94305
Associate Medical Director of ICUs
Stanford University Hospital
Stanford, California 94305
(*Orthopedic Surgery for Lower Extremities*)

**Steven R. Miller, PharmD**
Clinical Pharmacist
Department of Pharmacology
Stanford University Medical Center
Stanford, California 94305
(*Drug Interactions*)

**R. Scott Mitchell, MD**
Associate Professor of Cardiovascular Surgery
Stanford University School of Medicine
Stanford, California 94305
Chief, Division of Cardiac Surgery
Veterans Affairs Medical Center
Palo Alto, California 94304
(*Cardiac Surgery, Vascular Surgery*)

**Robert J. Moynihan, MD**
Medical Director
Department of Anesthesiology
Staff Physician
Departments of Anesthesia and Pediatrics
Sutter Memorial Hospital
Sacramento, California 95819
(*Pediatric Cardiovascular Surgery*)

**Harry A. Oberhelman, MD, FACS**
Chief, Division of Gastrointestinal Surgery
Professor of Gastrointestinal Surgery
Stanford University School of Medicine
Stanford, California 94305
(*Esophageal, Intestinal, Hepatic, Pancreatic, Peritoneal, Endocrine Surgery*)

**Ronald G. Pearl, MD, PhD**
Associate Professor of Anesthesia
Stanford University School of Medicine
Stanford, California 94305
(*Urology*)

**Kristi L. Peterson, MD**
Assistant Professor of Anesthesia
Stanford University School of Medicine
Stanford, California 94305
(*Vascular Surgery*)

**Barry Press, MD, FACS**
Assistant Professor of Plastic Surgery
Stanford, California 94305
Stanford University School of Medicine
Associate Chief and Director
Burn Center
Santa Clara Valley Medical Center
San Jose, California 95128
(*Burn Surgery*)

**Jon W. Propst, MD, PhD**
Attending Anesthesiologist
Marian Medical Center
Santa Maria, California 93454
(*Gynecological Oncology Surgery*)

**Emily Ratner, MD**
Assistant Professor of Anesthesia
Stanford University School of Medicine
Stanford, California 94305
(*Gynecology/Infertility Surgery*)

**Bruce A. Reitz, MD**
Professor and Chairman
Department of Cardiothoracic Surgery
Stanford University School of Medicine
Stanford, California 94305
Chief, Pediatric Cardiac Surgical Service
Lucile Salter Packard Children's Hospital at Stanford
Stanford, California 94305
(*Heart/Lung Transplantation, Pediatric Cardiovascular Surgery*)

**Lawrence A. Rinsky, MD**
Professor of Orthopedic Surgery
Stanford University School of Medicine
Stanford, California 94305
Chief, Pediatric Orthopedics
Lucile Salter Packard Children's Hospital at Stanford
Stanford, California 94305
(*Hand, Pediatric Orthopedic Surgery*)

**Myer H. Rosenthal, MD, FACCP**
Professor of Anesthesia
Medicine and Surgery
Stanford University School of Medicine
Medical Director of Intensive Care
Stanford University Hospital
Stanford, California 94305
(*Gynecological Oncology Surgery*)

**Jan T. Rydfors, MD**
Clinical Instructor
Department of Gynecology and Obstetrics
Stanford University School of Medicine
Stanford, California 94305

Department of Obstetrics and Gynecology
Palo Alto Medical Foundation
Palo Alto, California 94304
(*Gynecology/Infertility Surgery*)

**Stanley I. Samuels, MB, BCh**
Professor of Anesthesia
Stanford University School of Medicine
Stanford, California 94305
(*Dental, Ophthalmic, Restorative Surgery*)

**Stephen A. Schendel, MD, DDS**
Head
Division of Plastic and Reconstructive Surgery
Chief, Craniofacial Anomalies Center
Lucile Salter Packard Children's Hospital at Stanford
Stanford, California 94305
(*Dental, Restorative Surgery, Congenital Malformation Repair*)

**Velerig Selivanov, MD**
Attending Physician
Department of Surgery
Santa Teresa Community Hospital
San Jose, California 95119
(*Trauma Surgery*)

**Carol A. Shostak, RN, RTT, CMD**
Chief Medical Dosimetrist
Stanford University Medical Center
Stanford, California 94305
(*Pediatric Radiation Therapy*)

**Lawrence M. Shuer, MD**
Associate Professor, Acting Chair
Department of Neurosurgery
Stanford University School of Medicine
Stanford, California 94305
(*Neurosurgery, Pediatric Neurosurgery*)

**Norman E. Shumway, MD, PhD**
Professor of Cardiothoracic Surgery
Stanford University School of Medicine
Stanford, California 94305
(*Cardiac Surgery*)

**Lawrence Siegel, MD**
Assistant Professor of Anesthesia
Stanford University School of Medicine
Stanford, California 94305
(*Heart/Lung Transplantation*)

**Gary K. Steinberg, MD, PhD**
Associate Professor, Neurosurgery
Head, Cerebrovascular Surgery
Co-Director, Stanford Stroke Center
Stanford University School of Medicine
Stanford, California 94305
(*Neurosurgery, Pediatric Neurosurgery*)

**James M. Stone, MD**
Assistant Professor of Surgery
Stanford University School of Medicine
Stanford, California 94305
Director, Colon and Rectal Surgery
Division of Surgical Oncology
Stanford University Medical Center
Stanford, California 94305
(*Colorectal Surgery*)

**Price Stover, MD**
Fellow in Cardiovascular Anesthesia
Clinical Instructor of Anesthesia
Stanford University School of Medicine
Stanford, California 94305
(*Multi-organ Procurement for Transplantation*)

**Nelson Teng, MD, PhD**
Associate Professor, Department of Surgery
Stanford University School of Medicine
Stanford, California 94305
Director, Cancer Surgery Service
Stanford University Medical Center
Stanford, California 94305
(*Gynecological Oncology Surgery*)

**David J. Terris, MD**
Assistant Professor of Otolaryngology
Stanford University School of Medicine
Stanford, California 94305
(*Otolaryngology*)

**Mark A. Vierra, MD**
Assistant Professor of Surgery
Division of Gastrointestinal Surgery
Stanford University School of Medicine
Stanford, California 94305
(*Biliary Tract Surgery*)

**Lars M. Vistnes, MD, FRCS(C)**
Professor of Plastic and Reconstructive Surgery, Emeritus
Chairman, Department of Functional Restoration
Stanford University Medical Center
Stanford, California 94305
(*Aesthetic Surgery*)

# FOREWORD

During their training, it is perhaps inevitable that residents focus primarily on the dictates and options for administering anesthesia *to* the patient, as opposed to the equally important (*sine qua non*?) issue of administering it *for* the surgery. The experienced anesthesiologist learns the steps of and the requirements for the different types of surgery for which he/she provides anesthesia, and something of the indications and complications. This all-important aspect, however, is sometimes relatively overlooked and is very difficult for the inexperienced to assimilate into the intuitive database. This new book adopts a somewhat novel approach, and should fill a real need. It largely reflects the clinical practices of various clinicians at Stanford and, therefore, may in some details not exactly match those at other institutions. It should, however, provide an excellent reference source for a wide audience, not only of those in residency training programs, which served as the stimulus, but also for those in practice who are called upon to provide anesthesia for types of surgery with which they have no current experience.

It is a pleasure to see the labors of two of my stalwart clinician colleagues coming to fruition in print, following their conception during my years as department chairman.

*H.B. Fairley, MB, BS, FFARCS, FRCPC*
Stanford, California
September, 1993

# PREFACE

Frequently, anesthesiologists, from trainee to graybeard, may be taken aback when asked to perform anesthesia for a Cotrel-Dubousset or a Mustard's procedure. While much useful information can eventually be found through a diligent search of specialty texts, other key data are often difficult to find, necessitating last-minute consultations with colleagues who one hopes are more familiar with the surgery. Often, an arduous and usually time-consuming search of the literature may be required in order to gain a better understanding of the surgical and anesthetic implications of the operation. The purpose of this manual is to provide anesthesiologists with detailed information in a compact, easily assimilated format covering both the routine and many of the unusual surgical operations that they are likely to encounter during their professional lifetimes. This book is, we feel, unique in that it has been written primarily with emphasis on the surgical procedure itself, highlighting those aspects of the preoperative visit and anesthetic plan that are specifically relevant to that surgery. The cynical reader may well view this with a somewhat jaundiced eye as yet another anesthesia text in a world seemingly overloaded with worthwhile textbooks. First and foremost, this manual is not, and should not, be regarded as an anesthetic textbook in the standard sense. Rather, it should be regarded as a unique reference which may be used either by itself or in conjunction with a standard textbook of anesthesia or surgery.

The information provided for each operation is presented from both the surgeon's and the anesthesiologist's perspectives, with each section being co-authored by a surgeon and an anesthesiologist with a special interest in that field. In this way, we have attempted to provide both surgical and anesthetic considerations important for perioperative patient care.

In the first section, the salient features of the surgical procedure are presented in three subsections: (a) a brief description of the surgery itself, including common variant approaches; (b) a summary of the procedure; and (c) a description of the patient population characteristics. Within the Summary of Procedure the reader will find information on patient position, location of the incision, special instrumentation, antibiotics, and any intraoperative and postoperative considerations unique to the surgery. In addition, this section includes an estimate of surgical time and blood loss (which will, of course, vary from practice-to-practice and patient-to-patient). Finally, estimates of mortality and specific morbidities, listed in order of decreasing frequency, are provided. These figures are usually estimates gleaned from published data or based on the surgeon's experience and knowledge. Pain scores refer to the surgeon's estimate of the patient's pain in the first 24 hours following surgery. The common 0-10 scale, wherein 0 means no pain and 10 indicates the worst imaginable pain, is used. In the subsection on Patient Population Characteristics, we try to give the reader some idea of incidence of the proposed surgery. By incidence we mean how commonly the surgery is performed in a university hospital setting. The etiology, the predisposing factors that bring the patient to surgery, and any medical conditions associated with the primary condition are listed in order of decreasing frequency.

In the second section, anesthetic considerations are also presented in three subsections to assist the reader in the management of a patient, from the preoperative Anesthesia Assessment Clinic through the surgical procedure itself and on to the Post-Anesthesia Care Unit (or Intensive Care Unit). Preoperative Considerations includes a discussion of common characteristics of the patient populations presenting for the surgery, giving an indication of which organ systems may require special evaluation and what preoperative tests or further studies may be necessary prior to the surgery. Approaches to premedication also are discussed.

The subsection on Intraoperative Anesthetic Considerations will help guide the reader in the selection of an appropriate anesthetic technique and its subsequent management. This subsection includes a discussion of blood and fluid requirements, monitoring, patient positioning, intraoperative complications, and any other unique considerations pertaining to that surgery. Postoperative Considerations concludes with a discussion of complications common in the early postoperative period, as well as strategies for pain management.

Purists may quibble with our frequent reference to "standard techniques" for premedication, induction, intubation, maintenance, and emergence. The more querulous reader may well say there is no such thing as a standard anything, and that each patient should be individualized. While we agree with this concept in principle, for practical purposes it was necessary to provide standard, basic frameworks on which to build appropriately individualized anesthetic plans. It became obvious to us early on that it would be impossible to include specific details for each and every operation and their variants in combination with the nearly infinite permutations in patient pathology. It also became apparent that the common anesthetic considerations for some surgical procedures were so similar that a single discussion would be sufficient (e.g., anesthesia for surgery on the lower extremities). Finally, in the interest of brevity, we have used standard medical abbreviations in most of the subsections (with definitions in the Appendix).

All of these considerations had to be woven into a text considerably smaller than the Encyclopedia Britannica. How well we have done is left up to you, the Reader, to judge. It is our hope that with this manual in hand, anesthesiologists (and even our surgical colleagues) will speedily gain useful information on the myriad surgical operations and their attendant anesthetic concerns that we confront in our modern-day practice.

*Richard A. Jaffe*
*Stanley I. Samuels*
Stanford, California
September, 1993

## ACKNOWLEDGMENTS

The authors thankfully acknowledge the patient tolerance of family, friends and colleagues during the arduous gestation period of this project. We are especially grateful to our contributors; to our editor at Raven Press, Kathey Alexander, for her patience and continuing support; and to Audrey Stevens who assisted us so ably in the beginning of the project. Finally, our undying gratitude to our editorial assistant, Dee Mosteller, without whose relentless help this book would still be unfinished.

**Surgeons**

**Gary K. Steinberg, MD, PhD** *(Intracranial Neurosurgery)*
**Lawrence M. Shuer, MD** *(Intracranial, Spinal Neurosurgery)*
**John Adler, MD** *(Stereotactic Neurosurgery)*

# 1. NEUROSURGERY

**Anesthesiologist**

**C. Philip Larson, Jr, MD, MS**

**Surgeons**

**Gary K. Steinberg, MD, PhD**
**Lawrence M. Shuer, MD**
**John Adler, MD**

## 1.1 INTRACRANIAL NEUROSURGERY

**Anesthesiologist**

**C. Philip Larson, Jr, MS, MD**

# CRANIOTOMY FOR INTRACRANIAL ANEURYSMS

## SURGICAL CONSIDERATIONS

**Description:** Clipping of intracranial aneurysms is the treatment of choice for preventing aneurysmal rupture (with subarachnoid or intraparenchymal hemorrhage), aneurysmal enlargement or distal embolization from the aneurysm. **Hunt** and **Hess** described a clinical grading system for patients with ruptured intracranial aneurysms[4] that has prognostic value in terms of ultimate clinical outcome and is also used to determine the timing of surgery. Grading is based on the neurological examination and ranges from Grade I (minimal headache, no neurologic deficit) to Grade V (moribund). Common sites of aneurysms are shown in Fig 1.1-1.

Through a **craniotomy** or **craniectomy**, using microscopic techniques, the parent vessel giving rise to the aneurysm is identified. The aneurysm neck is isolated, and a small, non-ferromagnetic alloy spring clip is placed across the aneurysm neck, excluding it from the circulation. A **frontotemporal (pterional) craniotomy** normally is used to approach anterior circulation aneurysms. This requires extensive drilling of the medial sphenoid wing (pterion) and allows access to most aneurysms on the anterior and lateral Circle of Willis vessels: internal carotid-paraclinoid/superior hypophyseal artery; internal carotid-ophthalmic artery; posterior communicating artery; anterior choroidal artery; internal carotid artery bifurcation; middle cerebral artery; and anterior communicating artery. Posterior circulation aneurysms are approached via a subtemporal or pterional exposure (upper basilar artery, posterior cerebral artery, superior cerebellar artery), a suboccipital exposure (vertebral artery, posterior inferior cerebellar artery), or a combined subtemporal and suboccipital exposure (basilar trunk, vertebrobasilar junction). Circulatory arrest under CPB with deep hypothermia (16-20°C) is used for repairing some giant (>2.5 cm) aneurysms.

**Usual preop diagnosis**: Cerebral aneurysm; subarachnoid hemorrhage; intracerebral hemorrhage; progressive neurological deficits (mass effect on cranial nerves or CNS structures); TIAs; cerebral infarct

### SUMMARY OF PROCEDURE

| | Anterior Circulation Aneurysms | Posterior Circulation Aneurysms | Circulatory Arrest (CPB) W/Deep Hypothermia |
|---|---|---|---|
| **Position** | Supine, head in Mayfield headrest, turned 30-45° to side away from aneurysm, vertex dropped (Fig 1.1-4) | ⇐ Or lateral decubitus, head lateral in Mayfield headrest | ⇐ + Both groins must be accessible for arterial + venous cannulation; access to chest for defibrillation. |
| **Incision** | Frontotemporal | ⇐ Or temporal, temporosub-occipital or suboccipital | ⇐ |
| **Special instrumentation** | Operating microscope; aneurysm clips; radiolucent table and headrest for intraop angiography | ⇐ + Aperture clips to accommodate cranial nerves and critical vessels. | ⇐ + CPB pump; femoral cannulae; defibrillator; CUSA for partially thrombosed aneurysms |
| **Unique considerations** | Temporary arterial clipping; neuroprotective agents; mild hypothermia (30-33°C); intraop angiography with access to femoral artery; electrophysiological monitoring (SEPs, BAERs); brain relaxation; lumbar subarachnoid CSF drainage | ⇐ | ⇐ + No manipulation of brain retractors after systemic heparinization; attention to meticulous hemostasis |
| **Antibiotics** | Vancomycin (1 gm iv q 12 hrs) + cefotaxime (1 gm iv q 6 hrs) | ⇐ | ⇐ |
| **Surgical time** | 3 - 5 hrs | 3 - 6 hrs | 6 - 8 hrs |
| **Closing considerations** | Re-warming | ⇐ | ⇐ |
| **EBL** | 250-1000 cc | ⇐ | 2000-4000 cc |
| **Postop care** | ICU x 1-7 d; postop CBF monitoring | ⇐ | ⇐ + ICP monitoring |

| | Anterior Aneurysms | Posterior Aneurysms | Circulatory Arrest (CPB) |
|---|---|---|---|
| **Mortality** | Unruptured: 0.5% | 1.5% | 5-10% (giant aneurysms) |
| | Ruptured | | |
| | Hunt and Hess grades I-III: < 10% | < 15% | 5-15% |
| | Hunt and Hess grades IV-V: 20-40% | 20-50% | 15-50% |
| **Morbidity** | Neurological: 5-20% | 10-30% | 10-50% |
| | Cranial nerve injury | ⇐ | ⇐ |
| | Stroke | ⇐ | ⇐ |
| | Hydrocephalus | ⇐ | ⇐ |
| | Hyponatremia | ⇐ | ⇐ |
| | Respiratory failure: Rare | ⇐ | ⇐ |
| | Thromboembolism: Rare | ⇐ | ⇐ |
| | CSF leak: Rare | ⇐ | ⇐ |
| | Infection: Rare | ⇐ | ⇐ |
| | Massive blood loss: Rare | ⇐ | ⇐ |
| **Procedure code** | 61700 (intracranial aneurysm, carotid circulation) | 61702 (intracranial aneurysm, vertebral-basilar circulation | 61700 (intracranial aneurysm, carotid circulation) |
| | 61712 (aneurysm microdissection) | ⇐ | ⇐ |
| **Pain score** | 3-4 | 3-4 | 4-5 |

### PATIENT POPULATION CHARACTERISTICS

| | |
|---|---|
| **Age range** | 30-70 yrs |
| **Male:Female** | 44:56 |
| **Incidence** | 12/100,000/yr for ruptured aneurysms with subarachnoid hemorrhage |
| **Etiology** | Idiopathic (probably acquired and related to hemodynamic stress at arterial branch points, although may have congenital predisposition to loss of internal elastic lamina)<br>Traumatic<br>Infectious<br>Familial |
| **Associated conditions** | Polycystic kidney disease<br>Coarctation of the aorta<br>Marfan syndrome<br>Ehlers-Danlos syndrome<br>Intracranial arteriovenous malformations (AVMs)<br>Aortic aneurysm<br>Fibromuscular dysplasia<br>Pseudoxanthoma elastica<br>Rendu-Osler-Weber syndrome |

---

## ANESTHETIC CONSIDERATIONS

### PREOPERATIVE

Aneurysms may occur in any age group, although they generally become symptomatic and are diagnosed in young or middle-aged adults who are usually in otherwise good health. Most patients have warning Sx before the first major bleed, but these tend to be mild and nonspecific (e.g., headache, dizziness, orbital pain, slight motor or sensory disturbances). The symptoms are generally disregarded by both patients and physicians.

**Respiratory** Usually not significant unless the patient has Hx of smoking, or has pulmonary aspiration as a result of a neurological deficit from an intracranial hemorrhage.
**Tests:** As indicated from H&P.

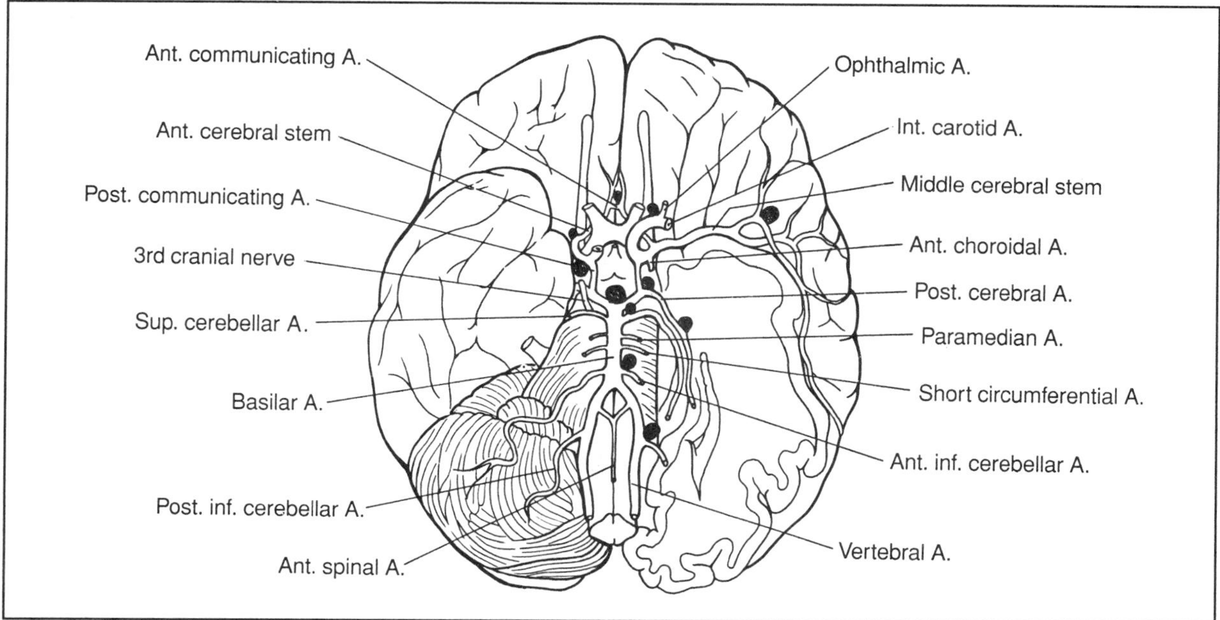


**Figure 1.1-1.** Cross-section of the Circle of Willis, showing sites of aneurysms; the majority (~90%) are located in the anterior half of the circle. (Reproduced with permission from Adams RD: *Principles of Neurology*, 4th edition. McGraw-Hill: 1989.)

**Cardiovascular** Generally, these patients do not have other cardiovascular diseases, although intracerebral aneurysms occur more commonly in patients with certain congenital disorders, such as polycystic disease of the kidneys, coarctation of the aorta, fibromuscular hyperplasia, Marfan and Ehlers-Danlos syndromes. Patients who have had a recent intracranial hemorrhage from leaking or rupture of a cerebral aneurysm are prone to develop systemic HTN, hypovolemia[8] and electrocardiographic abnormalities.[9] The HTN is thought to be due to autonomic hyperactivity, and is generally treated with anti-hypertensive medication, which should be continued up to the time of anesthesia and surgery. Why hypovolemia occurs following subarachnoid hemorrhage is not clear, but may be due in part to cerebral vasospasm, and to sustained bed rest. ECG abnormalities occur in 50-80% of patients who sustain an intracranial hemorrhage. Appropriate preop preparation includes ECG characterization of the abnormality. If patient has Hx of ischemic heart disease, then ECHO and cardiac enzyme studies may be helpful in determining whether ECG changes are due to heart disease or intracranial hemorrhage.

**Tests:** ECG; others as indicated from H&P.

**Neurological** Seldom do aneurysms produce neurological Sx by enlarging to the point that they compress adjacent neural tissue or cause ↑ICP. If an intracranial hemorrhage occurs, the neurological dysfunction will vary, depending on the site and extent of the hemorrhage. These patients may complain of severe headache, be confused and disoriented, have a motor deficit of one or more extremities, or be comatose. A major complication of an intracerebral hemorrhage is the development of cerebral vasospasm or vasoconstriction of cerebral vessels. The vasospasm may be local or diffuse, and may be mild or severe. If severe, it causes worsening of the neurological deficits. It usually occurs in the first wk after the bleed, peaks at ~10 d, and is usually resolved within 2-3 wks. The exact mechanism for the vasospasm is not known; but it is believed that the precipitating agent is free oxyhemoglobin which, in turn, may cause release of vasospastic substances such as serotonin, prostaglandins, or potassium from brain tissue. If the neurosurgeon suspects that the patient may have focal cerebral edema or vasospasm from an intracranial hemorrhage, surgery will generally be delayed until neurologic Sx have stabilized or resolved, and the CT scan is normal. Treatment during this waiting period usually involves support of BP and vigorous hydration to induce hypervolemic hemodilution, thereby increasing CBF and improving the rheological characteristics of the blood.

If a patient is evaluated by a neurosurgeon within 6-8 hrs of sustaining an intracranial hemorrhage, and if the severity of the neurological injury or deficit is minimal, the neurosurgeon may decide to ligate the aneurysm immediately. The rationale behind this approach is that failure to ligate promptly may result in an acute re-bleed and death. Although control of BP is important

**Neurological, continued** in all patients with aneurysms, it is particularly critical in this subset of patients. Any substantial increase in BP may cause a serious re-bleed, permanent neurological deficits or death; and any substantial decrease in BP may cause cerebral ischemia and infarction in the area of the original bleed. Arterial catheterization and continuous beat-to-beat monitoring of BP prior to induction of anesthesia is essential in these patients.

**Tests:** CT; MRI; cerebral angiogram, which the anesthesiologist should examine preop to identify the nature and site of the aneurysm.

**Hematologic** **Tests:** Hct; PT; PTT

**Laboratory** UA; electrolytes; CT or MRI scan; cerebral angiogram; others as indicated from H&P.

**Premedication** Seldom necessary; detailed discussion with the patient about the anesthetic plan, with appropriate reassurance, is usually enough. Should an intracranial aneurysm leak or rupture in the immediate preop period, its signs may be difficult to distinguish from those associated with excessive responses to premedication. If medication is desirable, small doses of sedative/hypnotics (e.g., midazolam 2-5 mg iv) are preferable to opiates.

## INTRAOPERATIVE

**Anesthetic technique:** GETA. The goals of anesthesia for this operation are to: (1) maintain optimum CPP (cerebral arterial pressure minus cerebral venous or intracranial pressure, whichever is greater), but be prepared to decrease CPP rapidly and profoundly if intracranial hemorrhage occurs during surgical clipping; (2) decrease intracranial volume (blood and tissue) to optimize working space for surgeons within the cranial compartment, thereby minimizing the need for surgical retraction of brain tissue; and (3) minimize metabolic rate and $CMRO_2$, with the expectation that the brain will tolerate severe hypotension and ischemia if sudden decreases in MAP and, hence, CPP become necessary.

**Induction** STP 5-10 mg/kg iv to provide amnesia and ↓cerebral blood volume by inducing cerebral vasoconstriction. Meperidine 1.5-2 mg/kg iv to provide analgesia for the first 2 hrs of surgery. Vecuronium 0.15 mg/kg; or a mixture of d-tubocurarine 0.3 mg/kg (7 ml) and pancuronium 0.04 mg/kg (3 ml) to provide muscle relaxation for tracheal intubation and positioning of the patient. This combination (labeled "curalon") has the advantages of being much less expensive and of longer duration than vecuronium, and is devoid of adverse cardiovascular effects.

Lidocaine administered either by topical spray (LTA spray) or iv in a dose of 1.5 mg/kg to lessen the cardiovascular responses to ET intubation.

**Maintenance** STP 15-20 mg/kg by continuous infusion to be completed within 1 hr from induction. When combined with induction dose, the total dose generally is ≤ 25 mg/kg. This dose provides additional amnesia, ↓cerebral blood volume, and ↓cerebral metabolism and $CMRO_2$ consumption. Isoflurane ≤ 1%, inspired with $O_2$. $N_2O$ is not used because of its potential for reversing protective effects of STP from focal ischemia at light-to-moderate levels of barbiturate anesthesia.[10,11] No additional neuromuscular blocking drugs are administered.

**Emergence** With this technique, patients will be sufficiently responsive within 30 min of conclusion of operation to permit gross neurological evaluation, and will not have any recall of the operative period. As recovery from anesthesia occurs, the patient's BP will generally increase in response to the emergence stimuli. Titration of ß-adrenergic blocking drugs such as esmolol and/or vasodilators such as SNP should be initiated, and the dose stabilized prior to transport to ICU. (See Control of BP, below.) If the brain has not been injured by the surgical procedure, patient should awaken from anesthetic within 30 min after cessation of isoflurane administration. As the patient is awakening, it is important to assure full reversal from neuromuscular blockade and close regulation of BP. If the patient begins to cough on ETT, either it should be removed or cough reflex suppressed with lidocaine sprayed down ETT while patient is still anesthetized. Patient is placed in bed in a 30° head-up position and transported to ICU for monitoring overnight. Supplemental $O_2$ should be administered and close regulation of BP maintained.

**Blood and fluid requirements**

IV: 16 ga x 2
NS/LR @ < 10 ml/kg + UO
Expand blood volume with albumin 5% if Hct >30%.
Albumin + PRBC if Hct < 30%
Avoid hetastarch; may → coagulopathy.[12]

What fluid and how much to give depends on patient's condition. If blood volume is normal, crystalloid fluid should not exceed 10 ml/kg beyond that required to replace UO. If blood volume is low because of vasospasm or prolonged bed rest, albumin 5% is given if Hct >30%; combinations of albumin and blood, if Hct is < 30%. Hetastarch 6% not recommended for these patients because of its potential for inducing a coagulopathy.

| | | |
|---|---|---|
| **Control of brain volume (ICP)** | Hyperventilate to $PaCO_2$ = 25-30 mmHg ($PETCO_2$=20-25 mmHg).<br>$PaO_2$ >100 mmHg<br>↓fluids < 10 ml/kg + UO<br>STP infusion<br>↓isoflurane < 1%<br>Mannitol 1 gm/kg<br>± Furosemide 0.3 mg/kg<br>Control BP & CVP: low normal.<br>± Steroids<br>± Lumbar CSF drain<br>Head up 20-30° | ↓$PaCO_2$ → ↓cerebral vascular volume (better surgical access) + ↑CBF to ischemic areas ("Robin Hood" effect) + ↓anesthetic requirements + ↑lactic acid buffering.<br><br>Mannitol/furosemide → ↓$K^+$; monitor level and replace as necessary. If mannitol is administered too rapidly, profound hypotension will occur, probably from peripheral vasodilation.<br>CSF drain often placed after induction of anesthesia, and may be opened as required. |
| **Monitoring** | Standard monitors (see Appendix).<br>± Bladder temperature<br>Arterial line (before induction)<br>CVP line<br>UO<br>± Evoked potentials[13] | Direct monitoring of arterial pressure is essential because of the marked fluctuations in BP that may occur, necessitating hypertensive or hypotensive drug therapy, as well as need for ABGs. Recording transducer should always be at the level of the head rather than the heart. Monitoring CVP via a right atrial catheter is desirable in virtually all patients to assess adequacy of fluid therapy intraop and postop. The catheter also is essential for infusion of vasoactive drugs commonly used during and/or after this operation. The ideal site for insertion of the catheter, in order of preference, is: right IJ, right subclavian, and right EJ vein. Localization of the catheter can be determined by CXR, ECG tracing (noting P-wave changes), or pressure-wave contour and value as the catheter is withdrawn from the RV into the right atrium. |
| **Hypothermia** | Ice packs<br>Thermal blanket<br>Cool air blower<br>Cold OR | Mild hypothermia (31°-33° C) is used in some centers during this operation for two purposes: 1) to ↓ $CMRO_2$ and 2) to decrease brain size[13]. $CMRO_2$ decreases about 7% for every degree C decrease in brain temperature; so at 31° C, cerebral metabolism is decreased about 40% below normal. From studies in animals, it is generally believed that this level of hypothermia is beneficial, although there are no studies in patients documenting decreased morbidity or mortality from its use. This level of hypothermia does not interfere appreciably with coagulation, nor it is generally associated with cardiac dysrhythmias. Warming is begun several hrs before the conclusion of the operation using thermal blanket, Bair Hugger®, and warming lights, by warming inspired gasses, and by increasing the ambient temperature in the OR. Usually by the time the operation is completed, patient temperature is near normal. |
| **Control of BP** | During application of head fixation device (Mayfield):<br>Prior to clipping: 80-100% of baseline MAP<br>Clipping of aneurysm, or in event of aneurysmal rupture: MAP ↓40-50 mmHg, if necessary<br>Post-clipping: usually MAP = 80-100 mmHg<br>If HR >80 bpm, esmolol 100-500 $\mu$g/kg/min to ↓HR to 50-60 bpm. | Control of BP is critical to the successful outcome of both anesthetic and operation. Substantial increases in BP will increase transmural pressure across the aneurysmal wall, and increase likelihood of rupture of the aneurysm. Substantial decreases in BP also are often desirable during clipping of the aneurysm to decrease transmural pressure and soften aneurysmal sac. BP may be reduced with isoflurane alone or in combination with a short-acting ß-adrenergic blocking drug such as esmolol. If a vasoconstrictor is needed, a pure $\alpha$-adrenergic stimulant such as phenylephrine is preferred because it |

| | | |
|---|---|---|
| **Control of BP, continued** | If HR already slow, or if esmolol alone does not produce satisfactory control of BP, administer SNP 0.1-0.5 μg/kg/min to desired effect.<br>Generally try to maintain postop BP at 80% of preop range. | has minimal dysrhythmogenic potential. Responses to vasoactive drugs are much easier to regulate if a normal blood volume has been established and maintained throughout the anesthetic period. |
| **Positioning** | For most aneurysms:<br>Supine, head turned<br>Three-point fixation (beware of marked ↑BP with use of pins).<br>Use shoulder roll.<br>✓ and pad pressure points.<br>✓ eyes. | Anesthetic gas hoses and all monitoring and vascular catheter lines are directed to patient's feet, where the anesthesiologist is positioned during surgery. In planning anesthetic equipment to be used, the anesthesiologist must make sure that all will reach the foot of operating table. Anti-embolism stockings and SCDs used to minimize DVT. |
| **Complications** | Hypothermia (mild) | |

## POSTOPERATIVE

| | | |
|---|---|---|
| **Complications** | Intracranial hemorrhage<br>Stroke<br>Cerebral vasospasm | If any of these complications occur, it is likely that the patient's trachea will have to be re-intubated and the patient transported to CT scanner for further neurological evaluation or possible re-operation. |
| **Pain management** | Meperidine (10 mg iv prn)<br>Codeine (30-60 mg im q 4 hrs prn) | |
| **Tests** | CT scan, if any change in neurological status | |


**References**

1. Schmidek HH, Sweet WH, eds: *Operative Neurosurgical Techniques: Indications, Methods, and Results*, Vols I-II. WB Saunders Co, Philadelphia: 1988.
2. Youmans JR, ed: *Neurological Surgery*, Vols 1-6. WB Saunders Co, Philadelphia: 1990.
3. Wilkins RH, Rengachary SS, eds: *Neurosurgery*, Vols 1-3. McGraw-Hill, New York: 1985.
4. Weir B: *Aneurysms Affecting the Nervous System*. Williams & Wilkins, Baltimore: 1987.
5. Ojemann RG, Heros RC, Crowell RM: *Surgical Management of Cerebrovascular Disease*. Williams & Wilkins, Baltimore: 1987.
6. Peerless SJ, Drake CG: Surgical management of posterior cerebral aneurysms. In *Operative Neurosurgical Techniques: Indications, Methods, and Results*, Vols I-II. Schmidek HH, Sweet WH, eds. WB Saunders Co, Philadelphia: 1988.
7. Sundt TM Jr: *Surgical Techniques for Saccular and Giant Intracranial Aneurysms*. Williams & Wilkins, Baltimore: 1990.
8. Brazenor GA, Chamberlain MJ, Gelb AW: Systemic hypovolemia after subarachnoid hemorrhage. *J Neurosurg Anesth* 1990; 2:42-9.
9. Andreoli A, dePasquale G, Pinelli G, et al: Subarachnoid hemorrhage: frequency and severity of cardiac arrhythmias. A survey of 70 cases studied in the acute phase. *Stroke* 1987; 18(3):558-64.
10. Hartung J, Cottrell JE: Nitrous oxide reduces STP-induced prolongation of survival in hypoxic and anoxic mice. *Anesth Analg* 1987; 66(1):47-52.
11. Warner DS, Zhou JG, Ramani R, Todd MM, McAllister A: Nitrous oxide does not alter infarct volume in rats undergoing reversible middle cerebral artery occlusion. *Anesthesiology* 1990; 73(4):686-93.
12. Cully MD, Larson CP Jr, Silverberg GD: Hetastarch coagulopathy in a neurosurgical patient. *Anesthesiology* 1987; 66(5):706-7.
13. Mooij JJ, Buchthal A, Belopavlovic M: Somatosensory evoked potential monitoring of temporary middle cerebral artery occlusion during aneurysm operation. *Neurosurgery* 1987; 21(4):492-96.

# ANESTHETIC CONSIDERATIONS FOR CRANIOTOMY FOR GIANT INTRACRANIAL ANEURYSMS

## PREOPERATIVE

Aneurysms are classified as "giant" when they are >2.5 cm in diameter. These giant aneurysms represent ~5% of all aneurysms. They occur twice as often in women, usually become symptomatic in the 4th or 5th decade of life, and present particularly difficult surgical challenges:[1,2] (1) their large size makes direct visualization of the vascular anatomy difficult; (2) vascular branches essential to maintaining flow to normal brain may be an integral part of the giant aneurysm, and cannot be included in the clipping without causing permanent neurological injury; (3) standard aneurysm clips may not occlude a large, turgid aneurysm, or may slip or move, once applied; and (4) giant aneurysms may rupture during dissection or clip application, resulting in severe neurological morbidity or mortality. A special anesthetic and surgical management, using deep hypothermia to 18°C, achieved with femoral-femoral CPB and temporary circulatory arrest, has evolved.[1,3] These techniques decompress the aneurysm, making it easier to clip, and protect the brain during circulatory arrest. The duration of cardiac arrest may be as long as 45 minutes.

**Respiratory** None unless patient has Hx of smoking, or has sustained pulmonary aspiration as a result of a neurological deficit from an intracranial hemorrhage.
**Tests:** CXR; others as indicated from H&P.

**Cardiovascular** Generally, these patients do not have other cardiovascular diseases. (See Anesthetic Considerations for "Ligation of Intracranial Aneurysms.")
**Tests:** ECG; others as indicated from H&P.

**Neurological** These patients usually present with complaints of intermittent or persistent headaches or visual disturbances which are probably due to aneurysmal compression of adjacent neural tissue or increased ICP. If an intracranial hemorrhage occurs, neurological dysfunction varies, depending on site and extent of the hemorrhage. Cerebral vasospasm is a major complication of intracranial hemorrhage (see discussion in Anesthetic Considerations for "Ligation of Intracranial Aneurysms," below).
**Tests:** CT; MRI; angiogram. The anesthesiologist should examine the cerebral angiogram preop to visualize the size and site of aneurysm.

**Hematologic** T&C for 6 U PRBCs.
**Tests:** Hct; PT; PTT; hemogram; others as indicated from H&P.

**Laboratory** UA; electrolyte panel

**Premedication** Premedication is seldom necessary in this procedure. Detailed discussion with patient about the anesthetic plan, with appropriate reassurance, is usually sufficient. Should an intracranial aneurysm leak or rupture in the immediate preop period, it may be difficult to distinguish this event from changes associated with excessive responses to premedication. If premedication is desirable, however, small doses of sedative/hypnotics (e.g., midazolam 2-5 mg) are preferable to opiates.

## INTRAOPERATIVE

**Anesthetic technique:** GETA. The goals of anesthesia for this procedure are to: (1) provide adequate surgical anesthesia; (2) decrease intracranial volume (blood and tissue) and optimize working space within the cranial compartment, thereby minimizing the need for surgical retraction of brain tissue; and (3) increase tolerance of the brain to ischemia by decreasing $CMRO_2$, which occurs with the use of deep hypothermia, barbiturate therapy and isovolemic hemodilution.

**Induction** STP 20 mg/kg iv to provide amnesia and decrease cerebral blood volume by inducing cerebral vasoconstriction. Meperidine 2 mg/kg iv to provide analgesia for the first 2 hrs. A long-acting muscle relaxant (e.g., mixture of d-tubocurarine 0.3 mg/kg [7 ml] and pancuronium 0.04 mg/kg [3 ml]) to provide relaxation for intubation and positioning. Lidocaine administered either by topical spray (LTA spray) or iv (1.5 mg/kg) to lessen cardiovascular responses to intubation.

**Maintenance** STP 20 mg/kg by continuous infusion, to be completed within 2 hrs of induction, for a total dose of 40 mg/kg. This dose provides additional amnesia and decreases cerebral blood volume and $CMRO_2$. The drug is most easily administered by constant infusion pump. Isoflurane $\leq$ 1%. $N_2O$ not used because of its potential for reversing protective effects of STP from focal ischemia.[3,4] An additional dose of neuromuscular blocking drugs is administered just prior to the start of CPB.

**Emergence** Because of the length and nature of the operation, and the potential for temporary neurological injury, it is advisable to leave the ETT in place immediately postop, and send patient to the ICU on controlled ventilation. If patient begins to cough, the reflex should be suppressed with opiates, neuromuscular blocking drugs, and/or LTA sprayed down the ETT. The patient is placed in bed in a 30° head-up position and transported to ICU for overnight monitoring. Supplemental $O_2$ should be administered, and close regulation of BP maintained.

| | | |
|---|---|---|
| **Blood and fluid requirements** | IV: 16 ga x 2<br>NS/LR @ 1-2 cc/kg/hr<br>PRBC 4-6 U | Cold NS up to 10 ml/kg, + a volume equal to UO, is administered during surgery. |
| **Isovolemic hemodilution** | CPD bags<br>5% albumin 8 x 250 cc<br>NS 4 x 1000 cc | Albumin and NS are placed in a refrigerator at 4°C the night before surgery to be used for cooling during isovolemic hemodilution. After induction of anesthesia, a 2nd arterial cannula is placed for removal of blood into CPD bags. Generally, about 1000 ml of blood are removed and replaced with 1 L of cold albumin 5%. This usually results in a decrease in Hct of 22-26%. Frequent intraop Hct checks are appropriate. The withdrawn blood is held at room temperature for reinfusion at the conclusion of operation. In addition, the perfusate from the CPB unit is spun down and packed cells returned to patient. |
| **Control of brain volume** | Hyperventilate to $PaCO_2$ = 25-30 mmHg.<br>Limit crystalloid < 10 ml/kg + UO.<br>Limit isoflurane ≤ 1%.<br>High-dose STP<br>Mannitol 1 gm/kg<br>± Furosemide 0.3 mg/kg<br>± Lumbar CSF drainage<br>Dexamethasone 8-12 mg | Ventilation is controlled and TV and RR adjusted such that $PaCO_2$ ranges from 25-30 mmHg. There are several advantages to hypocarbia, including: decreasing cerebral vascular volume to provide more surgical working space, thereby lessening need for vigorous retraction of brain tissue; improving regional distribution of CBF by preferentially diverting blood to potentially ischemic areas of the brain; better buffering of brain lactic acid that may form as a result of focal ischemia; and decreasing anesthetic requirement. |
| **Monitoring** | Standard monitors (see Appendix).<br>Temperature = esophageal, bladder and brain surface<br>Arterial line x 2<br>CVP (triple-lumen) line<br>UO | Once hemodilution is complete, a continuous ABG monitoring sensor (e.g., PB 3300) should be inserted into the 2nd arterial catheter for monitoring intraop and postop.[5] CVP (triple-lumen) with multiple stopcocks is used for infusions of esmolol, SNP and phenylephrine. Frequent checks are made of Hct, electrolytes, ACT values, before, during and after CPB. Keep UO > 0.5 cc/kg/hr. |
| **Control of BP** | Maintain BP normal-to-20% below normal with esmolol infusion, SNP or phenylephrine. | BP control is critical to successful surgery. ↑BP during induction or prior to CPB will increase transmural pressure across the aneurysmal wall, and increase likelihood of rupture. Prior to CPB, BP is generally kept to normal-to-20% below normal for patient, using anesthetic agents alone or with an esmolol infusion to ↓HR to a range of 50-60 bpm. If desired level of BP is not achieved with this combination, SNP infusion may be added. SNP also facilitates both cooling and rewarming because of its vasodilatory effect. If a vasoconstrictor is needed, particularly during CPB while patient is still cold, a pure α-adrenergic stimulant such as phenylephrine is preferred because of its minimal dysrhythmogenic potential. Responses to vasoactive drugs are much easier to regulate if normal blood volume has been established and maintained throughout the anesthetic period. |

| | | |
|---|---|---|
| **Positioning** | Shoulder roll<br>180° table rotation<br>√ and pad pressure points.<br>√ eyes.<br>Circuit extension tubes<br>Anti-embolism stockings and SCD | Anesthetic gas hoses and all monitoring and vascular catheter lines are directed to patient's feet, where the anesthesiologist is positioned during operation. In planning anesthetic equipment to be used, the anesthesiologist must make sure that all will reach the foot of operating table. Anti-embolism stockings and SCDs used to minimize DVT. |
| **Deep hypothermia and CPB** | Surface cooling<br>Thermal blanket<br>Ice packs<br>SNP infusion<br>Heparinization<br>Rewarming | Surface cooling is begun as soon as induction is complete, using thermal blankets above and below patient, ice packs and infusion of cold fluids during establishment of isovolemic hemodilution, and infusion of SNP, as tolerated, to induce cutaneous vasodilatation. Once the neurosurgeons have exposed the giant aneurysm and determined that it cannot be clipped without resorting to CPB, systemic **heparinization** (load: 300 U/kg; maintenance: 100 U/kg/hr) is established and patient is put on CPB using femoral-femoral bypass and cooled to ~18°C. During CPB cooling, the heart will usually fibrillate between 22-26°C. Once 18°C is reached, the CPB unit is shut off to deflate the aneurysm; it may be activated and shut off several times during clipping to evaluate adequacy of the surgical occlusion of the aneurysm and to apply additional clips. **Total circulatory arrest time should not exceed 45 min.** When clipping is complete, CPB is resumed and warming instituted. Partial CPB is continued until normal cardiac rhythm is established, and body temperature reaches ~36°C. Once partial CPB is D/C, patient will tend to cool unless vigorous efforts at warming are continued. Warming the OR and iv fluids, and use of warming lights and Bair Hugger® will facilitate the warming process. ACT analysis is performed to establish that heparin reversal is complete 5-10 min after protamine (1 mg/100 U heparin activity). If coagulation seems inadequate following heparin reversal, blood is sent for clotting studies, and platelets, FFP and calcium gluconate are administered as needed. Hetastarch 6% is not used in these patients because of its potential for inducing a coagulopathy.[4] |
| **Complications** | ↓↓BP 2° failure to maintain circulating volume<br>Dysrhythmias 2° ↓$K^+$ from diuresis and cold | |

## POSTOPERATIVE

| | | |
|---|---|---|
| **Complications** | HTN<br>Vasospasm<br>Intracranial hemorrhage and stroke<br>Coagulopathy<br>Hypothermia<br>Hypervolemia<br>DVT<br>Seizures<br>PE | HTN Rx: Esmolol + SNP titrated to effect<br>Vasospasm Rx: fluid-loading<br><br>Patient should be rewarmed to 36-37°C before terminating CPB. √ coagulation status.<br><br>Seizure Rx: Phenytoin (1 gm loading dose), **NB:** Incompatible with dextrose-containing solutions. |
| **Pain management** | Meperidine (10 mg iv prn)<br>Codeine (30-60 mg im q 4 hrs prn) | |

| | | |
|---|---|---|
| **Tests** | CT scan<br>Coagulation panel | If any question about neurological status arises, a CT scan is performed postop. Coagulation studies are needed early postop to assure normal coagulation. |


**References**

1. Silverberg GD, Reitz BA, Ream AK: Hypothermia and cardiac arrest in the treatment of giant aneurysms of the cerebral circulation and hemangioblastoma of the medulla. *J Neurosurg* 1981; 55(3):337-46.
2. Whittle IR, Dorsch NW, Besser M: Giant intracranial aneurysms: diagnosis, management, and outcome. *Surg Neurol* 1984; 21(3):218-30.
3. Silverberg GD: Giant aneurysms: surgical treatment. *Neurological Research* 1984; 6(1-2):57-63.
4. Cully MD, Larson CP Jr, Silverberg GD: Hetastarch coagulopathy in a neurosurgical patient. *Anesthesiology* 1987; 66(5):706-7.
5. Larson CP Jr: Clinical experience with an intra-arterial blood gas monitor. In *Electrolytes, Blood Gases and Other Critical Analyses: the Patient, the Measurement, and the Government.* D'Orazio P, Burritt MF, Sena SF, eds. Omnipress, Madison: 1992, 238-56.


# CRANIOTOMY FOR CEREBRAL EMBOLECTOMY

## SURGICAL CONSIDERATIONS

**Description:** This procedure is performed within 6 hours following the onset of a neurological deficit 2° a documented thrombotic or embolic occlusion of a major intracranial vessel. A craniotomy is fashioned and the occluded intracranial artery is exposed, using microscopic techniques. The involved arterial segment is isolated, temporarily occluded with miniature clips, and an **arteriotomy** is performed to remove the thrombus or embolus. Then the arteriotomy is closed. With the advent of intra-arterial or iv tissue plasminogen activator delivered by endovascular techniques, this procedure may become less frequently performed.

**Usual preop diagnosis**: Stroke; transient ischemic attack (TIA); intracranial arterial occlusion; catheter embolization to intracranial artery

### SUMMARY OF PROCEDURE

| | |
|---|---|
| **Position** | Supine or lateral decubitus |
| **Incision** | Frontal, temporal or occipital |
| **Special instrumentation** | Microscopic instruments (fine forceps, miniature vascular clips, operating microscope) |
| **Unique considerations** | Neuroprotective agents during arterial segment occlusion (barbiturates, mannitol), mild hypothermia (30-33°C) |
| **Antibiotics** | Vancomycin (1 gm iv q 12 hrs) + cefotaxime (1 gm iv q 6 hrs) |
| **Surgical time** | 3-4 hrs |
| **Closing considerations** | Avoid hypotension (MAP 80-100); induced mild HTN (MAP 90-110) during temporary arterial occlusion. |
| **EBL** | 100-250 cc |
| **Postop care** | Control BP (MAP 80-100 mmHg); start ASA postop d 1; ICU: 1-2 d. |
| **Mortality** | 5-10% |
| **Morbidity** | Intracerebral hemorrhage<br>Stroke<br>MI: Rare<br>Thromboembolism: Rare<br>Respiratory failure: Rare<br>Infection: Rare |
| **Procedure code** | 61711 (anastomosis, arterial, EC-IC arteries); 61712 (microdissection, intracranial or spinal) |
| **Pain score** | 3-4 |

### PATIENT POPULATION CHARACTERISTICS

| | |
|---|---|
| **Age range** | 50-80 yrs |
| **Male:Female** | 1:1 |
| **Incidence** | Rare |
| **Etiology** | Atherosclerosis<br>Carotid artery disease<br>Atrial fibrillation<br>Iatrogenic endovascular catheter complication |
| **Associated conditions** | HTN<br>CAD<br>Peripheral vascular disease<br>Carotid artery disease<br>Hyperlipidemia<br>Smoking<br>Alcohol abuse<br>Obesity<br>Atrial fibrillation |

## ANESTHETIC CONSIDERATIONS

See Anesthetic Considerations following "Craniotomy for Intracranial Aneurysms" (above).

**References**

1. Schmidek HH, Sweet WH, eds: *Operative Neurosurgical Techniques: Indications, Methods, and Results*, Vols I-II. WB Saunders Co, Philadelphia: 1988.
2. Youmans JR, ed: *Neurological Surgery*, Vols 1-6. WB Saunders Co, Philadelphia: 1990.
3. Wilkins RH, Rengachary SS, eds: *Neurosurgery*, Vols 1-3. McGraw-Hill, New York: 1985.
4. Sundt TM Jr: *Surgical Techniques for Saccular and Giant Intracranial Aneurysms*. Williams & Wilkins, Baltimore: 1990, 467-76.
5. Ojemann RG, Heros RC, Crowell RM: *Surgical Management of Cerebrovascular Disease*. Williams & Wilkins, Baltimore: 1987.

# CRANIOTOMY FOR INTRACRANIAL VASCULAR MALFORMATIONS

## SURGICAL CONSIDERATIONS

**Description:** Intracranial vascular malformations are congenital abnormalities that cause intracranial hemorrhage, seizures, headaches, progressive neurological deficits or audible bruits. Intracranial vascular malformations comprise high-flow, arteriovenous malformations (AVMs); low-flow, angiographically occult vascular malformations (AOVMs), including cavernous malformations, "cryptic" AVMs, capillary telangiectasias and transitional malformations; and low-flow, venous angiomas (developmental venous anomalies). **Microsurgical resection** is the optimal treatment for these lesions, although preop endovascular embolization and postop focused, stereotactic radiosurgery (heavy particle or photon) may be useful adjuncts.

Most moderate-size and large AVMs (> 3 cm diameter) are resected using a standard scalp flap and with craniotomy centered over the area of the AVM. The patient is positioned appropriately to place the craniotomy site uppermost in the field and parallel to the floor. For instance, a patient with a left frontal AVM would be positioned supine, head turned to the right, a left frontal or bicranial scalp flap raised and a left frontal craniotomy bone flap removed. A patient with a right medial occipital AVM would be positioned in the right lateral decubitus position with head turned semi-prone and a right occipital scalp flap and craniotomy performed. Smaller AVMs (< 3 cm diameter), many low-flow AOVMs, and many deep-seated vascular malformations (AVMs and AOVMs) require a small, stereotactic craniotomy (see "Stereotactic Neurosurgery"). This is performed by attaching a stereotactic base frame to the patient's skull, using local anesthetic and sedation, obtaining a CT scan or MRI scan with a rapid-opaque localizer fixed to the base frame and calculating the location of the AVM in relation to the frame, using a computer and stereotactic geometric principles. The patient is then taken to the OR, intubated fiber-optically (because of the frame position) and positioned for surgery. A three-dimensional arc frame is fixed to the base frame and coordinates appropriately set to localize the vascular malformation within the brain. A small scalp flap (a few inches in diameter) and a small craniotomy (a few cm in diameter) can be precisely fashioned for microscopic exposure of the malformation. Microsurgical resection of brain stem and thalamic vascular malformations often necessitate special positioning.

**Usual preop diagnosis:** Cerebral AVM; dural AVM; cavernous malformation; angiographically occult vascular malformation; intracerebral hemorrhage; subarachnoid hemorrhage; seizures; epilepsy; progressive neurological deficit; migraine or vascular headaches

## SUMMARY OF PROCEDURE

| | Standard Craniotomy (High-Flow AVM) | Stereotactic Craniotomy (Low-Flow AOVM) | Brain stem/Thalamic Vascular Malformations |
|---|---|---|---|
| **Position** | Supine, lateral, Concorde (modified prone) (Fig 1.1-2) | ⇐ | Lateral, Concorde, semi-sitting (Fig 1.1-3) |
| **Incision** | Frontal, temporal, parietal, occipital, suboccipital, or combination | ⇐ | Suboccipital (midline), paramedian or occipital |
| **Special instrumentation** | Operating microscope; irrigating bipolar coagulation; radiolucent table and headrest. Sundt mini aneurysm and micro AVM clips. Access to femoral artery for intraop angiography. | ⇐ | ⇐ |
| **Unique considerations** | Induced hypotension (MAP 60-65 mmHg) during resection, use of neuroprotective agents (see "Craniotomy for Aneurysms"). Relaxed brain. Mild hypothermia (30-33°C); ± lumbar CSF drain. | Use of neuroprotective agents and relaxed brain (see "Craniotomy for Aneurysms"). Mild hypothermia (30-33°C); ± lumbar CSF drain. | ⇐ |
| **Antibiotics** | Vancomycin (1 gm iv q 12 hrs) + cefotaxime (1 gm iv q 6 hrs) | ⇐ | ⇐ |
| **Surgical time** | 4 - 10 hrs | 2 - 5 hrs | 3 - 6 hrs |
| **Closing considerations** | Maintain MAP 60-65 mmHg. Avoid ↑venous pressure. | Avoid HTN (keep MAP 70-90 mmHg). | ⇐ |
| | For supratentorial vascular malformations, administer additional anticonvulsants; give loading dose of phenytoin (1 gm iv for adults) if not previously on anticonvulsants. | ⇐ | No anticonvulsants necessary |
| **EBL** | 500-3000 cc | < 250 cc | ⇐ |
| **Postop care** | ICU x 3-10 d. Maintain MAP 60-65 mmHg for 2-4 d. ICP monitoring, ventricular drain; fluid restriction in ICU. | ICU x 2 d; fluid restriction in ICU | ICU x 1-4 d; fluid restriction in ICU |
| **Mortality** | 1-10%, depending on AVM size, location, and venous drainage pattern | < 0.5% | < 2% |

| | Standard Craniotomy | Stereotactic Craniotomy | Brain stem/Thalamic |
|---|---|---|---|
| **Morbidity** | Overall: 5-30% | < 5% | 10-50% (transient) |
| | Neurological | ⇐ | ⇐ |
| | Intracranial hemorrhage | ⇐ | ⇐ |
| | Cerebral edema | ⇐ | ⇐ |
| | Stroke | ⇐ | ⇐ |
| | Hydrocephalus | ⇐ | ⇐ |
| | Massive blood loss: Occasional | ⇐ | ⇐ |
| | Thromboembolism: Rare | ⇐ | ⇐ |
| | Infection: Rare | ⇐ | ⇐ |
| **Procedure code** | 61680 (intracranial AVM; supratentorial, simple) | ⇐ | ⇐ |
| | 61682 (supratentorial complex) | ⇐ | ⇐ |
| | 61684 (infratentorial, simple) | | |
| | 61686 (infratentorial, complex) | | |
| | 61690 (dural, simple); 61692 (dural, complex) | | |
| | 61712 (microdissection, intracranial or spinal procedure) | | |
| **Pain score** | 3-4 | 3-4 | 3-4 |

## PATIENT POPULATION CHARACTERISTICS

| | |
|---|---|
| **Age range** | 15-40 yrs (most common), 41-60 yrs (less frequent) |
| **Male:Female** | 1:1 |
| **Incidence** | 0.5-1% of U.S. population |
| **Etiology** | Congenital<br>Traumatic for dural AVM |
| **Associated conditions** | Von Hippel-Lindau disease<br>Rendu-Osler-Weber syndrome<br>Familial cavernous malformation syndrome |

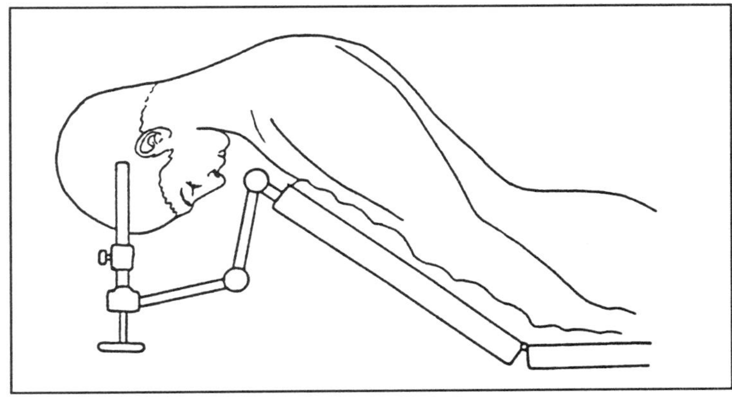

**Figure 1.1-2.** Concorde (modified prone) position for resection of posterior fossa vascular malformations. (Reproduced with permission from Sugita K: *Microsurgical Atlas*. Springer-Verlag Berlin Heidelberg: 1985.)

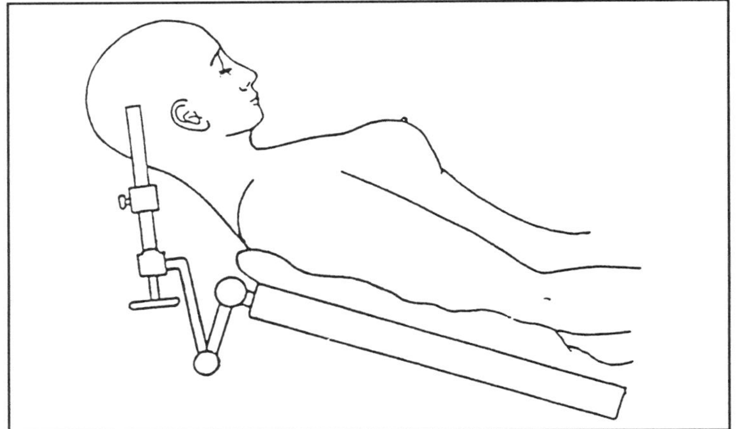

**Figure 1.1-3.** Semi-sitting position for resection of deep posterior corpus callosum or thalamic vascular malformations. (Reproduced with permission from Sugita K: *Microsurgical Atlas*. Springer-Verlag Berlin Heidelberg: 1985.)

# ANESTHETIC CONSIDERATIONS

## PREOPERATIVE

Arteriovenous malformations (AVMs) are direct arterial-to-venous communications without intervening capillary circulation.[7] With the gross and radiologic appearance of "a bag of worms," they can occur anywhere in the brain or spinal cord, varying in size from small lesions called "cryptic malformations" to very large lesions occupying a major portion of a cerebral hemisphere. Thought to be congenital, AVMs usually do not manifest themselves clinically until patients are in their late teens or 20's. Typically, these patients are otherwise healthy. On histological exam, the vessel walls are thin and lack a muscular layer; consequently, the vessels exhibit loss of normal vasomotor control or responsiveness to changes in $PaCO_2$. Treatment consists of surgical excision, radiologic embolization and/or Bragg peak proton beam therapy, alone or in combination.[8] **Stereotactic localization** is essential for safe excision of deep-seated AVMs (e.g. those located in the corona radiata, basal ganglia, visual center, cerebellar white matter or corpus callosum).

**Respiratory** — Not usually significant unless patient has Hx of smoking, or has pulmonary aspiration as a result of a neurological deficit from an intracranial hemorrhage.
**Tests:** As indicated from H&P.

**Cardiovascular** — Generally, these patients do not have other cardiovascular diseases. Occasionally, ECG changes are noted following intracranial hemorrhage, and may simply reflect the extent of brain injury.
**Tests:** ECG; others as indicated from H&P.

**Neurological** — Presenting Sx depend on location and size of AVM, and whether it is a low- or high-flow lesion. Hemorrhage with resultant neurological deficits is the most common Sx, although patients also may present with intractable seizure disorder, recurrent headaches or Sx of cerebral ischemia, including seizures 2° high-flow arteriovenous shunts, causing an intracerebral steal. Surgical treatment is vital not only to eliminate recurrent headaches or seizures but, more importantly, to prevent future hemorrhage (incidence of 2-3%/yr) and substantial mortality (6-30%) or severe morbidity (15-80%).[9] Hemorrhages from AVMs located deep in the brain (thalamus, caudate nucleus) or in the brain stem are particularly devastating. Unlike hemorrhages from an intracerebral aneurysm (generally intraventricular), hemorrhages from an AVM are usually intra-parenchymal; hence, they are seldom associated with cerebral vasospasm.
**Tests:** CT; MRI; cerebral angiogram. Preop cerebral angiogram indicates size and location of the AVM, and whether it is likely to be a low- or high-flow lesion.

**Hematologic** — After 7-8 hrs of surgery for AVM, it is fairly common for surrounding brain tissue to swell and vascular sites previously obliterated to bleed. The cause of this is unknown, but it may be related to the fact that the brain is rich in thromboplastin, which, in turn, may cause a local coagulopathy. Thus, it is advisable to obtain coagulation studies preop and stage excision over more than one sitting when AVM is large.
**Tests:** Hct; PT; PTT; platelet count; bleeding time

**Laboratory** — CBC; UA; electrolyte panel; and other tests as indicated from H&P.

**Premedication** — Seldom necessary; detailed discussion with patient about the anesthetic plan, with appropriate reassurance, is usually enough. If medication is desirable, small doses of sedative/hypnotic (e.g., midazolam 2-5 mg iv) are useful.

## INTRAOPERATIVE

**Anesthetic technique:** GETA. The goals of anesthesia for this operation are to: (1) maintain a somewhat decreased (10-20% below normal) CPP to lessen blood loss during excision of the AVM (CPP = cerebral arterial pressure minus cerebral venous or ICP, whichever is greater); (2) decrease intracranial volume (blood and tissue) to optimize surgical working space within the cranial compartment and minimize the need for surgical retraction of brain tissue; (3) decrease cerebral oxygen consumption ($CMRO_2$) to lessen the dependence, at least acutely, of normal brain on vessels feeding the AVM. For **stereotactic surgery**, a frame is placed on the patient's head under local anesthesia. The patient is then sent to CT where the exact coordinates defining the AVM and critical adjacent structures are established. The patient is brought to OR, anesthesia is induced with the frame in place and the frame is removed at the conclusion of operation, prior to emergence from anesthesia.

**Induction** — STP 5-10 mg/kg iv provides amnesia and decreases cerebral blood volume by inducing cerebral vasoconstriction. Meperidine 1.5-2 mg/kg iv provides analgesia for the first 2 hrs. Equivalent doses of other opiates work equally well. High-dose opiates used as a primary anesthetic technique do not alter CBF or $CMRO_2$ enough to provide any special benefits beyond their GA effects. Vecuronium 0.15 mg/kg, or a mixture of d-tubocurarine 0.3 mg/kg (7 ml) and pancuronium 0.04 mg/kg (3 ml), provide muscle relaxation for intubation and patient positioning.

**Induction, continued**

If patient is in a stereotactic frame, ET intubation must be accomplished before anesthesia is induced, because the frame partially occludes the mouth, making conventional laryngoscopy impossible. Oral fiber optic intubation of the trachea is the easiest method for accomplishing this. Following moderate sedation with meperidine (0.5-1 mg/kg) and midazolam (1-2 mg iv), the oropharynx is sprayed thoroughly several times with lidocaine 10% solution. Then a transtracheal injection of cocaine 4% (2-3 ml) is made, using a 3-ml syringe and 23-ga, 1" needle. Air is aspirated prior to injection to confirm the exact location of the needle. After insertion of a Tudor-Williams airway, the laryngoscopist stands beside the patient and inserts the FOL, on which is mounted a 7 or 8 ETT through the airway. Once the epiglottis is visualized, the scope is flexed about 20°, placing the tip at opening of the larynx. The scope is advanced into the airway; and, using it as a guide, the ETT is placed in airway. If the ETT does not advance easily through the glottic opening, rotating it counter-clockwise and asking the patient to take a deep breath facilitates insertion. The laryngoscopist also can place the scope in the airway by darkening the room and using the scope as a light wand, directing the light externally to the sternal notch and advancing it down the trachea.

**Maintenance**

STP 15-20 mg/kg by continuous infusion, to be completed within 1 hr from induction. Combined with the induction dose, total dose generally does not exceed 25 mg/kg. This dose is administered to provide additional amnesia, ↓cerebral blood volume and ↓$CMRO_2$. Isoflurane 1% or less with $O_2$. $N_2O$ is not used because of its potential for reversing protective effects of STP for focal ischemia at light-to-moderate levels of barbiturate anesthesia.[14] Mild hypothermia (32°C) may provide additional cerebral protection (see below). No additional neuromuscular blocking drugs are administered.

**Emergence**

If the brain has not been injured by the surgical procedure and patient is adequately rewarmed, awakening from the anesthetic should occur within 30 min after cessation of isoflurane administration. As patient is awakening, it is important to assure full reversal from neuromuscular blockade, and closely regulate BP. If the intubated patient begins to cough, either the ETT should be removed or the cough suppressed with lidocaine sprayed down the tube while patient is still anesthetized. Patient is placed in bed in a 30° head-up position and transported to ICU for overnight monitoring. Supplemental $O_2$ should be administered, and close regulation of BP maintained to prevent breakthrough bleeding from the raw surface areas left behind.

**Blood and fluid requirements**

IV: 16 ga x 2
NS/LR @ < 10 ml/kg + UO

If blood volume is normal, NS/LR – not to exceed 10 ml/kg beyond that required to replace UO – is given. If hypovolemic, albumin 5% is given if Hct >30%; combinations of albumin and blood, if Hct < 30%. Hetastarch is not recommended for these patients because of its potential for inducing a coagulopathy.[10]

**Hypothermia**

Ice packs
Thermal blanket
Cool air blower
Cold OR

Mild hypothermia (31°-33° C) is used in some centers during this operation to decrease $CMRO_2$ and brain size.[11] $CMRO_2$ decreases about 7% for every degree C decrease in brain temperature; so at 31° C, cerebral metabolism is decreased about 40% below normal. From studies in animals, it is generally believed that this level of hypothermia is beneficial,[13,14] although there are no studies in patients documenting decreased morbidity or mortality from its use. This level of hypothermia does not interfere appreciably with coagulation, nor is it generally associated with cardiac dysrhythmias. Warming is begun several hrs before the conclusion of surgery by using thermal blanket, Bair Hugger® and warming lights, by warming inspired gasses, and by increasing the ambient temperature in OR. Usually by the time the operation is completed, patient temperature is near normal.

**Control of brain volume**

Hyperventilate to $PaCO_2$ = 25-30 mmHg or $PETCO_2$=20-25 mmHg.
Limit isoflurane ≤ 1%.
Limit fluids.

↓$PaCO_2$ has several advantages, including ↓cerebral vascular volume, which provides surgeons more working space and lessens need for vigorous retraction of brain tissue. ↓$PaCO_2$ also improves the regional distribution of

| | | |
|---|---|---|
| **Control of brain volume, continued** | High-dose STP<br>Mannitol 1 gm/kg<br>Furosemide 0.3 mg/kg<br>Lumbar CSF drainage | CBF by: preferentially diverting blood to potentially ischemic areas of the brain; better buffering of the brain lactic acid that may form as a result of focal ischemia; and decreasing anesthetic requirement. If AVM is superficial, decreasing brain volume is less important, and the first 4 techniques listed (at left) are usually sufficient. If AVM is deep, the additional listed therapies may be needed. |
| **Monitoring** | Standard monitors (see Appendix).<br>+ Bladder temperature<br>Arterial line<br>CVP line<br>UO | Direct monitoring of arterial pressure prior to induction is essential for rapid control of BP. Transducer should always be placed at the level of the head rather than the heart, since CPP is arterial pressure at the brain level minus cerebral venous or ICP, whichever is higher. Monitoring CVP via a right atrial catheter is desirable in virtually all patients to assess adequacy of fluid therapy and for infusion of vasoactive drugs. The ideal site for insertion of the catheter, in order of preference, is: right IJ, right subclavian, and right EJ vein. Localization of the catheter can be determined by CXR, ECG tracing, noting P-wave changes, or pressure-wave contour and value as the catheter is withdrawn from the right ventricle into the right atrium. If patient has a high-flow AVM causing a large arteriovenous shunt, venous blood may appear arterialized (or bright red) during central venous catheterization, suggesting that the operator has punctured an artery rather than a central vein. |
| **Control of BP** | Isoflurane<br>Esmolol infusion<br>SNP infusion<br>Maintain normovolemia. | Close regulation of BP during induction and prior to excision of AVMs may be less critical than for aneurysmal surgery.[11] Once surgical excision is underway, however, modest decreases in MAP (≤ 20% below normal) using isoflurane, alone or in combination with esmolol and/or SNP, should be used to prevent excessive bleeding. Responses to vasoactive drugs are much easier to regulate if normal blood volume has been established and maintained throughout the anesthetic period. |
| **Positioning** | Shoulder roll<br>3-point fixation<br>✓ and pad pressure points.<br>✓ eyes.<br>180° rotation | For most AVMs, patient is positioned supine, head turned laterally in 3-point fixation and a roll under shoulder on the side of operation (Fig. 1.1-4). Anesthetic hoses and all monitoring and vascular catheter lines are directed to patient's feet where the anesthesiologist is positioned. In planning anesthetic equipment, make sure that all will reach the foot of operating table. Anti-embolism stockings and SCDs used to minimize DVT. |

**POSTOPERATIVE**

| | | |
|---|---|---|
| **Complications** | Neurological deficits<br>Cerebral edema and ↑ICP<br>Intracerebral hemorrhage | If any of these complications occur, it is likely that patient will have to be re-intubated and transported to the CT scanner for further neurological evaluation or possible re-operation. Careful regulation of BP is essential to avoid postop hemorrhage. |
| | Seizures | Seizure Rx: Phenytoin (1 gm loading dose). **NB:** Incompatible with dextrose-containing solutions. |
| **Pain management** | Codeine (30-60 mg im q 4 hrs prn) | |
| **Tests** | CT scan if neurological status changes. | |

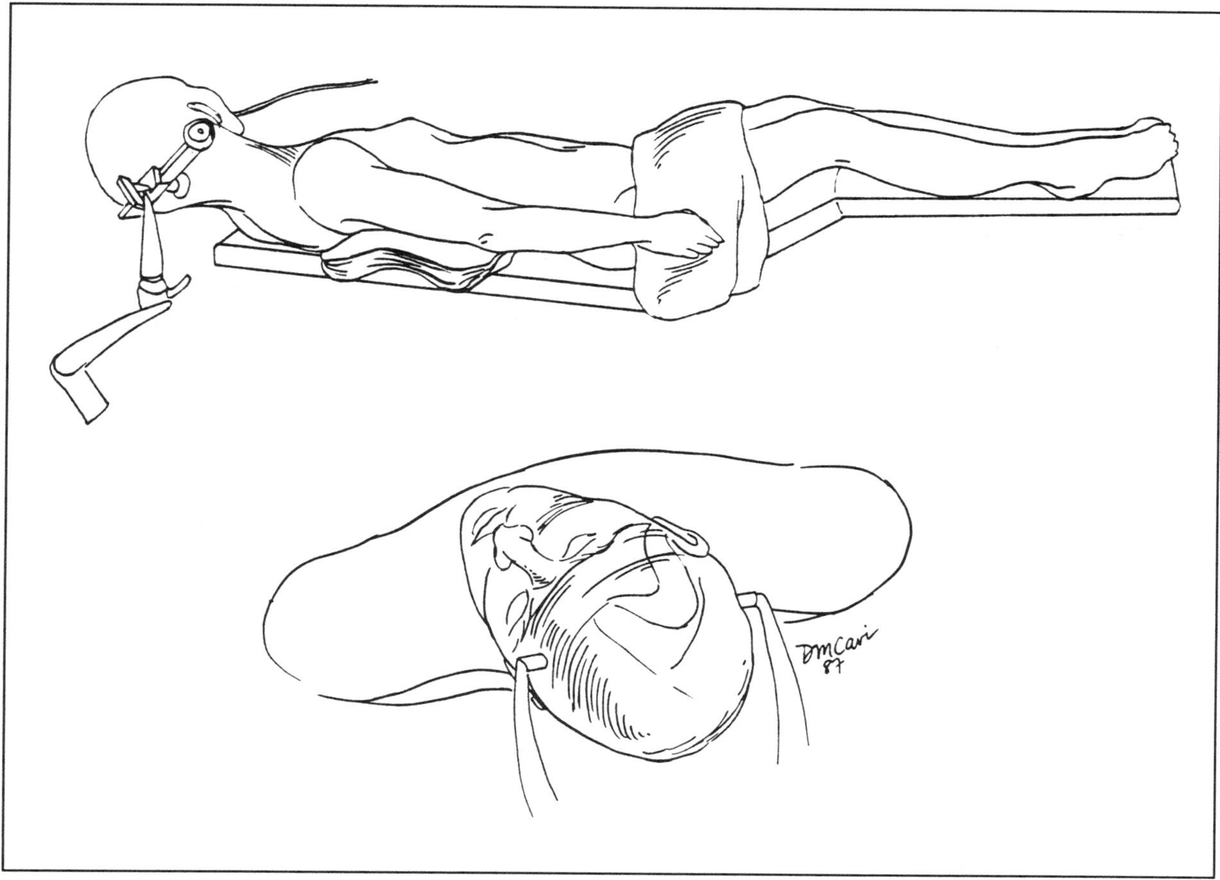


**Figure 1.1-4.** Supine position, head elevated above heart, turned 30-45° to side, vertex dropped for approach to anterior circulation aneurysms and frontal vascular malformations. (Reproduced with permission from Long DM: *Atlas of Operative Neurosurgical Technique*, Vol 1. Williams & Wilkins: 1989.)

**References**


1. Schmidek HH, Sweet WH, eds: *Operative Neurosurgical Techniques: Indications, Methods, and Results*, Vols I-II. WB Saunders Co, Philadelphia: 1988.
2. Youmans JR, ed: *Neurological Surgery*, Vols 1-6. WB Saunders Co, Philadelphia: 1990.
3. Wilkins RH, Rengachary SS, eds: *Neurosurgery*, Vols 1-3. McGraw-Hill, New York: 1985.
4. Ojemann RG, Heros RC, Crowell RM: *Surgical Management of Cerebrovascular Disease*. Williams & Wilkins, Baltimore: 1987.
5. Yasargil MG: *Microneurosurgery*. Thieme Medical Publishers Inc, New York: 1988.
6. Stein B, Soloman R. In *Neurological Surgery*, Vols 1-6. Youmans JR, ed. WB Saunders Co, Philadelphia: 1990.
7. Stein BM, Wolpert SM: Arteriovenous malformations of the brain. I: Current concepts and treatment. *Arch Neurol* 1980; 37(1):1-5.
8. Steinberg GK: Multimodality treatment of intracranial vascular malformations: Embolization, helium-ion radiosurgery, microsurgical resection. In *Arteriovenous Malformations in Functional Brain Areas*. Yamada S, ed. Futura Publishing Co, Mt. Kisco, NY: (In Press).
9. Wilkins RH: Natural history of intracranial vascular malformations: a review. *Neurosurgery* 1985; 16(3):421-30.
10. Cully MD, Larson CP Jr, Silverberg GD: Hetastarch coagulopathy in a neurosurgical patient. [Letter] *Anesthesiology* 1987; 66(5):706-7.
11. Szabo MD, Crosby G, Sundaram P, Dodson BA, Kjellberg RN: Hypertension does not cause spontaneous hemorrhage of intracranial arteriovenous malformations. *Anesthesiology* 1989; 70(5):761-3.
12. Smith RM, Stetson JB: Therapeutic hypothermia. *New Engl J Med* 1961; 265:1097-1103, 1147-51.
13. Berntman L, Welsh FA, Harp JR: Cerebral protective effect of low-grade hypothermia. *Anesthesiology* 1981; 55(5):495-98.
14. Sano T, Drummond JC, Patel PM, Grafe MR, Watson JC, Cole DJ: A comparison of the cerebral protective effects of isoflurane and mild hypothermia in a model of incomplete forebrain ischemia in the rat. *Anesthesiology* 1992; 76(2):221-28.

# CRANIOTOMY FOR EXTRACRANIAL-INTRACRANIAL REVASCULARIZATION (BYPASS)

## SURGICAL CONSIDERATIONS

**Description:** **Extracranial-intracranial (EC-IC) revascularization** procedures are performed when: (1) deliberate occlusion of a major cervical artery (carotid or vertebral) is necessary, and inadequate collateral CBF is available; or (2) stenosis or occlusion of major cervical or intracranial arteries causes transient ischemic attacks (TIAs) or stroke, despite the use of maximum medical therapy (ASA, heparin or Coumadin®). A donor extracranial scalp artery or interposition vein segment is sutured to a cervical artery and anastomosed to an intracranial artery, using microscopic techniques, through a **craniotomy**. The most common EC-IC procedure is a **superficial temporal artery (STA)-to-middle cerebral artery (MCA) branch anastomosis**. Other grafts include STA-to-posterior cerebral artery, STA-to-superior cerebellar artery, occipital artery-to-posterior inferior cerebral artery or interposition saphenous vein segment graft from the cervical external carotid artery to the middle cerebral artery, posterior cerebral artery or superior cerebellar artery.

**Variant procedure or approaches:** **Encephalo-duro-arterio-synangiosis (EDAS)** is a variant procedure wherein the STA is dissected circumferentially with its adventitia in the scalp, left in continuity and laid on the surface of the brain after opening the dura. **Omental-to-brain transposition** is another variant wherein the omentum, with its luxuriant blood supply, is lengthened, left attached to the right gastroepiploic artery, tunneled subcutaneously in the chest and neck, and laid over a large area of poorly vascularized cerebral cortex after opening the dura. Sometimes a free omental graft is transposed to the brain by anastomosing the omental gastroepiploic artery and vein to the superficial temporal artery and vein. Revascularization is induced by angiogenesis factors and growth substances secreted by the omentum.

**Usual preop diagnosis:** Stroke; TIA; carotid artery stenosis (inaccessible to carotid endarterectomy); carotid artery occlusion; middle cerebral artery stenosis or occlusion; vertebral artery stenosis or occlusion; basilar artery stenosis or occlusion; moyamoya disease (cerebral ischemia due to occlusion of vessels at base of the brain)

### SUMMARY OF PROCEDURE

| | EC-IC Bypass | EC-IC Bypass with Vein Graft | Omentum-to-Brain Transposition |
|---|---|---|---|
| **Position** | Supine or lateral decubitus | ⇐ | ⇐ |
| **Incision** | Frontal, parietal, temporal or occipital, or a combination of these, depending on area to be vascularized. | ⇐ + Medial aspect of leg and thigh for harvesting greater saphenous vein | ⇐ + Vertical abdominal incision for harvesting omentum; chest/neck incision for tunneling |
| **Special instrumentation** | Microscopic instruments; microvascular Doppler to identify scalp donor artery course and confirm graft patency. | ⇐ + Tunneling instruments | ⇐ |
| **Unique considerations** | Neuroprotective agents (barbiturates, mannitol) and induced mild HTN (MAP 90-110) during cross-clamp of recipient intracranial artery. Avoid excessive brain relaxation. | Attention to proper alignment of vein when tunneled, to avoid kinking; heparinization if major cervical artery (carotid, vertebral) is temporarily occluded. | ⇐ + Avoid devascularizing omentum during dissection and compromise to omental blood supply during tunneling and skin closure. |
| **Antibiotics** | Vancomycin (1 gm iv q 12 hrs) + cefotaxime (1 gm iv q 6 hrs) | ⇐ | ⇐ |
| **Surgical time** | 3-5 hrs | ⇐ | ⇐ |
| **Closing considerations** | Careful attention to hemostasis. Avoid compromise of graft with dural closure, bone replacement or scalp closure. | ⇐ | ⇐ |
| **EBL** | < 100 cc | ⇐ | 100-500 cc |

| | EC-IC Bypass | EC-IC with Vein Graft | Omentum-to-Brain |
|---|---|---|---|
| **Postop care** | Start ASA on postop d 1; monitor for subdural hygroma (CSF fluid collection in subdural space); ICU x 1 d. | ⇐ | ⇐ |
| **Mortality** | < 0.5% | ⇐ | ⇐ |
| **Morbidity** | Subdural hygroma: Rare | ⇐ | Abdominal hernia: Rare |
| | Wound infection: Rare | ⇐ | ⇐ |
| | Stroke: Rare | ⇐ | ⇐ |
| **Procedure code** | 61711, 61712 | ⇐ | ⇐ |
| **Pain score** | 3 | 3 | 3 |

### PATIENT POPULATION CHARACTERISTICS

**Age range** 40-80 yrs old (2-20 yrs for moyamoya disease)

**Male:Female** 1:1 for atherosclerotic disease; 1:1.4 for moyamoya disease

**Incidence** Thromboembolic stroke common, but indications for EC-IC bypass rare; 1/million/yr for moyamoya disease

**Etiology** Atherosclerosis
Embolism from heart or carotid artery

**Associated conditions** HTN
CAD
Peripheral vascular disease
Hyperlipidemia
Smoking
Alcohol abuse
Obesity
Moyamoya disease

---

## ANESTHETIC CONSIDERATIONS

### PREOPERATIVE

EC-IC bypass is used to make an anastomosis between external (usually superficial temporal artery) and internal carotid circulation. Patients with symptomatic moyamoya disease or bilateral carotid stenosis or occlusion also seem to be good candidates for EC-IC bypass, especially since there are no other forms of therapy which have proven to be effective.

**Respiratory** None unless patient has Hx of smoking, or has sustained pulmonary aspiration as a result of a neurological deficit.
**Tests:** CXR; others as indicated from H&P.

**Cardiovascular** These patients may have generalized vascular disease, including CAD, so a careful cardiac Hx, physical exam and ECG analysis should be done. If findings are positive, consider a more complete evaluation, including ECHO and coronary angiography. Be aware that cardiac insufficiency is the cause of about half of the deaths in patients with cerebrovascular disease.[11]
**Tests:** ECG; others as indicated from H&P.

**Neurological** Patients present with Sx of focal ischemic lesions. Cerebral angiography to rule out other causes of transient ischemic attacks and characterize collateral circulation. Regional CBF studies generally not helpful because measurement does not distinguish between low flow due to cerebrovascular obstruction from low flow due to low metabolic demands 2° prolonged cerebral ischemia.
**Tests:** CT; MRI; angiogram

**Hematologic** Anticoagulants or platelet-suppressive drugs such as NSAIDs should be D/C 2 wks before surgery to avoid excessive bleeding.
**Tests:** Hct; PT; PTT; hemogram

**Laboratory** UA; electrolyte panel; other tests as indicated from H&P.

**Premedication** Seldom necessary; detailed discussion with patient about the anesthetic plan, with appropriate reassurance, is usually enough. If premedication is desirable, small doses of sedative/hypnotics (e.g., midazolam 2-5 mg) are preferable to opiates.

## INTRAOPERATIVE

**Anesthetic technique:** GETA. The goals of anesthesia for this procedure are to: (1) provide adequate surgical anesthesia; (2) decrease intracranial volume (blood and tissue) to optimize working space within the cranial compartment, thereby minimizing the need for surgical retraction of brain tissue; and (3) increase tolerance of the brain to ischemia by decreasing $CMRO_2$ with the use of mild hypothermia (32-33°C) and barbiturate therapy, and maximizing flow to the ischemic area through collateral channels by maintaining BP at normal or somewhat elevated values.

**Induction** STP (20 mg/kg iv) provides amnesia and decreases cerebral blood volume by inducing cerebral vasoconstriction in the normally reactive vessels. Ischemic vessels will not contract in response to this drug. Meperidine 2 mg/kg or other equivalent opiate iv provides analgesia. A long-acting muscle relaxant (e.g., mixture of d-tubocurarine 0.3 mg/kg [7 ml] and pancuronium 0.04 mg/kg [3 ml]) for intubation and positioning of patient. Lidocaine 1.5 mg/kg administered either by LTA spray or iv to lessen cardiovascular responses to intubation.

**Maintenance** Isoflurane ≤ 1% inspired with $O_2$. $N_2O$ not used because of its potential for reversing the protective effects of STP for focal ischemia. STP (5-10 mg/kg) is given just prior to surgical occlusion of the cerebral vessel in preparation for anastomosis. This dose is given over 5-10 min to avoid sudden ↓BP. The concentration of isoflurane is decreased during STP administration.

**Emergence** Generally, ETT can be removed at the conclusion of anesthetic, unless operation has been particularly long or complex.

**Blood and fluid requirements**

IV: 16 ga x 2
NS/LR @ < 10 ml/kg + UO
CVP (triple-lumen)

Triple-lumen CVP with multiple stopcocks for connection of esmolol, SNP, phenylephrine infusions. One lumen is used for monitoring CVP.

**Control of brain volume**

Hyperventilate to $PaCO_2$ = 25-30 mmHg.
↓fluids < 10 ml/kg + UO
STP infusion
↓isoflurane < 1%
Mannitol 1 gm/kg
± Furosemide 0.3 mg/kg
± Lumbar CSF drain
Dexamethasone 8-12 mg

Generally, vigorous control of brain volume is not necessary since surgeon is working with cerebral vessels on the surface of the brain. If an omental graft is to be placed on the brain, however, additional brain shrinkage is useful. Ventilation is controlled and TV and RR are adjusted such that $PaCO_2$ ranges from 25-30 mmHg. Hypocarbia has several advantages, including decreasing cerebral vascular volume, providing more surgical working space and lessening need for vigorous retraction of brain tissue; improving the regional distribution of CBF by: preferentially diverting blood to potentially ischemic areas of the brain; better buffering of brain lactic acid that may form as a result of focal ischemia; and decreasing anesthetic requirement.

**Monitoring**

Standard monitors (see Appendix).
+ Bladder temperature
Arterial line
CVP (triple-lumen IJ catheter)
UO

**Control of BP**

Maintain normal BP.

Maintenance of normal BP is important because of the dependence of flow on collateral circulation, particularly during temporary occlusion of the surgical vessel being anastomosed. If a vasoconstrictor is needed, a pure α-adrenergic stimulant such as phenylephrine is preferred because it has minimal dysrhythmogenic potential. Responses to vasoactive drugs are much easier to regulate if a normal blood volume has been maintained throughout the anesthetic period.

**Positioning**

✓ and pad pressure points.
✓ eyes.
Shoulder roll
Anti-embolism stockings and SCDs

If omental graft is used, chest and abdomen must be clear of anesthetic apparatus. Anesthetic hoses and monitoring and vascular lines directed to patient's feet where the anesthesiologist is positioned during surgery. Anti-embolism stockings and SCDs used to minimize DVT.

| | | |
|---|---|---|
| **Deliberate hypothermia** | Thermal blanket, ice packs, Bair Hugger®<br>Maintain body temperature of ~32--33°C<br>Warm OR and fluids. | Surface cooling is begun as soon as induction of anesthesia is complete, using a thermal blanket underneath patient, ice packs and Bair Hugger® on top. When anastomosis is nearly complete, vigorous efforts at warming, including warming OR and iv fluids, are initiated. |
| **Complications** | Seizures<br>Stroke<br>Hemorrhage at anastomosis | Seizure Rx: Phenytoin (1 gm loading dose). **NB:** Incompatible with dextrose-containing solutions) |

### POSTOPERATIVE

| | | |
|---|---|---|
| **Complications** | Localized scalp necrosis | Major complications uncommon; localized scalp necrosis unique to this procedure. |
| **Pain management** | Meperidine (10 mg iv prn)<br>Codeine (30-60 mg im q 4 hrs prn) | |
| **Tests** | Cerebral angiogram<br>Regional blood flow studies<br>CT scan | Cerebral angiography documents patency of graft and collateral flow. Some centers have the capability of performing regional blood flow studies. If any question about neurological status, a CT scan is performed. |

**References**


1. Schmidek HH, Sweet WH, eds: *Operative Neurosurgical Techniques: Indications, Methods, and Results*, Vols I-II. WB Saunders Co, Philadelphia: 1988.
2. Youmans JR, ed: *Neurological Surgery*, Vols 1-6. WB Saunders Co, Philadelphia: 1990.
3. Wilkins RH, Rengachary SS, eds: *Neurosurgery*, Vols 1-3. McGraw-Hill, New York: 1985.
4. Sundt TM Jr: *Surgical Techniques for Saccular and Giant Intracranial Aneurysms*. Williams & Wilkins, Baltimore: 1990.
5. Ojemann RG, Heros RC, Crowell RM: *Surgical Management of Cerebrovascular Disease*. Williams & Wilkins, Baltimore: 1987.
6. Yonekawa Y, Gots Y, Ogata N: Moyamoya disease: diagnosis, treatment and recent achievement. In *Stroke: Pathophysiology, Diagnosis and Management*, 2nd edition. Barnett HJM, Mohr JP, Stein BM, Yabu F, eds. Churchill Livingstone, New York: 1992, 721-47.
7. Samson DS, Boone S: Extracranial-intracranial (EC-IC) arterial bypass: past performances and current concepts. *Neurosurgery* 1978; 3(1):79-86.
8. The EC/IC Bypass Study Group: Failure of extracranial-intracranial arterial bypass to reduce the risk of ischemic stroke. Results of an international randomized trial. *N Engl J Med* 1985; 313(19):1191-1200.
9. Ausman JI, Diaz FG: Critique of the extracranial-intracranial bypass study. *Surg Neurol* 1986; 26(3):218-21.
10. Day AL, Rhoton AL, Little JR: The extracranial-intracranial bypass study. *Surg Neurol* 1986; 26(3):222-26.
11. Fox JL, et al: Microsurgical treatment of neurovascular disease. *Neurosurgery* 1978; 3:285-337.


# CRANIOTOMY FOR TUMOR

## SURGICAL CONSIDERATIONS

**Description:** Tumors of the brain fall into various categories, which can be classified as: supratentorial and infratentorial, intra-axial (e.g., astrocytoma, oligodendroglioma, glioblastoma, etc.) and extra-axial (e.g., meningioma, acoustic neuroma, etc.). The surgical approach depends on the location of the lesion, whether there is a need for brain relaxation or not, or if exposure will require brain resection or incision. The positioning of the patient also depends on the location of tumor; e.g., the sitting position is often utilized for pineal tumors and for some other posterior fossa tumors (cerebellar tumors and acoustic neuromas) and the supine position is used for craniopharyngiomas and subfrontal tumors. Surgeons may prefer the lateral position for temporal lobe or parietal lobe lesions and the prone position for occipital lobe lesions and some cerebellar lesions. The prone or lateral position may be used for acoustic neuromas and the semi-sitting position may be used for occipital lesions. The patient's head is placed in a head holder (suction cup, horseshoe or Shea headrest). There are several common types of incisions, and the type used is customized to the lesion. The bone normally is removed by creating burr holes and then cutting a flap with the neuro bone saw. Some surgeons routinely use a "free-bone flap," in which the bone is completely removed and stored for the duration of the case. Other surgeons turn an osteoplastic flap, where the bone is left attached to muscle and/or pericranium to keep it partially vascularized. In the **suboccipital**, or **posterior fossa craniotomy**, the bone is often removed piecemeal, with either a drill or a series of rongeurs. Once the bone is removed, the dura is opened and, depending on tumor location and type, the surgeon either proceeds with tumor removal or obtains exposure within the brain in order to remove the tumor. Brain relaxation is requested if it is needed to expose and remove the lesion. When operating around the brain stem, vasomotor instability (bradycardia or HTN) may occur. The surgeon will need to know when these events occur, as they may signal injury to vital areas. Once the tumor is removed, the surgeon establishes hemostasis prior to dural closure. Occasionally, it is necessary to use a dural graft to close the dura. In supratentorial cases, the bone is usually replaced; however, the bone can be stored up to six months for subsequent replacement if swelling is anticipated. Patients undergoing this type of procedure usually require intensive postop care.

**Variant procedure or approaches:** Patient positioning varies from supine to prone to lateral to sitting, depending on surgeon's preference, as well as tumor location. Tumors on the convexity or close to the surface may not require much brain relaxation or exposure; however, tumors at the base of the brain may require extensive relaxation and exposure in order to be reached. Tumors at the base of the brain or deep within the ventricular system are usually removed with the aid of the operating microscope. Some are easily removed (e.g., convexity meningioma), while others are tedious and involve lengthy surgical time (e.g., craniopharyngioma and acoustic neuroma). Surgeons may use evoked potential monitoring techniques to aid in the removal of the tumors at the base of the brain in and about the cranial nerves.

**Usual preop diagnosis:** Brain tumor; glioma; glioblastoma; astrocytoma; oligodendroglioma; ependymoma; primitive neuroectodermal tumor; meningioma; craniopharyngioma; choroid plexus papilloma; hemangioblastoma; medulloblastoma; acoustic neuroma; pituitary adenoma

## SUMMARY OF PROCEDURE

| | |
|---|---|
| **Position** | Supine, lateral, prone or sitting |
| **Incision** | Dependent on location of tumor |
| **Special instrumentation** | Operating microscope; laser; CUSA; neuro drill (craniotome); ± evoked potential monitoring equipment |
| **Unique considerations** | ETT must be taped securely in a location satisfactory to the surgeon; anode or RAE® tube is helpful in certain situations. Brain relaxation techniques may be required. The patient with ↑ICP may require special consideration for induction of anesthesia. |
| **Antibiotics** | Cefotaxime 1 gm and vancomycin 1 gm (iv slowly) |
| **Surgical time** | 2.5 - 12 hrs |
| **Closing considerations** | Possible requirement for fascia lata graft or lyophilized (cadaveric) dura. Drain often left in epidural space. The surgeon often requests control of BP to avoid hemorrhage into bed of tumor. |
| **EBL** | 25-500 cc |
| **Postop care** | ICU or close observation unit x 1-3 d. Fluid and electrolytes require frequent monitoring, as the patient may develop SIADH following this procedure. BP may need to be controlled with hypotensive agents or ß-blockers. |
| **Mortality** | 0-5% (higher for tumors in critical locations) |
| **Morbidity** | Infection<br>Neurological: neurologic disability, nerve injury<br>Endocrine disorder: panhypopituitarism, diabetes insipidus (DI)<br>CSF leak<br>Massive blood loss: venous sinus injury |
| **Procedure code** | 61510-61530 (craniotomies for tumor); 61712 (microscopic) |
| **Pain score** | 2-6 |

## PATIENT POPULATION CHARACTERISTICS

| | |
|---|---|
| **Age range** | Infant - 85 yrs (usually 20-60 yrs) |
| **Male:Female** | ~1:1 |
| **Incidence** | Common neurosurgical procedure |
| **Etiology** | Neoplastic<br>Traumatic |

## ANESTHETIC CONSIDERATIONS

### PREOPERATIVE

Typically this is a healthy patient population, apart from Sx attributable to intracranial pathology (↑ICP, seizures, headache, N&V, visual disturbances, etc.).

**Respiratory** No special considerations, unless indicated from H&P.

**Cardiovascular** Benign or malignant brain tumors cause edema formation in adjacent normal brain tissue, which may lead to ↑ICP. If ICP increases sufficiently to cause herniation of the brain stem, patients develop the "Cushing triad" of HTN, bradycardia and ↓RR. These changes will resolve when ICP is reduced, so vigorous attempts to regulate BP and HR prior to craniotomy are not warranted. Once the diagnosis of brain tumor is made, most patients are placed on high-dose steroid therapy to lessen edema in surrounding normal brain. Steroids are extremely effective in this setting, and Sx of ↑ICP will often abate.

**Tests:** ECG; others as indicated from H&P.

**Neurological** Patients may present with complaints of headache, N&V, recent onset of seizures, visual changes or neurological deficits from compression of motor area, or as a result of hemorrhage from the tumor or edema in surrounding normal brain. Document preop physical findings.

**Tests:** A CT scan or MRI will delineate the site and size of the tumor, especially if iv contrast material, such as gadolinium, is administered to enhance the margins of the tumor.

**Laboratory** Other tests as indicated from H&P.

**Premedication** Standard premedication (except for patients with the possibility of ↑ICP → no sedation).

### INTRAOPERATIVE

**Anesthetic technique:** Small tumors, particularly those located in deeper brain structures, may be localized and resected using stereotactic and microsurgical techniques. Generally, the stereotactic frame is placed on patient's head under local anesthesia; then patient is taken to CT for determination of the coordinates to be used for stereotactic guidance to tumor site. In children, GETA may be needed both for placing the stereotactic frame and for completion of CT scan. GETA is almost invariably used for tumor removal, although MAC is used on rare occasions when the surgeon needs to assess motor or sensory function during resection of tumor adjacent to critical motor or sensory areas.

**Induction** If patient is in a stereotactic frame, or a difficult intubation is anticipated, orotracheal intubation will need to be accomplished before induction of GA. Awake fiber optic intubation is the best choice, since fitting a mask on the face with the stereotactic frame in place is impossible (see thoracolumbar procedures for technique). Once the airway is secured, anesthesia is usually induced with STP (3-5 mg/kg) and an opiate (e.g., meperidine 1.5-2 mg/kg), in combination with a non-depolarizing muscle relaxant (e.g., vecuronium 10 mg). To minimize ↑↑BP and ↑↑ICP with ET intubation, it is important that the patient be well-anesthetized (and paralyzed, if appropriate) before undertaking laryngoscopy. Induction doses of STP (8 mg/kg) or midazolam (0.4 mg/kg) may not be sufficient to abolish increases in MAP, CPP and, hence, ↑ICP associated with laryngoscopy and tracheal intubation.[8] Consideration should be given to using fentanyl (5-10 μg/kg) or lidocaine (1.5-2 mg/kg iv) as part of the induction technique. Once anesthesia is induced, a non-depolarizing neuromuscular blocking drug (vecuronium or atracurium 10 mg) is administered for ET intubation and subsequent positioning of the patient. Both of these non-depolarizing neuromuscular blocking drugs have been shown not to increase ICP in patients with brain tumors.[3,4] In contrast, both d-tubocurarine[5] and succinylcholine increase ICP in patients with brain tumors. The succinylcholine effect, however, can be abolished by a "defasciculating" dose of metocurine (0.03 mg/kg).[6] Since the same effect also can be achieved with incomplete neuromuscular blockade using other non-depolarizing drugs,[7] defasciculating doses of any non-depolarizing drug presumably will prevent ↑ICP with succinylcholine.

**Maintenance** The ideal drug for maintenance of anesthesia is one that decreases ICP and $CMRO_2$, maintains cerebral autoregulation, redistributes flow to the potentially ischemic areas and provides protection of the brain from focal ischemia. STP meets all of these criteria, and is an excellent anesthetic for this operation. An effective, safe and reliable method of delivery is a continuous infusion of STP, 0.5-1% solution administered at a rate of 0.2-0.3 mg/kg/min, to a total dose of 20-25 mg/kg. The administration should be complete by the time the dura is ready for opening. At these doses, CBF will be decreased by 50%, thereby decreasing cerebral blood volume and ICP and lessening need for brain retraction during operation. STP also may provide cerebral protection from focal

**Maintenance, continued**

ischemia by decreasing $CMRO_2$ (by ~50%), and by redistributing flow to potentially ischemic areas where surgical retraction is occurring. It is generally believed that cerebral reactivity to changes in $PaCO_2$ is preserved during STP anesthesia.

High-dose narcotic (e.g., fentanyl 10 μg/kg load + 2 μg/kg/hr infusion) has become an attractive technique for maintenance of anesthesia in patients undergoing craniotomy for tumor because of the circulatory stability these agents confer. Fentanyl does not have any direct effect on cerebral vasculature and, hence, does not increase ICP; but both alfentanil and sufentanil may cause mild cerebral vasodilatation and ↑ICP in patients with brain tumors, unless hypocarbia is instituted.[14] What evidence exists suggests that the opioids have minimal protective effect in the presence of focal cerebral ischemia.[16]

Isoflurane is regarded as the best volatile agent for patients undergoing neurosurgical procedures. Although isoflurane causes dose-dependent increases in CBF and volume and ↑ICP, these effects tend to be mitigated by the prior administration of STP, institution of hyperventilation, and limitation of the inspired isoflurane concentration to ≤ 1%.[17] If STP induction dose is low (5-6 mg/kg), however, and the inspired isoflurane concentration is ≥ 1%, some patients with supratentorial tumors will evidence ↑↑ICP, even if $PaCO_2$ is maintained at < 30 mmHg.[18] At inspired isoflurane concentrations of ≤ 1%, CBF responses to changes in $PaCO_2$ are maintained, and cerebral autoregulation remains intact.[19,20] Finally, isoflurane appears to provide protection from incomplete focal ischemia,[21,22] but whether it is as effective as STP in this regard remains controversial.

$N_2O$, a modest cerebrovascular dilator which increases ICP, does not appear to provide any cerebral protection in the presence of incomplete focal ischemia,[24] and, in fact, may attenuate the protective effects of STP or isoflurane.[25] Also, it has been suggested that $N_2O$ may increase likelihood of postop tension pneumocephalus, but this has recently been challenged.[26] Because the evidence relating to $N_2O$ is controversial and its risks and benefits unclear, its use is best left to the discretion of the anesthesiologist.

Generally, no further neuromuscular blocking drugs are administered beyond that used for tracheal intubation. With adequate anesthesia, and the head in Mayfield-Kees skeletal fixation, patient movement of any consequence is highly unlikely. Furthermore, it is useful to see movement of an extremity as an indicator of inadequate depth of anesthesia.

**Emergence**

It has been suggested that use of $N_2O$ during closure of a craniotomy may worsen a tension pneumocephalus, and that its use should be DC'd prior to closure; however, a recent study suggested that $N_2O$ did not increase ICP during closure.[26] With normal emergence, ETT should be removed before vigorous coughing ensues. If surgeon suspects that patient may have a slow recovery or a neurological injury from tumor removal, or if the anesthesiologist believes that recovery from anesthesia may be delayed, it is advisable to leave ETT in place at least overnight.

**Blood and fluid requirements**

IV: 16-18 ga x 2
NS/LR @ 2-3 cc/kg

Brain tumors can be highly vascular, so it is prudent to plan accordingly. To minimize postop cerebral edema, limit NS/LR to ≤ 10 ml/kg plus replacement of UO. If volume is needed, administer albumin 5% as required or hetastarch 6% ≤ 20 ml/kg. Transfuse for Hct < 25%. Controlled hypotension is generally not used in this operation unless bleeding becomes profuse, diffuse and difficult for the neurosurgeon to control.

**Monitoring**

Standard monitors (see Appendix).
Arterial line
CVP line
UO
± Doppler
± BAEP

If the tumor is in the posterior fossa and patient is in the seated position, a Doppler precordial chest stethoscope is necessary. If the tumor is an acoustic neuroma, the surgeon will request evoked potential monitoring, in which case the dose of barbiturate should be limited to ≤ 5 mg/kg to avoid interference with this monitoring.

**Positioning**

✓ and pad pressure points.
✓ eyes.

For brain tumors in the frontal, parietal or temporal lobes, patient will be supine with head in Mayfield-Kees skeletal fixation, turned to the side and a roll under the shoulder on the operative side (Fig 1.1-4). For occipital or posterior fossa tumors, patient may be prone or, preferably, sitting (see "Anesthetic Considerations for

| | | |
|---|---|---|
| **Positioning, continued** | | Cervical Neurosurgical Procedures"). Acoustic neuromas are generally most easily removed with patient in the lateral ("park-bench") position with a roll under the axilla. Patient generally lies on a bean bag which, when aspirated, holds her/him firmly in the lateral position. |
| **Control of ICP** | Control BP & CVP = low normal.<br>$PaO_2$ >100 mmHg<br>↓fluids < 10 ml/kg + UO<br>STP infusion<br>↓isoflurane < 1%<br>± Steroids | Patients with intracranial tumors may be on the steep portion of the intracranial compliance curve such that any increase in intracranial volume may cause ↑↑ICP. Transient increases in ICP – even up to 50-60 mmHg – are tolerated, provided they are promptly terminated. Sustained increases in ICP > 25-30 mmHg are associated with severe neurologic injury and poor outcome. |
| | Hyperventilate to $PaCO_2$ = 25-30 mmHg ($PETCO_2$=20-25 mmHg). | ↓$PaCO_2$ → ↓cerebral vascular volume (providing better surgical access) + ↑CBF to ischemic areas ("Robin Hood" effect) + ↓anesthetic requirements + ↑lactic acid buffering. |
| | Mannitol 1 gm/kg<br>± Furosemide 0.3 mg/kg | Mannitol/furosemide → ↓$K^+$; monitor level and replace as necessary. If mannitol is administered too rapidly, profound hypotension will occur, probably from peripheral vasodilation. |
| | ± Lumbar CSF drain<br>Head up 20-30° | CSF drain often placed after induction of anesthesia, and may be opened as required to ↓CSF volume. |

## POSTOPERATIVE

| | | |
|---|---|---|
| **Complications** | Seizures<br>Neurologic deficits<br>Hemorrhage requiring re-exploration<br>Edema and ↑ICP<br>Tension pneumocephalus | Seizure Rx: Phenytoin (1 gm loading dose). **NB:** Incompatible with dextrose-containing solutions.<br>In seated position, additional rare, but possible complications include quadriplegia from excessive flexion of head or tension pneumocephalus from air in cerebral cavities. Severe tension pneumocephalus may delay emergence from anesthesia, or cause postop neurologic deficits. |
| **Pain management** | Codeine (30-60 mg im q 4 hrs) | |
| **Tests** | CT scan | If patient exhibits any delay in emergence from anesthesia and surgery, or any new neurologic deficits emerge postop, a CT scan is invariably obtained. |

**References**


1. Apuzzo MLJ: *Brain Surgery: Complication, Avoidance and Management.* Churchill Livingstone, New York: 1993, 175-688.
2. Black PM: Brain tumors. *New Engl J Med* 1991; 324(21):1471-76, 1555-64.
3. Minton MD, Stirt JA, Bedford RF, Haworth C: Intracranial pressure after atracurium in neurosurgical patients. *Anesth Analg* 1985; 64(11):1113-16.
4. Stirt JA, Maggio W, Haworth C, Minton MD, Bedford RF: Vecuronium: effect on intracranial pressure and hemodynamics in neurosurgical patients. *Anesthesiology* 1987; 67(4):570-73.
5. Tarkkanen L, Laitinen L, Johansson G: Effects of d-tubocurarine on intracranial pressure and thalamic electrical impedance. *Anesthesiology* 1974; 40(3):247-51.
6. Stirt JA, Grosslight KR, Bedford RF, Vollmer D: "Defasciculation" with metocurine prevents succinylcholine-induced increases in intracranial pressure. *Anesthesiology* 1987; 67(1):50-53.
7. Minton MD, Grosslight KR, Stirt JA, Bedford RF: Increases in intracranial pressure from succinylcholine: prevention by prior nondepolarizing blockade. *Anesthesiology* 1986; 65(2):165-69.
8. Giffin JP, Cottrell JE, Shwiry B, Hartung J, Epstein J, Lim K: Intracranial pressure, mean arterial pressure, and heart rate following midazolam or STP in humans with brain tumors. *Anesthesiology* 1984; 60(5):491-94.
9. Pinaud M, Lelausque JN, Chetanneau A, Fauchoux N, Menegalli D, Souron R: Effects of propofol on cerebral hemodynamics and metabolism in patients with brain trauma. *Anesthesiology* 1990; 73(3):404-09.
10. Van Hemelrijck J, Fitch W, Mattheussen M, Van Aken H, Plets C, Lauwers T: Effect of propofol on cerebral circulation and autoregulation in the baboon. *Anesth Analg* 1990; 71(1):49-54.
11. Kochs E, Hoffman WE, Werner C, Thomas C, Albrecht RF, Schulte am Esch J: The effects of propofol on brain electrical activity, neurologic outcome, and neuronal damage following incomplete ischemia in rats. *Anesthesiology* 1992; 76(2):245-52.

12. Eng C, Lam AM, Mayberg TS, Lee C, Mathisen T: The influence of propofol with and without nitrous oxide on cerebral blood flow velocity and $CO_2$ reactivity in humans. *Anesthesiology* 1992; 77(5):872-79.
13. Ridenour TR, Warner DS, Todd MM, Gionet TX: Comparative effects of propofol and halothane on outcome from temporary middle cerebral artery occlusion in the rat. *Anesthesiology* 1992; 76(5):807-12.
14. Jung R, Shah N, Reinsel R, Marx W, Marshall W, Galicich J, Bedford R: Cerebrospinal fluid pressure in patients with brain tumors: impact of fentanyl versus alfentanil during nitrous oxide-oxygen anesthesia. *Anesth Analg* 1990; 71(4):419-22.
15. From RP, Warner DS, Todd MM, Sokoll MD: Anesthesia for craniotomy: a double-blind comparison of alfentanil, fentanyl, and sufentanil. *Anesthesiology* 1990; 73(5):896-904.
16. Nehls DG, Todd MM, Spetzler RF, Drummond JC, Thompson RA, Johnson PC: A comparison of the cerebral protective effects of isoflurane and barbiturates during temporary focal ischemia in primates. *Anesthesiology* 1987; 66(4):453-64.
17. Adams RW, Cucchiara RF, Gronert GA, Messick JM, Michenfelder JD: Isoflurane and cerebrospinal fluid pressure in neurosurgical patients. *Anesthesiology* 1981; 54(2):97-99.
18. Grosslight KR, Foster R, Colohan AR, Bedford RF: Isoflurane for neuroanesthesia: risk factors for increases in intracranial pressure. *Anesthesiology* 1985; 63(5):533-36.
19. McPherson RW, Traystman RJ: Effects of isoflurane on cerebral autoregulation in dogs. *Anesthesiology* 1988; 69(4):493-99.
20. Hoffman WE, Edelman G, Kochs E, Werner C, Segil L, Albrecht RF: Cerebral autoregulation in awake versus isoflurane-anesthetized rats. *Anesth Analg* 1991; 73(6):753-57.
21. Michenfelder JD, Sundt TM Jr, Fode N, Sharbrough FW: Isoflurane when compared to enflurane and halothane decreases the frequency of cerebral ischemia during carotid endarterectomy. *Anesthesiology* 1987; 67(3):336-40.
22. Baughman VL, Hoffman WE, Thomas C, Miletich DJ, Albrecht RF: Comparison of methohexital and isoflurane on neurologic outcome and histopathology following incomplete ischemia in rats. *Anesthesiology* 1990; 72(1):85-94.
23. Milde LN, Milde JH, Lanier WL, Michenfelder JD: Comparison of the effects of isoflurane and STP on neurologic outcome and neuropathology after temporary focal cerebral ischemia in primates. *Anesthesiology* 1988; 69(6):905-13.
24. Warner DS, Zhou J, Ramani R, Todd MM, McAllister A: Nitrous oxide does not alter infarct volume in rats undergoing reversible middle cerebral artery occlusion. *Anesthesiology* 1990; 73(4):686-93.
25. Hartung J, Cottrell JE: Nitrous oxide reduces STP-induced prolongation of survival in hypoxic and anoxic mice. *Anesth Analg* 1987; 66(1):47-52.
26. Domino KB, Hemstad JR, Lam AM, Laohaprasit V, Hamberg TA, Harrison SD, Grady MS, Winn HR: Effect of nitrous oxide on intracranial pressure after cranial-dural closure in patients undergoing craniotomy. *Anesthesiology* 1992; 77(3):421-25.
27. Nissenson AR, Weston RE, Kleeman CR: Mannitol. *West J Med* 1979; 131(4):277-84.
28. Domaingue CM, Nye DH: Hypotensive effect of mannitol administered rapidly. *Anaesth Intensive Care* 1985; 13(2):134-36.

# CRANIOTOMY FOR SKULL TUMOR

## SURGICAL CONSIDERATIONS

**Description:** Tumors of the skull fall into the classification of other bony tumors. Examples of types of skull tumors often requiring surgery include eosinophilic granuloma, histiocytosis, hemangioma, osteoma, epidermoid, dermoid tumor, metastatic tumors, osteosarcoma, fibrous dysplasia and meningioma. They may occur anywhere on the skull. The exact positioning of the patient depends on the location of tumor. For example, the sitting position is often used for tumors in the occipital or suboccipital regions and the supine position is used for frontal, temporal or parietal tumors. Some surgeons prefer the lateral position for temporal or parietal bone lesions and the prone position for occipital and some suboccipital bone lesions. The patient's head is placed in a head holder (either pins, suction cup, horseshoe or Shea headrest). The bone is usually removed by creating burr hole(s) and then cutting a flap with the neuro bone saw. In the suboccipital or posterior fossa craniotomy, the bone is often removed piecemeal with either a drill or a series of rongeurs. The dura usually is not opened unless it is involved with the tumor. The surgeon may elect to perform a **cranioplasty** to cover the defect, depending on size and location of the bone defect. The defect can be repaired using methylmethacrylate at the time of surgery, or bone may be harvested from either another location on the skull or another site (hip or rib) for reconstruction. Once the reconstruction is completed, the skin incision is closed. Occasionally, the tumor of the skull will be approached intracranially, if its location favors that approach. Examples include tumors of the petrous portion of the temporal bone or fibrous dysplasia involving the optic canal.

**Usual preop diagnosis**: Eosinophilic granuloma; histiocytosis; hemangioma; osteoma; epidermoid; dermoid tumor; metastatic tumors; osteosarcoma; fibrous dysplasia; meningioma

### SUMMARY OF PROCEDURE

| | |
|---|---|
| **Position** | Supine, lateral, prone or sitting |
| **Incision** | Dependent on location of tumor |
| **Special instrumentation** | Neuro drill |
| **Unique considerations** | ETT must be taped securely in a location satisfactory to the surgeon. Anode or RAE® tube may be helpful in certain situations. |
| **Antibiotics** | Cefazolin 1 gm iv |
| **Surgical time** | 1 - 4 hrs |
| **Closing considerations** | Drain often left in epidural space. Surgeon often requests control of BP to avoid hemorrhage into the bed of tumor. |
| **EBL** | 25-500 cc |
| **Postop care** | ICU or close observation unit |
| **Mortality** | 0-2% (higher for tumors in critical locations) |
| **Morbidity** | Usually < 5%:<br>Infection<br>Neurological disability<br>CSF leak<br>Massive blood loss - venous sinus injury |
| **Procedure code** | 61500 (removal of skull tumor); 62140-62141 (cranioplasty) |
| **Pain score** | 2-5 |

### PATIENT POPULATION CHARACTERISTICS

| | |
|---|---|
| **Age range** | Infant-85 yrs (usually 20-60 yrs) |
| **Male:Female** | ~1:1 |
| **Incidence** | Unknown |
| **Etiology** | Neoplastic<br>Traumatic |

## ANESTHETIC CONSIDERATIONS

See Anesthetic Considerations following "Craniotomy for Tumor" (above). Note, however, that patients with skull tumors rarely have problems with ICP.

**References**

1. Voorhies RM, Sundaresan N: Tumors of the skull. In *Neurosurgery*. Wilkins RH, Rengachary SS, eds. McGraw-Hill, New York: 1985, 984-1001.

# CRANIOTOMY FOR TRAUMA

## SURGICAL CONSIDERATIONS

**Description:** Head injuries occasionally require emergent surgical procedures to evacuate mass lesions or debride contused or contaminated brain. The majority of these injuries are supratentorial. The surgical procedure depends on the exact type and location of the injury (e.g., epidural, subdural, intracerebral hematomas or depressed skull fracture). Often the entire head is shaved and placed in a headrest (pins, suction cups or horseshoe). An incision is made according to the location and extent of the injury. The skin is incised and reflected and the skull is perforated with a cranial drill. If the abnormality is a chronic, subdural hematoma, it may be drained via burr holes. If there is a clot or depressed fracture or penetrating wound, a formal bone flap is elevated. Mass lesions are identified or removed, and the dura is repaired if lacerated. Depending on the injury and the presence of brain swelling, the dura may be patched and the bone flap replaced. An ICP monitor may be placed at the end of the procedure.

**Usual preop diagnosis:** Epidural hematoma; subdural hematoma; intracerebral hematoma; depressed skull fracture; cerebral contusions; gunshot wound of the brain

### SUMMARY OF PROCEDURE

| | |
|---|---|
| **Position** | Supine, lateral, prone or sitting, depending on site of injury |
| **Incision** | Varies with location of injury |
| **Unique considerations** | The patient may have ↑↑ICP. Because incipient herniation and/or associated injuries may be a concern, timing is critical. |
| **Antibiotics** | Vancomycin 1 gm iv slowly + cefotaxime 1 gm iv |
| **Surgical time** | 1.5 - 6 hrs |
| **Closing considerations** | Application of head dressing may jostle ETT at end of case → ↑BP. Patient may stay intubated postop. ICP monitor may be placed. Phenytoin may be given for seizure prophylaxis. |
| **EBL** | 25-500 cc |
| **Postop care** | ICU or close observation unit until stable. Fluid and electrolytes require frequent monitoring, as the patient may develop SIADH following this procedure. BP may need to be controlled with vasodilators and ß-blockers. |
| **Mortality** | 10-50%, depending on lesion; higher for acute subdural hematomas, lower for epidural hematomas. |
| **Morbidity** | Infection<br>Neurologic disability<br>Nerve injury<br>CSF leak<br>Endocrine disorder:<br>SIADH<br>Panhypopituitarism<br>Diabetes insipidus (DI)<br>Massive blood loss: venous sinus injury |
| **Procedure code** | 61304-61315 (craniotomy for hematomas); 62000-62010 (craniotomy for depressed fracture); 20922 (fascia lata graft) |
| **Pain score** | 2-4 |

### PATIENT POPULATION CHARACTERISTICS

| | |
|---|---|
| **Age range** | Infant-85 yrs (usually 15-40 yrs) |
| **Male:Female** | 2:1 |
| **Incidence** | Relatively common |
| **Etiology** | Trauma |
| **Associated conditions** | Abdominal injuries<br>Cervical spine fractures |

## ANESTHETIC CONSIDERATIONS

### PREOPERATIVE

Head injury is the leading cause of death of persons under 24 years of age.[1] A penetrating injury of the skull will usually cause major damage to the brain as a result of diffuse neuronal injury and hemorrhage into brain tissue. Surgery is necessary to control intracranial bleeding, to debride the wound, and to remove bone fragments, foreign material and damaged brain so that the cranial vault can better accommodate the brain swelling that inevitably occurs. Head injury also can be focal in nature, most commonly in the form of an epidural, subdural or intracranial hematoma. Epidural hematomas form between the skull and dura, and are usually due to bleeding from an artery (e.g., anterior cerebral or middle meningeal). Hence, time is of the essence and rapid evacuation and control of the bleeding is essential if permanent neurological injury is to be avoided. Subdural bleeding occurs between the dura and the leptomeninges lining the brain surface. This bleeding is usually venous in origin, and usually occurs more gradually. Focal intracranial hemorrhages may be either arterial or venous, and, as with subdural hematomas, must be evacuated if they are enlarging.

**Respiratory** Localized injuries to the frontal or parietal lobes may not cause any respiratory changes. If ↑ICP, respirations may become slow (< 10/min) and deep, and result in substantial hypocapnia. Many patients with head injuries demonstrate partial airway obstruction from the tongue falling back into the posterior pharyngeal space. If this occurs, or if the patient is comatose and unable to protect the airway and prevent aspiration of gastric contents, immediate tracheal intubation should be performed. Head injuries in the region of the occipital lobes may → apnea.
**Tests:** As indicated from H&P and as time allows.

**Cardiovascular** Most patients with head injuries evidence ↑BP and ↑HR. If ICP increases sufficiently to cause herniation of brain stem, patients develop the "Cushing triad" of ↑BP, ↓HR and ↓RR. These changes resolve when ↑ICP is relieved, so vigorous attempts to regulate BP and HR prior to craniotomy are not warranted. Patient, however, should be taken to OR as quickly as possible.
**Tests:** As indicated from H&P, and as time allows.

**Neurological** Neurological evaluation of the head-injured patient is based on the Glasgow Coma Scale (Table 1.1-1). The scale involves evaluation of three functions: eye opening, verbal response and motor response. Using this scoring system, the severity of brain injury may be classified as mild (13-15 points), moderate (9-12 points), or severe (8 points or less). By definition, any patient having 8 points or less is in coma. Additional useful neurological examinations include assessment of pupillary size and reactivity to the light, reflex responses, and evidence of asymmetry or flaccidity of the extremities or decerebrate or decorticate posturing. Head-injured patients whose neurological function is deteriorating rapidly, and in whom an epidural or subdural hemorrhage is suspected, should be taken to OR immediately without CT scan.
**Tests:** CT scan

**Table 1.1-1. Glasgow Coma Scale (GCS)**

| Category | Score |
|---|---|
| I. Eyes open: | |
| Never | 1 |
| To pain | 2 |
| To verbal stimuli | 3 |
| Spontaneously | 4 |
| II. Best verbal response: | |
| None | 1 |
| Incomprehensible sounds | 2 |
| Inappropriate words | 3 |
| Patient disoriented and converses | 4 |
| Patient oriented and converses | 5 |
| III. Best motor response: | |
| None | 1 |
| Extension (decerebrate rigidity) | 2 |
| Flexion abnormal (decorticate rigidity) | 3 |
| Flexion withdrawal | 4 |
| Patient localizes pain | 5 |
| Patient obeys | 6 |
| I + II + III Total = 3-15 | |

**Hematologic** Severe head injury may be associated with a progressively worsening coagulopathy, resulting in a clinical picture similar to that of DIC. The reason for this is not known, but the brain is rich in thromboplastin and other coagulation factors.
**Tests:** Hct; PT; PTT; others as indicated from H&P.

**Laboratory** Other tests as indicated from H&P, and as time permits.

**Premedication** Usually none

## INTRAOPERATIVE

**Anesthetic technique:** GETA

**Induction** ↑ICP is likely in most patients with head injury requiring operation, and induction of anesthesia is best-accomplished with drugs that ↓ICP. If patient is hemodynamically stable and not hypovolemic, induction with STP (≤ 10 mg/kg), propofol (1.5-3 mg/kg), ± opiate supplementation (meperidine 1.5-2 mg/kg, fentanyl 5 μg/kg) is satisfactory. If hemodynamically unstable, etomidate (0.1-0.4 mg/kg) is suitable for induction. Ketamine is not used because of its ability to ↑ICP. If patient is comatose, anesthetic requirement is less, needing only $O_2$ and muscle relaxant, or $N_2O$ 60% or low-dose isoflurane (≤ 0.5%). A non-depolarizing muscle relaxant (vecuronium or atracurium 10 mg) is administered for ET intubation.[2] Succinylcholine can be used if a "defasciculating" dose of a non-depolarizing neuromuscular blocking drug is administered first.[3] Nasotracheal intubation is not recommended for patients with maxillary and/or basilar skull fractures because of the potential for inserting the tube through the fracture site into the brain stem. To minimize ↑↑BP and ↑↑ICP with ET intubation, it is important that the patient be anesthetized and paralyzed before undertaking laryngoscopy. Induction doses of STP or propofol may not be sufficient to abolish increases in MAP, CPP and, hence, ICP associated with laryngoscopy and tracheal intubation.[4] In addition, consideration should be given to using lidocaine 2 mg/kg iv and fentanyl 5 μg/kg as part of the induction technique. Lidocaine has the amnesic effects of STP without the myocardial depressant effects. In hypovolemic patients, hydration with a mixture of crystalloid and colloid should be initiated prior to induction.

**Maintenance**

The ideal drug for maintenance of anesthesia decreases ICP and $CMRO_2$, maintains cerebral autoregulation, redistributes flow to potentially ischemic areas and provides protection of the brain from focal ischemia. STP meets these criteria, and is an excellent anesthetic for the head-trauma patient, provided the circulation tolerates the drug. A total dose of 15-20 mg/kg given by intermittent bolus injection or continuous infusion is sufficient. A continuous infusion of propofol 150 mg/kg/min to a total dose of 10 mg/kg can be used for the same purpose because it also decreases cerebral blood volume and ICP while maintaining cerebral autoregulation.[5,6]

Isoflurane is regarded as the best volatile agent for patients undergoing neurosurgical procedures. Although isoflurane causes dose-dependent increases in CBF and volume and, hence, ↑ICP, these effects tend to be mitigated by the prior administration of STP, hyperventilation, and by limiting the inspired isoflurane concentration to ≤ 1%. At < 1% isoflurane, CBF responses to changes in $PaCO_2$ are maintained, and cerebral autoregulation remains intact.[8,9] Finally, isoflurane appears to provide protection from incomplete focal ischemia.[10,11]

$N_2O$ may be administered, recognizing that it is a modest cerebrovascular dilator, thereby increasing ICP, an effect that would not be desirable in patients with a space-occupying lesion. Also, $N_2O$ does not appear to provide any cerebral protection in the presence of incomplete focal ischemia,[12] and, in fact, may attenuate the protective effects of STP or isoflurane.[13]

Generally, no further neuromuscular blocking drugs are administered beyond that used for tracheal intubation. With adequate anesthesia, and head in Mayfield-Kees skeletal fixation, patient movement of any consequence is highly unlikely. Furthermore, it is useful to see movement of an extremity as an indicator of inadequate depth of anesthesia.

**Emergence**

Because recovery from head injury is so unpredictable, it is generally advisable to leave the ETT in place and maintain controlled hyperventilation until there is sufficient clinical evidence that normal neurological recovery is occurring.

| | | |
|---|---|---|
| **Blood and fluid requirements** | Possible marked blood loss<br>IV: 16-18 ga x 1<br>NS @ 2-4 cc/kg/hr | Blood transfusion is often necessary. To minimize postop cerebral edema, total crystalloid volume should be limited to < 10 ml/kg plus replacement of UO. Glucose-containing solutions should be avoided; blood glucose levels should be maintained between 80-200 mg%. If volume is needed, albumin 5% (or hetastarch 6% up to 20 ml/kg) should be administered. |
| **Control of blood loss** | Low normal BP<br>HR = 50-70 | Blood loss is best minimized by maintaining MAP at low normal for that patient. Controlled hypotension generally is not used unless bleeding becomes profuse and difficult to control. HR is easily controlled with an esmolol infusion, and if additional ↓MAP is needed, SNP is begun. Hypotension is better treated with volume replacement than vasopressors. |
| **Monitoring** | Standard monitors (see Appendix).<br>± Arterial line<br>± CVP line<br>± UO | For minor head injuries, no special monitoring is needed. If the injury is extensive or unknown, or if the patient is unstable, invasive monitoring is mandatory. |
| **Positioning** | ✓ and pad pressure points.<br>✓ eyes. | For occipital or posterior fossa injuries, patient may be prone or sitting (see "Anesthetic Considerations for Cervical Neurosurgical Procedures"). Otherwise, patient will be supine with head in Mayfield-Kees skeletal fixation and turned to the side, and a roll placed under the shoulder on the operative side. |

| | | |
|---|---|---|
| **Control of ICP** | Adequate anesthesia<br>Head up 20-30°<br>STP infusion | Patients with skull fractures or intracranial bleeding may be on the steep portion of intracranial compliance curve such that any increase in intracranial volume may cause ↑↑ICP. Transient increases in ICP – even up to 50-60 mmHg – are tolerated, provided they are promptly terminated. Sustained increases in ICP > 25-30 mmHg are associated with severe neurologic injury and poor outcome. |
| | Hyperventilation to $PaCO_2$ = 25-30 mmHg<br>$PaO_2$ >100 mmHg | Hypocarbia is a potent cerebral vasoconstrictor, thereby decreasing cerebral blood volume and ICP. It should be recognized that some patients with diffuse brain injury will have lost cerebrovascular sensitivity to $PaCO_2$, such that hyperventilation will have little or no effect on vascular volume (or brain size). Maintaining $PaO_2$ will prevent cerebral vasodilatation from hypoxemia. Despite maintaining adequate ventilation, oxygenation and BP, patients with diffuse head injury often exhibit arterial and CSF lactic acidosis, a further indication of the metabolic derangement that exists in the brain from the injury.[16] |
| | Keep MAP low normal. | Control MAP and cerebral venous pressure so that CPP is maintained in the low normal range for that patient. Because most patients with head injury of any consequence lose cerebral autoregulation, ↑CPP → ↑cerebral blood volume and ↑ICP. Also, with loss of autoregulation, hypotension should be avoided to avoid cerebral ischemia. In severe, diffuse head injury with loss of autoregulation, some parts of the brain may exhibit "luxury perfusion," while other areas exhibit severe ischemia.[17] |
| | Mannitol 1 gm/kg<br>Furosemide 10-20 mg | With mannitol at a dose of 1 gm/kg, vigorous diuresis will commence in about 30 min (if blood volume is adequate), and brain shrinkage will follow. It is often necessary to provide supplemental potassium (20-30 mEq iv slowly). Simultaneous administration of furosemide (10-20 mg) is recommended to avoid the transient increases in cerebral blood volume and ICP that accompany mannitol administration. If mannitol is administered too rapidly, profound hypotension will occur, probably from peripheral vasodilatation.[15] |

## POSTOPERATIVE

| | | |
|---|---|---|
| **Complications** | Seizures<br>Neurologic deficits<br>Hemorrhage<br>Edema<br>↑ICP | Seizure Rx: Phenytoin (1 gm loading dose). **NB:** Incompatible with dextrose-containing solutions.<br>Some patients with severe head injury remain unconsciousness for weeks or months, without evidencing any substantial neurological recovery. A late complication of head injury is hydrocephalus requiring a shunt procedure. |
| **Pain management** | Codeine (30-60 mg im q 4 hrs) | |
| **Tests** | CT scan<br>ICP monitor | Unless neurological recovery is rapid, periodic CT scans are obtained postop to follow the intracranial changes. In addition, in many institutions, a device for monitoring ICP postop is placed at the time of operation. |

**References**

1. Cooper PR: Traumatic intracranial hematomas. In *Neurosurgery*. Wilkins RH, Rengachary SS, eds. McGraw-Hill, New York: 1985, 1657-69.

2. White RJ, Likavec MG: The diagnosis and initial management of head injury. *New Engl J Med* 1992; 327(21):1507-11.
3. Stirt JA, Maggio W, Haworth C, Minton MD, Bedford RF: Vecuronium: effect on intracranial pressure and hemodynamics in neurosurgical patients. *Anesthesiology* 1987; 67(4):570-73.
4. Stirt JA, Grosslight KR, Bedford RF, Vollmer D: "Defasciculation" with metocurine prevents succinylcholine-induced increases in intracranial pressure. *Anesthesiology* 1987; 67(1):50-53.
5. Giffin JP, Cottrell JE, Shwiry B, Hartung J, Epstein J, Lim K: Intracranial pressure, mean arterial pressure, and heart rate following midazolam or STP in humans with brain tumors. *Anesthesiology* 1984; 60(5):491-94.
6. Van Hemelrijck J, Fitch W, Mattheussen M, Van Aken H, Plets C, Lauwers T: Effect of propofol on cerebral circulation and autoregulation in the baboon. *Anesth Analg* 1990; 71(1):49-54.
7. Kochs E, Hoffman WE, Werner C, Thomas C, Albrecht RF, Schulte am Esch J: The effects of propofol on brain electrical activity, neurologic outcome, and neuronal damage following incomplete ischemia in rats. *Anesthesiology* 1992; 76(2):245-52.
8. Adams RW, Cucchiara RF, Gronert GA, Messick JM, Michenfelder JD: Isoflurane and cerebrospinal fluid pressure in neurosurgical patients. *Anesthesiology* 1981; 54(2):97-99.
9. McPherson RW, Traystman RJ: Effects of isoflurane on cerebral autoregulation in dogs. *Anesthesiology* 1988; 69(4):493-99.
10. Hoffman WE, Edelman G, Kochs E, Werner C, Segil L, Albrecht RF: Cerebral autoregulation in awake versus isoflurane-anesthetized rats. *Anesth Analg* 1991; 73(6):753-57.
11. Michenfelder JD, Sundt TM Jr, Fode N, Sharbrough FW: Isoflurane when compared to enflurane and halothane decreases the frequency of cerebral ischemia during carotid endarterectomy. *Anesthesiology* 1987; 67(3):336-40.
12. Baughman VL, Hoffman WE, Thomas C, Miletich DJ, Albrecht RF: Comparison of methohexital and isoflurane on neurologic outcome and histopathology following incomplete ischemia in rats. *Anesthesiology* 1990; 72(1):85-94.
13. Warner DS, Zhou J, Ramani R, Todd MM, McAllister A: Nitrous oxide does not alter infarct volume in rats undergoing reversible middle cerebral artery occlusion. *Anesthesiology* 1990; 73(4):686-93.
14. Hartung J, Cottrell JE: Nitrous oxide reduces STP-induced prolongation of survival in hypoxic and anoxic mice. *Anesth Analg* 1987; 66(1):47-52.
15. Nissenson AR, Weston RE, Kleeman CR: Mannitol. *West J Med* 1979; 131(4):277-84.
16. Domaingue CM, Nye DH: Hypotensive effect of mannitol administered rapidly. *Anaesth Intensive Care* 1985; 13(2):134-36.
17. King LR, McLaurin RL, Knowles HC Jr: Acid-base balance and arterial and CSF lactate levels following human head injury. *J Neurosurg* 1974; 40(5):617-25.
18. Overgaard J, Tweed WA: Cerebral circulation after head injury. Part 1: Cerebral blood flow and its regulation after closed head injury with emphasis on clinical correlations. *J Neurosurg* 1974; 41(5):531-41.

# MICROVASCULAR DECOMPRESSION OF CRANIAL NERVE

## SURGICAL CONSIDERATIONS

**Description:** Microvascular decompression is used to treat various disorders of the cranial nerves. The conditions in which this procedure is utilized most frequently include trigeminal neuralgia, hemifacial spasm and, more rarely, glossopharyngeal neuralgia. These conditions are thought to be caused by cross-compression of a cranial nerve by a vascular structure (usually an artery) A **craniectomy** is performed just behind the ear on the affected side. The dura at the junction of the transverse and sigmoid sinus is exposed. At this point, there is a risk of venous sinus bleeding. With brain relaxation, the cerebellum is retracted, exposing the cerebellopontine angle. The operating microscope allows the surgeon to explore the involved cranial nerve. If an offending vessel is identified, it is carefully dissected off the nerve and a pad (teflon sponge or muscle) is placed to keep the vessel from returning to its original position. In the case of trigeminal or glossopharyngeal neuralgia, occasionally a partial section of the nerve is performed, if no offending vessel is identified. With glossopharyngeal neuralgia, partial section of the 9th or 10th cranial nerve may cause some vasomotor instability. The main variations in this procedure are in patient positioning and surgeon's preference for various adjuncts. Patient positioning may be lateral, prone, supine or sitting. Intraop, mannitol (1 gm/kg) and a spinal drain (for CSF removal) may be needed for brain relaxation.

**Usual preop diagnosis:** Trigeminal neuralgia; tic douloureux; hemifacial spasm; tinnitus; glossopharyngeal neuralgia

### SUMMARY OF PROCEDURE

| | |
|---|---|
| **Position** | Normally, lateral ("park-bench"), head elevated 30°; less frequently, sitting, prone or supine |
| **Incision** | Retro-auricular (mastoid) |

| | |
|---|---|
| **Special instrumentation** | Operating microscope; cranial perforator; ± facial nerve monitoring; ± EMG; ± brain stem auditory evoked response (BAER) |
| **Unique considerations** | Risk of air embolus |
| **Antibiotics** | Cefotaxime 1 gm + vancomycin 1 gm iv slowly |
| **Surgical time** | 2 - 3 hrs |
| **EBL** | 25-250 cc |
| **Postop care** | ICU or close observation unit. Observe for change in neurologic status (e.g., level of alertness, response to commands), usually for 12-24 hrs. |
| **Mortality** | 0-3% |
| **Morbidity** | Usually < 5%:<br>Infection<br>Deafness<br>Facial weakness<br>Facial sensory deficit<br>CSF leak<br>Massive blood loss 2° vertebral artery injury |
| **Procedure code** | 61450-61460 (cranial nerve decompression or section codes); 61712 (microscopic) |
| **Pain score** | 4-6 |

### PATIENT POPULATION CHARACTERISTICS

| | |
|---|---|
| **Age range** | 40-85 yrs (usually 60-70 yrs) |
| **Male:Female** | ~2:3 |
| **Incidence** | Common |
| **Etiology** | Vascular compression of cranial nerve<br>Multiple sclerosis plaque |
| **Associated conditions** | HTN<br>Multiple sclerosis |

---

## ANESTHETIC CONSIDERATIONS

### PREOPERATIVE

Microvascular decompression involves a full craniotomy for decompression of a nerve which is causing facial pain and/or spasm of facial muscles. Generally, these patients have trigeminal neuralgia or tic douloureux which has not been responsive to medical management (carbamazepine [Tegretol®] therapy) and percutaneous rhizotomy or glycerol injection has failed.

| | |
|---|---|
| **Respiratory** | None unless the patient has a longstanding Hx of smoking, and has COPD. |
| **Cardiovascular** | Many patients will have Hx of idiopathic HTN and take any one of a variety of antihypertensive medications. Good control of BP preop is important because it will make intraop and postop management of BP easier. |
| **Neurological** | The presenting symptom is pain ± muscle spasm in the maxillary and/or mandibular division of the trigeminal nerve, unaccompanied by any motor or sensory deficits. |
| **Laboratory** | None, except for routine preop studies. |
| **Premedication** | Generally, patients for these procedures are elderly and do not require any special premedication. Midazolam 2-4 mg im will provide amnesia for the preop events, if that is desired by patient or surgeons. |

### INTRAOPERATIVE

**Anesthetic technique:** GA is necessary because a full craniotomy is performed. ICP is not increased in these patients, so special precautions in that regard are not necessary. Brain shrinkage, however, is important to provide the surgeon with sufficient space to identify and relieve the pressure on the offending nerve without requiring excessive brain retraction in the process.

**Induction** Induction is best accomplished with drugs that cause brain shrinkage, including STP (10 mg/kg) or propofol (1-2 mg/kg), followed by neuromuscular blockade and ET intubation.

**Maintenance** STP ≤ 20 mg/kg, or an equivalent dose of propofol, associated with an opiate such as fentanyl 2-3 μg/kg or meperidine 1.5 mg/kg, and isoflurane ≤ 1% concentration with $N_2O$ 60-70%, is satisfactory. BP is maintained in the normal range during the operation. Hyperventilation to achieve a $PaCO_2$ of 25-30 mmHg is helpful in decreasing brain size and providing adequate space for the surgeon to work. Once the nerve has been stented or transected, hyperventilation can be terminated and brain size can be allowed to return to normal. Sometimes the surgeon will also insert a spinal drain to remove CSF during the operation and improve exposure. The drain is usually opened at the time of dural opening and closed as soon as surgery on the nerve is complete.

**Emergence** The ETT is removed at the conclusion of operation. Postop HTN may need to be controlled with esmolol and/or SNP by continuous pump infusion.

**Blood and fluid requirements**

Minimal blood loss
IV: 18 ga x 1
NS @ 2-4 cc/kg/hr

Mannitol 1-1.5 mg/kg is sometimes necessary to provide sufficient brain shrinkage to permit adequate surgical exposure.

**Monitoring**

Standard monitors (see Appendix).
Arterial line
CVP line
± EMG and/or SSEP

Sometimes EMG and/or SSEP monitoring of the facial nerve is performed.

**Positioning**

✓ and pad pressure points.
✓ eyes.
Pillow between legs

Patients usually will be positioned laterally in the "park-bench" position. Padding of the axillae and elbows and placing a pillow between the legs are necessary. A bean bag is often used to hold patient stable in the lateral position.

## POSTOPERATIVE

**Complications**

Bleeding
Brain edema

Major complications from this operation are uncommon, and postop recovery is usually uneventful. On rare occasion, significant brain edema or bleeding may be experienced.

**Pain management** Codeine (30-60 mg im q 4 hrs)

**Tests** CT scan, if neurological recovery is delayed.

**References**

1. Jannetta PJ: Supralateral exposure of the trigeminal nerve in the cerebellopontine angle for microvascular decompression. In *Brain Surgery: Complication, Avoidance and Management.* Apuzzo MLJ, ed. Churchill Livingstone, New York: 1993, 2085-96.

# BIFRONTAL CRANIOTOMY FOR CSF LEAK

## SURGICAL CONSIDERATIONS

**Description:** CSF leaks may develop 2° trauma and, occasionally, to tumors or congenital malformations. Most of these leaks involve the floor of the anterior cranial fossa. The surgical repair for this type of problem is fairly standard: **bifrontal craniotomy** is performed with a bicoronal skin flap. The patient's head is stabilized with either suction cups or pins, and a bifrontal free-bone flap is used. Brain relaxation (minimum volume) is usually necessary for the procedure and may require placement of a spinal lumbar subarachnoid drain to remove CSF. The dura is opened across the sagittal sinus and an intradural exploration is undertaken to determine the site of the leak. The frontal lobes are elevated, and the olfactory tracts are often sacrificed. If the site of leak can be determined, the repair can be performed by use of some dura or graft material (either fascia lata, pericranium or cadaveric dura). It usually is necessary to strip the dura off the anterior cranial fossa to complete the repair. Defects in the bone can be plugged with some material (e.g., fat, muscle, bone or wax). Once the repair is complete, the dura can be closed and the bone flap replaced, often with a drain left in the epidural space. At this point, relaxation is no longer required; thus, if hyperventilation has been used, it can be reversed. The wound is closed with glial stitches and skin closure.

Another approach is used for dealing with CSF leaks 2° tumor at the base of the anterior cranial fossa which may invade dura and the cribriform plate region. In these cases, the procedure is often performed with an otorhinolaryngologist. This procedure is identical to bifrontal craniotomy, except that bone and tumor are removed at the floor of the anterior cranial fossa and the otorhinolaryngologist makes an incision on the face and performs surgery in the nasal cavity. A common space is created between the two operative fields. Closure involves isolating the two cavities once again. The dural repair is as above. The mucosa of the nasal cavity is recreated with use of a skin graft.

**Usual preop diagnosis:** CSF leak or rhinorrhea; fracture of the anterior cranial fossa; intra-nasal encephalocele; cribriform plate tumor; esthesioneurocytoma

### SUMMARY OF PROCEDURE

| | |
|---|---|
| **Position** | Supine |
| **Incision** | Bicoronal |
| **Special instrumentation** | Operating microscope (optional) |
| **Unique considerations** | Brain relaxation desired; lumbar subarachnoid catheter; fascia lata graft |
| **Antibiotics** | Cefotaxime 1 gm + vancomycin 1 gm iv slowly |
| **Surgical time** | 2 - 3.5 hrs, depending on extent of leak or lesion |
| **Closing considerations** | Drain often left in epidural space. Application of head dressing will jostle patient and ETT → ↑BP. |
| **EBL** | 75-500 cc |
| **Postop care** | ICU or close observation unit |
| **Mortality** | ≤ 5% |
| **Morbidity** | Infection<br>CSF leak<br>Neurologic disability<br>Nerve injury<br>Massive blood loss: venous sinus injury |
| **Procedure code** | 62100 (craniotomy for CSF leak); 61712 (microscopic) |
| **Pain score** | 3-5 |

### PATIENT POPULATION CHARACTERISTICS

| | |
|---|---|
| **Age range** | 15-65 yrs |
| **Male:Female** | ~3:2 |
| **Incidence** | Relatively rare neurosurgical procedure |
| **Etiology** | Traumatic<br>Congenital<br>Neoplastic |

## ANESTHETIC CONSIDERATIONS

See Anesthetic Considerations following "Transsphenoidal Resection of Pituitary Tumor" (below).

**References**


1. Couldwell WT, Weiss MH: Cerebrospinal fluid fistulas. In *Brain Surgery: Complication, Avoidance and Management.* Apuzzo MLJ, ed. Churchill Livingstone, New York: 1993, 2329-42.


# TRANSORAL RESECTION OF THE ODONTOID

## SURGICAL CONSIDERATIONS

**Description:** The transoral approach often provides excellent access to the odontoid process of the C2 vertebral body, as well as the skull base just anterior to the brain stem. This is important for conditions where there is pressure on the brain stem (such as in cases of basilar impression) or spinal cord (odontoid fractures or rheumatoid arthritis with pannus behind the odontoid). In these cases, the operation is performed through the oral cavity with an incision at the back of the mouth. Special retractors hold the mouth open and keep the tongue out of the way. Fluoroscopic guidance helps the surgeon maintain proper trajectory. Normally, drills are used to remove the bone of the basisphenoid or first and second vertebral bodies. Upon completion of the decompression, the mucosa is closed. It may be necessary to fuse the occiput to the upper cervical spine if the patient is made unstable by this procedure. This may take place at the same time, or at a later date. Cervical spine precautions normally are used during and after the case. The patient may be in traction with tongs or a halter and, thus, a fiber optic intubation may be required.

**Usual preop diagnosis:** Basilar impression (platybasia); odontoid fracture; rheumatoid arthritis with atlanto-axial instability and anterior impingement of the cord

### SUMMARY OF PROCEDURE

| | |
|---|---|
| **Position** | Supine; head in traction or pins |
| **Incision** | Back of oropharynx |
| **Special instrumentation** | Operating microscope; image intensifier; micro drill; intraoral retractors for exposure |
| **Unique considerations** | ETT must be taped securely in a location satisfactory to surgeon. Anode or RAE® tube may be helpful. Occasionally, a **tracheostomy** is performed in advance. |
| **Antibiotics** | Ampicillin (or vancomycin) 1 gm iv + cefotaxime 1 gm |
| **Surgical time** | 2.5 - 3 hrs |
| **Closing considerations** | Patient may remain intubated postop. |
| **EBL** | 25-250 cc |
| **Postop care** | ICU or close observation unit; monitor airway for swelling (✓ for stridor). |
| **Mortality** | 0-3% |
| **Morbidity** | All < 20%:<br>Infection<br>CSF leak<br>Neurological<br>Massive blood loss |
| **Procedure code** | 61575 (transoral approach to skull base or upper spine); 61676 (same, with tongue-splitting incision); 61712 (microscopic) |
| **Pain score** | 2-4 |

### PATIENT POPULATION CHARACTERISTICS

| | |
|---|---|
| **Age range** | 18-85 yrs (usually 20-60 yrs) |
| **Male:Female** | ~1:2 |
| **Incidence** | Rare |
| **Etiology** | Neoplastic<br>Traumatic<br>Congenital<br>Degenerative |
| **Associated conditions** | Rheumatoid arthritis<br>Traumatic injury |

## ANESTHETIC CONSIDERATIONS

See Anesthetic Considerations following "Transsphenoidal Resection of Pituitary Tumor" (below).

**References**

1. Menezes AH: Transoral approach to the clivus and upper cervical spine. In *Neurosurgery Update*, Vol I. Wilkins RH, Rengachary SS, eds. McGraw-Hill, New York: 1990, 306-313.
2. Crockard AH: Transoral approach to intra/extradural tumors. In *Surgery of Cranial Base Tumors*. Sekhar LN, Janecka ID, eds. Raven Press, New York: 1993, 225-34.

# TRANSSPHENOIDAL RESECTION OF PITUITARY TUMOR

## SURGICAL CONSIDERATIONS

**Description:** The transsphenoidal approach to the sella turcica is a direct procedure used to gain access to the pituitary gland and sella region and is associated with relatively fewer complications than a craniotomy. The procedure usually is performed through a sublabial incision in the maxillary gingiva or via an incision in or alongside the nose. An otorhinolaryngologist may participate in obtaining the exposure, which involves creating a tunnel to the sphenoid sinus through a plane between the septum of the nose and nasal mucosa. Once the sphenoid sinus is reached, it is entered by removing a portion of the vomer. The mucosa of the sphenoid sinus is stripped and the sella is entered by removing a portion of the sella floor. Under fluoroscopic guidance and with the aid of the operating microscope, the surgeon can operate safely within the region of the pituitary gland. The tumor is removed with a series of microdissectors and suctioned out with curettage. Following tumor removal, the surgeon may harvest fat from the thigh or abdomen to place in the sella to serve as a graft to seal the dura if CSF is found. The surgeon also may reconstruct the floor of the sella with bone salvaged from the exposure.

**Usual preop diagnosis:** Pituitary tumor; prolactin-secreting tumor; growth hormone-secreting tumor (acromegaly); ACTH-secreting tumor (Cushing's disease); visual compromise 2° intrasellar tumor; craniopharyngioma; occasionally, diabetes or prostate cancer; Forbes-Albright syndrome

### SUMMARY OF PROCEDURE

| | |
|---|---|
| **Position** | Supine, head elevated 30° |
| **Incision** | Sublabial, maxillary gingiva; abdomen or thigh for fat graft |
| **Special instrumentation** | Operating microscope; image intensifier; micro drill; laser (occasionally) |

| | |
|---|---|
| **Unique considerations** | ETT must be taped securely in a location satisfactory to surgeon. Anode or RAE® tube may be helpful. Dissection in the nasal cavity can be noxious stimulus, thus elevating BP, ICP, and risking air embolus. |
| **Antibiotics** | Ampicillin (or vancomycin) 1 gm iv + cefotaxime 1 gm iv |
| **Surgical time** | 2.5 - 3 hrs |
| **Closing considerations** | Possible abdominal or thigh-fat graft. Closure quite fast, requiring only gingival suture and nasal packs. |
| **EBL** | 25-250 cc |
| **Postop care** | ICU or close observation unit; fluid and electrolytes require frequent monitoring as the patient may develop diabetes insipidus (DI) transiently following this procedure. |
| **Mortality** | 0-3% |
| **Morbidity** | All < 5%:<br>Infection<br>CSF leak<br>Endocrine disorder: panhypopituitarism, DI<br>Cavernous sinus syndrome<br>Optic nerve injury<br>Massive blood loss: carotid injury |
| **Procedure code** | 61548 (transnasal removal of pituitary tumor); 61712 (microscopic) |
| **Pain score** | 2-4 |

### PATIENT POPULATION CHARACTERISTICS

| | |
|---|---|
| **Age range** | 18-85 yrs (usually 20-60 yrs) |
| **Male:Female** | ~1:2 |
| **Incidence** | Relatively uncommon |
| **Etiology** | Neoplastic<br>Traumatic |
| **Associated conditions** | Cushing's disease<br>Acromegaly<br>Amenorrhea/galactorrhea |

---

## ANESTHETIC CONSIDERATIONS

**(Procedures covered: bifrontal craniotomy for CSF leak; transoral resection of odontoid; transsphenoidal resection of pituitary tumor)**

### PREOPERATIVE

| | |
|---|---|
| **Endocrine** | Tumors of the pituitary gland are either nonfunctional or secretory. If nonfunctional, they will produce Sx either by their mass effect on adjacent pituitary tissue, or because of extension outside of the sella turcica. Rarely, the mass effect may cause the clinical picture of panhypopituitarism requiring preop treatment with thyroxine, glucocorticoid and vasopressin. Functional tumors secrete varying quantities of prolactin (→ lactation), growth hormone (→ acromegaly) and ACTH (→ adrenal hyperplasia).<br>**Tests:** Preop endocrine studies, including serum and urinary levels of pituitary, thyroid and adrenal hormones; appropriate replacement therapy established before proceeding with surgery.[2] |
| **Respiratory** | No special requirements, unless patient has acromegaly,[3] in which case large facial features, long neck, large tongue and redundant soft tissue in the oropharynx may make mask fit and ET intubation difficult. If these patients evidence hoarseness or inspiratory stridor, they should have a full clinical and radiological evaluation of the upper airway.<br>**Tests:** As indicated from H&P. |
| **Cardiovascular** | No special requirements unless patient has acromegaly, in which case they may have HTN, ischemic heart disease or diabetes.<br>**Tests:** As indicated from H&P. |

| | |
|---|---|
| **Neurological** | Secretory tumors of the pituitary are usually small, confined to the sella, rarely cause ↑ICP, and produce Sx of endocrine dysfunction early in their growth. In contrast, nonfunctional pituitary tumors may not produce Sx until they extend beyond the boundaries of the sella, causing headaches or pressure effects on the optic chiasm, producing visual field defects.<br>**Tests:** A CT or MRI will delineate the site and size of the tumor, especially if iv contrast material, such as gadolinium, is administered to enhance the margins of the tumor. |
| **Musculoskeletal** | If growth hormone is the primary secretant, patient will exhibit signs of acromegaly, including large hands, feet, head and tongue.<br>**Tests:** As indicated from H&P. |
| **Laboratory** | Hct and others as indicated from H&P. |

## INTRAOPERATIVE

**Anesthetic technique:** GETA is required for this operation, since the surgical approach is through the mouth above the maxillary gum line and behind the nose.

| | |
|---|---|
| **Induction** | If a difficult intubation is anticipated, orotracheal intubation will need to be accomplished before induction of GA. Awake FOL is the best choice (see "Anesthetic Considerations for Thoracolumbar Neurosurgical Procedures" for technique). Since these tumors are generally confined to the sella turcica and, hence, ICP is usually not increased, a standard induction technique is appropriate (see Appendix). If ↑ICP is of concern, induction should be similar to that used for patients with other kinds of brain tumors (see Anesthetic Considerations for "Craniotomy for Tumor"). To minimize the cardiovascular responses to ET intubation, it may be helpful to spray the larynx with lidocaine (4 cc, 4%; LTA kit), and then wait a few minutes before proceeding with ET intubation. Since the surgeon will be working from the patient's right side, the ETT and esophageal stethoscope must be positioned at the far side of the mouth. An oral airway should not be used. |
| **Maintenance** | Standard maintenance (see Appendix). Generally, no further neuromuscular-blocking drugs are administered beyond that used for ET intubation. With adequate anesthesia, and the head in Mayfield-Kees skeletal fixation, patient movement of any consequence is highly unlikely. Furthermore, it is useful to see movement of an extremity as an indicator of inadequate depth of anesthesia. Ventilation is controlled with $PaCO_2$ maintained in the normal range. Hyperventilation is not desired because it makes it more difficult for the neurosurgeon to locate the tumor in the sella, and establish that it has been removed in its entirety. |
| **Emergence** | At the conclusion of operation, a decision must be made regarding extubation of the trachea. If the patient evidences normal emergence from anesthesia, the ETT should be removed before vigorous coughing ensues. Before removing the ETT, however, the anesthesiologist must make certain that all blood accumulated in the back of the throat is suctioned out, and that oropharyngeal packs placed in the back of the throat by the surgeon have been removed. The surgeon will have packed the nose at the end of operation, forcing the patient to be an obligatory mouth breather until the nasal packs are removed. If there is any question about airway patency because of a large tongue, small mouth or soft-tissue redundancy in the oropharynx, the ETT should be left in place until patient is fully awake from anesthesia. |

| | | |
|---|---|---|
| **Blood and fluid requirements** | Minimal blood loss usual<br>Potential large blood loss<br>IV: 16-18 ga x 1<br>NS/LR @ 4-8 cc/kg/hr | Blood loss is minimal, unless the surgeon inadvertently enters the internal carotid artery or cavernous sinus during the course of dissection and drilling into the sella. |
| **Control of blood loss** | Deliberate hypotension | Controlled hypotension not used in this operation unless bleeding becomes profuse, diffuse or hard to control. |
| **Monitoring** | Standard monitors (see Appendix).<br>Arterial line<br>CVP line<br>UO<br>Doppler | Monitor for VAE in semi-sitting position. |
| **Positioning** | ✓ and pad pressure points.<br>✓ eyes.<br>Shoulder roll<br>Table turned 180° | The surgeon will use an operating microscope, which means that the anesthesiologist will be positioned near patient's feet. Anesthetic hoses and intravascular lines must be long enough to be accessible at patient's feet. |

## POSTOPERATIVE

| | | |
|---|---|---|
| **Complications** | Hypopituitarism<br>Diabetes insipidus (DI) | Replacement therapy with steroids is necessary until normal pituitary function returns. Occasionally, patients will develop DI postop, as evidenced by polyuria and decreased urine-specific gravity. Rarely, this may occur near the conclusion of anesthetic, necessitating vigorous fluid re-placement and vasopressin therapy (5-10 U sc or im bid). |
| **Pain management** | Codeine (30-60 mg im q 4 hrs) | |
| **Tests** | CT scan | If a patient exhibits any delay in emergence from anesthesia and surgery, or any new neurologic deficits emerge postop, a CT scan is invariably obtained. |

**References**

1. Hardy J: Transsphenoidal approach to the pituitary gland. In *Neurosurgery*. Wilkins RH, Rengachary SS, eds. McGraw-Hill, New York: 1985, 889-98.
2. Matjasko J: Perioperative management of patients with pituitary tumors. *Seminars in Anesth* 1984; 111:155-67.
3. Chan VWS, Tindal S: Anesthesia for transsphenoidal surgery in a patient with extreme giantism. *Br J Anaesth* 1988; 60:464-68.

# VENTRICULAR SHUNT PROCEDURES

## SURGICAL CONSIDERATIONS

**Description:** Many conditions exist whereby it is necessary to divert CSF from the ventricles to another body cavity for absorption. Most commonly, the patient has developed hydrocephalus where there is dilation of the ventricular system due to some blockage in the spinal fluid pathways or absorption of the fluid at the level of the arachnoid villi. The procedure involves shaving the scalp over either the parietal or the coronal region of the skull. A continuous surgical field is created from the cranium to the peritoneum in the case of a **VP shunt**. An incision is made over the intended region of cannulation of the ventricle. A burr hole is placed in the cranium, and a ventricular catheter is placed into the ventricle. A separate incision is made over the peritoneum and dissection is carried down to the level of the posterior rectus sheath or peritoneum. A length of catheter is then passed from the abdominal incision to the cranial incision in a subcutaneous tunnel created by a special tunneling instrument. It may be necessary to use one or more jump incisions between the head and abdominal incision. A pocket is created beneath the skin, usually behind the ear, for the valve. Connections are made between the ventricular catheter, valve and the peritoneal tubing. Once the system is found to be functioning satisfactorily, the peritoneal end is placed into the peritoneum and all wounds are closed. Any component of a shunt may malfunction; thus, it may be necessary to test each component at the time of the revision in order to identify the problem. Usually, the malfunctioning part is replaced. Valves usually are passive and have a preset pressure setting (e.g., low, medium, high).

**Variant procedure or approaches:** The ventricular catheter can be placed in either lateral ventricle; occasionally, both lateral ventricles are cannulated. This procedure is also used to shunt the fourth ventricle and, sometimes, subarachnoid cysts. The terminal end may alternatively be the right atrium (**VA shunt**) or the pleural cavity. To place the distal end into the atrium, a vein is cannulated in the neck (usually IJ or EJ), and the catheter is fed into the atrium under fluoroscopic guidance. It may be necessary to inject radiopaque contrast in order to verify proper placement. The pleural cavity is a less common site. The catheter is threaded into the pleural cavity, and a Valsalva maneuver is performed upon closure to reinflate the lung.

**Usual preop diagnosis:** Hydrocephalus; obstructive or communicating hydrocephalus; aqueductal stenosis; Dandy-Walker malformation; occult hydrocephalus; normal pressure hydrocephalus; subarachnoid cyst

### SUMMARY OF PROCEDURE

| | VP Shunt | VA Shunt |
|---|---|---|
| **Position** | Supine, with head turned | ⇐ |
| **Incision** | Scalp, either coronal and retro-auricular, or parietal; + neck and abdomen | Scalp, either coronal and retro-auricular or parietal; + neck |
| **Special instrumentation** | Ventricular endoscope (optional) | ⇐ + Image intensifier |
| **Unique considerations** | Patient to be treated as if there is ↑ICP. | ⇐ |
| **Antibiotics** | Cefotaxime 1 gm iv and vancomycin 1 gm iv | ⇐ |
| **Surgical time** | 1 hr | ⇐ |
| **EBL** | 5-25 cc | ⇐ |
| **Postop care** | PACU → room; usually kept flat for 24 hrs. | ⇐ |
| **Mortality** | < 1% | ⇐ |
| **Morbidity** | Infection: < 15%<br>Neurological:<br>Intracranial bleed: < 1%<br>Subdural hematoma: < 1%<br>Hardware failure: < 1% | ⇐ |
| **Procedure code** | 62223 | 62220 |
| **Pain score** | 4-6 | 2-4 |

### PATIENT POPULATION CHARACTERISTICS

| | |
|---|---|
| **Age range** | Newborn - elderly |
| **Male:Female** | 1:1 |
| **Incidence** | Common |
| **Etiology** | Congenital<br>Acquired<br>Neoplastic<br>Infectious<br>Post-hemorrhagic |
| **Associated conditions** | Myelodysplasia<br>Spina bifida<br>Intraventricular hemorrhage<br>Intraventricular tumor |

## ANESTHETIC CONSIDERATIONS

### PREOPERATIVE

Ventricular shunts are inserted to ameliorate hydrocephalus or cyst formations, which are either congenital or acquired.

**Cardiovascular** ↑ICP → ↑BP & ↓↓HR (Cushing's response)
**Tests:** As indicated from H&P.

**Neurological** The most common presenting Sx is headache. If hydrocephalus is severe, Sx of ↑ICP (>15 mmHg) (e.g., N&V, drowsiness, papilledema, seizures and focal neurological defects) develop.

**Laboratory** Tests as indicated by H&P.

**Premedication** Usually not required; should be avoided in patients with ↑ICP.

### INTRAOPERATIVE

**Anesthetic technique:** GETA

**Induction** If ↑ICP, iv induction with STP (3-5 mg/kg) or propofol (0.15-0.2 mg/kg) is preferred, because of their ability to decrease cerebral blood volume and, hence, ICP. ET intubation is accomplished with the use of a non-depolarizing neuromuscular blocking drug (e.g., vecuronium 0.1 mg/kg).

| | | |
|---|---|---|
| **Maintenance** | Isoflurane 1.5% or less, inspired with $N_2O/O_2$ mixture to maintain $O_2$ sat ~ 99%. Depending on duration of operation, additional doses of vecuronium (0.1 mg/kg) may be needed. Maintain normal temperature in children by keeping OR warm (78°F) and using warming lights as needed. Ventilation is controlled mechanically (ventilator) or manually from the start of anesthesia until the surgical wound is closed. TV and frequency are adjusted such that the $PETCO_2$ = 35-40 mmHg. Hyperventilation and hypocarbia are undesirable because they make cannulation of the ventricle(s) more difficult for the surgeon. Maintain normotension. | |
| **Emergence** | ETT is removed at the conclusion of the anesthetic. | |
| **Blood and fluid requirements** | IV: 18-20 ga x 1<br>NS/LR @ 4-6 ml/kg/hr | Administer crystalloid, usually NS (via measured volume system in a child). Blood is rarely, if ever, necessary. |
| **Monitoring** | Standard monitors (see Appendix). | |
| **Positioning** | Table turned 180°<br>✓ and pad pressure points.<br>✓ eyes. | Supine with a bolster under the shoulder on the operative side. The head, chest and abdomen are prepped, so all anesthesia equipment and lines must be at the sides of the patient. |
| **Special Drugs Administered** | Antibiotics, dexamethasone | |
| **Complications** | Infection<br>Valve malfunction | Major complications from this operation are uncommon, but include infection at the valve site or in the tubing, and malfunction of the valve, either draining too little or too much CSF. |

### POSTOPERATIVE

| | | |
|---|---|---|
| **Pain management** | Children < 2 yrs: Tylenol® suppositories (10-15 mg/kg q 4 hrs)<br>Adults: Fentanyl (25-75 kg q 30 min) | |


**References**

1. Ruge JR, McLone DG: Cerebrospinal fluid diversion procedures. In *Brain Surgery: Complication, Avoidance and Management.* Apuzzo MLJ, ed. Churchill Livingstone, New York: 1993, 1463-94.


# CRANIOCERVICAL DECOMPRESSION (CHIARI MALFORMATION)

## SURGICAL CONSIDERATIONS

**Description:** Certain congenital malformations known as **Chiari malformations** cause crowding of structures at the craniocervical junction. These are anomalies in which portions of the cerebellum protrude through the foramen magnum such that there is little room for the brain stem and upper cervical spinal cord at this level. Frequently, the malformation is accompanied by syringomyelia, a condition in which CSF is abnormally located within the spinal cord. The craniocervical decompression is designed to make room for the structures at this level. The foramen magnum is opened by removing bone from the suboccipital skull. The posterior arch of C1 is removed and as many upper cervical lamina as needed to fully decompress the malformation are removed. Next, the dura is opened; and, under microscopic guidance, the tonsils are dissected apart to gain an opening into the fourth ventricle. To make a patulous cisterna magna, the dura is patched with pericranium, fascia lata or tissue-bank dura. This procedure may be performed in either the prone or seated position. Some surgeons plug the foramen cecum with muscle or prosthetic material, which may lead to cardiorespiratory instability. A stent may be placed in the fourth ventricle and brought out to the subarachnoid space to ensure adequate drainage. At the same time, a shunt or stent may be placed into the syrinx cavity (see "Thoracic Laminectomy").

**Usual preop diagnosis:** Chiari Malformation I or II, Arnold-Chiari malformation; syringomyelia. (Chiari I malformations usually are not associated with conditions other than syringomyelia. Chiari II is commonly associated with spina bifida or myelodysplasia [Arnold-Chiari malformation]).

## SUMMARY OF PROCEDURE

| | |
|---|---|
| **Position** | Prone or sitting |
| **Incision** | Midline posterior, posterolateral thigh for fascia lata graft (optional) |
| **Special instrumentation** | Operating microscope |
| **Unique considerations** | Risk of air embolus; brain stem manipulation can cause BP and pulse instability. |
| **Antibiotics** | Cefotaxime 1 gm and vancomycin 1 gm iv slowly |
| **Surgical time** | 2.5 - 3.5 hrs |
| **Closing considerations** | Application of head dressing with consequent head movement → ↑BP and need for BP control. |
| **EBL** | 25-250 cc |
| **Postop care** | ICU or constant observation unit; neurological function monitored. |
| **Mortality** | 0-3% |
| **Morbidity** | All < 5%:<br>Infection<br>Neurological<br>Aseptic meningitis<br>CSF leak<br>Postop instability<br>Massive blood loss; vertebral artery injury |
| **Procedure code** | 61343; 61712 (microscopic); 20922 (fascia lata graft) |
| **Pain score** | 5-7 |

## PATIENT POPULATION CHARACTERISTICS

| | |
|---|---|
| **Age range** | Infant-70 yrs (usually 9-40) |
| **Male:Female** | ~1:1 |
| **Incidence** | Relatively rare neurosurgical procedure |
| **Etiology** | Congenital<br>Acquired, S/P lumboperitoneal shunting |
| **Associated conditions** | Hydrocephalus<br>Syringomyelia<br>Scoliosis<br>Myelodysplasia |

# ANESTHETIC CONSIDERATIONS

See Anesthetic Considerations following "Cervical or Craniocervical Fusion" (below).

**References**


1. Batzdorf U: *Syringomyelia: Current Concepts in Diagnosis and Treatment.* Williams & Wilkins, Baltimore: 1991.
2. Batzdorf U: Chiari malformation and syringomyelia. In *Brain Surgery: Complication, Avoidance and Management.* Apuzzo MLJ, ed. Churchill Livingstone, New York: 1993, 1985-2001.

# STEREOTACTIC SURGERY

## SURGICAL CONSIDERATIONS

**Description:** Stereotaxis is a set of neurosurgical techniques which apply simple rules of geometry to radiologic images. Stereotaxy is typically less invasive than conventional neurosurgery, and use of stereotactic instruments provides millimeter accuracy in certain intracranial operations. All current stereotaxic procedures begin with the attachment of a frame to the patient's head. The frame is anchored to the skull with either 4 pins or screws. This procedure typically is done outside the OR, using local anesthetic. In the cooperative adult, frame application takes only 5-10 min. For children, however, GA is used.

With the stereotactic frame in place, CT, MRI and cerebral angiography can all be utilized for stereotactic target identification and localization. During imaging, a set of fiducials (x-ray markers) is attached to the stereotaxic frame. These markers provide the geometric information needed for localization. Data from imaging studies are used to calculate, by hand or computer, the spatial coordinates of the target. In more complex stereotactic procedures, various points of interest, alternative trajectories or radiation dosimetry are also determined by computer. In nearly all cooperative patients, there is no need for sedation or analgesia throughout this stage of the procedure.

The spatial information determined from stereotaxy can be used to perform a number of markedly different operations. Except for radiosurgery, all are done in the OR and require additional anesthesia. The most common stereotaxic operations involve relatively minor "cutting" and can be done using light sedation and local anesthesia. These include biopsy, depth electrode placement, brain lesioning for Parkinson's disease or chronic pain and brachytherapy (the placement of radioactive implants). **Stereotaxic craniotomy**, however, is a major intracranial procedure – albeit through a smaller opening – and GA is needed.

After preparing and draping, stereotaxic procedures begin with the attachment of a specialized "operating" device to the stereotaxic frame. This instrument is used to provide spatial guidance throughout the surgical procedure. Minor stereotaxic operations generally require a burr hole for intracranial exposure. Maximal sedation is needed during drilling and dural opening. Patient oxygenation is frequently compromised by sterile draping.

**Radiosurgery** is a precision technique for ablating small tumors and malformations with large-dose radiation through the closed cranium. In contrast to other stereotaxic operations, radiosurgery is done outside the OR, using a linear accelerator or other specialized irradiation device. Cooperative adults need little, if any, sedation during the procedure. Children, however, almost always require GA from the beginning of frame placement through the actual treatment, which takes several hours. Thus, anesthesia must be administered at several locations, as well as during transport among these sites. Ideally, GA is initiated in the CT/MR suite and is maintained throughout stereotaxic frame placement and imaging. After transport to postop recovery, the child is kept asleep while radiosurgical treatment is being planned; this length of time ranges from 1 - 3 hours. The patient is then transported to the radiosurgical suite, still anesthetized, where treatment is performed. Depending on its complexity, radiosurgery lasts from 1 - 2 hours. Anesthetic monitoring can be particularly challenging in this environment. At the end of treatment, the stereotaxic frame is removed and the patient awakened.

**Variant procedure or approaches:** There are several different commercially available stereotactic systems, all of which utilize a frame anchored to the skull with pins or screws; also, frameless instruments are currently being introduced. All of these devices provide a frame of reference for both target localization and surgical therapy.

**Usual preop diagnosis:** Brain disease requiring biopsy; brain tumor; vascular malformation; Parkinson's disease

**SUMMARY OF PROCEDURE**

| | Biopsy, Functional Stereotaxis | Craniotomy | Pediatric Radiosurgery |
|---|---|---|---|
| **Position** | Supine or prone | Sitting, supine, prone, lateral, etc. | Supine or prone |
| **Incision** | 0.5 - 2 cm scalp incision | 5 - 12 cm scalp incision | None |
| **Special instrumentation** | Stereotactic treatment arc | ⇐ | ⇐ |
| **Unique considerations** | Incision infiltrated with local anesthesia and epinephrine: < 1 cc | Incision infiltrated with local anesthesia and epinephrine: 5-10 cc | Prolonged GA outside OR |

| | Biopsy, Functional | Craniotomy | Pediatric Radiosurgery |
|---|---|---|---|
| **Surgical time** | 0.5 - 1.5 hrs | 2 - 4 hrs | 5 - 8 hrs |
| **EBL** | < 10 cc | 20 - 1000 cc | None |
| **Postop care** | PACU → room | ICU | PACU → room |
| **Mortality** | < 0.5% | 1% | None |
| **Morbidity** | Overall: <1%<br>Symptomatic intracerebral hemorrhage (new neurologic deficits) | Overall 1-5% (same as standard craniotomy)<br>Infection<br>Hemorrhage | N&V: 10% |
| **Procedure code** | 61751 | 61795 | 61793 |
| **Pain score** | 2 | 4 | 2 |

### PATIENT POPULATION CHARACTERISTICS

| | |
|---|---|
| **Age range** | 1-80 |
| **Male:Female** | 1:1 |
| **Incidence** | 16.7/100,000 (35,000 new burn tumors annually in U.S.) |

---

## ANESTHETIC CONSIDERATIONS

### PREOPERATIVE

Neurosurgical procedures are performed using stereotactic control when the lesion is small and/or is located deep within brain tissue, or as a means of obtaining a biopsy of a lesion for diagnosis. For example, focal, deep-seated arteriovenous malformations (AVMs) may be resected under stereotactic control. More commonly, it is used to obtain a biopsy of a small tumor. These patients are often otherwise healthy.

**Neurological** — Neurological Sx vary, depending on site and size of the lesion; they should be carefully documented. In addition to the usual tests, a CT scan is obtained preop with the frame in place to determine stereotactic coordinates. Once the coordinates are established, the frame must not be moved on the head until the operation is complete.

**Laboratory** — Tests as indicated from H&P.

### INTRAOPERATIVE

**Anesthetic technique:** GETA or MAC. In adults, the stereotactic frame is placed the morning of operation under local anesthesia, and the patient is taken to the radiological suite for CT scan to determine stereotactic coordinates. The patient is then brought to OR with the frame still in place. If operation is to be a Bx, it is generally done under local anesthesia with MAC. If a complete resection is planned, such as in the removal of an AVM, GETA is used. In children, it is usually necessary to induce GA before placing the frame, thus necessitating the maintenance of GA during the CT scan. The child is then moved to OR, still anesthetized, and the operation is completed.

**Induction** — If MAC is planned, $O_2$ by nasal prongs is administered, and the patient is lightly sedated with combinations of droperidol 0.01 mg/kg to prevent N&V; midazolam 0.05 mg/kg in divided doses to provide amnesia; and meperidine 1.5 mg/kg or fentanyl 3.5 $\mu$g/kg in divided doses to provide analgesia. It is important that the patient be able to communicate with the surgeon as needed throughout the operation. If GETA is needed, FOL is necessary before inducing anesthesia because the frame precludes intubation by direct laryngoscopy (see Anesthetic Considerations for "Thoracolumbar Neurosurgical Procedures" for fiber optic technique). Once ET intubation is established, anesthesia may be induced with STP 5-10 mg/kg or propofol 1.5-2 mg/kg, followed by a non-depolarizing neuromuscular blocking drug to facilitate positioning of patient.

**Maintenance** — If GA is used, maintenance is the same as for a tumor (see Anesthetic Considerations for "Craniotomy for Tumor") or AVM (see Anesthetic Considerations for "Craniotomy for Intracranial Vascular Malformations"). If children are to be transported from the site of placement of the stereotactic frame to the radiological suite and then the OR, it is best to use inhalation anesthesia with isoflurane 1-1.5 in $O_2$ with spontaneous ventilation to assure adequate ventilation and oxygenation during transport and study. Opiates and non-depolarizing neuromuscular-blocking drugs should not be administered until the child is in the operating suite.

**Emergence** — ETT is generally removed at the conclusion of the operation.

| | | |
|---|---|---|
| **Blood and fluid requirements** | IV: 16-18 ga x 2 (adults);<br>20-22 ga (children)<br>NS/LR @ 4-6 ml/kg/hr | Blood loss is minimal since the volume of tissue removed is small. |
| **Monitoring** | If local anesthesia: standard monitors (see Appendix).<br>If GA:<br>Arterial line<br>CVP line<br>UO | |
| **Positioning** | √ and pad pressure points.<br>√ eyes. | |

**POSTOPERATIVE**

| | | |
|---|---|---|
| **Complications** | Bleeding | Focal bleeding may occur postop, causing onset of a neurological deficit. |
| **Pain management** | Vicodin® (1-2 mg po q 4 hrs prn) | |
| **Tests** | CT or MRI scan, if a new neurological deficit occurs. | |

**References**

1. Heilbrun MP, ed: *Stereotactic Neurosurgery.* Williams & Wilkins, Baltimore: 1988.

**Surgeon**

**Lawrence M. Shuer, MD**

## 1.2 SPINAL NEUROSURGERY

**Anesthesiologist**

**C. Philip Larson, Jr, MS, MD**

# LUMBAR FUSION

## SURGICAL CONSIDERATIONS

**Description:** The goal of a **lumbar spinal fusion** is to have two or more spinal segments unite as one over time. The procedure is often performed when there is instability of the spine, such as spondylolisthesis, or cases where the patient may have a known instability due to damage of the normal support structures (e.g., facets). Through a midline vertical incision, the paraspinal muscles are exposed and dissected off of the spinous processes, lamina and facets. Next, dissection is carried down to the transverse processes and/or sacral alae of the segments to be fused. Blood loss can be significant during this stage of surgery.

A **discectomy** or **nerve-root decompression** may be incorporated (see "Lumbar Laminotomy, Laminectomy," below). The bone surfaces are decorticated and bone graft material (usually harvested from the ilium) is placed in contact with them. Instrumentation may be used to achieve internal fixation. These types of hardware may include Knodt distraction rods, Harrington rods, or various types of pedicle screw and rod/plate combinations. Intraop x-rays may be taken to verify proper placement of the pedicle screws. The wound is closed in layers; and a drain is left in the wound at the end of the procedure.

**Variant procedure or approaches:** Some surgeons perform an **interbody lumbar fusion** following a **complete bilateral discectomy**. This procedure begins as a **lumbar laminectomy** and involves preparation of the vertebral body end plates for graft placement by the surgeon. This is achieved by removing the cartilaginous surface of the vertebral body. Rectangular bone grafts are shaped appropriately and countersunk into the disc space with retraction of the dural sack. The bone grafts may be taken from the patient's ilium or the tissue bank. This type of fusion also may be supplemented with some form of internal fixation as described above.

**Usual preop diagnosis:** Lumbar instability; spondylolisthesis; pseudospondylolisthesis; spondylolysis; mechanical back syndrome

**SUMMARY OF PROCEDURE**

| | Lateral Transverse Process | Posterior Lumbar Interbody |
|---|---|---|
| **Position** | Prone | ⇐ |
| **Incision** | Posterior midline | ⇐ |
| **Special instrumentation** | Drill for decortication; internal hardware, optional (see description of types of hardware, above) | ⇐ |
| **Unique considerations** | Localizing intraop spine x-ray is used to assess level for operation (optional); fluoroscopy or films for pedicle screw placement. | ⇐ |
| **Antibiotics** | Cefazolin 1 gm iv | ⇐ |
| **Surgical time** | 2 - 4 hrs for single level; additional levels, add 1 - 2 hrs each. | 2 - 3 hrs for single level; additional levels, add 0.5 hr each. |
| **Closing considerations** | No cast or brace | ⇐ |
| **EBL** | 250-500 cc | 50-300 cc |
| **Postop care** | PACU → room | ⇐ |
| **Mortality** | 0-5% | ⇐ |
| **Morbidity** | Infection<br>CSF leak<br>Nerve root injury<br>Postop instability<br>Massive blood loss: injury to retroperitoneal vessels | ⇐ |
| **Procedure code** | 22625-22650 (lumbar fusion codes)<br>22820 (harvesting bone graft)<br>22830 (instrumentation codes) | ⇐ |
| **Pain score** | 6-10 | 6-10 |

### PATIENT POPULATION CHARACTERISTICS

| | |
|---|---|
| **Age range** | 15-85 yrs (usually 30-60 yrs) |
| **Male:Female** | ~3:2 |
| **Incidence** | Common |
| **Etiology** | Degenerative<br>Congenital<br>Neoplastic<br>Traumatic<br>Infectious |

## ANESTHETIC CONSIDERATIONS

See Anesthetic Considerations following "Thoracic Laminectomy, Costotransversectomy" (below).

**References**

1. Dunsker SB: Lumbar spine stabilization: indications. *Clin Neurosurg* 1990; 36:147-58.
2. Egnatchik JG: Lumbar spine stabilization: techniques. *Clin Neurosurg* 1990; 36:159-67.

# LUMBAR LAMINOTOMY, LAMINECTOMY

## SURGICAL CONSIDERATIONS

**Description: Lumbar laminotomy** (partial removal of lamina) and **laminectomy** (complete removal of lamina) are procedures for decompressing the neural elements of the lumbar spine via a posterior approach. They can be used to treat lumbar radiculopathy 2° degenerative disc disease (e.g., herniated discs or osteophytes). **Decompressive laminectomy** can be used to treat compression of the cauda equina, usually 2° degenerative disease, congenital stenosis, neoplasm and, occasionally, trauma. Lumbar laminectomy is also used to gain access to the spinal canal for dealing with intradural tumors, etc.

Through a vertical midline incision, the lumbodorsal fascia is exposed and then the paraspinal muscles are dissected off of the spinous process and lamina of the segments intended for decompression. The level may need to be checked by intraop x-ray if the surgeon is not able to identify location based on visual confirmation of anatomic level. The bone landmarks are identified and ligamentous attachments are cut. The bone is removed piecemeal with either rongeurs, gouges or power drills. Care is taken not to injure the underlying dura. If a dural tear is made, it must be repaired. The surgeon may want a Valsalva-like maneuver (sustained inspiration at 30-40 cm $H_2O$) performed to test the integrity of the repair. If disc is to be removed, the dura is retracted and the annulus incised. The disc is removed piecemeal with a series of curettes and disc-biting rongeurs. There is a risk of damage to retroperitoneal structures (e.g., great vessels or intestines) during this portion of the procedure. More commonly, there may be troublesome epidural bleeding which may be difficult to control and will necessitate transfusion. Hemostasis is obtained prior to closure. The wound is closed in layers; a drain may be left in the epidural space. The patient is rolled onto his/her back on a hospital bed at the completion of the procedure.

**Variant procedure or approaches:** The extent of the procedure depends on the indications for treatment. When the patient has single nerve-root-compression syndrome, the laminotomy consists of decompressing that one root. When there is diffuse narrowing of the spinal canal, an extensive lumbar decompression over several segments may be indicated. The amount of bone removal varies from patient to patient and surgeon to surgeon. Occasionally, the procedure includes a fusion of some type, if it is felt that the patient has some instability.

**Usual preop diagnosis:** Lumbar radiculopathy (nerve-root compression); lumbar disc disease (herniation or degeneration of one or more lumbar discs); lateral recess stenosis; herniated disc, lumbar stenosis; neurogenic claudication; metastatic carcinoma or tumor to spine; lumbar spine tumor; spondylosis (arthritic degeneration); spondylolysis (structural defect in the pars interarticularis of the vertebra); spondylolisthesis (misalignment or slip of vertebra)

### SUMMARY OF PROCEDURE

| | Lumbar Laminotomy | Laminectomy |
|---|---|---|
| **Position** | Prone | ⇐ |
| **Incision** | Posterior midline | ⇐ |
| **Special instrumentation** | Operating microscope (optional) | ⇐ |
| **Unique considerations** | Localizing intraop spine x-ray taken to assess correct level for operation (optional) | ⇐ |
| **Antibiotics** | Cefazolin 1 gm iv | ⇐ |
| **Surgical time** | 1 - 2 hrs for single level; additional levels, add 0.5 - 1 hr each. | 2 hrs for single level; additional levels, add 0.5 hr each. |
| **EBL** | 25-500 cc | 50-1500 cc |
| **Postop care** | PACU → room | ⇐ |
| **Mortality** | 0.5% | ⇐ |
| **Morbidity** | The following usually occur in < 5% of cases: | ⇐ |
| | Infection | ⇐ |
| | CSF leak | ⇐ |
| | Nerve-root injury | ⇐ |
| | Postop instability | ⇐ |
| | Massive blood loss: injury to retroperitoneal vessels | ⇐ |
| **Procedure code** | 63030 (single level, single side)<br>63035 (additional levels)<br>63042 (re-exploration) | 63001 (1 or 2 levels)<br>63015 (>2 levels)<br>63045 (with foraminotomy)<br>63048 (additional levels) |
| **Pain score** | 4-10 | 4-10 |

### PATIENT POPULATION CHARACTERISTICS

| | |
|---|---|
| **Age range** | 15-85 yrs (usually 30-60 yrs) |
| **Male:Female** | ~3:2 |
| **Incidence** | Common |
| **Etiology** | Degenerative<br>Neoplastic<br>Traumatic<br>Infectious |

## ANESTHETIC CONSIDERATIONS

See Anesthetic Considerations following "Thoracic Laminectomy, Costotransversectomy" (below).

**References**

1. Rothman RH, Simeone FA: The operative treatment of lumbar disc disease. In *The Spine*. WB Saunders Co, Philadelphia: 1982, 601-29.

# THORACIC LAMINECTOMY, COSTOTRANSVERSECTOMY

## SURGICAL CONSIDERATIONS

**Description:** Thoracic laminectomy (midline removal of the lamina) and costotransversectomy (off midline removal of the rib head and transverse process) are procedures for decompressing the neural elements of the thoracic spine via a posterior approach. **Costotransversectomy** is used to treat thoracic radiculopathy 2° degenerative disc disease (e.g., herniated discs or osteophytes). **Decompressive thoracic laminectomy** is used to treat thoracic spinal cord compression usually 2° neoplasm and, occasionally, trauma. It is also used to gain access to the spinal canal or spinal cord for dealing with intradural or intramedullary tumors, etc. For the **laminectomy**, a midline incision is used to expose the thoracodorsal fascia. The paraspinal muscles are dissected off the spinous processes and lamina. The bone is then removed piecemeal with rongeurs or drills. The extent of the procedure depends on the indications for treatment. When there is diffuse narrowing of the spinal canal, an extensive thoracic decompression over several segments may be indicated. Hemostasis is achieved with bipolar cautery. The raw bone surfaces are sealed with bone wax. Topical hemostatic agents are used to aid in hemostasis in the epidural gutters. If the patient has an intradural tumor or process such as syringomyelia, the dura is opened and the operating microscope is used for this portion of the procedure. Once the intradural portion of the procedure is completed, the dura is closed. The surgeon may wish to test the integrity of the closure with a Valsalva-like maneuver (sustained inspiration at 30-40 cm $H_2O$). The wound is closed in layers; a drain may be left in the epidural space.

**Variant procedure or approaches:** When the patient has only a single nerve-root compression syndrome, the costotransversectomy consists of decompressing that one root. The spinal cord cannot be retracted, thus necessitating a lateral approach to the disc rather than the standard laminectomy. A paramedian approach is made to the junction of the rib head with the vertebral body. The paraspinal muscles are split on that side. Intraop x-rays are required to assess appropriate level. The rib head is dissected out and removed piecemeal with rongeurs. The transverse process is removed. This gives access to the lateral opening of the neural foramen. A thoracic disc can be removed with disc-biting rongeurs. Hemostasis is obtained and the wound is closed in layers.

**Usual preop diagnosis:** Thoracic radiculopathy (nerve-root compression); thoracic disc disease (herniation or degeneration of one or more thoracic discs); thoracic myelopathy (spinal-cord compression); metastatic carcinoma or tumor to spine; thoracic spine tumor; syringomyelia; intractable pain

### SUMMARY OF PROCEDURE

| | Thoracic Laminectomy | Costotransversectomy |
|---|---|---|
| **Position** | Prone; pin fixation or horseshoe headrest may be used. | ⇐ |
| **Incision** | Posterior midline | ⇐ + Paramedian |
| **Special instrumentation** | Operating microscope (optional); evoked potential monitoring equipment (optional) | ⇐ |
| **Unique considerations** | Localizing intraop spine x-ray taken to assess correct level for operation. | ⇐ |
| **Antibiotics** | Cefazolin 1 gm iv | ⇐ |
| **Surgical time** | 1.5 - 2 hrs for single level; additional levels, add 0.5 - 1 hr each. | 2 hrs for single level; additional levels, add 0.5 hr each. |
| **EBL** | 25-1500 cc | 50-500 cc |
| **Postop care** | PACU → room; neurologic monitoring to check for change | ⇐ |
| **Mortality** | 0-5% | ⇐ |
| **Morbidity** | All < 5%:<br>Infection<br>CSF leak<br>Neurological: myelopathy; root injury<br>Massive blood loss<br>Postop instability | ⇐ |
| **Procedure code** | 63003-63057 (thoracic laminectomy)<br>63172-63173 (syrinx procedures)<br>63195 (cordotomy-pain relief) | 63064-63066 (costotransversectomy) |

| | | |
|---|---|---|
| **Procedure code, continued** | 63251 (removal of AVM)<br>63266 (removal of intraspinal lesion other than tumor, extradural)<br>63271 (removal of intraspinal lesion other than tumor, intradural)<br>63276 (extradural, neoplasm)<br>63281 (intradural, extramedullary neoplasm)<br>63286 (intradural, intramedullary neoplasm) | |
| **Pain score** | 6-10 | 6-10 |

### PATIENT POPULATION CHARACTERISTICS

| | |
|---|---|
| **Age range** | 7-85 yrs (usually 30-60 yrs) |
| **Male:Female** | ~1:1 |
| **Incidence** | Relatively uncommon neurosurgical procedure |
| **Etiology** | Degenerative<br>Neoplastic<br>Traumatic<br>Infectious |
| **Associated conditions** | Paraplegia |

---

## ANESTHETIC CONSIDERATIONS FOR THORACOLUMBAR NEUROSURGICAL PROCEDURES

**(Procedures covered: lumbar fusion; laminectomy; laminotomy; thoracic laminectomy; costotransversectomy)**

### PREOPERATIVE

Surgery of the lumbar or thoracic spine is common, primarily because of the frequency of herniation of a lumbar or thoracic intervertebral disk causing compression of the adjacent spinal cord or nerve roots. In general, these patients are fit and healthy. Other, less frequent indications for thoracolumbar neurosurgery include: chronic instability of the back, either of congenital or acquired origin, requiring Knodt rod fusion, removal of a tumor of the spinal cord, or placement of a shunt from a spinal cord cyst into the subarachnoid or peritoneal spaces.

**Neurological** Patients with herniation of a thoracic or lumbar disk generally complain first of pain, usually radiating into the pelvis or down one or both legs. Temporary relief may be obtained by standing or lying down, in combination with the use of a back brace, local heat, and non-steroidal anti-inflammatory drugs. As nerve compression continues, patients begin to develop weakness and atrophy of specific leg muscle groups. These Sx, however, are not specific to herniation of a disk, and may be caused by a spinal cord tumor or cyst. Although myelography has been the standard method in the past for evaluating the presence of a herniated intervertebral disk, MRI of the spinal cord has virtually replaced it as the diagnostic test, because it will distinguish disk from tumor from cyst. The image may be enhanced by the use of gadolinium or other contrast material.

**Tests:** MRI

**Hematologic** None, unless anti-platelet agents have been used.

**Laboratory** Other tests as indicated from H&P.

**Premedication** Premedication is very useful in this patient population for purposes of relieving pain and lessening anxiety related to forthcoming surgery. Many of these patients have had prior back operations, and dread further surgery on their backs. Midazolam 2-4 mg iv and meperidine 20-40 mg iv in divided doses prior to entering the OR will make these patients amnestic and tractable.

### INTRAOPERATIVE

**Anesthetic technique:** GA is almost invariably used for these operations because it maximizes patient comfort, provides airway control and permits use of controlled hypotension. Spinal and epidural anesthesia are, in principle, excellent techniques for lumbar surgery, particularly for removal of a lumbar intervertebral disk, but they are seldom used because of the medicolegal concern that the regional anesthetic may be blamed for a new neurological deficit, if one should occur as a result of the surgery. Regional anesthesia is generally not suitable for lumbar fusion or removal of a spinal cord tumor or cyst because the duration of operation is usually unpredictable, and may be prolonged.

**Induction** Because the operation is performed with the patient in the prone position, it is desirable to place ETT under local anesthesia and have patient position him/herself prone before induction of GA. This technique eliminates the need for others to lift and position patient, and allows the anesthesiologist opportunity to confirm patient comfort, and that no pressure points exist before inducing GA. (See technique for fiber optic intubation below.) Once the intubated patient has moved into the prone position, and monitors have been reattached, anesthesia is induced with STP 3-5 mg/kg or propofol 2-3 mg/kg iv.

**Orotracheal fiber optic intubation** When premedication has been established, the oropharynx is sprayed vigorously ~6 times over a span of 10 min, using lidocaine 10% solution. Initially, the spray is directed at the front of the tongue; gradually, it is directed further back in the throat, until the entire oropharynx is numb. In reality, the lateral recesses of the oropharynx need not be anesthetized topically because both fiber optic laryngoscope and ETT are confined to the midline of the mouth. Next, a translaryngeal injection of cocaine 4% 2 ml is made, using a 3-ml syringe and a 23-ga, 3/4-inch needle. So that this injection can be made as rapidly as possible, it is important to use a small syringe, making certain that the connection between syringe and needle is tight. The patient is instructed not to cough until the injection is complete. Since this may be impossible for some patients, it is important that the operator's hand be fixed firmly against the patient's upper chest to assure that needle movement is minimized and that the full injection is made into the trachea. When the injection is complete, the patient is urged to cough vigorously.

Once the mouth and trachea are anesthetized with local anesthetic, an oral airway with a central orifice (i.e., Tudor Williams airway) is placed in the midline of the mouth. A 7-mm orotracheal tube, without connector attached, is placed over a fiber optic laryngoscope. With the operator at the patient's side near the waist, the fiber optic laryngoscope is introduced through the hole in the airway and advanced to end of airway. At this point, the epiglottis should be visible. The tip of the fiber optic scope is flexed toward the operator about 15°-20°, which should bring arytenoid cartilages and laryngeal opening into view. The scope is advanced into the larynx so that tracheal rings can be visualized. Often, the carina also can be visualized. The scope is placed on the patient's chest and, holding it so that it is not advanced further, the orotracheal tube is gently advanced into the trachea. To facilitate passage of the orotracheal tube past the arytenoid cartilages and into the larynx, it is often necessary to rotate the tube counterclockwise 90°, or even as much as 180°, several times as it is being advanced. Using this rotational movement, the operator should never need to push hard on the tube to position it in the larynx. Once the tube is in place, the fiber optic laryngoscope and oral airway are removed, and the 15-mm connector is reattached to the tube. To verify that the tube is properly positioned, a device can be attached to the connector and will make a distinct whistle as the patient exhales. The orotracheal tube is then firmly taped in place at one side of the mouth.

**Maintenance** Standard maintenance (see Appendix). It is helpful to surgeons if a single dose of neuromuscular-blocking drug (vecuronium 10 mg or a d-tubocurarine/pancuronium mix [21 mg/3 mg] 10 ml) is administered to relax the strap muscles of the back.

**Emergence** If an opiate-based anesthetic is used, the orotracheal tube often can be removed at the end of surgery while the patient is still in the prone position. This is not advisable if the original intubation was difficult, or if the operation was prolonged and airway edema or respiratory depression are likely.

| | | |
|---|---|---|
| **Blood and fluid requirements** | IV: 16-18 ga x 1-2 | Blood transfusion is rarely necessary for simple disk surgery. Autologous blood obtained preop and/or from a cell saver generally will be needed if an extensive laminectomy and fusion are performed. |
| **Control of blood loss** | Deliberate hypotension | Deliberate hypotension helps minimize blood loss when extensive laminectomy and fusion are performed. This is most easily achieved with a combination of esmolol and SNP administered by means of continuous infusion to achieve a HR of 50-70 bpm and MAP = 70-80 mmHg. |

| | | |
|---|---|---|
| **Monitoring** | Standard monitors (see Appendix).<br>± Arterial line<br>± CVP line<br>± Urinary catheter | For simple back surgery, standard monitors are sufficient. If deliberate hypotension is planned, an arterial catheter is necessary to monitor BP, and a CVP catheter is necessary for infusion of vasoactive drugs and monitoring of CVP. A urinary drainage catheter is also desirable if surgery is expected to last several hrs or substantial fluid shifts are anticipated. |
| **Positioning** | ✓ and pad pressure points.<br>✓ eyes and ears frequently.<br>✓ breasts and genitals.<br>✓ free abdominal movement.<br>Neutral C-spine | Except for syringoperitoneal shunts, which are performed with patient in lateral position, patients are positioned prone on a Wilson frame or on bolsters. Generally, the head is turned to one side on a pillow or towels or a Shea headrest. If patient has limited lateral movement of the head, or has cervical disk disease, placement of the head in the midline, using a horseshoe headrest or Gardner-Wells tongs, should be considered. Elbows and knees should be padded to avoid pressure sores. It is very useful to have patient position him/herself prior to induction of anesthesia to assure that all body parts are properly positioned and comfortable. |
| **Complications** | ↓BP<br>Bowel or ureteral injury<br>Hemorrhage | ↓BP may be 2° abdominal compression and ↓venous return.<br>↑blood loss may occur 2° epidural vein engorgement, abdominal compression or vascular injury. |

**POSTOPERATIVE**

| | | |
|---|---|---|
| **Complications** | Hemorrhage<br>↓BP<br>Nerve-root injury | If hypotension persists despite vigorous blood and fluid administration, the anesthesiologist should suspect bleeding into the retroperitoneal space or abdomen. Alert the surgeon of this possibility and prepare for immediate exploration of the abdomen. |
| **Tests** | Hct; document neurological status. | If postop bleeding is suspected, serial Hct determinations are useful. |

**References**

1. Sonntag VRH, Hadley MN: Surgical approaches to the thoracolumbar spine. In *Clinical Neurosurgery*, Vol 36. Williams & Wilkins, Baltimore: 1990, 168-85.

# CERVICAL LAMINECTOMY FOR TUMOR

## SURGICAL CONSIDERATIONS

**Description:** A **decompressive laminectomy** is used to expose a cervical tumor, which may be extradural, intradural, extramedullary or intramedullary. Depending on the location of the tumor, the surgeon may need to open the dura and/or spinal cord. Obviously, the intradural intramedullary tumors involve more risk and are more delicate to remove. Many lamina may be removed in order to expose and excise the tumor. Surgical adjunctive tools (e.g., CUSA, laser, surgical microscope, etc.) may be used to aid in removal of the tumor. Intraop evoked potential monitoring may be used during these procedures to test the integrity of the dorsal columns. Once the tumor has been removed, the wound is closed in layers, as in a simple laminectomy. These procedures may be performed in the prone or seated position.

**Usual preop diagnosis:** Cervical myelopathy (spinal-cord compression) 2° tumor; spinal tumor; spinal cord tumor; meningioma; schwannoma; ependymoma; astrocytoma; neurofibromatosis; von Hippel-Lindau disease; hemangioblastoma; metastatic tumor (carcinoma)

### SUMMARY OF PROCEDURE

| | |
|---|---|
| **Position** | Prone or seated, head in pin fixation |
| **Incision** | Posterior midline |
| **Special instrumentation** | Operating microscope; evoked potential monitoring (optional); laser; CUSA |
| **Unique considerations** | Fiber optic intubation occasionally indicated. Localizing intraop lateral cervical spine x-ray taken to assess correct level for operation. |
| **Antibiotics** | Vancomycin 1 gm iv slowly + cefotaxime 1 gm iv |
| **Surgical time** | 2.5 - 8 hrs |
| **Closing considerations** | Cervical orthosis (collar or halo vest) |
| **EBL** | 50-1000 cc |
| **Postop care** | PACU → room; occasionally patients may require ICU or constant observation. |
| **Mortality** | 0-5% |
| **Morbidity** | Infection<br>CSF leak<br>Myelopathy<br>Nerve injury<br>Postop instability<br>Massive blood loss; epidural ooze |
| **Procedure code** | 63275 (extradural tumor); 63280 (intradural, extramedullary); 63285 (intradural, intramedullary); 63290 (combined extradural and intradural); 61712 (microscopic) |
| **Pain score** | 5-7 |

### PATIENT POPULATION CHARACTERISTICS

| | |
|---|---|
| **Age range** | 5-85 yrs (usually 30-60) |
| **Male:Female** | 1:1 |
| **Incidence** | 3-10/100,000 |
| **Etiology** | Degenerative<br>Traumatic<br>Neoplastic: metastatic, primary CNS, known syndrome (e.g., neurofibromatosis)<br>Infectious |
| **Associated conditions** | Von Recklinghausen's disease<br>Neurofibromatosis<br>Von Hippel-Lindau disease |

## ANESTHETIC CONSIDERATIONS

See Anesthetic Considerations following "Cervical or Craniocervical Fusion" (below).

**References**

1. Wilkins RH, Rengachary SS, eds: Spinal tumors. In *Neurosurgery*. McGraw-Hill, New York: 1985, 1039-83.

# ANTERIOR CERVICAL DISCECTOMY, WITH OR WITHOUT FUSION

## SURGICAL CONSIDERATIONS

**Description: Anterior cervical discectomy** is a common procedure for excising herniated or degenerated discs and osteophytes which may be causing radiculopathy or myelopathy. Occasionally, the procedure is used for unstable conditions in which there is ligamentous laxity on either a degenerative or traumatic basis.

An incision is made in the anterolateral neck and dissection is carried down between the carotid sheath (carotid and jugular vessels) and the trachea and esophagus to the prevertebral fascia (Fig 1.2-1). At this point, the surgeon has exposed the anterior aspect of the vertebral bodies and discs. A lateral x-ray usually is taken to identify the appropriate levels. The disk is then removed via curettage. The posterior longitudinal ligament is often removed, along with any spurs compressing the spinal canal or nerve roots.

**Variant procedure or approaches:** This procedure can be performed with or without an **interbody fusion**, depending on surgeon's preference. Approximately 70% of patients who undergo an anterior discectomy without fusion will go on to fuse spontaneously (over 2-4 months) following the procedure. There are several variant approaches to surgical fusion. The fusion is usually performed by placing a bone graft into the disc space, after removal of the disc and osteophytes and after preparation of the graft recipient site. The bone grafts may be autologous (removed from the patient's iliac crest through a separate incision) or from a bone bank. Occasionally, the bone fusion may be supplemented by incorporating internal stabilizing hardware; for example, AO or Caspar stainless steel plates and screws.

**Usual preop diagnosis:** Cervical radiculopathy (nerve-root compression); cervical myelopathy (spinal cord compression); cervical instability (ligamentous laxity or disruption); cervical disc disease (herniation or degeneration of one or more cervical discs)

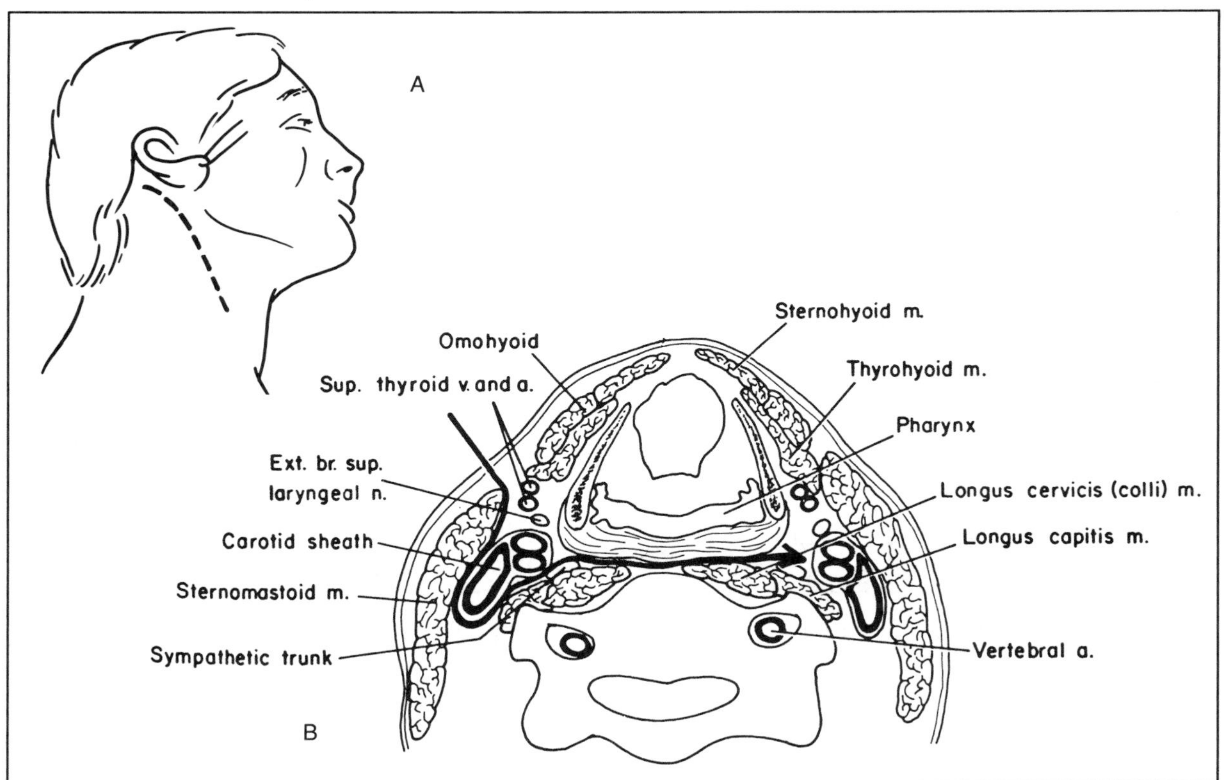


**Figure 1.2-1.** (A) Longitudinal incision along anterior border of sternomastoid muscle. (B) Cross-section of the neck at the level of the thyroid cartilage. Plane of dissection posterior to the carotid sheath and anterior to the sympathetic trunk is shown. (Reproduced with permission from Rothman RH, Simeone FA, eds: *The Spine*, 2nd edition. WB Saunders Co: 1982.)

### SUMMARY OF PROCEDURE

| | Simple Discectomy | Discectomy with Fusion |
|---|---|---|
| **Position** | Supine | ⇐ |
| **Incision** | Anterolateral neck | ⇐ + Anterolateral ilium, if autologous bone graft) |
| **Special instrumentation** | Operating microscope (optional) | ⇐ + Stainless steel plates and screws (optional) |
| **Unique considerations** | FOL occasionally indicated. Patient may be in cervical traction during procedure. Localizing intraop lateral cervical spine x-ray taken to assess correct level of operation. | ⇐ + Intraop x-rays may be taken to assess graft placement or instrumentation, if used. |
| **Antibiotics** | Cefazolin 1 gm iv | ⇐ |
| **Surgical time** | 1.5 - 2.5 hrs for single level; additional levels, add 0.5 - 1 hr for each. | 1.5 - 2.5 hrs for single level; add 0.5 hr for autologous graft; 0.5-1 hr for instrumentation. |
| **Closing considerations** | Cervical collar (optional) | Cervical orthosis collar; occasionally, halo vest |
| **EBL** | 25-250 cc | 50-500 cc |
| **Postop care** | PACU → room | ⇐ |
| **Mortality** | < 1% | ⇐ |
| **Morbidity** | Esophageal perforation: < 1% | ⇐ |
| | Infection: < 1% | ⇐ |
| | Massive blood loss - carotid or jugular injury, | ⇐ |
| | epidural ooze: < 1% | ⇐ |
| | Neurological myelopathy: < 1% | ⇐ |
| | Neurological nerve injury: | |
| | Root: < 1% | ⇐ |
| | Recurrent laryngeal nerve: 5% | ⇐ |
| | Sympathetic chain: < 1% | ⇐ |
| | Postop instability: < 1% | ⇐ |
| | | Instrument failure: < 1% |
| | | Slipped graft: < 1% |
| **Procedure code** | 63075, 63076 (additional level) | 63075, 22554, 22585 (additional level)<br>22845 (instrumentation)<br>22820 (harvest bone graft) |
| **Pain score** | 3-4 | 3-4 (6 if bone graft harvested from patient) |

### PATIENT POPULATION CHARACTERISTICS

| | |
|---|---|
| **Age range** | 18-85 yrs (usually 30-60) |
| **Male:Female** | 1:1 |
| **Incidence** | Common |
| **Etiology** | Degenerative<br>Traumatic<br>Infectious |

## ANESTHETIC CONSIDERATIONS

See Anesthetic Considerations following "Cervical or Craniocervical Fusion" (below).

**References**


1. Rothman RH, Simeone FA, eds: Surgical approaches to the cervical spine. In *The Spine*. WB Saunders Co, Philadelphia: 1982, 93-127.

# CERVICAL LAMINOTOMY, FORAMINOTOMY AND LAMINECTOMY

## SURGICAL CONSIDERATIONS

**Description:** Cervical laminotomy (removal of a portion of the lamina), foraminotomy (opening of the neural foramina), and laminectomy (removal of the lamina) are procedures for decompressing the neural elements of the cervical spine via a posterior approach. These procedures can be used to treat cervical radiculopathy 2° degenerative disc disease (i.e., herniated discs or osteophytes). **Decompressive laminectomy** can be used to treat cervical spine stenosis, which is present either on a congenital or degenerative basis, or to gain access to the spinal canal or spinal cord. The extent of the procedure depends on the indications for treatment. When the patient has only a single nerve-root-compression syndrome, the procedure may consist of decompressing that one root. When there is diffuse stenosis of the cervical canal, an extensive cervical decompression over several cervical vertebral segments may be indicated. The cervical dorsal fascia is exposed via a midline posterior incision. The paraspinal muscles are dissected off the spinous processes and lamina, and the bone is removed piecemeal with rongeurs or drills. The extent of the procedure depends on the indications for treatment. Hemostasis is achieved with bipolar cautery, and raw bone surfaces are sealed with bone wax. Topical hemostatic agents are used to aid in hemostasis in the epidural gutters. If the patient has an intradural tumor or process such as syringomyelia, the dura is opened and the operating microscope is used for this portion of the procedure. Once the intradural procedure is complete, the dura is closed, and the surgeon may wish to test the integrity of the closure with a Valsalva-like maneuver (sustained inspiration to 30-40 cm $H_2O$). The wound is closed in layers, and a drain may be left in the epidural space.

**Variant procedure or approaches:** The major variation in these procedures is patient position. Either prone or sitting position (using a pin fixation device with an overhead bar) may be used, depending on surgeon's preference.

**Usual preop diagnosis:** Cervical radiculopathy (nerve-root compression; cervical myelopathy (spinal cord compression; cervical disc disease (herniation or degeneration of one or more cervical discs)

### SUMMARY OF PROCEDURE

| | Cervical Laminotomy or Foraminotomy | Cervical Laminectomy |
|---|---|---|
| **Position** | Prone or sitting; pin fixation or horseshoe headrest | ⇐ |
| **Incision** | Posterior midline neck | ⇐ |
| **Special instrumentation** | Operating microscope (optional) | ⇐ |
| **Unique considerations** | Fiber optic intubation occasionally is indicated; a localizing intraop lateral cervical spine x-ray is taken to assess correct level for the operation. | ⇐ |
| **Antibiotics** | Cefazolin 1 gm (optional) | ⇐ |
| **Surgical time** | 1.5 - 2 hrs for single level; additional levels, add 0.5 - 1 hr for each. | 2 hrs for single level; additional levels, add 0.5 hr for each. |
| **EBL** | 25-250 cc | 50-500 cc |
| **postop care** | PACU → room | ⇐ |
| **Mortality** | 0-3% | ⇐ |
| **Morbidity** | All < 5%: | ⇐ |
| | Infection | ⇐ |
| | Neurological: myelopathy; root injury | ⇐ |
| | CSF leak | ⇐ |
| | Postop instability | ⇐ |
| | Air embolism | ⇐ |
| | Massive blood loss | ⇐ |
| **Procedure code** | 63020 (single-level, single-side)<br>63035.(additional levels)<br>63040 (re-exploration) | 63001 (1 or 2 levels)<br>63015 (>2 levels)<br>63045 (with foraminotomy)<br>63048 (additional levels) |
| **Pain score** | 7-10 | 7-10 |

### PATIENT POPULATION CHARACTERISTICS

| | |
|---|---|
| **Age range** | 18-85 yrs (usually 30-60 yrs) |
| **Male:Female** | ~1:1 |
| **Incidence** | Common |
| **Etiology** | Degenerative<br>Traumatic<br>Infectious |

---

## ANESTHETIC CONSIDERATIONS

See Anesthetic Considerations following "Cervical or Craniocervical Fusion" (below).

**References**

1. Ehni G: Extradural spinal cord and nerve root compression from benign lesions of the cervical area. In *Neurological Surgery*. Youmans JR, ed. WB Saunders Co, Philadelphia: 1982, 2574-2612.

# VERTEBRAL CORPECTOMY WITH STRUT FUSION

## SURGICAL CONSIDERATIONS

**Description: Vertebral corpectomy** (removal of vertebral body) with fusion is used to treat conditions in which there is anterior impingement of the spinal cord or narrowing of the spinal canal at the level of the vertebral body (not just the disc). This is utilized for pathologic fractures of the spine (e.g., metastatic carcinoma), or certain infections of the vertebral body. Conditions such as ossification of the posterior longitudinal ligament (OPLL) are best treated in this manner. This procedure is also used to treat some fractures of the cervical spine. Occasionally, this approach may be used to remove intradural lesions anterior to the spinal cord. The vertebral body or bodies can be removed, allowing for decompression of the anterior spinal canal. The spine must be stabilized following corpectomy, usually with a bone graft (autologous ilium, fibula or bone-bank bone). This procedure is performed using the same exposure as described in the section on **anterior cervical discectomy**. In this case, however, the exposure is more generous. More bone is removed and a fusion is performed at the completion of bone removal. Some patients with limited life expectancy may be candidates for use of a prosthesis instead of bone graft. This may involve use of a polymerizing acrylic to replace bone. Occasionally, the bone fusion may be supplemented by incorporating internal stabilizing hardware (e.g., AO or Caspar stainless steel plates and screws).

**Usual preop diagnosis:** Cervical myelopathy (spinal cord compression) 2° fracture of the cervical spine (traumatic or pathologic); narrowing of the spinal canal due to congenital conditions; degenerative conditions such as severe disc disease with osteophyte formation; OPLL; cervical instability (ligamentous laxity or disruption or destruction of bone due to tumor or infection); failed previous spinal fusion

### SUMMARY OF PROCEDURE

| | |
|---|---|
| **Position** | Supine |
| **Incision** | Anterolateral neck; anterolateral ilium, or possibly lateral lower leg for bone graft |
| **Special instrumentation** | Operating microscope (optional); stainless steel plates and screws (optional) |
| **Unique considerations** | Fiber optic intubation occasionally indicated. Patient may be in cervical traction during the procedure. Localizing intraop lateral cervical spine x-ray taken to assess correct level for operation. Intraop x-rays may be taken to assess graft placement or instrumentation. |

| | |
|---|---|
| **Antibiotics** | Cefazolin 1 gm |
| **Surgical time** | 2.5 - 3 hrs for single level; additional levels, add 0.5 - 1 hr for each; add 0.5 - 1 hr for instrumentation; add 0.5 hr for harvesting autologous bone. |
| **Closing considerations** | Cervical orthosis (collar or halo vest) |
| **EBL** | 50-1000 cc |
| **Postop care** | PACU → room |
| **Mortality** | 0-5% |
| **Morbidity** | Infection<br>Neurological: myelopathy; nerve-root injury<br>Recurrent laryngeal nerve injury<br>Sympathetic chain<br>Esophageal perforation<br>Postop instability<br>Slipped graft<br>Instrument failure<br>CSF leak<br>Massive blood loss: carotid or jugular injury, epidural ooze |
| **Procedure code** | 63081 (single segment); 63082 (each additional segment); 22140 (reconstruction of spine, single segment); 22145 (reconstruction, additional segments); 22845 (instrumentation); 22820 (harvest bone graft) |
| **Pain score** | 4-7 |

### PATIENT POPULATION CHARACTERISTICS

| | |
|---|---|
| **Age range** | 18-85 yrs (usually 30-60 yrs) |
| **Male:Female** | 1:1 |
| **Incidence** | Relatively common |
| **Etiology** | Degenerative<br>Traumatic<br>OPLL<br>Neoplastic<br>Infectious |

---

## ANESTHETIC CONSIDERATIONS

See Anesthetic Considerations following "Cervical or Craniocervical Fusion" (below).

**References**

1. Rengachary SS, Redford JB: Partial median corpectomy for cervical spondylotic myelopathy. In *Neurosurgery Update*, Vol II. Wilkins RH, Rengachary SS, eds. McGraw-Hill, New York: 1991, 356-59.

# CERVICAL OR CRANIOCERVICAL FUSION

## SURGICAL CONSIDERATIONS

**Description:** Certain conditions, including those where there is instability of the spine due to traumatic, degenerative and certain neoplastic conditions, require posterior fusion of the cervical spine. The fusion usually involves two, or possibly three vertebral segments. Occasionally, it is necessary to fuse the occiput to the upper cervical spine.

The operation involves exposing the spinous processes, lamina and facets of the levels to be fused. A bone graft will be harvested from the posterior iliac crest and fashioned appropriately. The bone graft is secured with wire to the decorticated segments to be fused. The wire will be either sublaminar, through the base of the spinous process or lamina, or through the facet. X-rays may be taken to verify alignment. The wound is closed in layers, possibly with a drain in place. Some of the fusions will be supplemented with instrumentation. Luque rectangles with sublaminar wires or lateral mass plate and screws may be incorporated to internally fixate a fusion. An orthopedic surgeon may be co-surgeon on some of these procedures.

**Usual preop diagnosis:** Spinal fracture; cervical instability; atlanto-axial instability; odontoid fracture; pseudarthrosis

### SUMMARY OF PROCEDURE

| | |
|---|---|
| **Position** | Prone, head in tong traction or pins |
| **Incision** | Midline posterior, posterior ilium for graft |
| **Special instrumentation** | Luque rectangles and other hardware for fixation |
| **Unique considerations** | Unstable cervical spine preop may require fiber optic intubation. |
| **Antibiotics** | Cefazolin 1-2 gm iv |
| **Surgical time** | 2.5 - 3.5+ hrs (longer for complicated cases) |
| **Closing considerations** | Possible need for halo vest placement or other cervical brace upon closure |
| **EBL** | 100-500 cc |
| **Postop care** | Patient to PACU; then close observation unit or routine floor; neurological function monitoring during observation |
| **Mortality** | 0.3% |
| **Morbidity** | Infection<br>Neurological impairment<br>CSF leak<br>Massive blood loss |
| **Procedure code** | 22590-22600 (cervical and craniocervical fusion); 22650 (additional levels); 22840-22842 (instrumentation) |
| **Pain score** | 5-9 |

### PATIENT POPULATION CHARACTERISTICS

| | |
|---|---|
| **Age range** | 3-70 yrs (usually 9-40) |
| **Male:Female** | ~2:1 |
| **Incidence** | Relatively common |
| **Etiology** | Congenital<br>Traumatic<br>Degenerative<br>Inflammatory<br>Rheumatic<br>Neoplastic |
| **Associated conditions** | Spinal cord injury<br>Rheumatoid arthritis |

# ANESTHETIC CONSIDERATIONS FOR CERVICAL NEUROSURGICAL PROCEDURES

**(Procedures covered: cervical laminectomy for tumor; anterior cervical discectomy; cervical laminotomy, foraminotomy, laminectomy; vertebral corpectomy; cervical or craniocervical fusion; craniocervical decompression)**

## PREOPERATIVE

Surgery of the cervical spine is common, primarily because of the frequency of herniation of a cervical intervertebral disk causing compression of the adjacent spinal nerve roots. Other, less frequent indications for cervical surgery include: acute or chronic instability of the neck, either of congenital or acquired origin, requiring fusion; removal of a tumor of the spinal cord; or craniocervical decompression for Arnold-Chiari malformation.

**Respiratory** Acute fractures of the cervical spine may be associated with sufficient trauma to the spinal cord to cause acute respiratory insufficiency and inability to handle oropharyngeal secretions. If this occurs, immediate tracheal intubation is necessary. Before initiating intubation, the neck must be stabilized, preferably in Gardner-Wells tongs or a body jacket; lacking those, a tight neck collar with sandbags on each side of the head will suffice. The objective is to **not flex or extend the head or move it laterally** during the course of tracheal intubation.

**Tests:** ABG to substantiate degree of respiratory impairment

**Cardiovascular** Acute fractures of the cervical spine and associated spinal cord trauma may result in loss of sympathetic tone, which, in turn, may cause peripheral vasodilation and bradycardia. Generally, this condition can be treated effectively with crystalloid and/or colloid infusion, and atropine to ↑HR. Rarely is it necessary to use vasopressors to maintain BP or HR.

**Tests:** As indicated from H&P.

**Neurological** Patients with herniation of a cervical disk generally complain first of pain in the neck, particularly with lateral rotation of the head. The pain may radiate down one or, rarely, both arms. As nerve compression continues, patients begin to develop weakness and atrophy of specific muscle groups in the arm. These Sx, however, are not specific to herniation of a disk, and may be caused by a spinal cord tumor or cyst. Patients with acute fractures of the neck and attendant spinal cord trauma at T1 level will be paraplegic, while fractures above C5 may result in quadriplegia and loss of phrenic nerve function. Injuries between these two levels result in variable loss of motor and sensory functions in the upper extremities. A careful documentation of preop sensory and motor deficits is important.

**Tests:** MRI has replaced myelography as the primary diagnostic test, because it distinguishes disk from tumor from cyst. Emergency CT is invaluable in the assessment of patients with acute neck injuries and suspected cervical fracture; if not available, A-P and lateral x-rays of the neck generally will reveal the site and extent of bony injury.

**Hematologic** Anti-platelet agents should be stopped 10 d before surgery.

**Tests:** Hct; others as indicated from H&P.

**Laboratory** Other tests as indicated from H&P.

**Premedication** Premedication is very useful in this patient population. Midazolam 2-4 mg iv and meperidine 20-40 mg iv in divided doses prior to entering the OR makes patients amnestic and tractable.

## INTRAOPERATIVE

**Anesthetic technique:** GETA

**Induction** For patient with stable neck, orotracheal intubation using standard laryngoscopy, if possible, is acceptable. If patient's neck is unstable, with head in tongs, a halo device or a body jacket, or if findings on H&P suggest that tracheal intubation may be difficult, it is preferable to place ETT with FOL under local anesthesia before induction of GA. In skilled hands, **orotracheal fiber optic intubation** is the easiest, quickest and most pleasant method for placing the ETT. Nasotracheal intubation is rarely, if ever, needed for this type of surgery. (For details of fiber optic intubation, see "Anesthetic Considerations for Thoracolumbar Neurosurgical Procedures.") Once ETT is in place, anesthesia is induced with STP 3-5 mg/kg or propofol 1.5-2.5 mg/kg iv.

**Maintenance** Standard maintenance (see Appendix). It is helpful to surgeons if a single dose of neuromuscular blocking drug – vecuronium 10 mg or a d-tubocurarine/pancuronium mix (21 mg/3 mg) 10 ml – is administered to relax neck muscles. Additional doses of relaxants are rarely necessary.

| | | |
|---|---|---|
| **Emergence** | If a cervical fusion has been performed, and the patient is returned to a halo device or body jacket, it is desirable to leave ETT in place until patient is fully awake and able to manage his/her own airway. To permit tolerance of the ETT and minimize coughing during emergence, it is useful to spray lidocaine (4 cc 4%) down the orotracheal tube, or inject the same dose of lidocaine through the secondary port of a cuff system designed for this purpose. **NB:** Immediate airway obstruction 2° soft-tissue occlusion or superior laryngeal nerve damage may occur on extubation. A useful way to test for airway patency is to deflate the cuff of the tracheal tube and determine that patient is able to breathe around the tube as well as through it. | |
| **Blood and fluid requirements** | IV: 16-18 ga x 1<br>NS/LR @ 4-6 cc/kg/hr | Blood transfusion is rarely needed for operations on the cervical spine. |
| **Monitoring** | Standard monitors (see Appendix).<br>± Arterial line<br>± CVP line<br>± Doppler<br>± Urinary catheter | If a posterior surgical approach with patient in seated position is planned, an arterial catheter is useful for monitoring BP, and a CVP catheter is necessary for monitoring CVP and aspiration of air, should an air embolism occur. If patient is seated, an ultrasonic Doppler flow probe also should be placed on the anterior chest wall with confirmation of its performance by injecting 1 ml of agitated NS into CVP line and listening for the change in Doppler sound. |
| **Positioning** | Supine:<br>✓ and pad pressure points.<br>✓ eyes.<br>Shoulder roll<br>Cervical traction | For **anterior cervical discectomy** and/or fusion, patient is positioned supine with a roll under the shoulders and head is moderately hyperextended. A cervical strap is placed below the chin and behind the occiput, and attached to a weight of 5-10 lbs hung over the head of the bed. If patient is in a halo or tongs, 5-10 lbs of weight are attached to the device. The surgical incision is made in the right side of the neck. |
| | Prone:<br>✓ and pad pressure points.<br>✓ eyes.<br>✓ genitalia. | A **posterior approach** is used if the operation is for spinal stenosis or craniocervical decompression. With this approach, patient is positioned either prone (on a Wilson frame or on bolsters), or sitting, with the head in 3-point fixation. |
| | Sitting:<br>✓ and pad pressure points.<br>✓ eyes.<br>VAE monitoring<br>✓ ETT position. | There are advantages to both neurosurgeon and anesthesiologist, as well as the patient for using a seated position. For the neurosurgeon: (1) easier access to the lesion; (2) less blood loss, since both arterial and venous pressures are lower than if patient were prone;[2] (3) less interference from CSF, since it readily drains away from the operative site; and (4) lower incidence of postop neurological injury.[2] Advantages to the anesthesiologist are: (1) less chance that ETT and other arterial and venous catheters will become dislodged than with patient prone; (2) less chance for inadvertent pressure injury; (3) easier assessment and management of ventilation; and (4) easier access to patient for insertion of additional catheters, if necessary. |
| **Complications** | VAE | The major disadvantage of the sitting position is the risk of VAE, particularly paradoxical air embolism to the left side of the heart through a PFO (or, rarely, through the pulmonary circulation) → CNS or coronary emboli. Incidence of VAE is 25-45% in patients operated on in the seated position.[2,3] VAE is easily detected using a combination of Doppler, $ETCO_2$ and $ETN_2$ analysis; and complications are rare.[2,4] If VAE is suspected (Sx = ↓$ETCO_2$, ↑$ETN_2$, ↓BP, dysrhythmias), notify the surgeon and aspirate the right atrial catheter using a 10 ml |

| | | |
|---|---|---|
| **Complications, continued** | | syringe. This generally will confirm the diagnosis as well as provide treatment. If VAE continues, and the surgeon has difficulty identifying the site of air entrainment, consider using PEEP $\leq$ 10 cm $H_2O$ or bilateral jugular compression to increase CVP and cerebral venous pressure. Low levels of PEEP applied and released gradually will not promote paradoxical air embolism.[5,6] |
| | ↓BP | Hypotension caused by venous pooling, inadequate venous return to the heart, and decreased cardiac output can be treated by wrapping lower extremities while patient is supine, infusing adequate fluid volume to maintain right heart filling pressure, and avoiding excessive depth of anesthesia. |

## POSTOPERATIVE

| | | |
|---|---|---|
| **Complications** | Airway obstruction<br>Hematoma<br>Neurologic deficit | The cause of the airway obstruction is usually from soft tissue falling back against the posterior pharyngeal wall which cannot be corrected by forward displacement of the mandible because of the neck fusion or postop traction/stabilization device (halo or body jacket). May require oral or nasal airway. |
| | Tension pneumothorax | Delayed respiratory insufficiency is usually caused by either development of a tension pneumothorax from entrainment of air via the surgical wound or an unsuspected oropharyngeal laceration during tracheal intubation, or from bleeding into the neck at the surgical site, with progressive compression and occlusion of the airway. If a tension pneumothorax is suspected and circulatory signs are stable, immediate CXR should confirm the diagnosis. If circulation is failing, an 18- or 20-ga needle catheter should be inserted immediately anteriorly at the 2nd intercostal space on the suspected side to relieve the pneumothorax. If the diagnosis is airway obstruction from bleeding into the neck, the wound should be opened immediately, and clots and blood removed. This should be done **before attempting tracheal intubation**. Intubation of the airway is futile and wastes valuable time if the cause is airway compression by blood in the wound. It is sometimes difficult to distinguish airway obstruction from tension pneumothorax by physical signs. One useful way is to check for the "puff sign." With airway obstruction from any cause, what gas moves in and out of the airway does so very slowly because of the obstruction. In contrast, with tension pneumothorax, gas moves in and out of airway with great speed because of high intrapleural pressure. By applying positive pressure to airway and listening at patient's mouth for the sound of gas escaping as airway pressure is released, one hears either a puff or jet of air escaping (tension pneumothorax) or slow, gradual exit of air (airway obstruction). |
| **Pain management** | Meperidine (10 mg iv prn)<br>Codeine (20 mg iv or po prn) | |
| **Tests** | CXR<br>Hct | Repeat neurological exam prior to discharge from PACU. |

**References**

1. Sonntag VKH, Hadley MN: Management of upper cervical spinal instability. In *Neurosurgery Update*, Vol II. Wilkins RH, Rengachary SS, eds. McGraw-Hill, New York: 1991, 222-33.
2. Black S, Ockert DB, Oliver WC Jr, Cucchiara RF: Outcome following posterior fossa craniectomy in patients in the sitting or horizontal positions. *Anesthesiology* 1988; 69(1):49-56.
3. Cucchiara RF, Nugent M, Seward JB, Messick JM: Air embolism in upright neurosurgical patients: Detection and localization by two-dimensional transesophageal echocardiography. *Anesthesiology* 1984; 60(4):353-55.
4. Black S, Cucchiara RF, Nishimura RA, Michenfelder JD: Parameters affecting occurrence of paradoxical air embolism. *Anesthesiology* 1989; 71(2):235-41.
5. Pearl RG, Larson CP Jr: Hemodynamic effects of positive end-expiratory pressure during continuous venous air embolism in the dog. *Anesthesiology* 1986; 64(6):724-29.
6. Zasslow MA, Pearl RG, Larson CP Jr, Silverberg G, Shuer LF: PEEP does not affect left atrial-right atrial pressure difference in neurosurgical patients. *Anesthesiology* 1988; 68(5):760-63.

# SURGERY FOR SPASTICITY

## SURGICAL CONSIDERATIONS

**Description:** Neurologic conditions associated with spasticity of the extremities include spinal cord injury, multiple sclerosis, stroke, etc. The spasticity is often managed with oral medications. An alternative approach is to infuse baclofen (GABA-agonist that decreases frequency and amplitude of tonic impulses to the muscle spindles) into the subarachnoid space via an implanted pump. When these therapeutic modalities fail, it may be necessary to perform surgery. Some of the procedures are destructive in that a lesion is placed in certain nerves or the spinal cord to destroy the reflex arc which is contributing to the spasticity. There are both percutaneous and open techniques for placing the lesion. In the **open procedures**, a **laminectomy** is performed (see "Lumbar Laminotomy, Laminectomy"). In a case where a **myelotomy** is to be performed, the lower spinal cord is exposed and incised at the appropriate location to interrupt the reflex arc. In certain cases, selective electrical stimulation can be performed on isolated dorsal rootlets from the involved extremity. Abnormal responses in the extremities are monitored via EMG and direct observation. When abnormal responses are detected, that particular rootlet is divided (dorsal rhizotomy). This procedure is somewhat tedious and requires that stable anesthetic conditions be maintained so that appropriate monitoring can be carried out during the procedure. The surgeon usually must sacrifice 40-60% of the dorsal rootlets in cases of spastic diplegia found in cerebral palsy.

**Variant procedure or approaches:** Percutaneous **radiofrequency rhizotomy** is another procedure used for spasticity. A thermal lesion is placed in the appropriate dorsal roots with a radiofrequency generator. Needles are passed into the neural foramen via a posterolateral trajectory for levels L1-L5, and then from a midline approach to the S1 root. The needle position is determined by A-P and lateral fluoroscopy and by stimulus mapping. Stimulating current is delivered via an electrode passed through the needle. A low-level stimulating current causes muscle twitching in the appropriate leg if the needle is in the proper location. Once placed and verified, the radiofrequency generator is used to produce the lesion. At the termination of this procedure, the patient's legs should be flaccid. Patients with spinal cord injury-producing anesthesia below T10 may not require additional anesthetic for the procedure.

**Usual preop diagnosis:** Spasticity; multiple sclerosis; spinal cord injury

**SUMMARY OF PROCEDURE**

| | Open Rhizotomy or Myelotomy | Radiofrequency Rhizotomy |
|---|---|---|
| **Position** | Prone | ⇐ |
| **Incision** | Midline | Needles placed in lumbar region |
| **Special instrumentation** | EMG monitor; nerve stimulator | Radiofrequency generator; fluoroscope |

| | Open Rhizotomy or Myelotomy | Radiofrequency Rhizotomy |
|---|---|---|
| **Unique considerations** | Anesthetic which allows EMG recordings | May not require anesthesia if anesthetic below waist (spinal cord surgery). |
| **Antibiotics** | Cefotaxime 1 gm iv; vancomycin 1 gm iv, slowly | None |
| **Surgical time** | 4 hrs | 2 hrs |
| **Closing considerations** | Surgeon may wish to test dural closure with Valsalva maneuver. | Remove needle. |
| **EBL** | 50-250 cc | Negligible |
| **Postop care** | Head flat; PACU → room | ⇐ |
| **Mortality** | < 1% | ⇐ |
| **Morbidity** | All < 5%:<br>CSF leak<br>Infection<br>Hemorrhage<br>Neurological impairment | ⇐ |
| **Procedure code** | 63185-63190 (laminectomy for rhizotomy)<br>61712 (operating microscope) | 63600 (percutaneous procedure) |
| **Pain score** | 4 | 2 |

### PATIENT POPULATION CHARACTERISTICS

| | |
|---|---|
| **Age range** | 3-55 yrs |
| **Male:Female** | ~3:2 |
| **Incidence** | Relatively uncommon neurosurgical procedure |
| **Etiology** | Hyperactivity of gamma stretch reflex |
| **Associated conditions** | Multiple sclerosis<br>Cerebral palsy<br>Spinal cord injury |

## ANESTHETIC CONSIDERATIONS

See Anesthetic Considerations following "Surgical Correction of Spinal Dysraphism," in Pediatric Surgery section.

**References**


1. Peacock WJ, Staudt LA, Nuwer MR: A neurosurgical approach to spasticity: selective posterior rhizotomy. In *Neurosurgery Update*, Vol II. Wilkins RH, Rengachary SS, eds. McGraw-Hill, New York: 1991, 403-7.
2. Kennemore DE: Percutaneous electrocoagulation of spinal nerves for the relief of pain and spasticity. In *Radionics Procedure Technique Series*. Radionics, Burlington MA: 1978.

**Surgeon**

**Lawrence M. Shuer, MD**
**Gary K. Steinberg, MD, PhD**

## 1.3 OTHER NEUROSURGERY

**Anesthesiologist**

**C. Philip Larson, Jr, MS, MD**

# CAROTID THROMBOENDARTERECTOMY

## SURGICAL CONSIDERATIONS

**Description:** Carotid thromboendarterectomy (TEA) is frequently used to treat severe atherosclerotic occlusive disease involving internal carotid arteries at the common carotid artery bifurcation. Atherosclerotic carotid artery disease commonly causes thromboembolic or hemodynamic stroke and transient ischemic attacks (TIAs). Recent studies[4] proved the efficacy of this operation, compared with medical treatment for symptomatic high-grade stenoses (>70%), and ongoing studies are evaluating its benefit for asymptomatic lesions and symptomatic lesions of moderate stenoses (50-70%).

The operation involves opening the common carotid arteries and the proximal internal carotid arteries in the neck (Fig 1.3-1), removing atherosclerotic plaque from the inside of the artery, and resuturing the wall of the arteries (media and adventitia). Opening the carotid artery (**arteriotomy**) requires temporary occlusion of the proximal common carotid artery, distal internal carotid artery, external carotid artery and usually its first branch, the superior thyroid artery. The entire procedure can be achieved under continued occlusion of these vessels, if the collateral blood flow to the territory supplied by the occluded internal carotid is deemed adequate (on the basis of intraop EEG monitoring, internal carotid artery back-bleeding, stump pressures, CBF studies, or angiography). Alternatively, an internal shunt between the proximal common carotid artery and distal internal carotid artery can be placed after the arteriotomy for use during the endarterectomy. Sometimes a vein graft or synthetic graft (Gortex®, Dacron®) is used to reconstruct ("patch") the arteriotomy site.

**Usual preop diagnosis:** Stroke; TIAs; carotid artery stenosis; carotid artery dissection

### SUMMARY OF PROCEDURE

| | |
|---|---|
| **Position** | Supine |
| **Incision** | Anterolateral neck; occasionally if "patching" arteriotomy, may have to harvest portion of greater saphenous vein from leg |
| **Special instrumentation** | Magnification loupes; vascular instruments ± shunt (Bard, Javid, Pruitt-Inahara) |
| **Unique considerations** | Techniques for monitoring collateral blood flow: EEG-spectral analysis or raw EEG, back-bleeding or internal carotid artery stump pressure (>50 mmHg); CBF measurements using Xenon; transcranial Doppler; full anticoagulation with heparin (10,000 U iv) during arterial occlusion ± reversal with protamine (50-100 mg iv) at end of arteriotomy repair and 10 min after reopening of carotid arteries; maintaining mild HTN during internal carotid artery occlusion (MAP 90-110); use of intraop neuroprotective agents during internal carotid artery occlusion (e.g., iv STP 4-5 mg/kg). |
| **Antibiotics** | Cefazolin (1 gm iv q 6 hrs) |
| **Surgical time** | 2 - 2.5 hrs |
| **Closing considerations** | Avoid HTN or hypotension (MAP 80-110); meticulous hemostasis. |
| **EBL** | 50-150 cc |
| **Postop care** | Control of BP (MAP 80-100 mmHg); start ASA on postop d 1; ICU x 1 d. |
| **Mortality** | 0.5-1% |
| **Morbidity** | Cranial nerve injury: Up to 39%<br>Stroke: 1-2%<br>MI: < 1%<br>Wound infection: Rare |
| **Procedure code** | 35301 |
| **Pain score** | 3 |

### PATIENT POPULATION CHARACTERISTICS

| | |
|---|---|
| **Age range** | 50-80 yrs |
| **Male:Female** | 1:1 |
| **Incidence** | 100,000 carotid endarterectomies/yr in U.S. |
| **Etiology** | Atherosclerosis<br>Occasionally, traumatic (dissection) |

**Associated conditions**

HTN
CAD
Peripheral vascular disease
Smoking
Obesity
Alcohol abuse
Hyperlipidemia

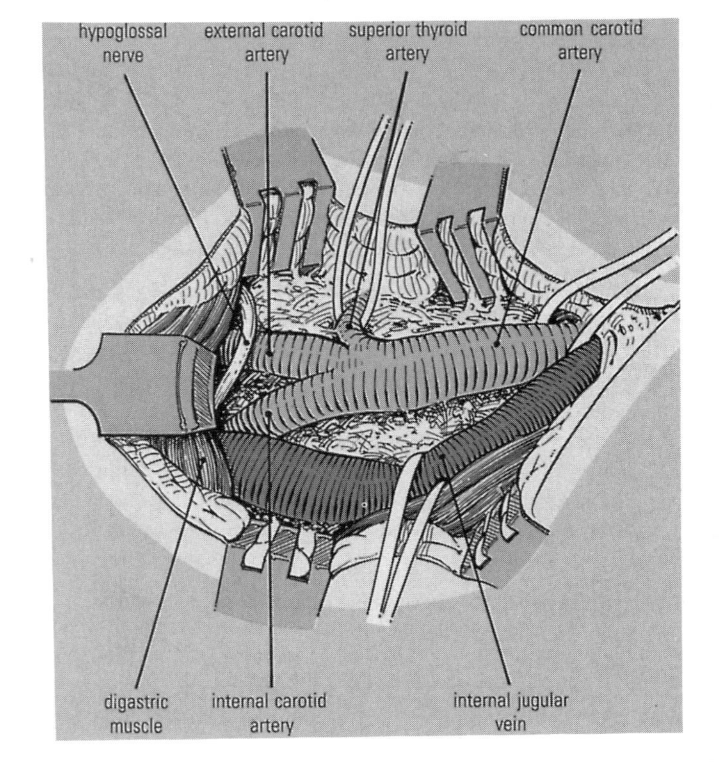


**Figure 1.3-1.** Exposure and control of carotid artery. (Reproduced with permission from Calne R, Pollard SG: *Operative Surgery*. Gower Medical Pub: 1992.)

---

## ANESTHETIC CONSIDERATIONS

**(Procedures covered: carotid thromboendarterectomy, carotid endarterectomy)**

### PREOPERATIVE

The incidence of occlusive or ulcerative lesions of the extracranial or intracranial vasculature increases with advancing years. Generally, these lesions are asymptomatic until the cross-sectional area of the vessel is decreased by at least 50%.[8] This is because the cerebral vasculature has excellent collateral circulation, most importantly the Circle of Willis, but also the carotid-basilar anastomosis via the trigeminal artery and the extra- to intracranial collateral flow via the ophthalmic artery or branches of the vertebral artery. Systemic hypotension such as that arising from a cardiac dysrhythmia may be a cause of cerebral ischemia in some patients with carotid stenosis. Patients presenting for carotid endarterectomy generally fall into one of three categories: (1) Those with transient ischemic attacks (TIAs), presenting with symptoms that may be focal or generalized. Two recent clinical trials[9,10] clearly document that carotid endarterectomy is superior to medical management in preventing the development of strokes in patients who are symptomatic from carotid stenosis of >70%. (2) Patients with completed stroke. If the stroke is fresh (having occurred within 2-4 weeks), most surgeons will not operate on the patient for fear of converting an ischemic infarct into a hemorrhagic infarct. Angiographic evaluation following recovery from an acute stroke usually demonstrates a stenotic and/or ulcerative lesion at the carotid bifurcation. (3) Patients with asymptomatic bruit, which usually is found during a routine physical examination of the neck. These are of concern because they may signal the development of carotid stenosis.[11]

**Respiratory**

Hx of pulmonary disease should be evaluated with spirometry, ABGs and CXR. If there is evidence of pulmonary infection, appropriate antibiotic therapy should be instituted. If secretions are excessive, preop pulmonary physiotherapy, including bronchodilator therapy, may be indicated. Patients should be asked to stop smoking prior to anesthesia, even if only the night before. While cessation of smoking for such a short time will not lessen the volume of secretions appreciably, or make the airways less irritable to a foreign body such as an ETT, it will provide sufficient time for the carbon monoxide levels in the blood to decrease, thereby enhancing $O_2$-carrying capacity. **Tests:** ABGs; spirometry; CXR, as indicated from H&P.

**Cardiovascular** In addition to the usual measures taken in preop evaluation of any patient undergoing anesthesia, there are special considerations that relate to patients who are to undergo a carotid endarterectomy. Most important is a careful evaluation of cardiovascular status, including a detailed Hx of cardiovascular function and serial determinations of BP in both arms to establish the range of pressures that normally occur, and whether there are regional differences. If BP is different in the two arms, it should be measured intraop and postop in the arm with the higher values. Also, a preop ECG is mandatory. The reason for concern about cardiovascular function is twofold: (1) It is often necessary to administer vasoactive drugs to artificially regulate BP during carotid endarterectomy, either to maintain it at a normal value, or sometimes to increase it as much as 20% above the highest resting pressure to maintain optimal collateral circulation during surgical carotid occlusion. (2) The incidence of perioperative MI in this surgical population is at least 1%, and represents the most common major postop complication in this operation. Except in the case of emergencies, anesthesia and operation should not proceed in the face of severe, uncontrolled HTN or diabetes or a MI within the last 3 mo. Antihypertensive medications should be continued up to the time of anesthesia.

**Tests:** ECG; others as indicated from H&P.

**Neurological** The Sx of cerebrovascular insufficiency are due to either critical stenosis or occlusion of cerebral vessels, combined with inadequate collateral circulation, or the development of ulcerative lesions at arterial branch points. The degenerative plaques or mural thrombi readily break off from the vessel wall and cause focal ischemic lesions. Manual occlusion of the carotid arteries is not an appropriate test of tolerance to temporary circulatory occlusion, as it may endanger the patient by precipitating embolization from an ulcerative lesion or by inducing bradycardia and hypotension from activation of the carotid sinus reflex. It is desirable, however, to position the patient's head in the operative position as a test of the effect of that position on CBF. It is well-documented that hyperextension and lateral rotation of the head may occlude vertebral-basilar flow between the scalenus anticus and longus coli muscles and, if sustained, contribute to postop cerebral ischemia. Sx of dizziness or diplopia will emerge with this maneuver if CBF is compromised.

**Hematologic** If a patient is on long-term ASA therapy to minimize platelet aggregation and thrombus formation, it should be stopped at least 2 wks prior to surgery.

**Tests:** Bleeding time; PT; PTT.

**Laboratory** Cerebral angiography will identify type of lesion (ulcerative or stenotic), its location, and extent of collateral circulation. Another commonly used technique, digital subtraction angiography (DSA), involves iv injection of a contrast agent. Through use of computer reconstruction, a vascular image is formed. This circumvents the need for arterial catheterization, but does not give as clear or detailed an image as conventional angiography. As part of the preop evaluation, anesthesiologists should take time to examine the angiograms of the patient to familiarize themselves with the type, location and extent of the lesion.

**Premedication** Use of premedication in patients undergoing carotid endarterectomy is controversial. Should a new TIA or stroke occur in the immediate preop period, its Sx may be difficult to distinguish from those associated with excessive responses to premedication. In this population, detailed discussion about the anesthetic and surgical plan, with appropriate reassurance, is usually enough. If medication is desired, small doses of sedative/hypnotic (e.g., midazolam 1-3 mg or diazepam 5-10 mg) are preferable to opiates.

## INTRAOPERATIVE

**Anesthetic technique:** GETA is preferred as it offers several advantages. Direct advantages are: protection of ischemic brain by decreasing $CMRO_2$ and redistributing flow toward the potentially ischemic area. Indirect advantages are: greater patient comfort and, more importantly, ability to regulate $PaO_2$, $PaCO_2$ and BP to maximize oxygenation and perfusion to potentially ischemic brain. This is important because the brain has a high rate of metabolism with essentially no $O_2$ storage capacity. Consequently, ↓CBF without corresponding ↓$CMRO_2$ can produce neurologic sequelae. There is evidence that barbiturates are superior to other agents in protecting the brain from focal ischemia induced by temporary carotid occlusion during this procedure.[15,16,17] Local anesthesia (field or cervical plexus block) was considered advantageous because it allowed surgeons to evaluate cerebral function during surgical carotid occlusion. Though still used in some centers with success, local anesthesia has theoretical and practical disadvantages. Theoretically, local anesthesia provides no protection to the brain if ischemia ensues. Practically, this technique does not eliminate the occurrence of operative neurological deficits and also is unacceptable to many patients. Once a carotid endarterectomy has begun under local anesthesia, it is technically difficult and potentially hazardous to patient to convert quickly to GA.

**Induction** Induction is begun with meperidine 1.5 mg/kg and STP 10 mg/kg, the latter given slowly by continuous infusion, using a pump to allow time for assessment of cardiovascular responses. As patient consciousness is lost, a muscle relaxant, a 10 ml mixture of d-tubocurarine 7 ml (2.1 mg/ml) and pancuronium 3 ml (0.3 mg/ml) is given. If there is concern about the possibility of hypotension from this dose of STP, lidocaine 1.5 mg/kg iv can be combined with a lower dose of STP, recognizing that lidocaine is acting as a GA in the same manner as STP, but without the myocardial depressant effects.

**Maintenance** Anesthesia is maintained with $N_2O$ 60%, $O_2$ 40%, and isoflurane up to 1%. Isoflurane is clearly superior to either enflurane or halothane for this operation because of its relative protective effect in focal cerebral ischemia. Critical CBF, or blood flow below which EEG changes indicative of cerebral ischemia during carotid cross-clamp appear, is significantly lower (10 ml/100 gm/min) for isoflurane than for halothane (20 ml/100 gm/min) or enflurane (15 ml/100 gm/min).[18] VT and frequency are adjusted so that $PaCO_2$ = 25-30 mmHg and $PaO_2$ = 100-150 mmHg. Hypocarbia may divert CBF preferentially to potentially ischemic areas of the brain by constricting the non-ischemic, normally reactive vessels. Heparin 10,000 U is administered iv and allowed 3-5 min to recirculate before surgical cross-clamping of the carotid circulation is performed. Just prior to surgical cross-clamping of the carotid artery, an additional dose of STP sufficient to produce burst suppression on the EEG (usually about 5 mg/kg) may be administered for its cerebral-protective effect.

**Emergence** Upon removal of the carotid cross-clamps, total carotid occlusion time should be noted on the anesthetic record. Once bleeding from the arteriotomy site has been controlled, protamine (50-100 mg) is administered iv slowly over at least 10 min. If ↓BP occurs, rate of protamine administration is slowed. If vasopressors were used during operation, patient should be weaned from them during emergence, because HTN is likely as patient awakens from anesthesia. The need to control BP with a combination of esmolol and sodium NTP is likely in the emergence phase.

| | | |
|---|---|---|
| **Blood and fluid requirements** | IV: 18 ga x 2<br>NS/LR @ 5-10 cc/kg/hr | Blood replacement is seldom an issue. Studies in rats[19] and monkeys[20] indicate that glucose may worsen the tolerance of brain to global ischemia. In contrast, glucose may be beneficial in focal ischemia.[21,22] Because of conflicting evidence, it is prudent to avoid glucose-containing solutions. |
| **Monitoring** | Standard monitors (see Appendix).<br>Arterial line<br>UO | Marked fluctuations in BP may occur, necessitating hypertensive or hypotensive drug therapy. The arterial pressure transducer should be placed at the level of the head to accurately assess CPP. A CVP catheter is seldom necessary. Vasoactive drugs can be given quickly and safely through a cannula placed in the arm. |
| **Cerebral perfusion monitoring** | rCBF | Regional CBF (rCBF) >24 ml/min/100 gm brain is satisfactory, and < 18 ml/min/100 gm indicates potential for cerebral ischemia; however, capability for making rCBF measurements is not generally available in OR. |
| | EEG | A variety of new spectral compression EEG techniques permit computerized EEG analysis in OR. The major disadvantages of this analysis are: the EEG usually does not change until severe cerebral ischemia occurs, so it is not a good prodromal indicator of ischemia; the EEG may not identify small focal areas of ischemia; and the depth of anesthesia and level of ventilation must be held stable or the EEG will not be interpretable. |
| | Stump pressure | Stump pressure (pressure distal to the carotid clamp – also called "back pressure") is used to evaluate the adequacy of cerebral perfusion. Cerebral ischemia rarely occurs at stump pressures >60 mmHg. The major criticism of stump pressure is the large number of false positives; that is, a stump pressure < 60 mmHg and a rCBF >24 ml/min/100 gm brain. This occurs in about a |

| | | |
|---|---|---|
| **Cerebral perfusion monitoring, continued** | | third of patients[23] and results in a shunt being placed when none is needed. The simplicity of the measurement and its validity when pressure >60 mmHg still make it the most useful clinical method for assuring adequate perfusion during CEA. |
| **Control of BP** | Keep MAP ≥ awake levels.<br>Autoregulation<br>Vasopressors | It is highly desirable to maintain MAP at or slightly above the patient's highest recorded resting pressure while awake. Surgical occlusion of the carotid artery will often decrease distal perfusion pressure (stump pressure) < 60 mmHg. Volatile anesthetics impair autoregulation; therefore, the higher the pressure, the more likely it is that cerebral perfusion will be adequate during surgical occlusion. A pure $\alpha$-adrenergic agonist (e.g., phenylephrine) is ideal to support BP because it has minimal dysrhythmogenic potential. The modified V-5 lead will usually indicate if the ↑BP is causing myocardial ischemia. If hypertensive episodes occur during surgery, esmolol ± SNP works well. |
| **Positioning** | √ and pad pressure points.<br>√ eyes. | |

## POSTOPERATIVE

| | | |
|---|---|---|
| **Complications** | Circulatory instability | Circulatory instability is common.[24] Hypotension may be due to hypovolemia, depression of circulation by anesthetic or other drugs, dysrhythmias, or exposure of the baroreceptor mechanism to a new higher pressure, causing an exaggerated reflex response. Rx by volume expansion and pressors. |
| | HTN<br><br>MI | HTN may be due to loss of the normal carotid baroreceptor mechanism. It may → excessive bleeding, increased myocardial $O_2$ consumption or dysrhythmias and MI, intracerebral hemorrhage and increased ICP from cerebral edema. |
| | Loss of carotid body function | Chemoreceptor function is lost in most patients after CEA, as evidenced by a loss of ventilatory and circulatory responses to hypoxia and a modest increase in resting arterial $PaCO_2$.[24] These patients should be given supplemental $O_2$ postop. Special attention must be directed toward preventing atelectasis or other pulmonary or circulatory abnormalities that might cause hypoxemia, and to which the patient could only respond by further respiratory and circulatory depression and loss of consciousness. |
| | Respiratory insufficiency | Acute respiratory insufficiency may occur 2° hematoma formation with tracheal deviation, vocal cord paralysis from surgical traction on laryngeal nerves, or tension pneumothorax from dissection of air through the wound into the mediastinum and pleural space. Unexpected respiratory distress should immediately bring these 3 possibilities to mind with appropriate diagnosis and therapy. A hematoma which causes respiratory distress always should be evacuated before reintubation is attempted. |
| | Tension pneumothorax | Likewise, if there is evidence of circulatory insufficiency, a tension pneumothorax should be relieved immediately by needle evacuation. |

| | | |
|---|---|---|
| **Complications, continued** | Intimal flap → stroke | Should a patient emerge from anesthesia with a new neurological deficit, immediate cerebral angiography should be performed to determine if an intimal flap has formed at the site of operation. This is a surgically correctable lesion and, if corrected immediately, may lessen the severity of the subsequent neurological deficit. |
| **Pain management** | Meperidine (10 mg iv prn)<br>Codeine (30-60 mg im q 4 hrs) | |
| **Tests** | Cerebral angiography | Emerging stroke → suspect intimal flap → emergency cerebral angiography or immediate surgical exploration of operative site. |

## References


1. Schmidek HH, Sweet WH, eds: *OperativeNeurosurgicalTechniques, Indications, Methods, Results*, Vol I-II. Grune & Stratton, Orlando: 1988.
2. Youmans JR, ed: *Neurological Surgery*, Vol 1-6. WB Saunders Co, Philadelphia: 1990.
3. Wilkins RL, Rengachary SS, eds: *Neurosurgery*, Vol 1-3. McGraw-Hill, New York: 1985.
4. Steinberg GK, Anson JA: Carotid endarterectomy: update. *Western J Med* 1992; 158:64-65.
5. Ferguson GG: Extracranial carotid artery surgery. *Clin Neurosurg* 1992; 29:543-79.
6. Sundt TM: *Surgical Techniques for Saccular and Giant Intracranial Aneurysms*. Williams & Wilkins, Baltimore: 1990.
7. Ojemann RG, Heros RC, Crowell RM: *Surgical Management of CerebrovascularDisease*. Williams & Wilkins, Baltimore: 1988.
9. Wylie EJ, Ehrenfeld WK, eds: *Extracranial Occlusive CerebrovascularDisease; Diagnosis and Management*. WB Saunders Co, Philadelphia: 1970.
9. North American Symptomatic Carotid Endarterectomy Trial Collaborators: Beneficial effect of carotid endarterectomy in symptomatic patients with high-grade carotid stenosis. *N Engl J Med* 1991; 325(7):445-53.
10. European Carotid Surgery Trialists' Collaborative Group: MCR European carotid surgery trial: interim results for symptomatic patients with severe (70-99%) or with mild (0-29%) carotid stenosis. *Lancet* 1991; 337:1235-43.
11. Wolf PA, Kannel WB, Sorlie P, McNamara P: Asymptomatic carotid bruit and risk of stroke. The Framingham Study. *JAMA* 1981; 245(14):1442-45.
12. Hobson RW II, Weiss DG, Fields WS, Goldstone J, Moore WS, Towne JB, Wright CB: Efficacy of carotid endarterectomy for asymptomatic carotid stenosis. The Veterans Affairs Cooperative Study Group. *N Engl J Med* 1993; 328(4):221-27.
13. Ropper AH, Wechsler LR, Wilson LS: Carotid bruit and the risk of stroke in elective surgery. *N Engl J Med* 1982; 307(22):1388-90.
14. Bandyk DF, Thiele BL: Noninvasive assessment of carotid artery disease. *West J Med* 1983; 139(4):486-501.
15. Smith A, Hoff JT, Nielsen SL, Larson CP Jr: Barbiturate protection in acute focal cerebral ischemia. *Stroke* 1974; 5(1):1-7.
16. Michenfelder JD, Milde JH, Sundt TM Jr: Cerebral protection by barbiturate anesthesia. Use after middle cerebral artery occlusion in Java monkeys. *Arch Neurol* 1976; 33(5):345-50.
17. Nehls DG, Todd MM, Spetzler RF, Drummond JC, Thompson RA, Johnson PC: A comparison of the cerebral protective effects of isoflurane and barbiturates during temporary focal ischemia in primates. *Anesthesiology* 1987; 66(4):453-64.
18. Michenfelder JD, Sundt TM, Fode N, Sharbrough FW: Isoflurane when compared to enflurane and halothane decreases the frequency of cerebral ischemia during carotid endarterectomy. *Anesthesiology* 1987; 67(3):336-40.
19. Pulsinelli WA, et al: Moderate hyperglycemia augments ischemic brain damage: a neuropathologic study in the rat. *Neurology* 1982; 32(11):1239-46.
20. Lanier WL, Stangland KJ, Scheithauer BW, Milde JH, Michenfelder JD: The effects of dextrose infusion and head position on neurologic outcome after complete cerebral ischemia in primates: examination of a model. *Anesthesiology* 1987; 66(1):39-48.
21. Zasslow MA, Pearl RG, Shuer LM, Steinberg GK, Lieberson RE, Larson CP Jr: Hyperglycemia decreases acute neuronal ischemic changes after middle cerebral artery occlusion in cats. *Stroke* 1989; 20(4):519-23.
22. Kraft SA, Larson CP Jr, Shuer LM, Steinberg GK, Benson GV, Pearl RG: Effect of hyperglycemia on neuronal changes in a rabbit model of focal cerebral ischemia. *Stroke* 199; 21(3):447-50.
23. McKay RD, Sundt TM, Michenfelder JD, et al: Internal carotid artery stump pressure and cerebral blood flow during carotid endarterectomy: modification by halothane, enflurane, and Innovar®. *Anesthesiology* 1976; 45(4):390-99.
24. Wade, JG, Larson CP Jr, Hickey RF, Ehrenfeld WK, Severinghaus JW: Effect of carotid endarterectomy on carotid chemoreceptor and baroreceptor function in man. *N Engl J Med* 1970; 282(15):823-29.

# PERCUTANEOUS PROCEDURES FOR TRIGEMINAL NEURALGIA

## SURGICAL CONSIDERATIONS

**Description:** Two percutaneous procedures are commonly used to treat trigeminal neuralgia (a well-defined pain disorder of the face). Each involves placing a needle percutaneously from the cheek into the foramen ovale at the base of the skull under a light iv anesthetic. For the **glycerol injection**, it is necessary for the surgeon to verify that the needle is placed in the cistern of the trigeminal nerve gasserian or ganglion. This is usually done via image intensification or x-ray films. There should be free flow of CSF through the needle. The patient is placed in the seated position, with head flexed, and sterile glycerol is injected into the cistern. The patient is taken to the recovery room, with the head still flexed, for an hour. The glycerol damages neurons in the ganglion, which usually causes mild sensory loss and relieves the tic pain in most cases. Injection of the glycerol is often very painful.

**Radiofrequency rhizotomy** is the other percutaneous procedure used for trigeminal neuralgia. This procedure differs from glycerol injection in that a radiofrequency generator is used to place a thermal lesion in the appropriate portion of the gasserian ganglion. The needle is actually an insulated electrode with a portion of the tip exposed. The proper needle position is determined by applying stimulating current, with the patient awake, while assessing patient's responses. Multiple brief periods of anesthesia may be required to adjust needle position or to lesion the nerve. It is important for the patient to awaken quickly and be able to cooperate with the stimulus localization throughout this procedure.

**Usual preop diagnosis:** Trigeminal neuralgia; tic douloureux

### SUMMARY OF PROCEDURE

| | Glycerol Injection | Radiofrequency Rhizotomy |
|---|---|---|
| **Position** | Supine | ⇐ |
| **Incision** | Needle placed lateral to mouth on cheek | ⇐ |
| **Special instrumentation** | Image intensifier | ⇐ + Radiofrequency generator |
| **Unique considerations** | Hypertensive response to needle placement | ⇐ + Requirement for periodic deep sedation with rapid awakening for radiofrequency lesioning. |
| **Antibiotics** | Usually none | ⇐ |
| **Surgical time** | 0.5 hrs | 1 - 1.5 hrs |
| **EBL** | None | ⇐ |
| **Postop care** | Seated position with head flexed for 1 hr | None |
| **Mortality** | < 1% | ⇐ |
| **Morbidity** | Usually < 5%:<br>Infection<br>Complete facial numbness (anesthesia dolorosa)<br>Extraocular muscle paresis<br>CSF leak<br>Carotid puncture<br>Facial hematoma | ⇐ |
| **Procedure code** | 61790 (percutaneous procedures) | ⇐ |
| **Pain score** | 2-4 | 2-4 |

### PATIENT POPULATION CHARACTERISTICS

| | |
|---|---|
| **Age range** | 40-85 yrs (usually 60-70 yrs) |
| **Male:Female** | ~2:3 |
| **Incidence** | Relatively common neurosurgical procedure |
| **Etiology** | Vascular compression of a cranial nerve<br>Multiple sclerosis plaque |
| **Associated conditions** | HTN<br>Multiple sclerosis |

# ANESTHETIC CONSIDERATIONS

## PREOPERATIVE

Trigeminal neuralgia, or tic douloureux, is a condition that develops in adults usually over the age of 60 years. It is more common in women in whom an intermittent, severe, lancinating pain arises over the maxillary and/or mandibular divisions of the trigeminal nerve. The ophthalmic division of the trigeminal nerve is rarely involved. The pain is unilateral, and often can be precipitated by stimulating a trigger point, such as by rubbing the cheek, mastication or brushing the teeth. The cause of this condition is not known. Medical management consists of therapy with carbamazepine (Tegretol®), an anticonvulsant and analgesic specific for this condition. Surgery is considered when medical management fails to control pain, or complications of drug therapy develop (anemia, bleeding disorders, dizziness, etc.). One of two types of percutaneous procedures is performed: either **glycerol injection** or **radiofrequency rhizotomy** of the symptomatic branches of the trigeminal ganglion. If these treatments fail, surgical exploration of the trigeminal ganglion is considered.

**Respiratory** No special considerations, unless patient has a longstanding Hx of smoking and has COPD.
**Tests:** CXR; others as indicated from H&P.

**Cardiovascular** Most patients have Hx of idiopathic HTN and take any one of a variety of antihypertensive medications. Good control of BP preop is important because most patients become hypertensive during the operative procedure. Intraop HTN is unavoidable because of the surgical need to have the patient awake during much of the procedure.
**Tests:** ECG; others as indicated by H&P.

**Neurological** The presenting symptom is pain in the maxillary and/or mandibular division of the trigeminal nerve, unaccompanied by motor or sensory deficits.

**Laboratory** Hct; UA; other tests as indicated from H&P.

**Premedication** None, except for atropine 0.5 mg or glycopyrrolate 0.2 mg iv shortly before induction of anesthesia to minimize oral secretions while the surgeon is working in the mouth positioning the needle.

## INTRAOPERATIVE

**Anesthetic technique:** GA, regardless of which percutaneous technique is to be used. $O_2$ by nasal cannula should be administered before induction of anesthesia. To keep the cannula out of the surgeon's field, it must be taped above the eye on the side of operation.

**Induction** Because the surgeon will want the patient awake as soon as the needle is in place to check for symptoms of pain, the induction drug must be potent, but short-acting. Either methohexital 1-1.5 mg/kg or propofol (1-2 mg/kg) are suitable for this purpose. The drug should be injected by bolus into a rapidly flowing iv to achieve a high concentration of drug in the brain quickly. Continuous infusion of the drug is not satisfactory, because it either fails to achieve a high brain concentration quickly, or its continuous administration prolongs the time before the patient is sufficiently arousable to communicate with the surgeon. In experienced hands, the needle is placed within a matter of 2-3 min. If difficulty is encountered in placing the needle, additional doses of induction drug may be needed. Patients invariably develop apnea for 1-2 min, followed by partial or total airway obstruction, while the surgeon has his hand in the mouth positioning the needle. Prior to induction of anesthesia, therefore, it is essential that the anesthesiologist optimize ventilation and oxygenation by asking patient to take a series of deep breaths through the nose with the mouth closed. This will increase the $O_2$ level and decrease the $CO_2$ level in the lungs prior to induction. To maintain adequate spontaneous ventilation and oxygenation, it is usually necessary to institute forward displacement of the mandible while the surgeon inserts the needle. Another alternative is to insert a nasal airway.

If **glycerol injection** is used, needle position is verified by radiological imaging, using a radio-opaque dye. Patient is awakened and placed in a seated position with head flexed. The glycerol is injected, causing severe pain. Patient is then moved to recovery room still in seated position with the head forward to keep the glycerol localized to the region of the trigeminal ganglion.

If **radiofrequency rhizotomy** is performed, the patient is awakened and the position of the needle is verified by stimulating the ganglion with heat and determining the site of pain. The patient is then re-anesthetized with a smaller bolus of the same drug to permit high-intensity heat stimulation for ~1 min. This procedure may be repeated several times. Each time, the patient needs less anesthetic, because of both the cumulative effects of the drug, and the fact that the trigeminal ganglion is becoming permanently damaged by the heat.

| | | |
|---|---|---|
| **Emergence** | In the recovery room, patients are maintained in a seated position with an ice pack on the cheek at the site of needle insertion to minimize postop bleeding and swelling. Following glycerol injection, patients often complain of pain in the face, requiring opiate analgesics. Following radiofrequency rhizotomy, the face is usually numb, the end point for concluding the operation. | |
| **Blood and fluid requirements** | IV: 18 ga x 1<br>NS/LR @ 4-6 ml/kg/hr | |
| **Monitoring** | Standard monitors (see Appendix). | |
| **Control of BP** | Clonidine patch<br>Labetalol | Patients almost invariably become hypertensive during this therapy. Attempts to lessen these episodes with a clonidine patch preop or use of intermittent doses of labetalol prophylactically or therapeutically are only partially successful. |
| **Positioning** | Table turned 180°<br>✓ and pad pressure points.<br>✓ eyes. | Patient supine with head in the midline. |
| **Complications** | Failure of needle placement<br>Bleeding<br>Respiratory arrest | Major complications from this operation are uncommon, but include: (1) Failure to identify the foramen ovale, through which the needle must be inserted to reach the trigeminal ganglion. If the needle cannot be placed within 30-40 min, the procedure is usually aborted until another day. (2) Bleeding into cheek from puncture of a branch of the facial artery. (3) Apnea from spillover of the neurolytic solution into circulating CSF, presumably affecting the respiratory center in the 4th ventricle. |

## POSTOPERATIVE

**Pain management** Parenteral opiates (see Appendix).

### References

1. Young RF: Stereotactic procedures for facial pain. In *Brain Surgery: Complication, Avoidance and Management*. Apuzzo MLJ, ed. Churchill Livingstone, New York: 1993, 2097-113.

**Surgeons**

**Sally Byrd, MD** *(Ophthalmic Surgery)*
**Peter R. Egbert, MD** *(Ophthalmic Surgery)*
**Michael W. Gaynon, MD** *(Retinal Surgery)*

# 2. OPHTHALMIC SURGERY

**Anesthesiologists**

**Jayshree Desai, MD**
**Stanley I. Samuels, MB, BCh, FFARCS**
**Richard A. Jaffe, MD, PhD**

# CATARACT EXTRACTION WITH INTRAOCULAR LENS INSERTION

## SURGICAL CONSIDERATIONS

**Description:** The **extracapsular cataract technique** involves removing the lens in pieces. A small (3-10 mm) incision is made at the superior corneal scleral junction. The anterior capsule of the lens is removed, and the nucleus is then either expressed intact or is emulsified and sucked out by the **phacoemulsification technique (ultrasonic fragmentation)**. Finally, the cortex is aspirated using a manual irrigation aspirating needle or the automatic aspiration device attached to the phacoemulsification machine. A plastic intraocular lens is placed behind the iris and supported by the remaining intact posterior capsule of the natural lens or placed directly into the capsular bag (Fig 2-1). The wound is closed with multiple 10-0 nylon sutures.

**Variant procedure or approaches**: **Intracapsular cataract extraction** is rarely done anymore due to the superior results of extracapsular surgery. In intracapsular extraction, the entire lens is removed intact by application of a cryoprobe. It is most commonly done when the lens has lost its zonular support 2° trauma or a genetic condition.

**Usual preop diagnosis**: Cataract

### SUMMARY OF PROCEDURE

| | |
|---|---|
| **Position** | Supine |
| **Incision** | 3-10 mm at periphery of cornea |
| **Special instrumentation** | Surgical microscope; automated irrigation/aspiration machine; sometimes phacoemulsification machine |
| **Antibiotics** | Subconjunctival cefazolin (50-100 mg) or gentamicin (20-40 mg) |
| **Surgical time** | 30 - 60 min |
| **EBL** | None |
| **Mortality** | Minimal |
| **Morbidity** | Corneal edema: 1%<br>Retinal detachment: < 1%<br>Wound rupture: < 1%<br>Infection: < 0.1% |
| **Procedure code** | 66840-66984 |
| **Pain score** | 1 |

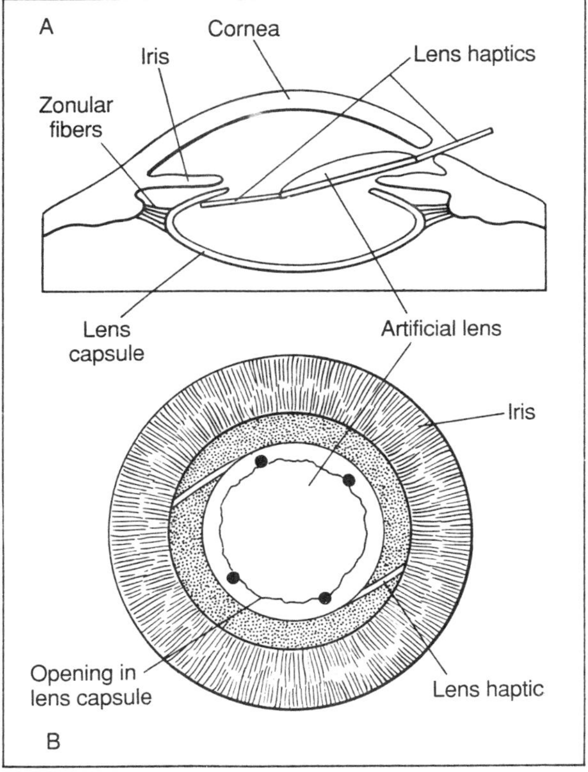


**Figure 2-1.** (A) Placement of intraocular lens into remaining capsular bay. (B) "In-the-bag" insertion. (Reproduced with permission from Spaeth GL, ed: *Ophthalmic Surgery: Principles & Practice*, 2nd edition. WB Saunders: 1990.)

### PATIENT POPULATION CHARACTERISTICS

| | |
|---|---|
| **Age range** | 50-90 yrs, usually elderly |
| **Male:Female** | 1:1 |
| **Incidence** | 1,000,000/yr in U.S. |
| **Etiology** | Formation may be accelerated by poor nutrition, UV light exposure. Steroids may speed development. |
| **Associated conditions** | Associated systemic diseases of the elderly: Common<br>HTN<br>Diabetes<br>Heart disease |

## ANESTHETIC CONSIDERATIONS

See "Anesthetic Considerations for Ophthalmic Surgical Procedures under MAC" following "Pterygium Excision."

**References**

See General References following "Ophthalmic Surgery" section.

# CORNEAL TRANSPLANT

## SURGICAL CONSIDERATIONS

**Description**: The eye may be removed from a suitable donor up to a maximum of 24 hours before transplantation; the cornea is removed from the donor eye in the OR just before transplantation. The central portion of the recipient's cornea (generally an 8 mm button) is removed, using a round trephine, followed by corneal scissors. At this time, there is a large hole in the patient's eye and pressure on the eye must be avoided. If the patient needs a cataract extraction, a plastic **intraocular lens insertion** or **anterior vitrectomy** may be done concurrently. The donor cornea is sutured into place with multiple 10-0 nylon sutures in order to achieve a water-tight closure (Fig 2-2).

**Usual preop diagnosis**: Corneal scar; corneal dystrophy; keratoconus

### SUMMARY OF PROCEDURE

| | |
|---|---|
| **Position** | Supine |
| **Incision** | Corneal |
| **Special instrumentation** | Surgical microscope |
| **Unique considerations** | Open-globe precautions |
| **Antibiotics** | Subconjunctival gentamicin (20-40 mg) or cefazolin (50-100 mg) |
| **Surgical time** | 60 - 90 min |
| **EBL** | Minimal |
| **Postop care** | Patients must be followed closely for evidence of tissue rejection in immediate postop period. |
| **Mortality** | Minimal |
| **Morbidity** | Graft rejection: 5%<br>Infection: < 1%<br>Wound dehiscence |
| **Procedure code** | 65730-65755 |
| **Pain score** | 2 |

### PATIENT POPULATION CHARACTERISTICS

| | |
|---|---|
| **Age range** | Any age |
| **Male:Female** | 1:1 |
| **Incidence** | 1,000/yr in U.S. |
| **Etiology** | Scarring, infection or trauma<br>Various inheritable conditions<br>Damage to the cornea (decompensation) 2° cataract surgery: Rare |
| **Associated conditions** | Trauma<br>Infection<br>Corneal dystrophies<br>Congenital malformations which may involve cornea: Rare |

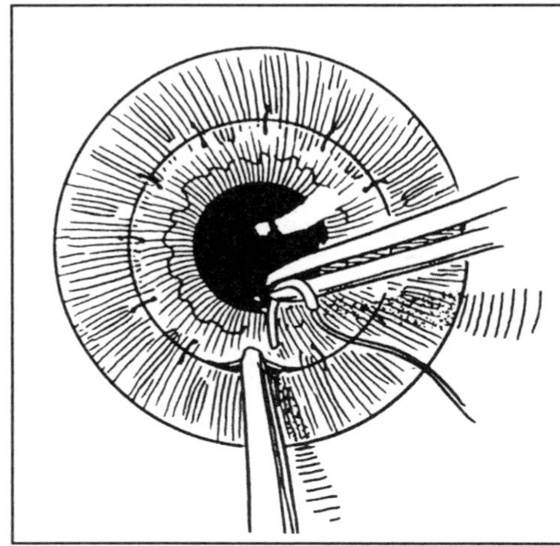

**Figure 2-2.** Suturing donor cornea on recipient eye. (Reproduced with permission from Phelps CD, ed: *Manual of Common Ophthalmic Surgical Procedures*. Churchill Livingstone: 1986.)

## ANESTHETIC CONSIDERATIONS

See "Anesthetic Considerations for Ophthalmic Surgical Procedures under MAC" following "Pterygium Excision" (below).

**References**

See General References following "Ophthalmic Surgery" section.

# TRABECULECTOMY

## SURGICAL CONSIDERATIONS

**Description**: Trabeculectomy is the most commonly performed surgery to lower intraocular pressure (IOP) in patients with glaucoma. The goal is to create a fistula from the anterior chamber to the subconjunctival space, thus giving the intraocular fluid an alternate exit route and lowering eye pressure. The conjunctiva near the cornea is reflected back from the sclera. An opening approximately 2 x 2 mm is made into the anterior chamber under a partial-thickness scleral flap (Fig 2-3), and an **iridectomy** is performed. The scleral flap partially retards leakage of aqueous from the anterior chamber through the subconjunctival space and decreases the amount of postop hypotony. The sclera is closed and the conjunctiva sutured. A full-thickness procedure varies only in the absence of a scleral flap.

**Variant procedure or approaches**: In certain patients for whom glaucoma surgery has failed, or who have particularly refractive glaucoma, a **glaucoma seton implant** (e.g., **Molteno** or **Baerveldt**) may be used to maintain drainage fistulas. This involves dissecting the conjunctiva away from sclera and inserting a small tube (usually Silastic®) directly into the anterior chamber from the corneal limbus. The tube is connected to one or two small plates which are sewn to the sclera. Exposed tube is covered by sclera, usually from a donor eye, and then the conjunctiva is brought back down and sewn into place. The plates prevent conjunctiva from scarring back down to sclera, thus allowing the fluid draining from the anterior chamber to collect and then reabsorb.

In infants and children with congenital glaucoma, the procedures of choice involve making a long opening directly into the drainage angle of the anterior chamber, either as a goniotomy or trabeculotomy. A **goniotomy** is performed by passing a small knife across the anterior chamber into the angle and then, under direct visualization with a goniotomy lens, making an incision over trabecular meshwork extending 1-2 quadrants. In a **trabeculotomy,** a cutdown is made at the limbus and Schlemm's canal is identified. A special instrument is passed into Schlemm's canal and rotated into the anterior chamber, opening the canal directly to the anterior chamber.

**Usual preop diagnosis**: Glaucoma

### SUMMARY OF PROCEDURE

| | |
|---|---|
| **Position** | Supine |
| **Incision** | Superior portion of eye |
| **Special instrumentation** | Surgical microscope |
| **Antibiotics** | Subconjunctival cefazolin (50-100 mg), gentamicin (20-40 mg), and dexamethasone (2-4 mg) |
| **Surgical time** | 30 - 60 min |
| **EBL** | Minimal |
| **Postop care** | May involve treatment with antimetabolite drugs (e.g., fluorouracil) to retard scarring; also may involve cutting scleral flap sutures with laser to control postop pressure. |
| **Mortality** | Minimal |
| **Morbidity** | Excessive drainage with low IOP: 5% |
| **Procedure code** | 65820, 65850, 66150-66180 |
| **Pain score** | 1 |

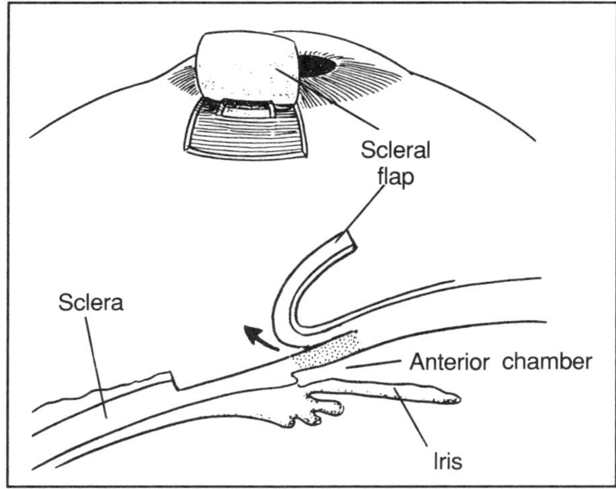


**Figure 2-3.** Small opening made in anterior chamber under a scleral flap. Opening corresponds to shaded area in lower diagram. (Reproduced with permission from Phelps CD, ed: *Manual of Common Ophthalmic Surgical Procedures.* Churchill Livingstone: 1986.)

### PATIENT POPULATION CHARACTERISTICS

| | |
|---|---|
| **Age range** | Infants-adults |
| **Male:Female** | 1:1 |
| **Incidence** | 10,000/yr in U.S. |
| **Etiology** | Unknown for most part; occasionally results from eye trauma, inflammation, abnormal vascular growth or certain congenital anomalies with abnormal eye development. |

| | |
|---|---|
| **Associated conditions** | Congenital glaucoma may be associated with other congenital syndromes:<br>Rieger's syndrome<br>Neurofibromatosis<br>Sturge-Weber syndrome |

## ANESTHETIC CONSIDERATIONS

See "Anesthetic Considerations for Ophthalmic Surgical Procedures under MAC" following "Pterygium Excision" (below).

**References**

See General References following "Ophthalmic Surgery" section.

# ECTROPION REPAIR

## SURGICAL CONSIDERATIONS

**Description:** Ectropion is a malposition of either the upper or lower eyelid in which the lid margin is everted away from the globe. Surgical repair can be approached in a variety of ways, depending on the underlying pathology. Generally speaking, ectropion involves either loose or excess lid tissue which causes the lid to fall away from the eye, or scarring (cicatrix) of the skin of the lid which pulls it away from the globe. In the first case, a lid-tightening procedure is performed, either by simply removing a full-thickness wedge of lid and re-approximating the cut edges, or with the "lateral canthal strip" procedure. In this operation, the inferior cruz of the lateral canthal tendon is disinserted (Fig 2-4) and a strip of lateral tarsus is isolated by dissecting it free from overlying skin and orbicularis muscle and then by removing conjunctiva from the posterior surface. This strip of tarsus is then shortened to a length necessary to restore proper lid tension and sutured in place to the periosteum of the lateral orbital rim. Excess skin is excised and the defect closed.

**Variant procedure or approaches:** In the case of cicatricial ectropion, the contracted scar can sometimes be released by using a z-plasty technique to release vertical tension. Alternatively, a full-thickness skin graft taken from upper lid or the postauricular or supraclavicular regions is used to fill in any defects after all scar bands have been lysed.

**Usual preop diagnosis:** Ectropion of the eyelid

### SUMMARY OF PROCEDURE

| | |
|---|---|
| **Position** | Supine |
| **Incision** | Generally at lateral canthus for involutional ectropion; in area of scarring. |
| **Antibiotics** | Postop topical antibiotics |
| **Surgical time** | 0.5 - 1 hr |
| **EBL** | Minimal |
| **Mortality** | Minimal |
| **Morbidity** | Infection: < 1% |
| **Procedure Code** | 67916-7, 67961 |
| **Pain score** | 2 |

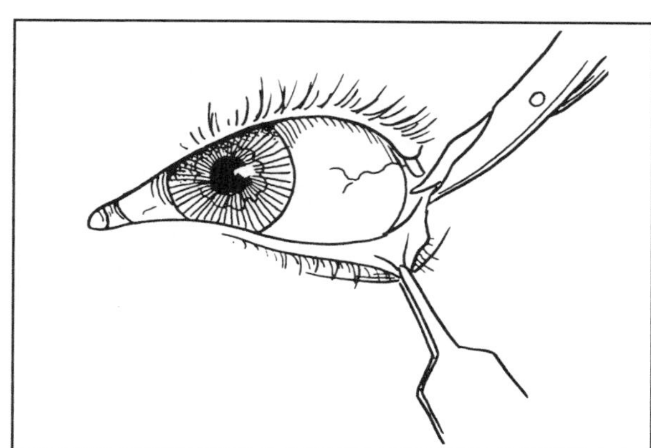

**Figure 2-4.** Disinsertion of the inferior cruz of the lateral canthal tendon. (Reproduced with permission from Phelps CD, ed: *Manual of Common Ophthalmic Surgery*. Churchill Livingstone: 1986.)

### PATIENT POPULATION CHARACTERISTICS

| | |
|---|---|
| **Age range** | Elderly; cicatricial ectropion may occur in younger patients 2° trauma or burns. |
| **Male:Female** | 1:1 |
| **Incidence** | Common |
| **Etiology** | Aging |

## ANESTHETIC CONSIDERATIONS

See "Anesthetic Considerations for Ophthalmic Surgical Procedures Under MAC" following "Pterygium Excision" (below).

**References**

See General References following "Ophthalmic Surgery" section.

# ENTROPION REPAIR

## SURGICAL CONSIDERATIONS

**Description:** Entropion involves the inward rotation of the eyelid toward the globe. As with ectropion repair, multiple procedures have been described, their use depending on concomitant lid findings and surgeon's preference. In senile or involutional entropion, which involves primarily the lower lids, the most common underlying pathology is dehiscence or weakening of the lower lid retractor muscles, often in combination with horizontal lid laxity. One approach is to make a horizontal lid incision through skin and orbicularis muscle approximately 2 mm from the lashes. Orbital septum is then incised and the lower lid retractor muscles identified and sewn back onto the inferior tarsal border. Skin is closed after excising redundant tissue. If horizontal lid laxity also exists, a lateral tarsal strip procedure, similar to that described for ectropion repair, can also be done.

**Variant procedure or approaches:** In the case of cicatricial entropion, involving either the upper or lower lids, there is scarring or shrinkage of the conjunctival tarsal surface. This pulls the lid margin inward toward the globe. In mild cases, a **Weis procedure** may be performed. This involves making a full-thickness horizontal lid incision, fracturing the tarsus and everting it with carefully placed sutures and reclosing the skin. For more severe cicatricial entropion, a full-thickness mucosal graft may be needed on the inner lid surface. This is commonly taken from the lower lip.

**Usual preop diagnosis:** Entropion of eyelid

### SUMMARY OF PROCEDURE

| | |
|---|---|
| **Position** | Supine |
| **Antibiotics** | Topical antibiotics postop |
| **Surgical time** | 0.5 - 1.5 hr |
| **EBL** | Minimal |
| **Mortality** | Minimal |
| **Morbidity** | Infection: < 1% |
| **Procedure code** | 67923-67924, 67961 |
| **Pain score** | 2 |

### PATIENT POPULATION CHARACTERISTICS

| | |
|---|---|
| **Age range** | Involutional entropion, primarily in elderly; cicatricial entropion, any age |
| **Male:Female** | 1:1 |
| **Incidence** | Common |

| | |
|---|---|
| **Etiology** | Cicatricial entropion associated with trauma, chemical injury or chronic infection or inflammation |
| **Associated conditions** | Stevens-Johnson syndrome<br>Cicatricial pemphigoid<br>Trachoma |

## ANESTHETIC CONSIDERATIONS

See "Anesthetic Considerations for Ophthalmic Surgical Procedures under MAC" following "Pterygium Excision" (below).

**References**

See General References following "Ophthalmic Surgery" section.

# PTOSIS SURGERY

## SURGICAL CONSIDERATIONS

**Description:** The most frequently performed procedure for ptosis correction involves shortening, or simply reattaching, the levator palpebrae aponeurosis at its site of insertion on the superior tarsus. **Levator aponeurosis surgery** in adults is performed preferably under local anesthesia so that lid position with eyes open can be adequately assessed and adjusted. An incision is made through the skin along the upper eyelid crease, and the dissection is carried down through the orbicularis muscle and orbital septum until the levator aponeurosis is isolated and sewn to the superior tarsus. The exact position is adjusted according to lid height and contour. The skin incision is closed, with any excess being excised.

**Variant procedure or approaches:** Patients with little or no levator function, as assessed by their preop eyelid excursion, may require a **frontalis suspension** operation. This involves suspending the upper lid from the brow so that the lid is opened by raising the brow and closed by contracting the orbicularis muscle. For this purpose, autogenous, or cadaver fascia lata or an alloplastic material (e.g., silicone rod) is tunneled beneath the skin and muscle from the brow to the upper lid margin and then tied at a length appropriate for the desired lid height. Frontalis suspension in both children and adults is done under GA.

**Usual preop diagnosis:** Congenital or acquired ptosis

### SUMMARY OF PROCEDURE

| | Ptosis Corrections | Frontalis Suspension |
|---|---|---|
| **Position** | Supine. When levator surgery is performed under local anesthesia, patient may be required to sit upright for more accurate assessment of lid position. | Supine |
| **Incision** | Generally through upper lid crease | Small incisions above lid margin and brow |
| **Antibiotics** | Topical antibiotics postop | ⇐ |
| **Surgical time** | 1 - 1.5 hrs | 1 hr |
| **EBL** | Minimal | ⇐ |
| **Mortality** | Minimal | ⇐ |
| **Morbidity** | Infection: < 1% | ⇐ |
| | Corneal exposure from over-correction | ⇐ |
| **Procedure code** | 67901-67904 | ⇐ |
| **Pain score** | 3 | 3 |

### PATIENT POPULATION CHARACTERISTICS

| | |
|---|---|
| **Age range** | Generally elderly unless congenital |
| **Male:Female** | 1:1 |
| **Incidence** | Common |
| **Etiology** | Stretching or dehiscence of the levator aponeurosis associated with aging: Common<br>Neurogenic (e.g., 3rd nerve palsy) or congenital ptosis |
| **Associated conditions** | Systemic disorders such as myasthenia gravis, myotonic dystrophy or progressive external ophthalmoplegia |

## ANESTHETIC CONSIDERATIONS

See "Anesthetic Considerations for Ophthalmic Surgical Procedures under MAC" following "Pterygium Excision" (below).

**References**

See General References following "Ophthalmic Surgery" section.

# EYELID RECONSTRUCTION

## SURGICAL CONSIDERATIONS

**Description:** Tumors of the lids, both benign and malignant, frequently need to be excised, making it necessary to reconstruct the lid to protect and maintain eye function and give the best cosmetic results. When a tumor is known to be malignant, resection is usually carried out under frozen section control. In some instances, however, particularly with tumors involving the medial canthal area, resection is first done by a Mohs surgeon (a dermatologist trained in this technique) with reconstruction being undertaken during a separate operation. Mohs surgery involves horizontal sectioning of tumor under microscopic control, allowing the tumor to be completely removed with the least sacrifice of normal tissue. If the remaining defect is 25% or less of the total lid length, closure can be accomplished often by simply closing the defect. Deep bites are taken through tarsus before closing the skin, and special care is taken in re-approximating the lid margin so as not to leave a notch or step.

**Variant procedure or approaches:** If the lid defect cannot be pulled together, but is lacking only a few millimeters, a **lateral canthotomy** may be performed with lysis of the corresponding branch of the lateral canthal tendon. For larger defects affecting up to 40-50% of the medial or central lids, a **semicircular flap** is often utilized. This is made laterally, extensively undermined and used in conjunction with lateral canthal lysis. For larger lid defects, a variety of full- and partial-thickness flaps and grafts can be used, depending on the location of the defect and surgeon's preference. Some procedures involve using a tunnel flap, which advances tissue from one lid to another, and closing the eye for 3-12 weeks, at which time the flap can be separated from its pedicle.

**Usual preop diagnosis:** Basal-cell carcinoma; malignant tumor; squamous-cell carcinoma; sebaceous-cell carcinoma; malignant melanoma; nevi

### SUMMARY OF PROCEDURE

| | |
|---|---|
| **Position** | Supine |
| **Incision** | Variable, depending on tumor location |
| **Antibiotics** | Topical, following surgery |
| **Surgical time** | 0.5 - 2 hrs |

| | |
|---|---|
| **EBL** | Minimal |
| **Mortality** | Minimal |
| **Morbidity** | Infection: < 1%<br>Dry eye<br>Secondary lid deformity |
| **Procedure code** | 67840, 67961-67975 |
| **Pain score** | 3 |

### PATIENT POPULATION CHARACTERISTICS

| | |
|---|---|
| **Age range** | More common in elderly, but young adults included |
| **Male:Female** | 1:1 |
| **Incidence** | Common |
| **Etiology** | Skin cancers related to sun exposure |

## ANESTHETIC CONSIDERATIONS

See "Anesthetic Considerations for Ophthalmic Surgical Procedures under MAC" following "Pterygium Excision" (below).

**References**

See General References following "Ophthalmic Surgery" section.

# PTERYGIUM EXCISION

## SURGICAL CONSIDERATIONS

**Description:** Pterygia are vascular fleshy growths arising from the conjunctiva and extending onto the cornea. Pterygium removal is often performed under local anesthetic with a subconjectival, rather than a retrobulbar injection. It is frequently done in the clinic setting, with an operating microscope, if the planned dissection is not too extensive. They are removed by carefully dissecting the head from the cornea, undermining and excising a portion of the body, and leaving an area of bare sclera or relaxing the adjacent conjunctiva and pulling it closed. The defect also may be covered with a conjunctival graft taken from the same or opposite eye.

**Variant procedure or approaches:** Due to the general high recurrence rate, many minor variations in the approach have been attempted, including folding part of the pterygium under itself and applying β-radiation at the limbus to prevent it from growing back.

**Preop diagnosis or indications:** Pterygium causing decreased vision or motility, excessive irritation or cosmetic disfigurement

### SUMMARY OF PROCEDURE

| | |
|---|---|
| **Position** | Supine |
| **Incision** | In area of pterygium – most commonly medial interpalpebral region |
| **Antibiotics** | Topical antibiotics postop |
| **Surgical time** | 15 - 45 min |
| **EBL** | None |
| **Mortality** | Minimal |
| **Morbidity** | High recurrence rate, often in more aggressive form |
| **Procedure code** | 65420-65426 |
| **Pain score** | 2-3 |

## PATIENT POPULATION CHARACTERISTICS

| | |
|---|---|
| **Age range** | Young-to-middle-age adults |
| **Male:Female** | 1:1 |
| **Incidence** | Common in tropical regions; unusual in temperate climates |
| **Etiology** | Related to solar exposure |

---

# ANESTHETIC CONSIDERATIONS FOR OPHTHALMIC SURGICAL PROCEDURES UNDER MAC

**(Procedures covered: cataract extraction and other procedures; corneal transplant; trabeculectomy; ectropion-entropion repair; ptosis surgery; eyelid reconstruction; pterygium excision)**

## PREOPERATIVE

Surgical procedures that are of relatively short duration and those that result in minimal blood loss and fluid shifts are being performed increasingly more often on an outpatient basis, usually with local anesthesia (e.g., retrobulbar or peribulbar blocks) under MAC (see Appendix). The majority of these ocular procedures are performed on elderly patients who usually have multiple medical problems; thus, anesthesiologists are faced with monitoring and managing these potentially challenging patients. A thorough preop H&P, along with appropriate lab workup, are mandatory, even if local anesthesia/MAC is to be used. Contraindications to use of local anesthesia for ocular surgery include: coagulation abnormalities; open-eye injuries; patients with chronic cough or claustrophobia, or who are unable to lie flat; and patients who refuse local anesthesia.

| | |
|---|---|
| **Respiratory** | Elderly patients have increased incidence of hiatal hernia and, therefore, are at increased risk for pulmonary aspiration. Patients with severe COPD should have recent PFTs. Assess the patient's ability to lie flat for the duration of the procedure.<br>**Tests:** CXR; PFTs; others as indicated from H&P. |
| **Cardiovascular** | Hx of HTN, CAD, CHF, or poor exercise tolerance should prompt a thorough investigation into the patient's cardiac status, including efficacy of current medications and recent ECG (compared with previous ECGs). Consultation with a cardiologist may be appropriate to optimize the patient's condition before surgery.<br>**Tests:** ECG; others (e.g., ECHO) as indicated from H&P. |
| **Diabetes** | Diabetic patients are at increased risk for silent myocardial ischemia. Pulmonary aspiration 2° diabetic gastroparesis is also a risk in this population. Patients usually take 1/2 or 1/3 of their normal NPH insulin dose (on the morning of surgery); fasting blood sugar is checked; and an iv infusion of D5 LR is started if glucose < 90 mg/dl, or treated with regular insulin if glucose >200 mg/dl. Blood sugar is checked intraop and postop. |
| **Musculoskeletal** | Arthritic changes make lying flat difficult for some patients. |
| **Hematologic** | ✓ for recent ASA use, particularly in patients undergoing lid or orbital procedures; if necessary, ✓ bleeding time (normal = < 8 min) to evaluate platelet function.<br>**Tests:** CBC; bleeding time; others as indicated from H&P. |
| **Laboratory** | Electrolytes, BUN, creatinine are usual in patients >70 yrs; in other patients, as indicated from H&P. |
| **Premedication** | For patients with increased risk of aspiration (e.g., with hiatal hernia or diabetic gastroparesis) and for the obese and very anxious patients, metoclopramide 10 mg iv may enhance gastric emptying. Patients will benefit from a detailed explanation of events prior to surgery (including iv placement, application of monitors, performance of local block by the ophthalmologist, ocular pressure, prepping eye and draping of the whole face, provision of supplemental $O_2$ and the assurance that the anesthesiologist will always be nearby, monitoring the patient. |

## INTRAOPERATIVE

**Anesthetic technique:** MAC (see Appendix). Placement of the retrobulbar or peribulbar blocks may be painful and very short-acting agents (e.g., thiopental 25-75 mg, propofol 30-50 mg or alfentanil 5-7 mg/kg) should be administered to minimize patient discomfort. Doses vary significantly among patients, and should be administered in small increments. Deep sedation and apnea should be avoided. The patient must be awake enough to have control over his or her actions. Usually further sedation is unnecessary and may interfere with patient cooperation during the surgery.

Coughing or Valsalva maneuver must be avoided during the procedure, and the anesthesiologist should always be prepared to administer GA if necessary. Coughing or sneezing is usually not a problem postop.

| | | |
|---|---|---|
| **Blood and fluid requirements** | IV: 18 ga x 1<br>NS/LR @ 5-10 cc/kg/hr | |
| **Monitoring** | Standard monitors (see Appendix).<br>Verbal response | It is important to remain in communication with the patient throughout the procedure. (Take care to avoid evoking head movement.) |
| **Positioning** | √ and pad pressure points.<br>√ eyes. | Pillows under knees to relieve back strain. |
| **Complications** | Dysrhythmias, especially ↓HR<br>↑BP<br>Retrobulbar hemorrhage<br>Globe perforation | See Anesthetic Considerations for "Strabismus Surgery" (below). |
| | Convulsions 2° iv local anesthetic<br>Respiratory arrest | Supportive treatment with IPPV |
| | Oculocardiac reflex (OCR) → ↓↓HR, ↓↓BP | Rx: Stop stimulation; use atropine. |

### POSTOPERATIVE

| | | |
|---|---|---|
| **Complications** | Myocardial ischemia | Rx: Provide $O_2$; √ BP; sublingual NTG; √ ECG; cardiology consultation. |
| | Corneal abrasion<br>Photophobia | |
| | N&V<br>Diplopia | Rx: Metoclopramide 10 mg iv, droperidol 0.625 mg iv, ondansetron 4 mg iv. |
| **Pain management** | Acetaminophen 325-1000 mg po | |

**Table 2-1. Commonly used ophthalmic drugs and their systemic effects**

| | |
|---|---|
| **Phenylephrine** | An α-adrenergic agonist which causes mydriasis (pupillary dilation) and vasoconstriction to aid ocular surgery; however, it also can precipitate significant HTN and dysrhythmias. |
| **Echothiophate** | An irreversible cholinesterase inhibitor used in glaucoma treatment to cause miosis and ↓IOP. Its systemic absorption can reduce plasma cholinesterase activity and thereby prolong paralysis 2° to succinylcholine (usually not more than 20-30 min). |
| **Timolol** | A non-selective β-adrenergic antagonist which decreases production of aqueous humor → ↓IOP. Rarely it may be associated with atropine-resistant bradycardia, asthma, CHF and hypotension. |
| **Acetazolamide** | A carbonic anhydrase inhibitor used to ↓IOP. It also can cause diuresis and a hypokalemic metabolic acidosis. |
| **Atropine** | An anti-cholinergic which produces mydriasis to aid with ocular examination and surgery. It also can precipitate central anti-cholinergic syndrome. (Sx range from dry mouth, tachycardia, agitation, delirium and hallucinations to unconsciousness.) Physostigmine 0.01-0.03 mg/kg will increase central acetylcholine and reverse the symptoms. (It may be repeated after 15-30 min.) |

**References**


1. Barash PG, Cullen BF, Stoelting RK, eds: *Clinical Anesthesia.* JB Lippincott, Philadelphia: 1989, 1062.
2. McGoldrick KE, ed: *Anesthesia for Ophthalmic and Otolaryngologic Surgery.* WB Saunders Co, Philadelphia: 1992.

# REPAIR OF RUPTURED OR LACERATED GLOBE

## SURGICAL CONSIDERATIONS

**Description**: The goal of this surgery is to repair the cornea and sclera sufficiently to create a water-tight wound. The laceration often contains a prolapsed iris, which must be removed or reposited. The cornea is then carefully closed with 10-0 nylon suture. An associated cataract may need to be removed and the associated scleral laceration may need to be closed. Lacerations extending beyond the equator of the globe, however, are generally inaccessible to closure. At times, a laceration may involve one of the extraocular muscle tendons, necessitating reattachment to the globe.

**Usual preop diagnosis**: Ruptured or lacerated globe

### SUMMARY OF PROCEDURE

| | |
|---|---|
| **Position** | Supine |
| **Incision** | A conjunctival incision may be indicated to improve exposure, if the laceration extends past the corneal limbus onto the sclera |
| **Special instrumentation** | Surgical microscope |
| **Antibiotics** | Subconjunctival cefazolin 100 mg or gentamicin 20-40 mg; iv broad spectrum antibiotics (cephalosporin or vancomycin, and an aminoglycoside) |
| **Closing considerations** | Once wound is closed, avoid coughing, bucking, etc. |
| **Surgical time** | 0.5 - 2 hrs |
| **EBL** | Minimal |
| **Postop care** | IV antibiotics are usually continued 5 d |
| **Mortality** | Minimal |
| **Morbidity** | Infection-variable, depending on type of injury<br>Wound leak: 5%<br>Sympathetic ophthalmia: < 1% |
| **Procedure code** | 65280-65290 |
| **Pain score** | 4 |

### PATIENT POPULATION CHARACTERISTICS

| | |
|---|---|
| **Age range** | Any age |
| **Male:Female** | 2:1 |
| **Incidence** | Fairly common, but depends on patient population. |
| **Etiology** | Trauma |
| **Associated conditions** | May be associated with orbital or facial trauma. |

---

## ANESTHETIC CONSIDERATIONS

### PREOPERATIVE

This is a generally healthy patient population; however, patients with penetrating eye injuries present the anesthesiologist with two special challenges: (1) They invariably have full stomachs, resulting in risk of aspiration. (2) They are at risk of blindness 2° increased intraocular pressure (IOP) and loss of ocular contents. This may be a result of coughing, crying and/or struggling during induction. Normal IOP ranges from 10-22 mmHg, depending on the rate of formation and drainage of aqueous humor, choroidal blood volume, scleral rigidity, extraocular muscle tone, as well as extrinsic pressure on the eye (e.g., a poorly fitting mask or retrobulbar hematoma). Patient movement, coughing, straining, vomiting, hypercarbia, HTN and ET intubation may also increase IOP as much as 40 mmHg or more. Obtain H&P and establish patient's last oral intake.

| | |
|---|---|
| **Full-stomach precautions** | Consider patient to have a full stomach if the injury occurred within 8 hrs of the last meal. Pain and anxiety due to trauma will delay gastric emptying. Goal is to minimize risk of aspiration pneumonitis by decreasing gastric volume and acidity. Consider premedication with metoclopramide (10-20 mg iv), antacids such as Na citrate (15-30 ml orally immediately prior to induction) |

and $H_2$-histamine receptor antagonists (ranitidine [50 mg iv]). $H_2$-histamine receptor antagonists, however, have no effect on the pH of gastric secretions present in the stomach prior to administration, and are, therefore, of limited value in patients presenting for emergency surgery. If patient has Hx of smoking or is an asthmatic, consider preop use of inhalers such as albuterol (2-4 puffs).

**Tests:** As indicated from H&P, and time permitting.

**Laboratory** Other tests as indicated from H&P.

**Premedication** Patients often are very anxious and may benefit from benzodiazepines (e.g., midazolam 0.5-0.7 mg/kg po in cola or apple juice, 30 cc for pediatric population). Avoid narcotic premedication, which may increase nausea and possibility of emesis.

## INTRAOPERATIVE

**Anesthetic technique:** GETA. Regional anesthesia (e.g., retrobulbar block) is contraindicated in patients with open-eye injury because of ↑IOP, which may accompany injection of local anesthetic behind the globe. Thus, in spite of the increased risk of aspiration from a full stomach, GETA is recommended.

**Induction** To protect the airway and prevent ↑IOP, a rapid-sequence induction with cricoid pressure and a smooth intubation are required. While the choice of induction agent is relatively straightforward – thiopental 3-5 mg/kg or propofol 1-2 mg/kg – the choice of neuromuscular blocking agents for facilitating intubation is controversial. Succinylcholine provides a rapid onset, short duration of action and excellent intubating conditions, but it also transiently increases IOP. This ↑IOP is not always attenuated by pretreatment with a non-depolarizing agent (e.g., d-tubocurarine or pancuronium). The use of an intubating dose of a non-depolarizing muscle relaxant (e.g., vecuronium or atracurium), however, also has disadvantages: the airway is unprotected for up to 3 min, increasing risk of aspiration, and an early attempt at intubation may significantly ↑IOP as a result of coughing and straining. There are no reports in the literature documenting exacerbation of eye injuries with the use of succinylcholine following pretreatment of a non-depolarizing muscle relaxant. Given that the anesthesiologist's main concern is safe airway management, the following is a suggested induction plan:

(1) Preoxygenation, avoiding external pressure on the eye from face mask.

(2) Pretreatment with a non-depolarizing relaxant (e.g., d-tubocurarine 0.06 mg/kg), followed by iv lidocaine (1 mg/kg) and fentanyl (2-3 $\mu$g/kg) to blunt the cardiovascular response to laryngoscopy and intubation.

(3) Consider 5-10 mg labetalol, also to blunt cardiovascular response to laryngoscopy and intubation (if patient does not have reactive airway disease).

(4) 4 min later, while maintaining cricoid pressure, induce with thiopental (4-6 mg/kg) and succinylcholine (1.5 mg/kg). Note: for pediatric patients, it might be appropriate to induce with halothane while maintaining cricoid pressure and intubating while patient is deeply anesthetized with the inhalational agent. Trying to start an iv prior to induction may precipitate struggling and crying, leading to further eye injury.

**Maintenance** Standard maintenance (see Appendix). Avoid hypercapnia, which increases IOP. Muscle relaxation (vecuronium or atracurium) is mandatory until the eye is surgically closed. Humidify gasses for pediatric patients.

**Emergence** 30 min before conclusion of surgery, give iv anti-emetic (e.g., metoclopramide 0.1 mg/kg iv). Decompress the stomach with OG tube. Goal is smooth emergence and extubation with patient awake with intact airway reflexes. IV lidocaine (1.5 mg/kg) 5 min before extubation; posterior pharyngeal suctioning with patient deeply anesthetized, combined with a small amount of narcotic (fentanyl 1-2 $\mu$g/kg), may blunt cough reflex prior to extubation. The common occurrence of postop N&V requires administration of intraop anti-emetics (e.g., metoclopramide 10 mg iv, droperidol 0.625 mg iv or ondansetron 4 mg iv).

**Blood and fluid requirements** IV: 18 ga x 1 (adult)
20 ga x 1 (child)
NS/LR @ 5-10 cc/kg/hr
Warm fluids.

**Monitoring** Standard monitors (see Appendix). Neuromuscular blockade must be monitored closely and additional relaxant given as necessary to prevent patient movement during surgery.

| | | |
|---|---|---|
| **Positioning** | √ and pad pressure points.<br>√ eyes. | |
| **Complications** | ↑IOP with extrusion of intraocular contents<br>Aspiration of gastric contents | |

### POSTOPERATIVE

| | | |
|---|---|---|
| **Complications** | N&V<br>Corneal abrasion<br>Aspiration pneumonitis<br>Photophobia<br>Diplopia<br>Hemorrhagic retinopathy | Rx: Metoclopramide 10 mg iv, droperidol 0.625, ondansetron 4 mg iv.<br>Provide $O_2$ by face mask, if not intubated. Follow $O_2$ saturation. √ CXR. |
| **Pain management** | Parenteral opiates (see Appendix). | |

**References**

1. Barash PG, Cullen BF, Stoelting RK, eds: *Clinical Anesthesia.* JB Lippincott, Philadelphia: 1989, 1062.
2. McGoldrick KE, ed: *Anesthesia for Ophthalmic and Otolaryngologic Surgery.* WB Saunders Co, Philadelphia: 1992.


Also see General References following "Ophthalmic Surgery" section.

# STRABISMUS SURGERY

## SURGICAL CONSIDERATIONS

**Description:** Strabismus surgery is performed on patients with ocular malalignment, and involves lengthening or shortening individual muscles or pairs of muscles with an eventual goal of straightening the eyes cosmetically and allowing binocular vision. An incision is made transconjunctivally in the proximity of the muscle being worked on (Fig 2-5A). The muscle is then isolated and either recessed by disinserting it and sewing it further back on the globe, which effectively decreases the muscle tension, or resected (Fig 2-5B) by removing a segment of muscle, which increases its tension. Depending on the pattern of strabismus, oblique muscles are sometimes totally disinserted or partially transected to weaken their action.

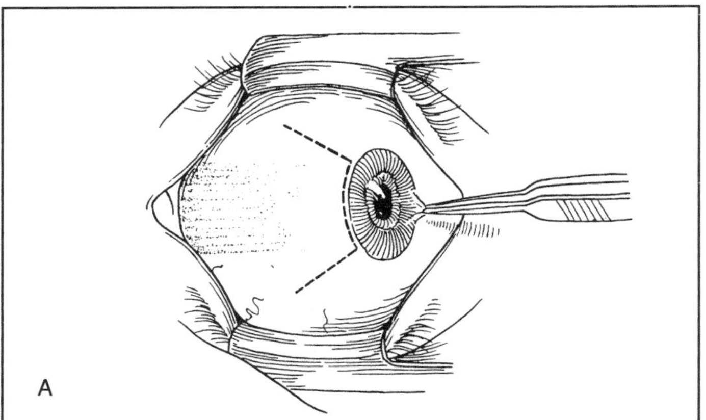


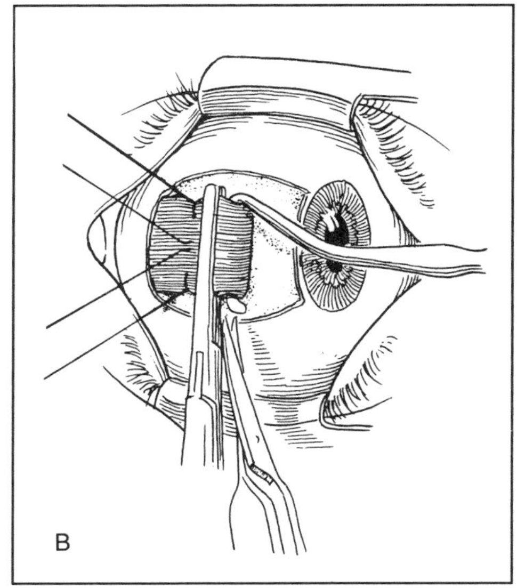


**Figure 2-5.** (A) Conjuntival incision in region of horizontal rectus muscle. (B) Resection of horizontal rectus muscle – sutures have been passed through muscle prior to its disinsertion from the globe. (Reproduced with permission from Phelps CD: *Manual of Common Ophthalmic Surgical Procedures.* Churchill Livingstone: 1986.)

**Variant procedure or approaches:** In adults and very cooperative older children, an **adjustable suture approach** is sometimes used. The muscle is tied in such a way that it can be either lengthened or shortened postop before being tied securely in place.

**Usual preop diagnosis:** Strabismus

### SUMMARY OF PROCEDURE

| | |
|---|---|
| **Position** | Supine |
| **Incision** | Transconjunctival (Fig 2-5A) |
| **Antibiotics** | Topical antibiotics at end of surgery |
| **Surgical time** | 0.5 – 1 hr |
| **EBL** | Minimal |
| **Mortality** | Minimal |
| **Morbidity** | Continued malalignment: 30%<br>Infection: < 1% |
| **Procedure code** | 67311–67335 |
| **Pain score** | 3–4 |

### PATIENT POPULATION CHARACTERISTICS

| | |
|---|---|
| **Age range** | Children (most common) |
| **Male:Female** | 1:1 |
| **Incidence** | Relatively common |
| **Etiology** | Generally idiopathic<br>Ocular muscle palsies may be associated with trauma, inflammation, tumors and local ischemia. |
| **Associated conditions** | Higher incidence in premature infants and certain congenital syndromes |

## ANESTHETIC CONSIDERATIONS

### PREOPERATIVE

In children, strabismus is the most frequent ophthalmic condition requiring surgical repair. Although most patients with this condition are otherwise healthy, there is an increased incidence of strabismus in children with cerebral palsy or meningomyelocele with hydrocephalus. Unlike many adult eye surgeries, which can be performed under regional anesthesia (retrobulbar or peribulbar block), in children, GA is almost always required to ensure good surgical conditions. The anesthesiologist should be aware of the potential problems that are associated with strabismus surgery, including: increased risk of malignant hyperthermia (MH); occurrence of the oculocardiac reflex (OCR); and increased incidence of postop N&V. It has been noted that individuals at risk for MH often have musculoskeletal abnormalities, such as strabismus or ptosis. It is, therefore, important to obtain a thorough family history of anesthetic problems. Avoid the use of succinylcholine since it can induce a tonic contracture of the extraocular muscles, which can interfere with the forced duction test (FDT). The surgeon performs the FDT by grasping the sclera of the operative eye and moving it into each field of gaze in order to determine if the strabismus is a result of paretic or restrictive extraocular muscles. This helps in forming the surgical plan.

| | |
|---|---|
| **Respiratory** | Surgery should be postponed for patients presenting with Sx of acute RTI, and recent fever or chills. These patients may be predisposed to bronchospasm and laryngospasm → difficulty with ventilation and oxygenation. A thorough H&P should be performed.<br>**Tests:** As indicated from H&P. |
| **Malignant hyperthermia** | ✓ for personal or family Hx of MH. If patient is MH-susceptible (had previous episodes of MH or had developed masseter spasm [trismus] with succinylcholine), avoid succinylcholine and other triggering agents, including halothane, enflurane and isoflurane. $N_2O$ also may be a weak triggering agent. "Safe" agents include thiopental, pancuronium, droperidol, opiates and benzodiazepines. A "clean" anesthetic machine without vaporizers or one that was flushed overnight with $O_2$ and has fresh $CO_2$ absorbent should be used. Dantrolene and ice should be readily available.<br>**Tests:** Halothane and caffeine contracture test of skeletal muscle Bx if indicated from H&P. |
| **Laboratory** | Other tests as indicated from H&P. |

**Premedication** Use midazolam 0.5-0.7 mg/kg po in apple juice or cola (20-30 cc). The child should be made aware that one or both eyes may have patches on them after the surgery, so that blurred or diminished vision may be present during emergence.

## INTRAOPERATIVE

**Anesthetic technique:** GETA

**Induction** Standard mask induction (see Appendix). Following induction, give atropine 0.02 mg/kg or glycopyrrolate 0.01 mg/kg iv to offset the vagal response to intubation and, thus, bradycardia seen with oculocardiac reflex (OCR). Surgeons will perform the FDT, and then the patient is intubated with a non-depolarizing neuromuscular blocker.

**Maintenance** Standard maintenance (see Appendix).

**Emergence** To decrease incidence of postop emesis, administer metoclopramide 0.1 mg/kg iv about 30 min prior to end of surgery; suction stomach while patient is deeply anesthetized. The common occurrence of postop N&V requires the administration of intraop anti-emetics.

**Blood and fluid requirements** IV: 20 or 22 ga x 1
NS/LR @ 5-10 cc/kg/hr
Warm fluids, humidify gasses.

**Monitoring** Standard monitors (see Appendix).

**Positioning** ✓ and pad pressure points.
✓ eyes.

**Complications** Oculocardiac reflex (OCR) → ↓↓HR, ↓↓BP

OCR is triggered by direct eye pressure, pain and/or traction on the extrinsic eye muscles. It has both trigeminal afferent pathway and vagal efferent path. The most common cardiac dysrhythmia is bradycardia. Others that are seen incude junctional rhythm, multifocal PVCs, AV block, VT and asystole. Rx: D/C stimulus and provide adequate depth of anesthesia. Do not give atropine during a dysrhythmia because of the possibility that it may precipitate a dangerous rhythm. Lidocaine infiltration near the eye muscles may be helpful. Fortunately, with repeated manipulation, the OCR quickly fatigues.

Malignant hyperthermia

Consider MH if the following are noted: unexplained tachycardia; ↑$ETCO_2$; muscular rigidity, masseter spasm; ↑temperature (a late sign). To evaluate, obtain ABGs. MH produces ↓$PaO_2$, ↑$PaCO_2$, ↑$K^+$ and acidosis. If MH is suspected, stop anesthetics and change anesthetic tubing and $CO_2$ absorbent. Stop surgery as soon as possible, hyperventilate patient with 100% $O_2$, treat acidosis with bicarbonate, and treat hyperkalemia with 1 U regular insulin/3 gm glucose. Give dantrolene 2.5 mg/kg iv as soon as possible. Also cool the patient and maintain UO. Further doses of dantrolene may be necessary (can give up to 10 mg/kg).

## POSTOPERATIVE

**Complications** N&V
MH

Rx: Metoclopramide 10 mg iv, droperidol 0.625 mg iv, ondansetron 4 mg iv.

**Pain management** Acetaminophen suppositories 15-20 mg/kg q 4-6 hrs

**References**


1. Barash PG, Cullen BF, Stoelting RK, eds: *Clinical Anesthesia.* JB Lippincott, Philadelphia: 1989, 1062.
2. McGoldrick KE, ed: *Anesthesia for Ophthalmic and Otolaryngologic Surgery.* WB Saunders Co, Philadelphia: 1992.

# DACRYOCYSTORHINOSTOMY (DCR)

## SURGICAL CONSIDERATIONS

**Description**: DCR is performed in patients who have chronic epiphora or dacryocystitis 2° obstruction at the level of the nasolacrimal duct. The goal is to create a new drainage path for tears from the lids to the nose. A 15 mm incision is made on the side of the nose near the medial canthus (Fig 2-6). A subperiosteal dissection is made to the lacrimal sac and the lacrimal sac is identified. The thin bone separating the lacrimal fossa from the middle fossa of the nose is broken and rongeured to make a 10-15 mm-diameter opening. The mucosa of the lacrimal sac is then anastomosed to the mucosa of the nose. Sometimes a silicone tube is placed through the lacrimal canaliculi through the anastomosis and tied in the nose to prevent closure by scarring. The wound closure is a simple skin closure.

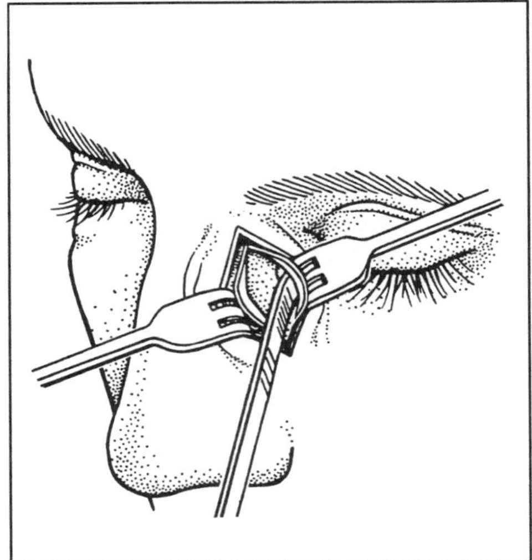

**Figure 2-6.** Incision site. (Reproduced with permission from Levine MR, ed: *Manual of Oculoplastic Surgery*. Churchill Livingstone: 1988.)

**Variant procedure or approaches**: In certain older patients with recurrent dacryocystitis 2° nasolacrimal duct (NLD) blockage, epiphora may not be a problem because of concomitant low-tear production. In these cases, it may be possible to do a **dacryocystectomy** or **tear-sack resection** without making a new passage into the nose. When blockage to tear drainage is at the level of the canaliculi, it may be necessary to do a **conjunctivorhinostomy** with insertion of a Jone's tube (Fig 2-7). The initial steps for this procedure are essentially the same as those for the DCR; however, the canaliculi are bypassed by inserting a small Pyrex® tube through the conjunctiva in the region of the caruncle (which is excised) so that it passes through the bony opening, with the nasal-to-lacrimal-sac anastomosis and into the nose. There is a congenital form of NLD obstruction which generally occurs at the level of the nose. Often the obstruction will decrease with time; however, if it persists, a **NLD probing** may be done. This involves passing a bent wire from the upper and lower puncti through the canaliculi, tear sac, nasolacrimal duct and then into the nose. At times, a Silastic® stent is also passed through the lacrimal drainage tract and left in place for several months.

**Usual preop diagnosis:** Occlusion of the nasal lacrimal duct

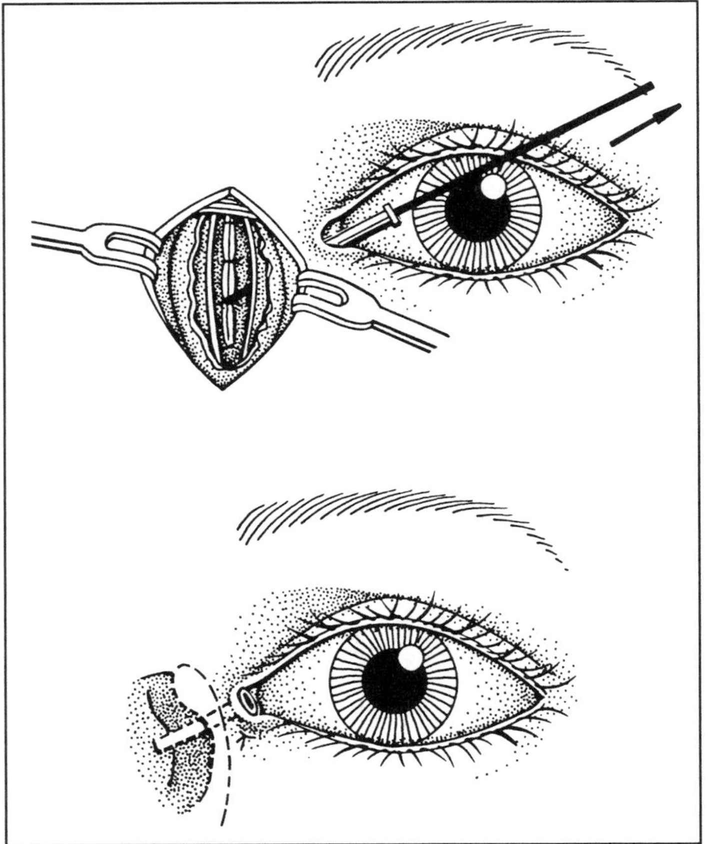

**Figure 2-7.** Insertion of a Pyrex® Jone's tube into the region of the caruncle for **conjunctivorhinostomy** procedure. (Reproduced with permission from Levine MR: *Manual of Oculoplastic Surgery*. Churchill Livingstone: 1988.)

### SUMMARY OF PROCEDURE

| | |
|---|---|
| **Position** | Supine |
| **Incision** | 2 cm at side of nose (Fig 2-6) |
| **Special instrumentation** | Headlight; bone equipment |
| **Unique considerations** | Nasal pack with vasoconstrictor used at start of procedure. Blood often drains into throat during surgery. |
| **Antibiotics** | IV antibiotics at time of surgery, followed by a short course of oral antibiotics, used by some surgeons. |
| **Surgical time** | 1 - 1.5 hrs |
| **EBL** | 100 cc; may be considerably larger from unusual nasal or ethmoid bleeding that is difficult to stop. |
| **Postop care** | Usually outpatient; may have bleeding from nose, especially in children. |
| **Mortality** | Minimal |
| **Morbidity** | Bleeding from nose: 5%<br>Infection: < 1% |
| **Procedure code** | 68520, 68720, 68820-68830, 68750 |
| **Pain score** | 2 |

### PATIENT POPULATION CHARACTERISTICS

| | |
|---|---|
| **Age range** | 30-70 yrs |
| **Male:Female** | 1:1 |
| **Incidence** | Fairly common |
| **Etiology** | Infection in nasolacrimal duct |

## ANESTHETIC CONSIDERATIONS

See Anesthetic Considerations following "Orbitotomy – Anterior and Lateral" (below).

**References**

See General References following "Ophthalmic Surgery" section.

# ENUCLEATION

## SURGICAL CONSIDERATIONS

**Description:** Enucleation involves removal of the entire globe and a portion of the optic nerve. The overlying conjunctiva, Tenon's fascia and extraocular muscles are left behind and then sewn over the orbital implant to keep it in position and give it motility. The procedure starts with a 360° conjunctival incision adjacent to the cornea. The conjunctiva and Tenon's fascia are dissected from the sclera and the four rectus muscles are cut from the globe, passing suture through the cut ends so that the muscles may be sewn over or onto the implant later. With outward traction on the eye, the oblique muscles are cut, the optic nerve is sectioned and the globe is removed. The empty socket is tamponaded for 2-5 minutes or until all bleeding has stopped. An implant, commonly a polyethylene sphere, is selected and Tenon's fascia and conjunctiva, along with the recti muscles, are sewn securely closed over it. An alternative implant is a hydroxyapatite (coral) sphere which, because of its roughness, is frequently covered with eye bank sclera or temporalis fascia harvested at the time of enucleation.

**Variant procedure or approaches:** Evisceration involves removing the intraocular contents and leaving behind the scleral shell with the attached extraocular muscles. It affords better motility but there is increased risk of sympathetic ophthalmia (an autoimmune condition which may affect the remaining eye, causing severe inflammation) and it should not be performed for tumor removal because of the increased chances of incomplete removal.

**Usual preop diagnosis:** Blind eye 2° to trauma or end-stage glaucoma; procedure to decrease risk of sympathetic ophthalmia or for pain relief; intraocular tumors such as melanoma or retinoblastoma; endophthalmitis with total loss of vision

### SUMMARY OF PROCEDURE

| | |
|---|---|
| **Position** | Supine |
| **Incision** | 360° conjunctival incision |
| **Antibiotics** | Topical antibiotics at end of case |
| **Surgical time** | 1 - 1.5 hr |
| **EBL** | Approx 20 cc |
| **Mortality** | Minimal |
| **Morbidity** | Infection: < 1% |
| **Procedure code** | 65091 - 65105 |
| **Pain score** | 6 |

### PATIENT POPULATION CHARACTERISTICS

| | |
|---|---|
| **Age range** | Any age, although trauma requiring enucleation is more frequent in young males |
| **Male:Female** | Male > Female |
| **Incidence** | Relatively common |
| **Etiology** | Trauma<br>Ocular tumors<br>Phthisis (TB) |
| **Associated conditions** | In the past, rubeotic glaucoma in patients with diabetes mellitus was a common cause for enucleation; fortunately, this complication is less frequently found. |

## ANESTHETIC CONSIDERATIONS

See Anesthetic Considerations following "Orbitotomy – Anterior and Lateral" (below).

**References**

See General References following "Ophthalmic Surgery" section.

# ORBITOTOMY – ANTERIOR AND LATERAL

## SURGICAL CONSIDERATIONS

**Description:** Surgical access to the orbit may be necessary to biopsy or remove an orbital tumor, repair orbital fractures, drain an orbital abscess or remove a foreign body. For the purpose of surgery, the orbit may be divided into several compartments (Fig 2-8), including the peripheral surgical space, subperiosteal space, sub-Tenon's space and central surgical space. The particular approach to the orbit depends on the lesion's location, size and suspected pathology. In general, anterior orbitotomy is used to biopsy lesions throughout the orbit or remove small tumors from the anterior orbit. A lateral orbitotomy is generally required for larger, more posteriorly located tumors, and when complete exposure of the lacrimal gland is required. Occasionally, a combined anterior and lateral approach is used for very extensive lesions.

**Anterior orbitotomies** are generally approached in three basic ways. The **trans-conjunctival approach** is used for lesions in the sub-Tenon's space. The area within the muscle cone also can be reached by disinserting the lateral or medial rectus muscles. This, for example, would be a common approach for biopsy or decompression of the optic nerve. The **transseptal approach** is particularly useful for anteriorly located tumors palpable through the eyelids. The incision is made through the skin and orbital septum directly into the peripheral orbital space. It is often used for lesions such as hemangiomas, lymphomas and dermoids. Finally, the **transperiosteal**, or **extraperiosteal approach** is used primarily for lesions along the superior, medial or inferior orbital walls or within the frontal or ethmoid sinuses. A skin incision is made just outside the orbital rim in the desired quadrant. Periosteum is identified and incised and then reflected from the orbital margin and wall. It is the common approach for orbital wall fractures, and mucoceles of the frontal or ethmoid sinuses. It is also used for drainage of subperiosteal hematomas or abscesses and for orbital decompression in thyroid disease.

**Variant procedure or approaches:** Lateral orbitotomies involve removing a portion of the bone from the lateral wall to give access to the retrobulbar space. It is also the only approach which gives complete exposure of the lacrimal gland, a necessity in removing certain tumors. A skin incision is made over the lateral brow and extended to the zygomatic arch. Dissection is carried out down to the periosteum, which is then incised along the lateral orbital rim and reflected. The lateral bony wall is removed using a saw and rongeurs, and the inner periosteum (periorbital) is opened to expose the orbit. After removal or biopsy of the lesion, the bone is wired back into place and the wound closed in layers.

**Usual preop diagnosis:** Tumors such as hemangiomas, inflammatory pseudotumors, lymphomas, lacrimal gland tumors, rhabdomyosarcoma; trauma resulting in orbital wall fractures or retained foreign body; infection with abscess formation

## SUMMARY OF PROCEDURE

| | |
|---|---|
| **Position** | Generally supine. May have head slightly elevated to reduce venous pressure and rotate face away from the operative site when using the lateral approach. |
| **Incision** | Variable (see above). |
| **Special instrumentation** | Operating microscope sometimes used for deep orbitotomies, especially when working around optic nerve. |
| **Antibiotics** | Variable; some surgeons use iv antibiotics both prophylactically and following surgery. |
| **Surgical time** | 1-3 hrs |
| **EBL** | Usually minimal; may be considerable if vascular tumor and extensive dissection are involved. |
| **Mortality** | Minimal |
| **Morbidity** | Decreased ocular motility<br>Secondary infection<br>Loss of vision |
| **Procedure code** | 67400-67450 |
| **Pain score** | 3-6 |

## PATIENT POPULATION CHARACTERISTICS

| | |
|---|---|
| **Age range** | Any age |
| **Male:Female** | 1:1 |
| **Incidence** | Rare |
| **Etiology** | Tumor<br>Trauma<br>Infection |

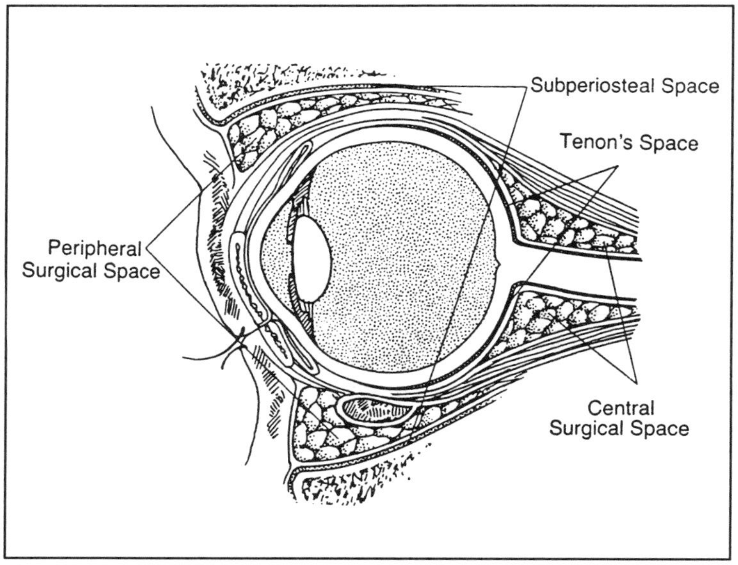

**Figure 2-8.** Orbital compartments. (Reproduced with permission from Levine MR: *Manual of Oculoplastic Surgery*. Churchill Livingstone, 1988.)

## ANESTHETIC CONSIDERATIONS

**(Procedures covered: dacryorhinocystorhinostomy (DCR); enucleation; anterior and lateral orbitotomy.)**

### PREOPERATIVE

Patients presenting for DCR, enucleation and orbitotomy represent a diverse population. These patients are generally healthy, aside from the infection, tumor or trauma underlying their ocular or periocular pathology. Preop evaluation should focus on possible co-existing disease and the systemic manifestations of previous therapeutic intervention (e.g., chemotherapy and drugs used to treat glaucoma).

**Laboratory** Tests as indicated from H&P.
**Premedication** Standard premedication (see Appendix).

### INTRAOPERATIVE

**Anesthetic technique:** GETA.

**Induction** Standard induction (see Appendix). An oral RAE® ETT may be preferred.
**Maintenance** Standard maintenance (see Appendix). Muscle relaxation is not required.
**Emergence** No special considerations. The common occurrence of postop N&V requires the administration of intraop anti-emetics (e.g., metoclopramide 10 mg iv, droperidol 0.625 mg iv or ondansetron 4 mg iv).

**Blood and fluid requirements** Blood loss variable
IV: 18 ga x 1
NS/LR @ 4-6 cc/kg/hr

**Monitoring** Standard monitors (see Appendix).

**Positioning** Table rotated 90°
✓ and pad pressure points.
✓ eyes.

**Complications** Oculocardiac reflex (OCR) → ↓↓HR
Rx: atropine
See discussion in Anesthetic Considerations for "Strabismus Surgery" (above).

### POSTOPERATIVE

**Complications** N&V — Rx: Metoclopramide 10 mg iv, droperidol 0.625 mg iv, ondansetron 4 mg iv.

**Pain management** Parenteral opiates (see Appendix).

---

# RETINAL SURGERY

---

## SURGICAL CONSIDERATIONS

**Description**: Retinal surgery is performed for: retinal detachment; vitreous hemorrhage or opacification; macular epiretinal membranes or other surgically correctable macular conditions; dislocated intraocular lenses; and posterior segment trauma, including repair of ruptured globes and removal of intraocular foreign bodies. Most retinal detachments are due to one or more small tears in the retina caused by traction following a vitreous separation. Less commonly, retinal detachments are induced by trauma, which may involve an open globe. Care must be taken to avoid any increase in intraocular pressure (IOP) in an eye which may harbor a rupture. On rare occasion, a retinal detachment is due to the formation of a giant retinal tear. Just as rarely, retinal surgery is done on premature infants in an effort to prevent or repair retinal detachments. The ultimate aim of retinal surgery is the preservation or recovery of vision through the restoration of normal posterior segment anatomy. (Anatomy of the eye shown in Fig 2-9.)

Retinal surgery may involve various procedures alone or in combination, including scleral buckling, vitrectomy, gas-fluid exchange, and injection of vitreous substitutes. **Scleral buckles** are silicone rubber appliances sutured to the sclera to indent the eye wall, thereby relieving vitreous traction and functionally closing retinal tears. This is an external procedure in which the eye may either not be entered at all or entered with a small needle puncture through the sclera for drainage of subretinal fluid.

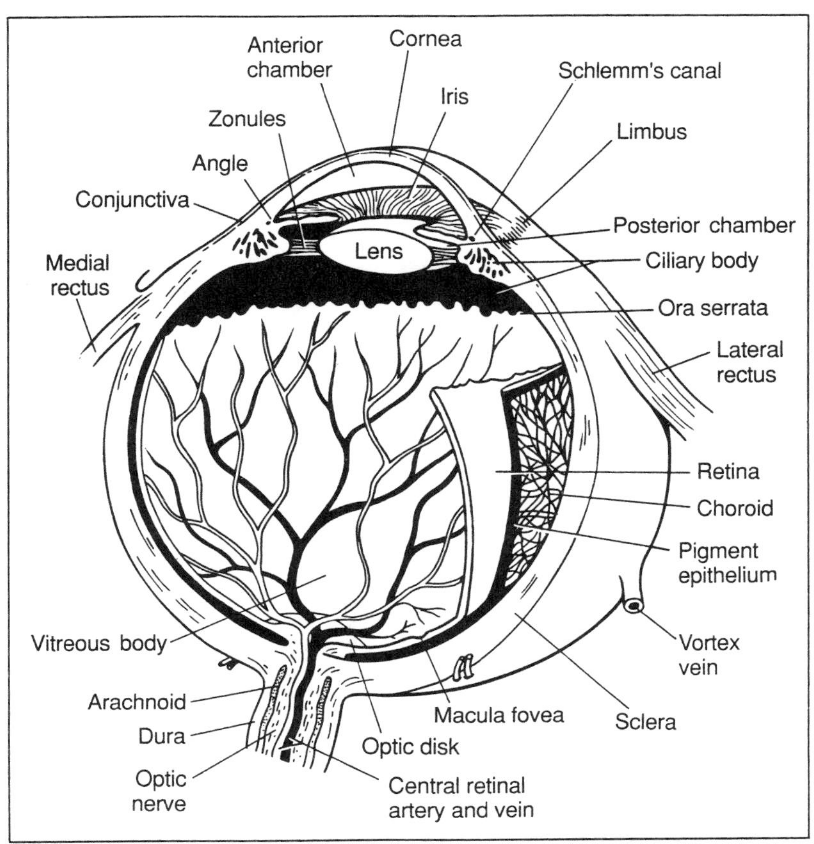


**Figure 2-9.** Eye anatomy. (Reproduced with permission from Langstom D, ed: *Manual of Ocular Diagnosis and Therapy*. Little, Brown, New York: 1985. Adapted from Peck P: *Anatomy of the Eye*. Lederle Laboratories, Pearl River, NY.)

**Vitrectomy** is an intraocular procedure in which three 20-ga openings are made into the vitreous cavity with a myringotomy blade 3 - 4 mm posterior to the limbus (the junction of the cornea and the sclera.) One of these openings in the inferotemporal quadrant is used for infusion of balanced salt solution via a sutured cannula. The remaining openings are at the 9:30 and 2:30 o'clock positions. One is used for a hand-held fiber optic light; the other, for insertion of a variety of manual and automated instruments, including suction cutters, scissors and forceps used to remove and section abnormal tissue within the vitreous cavity. Visualization of the retina during vitrectomy is made possible by a flat contact lens, which is either sutured to the eye or held in position by the assistant. Balanced salt solution replaces the vitreous and other tissues removed during the operation. A bubble of gas is sometimes introduced into the vitreous cavity during a scleral buckle or a vitrectomy when the surgeon wants an internal tamponade of retinal tears which cannot be adequately closed by a scleral buckle alone.

In the case of a giant retinal tear, a **gas-fluid exchange** is performed with the patient in the prone position toward the end of the operation. This requires that the patient be on a Stryker frame, so that he or she can be moved from the supine to the prone position for the gas-fluid exchange.

**Liquid vitreous substitutes**, such as perfluorocarbon liquids or silicone oil, are sometimes introduced into the vitreous cavity during a vitrectomy. Perfluorocarbon liquids are heavier than water, and are used as an intraop tool to unfold the detached retina; they are then removed at the end of the procedure. Perfluorocarbon liquids make possible repair of giant retinal tears in the supine position, thus eliminating the need for a Stryker frame. They are not FDA-approved and, therefore, not widely available at this time. Silicone oil is used for complex detachments in which a long-term, internal tamponade of retinal tears is deemed necessary to prevent re-detachment. It sometimes is removed a few months postop with a second operation. Cryotherapy or lasers are used frequently to establish chorioretinal adhesions around retinal tears. Cryotherapy is applied to the sclera; a laser is applied with a fiber optic cable introduced into the vitreous cavity during vitrectomy surgery. It also can be administered with an indirect ophthalmoscope delivery system for those eyes not undergoing vitrectomy.

Simple detachments frequently can be repaired by a **pneumatic retinopexy**, in which retinal tears are treated with cryotherapy or laser and an expanding gas is injected into the vitreous cavity. This technique is usually done in phakic eyes (which have not undergone cataract extraction) with tears in the superior 8 clock hours (clockwise from 8-4 o'clock). Pneumatic retinopexy is sometimes done as an outpatient office procedure, with local anesthesia or MAC. The other procedures discussed are done with MAC or GA, according to surgeon's preference and patient's systemic condition. Some surgeons inject retrobulbar or subconjunctival bupivacaine at the end of a procedure done under GA to decrease postop pain.

**Usual preop diagnosis**: Retinal detachment; diabetic retinopathy; vitreous hemorrhage or opacification; epiretinal membrane; ruptured globe; retinopathy of prematurity (ROP)

### SUMMARY OF PROCEDURE

| | |
|---|---|
| **Position** | Supine, on Stryker frame (prone) for giant retinal tear |
| **Incision** | Transconjunctival |
| **Special instrumentation** | Vitrectomy machine; cryoprobe; laser; indirect ophthalmoscope; microscope; Stryker frame (giant retinal tear) |
| **Unique considerations** | Ruptured globe – avoid increased IOP. Stop $N_2O$ 5-10 min before a gas-fluid exchange. |
| **Antibiotics** | May use iv antibiotics in addition to subconjunctival antibiotics at conclusion of surgery. |
| **Surgical time** | Pneumatic retinopexy: 1 hr<br>Scleral buckle: 1 - 3 hrs<br>Vitrectomy: 1 - 4+ hrs<br>Giant tear: 2 - 4+ hrs |
| **Closing considerations** | Try to avoid postop bucking or vomiting. |
| **EBL** | None |
| **Postop care** | Prone positioning, if gas was injected. |
| **Mortality** | Extremely rare |
| **Morbidity** | Hemorrhage: < 5%<br>Retinal detachment: < 5%<br>Infection: < 1% |
| **Procedure code** | 67103-67108 |
| **Pain score** | 6 |

### PATIENT POPULATION CHARACTERISTICS

| | |
|---|---|
| **Age range** | Usually adults; occasionally premature infants (ROP) and children (retinal detachment or trauma) |
| **Male:Female** | 1:1 |
| **Incidence** | 1/20,000 phakic; 1/250 pseudophakic (post-cataract extraction with placement of intraocular lens) |
| **Etiology** | Majority idiopathic; some induced by trauma |
| **Associated conditions** | Idiopathic: retinal detachment, epiretinal membrane, macular hole<br>Diabetic retinopathy<br>Prior eye surgery: retinal detachment<br>Trauma: vitreous hemorrhage, retinal detachment, ruptured globe<br>HTN: vitreous hemorrhage<br>Extreme prematurity: ROP |

---

## ANESTHETIC CONSIDERATIONS

### PREOPERATIVE

Retinal detachments are classified as traction, exudative or rhegmatogenous (rupture, tear). Children, especially those with retinopathy of prematurity, sickle-cell retinopathy, retinoblastoma and those with severe renal disease or diabetes are prone to developing retinal detachments. In adults, retinal detachments are most frequently associated with diabetes, sickle-cell retinopathy, metastatic lung or breast cancer, myopia, trauma and previous cataract surgery. Rhegmatogenous retinal detachments (more common in adults) start off with a small retinal tear, which allows the vitreous to seep in between the retina and pigment epithelium, forcing retinal separation. Symptoms range from floaters and flashes to showers of black specks, and, ultimately, to a dark shadow that impinges on the field of vision. Surgeons prefer a "soft" eye during retinal reattachment surgery and, therefore, patients may be given acetazolamide or mannitol to decrease IOP.

**Respiratory** **Tests:** As indicated from H&P.

**Cardiovascular** Mannitol decreases IOP by increasing plasma oncotic pressure relative to aqueous humor pressure. It is usually given just prior to or during surgery. Total dosage should not exceed 1.5-2 gm/kg iv over a 30-60 min period. Rapid infusion of large doses of mannitol may precipitate CHF, pulmonary edema, electrolyte abnormalities, HTN and, possibly, myocardial ischemia; hence, the importance of a thorough evaluation of the patient's renal and cardiovascular status prior to administering mannitol.
**Tests:** ECG, others as indicated from H&P.

**Diabetes** Diabetic patients are at increased risk for silent myocardial ischemia. Pulmonary aspiration 2° diabetic gastroparesis is also a risk in this population. Patients usually take 1/2 or 1/3 of their normal NPH insulin dose (on the morning of surgery); fasting blood sugar is checked; and an iv infusion of D5 LR is started if glucose < 90 mg/dl, or treated with regular insulin if glucose >200 mg/dl. Blood sugar is checked intraop and postop.

**Renal** Acetazolamide, a carbonic anhydrase inhibitor, decreases secretion of aqueous humor. It also inhibits renal carbonic anhydrase, thereby facilitating the loss of $HCO_3$, $Na^+$, $K^+$ and water. Thus, patients on chronic therapy may be acidotic, hypokalemic and hyponatremic.
**Tests:** Electrolytes; others as indicated from H&P.

**Hematologic** ✓ for sickle-cell disease. Sickle-cell trait is not commonly associated with perioperative complications. Patients with sickle-cell anemia should be well-hydrated and transfused preop, as necessary to increase HbA concentration >40%.

**Laboratory** Tests as indicated from H&P.

**Premedication** Midazolam 0.5 mg po for pediatric patients, and midazolam 1-2 mg iv incrementally for adults, to alleviate anxiety. Avoid excessive sedation (respiratory depression) in sickle-cell patients.

## INTRAOPERATIVE

**Anesthetic technique:** GETA. Retinal detachment surgery may be performed under regional anesthesia, but most anesthesiologists prefer GETA, especially if the surgery is expected to be > 2 hrs.

**Induction** Standard induction (see Appendix) is appropriate for these patients, with care being taken not to put pressure on the affected eye with the face mask.

**Maintenance** Standard maintenance (see Appendix). Ophthalmologists, however, may use expanding gasses such as sulfur hexafluoride ($SF_6$), perfluropropane ($C_3F_8$) or octafluorocyclobutane ($C_4F_8$) for internal tamponade of the retinal breaks; and if $N_2O$ is used, the injected bubble may expand rapidly, causing a dramatic rise in IOP. This can impair retinal blood flow. $N_2O$ should be discontinued at least 15 min before gas injection. If patient needs a second surgery and GA after the first gas injection, $N_2O$ should be avoided for 5 d for air injection, 10 d for $SF_6$ injection, 13-15 d for $C_4F_8$, and approximately 30 d for $C_3F_8$. Non-depolarizing muscle relaxants may be advantageous, especially if $N_2O$ is discontinued. Consider droperidol 15 $\mu$g/kg iv or metoclopramide 0.15 mg/kg iv to decrease postop nausea.

**Emergence** Use narcotics for pain control and iv lidocaine 1.0-1.5 mg/kg 5 min prior to extubation to provide smooth emergence. The common occurrence of postop N&V requires the administration of intraop anti-emetics (e.g., metoclopramide 10 mg iv, droperidol 0.625 mg iv or ondansetron 4 mg iv).

| | | |
|---|---|---|
| **Blood and fluid requirements** | IV: 18 ga x 1 (adult)<br>20 ga x 1 (child)<br>NS/LR @ 5-10 cc/kg/hr<br>Hydrate, oxygenate and warm patients | Keep sickle-cell patients well-hydrated, oxygenated and warm to avoid sickle-cell crisis. |
| **Monitoring** | Standard monitors (see Appendix). | |
| **Positioning** | ✓ and pad pressure points.<br>✓ and pad non-surgical eye. | Careful padding and frequent repositioning will help avoid circulatory stasis in sickle-cell patients. |
| **Complications** | Oculocardiac reflex (OCR) | See Intraoperative Complications under Anesthetic Considerations for "Strabismus Surgery" (above). |

## POSTOPERATIVE

| | | |
|---|---|---|
| **Complications** | N&V<br>Corneal abrasion<br>Vitreous hemorrhage<br>Glaucoma<br>Ptosis<br>Diplopia<br>Loss of vision | Rx: Metoclopramide 10 mg iv, droperidol 0.625 iv, or ondansetron 4 mg iv; however, eye pain (e.g., 2° to corneal abrasion) may also cause N&V. If this is the case, treat pain also. |
| **Pain management** | Meperidine 0.5-1 mg/kg/hr iv | Avoid excessive sedation in sickle-cell patients. |
| **Tests** | None routinely required. | |

**References**

1. Benson WE: *Retinal Detachment, Diagnosis and Management*, 2nd edition. JB Lippincott Co, Philadelphia: 1988.
2. McGoldrick KE, ed: *Anesthesia for Ophthalmic and Otolaryngologic Surgery*. WB Saunders Co, Philadelphia: 1992.
3. Barash PG, Cullen BF, Stoelting RK, eds: *Clinical Anesthesia*. JB Lippincott, Philadelphia: 1989, 1062.

**General References**

1. Phelps CD, ed: *Manual of Common Ophthalmic Surgical Procedures*. Churchill Livingstone, New York: 1986.
2. Levine MR, ed: *Manual of Oculoplastic Surgery*. Churchill Livingstone, New York: 1988.
3. Spaeth GL, ed: *Ophthalmic Surgery: Principles and Practice*, 2nd edition. WB Saunders Co, Philadelphia: 1990.
4. Stewart WB, ed: *Ophthalmic Plastic and Reconstructive Surgery*. American Academy of Ophthalmology, [CITY?]: 1984.
5. Waltman SR, Keates RH, Hoyt CS, Frueh BR, Herschler J, Carroll DM, eds: *Surgery of the Eye*. Churchill Livingstone, New York: 1988.

**Surgeons**

**Amar Kaur, MD**
**David J. Terris, MD**
**Willard E. Fee, Jr, MD**

# 3. OTOLARYNGOLOGY - HEAD AND NECK SURGERY

**Anesthesiologists**

**Raymond R. Gaeta, MD**
**John G. Brock-Utne, MD(Bergen), MA, MB, BCh(TCD), FFA(SA)**

# OTOLARYNGOLOGY - HEAD AND NECK SURGERY

## INTRODUCTION – SURGEON'S PERSPECTIVE

### AIRWAY COMPETITION

Induction and maintenance of anesthesia for surgery of the head and neck requires interdisciplinary cooperation. Thorough communication both preop and intraop is required for a satisfactory outcome. Of necessity, anesthesiologists cannot have control of the head for many of the cases and competition for the airway produces some anxiety on the part of both physicians. For many procedures, head movement is the norm and unless the tube is properly secured, extubation can occur. Inflammatory or neoplastic lesions of the upper aerodigestive tract produce some degree of airway obstruction and may make intubation extremely difficult – in some cases impossible, necessitating tracheostomy under local anesthesia before induction of GA. Airway obstruction upon induction of anesthesia can occur even with seemingly simple procedures such as tonsillectomy.

### PREMEDICATION

There are few areas in surgery that have as many functional and/or cosmetic consequences as surgery of the head and neck. The properly informed patient understands the consequences and comes to the OR with a certain degree of anxiety. For oral cavity procedures or endoscopy, a drying agent facilitates performance of the procedure, making a combination of morphine or meperidine and scopolamine the agents of choice for people < 70 years. A small percentage of patients > 70 years of age will have a post-scopolamine psychosis that will be unpleasant for all concerned. For that reason, atropine or glycopyrrolate is substituted.

### TUBES AND TUBE SIZE

Seldom is there a need for anything larger than a size 6.0 mm ETT. The surgeon may need to lift the tube to examine the larynx adequately, and having to move a larger tube around can be difficult. For procedures on the oral cavity and pharynx, or for endoscopy, a cuffed tube is required to prevent anesthesia blow-by or aspiration of blood into the tracheobronchial tree. If a mouth gag is utilized, an anode or armored tube should be used to prevent compression of the tube by the gag. Although rare, anode tube obstruction does occur, and constant vigilance is required. If intra-oral or laryngeal surgery is performed with the laser, compatible ETTs must be used to prevent ignition of the tubes, resulting in intratracheal or laryngeal fires. Maintenance of anesthesia for laser cases should be performed without $N_2O$ and with $FiO_2 < 0.3$. If $FiO_2$ must be raised beyond that for any reason, the laser should not be used until the $FiO_2 < 0.3$.

### MUSCLE RELAXATION

In some cases, muscle relaxation is mandatory; in others, it is contraindicated. In the case of parotidectomy, visual or monitored facial muscle movements are required; thus, no muscle relaxant is indicated. In the case of rigid esophagoscopy, muscle relaxation is often helpful in passing through the cricopharyngeal muscle. As a matter of habit, it is best to ask, as there is nothing more frustrating than having to wait for muscle relaxation to wear off before proceeding.

### PATIENT POSITIONING

It is rare that anything other than the supine position is used. Prior to induction, the shoulders should always be at the break in the table so that head and neck can be flexed and/or extended as required intraop. This is especially true for endoscopy. Reverse Trendelenburg position is utilized for esophagoscopy to prevent gastric contents from seeping into the esophagus and slowing down the performance of the procedure. For most major head and neck procedures, elevating the head to ~30° increases venous return, decreases blood loss and expedites the procedure.

### HYPOTENSIVE ANESTHESIA

Anything that can be done to reduce blood loss results in faster surgery and less morbidity to the patient. One-third of the anatomy of the entire body is concentrated in the head and neck, and most surgical procedures are designed to preserve function, making some dissections quite tedious. Anything that can be done to maintain relative hypotension is very much appreciated by the surgeon. True hypotensive anesthesia is usually only required for excisions of angiofibromas, AV malformations, hemangiomas or glomus tumors.

# TONSILLECTOMY AND/OR ADENOIDECTOMY

## SURGICAL CONSIDERATIONS

**Description:** The dissection is carried out with the patient lying supine, shoulders elevated on a small pillow (Fig 3-1). A mouth gag is inserted; and, if an adenoidectomy is being done concurrently, adenoids are removed first, with a curette, and the nasopharynx packed. The tonsillectomy is then accomplished by firmly grasping the upper pole of the tonsil and drawing it medially, allowing a mucosal incision to be made over the anterior faucial pillar. The tonsil is dissected from its bed and removed. A snare may be used to snip the dissected tonsil off at the lower pole. Hemostasis is secured with gauze packs and the use of electrocautery. Packs are removed from the nasopharynx and tonsillar beds before extubation. Tonsillectomy may be combined with **palatopharyngoplasty** in cases of sleep apnea or stertorous breathing.

**Variant procedure or approaches:** **Guillotine technique** (rarely used)

**Usual preop diagnosis:** Chronic tonsillitis and/or adenoiditis (most common); sleep apnea; asymmetric enlargement of tonsils (to rule out cancer); nasal airway obstruction; snoring; peritonsillar abscess

### SUMMARY OF PROCEDURE

| | |
|---|---|
| **Position** | "Rose" (supine, shoulder roll, head extended); surgeon at head of table (turned 90-180°) |
| **Incision** | Intraoral mucosal |
| **Special instrumentation** | Mouth gag (McIvor) |
| **Unique considerations** | Use of armored ETT prevents compression of tube by mouth gag. |
| **Antibiotics** | Not used routinely. |
| **Surgical time** | 30 min - 1 hr |
| **Closing considerations** | If patient has sleep apnea, heightened sensitivity to narcotics and sedatives may make emergence difficult. Avoid hypercapnia on emergence to prevent vasodilation and resultant bleeding. Awake extubation provides maximum airway protection. |
| **EBL** | 25-200 cc. Monitor suction bottle contents and irrigation as an indication of blood loss. |
| **Postop care** | Lateral position; head down; gentle suctioning |
| **Mortality** | Rare |
| **Morbidity** | Bleeding: 4%[1]<br>Delayed bleeding: 3.2%<br>Infection: 4%<br>Aspiration: Rare<br>Tooth damage: Rare |
| **Procedure code** | 42820 (tonsillectomy); 42821 (adenoidectomy) |
| **Pain score** | 4-6 |

### PATIENT POPULATION CHARACTERISTICS

| | |
|---|---|
| **Age range** | 2+ yrs |
| **Male:Female** | 1:1 |
| **Incidence** | 750,000 cases/yr in U.S. |
| **Etiology** | Chronic infection<br>Sleep apnea<br>Peritonsillar abscess<br>Snoring<br>Cancer |
| **Associated conditions** | Non-specific |

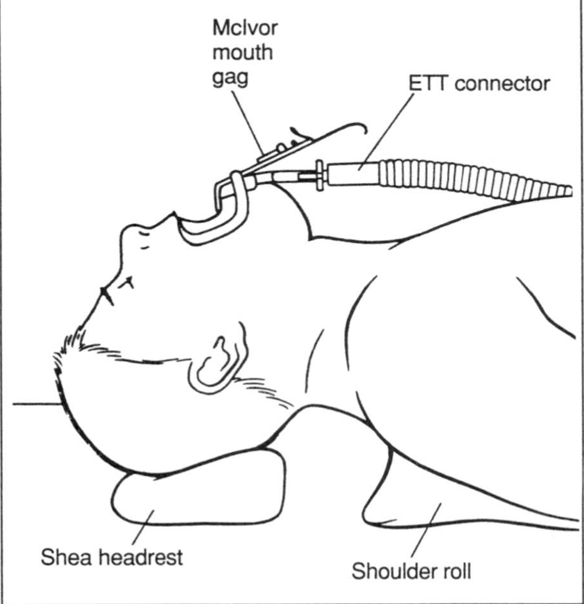


**Figure 3-1.** The "Rose" position for tonsillectomy.

# ANESTHETIC CONSIDERATIONS

## PREOPERATIVE

Most T/A patients are young and otherwise healthy; however, a subset of both pediatric and adult patients may present with Sx of obstructive sleep apnea (OSA) or upper RTI. It is important to distinguish between a child with chronic sniffles and one who presents with an acute RTI, which may necessitate postponing an elective surgical procedure. For many children, this is their first anesthetic; therefore, it is imperative to check family history for anesthetic problems.

**Respiratory** In patients presenting with Sx of acute RTI (purulent sputum or nasal secretions, fever, etc.), the general recommendation is to postpone any elective procedure until symptoms have abated, usually within 7-14 d. The rationale for postponing surgery includes: the possibility of progression from an upper RTI to a lower RTI; presence of secretions which may obstruct the ETT and plug small airways; predisposition to laryngospasm, and ↓respiratory reserve. The patient with OSA is often obese, with a potentially difficult airway, consequent to a short, thick neck, large tongue and redundant pharyngeal tissue. These patients may require an awake FOL.
**Tests:** As indicated from H&P.

**Dental** Parents should be informed that loose teeth in pediatric patients may be dislodged/damaged. Physical exam should include a careful dental assessment.

**Cardiovascular** Rarely, chronic airway obstruction may lead to pulmonary HTN and heart failure.
**Tests:** As indicated from H&P.

**Hematologic** √ for recent ASA use and Hx of excessive bleeding following minor trauma or tooth extraction.

**Laboratory** Other tests as indicated from H&P.

**Premedication** Sedative premedication should be avoided in OSA patients because of their sensitivity to sedative drugs. Otherwise, midazolam iv 0.5 mg/kg po will provide satisfactory preop sedation.

## INTRAOPERATIVE

**Anesthetic technique:** GETA

**Induction** A standard induction (see Appendix) is suitable for many of these patients; however, in patients with chronic upper airway obstruction, the airway may obstruct following inhalation induction and anesthesia. Use of an oral airway or nasal airway frequently resolves the problem (especially if the mouth is sprayed with local anesthetic prior to induction). In adults with OSA, an awake FOL is usually indicated. Typically, an oral RAE tube should be used, held in place by means of a mouth gag. Following placement of the gag, the ETT may be dislodged, kinked or inadvertently advanced into a mainstem bronchus. Thus, it is essential to verify tube placement (e.g., chest movement, bilateral and equal breath sounds and normal PIP).

**Maintenance** Standard maintenance (see Appendix). Muscle relaxation not required.

**Emergence** At the end of the procedure, the patient should be turned onto the side in the tonsillar position (semi-prone, with head down). Patient can be prevented from rolling onto his/her face by using a large pillow beneath the chest, and from rolling supine by extending the lower arm behind the body. Patients are usually extubated awake when protective airway reflexes have returned. Remember to verify removal of throat pack before extubation. Use care when suctioning pharynx.

| | | |
|---|---|---|
| **Blood and fluid requirements** | IV: 18 ga x 1 (adult)<br>20 ga x 1 (child)<br>NS/LR @ 5-10 cc/kg/hr | Blood loss typically averages 4 cc/kg. |
| **Monitoring** | Standard monitors (see Appendix). | Careful monitoring of blood loss is important in the pediatric population. |
| **Positioning** | √ and pad pressure points.<br>√ eyes. | |
| **Complications** | ETT damage<br>ETT dislodgement | ETTs (with stylet) of different sizes should be readily available. |

## POSTOPERATIVE

| | | |
|---|---|---|
| **Complications** | Retention of throat pack | Manifested by severe postop respiratory distress. Under direct laryngoscopy, remove pack with Magill forceps. |

| | | |
|---|---|---|
| **Complications, cont.** | Laryngospasm and/or bronchospasm | A relatively common complication. Rx: 100% $O_2$ via mask ventilation with jaw thrust and CPAP is generally sufficient. Rapid-sequence induction and direct laryngoscopy/intubation for persistent spasm. |
| | Bleeding tonsil | This is a serious complication and common cause of mortality following tonsillectomy in children. Sx include ↑HR, ↑RR, ↓BP and pallor. The patient may swallow most of the blood being lost and should be treated as a high risk for aspiration. Blood loss (Hct < 25%) should be replaced, if possible, before reinduction of anesthesia. Following volume resuscitation, anesthesia (etomidate 0.2-0.3 ml/kg or ketamine 1-2 mg/kg) should be induced by rapid-sequence technique with cricoid pressure. Suction must always be available. Before extubation, NG tube should be passed and stomach contents aspirated. |
| **Pain management** | Meperidine 0.5-1 mg/kg/hr iv<br>Acetaminophen suppositories q 4-6 hrs, 240 mg (4-5 yrs), 325-650 mg (10-11 yrs) | |
| **Tests** | Hct (if blood loss suspected). | Frequent swallowing, especially in children, may be a sign of ongoing hemorrhage. |

**References**

1. Breson K, Diepeveen J: Dissection tonsillectomy — complications and follow-up. *J Laryngol Otol* 1969; 83(6):601-8.
2. Brown BR Jr: *Anesthesia and ENT Surgery*. FA Davis Co, Philadelphia: 1987.
3. Morrison JD: *Anesthesia for Eye, Ear, Nose and Throat Surgery*, 2nd edition. Morrison JD, Mirakhur RK, Craig HJL, eds. Churchill Livingstone, New York: 1985.

# LARYNGOSCOPY/BRONCHOSCOPY/ESOPHAGOSCOPY

## SURGICAL CONSIDERATIONS

**Description: Laryngoscopy** is used for visualization of the pharynx, hypopharynx or larynx for diagnostic and/or therapeutic benefit. The patient lies supine with cervical spine flexed and atlantoaxial joint extended (this position is best achieved with a headrest); and the teeth are protected with a mouth guard. The laryngoscope is introduced (Fig 3-2) and, with a lifting motion, a thorough examination of the oropharynx, hypopharynx, laryngopharynx and larynx is carried out; and biopsies can be taken. Any bleeding encountered normally can be controlled easily with pressure. Laryngoscopy is often combined with esophagoscopy, bronchoscopy or direct nasopharyngoscopy to survey the aero-digestive tract for malignancy. If diagnostic, the surgeon may need to visualize the airway prior to intubation and/or muscle relaxation. If a laser is to be utilized, use of a special laser ETT, < 30% $O_2$ concentration, and avoidance of $N_2O$ are required.

**Usual preop diagnosis:** Oropharyngeal, hypopharyngeal or laryngeal tumors

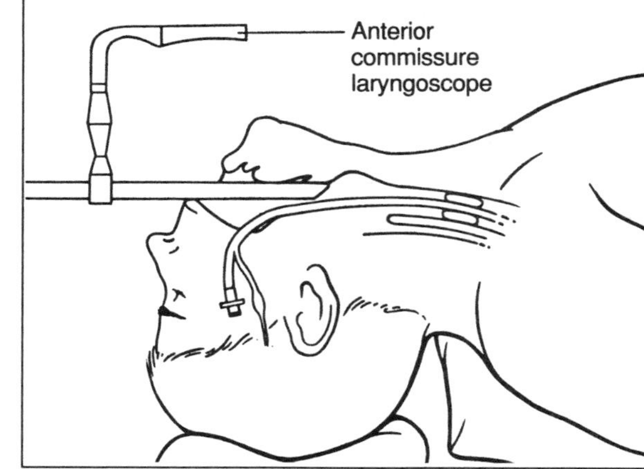

**Figure 3-2.** Placement of anterior commissure laryngoscope for laryngoscopy.

**Bronchoscopy** is used for visualization of the tracheobronchial tree for both diagnostic and therapeutic purposes. The patient lies supine with head elevated and neck

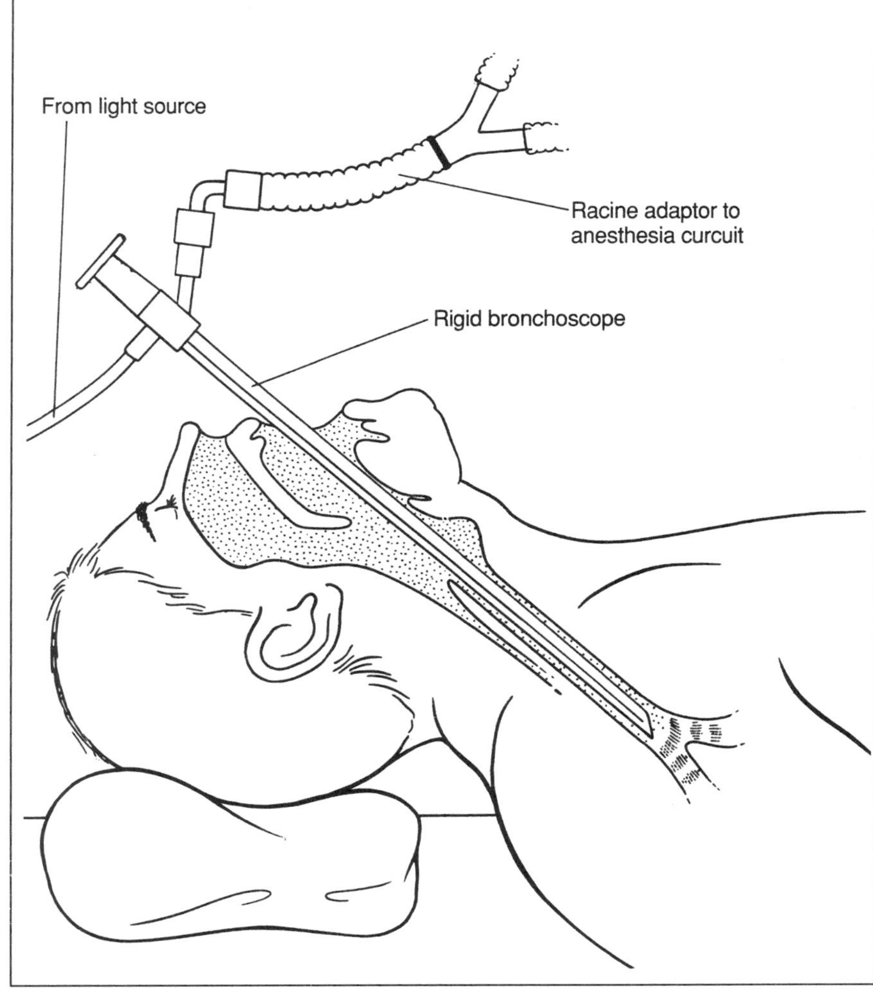


**Figure 3-3.** Rigid bronchoscopy showing adaptor (Racine) for anesthesia machine. Note neck flexion and head extension to align oropharyngeal and tracheal axes.

extended at the upper cervical level. The bronchoscope is directed along the right side of the tongue forward toward the midline to visualize the epiglottis. Next, the bronchoscope tip is used to lift the epiglottis and advance the bronchoscope through the vocal cords, into the trachea and bronchus (Fig 3-3). The scope can be directed for inspection of the carina, main bronchi and, with the aid of telescopes, the segmental bronchi. This is often performed with direct laryngoscopy, esophagoscopy, or as part of **panendoscopy**.

**Usual preop diagnosis:** Head and neck squamous-cell carcinoma; foreign body in bronchus

**Esophagoscopy** is used for visualization of the esophagus for either diagnostic or therapeutic benefit. The patient is supine with head elevated and neck extended at the upper cervical level. The esophagoscope (held in the right hand) is advanced through the mouth behind the arytenoids, gently using the left thumb. The bevel of the scope is then used to advance through the cricopharyngeus muscle (upper esophageal sphincter) with an upward lifting movement, entering the cervical esophagus. As the scope advances, the head may have to be lowered or the neck extended and the scope directed slightly toward the left. It should be advanced only when a visible lumen is seen all the way down to the cardia. A biopsy may be taken through the scope. Esophagoscopy also is often performed as part of **panendoscopy**.

**Usual preop diagnosis:** Head and neck squamous-cell carcinoma; foreign body ingestion

## SUMMARY OF PROCEDURE

| | Laryngoscopy | Bronchoscopy | Esophagoscopy |
|---|---|---|---|
| **Position** | Supine; table 90° | ⇐ | ⇐ + Reverse Trendelenburg or head up 30° to prevent gastric reflux. |
| **Special instrumentation** | Laser ETT; microscope (both used occasionally). | Rigid or flexible bronchoscopes of various sizes. If rigid scope used, an adaptor connects it to anesthesia tubing. If flexible scope used, accessory port adaptor should be connected to the ETT. | Rigid esophagoscope or flexible gastroscope |

| | **Laryngoscopy** | **Bronchoscopy** | **Esophagoscopy** |
|---|---|---|---|
| **Unique considerations** | Steroids (dexamethasone 4-12 mg) may be helpful if airway is compromised and extensive manipulation or therapeutic procedure required. | With laser ablation, keep $O_2$ < 30%, avoid $N_2O$. Bleeding following Bx or removal of tumors is rare, but may require re-bronchoscopy and suctioning to adequately ventilate the patient. | May need to deflate ETT cuff to introduce scope or retrieve foreign body. |
| **Antibiotics** | None | Usually none | None |
| **Surgical time** | 10 min - 1.5 hrs (diagnostic vs therapeutic) | 10 - 60 min | ⇐ |
| **EBL** | Minimal | ⇐ | ⇐ |
| **Postop care** | Rarely may require overnight ICU monitoring if airway compromised and no tracheostomy performed. | Usually PACU. If surgery 2° airway obstruction, it may worsen immediately postop, requiring ICU observation. | PACU; may require overnight observation to rule out perforation. |
| **Mortality** | < 1% | ⇐ | < 0.1% |
| **Morbidity** | Laryngospasm: < 5% | – | ⇐ |
| | Airway obstruction upon induction: 1% | ⇐ | < 1% |
| | Damaged teeth: < 1% | 1% | ⇐ |
| | Laryngeal edema requiring tracheostomy or reintubation: < 1% | Pneumonia: 1% | Perforation of esophagus: 1% |
| **Procedure code** | 31515-31535 | 31622 | 43200-43202 |
| **Pain score** | 1-2 | 1-2 | 1-2 |

### PATIENT POPULATION CHARACTERISTICS

| | | | |
|---|---|---|---|
| **Age range** | Newborn - old age | ⇐ | ⇐ |
| **Male:Female** | 1:1 | ⇐ | ⇐ |
| **Incidence** | Common | ⇐ | ⇐ |
| **Etiology** | Neoplasia | ⇐ | ⇐ |
| | Foreign bodies | ⇐ | ⇐ |
| | Congenital webs/cysts | ⇐ | ⇐ |

---

## ANESTHETIC CONSIDERATIONS

**(Procedures covered: direct laryngoscopy, bronchoscopy, esophagoscopy)**

### PREOPERATIVE

Close attention to airway management is paramount in this procedure. Surgeons and anesthesiologists must share the airway; hence, close communication is essential.

**Airway** Patients with lesions in the mediastinum may have involvement of the recurrent laryngeal nerve, with hoarseness, and potential airway management problems (e.g., difficult mask ventilation, difficult intubation, ↑aspiration risk). (See Anesthetic Considerations for "Mediastinoscopy.")

**Respiratory** In laryngoscopy/bronchoscopy patients, respiratory function may be impaired. COPD and tobacco use are common. PFTs may show ↓$FEV_1$, ↓FVC, or ↓$FEV_1$/FVC ratio. ABGs may demonstrate ↓$PaO_2$ and/or ↑$PaCO_2$. Lesions of the upper airway may impede intubation and ventilation. For esophagoscopy patients, obstructing lesions of the esophagus can be associated with regurgitation of fluid or particulate matter on induction. Patients requiring urgent endoscopy for GI bleeds or foreign bodies should be considered at risk for aspiration.

**Tests:** CXR; ABG; PFTs – as indicated from H&P.

**Dental** Patients (or parents, as appropriate) should be informed that loose teeth may be dislodged/damaged. Physical exam should include a careful dental assessment.

**Cardiovascular** Tobacco use (>40 pack-years) increases the incidence of heart disease. Carefully assess patient, including exercise tolerance. Look for Sx of CAD (e.g., angina) and CHF (e.g., orthopnea, PND, peripheral edema) in patients with cardiac risk factors (including age >40 yrs, male, HTN, hypercholesteremia, long Hx of smoking, obesity and family Hx). The volume status of debilitated patients who are unable to eat because of obstructing lesions of the esophagus should be assessed. **Tests:** ECG; CXR; treadmill stress test; ECHO, if indicated from H&P. Orthostatic BP and HR changes >10 mmHg, ↓SBP, and/or 15 beat/min ↑HR suggest significant (>20%) hypovolemia.

**Neurologic** Some patients may have Hx of alcohol abuse which may result in increased anesthetic requirements because of hepatic enzyme induction.

**Hematologic** Patients with malignancy or chronic disease may have evidence of anemia or coagulopathy. **Tests:** CBC; PT; PTT, platelets – as indicated from H&P.

**Gastrointestinal** In obstructing lesions, a CXR should be obtained for evidence of esophageal dilatation and retained fluids, which may be regurgitated during induction. Hypokalemia and hypomagnesemia should be corrected preop. Patients with malignant tumors may be malnourished. **Tests:** CXR; electrolytes

**Laboratory** LFTs, and others, if indicated from H&P.

**Premedication** A drying agent (e.g., glycopyrrolate 0.2 mg iv) given pre-induction, facilitates panendoscopy; however, ↑HR may be detrimental in those with CAD. Benzodiazepines and/or opiates may be appropriate (see "Standard Premedication," Appendix). Care must be taken not to oversedate these patients.

## INTRAOPERATIVE

**Anesthetic technique:** GETA. The challenge of airway management in these cases requires careful planning and continuous communication with the surgeon. Fiber optic esophagoscopy can be performed under MAC (see Appendix) with appropriate sedation, using short-acting agents, including midazolam, fentanyl or propofol. Rigid esophagoscopy requires GA to provide adequate anesthesia and muscle relaxation.

**Induction** With a normal airway, standard induction (see Appendix) is appropriate. Any patient at risk for aspiration, however, requires rapid-sequence induction with cricoid pressure. A cuffed ETT should be placed and cricoid pressure released only after the airway is secured. In cases where there is the potential for airway obstruction, an awake fiber optic intubation under topical and transtracheal anesthesia should be performed. Generally, small ETTs (~5-6 mm) are used to facilitate visualization of the larynx by the surgical team. For laser cases, a shielded tube manufactured specifically for laser surgery is required. The cuff should be filled with NS, rather than air.

**Maintenance** Standard maintenance (see Appendix) with muscle relaxation and 100% $O_2$. Anesthesia may be supplemented with iv agent (e.g., fentanyl or meperidine titrated to effect). Ventilation can be achieved by a variety of methods; see discussion below. For laser cases, dilute $O_2$ with air, $N_2$ or helium. High $FiO_2$ and $FiN_2O$ support combustion. Cover patient's eyes with protective glasses. Complete muscle relaxation is essential during rigid esophagoscopy to prevent esophageal perforation. ETT should be firmly secured and held manually throughout the procedure, as movement of the esophagoscope may dislodge the ETT. Hand ventilation will allow detection of disconnects and/or airway occlusion related to procedure.

**Emergence** Patient should have full return of protective airway reflexes prior to extubation.

| | | |
|---|---|---|
| **Blood and fluid requirements** | IV: GI bleeder: 14-16 ga x 2<br>Others: 18 ga x 1<br>NS/LR @ 3-5 cc/kg/hr<br>For esophagoscopy: NS/LR @ 4-6 ml/kg/hr | Blood loss is usually minimal; however, in case of GI bleed, blood loss may be massive. T&C patient for 2 U PRBC, with blood immediately available in OR. |
| **Monitoring** | Standard monitors (see Appendix).<br>± Arterial line | + Other monitors as indicated by patient condition. In cases of potential hemorrhage, an arterial line is desirable. |
| **Positioning** | Table rotated 90°<br>✓ and pad pressure points.<br>✓ eyes. | Patient should have a shoulder roll with neck extension to facilitate endoscopy. For flexible fiber optic endoscopy, patients will generally be in the lateral decubitus position. |

| | | |
|---|---|---|
| **Ventilation** | Small cuffed ETT<br>Apneic oxygenation<br>Jet ventilation (Saunders attachment)<br>Racine adapter (rigid bronchoscopy) (Fig 3-3) | The use of a small, cuffed ETT offers the usual advantages of airway protection, controlled ventilation and ease of respiratory gas monitoring. The potential for interfering with surgical visualization, however, may preclude its use. Jet ventilation in patients with adequate pulmonary compliance will provide good surgical visibility, but it requires special equipment and can cause barotrauma. Apneic oxygenation is limited by ↑$PaCO_2$ (~3 mmHg/mm) producing acidosis and dysrhythmias. Apnea periods should be < 5 min. |
| **Complications** | Inadequate ventilation<br>Loss of airway<br>Perforation of airway<br>Pneumothorax<br>Dysrhythmias<br>Eye trauma<br>Bleeding post-Bx | Inadequate ventilation → ↑$PaCO_2$ ↓$PaO_2$ → dysrhythmias.<br>Mechanical or laser perforation of the airway may lead to bronchospasm or uncontrollable hemorrhage.<br>Eye trauma from surgical instruments used during endoscopy may require ophthalmology consult. |
| **Airway fire** | Stop ventilation.<br>Remove ETT.<br>Extinguish fire with NS.<br>Re-establish airway.<br>Resume ventilation with air until all burning is stopped.<br>Resume 100% $FiO_2$.<br>✓ airway for extent of damage.<br>Save tube for later examination. | This is an acute, life-threatening emergency requiring prompt treatment. $O_2$ and $N_2O$ both support combustion; hence, these need to be turned off while the fire is extinguished. Once the fire is out, ventilation should be resumed with 100% $O_2$. Bronchoscopy is required to ✓ extent of damage. |

## POSTOPERATIVE

| | | |
|---|---|---|
| **Complications** | Dental trauma<br>Massive bleeding<br>Eye trauma<br>Esophageal rupture<br>Pneumothorax<br>Pneumomediastinum<br>Hemothorax | Dental trauma may result from surgical manipulation of the airway.<br>Pneumothorax, mediastinal air or hemothorax from esophageal rupture may present as hypotension, cardiovascular collapse or increased airway pressures. |
| **Pain management** | Acetaminophen ± opiates<br>Generally, mild analgesics or no medication is required after a simple esophagoscopy. | |
| **Tests** | CXR<br>Hct | For evidence of pneumothorax, hemothorax, mediastinal air. |


**References**

1. Lore JM: *An Atlas of Head and Neck Surgery*, 3rd edition. WB Saunders Co, Philadelphia: 1988.
2. Brown BR Jr: *Anesthesia and ENT Surgery*. FA Davis Co, Philadelphia: 1987.
3. Morrison JD: *Anesthesia for Eye, Ear, Nose and Throat Surgery*, 2nd edition. Morrison JD, Mirakhur RK, Craig HJL, eds. Churchill Livingstone, New York: 1985.

# NASAL SURGERY

## (RHINOPLASTY, SEPTOPLASTY, SEPTORHINOPLASTY)

## SURGICAL CONSIDERATIONS

**Description:** Nasal surgery is performed for either cosmetic or functional restoration of the airway, or both. Functional restoration is usually performed for either congenital or post-traumatic deviations of the septum. The procedure varies in each individual case, although in all nasal surgery, the nasal cavity is first cocainized with 4% cocaine-soaked pledgets placed in each nostril for 5-10 min. **Septoplasty** can usually be carried out under sedation with local anesthesia, using 1% lidocaine with 1:100,000 epinephrine. **Rhinoplasty-septorhinoplasty** is usually carried out under local anesthesia, but if GA is used, a mouth pack is inserted. Local infiltration with 1% lidocaine with 1:100,000 epinephrine is used to ensure vasoconstriction and to minimize bleeding. Intranasal incisions are made and septal problems corrected. Generally, an anterior hemitransfixion incision is made down to the cartilage, and a submucoperichondrial flap is elevated the length of the septum. A similar flap may be elevated on the contralateral side. Bony deformities are resected with an osteotome, while cartilaginous deformities are either resected or weakened by morselizing, either *in situ* or after removal, and then replaced. The incision is closed with interrupted absorbable sutures. In **rhinoplasty**, tip remodelling, hump reduction and bony osteotomies are done to remodel the nasal contour. Surgery on the inferior turbinates in the form of intramural cautery, resection of turbinate bone, resection of turbinate mucosa or, in some cases, complete turbinectomy may be required to produce a satisfactory airway. After the surgery is complete, both nasal cavities are packed and external splints may be used for rhinoplasty and septorhinoplasty cases.

**Usual preop diagnosis:** Nasal deformity or deviation; deviated septum

### SUMMARY OF PROCEDURE

| | |
|---|---|
| **Position** | Head up 30° to decrease bleeding. Table may be turned 90-180°. |
| **Incision** | Intranasal, usually; extended only in open septorhinoplasty |
| **Unique considerations** | Nose initially cocainized; use of 1% lidocaine with 1:100,000 epinephrine to decrease bleeding. |
| **Antibiotics** | Cefazolin 1 gm iv; routinely used as long as nasal packs are in place. |
| **Surgical time** | 1 - 2.5 hrs |
| **Closing considerations** | Nose often packed postop, necessitating oral airway after extubation. |
| **EBL** | 50-100 cc (excessive blood loss rare) |
| **Postop care** | PACU |
| **Mortality** | Minimal |
| **Morbidity** | Septal perforation: 5%<br>Bleeding: 4%<br>Infection: 4% |
| **Procedure code** | 30520 (septoplasty); 30400-30450 (rhinoplasty) |
| **Pain score** | 4-6 |

### PATIENT POPULATION CHARACTERISTICS

| | |
|---|---|
| **Age range** | Young teens - young adults |
| **Male:Female** | 1:1 |
| **Incidence** | Common |
| **Etiology** | Congenital/traumatic septal and/or nasal deviation |

## ANESTHETIC CONSIDERATIONS

See Anesthetic Considerations following "Sinus Surgery" (below).

**References**

1. Sheen JH: *Aesthetic Rhinoplasty*, 2nd edition. Sheen JH, Sheen AD, eds. CV Mosby, St. Louis: 1987.

# SINUS SURGERY

## (EXTERNAL OR ENDOSCOPIC)

## SURGICAL CONSIDERATIONS

**Description:** Sinus surgery is performed to eliminate infection, polyps or neoplastic conditions that result in obstruction of the sinuses → secondary infection. Providing aeration of the sinuses so that mucous secretion can adequately drain into the nose and nasopharynx is the goal. The patient should be intubated orally and pharynx packed. Nasal mucosa is cocainized with 4% cocaine, and a local injection of 1% lidocaine with 1:100,000 epinephrine is used before making incisions. **Endoscopic sinus surgery** is carried out intranasally using endoscopes with a video monitor. Biting forceps are used to remove polyps, diseased mucosa or biopsy material. **External approaches** include: **Caldwell-Luc** (a sublabial approach to the maxillary sinus), **transantral ethmoidectomy**, **external ethmoidectomy**, **transseptal sphenoidectomy**, and **frontal osteoplastic flap** via coronal or brow incision. These procedures accomplish the same end as endoscopic sinus surgery. They involve external incisions and tend to be done for persistent diseases that recur despite intranasal surgery. The **Caldwell-Luc** is performed through an intra-oral incision placed in the gingival-buccal sulcus just posterior to the canine fossa. A submucoperiosteal flap is elevated superiorly, exposing the infraorbital nerve. The sinus is entered just inferior to this nerve using a small osteotome. The opening is widened with biting forceps, and the mucosal lining of the diseased sinus is usually exenterated. Typically, a nasoantral window is placed through the inferior meatus to allow additional drainage. The gingival-buccal incision is then closed with interrupted absorbable sutures. The external methods are also the preferred approaches to deal with neoplastic conditions. A craniofacial **combined neurosurgical-external sinus approach** is occasionally required to clear neoplastic nasal and sinus disease. After endoscopic or external sinus surgery, the nose/sinus is usually packed; thus, an oral airway will aid postop mouth breathing on extubation until patient is fully awake.

**Usual preop diagnosis:** Infection; nasal polyps; neoplasia (benign or malignant)

### SUMMARY OF PROCEDURE

| | |
|---|---|
| **Position** | Head up 30° (minimizes bleeding). Table may be turned 90-180°. |
| **Incision** | Endoscopic: intranasal. External: sublabial, medial orbital or bicoronal. |
| **Special instrumentation** | Nasal endoscopes; video monitor setup; microscope (may be used for external approaches). |
| **Unique considerations** | Nose may be packed bilaterally, necessitating use of oral airway on emergence. 1% lidocaine with 1:100,000 epinephrine normally used to decrease bleeding. |
| **Antibiotics** | Cefazolin 1 gm iv |
| **Surgical time** | 1 - 3 hrs |
| **EBL** | 50-300 cc (excessive blood loss rarely anticipated). Watch suction bottle and measure irrigation. |
| **Postop care** | PACU |
| **Mortality** | Minimal |
| **Morbidity** | Bleeding: 4%<br>Infection: 4% |
| **Procedure code** | 31250-31285 (endoscopic procedures); 31020-31090 (external procedures) |
| **Pain score** | 2-4 (4-6 for external approaches) |

### PATIENT POPULATION CHARACTERISTICS

| | |
|---|---|
| **Age range** | Children - adults |
| **Male:Female** | 1:1 |
| **Incidence** | Common |
| **Etiology** | Infectious<br>Allergic<br>Neoplastic |
| **Associated conditions** | Asthma: most patients who have asthma will benefit from sinus surgery with reduction in the incidence and/or severity of asthmatic attacks. Rarely, surgery itself may precipitate an asthmatic attack upon emergence or in the immediate postop period.<br>Cystic fibrosis patients are generally assisted by performing postop bronchoscopy at the termination of procedure to facilitate pulmonary toilet in the immediate postop period. |

# ANESTHETIC CONSIDERATIONS FOR NASAL & SINUS SURGERY

## PREOPERATIVE

These cases are typically elective and can be performed on an outpatient basis.

**Respiratory** — Patients with nasal polyps and asthma often have a hypersensitivity to ASA, which can precipitate bronchospasm; hence, NSAIDs, including ketorolac, should be avoided. Some patients undergoing nasal surgery may have obstructive sleep apnea (OSA), which can be associated with redundant pharyngeal tissues and/or chronic airway obstruction. (See Anesthetic Considerations for "Tonsillectomy and/or Adenoidectomy.")
**Tests:** ABGs, PFTs with flow-volume loops in patients with sleep apnea or asthma

**Cardiovascular** — The intraop use of topical vasoconstrictors, including cocaine, to control bleeding may result in ↑BP, dysrhythmias, coronary artery spasm and seizures; therefore, a careful evaluation of the cardiovascular system is essential. Patients with obstructive sleep apnea (OSA) may have evidence of cor pulmonale.
**Tests:** ECG; ECHO, if indicated from H&P.

**Premedication** — Standard premedication (see Appendix). Sedation should be avoided in patients with Hx of OSA.

## INTRAOPERATIVE

**Anesthetic technique:** Rhinoplasty or repair of septal defects is commonly performed under local anesthesia with MAC (see Appendix) and sedation. Other types of nasal and sinus surgery may require GA.

**Induction** — For those procedures done under GA, standard induction (see Appendix) is appropriate. ETT may be taped to one side; if a RAE tube is used, it should be taped in the midline.

**Maintenance** — Standard maintenance (see Appendix).

**Emergence** — The oropharynx should be suctioned carefully to avoid aspiration. These patients may have a nasal or pharyngeal pack, which must be removed prior to emergence. Also, patients may have surgical packs placed in the nares, which makes them obligate mouth breathers. Patients should have return of full airway reflexes before extubation.

| | | |
|---|---|---|
| **Blood and fluid requirements** | Blood loss generally minimal<br>IV: 18 ga x 1<br>NS/LR @ 4-6 cc/kg/hr | Blood loss controlled with surgical hemostasis and topical applications of vasoconstrictors, including cocaine or epinephrine. |
| **Monitoring** | Standard monitors (see Appendix). | |
| **Positioning** | Head elevated 30°<br>Table turned 90°-180°<br>✓ and pad pressure points.<br>✓ eyes. | Extension tubing for the anesthesia circuit should be available. |
| **Complications** | Dysrhythmias | Dysrhythmias related to vasoconstrictor agents may be a problem, particularly in patients with CAD. Halothane should be avoided, if possible, as dysrhythmias may occur with low doses of epinephrine. |

## POSTOPERATIVE

| | | |
|---|---|---|
| **Complications** | Occult postop bleeding | Occult postop bleeding may cause the patient to swallow large quantities of blood, which may be aspirated if a second anesthetic induction is required. |
| **Pain management** | Acetaminophen ± codeine or hydrocodone | |


**References**

1. Rice DH: *Endoscopic Paranasal Surgery.* Rice DH, Schaefer SD, eds. Raven Press, New York: 1988.
2. Brown BR Jr: *Anesthesia and ENT Surgery.* FA Davis Co, Philadelphia: 1987.
3. Morrison JD: *Anesthesia for Eye, Ear, Nose and Throat Surgery*, 2nd edition. Morrison JD, Mirakhur RK, Craig HJL, eds. Churchill Livingstone, New York: 1985.

# EAR SURGERY

## SURGICAL CONSIDERATIONS

**Description:** Surgery on the external ear is performed for reconstruction of a congenitally deformed ear or following trauma, and may therefore involve multiple cosmetic procedures. More commonly, surgery is performed to restore hearing, eliminate infections, remove cholesteatoma or for neoplastic conditions. The surgical approaches, techniques, and instrumentation are highly variable and individualized according to the surgeon; however, anesthesia for ear surgery is relatively generic. Since the facial nerve travels in the temporal bone, most surgeons do not want the patient paralyzed, so that they can either observe or monitor facial nerve function intraop. If **tympanoplasty** (repair of the ear drum) or a **tympanomeatal flap** is being created (as in the case of **stapedotomy** or **stapedectomy**) $N_2O$ is not used. This is to prevent pressurization of the middle ear space, which leads to displacement of either the tympanic membrane or the graft. There are many approaches to the middle ear, but, basically, the procedures are performed via a **transcanal approach**, using the microscope, or from a **post-auricular approach**, through the mastoid. A **myringotomy** typically is made in radial fashion in the anterior/inferior quadrant of the tympanic membrane and fluid liberated with a suction. If long-term ventilation is indicated, a tympanostomy tube is placed with the flange on the medial and lateral surface of the tympanic membrane. In most cases, these procedures can be performed using mask GA. **Exploratory tympanotomy** begins with injection of 2% lidocaine, **1:20,000** of epinephrine, followed by a curved incision along the posterior external auditory canal. The canal skin and the tympanic membrane are elevated forward to expose the middle ear contents, which can be approached either through the canal, or by a post-auricular approach. A tympanic membrane perforation can be repaired by placing a temporalis fascia graft, while abnormalities in the ossicular chain can be repaired with prosthesis. Gelfoam® is frequently placed in the middle ear, and the tympanic membrane is returned to its anatomic position. The external canal is likewise packed with Gelfoam®. A post-auricular approach is usually employed for a **simple mastoidectomy**. After gaining exposure of the mastoid cortex, a large burr is used to drill away the diseased mastoid air cells, exposing the facial nerve, the semicircular canals, and the middle ear space. The incision is then closed and a mastoid dressing applied. A **modified radical mastoidectomy** is similar to a simple mastoidectomy, except that the posterior external canal is removed, so that the mastoid can be visualized through the external canal during postop visits. Finally, a **radical mastoidectomy** includes not only removal of the posterior external canal, but removal of the tympanic membrane, malleus, and incus as well. This surgery is rarely performed. Glomus tumors may extend into the neck and require both a transmastoid and a transcervical approach. Removal of large glomus tumors may result in rapid and profound blood loss (>1000 cc) and require intra-arterial monitoring and the ability to provide rapid transfusion. (Middle ear anatomy is shown in Fig 3-4.)

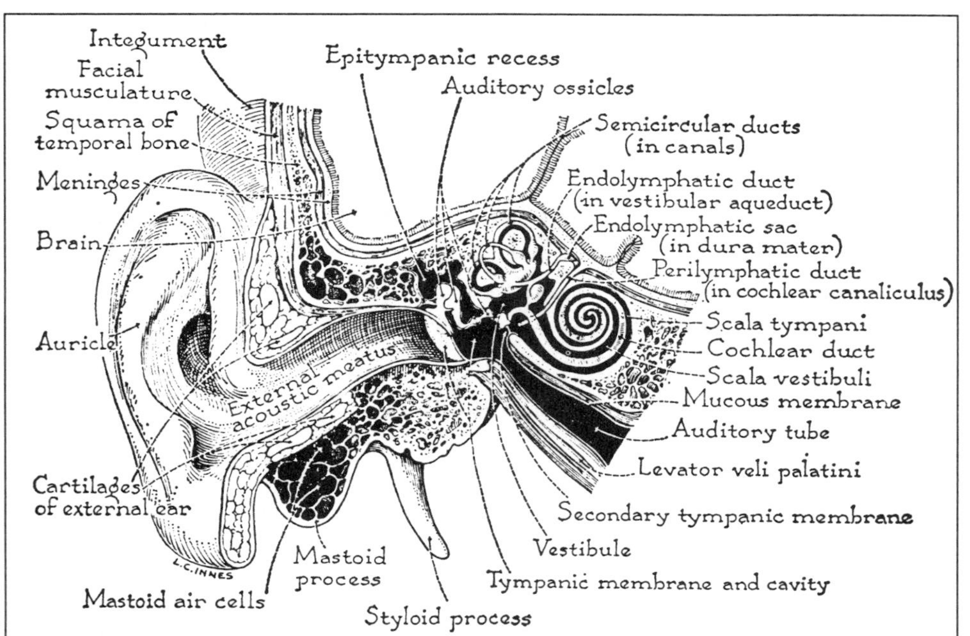

**Figure 3-4.** Middle ear anatomy. (Reproduced with permission from Anson BJ, McVay CB: *Surgical Anatomy*, 5th edition. WB Saunders Co: 1981.)

**Usual preop diagnosis:** Congenitally deformed ear; conductive hearing loss; chronic otitis media ± perforation of the tympanic membrane; cholesteatoma; neoplasia; trauma

## SUMMARY OF PROCEDURE

| | |
|---|---|
| **Position** | Supine |
| **Incision** | Post-auricular, endaural or transcanal |
| **Special instrumentation** | Ear instruments; microscope; occasionally laser; micro-drill |
| **Unique considerations** | Facial nerve monitoring or observation; therefore, no muscle relaxation. D/C $N_2O$ 30 min before laying down tympanic membrane graft. |
| **Antibiotics** | Varies with situation and type of surgery. |
| **Surgical time** | 1.5 - 4 hrs |
| **EBL** | Negligible for most; the rare exception is excision of glomus tumors (mentioned above). |
| **Mortality** | Minimal |
| **Morbidity** | The incidence of these complications varies according to type of surgery and primary pathology:<br>Infection<br>Vertigo<br>Sensorineural hearing loss<br>Facial nerve paralysis<br>Perilymph fistula |
| **Pain score** | 2-6, depending on extent of surgery |

## PATIENT POPULATION CHARACTERISTICS

| | |
|---|---|
| **Age range** | Infants - adults |
| **Male:Female** | 1:1 |
| **Incidence** | Common |
| **Etiology** | Infectious<br>Trauma<br>Congenital<br>Neoplastic |

---

# ANESTHETIC CONSIDERATIONS

**(Procedures covered: ear surgery, otoplasty)**

## PREOPERATIVE

This patient population is generally young and healthy. Myringotomy and pressure equalization tube insertion are generally very short procedures. In contrast, ossicular and tympanic membrane reconstruction are much longer. External ear reconstructions may be associated with other congenital abnormalities, which should be considered preop.

**Respiratory** Many pediatric patients present with concurrent Sx of upper RTI. These patients may have a predisposition to laryngospasm intraop and postop. In patients presenting with Sx of acute RTI (purulent sputum or nasal secretions, fever, etc), the general recommendation is to postpone any elective procedure until symptoms have abated, usually within 7-14 d. The rationale for postponing surgery includes: the possibility of progression to a lower RTI; secretions which may obstruct the ETT and plug small airways; a predisposition to laryngospasm; and ↓respiratory reserve.

**Tests:** As indicated from H&P.

**Dental** Any loose teeth in young children should be identified preop.

**Premedication** Standard premedication (see Appendix).

## INTRAOPERATIVE

**Anesthetic technique:** GETA, or mask GA (for uncomplicated pressure equalization tube placement or myringotomy).

**Induction** In children, inhalation induction with $N_2O$, $O_2$ and halothane is appropriate. In adults or pediatric patients with an established iv line, standard induction (see Appendix) may be used. A RAE tube is helpful in avoiding intrusion onto the surgical field.

**Maintenance** For short cases where an adequate airway can be maintained, use of face mask (or laryngeal mask airway) anesthesia with volatile agents is desirable; otherwise, standard maintenance (see Appendix) is appropriate. In longer cases, opiates may be administered, provided an anti-emetic is used to avoid postop nausea. $N_2O$ should be discontinued at least 1/2 hr before placement of a tympanic membrane graft, as the diffusion of $N_2O$ into closed spaces may unseat the graft. Muscle relaxants should be used to eliminate patient movement during microscopic surgery. In some cases, however, the surgeon may wish to use a nerve stimulator and muscle relaxants should be avoided.

**Emergence** Extubation should be smooth to avoid straining, which may unseat the tympanic membrane graft or disrupt other repairs; hence, deep extubation should be considered in this patient population. This consists of giving a spontaneously breathing patient 3-4% halothane or 2-3% isoflurane or 2-3% desflurane in 100% $O_2$ for 3-5 min; then the airway is inspected using a laryngoscope. If clear, the trachea is extubated with the patient in the tonsillar (lateral) position; and 100% $O_2$ is administered by mask. The anesthesiologist maintains the airway until patient is fully awake. Anti-emetics (e.g., metoclopramide 0.15 mg/kg iv) should be used in cases of middle-ear surgery.

**Blood and fluid requirements** IV: 18 ga x 1 (adult)
20 - 22 ga x 1 (child)
NS/LR @ 2-4 cc/kg/hr

In small children, initial fluid deficit should be replaced with a dextrose-containing solution (e.g., D5 ¼ NS). Blood loss is minimal in these cases.

**Control of bleeding** Head-up position
Injection of epinephrine-containing solutions by surgeon
Deliberate hypotension

These special considerations are applicable to microscopic surgical procedures, where even the smallest quantity of blood may interfere with visualization.

**Monitoring** Standard monitors (see Appendix).

**Positioning** ✓ and pad pressure points.
✓ eyes.
✓ opposite ear.

Surgeon may request unobstructed access to the head. Under those circumstances, a RAE or anode tube should be used to secure airway.

### POSTOPERATIVE

**Complications** N&V
Facial nerve injury

Liberal prophylactic use of anti-emetics is indicated.

**Pain management** Pedi: acetaminophen 15 mg/kg pr
Adult: acetaminophen + codeine po

If patient is npo, the use of iv PCA (morphine sulfate 2-5 mg iv every 10-15 min) is appropriate.

**References**

1. Glasscock ME: *Surgery of the Ear*, 4th edition. Glasscock ME, Shambaugh GE, eds. WB Saunders Co, Philadelphia: 1990.
2. Goycoolea MV, Paparella MM, Nissen RL, eds: *Atlas of Otologic Surgery*. WB Saunders Co, Philadelphia: 1989.
3. Brown BR Jr: *Anesthesia and ENT Surgery*. FA Davis Co, Philadelphia: 1987.
4. Morrison JD: *Anesthesia for Eye, Ear, Nose and Throat Surgery*, 2nd edition. Morrison JD, Mirakhur RK, Craig HJL, eds. Churchill Livingstone, New York: 1985.

# REPAIR OF MAXILLOFACIAL FRACTURES

## SURGICAL CONSIDERATIONS

**Description:** The forces required to produce facial fractures are considerable, and frequently result in other associated trauma (e.g., cervical spine injury, subdural hematoma, pneumothorax, intra-abdominal bleeding). Soft tissue injury to the tongue or larynx can make airway management difficult. When in doubt, a **tracheostomy** under local anesthesia or awake intubation should be considered. In mandible or maxillary fractures, nasal intubation is usually best, because the patient will be placed in intermaxillary fixation (IMF) (teeth brought together via wires or rubber bands) at the conclusion of the procedure. In malar or nasal bone fractures, the fixation may be precarious, making it undesirable to use masked ventilation at the termination of the procedure and necessitating awake extubation. Facial nerve monitoring or observation may be required, contraindicating the use of muscle relaxants. The surgical approach depends very much on the complexity of the fracture. Simple nasal fractures are easily reduced, whereas orbital floor fractures may need a subciliary lower eyelid incision and require an additional **Caldwell-Luc approach** when associated with extensive maxillary bone fractures. Zygomatic and maxillary fractures, commonly fixed with mini-plates, may require IMF. Mandibular fractures are usually reduced and fixed with either wires or dynamic compression plates. When wires are used, the patient is put into IMF postop. If rigid fixation is used for the fracture, one can do away with IMF.

**Usual preop diagnosis:** Facial bone fracture

### SUMMARY OF PROCEDURE

| | |
|---|---|
| **Position** | Supine |
| **Incision** | Depends on facial bones involved in fracture |
| **Special instrumentation** | Wires; plating system; drill |
| **Unique considerations** | ETT needs to be securely anchored, as manipulations may dislodge it. Nasal intubation usually required for maxillary, complex and mandibular fractures, as patient may be fixed in IMF preop. |
| **Antibiotics** | Cefazolin 1 gm, metronidazole 500 mg |
| **Surgical time** | 30 min (for simple manipulations); 2 - 4 hrs (for multiple fractures) |
| **Closing considerations** | May need awake extubation. |
| **EBL** | Minimal – 200-400 cc (if major vessels lacerated by fractures of maxilla) |
| **Postop care** | If patient extubated after procedure and fixed in IMF, wire scissors must be available at all times by patient's bed to release IMF in case of respiratory embarrassment. |
| **Mortality** | Not usually associated unless other major trauma (e.g., base-of-skull fracture, etc.) involved. |
| **Morbidity** | Bleeding: 2-4%<br>Infection: 2%<br>Malocclusion: Uncommon<br>Malunion: Uncommon |
| **Procedure code** | Variable |
| **Pain score** | 2-4, depending on extent of injury and repair |

### PATIENT POPULATION CHARACTERISTICS

| | |
|---|---|
| **Age range** | Children - adults |
| **Male:Female** | 2:1 |
| **Incidence** | Common in urban setting/county hospitals |
| **Etiology** | Trauma: Mostly fights and gunshot wounds |
| **Associated conditions** | Head injury<br>Cervical spine injury<br>Abdominal and limb injury |

## ANESTHETIC CONSIDERATIONS

**(Procedures covered: facial fractures, LeFort ostomies)**

### PREOPERATIVE

Typically, there are two patient populations: 1) healthy, presenting for correction of malocclusion and facial deformities (orthognathic surgery); and 2) trauma patients usually presenting >24 hrs after initial injury. Both groups may present problems with airway management and, therefore, may require awake fiber optic intubation (difficult in the presence of oropharyngeal bleeding). In trauma patients, other injuries should be sought and corrected preop, as appropriate.

| | |
|---|---|
| **Respiratory** | Airway and nasal obstruction following trauma can be extreme, as a result of soft-tissue swelling, and accumulated blood and secretions. The extent of facial fractures, particularly in the mid-face, should be identified as they may preclude nasal intubation. Mandibular fractures may make access to the oropharynx difficult. In the case of massive trauma to the face, urgent tracheostomy should be considered.<br>**Tests:** As indicated from H&P. |

| | | |
|---|---|---|
| **Neurologic** | Intracranial injury may be associated with facial fractures. Patients with head trauma may have ↑ICP; therefore, appropriate methods (e.g., $CO_2$↓, fluid↓, smooth induction/intubation) are used to prevent further ↑ICP. Basilar skull fractures preclude passage of nasotracheal and NG tubes. In the presence of otorrhea or rhinorrhea, positive-pressure mask ventilation is inadvisable, due to the potential for causing pneumocephalus.<br>**Tests:** Review skull and C-spine x-rays. | |
| **Musculoskeletal** | Cervical spine injuries are commonly associated with facial injuries. The C-spine should be cleared by x-ray exam prior to transport to OR. If C-spine cannot be cleared, intubation should be done with the head in a neutral position (splinted or with axial traction), using direct FOL. | |
| **Hematologic** | Maxillary surgery may be associated with major blood loss and, for elective cases, autologous donation should be encouraged.<br>**Tests:** Hct | |
| **Laboratory** | Tests as indicated from H&P. | |
| **Premedication** | Trauma patients should be considered to have full stomachs, and sedative premedications are best avoided. Aspiration prophylaxis with 0.3 M Na citrate (30 cc po), ± metoclopramide 10 mg iv ± ranitidine 50 mg iv, should be considered. Standard premedication (see Appendix) is appropriate for non-trauma patients with normal airways. | |

## INTRAOPERATIVE

**Anesthetic technique:** The majority of patients presenting for elective procedures are healthy and have normal airways. In the case of facial trauma, however, intubation of the trachea may be impossible. Hence, a tracheostomy under local anesthesia may be life-saving.

| | |
|---|---|
| **Induction** | For elective cases, use standard induction (see Appendix). Under emergent circumstances, a rapid-sequence induction with cricoid pressure should be used, if the airway is easy to manage; otherwise, an awake FOL is indicated. |
| **Maintenance** | Standard maintenance (see Appendix). |
| **Emergence** | The return of airway reflexes is mandatory before extubation. In some cases, the patient may have the mandible and maxilla wired together, making airway access difficult. Wire cutters should be readily available. Use of an anti-emetic (e.g., metoclopramide 10 mg iv, ondansetron 4 mg iv or droperidol 0.625 mg iv) to avoid postop N&V is important. |

| | | |
|---|---|---|
| **Blood and fluid requirements** | 1° iv: 16-18 ga<br>2° iv: 18 ga or larger<br>NS/LR @ 2-4 cc/kg/hr<br>Trauma: NS/LR @ 6-8 cc/kg/hr | Blood loss from facial fractures or orthognathic procedures can be extensive. T&C patient so blood is immediately available in OR. |
| **Control of blood loss** | Surgical hemostasis<br>Topical vasoconstrictors<br>Posterior oropharyngeal packing<br>Controlled hypotension | Surgical hemostasis should control most bleeding in these procedures. Topical vasoconstrictors such as phenylephrine or cocaine can be applied on the surgical field. Posterior oropharyngeal packing can keep blood from passing undetected into the upper GI tract. Controlled ↓BP can be achieved simply by increasing volatile anesthetic levels. |
| **Monitoring** | Standard monitors (see Appendix).<br>± Arterial line | An arterial line is required for controlled hypotension, and may be useful in emergency cases. |
| **Complications** | ETT damage 2° surgical manipulation | In case of ETT damage, be prepared to reestablish the airway rapidly by re-intubation, usually over an intubating stylet or gum elastic bougie. |

## POSTOPERATIVE

| | | |
|---|---|---|
| **Complications** | Need for airway access | Wire cutters should be available for patients whose jaws are wired together. |
| | Ingestion of blood with subsequent vomiting and aspiration | Vomiting and aspiration of swallowed blood can complicate postop period. Anti-emetics should be used. |
| **Pain management** | PCA (see Appendix). | |

References

1. Meyerhoff WL, Maisel RH, Hilger PA: *Fractures of the Facial Skeleton: A Manual.* American Academy of Otolaryngology, Rochester, MN: 1980.
2. Brown BR Jr: *Anesthesia and ENT Surgery.* FA Davis Co, Philadelphia: 1987.
3. Morrison JD: *Anesthesia for Eye, Ear, Nose and Throat Surgery*, 2nd edition. Morrison JD, Mirakhur RK, Craig HJL, eds. Churchill Livingstone, New York: 1985.

# PAROTIDECTOMY: SUPERFICIAL, TOTAL, RADICAL

## SURGICAL CONSIDERATIONS

**Description:** A **superficial parotidectomy** (better called a **supra-neural parotidectomy**) removes all of the parotid gland lateral to the facial nerve, dissecting and protecting the facial nerve (Fig 3-5). It is usually performed for a tumor, but occasionally is performed for infectious disorders or to enable the surgeon to approach tumors of the deep lobe.

A **total parotidectomy** is performed for either infectious disorders or for tumors that arise in the parotid gland medial to the facial nerve. The integrity of the facial nerve is preserved during total parotidectomy, as long as it is not involved with malignancy. It may be combined with neck dissection (radical or functional) or with modified temporal bone resections when the tumor extends into the ear canal or middle ear or invades the facial nerve at the base of the skull.

A **radical parotidectomy** removes the total parotid gland, together with the facial nerve, which usually is reconstructed with a facial-nerve graft. The mastoid may have to be drilled to get a healthy proximal end of the facial nerve. **Microsurgical techniques** are then used to graft the resected nerve. The graft may be harvested from the opposite greater auricular nerve or the sural nerve may be used.

**Usual preop diagnosis**: Superficial parotidectomy: benign or malignant tumor of the superficial lobe of the parotid gland; infectious disorders. Total parotidectomy: malignant tumors or benign tumors of the deep lobe of the parotid gland. Radical parotidectomy: invasive malignant parotid tumors.

### SUMMARY OF PROCEDURE

| | Superficial | Total | Radical |
|---|---|---|---|
| **Position** | Supine; head turned slightly to opposite side | ⇐ | ⇐ |
| **Incision** | Pre-auricular, extending into neck; has many variations, including modified face-lift incision. | ⇐ | May require post-aural extension for mastoid access. |
| **Special instrumentation** | Facial nerve stimulator, facial nerve monitor | ⇐ | ⇐ + Drill for mastoidectomy; microscope/microsurgical instruments and 9-0 nylon for nerve re-anastomosis |
| **Unique considerations** | Muscle relaxation is not indicated 2° facial nerve identification. Tape oral ETT to the opposite side of the mandible. | Nasal intubation may be necessary to dislocate mandible anteriorly. Be certain that the ETT is well below vocal cords to allow for anterior dislocation → 1-2 cm of superior ascent of ETT. | ⇐ |
| **Antibiotics** | None or cefazolin 1 gm | Cefazolin 1 gm | ⇐ |
| **Surgical time** | 1.5 - 2 hrs | 2 - 4 hrs | 4 - 6 hrs |

| | Superficial | Total | Radical |
|---|---|---|---|
| **EBL** | 25-200 cc | 200-300 cc | 500-700 cc for total parotidectomy, neck dissection and modified temporal bone resection. Sudden, large blood losses do not occur; transfusion usually not necessary. |
| **Mortality** | Very rare | ⇐ | ⇐ |
| **Morbidity** | Dysesthesia or anesthesia of the greater auricular nerve: 100% (almost all will recover within 1 yr).<br>Facial nerve weakness (temporary): 20-50%<br>Frey's syndrome: 35% will have measurable gustatory sweating, but only 5% will have clinical symptoms.<br>Bleeding: 4%<br>Infection: 4%<br>Permanent facial nerve paralysis: < 1% | ⇐ | Facial nerve loss: With graft, function returns slowly over 1 yr. |
| **Procedure code** | 42415 | 42420 | 42425; 64864/42420 (includes facial nerve grafting) |
| **Pain score** | 2-3 | 3-4 | 4-6 |

### PATIENT POPULATION CHARACTERISTICS

| | |
|---|---|
| **Age range** | Infants - old age |
| **Male:Female** | 1:1 |
| **Incidence** | Common |
| **Etiology** | Benign mixed tumor (pleomorphic adenoma): 75%<br>Variety of low- to high-grade malignant cancers: 25%<br>Chronic sialoadenitis (results from ductal strictures and/or stones): Rare |
| **Associated conditions** | Non-specific |

---

## ANESTHETIC CONSIDERATIONS

See Anesthetic Considerations following "Submandibular Gland Excision" (below).

---

**References**

1. Thawley SE, Panje WR, eds: *Comprehensive Management of Head and Neck Tumors*. WB Saunders Co, Philadelphia: 1987.
2. Terris DJ, Fee WE: Current Issues in Nerve Repair. *Arch Otolaryngol. Head Neck Surg* (In Press).

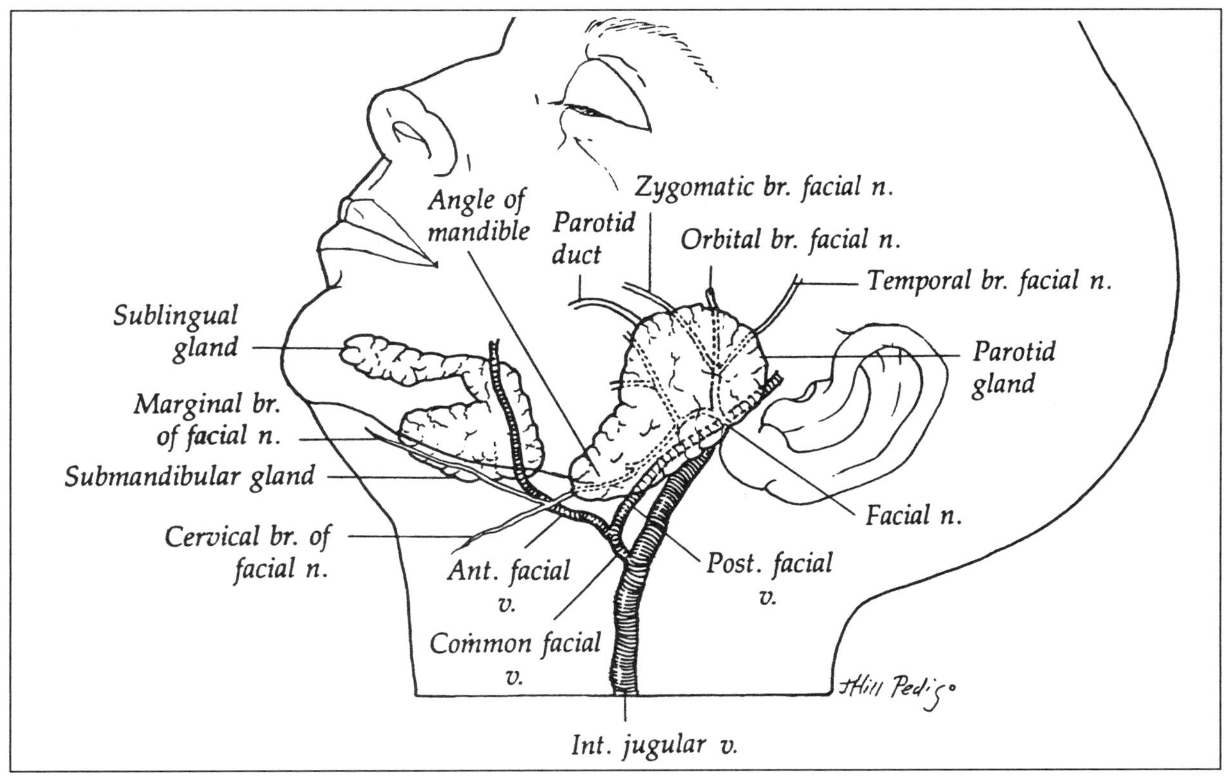


**Figure 3-5.** Relationship of parotid gland and neurovascular structures. (Reproduced with permission from Ballenger JJ: *Diseases of the Nose, Throat, Ear, Head & Neck.* Lea & Febiger: 1991.)

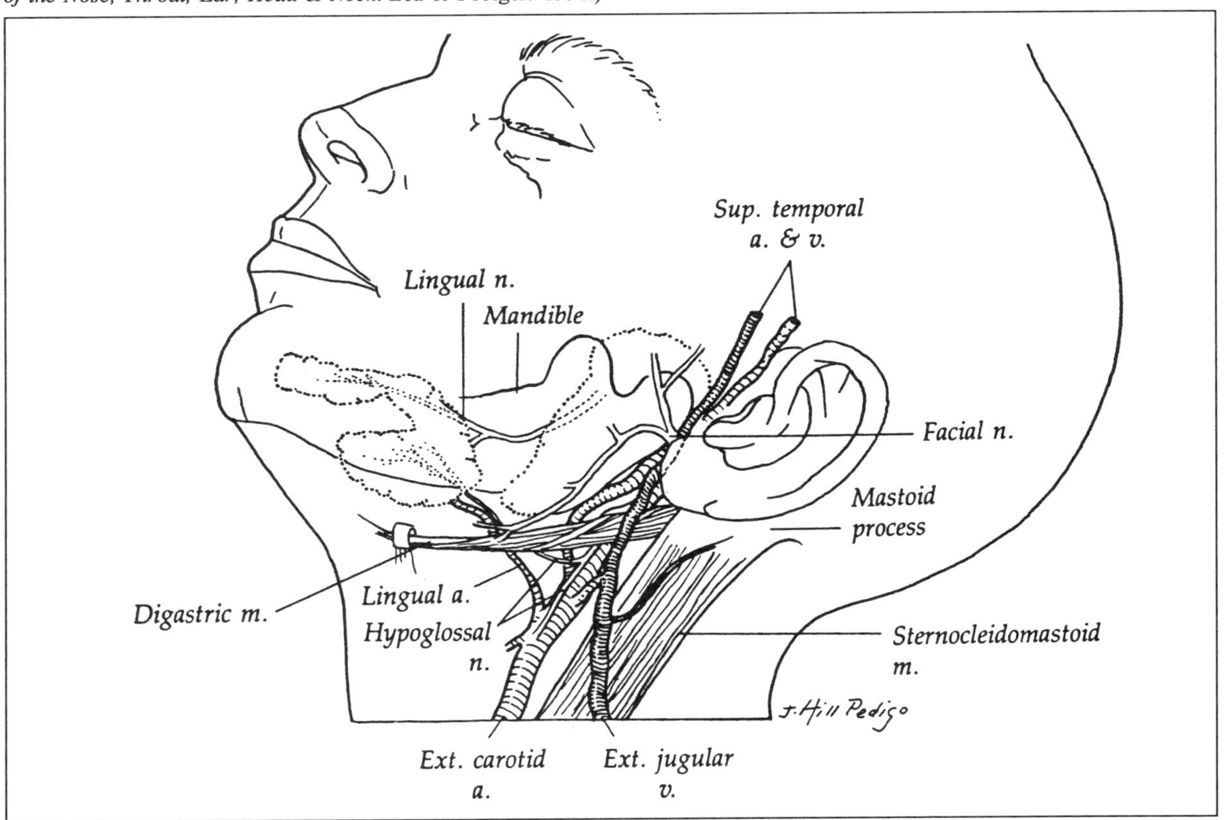


**Figure 3-6.** Relationship of submandibular gland and adjunct structures. (Reproduced with permission from Ballenger JJ: *Diseases of the Nose, Throat, Ear, Head & Neck.* Lea & Febiger: 1991.)

# SUBMANDIBULAR GLAND EXCISION

## SURGICAL CONSIDERATIONS

**Description:** Removal of the submandibular gland is performed for either chronic sialoadenitis due to ductal strictures and/or stones or benign or malignant tumors of the submandibular gland. (General anatomy of the area is shown in Fig 3-6.) The patient lies supine with a pillow under the shoulder and head turned slightly to the opposite side. A skin crease incision is made below the mandible and skin flaps elevated. The marginal mandibular nerve is usually carefully identified or may be avoided by identifying the facial vein and dissecting deep to its plane, employing the so-called **Hayes-Martin maneuver**. Dissection is carried out within the capsule of the submandibular gland, which is then excised and removed. Frozen section usually is performed and, if necessary, further excision, including a neck dissection for high-grade malignancies, is done.

**Variant procedure or approaches:** Occasionally, it may be necessary to perform a **neck dissection** (radical or functional) in the case of high-grade malignancy.

**Usual preop diagnosis:** Chronic sialoadenitis; stones; benign or malignant tumors

### SUMMARY OF PROCEDURE

| | |
|---|---|
| **Position** | Supine |
| **Incision** | Upper neck skin crease |
| **Special instrumentation** | Occasionally, facial nerve stimulator |
| **Unique considerations** | If surgeon plans to use facial nerve stimulator, muscle relaxation is not indicated. |
| **Antibiotics** | Usually not indicated |
| **Surgical time** | 0.5 - 1 hr |
| **EBL** | 25 cc (400 cc if neck dissection is done) |
| **Postop care** | PACU → room or home |
| **Mortality** | Minimal |
| **Morbidity** | Marginal mandibular nerve paresis or paralysis: 20%<br>Bleeding: 4%<br>Infection: 4%<br>Lingual dysesthesia: 1%<br>XIIth nerve paresis or paralysis: < 1% |
| **Procedure code** | 42440 |
| **Pain score** | 2-4 |

### PATIENT POPULATION CHARACTERISTICS

| | |
|---|---|
| **Age range** | Unlimited |
| **Male:Female** | 1:1 |
| **Incidence** | Rare |
| **Etiology** | Chronic infection<br>Neoplasia: ~60% of tumors are benign, with the remaining being low- and high-grade malignancies. |
| **Associated conditions** | Non-specific |

---

## ANESTHETIC CONSIDERATIONS

**(Procedures covered: parotidectomy, submandibular gland excision)**

### PREOPERATIVE

Diseases of the parotid gland have been associated with the use of alcohol and autoimmune disease; therefore, Sx of alcohol abuse and alcohol-related diseases should be sought.

| | |
|---|---|
| **Respiratory** | Rarely, the submandibular gland may be enlarged enough to cause upper respiratory tract obstruction. Evaluate airway carefully and consider FOL.<br>**Tests:** As indicated from H&P. |
| **Neurological** | Surgical approach to the parotid gland will place the facial nerve at jeopardy; thus, all preop facial nerve deficits should be documented. Note Sx of alcohol abuse, since chronic alcohol intake may cause hepatic enzyme induction with increased anesthetic requirement. Sx of alcohol withdrawal should be controlled prior to surgery in consultation with the patient's primary physician. |
| **Hematologic** | Submandibular and parotid malignancies may be associated with chronic debilitation and anemia.<br>**Tests:** Hb |
| **Laboratory** | Other tests as indicated from H&P. |
| **Premedication** | Standard premedication (see Appendix). |

### INTRAOPERATIVE

**Anesthetic technique:** GETA

| | | |
|---|---|---|
| **Induction** | Standard induction (see Appendix). Should tumor extend into upper respiratory tract, however, a tracheostomy under local anesthesia or fiber optic intubation should be considered. ETT should be secured on the non-operative side. | |
| **Maintenance** | Standard maintenance (see Appendix). Muscle relaxants should be avoided if nerve stimulation is done for facial nerve preservation. If muscle relaxants are used, very short-acting agents, such as mivacurium (0.15 mg/kg), should be used and coordinated with the surgeons so that adequate nerve-stimulation tests can be performed. | |
| **Emergence** | No special considerations | |
| **Blood and fluid requirements** | IV: 18 ga x 1<br>NS/LR @ 3-6 ml/kg/hr | |
| **Monitoring** | Standard monitors (see Appendix). | Invasive monitoring may be indicated, depending on patient's general health. |
| **Positioning** | Table may be rotated 90°-180°. | Extension tubes for the anesthesia circuit should be available. |

### POSTOPERATIVE

| | | |
|---|---|---|
| **Complications** | Facial paralysis 2° surgical trauma | Notify surgeons. |
| **Pain management** | PCA (see Appendix).<br>Parenteral opiates (see Appendix). | |


**References**

1. Johns ME, Price JC, Mattox DE: *Atlas of Head and Neck Surgery.* BC Decker, Philadelphia: 1990.
2. Brown BR Jr: *Anesthesia and ENT Surgery.* FA Davis Co, Philadelphia: 1987.
3. Morrison JD: *Anesthesia for Eye, Ear, Nose and Throat Surgery*, 2nd edition. Morrison JD, Mirakhur RK, Craig HJL, eds. Churchill Livingstone, New York: 1985.


# NECK DISSECTION: FUNCTIONAL, MODIFIED RADICAL, RADICAL

## SURGICAL CONSIDERATIONS

**Description:** A **radical neck dissection** consists of a complete **cervical lymphadenectomy**, together with the resection of the sternocleidomastoid muscle, IJ vein and cranial nerve XI. A **modified neck dissection** is a variation between a functional neck dissection and a radical neck dissection, and includes supraomohyoid neck dissection, posterior neck dissection, anterior neck dissection, etc. A **functional neck dissection** is a complete cervical lymphadenectomy, preserving the sternocleidomastoid muscle, IJ vein and cranial nerve XI. Neck dissections are seldom performed as isolated surgical procedures; usually they are combined with resection of the primary lesion such as tongue, pharynx, larynx, etc.

Typically, the neck dissection is performed through 1 or 2 horizontal neck incisions – occasionally extending vertically to expose the neck from the mandible down to the clavicle. The procedure usually begins with transection of the sternocleidomastoid muscle at its sternal attachment, if this muscle is to be removed. The IJ vein is isolated, cut and tied (again, if it is to be removed). The inferior portion of the dissection includes identification and preservation of the brachial plexus, the phrenic nerve, the vagus nerve and the carotid artery. As the dissection specimen is swept superiorly, cervical sensory branches are divided. The accessory nerve (XI) is identified and carefully preserved. When the digastric muscle is encountered, the submandibular portion of the dissection is complete. The hypoglossal nerve (XII) and lingual nerve are identified and preserved. The submental triangle may or may not be resected. The specimen is attached at the skull base and after retraction of the digastric muscle, the IJ vein is ligated and cut at the skull base. The sternocleidomastoid muscle is divided at the mastoid and the specimen is removed. Drains are placed posteriorly, and the wound is closed in layers.

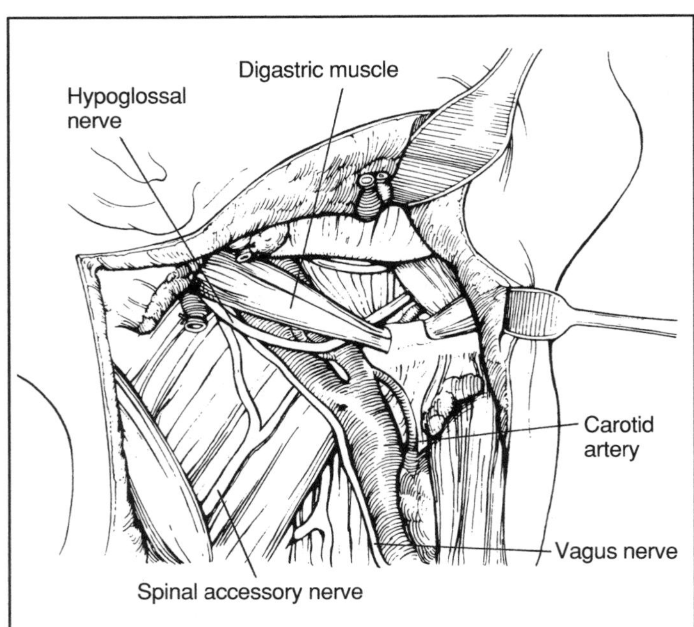


**Figure 3-7.** Surgical field after completion of accessory nerve-sparing neck dissection. (Reproduced with permission from Thawley SE, Panje WR, et al, eds: *Comprehensive Management of Head and Neck Tumors*. WB Saunders Co: 1987.)

**Variant procedure or approaches:** In a **composite resection ("commando,"** a radical neck dissection + partial mandibulectomy ± partial glossectomy), the neck dissection normally is done first, and an attempt is made to keep the neck specimen in continuity with the primary resection. Although the upper limb of the neck incision is commonly extended through the chin and lip to gain exposure to the oral cavity and oropharynx, this is not necessary. A combination of intraoral exposure and external approach through the neck incision is sufficient to visualize the primary lesion, and resect it, usually with a segment of mandible. The resultant defect is closed either primarily, with a split-thickness skin graft, or with a chest flap (pectoralis major or deltopectoral). More recently, free flaps may be brought in for closure and revascularized using the facial artery or superior thyroid artery. A **tracheostomy** is almost always performed as part of a composite resection.

**Usual preop diagnosis:** Cancer of the mouth, oropharynx or tonsil, with documented or suspected spread from a primary source to the cervical lymph nodes

**SUMMARY OF PROCEDURE**

| | Functional | Modified Radical | Radical |
|---|---|---|---|
| **Position** | Supine; head turned to opposite side; pillow below shoulders | ⇐ | ⇐ |
| **Incision** | Various neck incisions (e.g., utility, McFee, lip split, etc.), depending on site of primary. | ⇐ | ⇐ |
| **Unique considerations** | If neck dissection performed on opposite side, significant laryngeal edema may ensue, necessitating tracheostomy. | If cranial nerve XI is dissected/preserved, nerve stimulator may be needed, so muscle relaxation is undesirable. | Rarely, carotid artery needs to be resected or resected/reconstructed, making vascular instruments desirable. |

| | Functional | Modified Radical | Radical |
|---|---|---|---|
| | Dissection around the carotid bulb may result in profound bradycardia, responsive to local anesthetic injection of the bulb and/or iv atropine. | ⇐ | ⇐ |
| **Antibiotics** | Cefazolin 1 gm iv (+ metronidazole 500 mg if aerodigestive mucosa is involved). | ⇐ | ⇐ |
| **Surgical time** | Neck dissection: 1.5 - 3 hrs<br>With resection of primary and reconstruction: 3 - 6 hrs | ⇐ | ⇐ |
| **EBL** | Neck dissection: 150-200 cc | ⇐ | ⇐ |
| | Post-radiated patients: 200-400 cc | ⇐ | ⇐ |
| | If primary is also resected: 400-700 cc | ⇐ | ⇐ |
| | If flap reconstructions are required: 700-1200 cc | ⇐ | ⇐<br>Uncontrolled bleeding of IJ vein at skull base (rare) can be problematic, resulting in sudden large blood losses. Usually can be controlled by surgeon with digital pressure, allowing anesthesiologist to prepare for increasing fluid volume or transfusion. |
| **Postop care** | Routine ward care for neck dissection; tracheostomy care if opposite neck also dissected. ICU overnight if 6-8 hrs' operating time. | ⇐ | ⇐ |
| **Mortality** | Rare | ⇐ | ⇐ |
| **Morbidity** | Bleeding | ⇐ | ⇐ |
| | Infection | ⇐ | Painful shoulder syndrome: 20% |
| | Cranial nerve injury | ⇐ | |
| | Chyle leak | ⇐ | |
| **Procedure code** | 38700 | 38724 | 38720 |
| **Pain score** | 4-6 (Depending on 1° site, pain score may be 6-8.) | 6-8 | 6-8 |

### PATIENT POPULATION CHARACTERISTICS

| | |
|---|---|
| **Age range** | Adults |
| **Male:Female** | 3:1 |
| **Incidence** | Common |
| **Etiology** | Head and neck tumors |
| **Associated conditions** | COPD<br>Atherosclerosis |

## ANESTHETIC CONSIDERATIONS

See Anesthetic Considerations following "Glossectomy" (below).

**References**

1. MacComb WS: Mortality from radical neck dissection. *Am J Surg* 1968; 115(3):352-54.
2. Reed GF, Rabuzzi DD: Neck dissection. *Otolaryngol Clin North Am* 1969; 2:547-63.

# LARYNGECTOMY: TOTAL, SUPRAGLOTTIC, HEMI

## SURGICAL CONSIDERATIONS

**Description:** A **total laryngectomy** involves removal of the vallecula (or, if necessary, the posterior third of the tongue) to the first or second tracheal rings. An apron flap incision allows exposure in a subplatysmal plane from the hyoid bone to the clavicle. A **tracheostomy** is performed and an anode tube placed. The strap muscles are divided inferiorly and the hyoid bone is skeletonized. The thyroid gland is resected away from the trachea, unless it is to be included in the specimen. Typically, the larynx is transected just above the hyoid bone, and the specimen is removed. The pharynx is closed in a T-shape and the trachea is brought out to the skin as an end-tracheostomy. No ET or tracheostomy tube is required.

A **supraglottic laryngectomy** involves resection of the larynx from the ventricle to the base of tongue, leaving the true cords. The exposure is similar to that for a total laryngectomy; however, the strap muscles are preserved intact. Once the thyroid cartilage is exposed, subperichondrial flaps are elevated off of the thyroid lamina, and used later for reconstruction. Cuts are made either with a knife or saw through the mid-thyroid cartilage at a level just above the true vocal cords and completed at the base of tongue. The specimen includes the false vocal cords and supraglottic larynx, the epiglottis and a portion of the base of tongue. Closure is obtained by approximating the thyroid perichondrium to the base of tongue and then the strap muscles also to the base of tongue. A temporary tracheostomy is required.

A **hemilaryngectomy** (also called a **vertical partial laryngectomy**) involves removal of a unilateral true and false cord, retaining the epiglottis and opposite side true and false cord, with various methods of reconstruction. The exposure required for a hemilaryngectomy is similar to that for a supraglottic laryngectomy. A perichondrial flap is similarly raised; however, it is limited to the ipsilateral thyroid lamina. Cuts on the ipsilateral thyroid cartilage are made with either a knife or saw and the anterior commissure is divided with Pott's scissors. After the tumor is resected, closure is obtained utilizing the thyroid perichondrium. Typically, the sternohyoid muscle is used to reconstruct the vocal cord. The wound is then closed in layers and drains are placed. Again, a tracheostomy is required.

A **near-total laryngectomy** involves removal of all of the larynx except for one arytenoid in constructing a phonatory shunt for speaking. All of the techniques involve creation of a temporary or permanent **tracheostomy**, and may be combined with **neck dissection** (radical or functional) and with partial or total **pharyngectomy**, which necessitates flap reconstruction.

**Usual preop diagnosis:** Cancer of larynx; intractable aspiration, with resultant pneumonia unresponsive to other techniques

**SUMMARY OF PROCEDURE**

| | Total | Supraglottic | Hemi |
|---|---|---|---|
| **Position** | Supine | ⇐ | ⇐ |
| **Incision** | Various neck incisions, depending on whether or not reconstruction is anticipated, and requirements of neck dissection. | Horizontal | ⇐ |
| **Special instrumentation** | Major head/neck set; headlights; sterile anesthesia connecting tubes; 6 Fr anode tube; No 8 and No 10 cuffed laryngectomy tubes | ⇐ | Newborn Finochetto rib retractor |

| | Total | Supraglottic | Hemi |
|---|---|---|---|
| **Unique considerations** | Tumors of the larynx necessarily produce distortion of the airway and, occasionally, a compromised airway prior to onset of anesthesia. A patient with compromised airway is probably best-treated by tracheostomy under local anesthesia prior to the start of GA. Intubation can be exceedingly difficult. | ⇐ | ⇐ |
| **Antibiotics** | Cefazolin 1 gm; metronidazole 500 mg | ⇐ | ⇐ |
| **Surgical time** | 2 - 6 hrs | ⇐ | Rarely is neck dissection necessary. |
| **EBL** | Total laryngectomy: 200-300 cc<br>Total laryngectomy with neck dissection: 500-700 cc<br>Total laryngectomy, pharyngectomy and flap reconstruction: 700-1200 cc.<br>Sudden large blood losses do not occur; transfusion usually is not necessary. | ⇐ | 25-100 cc |
| **Postop care** | Suctioning of tracheal secretions as in tracheostomy. | ⇐ | ⇐ |
| **Mortality** | < 1% | ⇐ | ⇐ |
| **Morbidity** | Fistula (radiation salvage): 20% | 1% | ⇐ |
| | Fistula formation (un-irradiated): 5% | – | |
| | Bleeding: 4% | ⇐ | |
| | Infection: 4% | ⇐ | |
| **Procedure code** | 31360 | 31367 | 31370 |
| **Pain score** | 4-6 | 4-6 | 4-6 |

### PATIENT POPULATION CHARACTERISTICS

| | |
|---|---|
| **Age range** | 40-80 yrs |
| **Male:Female** | 3:1 |
| **Incidence** | Common |
| **Etiology** | Smoking<br>Alcohol |
| **Associated conditions** | COPD<br>Atherosclerosis |

## ANESTHETIC CONSIDERATIONS

See Anesthetic Considerations following "Glossectomy" (below).

**References**


1. Roberson JB Jr, Fee WE Jr: Conservation surgery for laryngeal carcinoma. *Ann Acad Med Singapore* 1991; 20(5):656-64.
2. Friedman M, ed: Laryngeal Surgery. *Operative Techniques in Otolaryngology/Head and Neck Surgery* 1990; 1(1):1-82.

# GLOSSECTOMY

## SURGICAL CONSIDERATIONS

**Description:** **Glossectomy**, either **partial** or **total**, is performed for neoplastic lesions of the tongue. During this procedure, nasal intubation is helpful, but not mandatory. On the other hand, complete relaxation, is necessary. Additionally, a drying agent such as scopolamine or glycopyrrolate helps reduce oral secretions and facilitates surgery. A side-biting or Dingman mouth gag is used to gain adequate surgical exposure. The lesion is resected with electrocautery and can usually be closed primarily. Depending on the extent of resection, and location on the tongue, a **tracheostomy** may be indicated, or oral intubation alone may suffice, for a period of 24-48 hrs. If neither is done, a short course of steroids helps reduce the lingual edema. A NG tube is placed for postop feeding. A **total glossectomy** is performed in similar fashion, but is frequently combined with a **laryngectomy** because of the aspiration that ensues.

**Variant procedure or approaches:** Glossectomy may be done with a **neck dissection** or **mandibulectomy** and, on occasion, also may be combined with a **total laryngectomy**.

**Usual preop diagnosis:** Neoplastic disease of the tongue or adjacent structures (e.g., alveolus, floor of mouth), with involvement of the tongue

### SUMMARY OF PROCEDURE

| | Partial | Total |
|---|---|---|
| **Position** | Supine | ⇐ |
| **Incision** | Intra-oral | ⇐ + Suprahyoid approach/neck approach |
| **Special instrumentation** | Dingman mouth gag | ⇐ |
| **Unique considerations** | Hypotensive anesthesia<br>Nasal intubation<br>Postop tracheostomy<br>Steroids, if a tracheostomy will not be performed. | ⇐ |
| **Antibiotics** | Cefazolin 1 gm, metronidazole 500 mg | ⇐ |
| **Surgical time** | 30 min - 1 hr | 2 - 4 hrs |
| **Closing considerations** | Usually primary closure. May keep patient intubated 24-48 hrs if minimal tongue edema expected. | Flap repair required; laryngeal suspension usually required. Tracheostomy mandatory postop. |
| **EBL** | 50-100 cc | 200-400 cc |
| **Postop care** | Intubated 24-48 hrs | Tracheostomy care |
| **Mortality** | < 1% | ⇐ |
| **Morbidity** | Bleeding<br>Infection<br>Aspiration | Aspiration<br>Bleeding<br>Infection |
| **Procedure code** | 41120 (partial glossectomy); 41130 (hemiglossectomy) | 41140 |
| **Pain score** | 1-2 | 2-4 |

### PATIENT POPULATION CHARACTERISTICS

| | |
|---|---|
| **Age range** | Adults |
| **Male:Female** | 3:1 |
| **Incidence** | Uncommon |
| **Etiology** | Neoplasia |
| **Associated conditions** | Non-specific |

# ANESTHETIC CONSIDERATIONS

**(Procedures covered: radial neck dissection, laryngectomy, glossectomy)**

## PREOPERATIVE

A radical neck dissection generally is done for carcinomas of the head and neck. Since ENT malignancies are commonly associated with the chronic use of tobacco and alcohol, which may lead to significant cardiopulmonary disorders, evidence of physiologic alterations related to this abuse should be sought. In addition, these patients may be malnourished, suffer from Sx of alcohol withdrawal, and present problems in airway management. A laryngectomy is frequently preceded by panendoscopy and tracheostomy (see appropriate sections).

**Airway** Tumor or edema may distort normal anatomy and compromise the airway. These changes may become more pronounced with the induction of anesthesia. A CXR may show tracheal deviation. Flow volume loops can show characteristic patterns of obstruction. Lesions of the upper airway, previous surgery and prior XRT may impede intubation and ventilation. Review of preop indirect and direct laryngoscopies and/or CT scan may be helpful in planning intubation. Preliminary tracheostomy may be required in cases of significant compromise.

**Respiratory** Smoking (>40 pack-years) may cause impaired respiratory function, and COPD is common, with ↓$FEV_1$, ↓FVC or $FEV_1$/FVC ratio; and ABGs may demonstrate hypoxemia and/or $CO_2$ retention.
**Tests:** CXR; PFT; baseline ABG – as indicated from H&P.

**Cardiovascular** Since tobacco use raises incidence of heart disease, assess exercise tolerance. Note Sx of CAD (e.g., angina) and CHF (e.g., orthopnea, PND, peripheral edema) in patients with cardiac risk factors (e.g., age >40 yrs, male gender, HTN, hypercholesteremia, smoking, obesity, family Hx).
**Tests:** ECG; CXR; treadmill stress test; ECHO, if indicated.

**Neurologic** Look for Sx of alcohol abuse. Patients may have increased anesthetic requirements because of hepatic enzyme induction. Alcohol withdrawal seizures may occur. Signs of alcohol withdrawal (e.g., tremulousness, increased sympathetic activity and altered mental status) should be sought.
**Tests:** Hepatic function tests, if indicated from H&P.

**Hematologic** In cases of malignancy or chronic disease, anemia or coagulopathies may be present.
**Tests:** Hb; PT; PTT; platelet count

**Laboratory** Other tests as indicated from H&P.

**Premedication** Standard premedication (see Appendix). A pre-induction drying agent (e.g., glycopyrrolate 0.2 mg iv) facilitates panendoscopy prior to a laryngectomy. Consider contraindications such as ↑HR in patients with CAD.

## INTRAOPERATIVE

**Anesthetic technique:** GETA

**Induction** With a normal airway, standard induction (see Appendix) is appropriate. In cases with the potential for airway obstruction, an awake FOL under topical and transtracheal anesthesia should be performed. Efforts to maintain spontaneous ventilation prior to intubation are paramount. Occasionally, a tracheostomy under local anesthesia may be necessary to manage a severely compromised airway.

**Maintenance** Standard maintenance (see Appendix). Muscle relaxants should be avoided if nerve stimulation is done for facial nerve localization. If muscle relaxants are used, short-acting agents, such as atracurium or mivacurium, are indicated and coordinated with the surgeons so that adequate nerve stimulation tests can be performed. If the procedure includes a tracheostomy or laryngectomy, it is prudent to give the patient 100% $O_2$ before removing the oral ETT. Following tracheostomy, a sterile anode tube with breathing circuit is inserted and connected by the surgeon. The anode tube is frequently sutured to the chest wall to ensure stability. ✓ bilateral breath sounds, airway compliance and $ETCO_2$ waveform to ensure correct placement of tube.

**Emergence** Typically no special considerations. Many patients will have a tracheostomy. Gradual emergence allows maintenance of baseline hemodynamic parameters, very important in patients with CAD.

**Blood and fluid requirements**

Moderate blood loss
1° iv: 16 ga or larger
2° iv: 18 ga or larger
NS/LR @ 3-5 cc/kg/hr
Fluid warmer and humidifier

Blood loss may be massive if the jugular vein or carotid artery are damaged. T&C patient so blood will be immediately available in OR. Initial blood loss may be replaced with NS/LR.

| | | |
|---|---|---|
| **Control of blood loss** | Surgical hemostasis<br>Topical vasoconstrictors<br>Deliberate hypotension<br>Head-up tilt 30° | Hemostasis is the primary means of blood-loss control. Vasoconstrictive agents (e.g., phenylephrine or epinephrine) used topically, can be helpful. Deliberate hypotension utilizing a volatile anesthetic or SNP may be useful. |
| **Monitoring** | Standard monitors (see Appendix).<br>± Arterial line<br>Foley catheter<br>CVP line | An arterial line is useful in the course of a neck dissection (serial Hct, ABG, electrolytes, etc.); it is required for the use of deliberate hypotension. CVP, if indicted by coexisting disease (basilic/cephalic vein preferred). |
| **Positioning** | Usually supine, head elevated 30°.<br>Table turned 180°<br>✓ and pad pressure points.<br>✓ and pad eyes. | Extension tubes should be available. |
| **Complications** | Vagal reflexes → ↓HR and ↓BP | Rx: stop surgery; iv atropine; lidocaine infiltration by surgeons. Prepare for CPR. |
| | Dysrhythmias | When dysrhythmias are detected, surgeon should stop manipulation of the carotid sinus region. Atropine may be used for marked bradycardia. Infiltration of the surgical field with local anesthetic may blunt or ablate further episodes. |
| | ↑Q-T interval | Interruption of cervical sympathetic outflow to heart (with right radical neck dissection) → ECG changes. |
| **VAE** | ↓$ETCO_2$<br>↓BP<br>↓ST segment<br>"Mill wheel" murmur<br>Dysrhythmias | With large veins open in the neck, VAE is possible, and may account for unexplained hypotension and/or dysrhythmia. Rx: notify surgeon, flood field with NS, head down, aspirate CVP, 100% $O_2$ circulatory support (fluid, pressors, as required). |

## POSTOPERATIVE

| | | |
|---|---|---|
| **Complications** | Nerve injury | Facial nerve injury can cause facial droop. Recurrent laryngeal nerve injury can result in vocal cord dysfunction. The phrenic nerve also may pass in the surgical |
| | Diaphragmatic paralysis | field and respiratory problems may develop if diaphragmatic paralysis occurs. |
| | Pneumothorax | Pneumothorax may occur with low neck dissection. Dx: ↑RR, ↓BP, ↑CVP, wheezing, ↓$O_2$ saturation, SOB, chest pain, ↓breath sounds, ↓ECG amplitude, dullness on percussion CXR. Rx: chest tube or needle aspiration, 100% $O_2$, ventilation and volume expansion.<br>Agitation ↑$PaCO_2$, ↓$PaO_2$, ↑HR. Rx: ✓ restrictive neck dressings; evacuate hematoma; reestablish airway with ETT; 100% $O_2$; ventilate patient as required. |
| **Pain management** | PCA (see Appendix).<br>Parenteral opiates (see Appendix). | |
| **Tests** | CXR<br>ECG | CXR for position of tracheostomy tube and evidence of pneumothorax; ECG for diagnosis of rhythm disturbances. |

### References


1. Brown BR Jr: *Anesthesia and ENT Surgery*. FA Davis Co, Philadelphia: 1987.
2. Morrison JD: *Anesthesia for Eye, Ear, Nose and Throat Surgery*, 2nd edition. Morrison JD, Mirakhur RK, Craig HJL, eds. Churchill Livingstone, New York: 1985.

# MAXILLECTOMY

## SURGICAL CONSIDERATIONS

**Description:** Maxillectomy is performed for benign or malignant neoplastic lesions of the maxillary sinuses. There are two basic types of this procedure: (1) **partial maxillectomy** and (2) **total maxillectomy**, with or without orbital exenteration, depending on tumor extent. Dental obturator is usually fitted immediately after the surgical resection. A Weber-Ferguson incision is made along the nasofacial groove and ala, exposing the face of the maxilla. An intraoral Caldwell-Luc incision is made and connected with the Weber-Ferguson incision. An **external ethmoidectomy** is usually performed at this time. The proposed osteotomy sites are then outlined with electrocautery and the bone is exposed. A sagittal saw or osteotome is used to make the bony cuts through the palate, maxillary tuberosity, and maxilla at a point dictated by the tumor. Frequently, the specimen must be dissected away from the pterygoid musculature and the internal maxillary artery. After bleeding is controlled, the defect is lined with a split-thickness skin graft and packed with gauze, which is held in place by a dental obturator. For a partial or medial maxillectomy, the palate and lateral maxilla are preserved intact, so that a split-thickness skin graft and dental obturator are thus not necessary.

**Variant procedure or approaches:** Maxillectomy may be included in a **craniofacial *en-bloc* resection**.

**Usual preop diagnosis:** Neoplastic disease of maxillary sinus or lateral wall of nose

**SUMMARY OF PROCEDURE**

| | Partial Maxillectomy | Total Maxillectomy |
|---|---|---|
| **Position** | Supine, with head elevated 30° | ⇐ |
| **Incision** | Oral approach for partial palatal resections. Weber-Ferguson incision for medial maxillectomy. | Weber-Ferguson, with extension around eyelids if orbital exenteration involved. |
| **Special instrumentation** | Power saw, drill; dermatome; nasal osteotomes; curved Lambottes osteotomes; dental instruments for tooth extraction | ⇐ |
| **Unique considerations** | Hypotensive anesthesia during procedure to reduce blood loss | ⇐ |
| **Antibiotics** | Routine, broad-spectrum – cefazolin 1 gm + metronidazole 500 mg | ⇐ |
| **Surgical time** | 1 - 2 hrs | 2 - 4 hrs |
| **Closing considerations** | Nose may be packed, mandating oral airway upon extubation. | ⇐ |
| **EBL** | 100-200 cc. Sudden brisk bleeding due to transection of internal maxillary artery occurs when posterior maxillary cut is made with curved osteotome. Control of this bleeding often cannot be achieved until maxillectomy specimen is removed. A 200-300 cc blood loss within 5 min is not unusual. Although not often needed, T&C for 1-2 U PRBCs is wise. Watch suction bottle and measure irrigation. | 200-700 cc |
| **Postop care** | Mist via face mask is helpful (especially if the nose is packed) to prevent drying of oral mucous membranes immediately postop. | ⇐ |
| **Mortality** | < 1% | ⇐ |
| **Morbidity** | Bleeding: 5%<br>Diplopia (if eye saved): 5%<br>Infection: 4% | ⇐ |
| **Procedure code** | 31225-52 | 31225 or 31230 (with orbital exenteration) |
| **Pain score** | 2-3 | 3-6 |

### PATIENT POPULATION CHARACTERISTICS

| | |
|---|---|
| **Age range** | Usually 6th-7th decade |
| **Male:Female** | 3:1 |
| **Incidence** | Common |
| **Etiology** | Benign and malignant paranasal sinus and nasal neoplasia<br>Inverting papilloma |

## ANESTHETIC CONSIDERATIONS

### PREOPERATIVE

Typically, these patients are in relatively good health, apart from some symptoms referable to nose and sinuses.

| | |
|---|---|
| **Airway** | A careful inspection is warranted, although it is unlikely that the disease process will result in airway compromise. XRT is typically done postop. |
| **Laboratory** | Tests as indicated from H&P. |
| **Premedication** | Standard premedication (see Appendix). |

### INTRAOPERATIVE

**Anesthetic technique:** GETA

| | |
|---|---|
| **Induction** | Standard induction (see Appendix). |
| **Maintenance** | Standard maintenance (see Appendix). Deliberate hypotension may be beneficial during a maxillectomy (if patient's medical condition permits), to minimize blood loss and improve visibility within the surgical field. |
| **Emergence** | The oropharynx should be suctioned carefully to avoid aspiration of pharyngeal contents. The patient may have a pharyngeal pack in place which must be removed prior to emergence. They may also have surgical packs, sutured to the nose at the conclusion of surgery. Patients should have return of airway reflexes before extubation. |

| | | |
|---|---|---|
| **Blood and fluid requirements** | Blood loss moderate-to-severe<br>IV: 16 ga x 1-2 | Blood loss controlled with surgical hemostasis, topical applications of vasoconstrictors (cocaine or epinephrine) and perhaps deliberate hypotension. |
| **Monitoring** | Standard monitors (see Appendix).<br>± Arterial line<br>± CVP line | Invasive monitoring may be necessary for deliberate hypotension; otherwise, as indicated from patient's medical condition. |
| **Positioning** | Head elevated 30°<br>Table turned 90-180°<br>✓ and pad pressure points.<br>✓ eyes. | |
| **Complications** | Dysrhythmias | Dysrhythmias 2° to vasoconstrictor agents may be a problem, particularly in those patients with CAD. |

### POSTOPERATIVE

| | | |
|---|---|---|
| **Complications** | Occult postop bleeding | Postop bleeding may cause the patient to swallow large quantities of blood, which may be aspirated, especially if patient needs to be reanesthetized to obtain hemostasis. |
| **Pain management** | PCA (see Appendix).<br>Other analgesia | |

**References**

1. Lore JM: *An Atlas of Head and Neck Surgery.* WB Saunders Co, Philadelphia: 1988.
2. Brown BR Jr: *Anesthesia and ENT Surgery.* FA Davis Co, Philadelphia: 1987.
3. Morrison JD: *Anesthesia for Eye, Ear, Nose and Throat Surgery,* 2nd edition. Morrison JD, Mirakhur RK, Craig HJL, eds. Churchill Livingstone, New York: 1985.

# TRACHEOSTOMY

## SURGICAL CONSIDERATIONS

**Description:** Tracheostomy is performed either prophylactically in anticipation of upper airway obstruction due to major head and neck surgery, or to establish an airway in acute infectious processes of the head and neck associated with airway obstruction. Other indications are: laryngeal fractures, sleep apnea, inability to intubate for various reasons, requirements for prolonged ventilatory assistance, etc. A tracheostomy tube is placed, or a permanent tracheostomy can be fashioned by using interdigitating neck skin flaps and tracheal flaps. Rarely, an ETT may serve as a tracheostomy securing an airway. Tracheostomy under local anesthesia is the preferred technique for anyone with upper airway obstruction. After infiltrating the operative site with 1% lidocaine, with 1:100,000 epinephrine, a horizontal incision is made 1 cm below the cricoid, exposing the strap muscles, which are separated in the midline. The thyroid isthmus is encountered and divided with electrocautery. The pretracheal fascia is removed, and the cricoid cartilage identified. The trachea is entered, usually at the 2nd or 3rd ring, with either a horizontal or cruciate incision, or a segment of tracheal wall may be removed. In infants, a vertical incision is used with stay sutures attached to each flap. The tracheotomy tube is introduced and secured with trach ties and/or sutures.

**Variant procedure or approaches: Cricothyroidotomy** (incision placed just over the cricothyroid membrane into the subglottic larynx) is the preferred technique to obtain a rapid airway in an emergency. Conversion to a conventional tracheostomy should be performed either immediately or within the first 24 hours to prevent development of cricoid cartilage chondritis with resultant subglottic stenosis.

**Usual preop diagnosis:** Acute upper airway obstruction

### SUMMARY OF PROCEDURE

| | Tracheostomy | Cricothyrotomy |
|---|---|---|
| **Position** | Supine; head extended; sandbag under shoulder, if tolerated. | ⇐ |
| **Incision** | Transverse skin crease, midway between thyroid notch and suprasternal notch | Transverse skin crease between thyroid and cricoid cartilage |
| **Special instrumentation** | None | Cricothyrotome or mini-tracheostomy set |
| **Unique considerations** | Most often performed under controlled conditions, if possible with patient intubated. Can be performed under local anesthesia. | Usually performed in acute emergency situations and converted to standard tracheostomy when patient stabilized. |
| **Antibiotics** | None | ⇐ |
| **Surgical time** | 3 - 20 min | 3 - 5 min |
| **EBL** | 5-25 cc | Minimal |
| **Postop care** | Warm mist to replace humidification, warm inhaled air. Hospitals should have full protocol for tracheostomy suctioning and cleaning. | ⇐ |
| **Mortality** | < 1% | ⇐ |
| **Morbidity** | Bleeding: < 5% | ⇐ |
| | Infection: < 5% | Subglottic stenosis |
| | Tracheomalacia: 1% | |
| | Tracheostenosis: 1% | |
| **Procedure code** | 31605 | 31600 |
| **Pain score** | 1-2 | 2-3 |

### PATIENT POPULATION CHARACTERISTICS

| | |
|---|---|
| **Age range** | Adults |
| **Male:Female** | 2:1 |
| **Incidence** | Common |
| **Etiology** | Upper airway obstruction<br>Prolonged intubation<br>Airway toilet |

## ANESTHETIC CONSIDERATIONS

### PREOPERATIVE

Typically, there are 3 patient populations presenting for tracheostomy: (1) intubated patients in chronic respiratory failure or following major trauma; (2) patients for whom tracheostomy is part of a scheduled procedure (e.g., radical neck dissection); and (3) the rare patient who, having failed intubation, presents in respiratory distress for emergency tracheostomy. These patients are in acute respiratory distress and may require immediate transtracheal jet ventilation and subsequent tracheostomy. An example of this group is the patient presenting with Ludwig's angina, a severe indurated cellulitis resembling an abscess of the sublingual and submaxillary spaces of the floor of the mouth. The tongue may be elevated against the roof of the mouth and the airway may become obstructed rapidly. An emergency tracheostomy under local anesthetic may be necessary. Primary treatment of Ludwig's angina includes antibiotics and, if necessary, incision and drainage under local anesthesia. The following preop considerations apply only to patients in groups 1 and 2. Of these, the first group presents little or no airway challenge to the anesthesiologist; however, the second group does. Thus, the focus of the preop evaluation in group 2 is to identify those patients who may prove to be difficult or impossible to ventilate or intubate. Features of the H&P which may be associated with a difficult airway include: (1) specific anatomic characteristics (e.g., bull neck, large tongue, receding jaw, limited mouth opening, difficulty visualizing posterior pharynx, ↓C-spine ROM and obesity); (2) stridor (inspiratory = obstruction at or above larynx; expiratory = subglottic or intrathoracic obstruction). (3) Hoarseness (vocal cord lesion or dysfunction); (4) tachypnea; (5) marked respiratory effort; (6) dyspnea; (7) previous Hx of gland and neck surgery, trauma or XRT; (8) Hx of previous difficult intubation, vocal cord paralysis; and (9) infections such as epiglottitis or Ludwig's angina.

**Respiratory** — Patients in group 1 may have respiratory insufficiency, requiring mechanical ventilation with PEEP to maintain adequate oxygenation. The continued application of PEEP may be an important consideration during transport from ICU to OR. Patients in group 2 require a careful airway evaluation as outlined above. Based on the assessment, the anesthesiologist must decide whether to choose a direct laryngoscopy, an awake FOL or a tracheostomy under local anesthesia to secure the airway. These patients often have a long Hx of smoking, with consequent COPD.
**Tests:** CXR; PFT (if Sx of pulmonary dysfunction); ABG

**Cardiovascular** — Patients in group 2 may have significant cardiac risk factors, including smoking (>40-pack-years Hx), alcohol abuse, male gender, ↑cholesterol, family Hx and HTN). Assess exercise tolerance. Look for Sx of CAD (e.g., angina) and CHF (e.g., orthopnea, PND, edema, DOE).
**Tests:** ECG in patient with cardiac risk factors

**Neurological** — Look for Sx of ETOH abuse. These patients may require more anesthetic because of hepatic enzyme induction. The perioperative period may be complicated by Sx of ETOH withdrawal.

**Hematologic** — In cases of malignancy or chronic disease, coagulopathies or anemia may be present.
**Tests:** Hb; PT; PTT; platelet count

**Laboratory** — Other tests as indicated from H&P.

**Premedication** — Standard premedication (see Appendix) in elective cases. Premedication is best avoided if airway is compromised, or in emergencies.

### INTRAOPERATIVE

**Anesthetic technique:** GETA (intubated or intubatable patients) or local anesthesia (in the presence of airway compromise or anticipated difficult intubation).

**Induction** — If already intubated, convert pre-existing sedation to GA using carefully titrated induction agents (e.g., etomidate 0.3 mg/kg iv). If not intubated and no airway problems are anticipated, a standard induction (see Appendix) may be appropriate. If airway problems are anticipated, an awake fiber optic intubation is the method of choice. In any event, the anesthesiologist should be prepared to deal with a failed intubation and have a surgeon immediately available to perform a tracheostomy if ventilation proves impossible.

**Maintenance** — Standard maintenance (see Appendix).

**Emergence** — No special considerations

| | | |
|---|---|---|
| **Blood and fluid requirements** | IV: 18 ga x 1<br>NS/LR @ 1-2 ml/kg/hr | Generally, little blood loss when done as an isolated procedure. |
| **Monitoring** | Standard monitors (see Appendix). | Avoid monitor placement in prepped area. Invasive monitoring may be appropriate, depending on patient condition. |

| | | |
|---|---|---|
| **Positioning** | ✓ and pad pressure points.<br>✓ eyes.<br>Shoulder roll | Generally, patient will have a shoulder roll with neck extension to optimize surgical field. |
| **Airway management** | 100% $O_2$ prior to tracheostomy<br>Sterile ventilation hoses | Frequently, when the tracheostomy is a prelude to a more major procedure, an anode tube is inserted through the tracheostomy by surgeons and sutured in place. It is replaced at the end of surgery by a cuffed tracheostomy tube. |
| **Complications** | Pneumothorax<br>Hemorrhage<br>Aspiration of blood<br>Difficult ETT insertion/reinsertion<br>Pneumomediastinum | Pneumothorax may occur with low neck dissection. Dx: ↑RR, ↓BP, ↑CVP, wheezing, ↓$O_2$ saturation, SOB, chest pain, ↓breath sounds, ↓ECG amplitude, dullness on percussion CXR. RX: chest tube or needle aspiration, 100% $O_2$, ventilation and volume expansion. |

### POSTOPERATIVE

| | | |
|---|---|---|
| **Complications** | Pneumothorax | (See pneumothorax Dx/Rx in Intraoperative Complications, above.) |
| | Recurrent laryngeal nerve damage<br>Airway compromise<br>Blood loss | Bilateral recurrent laryngeal nerve injury → airway obstruction, necessitating reintubation. Airway compromise may also be the result of a hematoma, requiring emergent evacuation and reintubation. |
| **Pain management** | IV opiates, as patient will remain npo postop.<br>PCA (see Appendix). | |
| **Tests** | CXR | For position of tracheostomy tube, evidence of pneumothorax, pneumomediastinum |

**References**

1. Pemberton LB: A comprehensive view of tracheostomy. *Am Surg* 1972; 38(5):251-56.
2. Peterson LJ: Odontogenic Infections. In *Otolaryngology-Head & Neck Surgery.* Cummings CW, Fredrickson JM, Hanker LA, Krause CJ, Schuller DE, eds. CV Mosby Co, St Louis: 1986, Vol 2, 1213-30.
3. Brown BR Jr: *Anesthesia and ENT Surgery.* FA Davis Co, Philadelphia: 1987.
4. Morrison JD: *Anesthesia for Eye, Ear, Nose and Throat Surgery*, 2nd edition. Morrison JD, Mirakhur RK, Craig HJL, eds. Churchill Livingstone, New York: 1985.

# INTUBATION FOR EPIGLOTTITIS

## ANESTHETIC CONSIDERATIONS

### PREOPERATIVE

Epiglottitis is an acute inflammation and swelling of the epiglottis associated with a generalized systemic toxicity, usually due to hemophilus influenza Type B. It also can be caused by ß-hemolytic streptococci, staphylococci or pneumococci. It occasionally results in total laryngeal obstruction and death due to asphyxia. The typical patient is a previously healthy child between 1-4 years of age, but adults can be affected as well. In both, the treatment of choice is ET intubation and antibiotics. About 80% of hemophilus influenza infections are sensitive to ampicillin. Steroids also have been recommended, but no difference in outcome has been reported.

**Respiratory** Symptoms may be sore throat, fever, muffled voice, dysphagia and rapidly increasing stridor. The child sits upright, leaning forward and drools saliva. It is imperative to realize that total airway obstruction can occur suddenly and without warning. Rapid treatment should be instituted instead

| | | |
|---|---|---|
| | of performing time-consuming investigations. The sudden development of respiratory obstruction in the x-ray suite could have a disastrous outcome. | |
| **Hematologic** | A high leukocyte count is usually found in these patients.<br>**Tests:** Blood drawing before the airway is secured may be inadvisable. | |
| **Premedication** | None | |

## INTRAOPERATIVE

**Anesthetic technique:** GETA. It is essential that an experienced anesthesiologist be present for this procedure. It is important that no exam of the throat be made (as this may precipitate complete airway obstruction) except under an anesthetic. In adults, it has been suggested that indirect laryngoscopy or FOB may be performed without the risk of precipitating complete laryngeal obstruction, although this is controversial.

| | | |
|---|---|---|
| **Induction** | While the patient is breathing spontaneously, atropine 0.02 mg/kg is given to prevent vagal reflexes and bradycardia from manipulation of the inflamed epiglottis. An experienced ENT surgeon with an emergency tracheostomy set must be available. Inhalation induction, with halothane and 100% $O_2$, is used, with patient sitting. Induction may be prolonged and intubation extremely difficult. Smaller than usual oral ETT is used initially, then may be changed to a nasal tube at the end of the procedure; however, this may prove hazardous. | |
| **Maintenance** | Standard maintenance (see Appendix). | |
| **Emergence** | The patient will remain intubated for 24-48 hrs and should be kept sedated and restrained to prevent accidental extubation. (The mean duration of intubation in one series was 36 hrs.) It is believed that direct observation of the epiglottis is the only reliable way to determine the stage at which the ETT is no longer necessary. | |
| **Blood and fluid requirements** | Minimal blood loss<br>IV: 18 ga (adult)<br>22-26 ga (child)<br>NS/LR @ 4-7 ml/kg/hr (adult)<br>@ 2-3 ml/kg/hr (child) | If possible, the iv should be placed following induction of anesthesia because subsequent crying and struggling may → acute respiratory obstruction. |
| **Monitoring** | Standard monitors (see Appendix). | |
| **Positioning** | ✓ and pad pressure points.<br>✓ eyes. | |
| **Complications** | Pulmonary edema | A short-lived pulmonary edema occasionally occurs after relief of the obstruction and must be treated with IPPV. |

## POSTOPERATIVE

| | | |
|---|---|---|
| **Complications** | Accidental extubation<br>ETT blockage | Accidental extubation and ETT blockage are serious complications that can prove fatal. The blockages are sometimes due to crusting of the ETT because of insufficient humidification. The tube should be changed after 24 hrs. |
| | PCA (see Appendix). | Postop sedation and manual restraints |

**References**

1. Brown BR Jr: *Anesthesia and ENT Surgery*. FA Davis Co, Philadelphia: 1987.
2. Morrison JD: *Anesthesia for Eye, Ear, Nose and Throat Surgery*, 2nd edition. Morrison JD, Mirakhur RK, Craig HJL, eds. Churchill Livingstone, New York: 1985.

**Surgeon**

**Stephen A. Schendel, MD, DDS**

# 4. DENTAL SURGERY

**Anesthesiologists**

**Richard A. Jaffe, MD, PhD**
**Stanley I. Samuels, MB, BCh, FFARCS**

# TEMPOROMANDIBULAR JOINT ARTHROSCOPY/ARTHROPLASTY

## SURGICAL CONSIDERATIONS

**Description:** **Temporomandibular joint (TMJ) arthroplasty** is a common procedure which is usually performed bilaterally. This involves a preauricular incision with opening of the joint compartment and, usually, a repositioning of the disc. Severely damaged discs require removal and replacement. When a disc removal is required, a substitute material, consisting chiefly of temporalis fascia flaps, free dermagrafts or auricular cartilage grafts, is usually placed. Associated with this may be procedures to smooth and reshape the condylar head and eminence of the glenoid fossa. **TMJ arthroscopy** may be performed prior to the actual arthroplasty, or as a separate procedure. This involves placing a scope into the joint from a preauricular approach and visualizing the internal structures of the superior compartment for the purpose of irrigation and debridement.

**Usual preop diagnosis:** Internal derangement, subluxation and ankylosis of TMJ

### SUMMARY OF PROCEDURE

| | Arthroscopy | Arthroplasty |
|---|---|---|
| **Position** | Supine | ⇐ |
| **Incision** | Preauricular | ⇐ |
| **Special instrumentation** | Arthroscope | Air power tools (may have limited opening) |
| **Antibiotics** | Penicillin 2 million U q 6 hr | ⇐ |
| **Surgical time** | 0.5 hr | 1.5 hrs/side |
| **EBL** | Minimal | ⇐ |
| **Postop care** | May be an out-patient procedure; PACU → room. | ⇐ |
| **Mortality** | Minimal | ⇐ |
| **Morbidity** | VII nerve damage: 7-32%[1,2] | ⇐ |
| **Procedure code** | 21010 | 21240, 21242, 21243 |
| **Pain score** | 5 | 6 |

### PATIENT POPULATION CHARACTERISTICS

| | |
|---|---|
| **Age range** | 20-40 yrs |
| **Male:Female** | 1:9 |
| **Incidence** | Up to 17% of the population suffers from TMJ dysfunction (TMJD). |
| **Etiology** | TMJD<br>Idiopathic<br>Trauma |

## ANESTHETIC CONSIDERATIONS

See "Anesthetic Considerations for Dental/Oral Surgery" following "Restorative Dentistry" (below).

# ORAL SURGERY

## SURGICAL CONSIDERATIONS

**Description:** Surgery of the oral cavity, frequently performed under GA, includes the removal of impacted teeth, multiple dental extractions, pre-prosthetic surgery (e.g., vestibuloplasties [surgical modifications of the gingival mucous membrane relationships]) and the insertion of osteointegrated implants.

SUMMARY OF PROCEDURE

| | Surgical Removal of Teeth | Pre-Prosthetic Surgery | Dental Implants |
|---|---|---|---|
| **Position** | Supine | ⇐ | ⇐ |
| **Incision** | Intraoral | ⇐ | ⇐ |
| **Special instrumentation** | None | ⇐ | Specific dental implant insertion kit and implants |
| **Unique considerations** | Nasal intubation; throat pack used. | ⇐ | ⇐ |
| **Antibiotics** | Penicillin x 5 d po | ⇐ | ⇐ |
| **Surgical time** | 0.5 - 1 hr | 1 - 2 hrs | 0.5 - 2 hrs |
| **EBL** | Minimal | ⇐ | ⇐ |
| **Postop care** | PACU → home | ⇐ | ⇐ |
| **Mortality** | Minimal | ⇐ | ⇐ |
| **Morbidity** | Pain | ⇐ | ⇐ |
| | Swelling | – | ⇐ |
| | Infection | – | Loss of implant |
| **Procedure code** | 41899 | ⇐ | 21248 |
| **Pain score** | 3 | 3 | 2 |

PATIENT POPULATION CHARACTERISTICS

| | | | |
|---|---|---|---|
| **Age range** | 15-20 yrs | >40 yrs | ⇐ |
| **Male:Female** | 1:1 | ⇐ | ⇐ |
| **Incidence** | Unknown | ⇐ | ⇐ |
| **Etiology** | Congenital | ⇐ | ⇐ |
| | Idiopathic | ⇐ | ⇐ |
| **Associated conditions** | Loose teeth | ⇐ | |

## ANESTHETIC CONSIDERATIONS

See "Anesthetic Considerations for Dental/Oral Surgery" following "Restorative Dentistry" (below).

# RESTORATIVE DENTISTRY

## SURGICAL CONSIDERATIONS

**Description**: Multiple dental restorative procedures are performed under GA when there is rampant caries, and an extensive amount of dental work must be performed at one time. The second most common indication for GA is for procedures that need to be performed on mentally retarded patients who are not candidates for a local anesthetic. The actual amount of restorative dentistry is quite variable, depending on the individual case; and no two are exactly the same. Thus, depending on the procedures that need to be performed, the length of the case can be quite variable. Generally, blood loss is not a problem.

### SUMMARY OF PROCEDURE

| | |
|---|---|
| **Position** | Supine |
| **Incision** | Teeth, gingiva |
| **Special instrumentation** | Dental armamentarium |
| **Unique considerations** | Nasal intubation |
| **Surgical time** | 0.5 - 3 hrs |
| **EBL** | Minimal |
| **Postop care** | PACU → home |
| **Mortality** | Minimal |
| **Morbidity** | Pain<br>Swelling |
| **Procedure code** | 41899 |
| **Pain score** | 1-3 |

### PATIENT POPULATION CHARACTERISTICS

| | |
|---|---|
| **Age range** | 2 yrs - adult |
| **Male:Female** | 1:1 |
| **Incidence** | Unknown |
| **Etiology** | Idiopathic or congenital anomalies |
| **Associated conditions** | Mental retardation (majority)<br>Down syndrome<br>Seizures |

## ANESTHETIC CONSIDERATIONS FOR DENTAL/ORAL SURGERY

### PREOPERATIVE

Most patients presenting for dental or oral surgery will usually require only local anesthesia provided by the dentist/oral surgeon. GA may be required, however, for several unique patient groups: (1) young children (some with systemic diseases such as CHD, hemophilia); (2) the mentally retarded; (3) those with poorly controlled seizure disorders; (4) those presenting for TMJ procedures; and (5) those with an oral septic focus who may be quite ill. If the patient does not fall into one of these readily identifiable categories, the reasons for GA should be ascertained.

**Airway** Patients presenting for TMJ procedures may have problems with mouth opening (2° pain, arthritis), making airway examination difficult. Nasotracheal intubation using FOL should be planned. Examine nares for patency.

**Respiratory** Surgery should be postponed (2-6 wk) in patients presenting with Sx of acute RTI (fever, coughing, purulent sputum, etc.). Sx of chronic respiratory disease should be sought and treated before surgery.

**Tests:** As indicated from H&P.

**Cardiovascular** Patients with dysrhythmias may be sensitive to the epinephrine used in local anesthetic solutions administered intraop. As with other types of elective surgery, pre-existing cardiovascular problems should be treated before inducing anesthesia. Prophylactic antibiotics for endocarditis may be required in some patients.

**Tests:** As indicated from H&P.

**Neurological** Patients with seizure disorders should be on optimal medical therapy before surgery. Discuss precipitating factors and prodromal Sx with the patient.

**Tests:** ✓ therapeutic levels of anticonvulsant (e.g., phenytoin=10-20 μg/cc; carbamazepine=3-12 μg/cc; phenobarbital=10-40 μg/cc).

**Musculoskeletal** In addition to TMJ problems, rheumatoid arthritis is associated with cricoarytenoid joint immobility and cervical spine immobility/instability that may complicate intubation.

**Laboratory** Other tests as indicated from H&P.

**Premedication** Standard premedication (see Appendix) usually is appropriate.

## INTRAOPERATIVE

**Anesthetic technique:** GETA. Typically a nasotracheal intubation is required, using an ET tube 0.5-1 mm smaller than for oral intubation. In patients with difficult airways, an awake nasal FOL is indicated. (See general discussion of awake FOL in Anesthetic Considerations following section on thoracic laminectomy.)

| | |
|---|---|
| **Induction** | In patients with normal airways, anesthesia may be induced in the usual fashion (see Appendix). Following loss of consciousness, topical intranasal cocaine is applied (4% on pledgets, 4 cc maximum) to shrink the nasal mucosa and for vasoconstriction. The well-lubricated ETT is passed through the nose into the trachea, either blindly or assisted by McGill's forceps under direct laryngoscopy. |
| **Maintenance** | Standard maintenance (see Appendix). |
| **Emergence** | No special considerations except that throat packs must be removed prior to extubation. |
| **Blood and fluid requirements** | IV: 18 ga x 1<br>NS/LR @ 4-6 ml/kg/hr |
| **Monitoring** | Standard monitors (see Appendix). |
| **Positioning** | √ and pad pressure points.<br>√ eyes. |

## POSTOPERATIVE

| | | |
|---|---|---|
| **Complications** | Airway obstruction 2° retained throat pack<br>N&V | These patients may swallow blood, with consequent N&V. Rx: metoclopramide 10 mg iv. |
| **Pain management** | Oral analgesics (see Appendix). | |

**References for Dental/Oral Surgery**

1. Dolwick MF, Kretzschmar DP: Morbidity associated with the preauricular and perimeatal approaches to the temporomandibular joint. *J Oral Maxillofac Surg* 1982; 40(11):699-700.
2. Zide BM: The temporomandibular joint. In *Plastic Surgery*, Vol 2. McCarthy JG, ed. WB Saunders Co, Philadelphia: 1990, 1475-1513.
3. Coplans MP, Green RA: *Anesthesia and Sedation in Dentistry*. Elsevier Science Pub Co, New York: 1983.

**Surgeon**

**James B.D. Mark, MD**

# 5. THORACIC SURGERY

**Anesthesiologist**

**Jay B. Brodsky, MD**

# LOBECTOMY, PNEUMONECTOMY

## SURGICAL CONSIDERATIONS

**Description:** It is generally agreed that appropriate pulmonary resection, including lymph node dissection, is the mainstay of treatment for a curable carcinoma of the lung. The operations most often carried out are **lobectomy** (or **bilobectomy** on the right) or **pneumonectomy**, depending on the extent of the disease. (Fig 5-1 shows segmental anatomy of the lung.) If the cancer is encompassable and entirely removable by lobectomy, then pneumonectomy is not necessary. There is some enthusiasm for even more conservative resection of lung cancers with curative intent. (See "Wedge Resection of Lung Lesion" and "Thoracoscopy.")

The standard incision for lobectomy or pneumonectomy, or for any operation requiring safe access to the pulmonary hilar structures, is posterolateral with the patient in the lateral decubitus position. Latissimus dorsi and serratus anterior muscles are divided, and a rib may or may not be resected. Exploration of the pleural cavity is carried out in order to determine resectability in the case of lung cancer and to further assess the pathologic process which is present. Safe dissection and division of appropriate hilar vessels and bronchi depend on the surgeon having a thorough knowledge of hilar anatomy, including its important variations (of which there are many). Complications are far better prevented than treated. Specific techniques of division of vessels and bronchi vary among surgeons. For the main PA or the main veins, staplers are widely used. Some thoracic surgeons still ligate vessels and staple bronchi. Fewer suture bronchi.

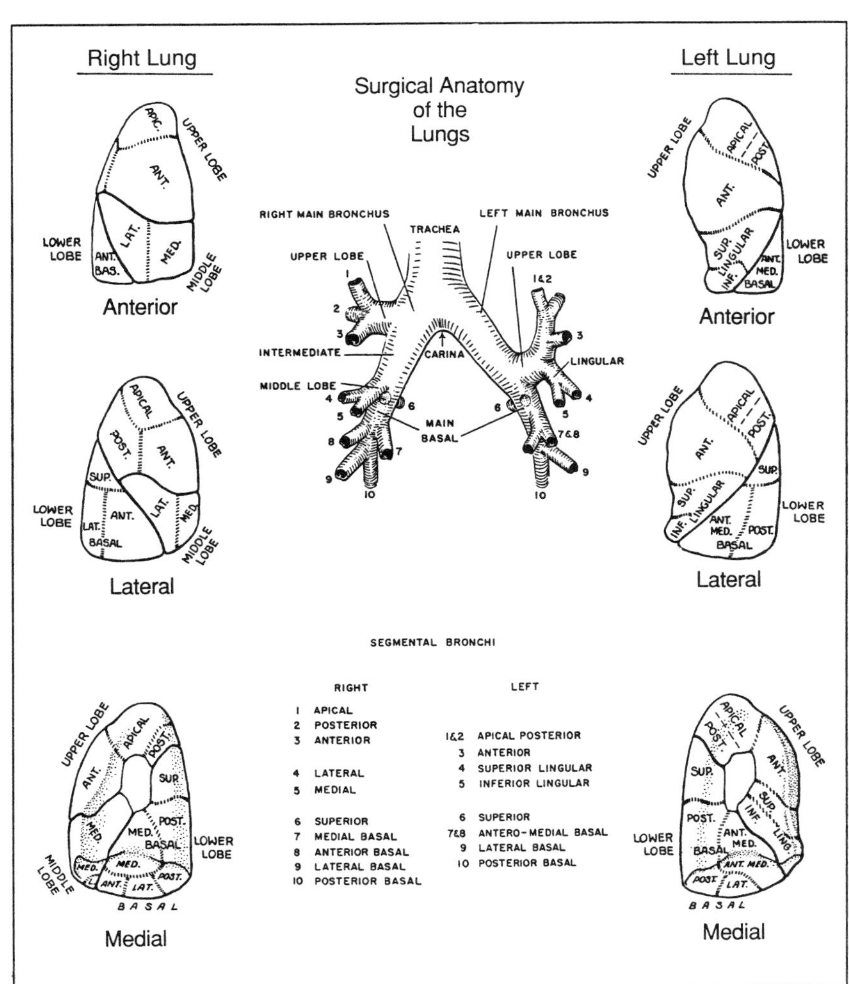


**Figure 5-1.** Segmental anatomy of the lungs. (Reproduced with permission from Waldhausen JA, Pierce WS: *Johnson's Surgery of the Chest.* Hill E, Beisel D, illustrators. Year Book Medical Pub: 1965.)

Standard chest drainage following lobectomy calls for the use of two tubes, usually 28-32 Fr, one positioned anteriorly and one posteriorly. The tubes are attached to an underwater seal apparatus. Suction is employed (usually at –20 cm $H_2O$) to encourage expansion of the remaining lobe or lobes, in addition to improving drainage of air and fluid. Pleural drainage following pneumonectomy is not practiced uniformly. A small (16 Fr) tube may be placed while closing in order to establish an intrapleural pressure of about –5 cm $H_2O$ by removal of or instillation of air. At this point, the tube is removed. Our preference is to leave a 24-28 Fr tube in the empty pleural cavity for 18-24 hrs with the tube attached to a special pneumonectomy Pleurevac®, which balances the intrapleural pressures appropriately and does not allow suction. A more limited, muscle-sparing incision is sometimes used in an effort to cause less pain and consequently fewer postop pulmonary problems. Pain generally can be well-controlled with epidural analgesia postop and the standard incision provides the safest access to structures deep in the chest. Median sternotomy can be used for pneumonectomy or lobectomy, although it has the disadvantage of providing less access to the posteriorly placed structures and particularly difficult access to the left inferior pulmonary vein.

Lobectomy and, less often, pneumonectomy, are occasionally accompanied by bronchoplasty in order to preserve functioning pulmonary tissue while still completely removing the cancer. In special circumstances a median sternotomy approach is used for lobectomy or pneumonectomy.

**Usual preop diagnosis**: Carcinoma of the lung

**SUMMARY OF PROCEDURE**

| | Lobectomy | Pneumonectomy |
|---|---|---|
| **Position** | Lateral/supine | ⇐ |
| **Incision** | Posterolateral/median sternotomy | ⇐ |
| **Special instrumentation** | DLT | ⇐ |
| **Surgical time** | 2 - 3 hrs | ⇐ |
| **EBL** | < 500 cc (more in re-do or inflammatory cases) | ⇐ |
| **Postop care** | ICU; careful attention to pulmonary toilet; chest tube output – 2 tubes | Special balanced drainage – 1 tube |
| **Mortality** | ± 1% | ± 5% |
| **Morbidity** | Dysrhythmias: 20-30%<br>Pain<br>PE<br>MI<br>Bronchopleural fistula<br>Chylothorax<br>Subcutaneous emphysema<br>Phrenic nerve injury<br>Recurrent laryngeal nerve injury | ⇐ |
| **Procedure code** | 32480 | 32440 |
| **Pain score** | 7-8 | 7-8 |

**PATIENT POPULATION CHARACTERISTICS**

| | |
|---|---|
| **Age range** | 40-80 yrs |
| **Male:Female** | 1.5:1 |
| **Incidence** | Common thoracic procedure; increasing in females. |
| **Etiology** | Smoking |
| **Associated conditions** | Cardiopulmonary disease |

---

## ANESTHETIC CONSIDERATIONS

### PREOPERATIVE

**Respiratory**: Question patient about dyspnea, productive cough and cigarette smoking. Examine patient for cyanosis, clubbing, RR and pattern. Listen to chest for wheezes, rhonchi, rales. Morbidity and mortality following thoracotomy increased with pre-existing pulmonary, cardiovascular and neurologic disease.

**Tests:** PFT (see below); CXR; if chest CT available, look for airway obstruction that could interfere with DLT placement; ABG.

**Pulmonary function**: Establish a baseline and identify patients with advanced pulmonary disease who are unable to tolerate planned operation. Whole-lung tests (ABG), single-lung tests (split-function lung tests = ventilation/perfusion studies) if pneumonectomy planned. A VC at least 3 x TV is necessary for effective cough postop. A VC < 50% predicted or < 1500 ml predicts increased risk for postop complications following pulmonary resection. Operative risk for pneumonectomy increases if patient is hypercapnic ($PaCO_2$ >45 mmHg) on room air, $FEV_1$/FVC < 50% of predicted, $FEV_1$ < 2 L, if >60-70% blood flow is to diseased lung, and if mean PA pressure increases >30 mmHg with occlusion of PA. Mimic post-pneumonectomy conditions by temporary unilateral occlusion of main PA. Patient may show improvement in PFTs following bronchodilator therapy.

**Table 5-1. Classification of risk of pulmonary complications of thoracic and abdominal procedures**

| Category | Point |
|---|---|
| I. Expiratory Spirogram | |
| a. Normal (%FVC + %$FEV^1$/FVC >150) | 0 |
| b. %FVC + %$FEV^1$/FVC=100-150 | 1 |
| c. %FVC + %$FEV^1$/FVC < 100 | 2 |
| d. Preop FVC < 20 ml/kg | 3 |
| e. Post-bronchodilator $FEV^1$/FVC < 50% | 3 |
| II. Cardiovascular System | |
| a. Normal | 0 |
| b. Controlled HTN, MI sequelae for more than 2 yrs | 0 |
| c. Dyspnea on exertion, orthopnea, paroxysmal nocturnal dyspnea, dependent edema, CHF, angina | 1 |
| III. ABGs | |
| a. Acceptable | 0 |
| b. $PaCO_2$ >50 mm Hg or $PaCO_2$ < 60 mmHg on room air | 1 |
| c. Metabolic pH abnormality >7.50 or < 7.30 | 1 |
| IV. Nervous System | |
| a. Normal | 0 |
| b. Confusion, obtundation, agitation, spasticity, discoordination, bulbar malfunction | 1 |
| c. Significant muscular weakness | 1 |
| V. Postop Ambulation | |
| a. Expected ambulation (minimum, sitting at bedside) within 36 hrs | 0 |
| b. Expected complete bed confinement for at least 36 hrs | 1 |

0 Points = Low Risk    1-2 Points = Moderate Risk    3 Points = High Risk

Shapira BA, Harrison RA, Kacmarek RM, Cane RD: *Clinical Application of Respiratory Care*, 3rd edition. Year Book Medical Publishers, Chicago: 1985. (With permission.)

**Cardiovascular** Prophylactic digitalization to reduce risk of postop heart failure is recommended prior to pneumonectomy.

**Tests:** ECG – look for evidence of RV hypertrophy, conduction problems and prior ischemia; others as indicated from H&P.

**Neurological** ✓ Hx of previous back surgery, peripheral neuropathy. Examine lumbar area for skin lesions, infection, deformities. Avoid placement of epidural catheter in patient with neurologic problems.

**Musculoskeletal** Patients with lung cancer may have myasthenic (Eaton-Lambert) syndrome with increased sensitivity to non-depolarizing muscle relaxants. Monitor relaxation with peripheral nerve stimulator.

**Hematologic** Transfuse patient with preop Hct < 25%. Adequate $O_2$-carrying capacity essential. T&C 2-4 U of blood, or obtain 1-3 U of autologous blood during the month before surgery.

**Tests:** Hct; PT; PTT (if epidural anesthesia planned)

**Laboratory** Other tests as indicated from H&P.

**Premedication** Midazolam 1-2 mg iv if patient anxious. When epidural opioids are planned, avoid opioid or sedative premedication which can potentiate postop respiratory effects of spinal opioids.

## INTRAOPERATIVE

**Anesthetic technique:** Combined epidural and inhalational agent.

**Preinduction** Place lumbar epidural catheter and advance catheter 4-6 cm past needle in epidural space; secure with tape. Administer test dose: 3 ml lidocaine (1.5%) + 1:200,000 epinephrine. If no hypotension or tachycardia, administer 12-18 ml lidocaine (1.5-2.0%) and record evidence of anesthetic level. Confirm functioning epidural catheter preop to ensure predictable postop analgesia. Giving local anesthetics through the epidural catheter intraop reduces the amounts of general anesthetics and muscle relaxants required. Post-thoracotomy analgesia is excellent with lumbar epidural opioids. Placement of lumbar catheter is safer than thoracic catheter.

**Induction** Standard induction (see Appendix).

**Maintenance** $O_2$ and isoflurane (1.0-1.5%); less anesthetic required when epidural local anesthetics used. Avoid $N_2O$, especially during OLV, since hypoxemia is unpredictable; use $FiO_2 = 1.0$. Lidocaine (1.5% or 2.0%) 10-12 ml, administered via epidural every 45 min, or bupivacaine (0.5%) 10-12 ml every 1.5-2 hrs. Hydromorphone (Dilaudid®) (1.0-1.5 mg) or morphine (5.0-7.5 mg) in 10 ml NS through epidural during case. Epidural hydromorphone is preferred since, in equipotent doses, analgesia is equivalent to that with morphine, but with fewer side effects. Lung manipulation during surgery releases vasoactive substances that interfere with hypoxic pulmonary vasoconstrictive (HPV) reflex. Thus, clinically, the choice of anesthetic agent should not be influenced by experimental studies which indicated that the HPV reflex is maintained with iv agents, but may not be with inhalational agents. Inhalational anesthetics are potent bronchodilators and depress airway reflexes.

**Emergence** Prior to closing chest, lungs are inflated to 30 cm $H_2O$ pressure to re-inflate atelectatic areas and to check for significant air leaks. Surgeon inserts chest tubes to drain pleural cavity and aid lung re-expansion. Patient is extubated in OR. If postop ventilation is required (rare), DLT exchanged for ETT. Patient transferred in head-elevated position to PACU or ICU breathing mask $O_2$. If hemodynamically unstable, monitor ECG, pulse oximetry and arterial pressure during transfer.

**Blood and fluid requirements**

IV: 18 ga x 1 + 16 ga x 1
Restrict iv fluids; usually administer 1000-1500 ml NS/LR total.
Blood: ± 1 U autologous blood if available; use vasopressor (ephedrine 5-10 mg iv bolus or phenylephrine 50-100 $\mu$g iv bolus) if hypotensive.

Postop, PVR is increased proportionate to the amount of lung tissue removed. An overhydrated patient is at increased risk of right heart failure. Use of epidural local anesthetics can cause hypotension in a volume-restricted patient; vasopressor often needed.

**Monitoring**

Standard monitors (see Appendix).
Arterial line
Urinary catheter
± CVP line
± PA line

It is mandatory to follow oxygenation continuously during OLV. Currently this can be done only with pulse oximetry, although continuous intra-arterial $PO_2$ monitoring may soon be commercially available. CVP and/or PA line optional for pneumonectomy and for patients with co-existing cardiac disease. During open thoracotomy, CVP monitoring may be inaccurate. A PA line, placed immediately preop in the operated PA, may interfere with pneumonectomy. Central volume monitoring is useful for postop management.

**Positioning**

Axillary roll, "airplane" for upper arm; avoid hyperextending arms.
√ and pad pressure points.
√ eyes.

**Fiber optic bronchoscopy**

FOB performed immediately prior to thoracotomy to evaluate resectability of lesion. Patient intubated with large ETT (≥ 8 mm), replaced with DLT or BB following bronchoscopy (see "Bronchoscopy").

Use the largest plastic DLT that atraumatically passes through the glottis (41 Fr for men, 39 Fr for women). DLT can be placed accurately by careful auscultation ± confirmation by FOB. If FOB is used, pass down tracheal lumen. Top of blue endobronchial cuff should be visible below carina in bronchus. For small children, the balloon of a Fogarty embolectomy catheter is used as a BB; for adults, use a Univent® tube. FOB always needed to confirm BB placement. With BB, operated lung cannot safely be re-inflated and collapsed periodically during surgery.

**Lung isolation** — Separate lungs to prevent contralateral contamination (infection, pus, blood, tumor), allow selective ventilation and facilitate operation.

**One-lung ventilation** — Use large TV (12-15 ml/kg/hr) during two-lung ventilation; do not change TV when OLV instituted.

Large TV during OLV prevents atelectasis of the dependent ("down," ventilated) lung. Ventilation rate adjusted to avoid hyperventilation. Compliance is reduced (same TV to one lung) and resistance is increased (1 lumen instead of 2); PIPs will be higher. Intraop hypoxemia during OLV is uncommon when $FiO_2 = 1.0$ and large TV used. If pulse oximetry < 94% or $PO_2$ < 100, recheck position of DLT or BB. The DLT endobronchial cuff can obstruct the upper lobe bronchus of the ventilated lung or the DLT or BB balloon can herniate into the carina, obstructing both lungs. PEEP to ventilated lung can be used, but with caution since overdistention of alveoli will increase shunt to the "up" lung, worsening hypoxemia. If hypoxemia persists, insufflate operated ("up," collapsed) lung with 100% $O_2$ and apply CPAP (5-10 cm $H_2O$) to the "up" lung to improve oxygenation without interfering with surgical field. The PA of the operated lung during pneumonectomy can be clamped completely, eliminating shunt.

## POSTOPERATIVE

| | | |
|---|---|---|
| **Complications** | Airway trauma from intubation, tracheobronchial rupture | Do not overdistend bronchial balloon or DLT cuffs. DLT bronchial cuff usually requires < 2 ml air for airtight seal. |
| | Injuries related to lateral positioning | Pressure damage to ear, eye, nose, deltoid muscle, iliac crest, brachial plexus, and radial, ulnar, common peroneal and sciatic nerves have all been reported. |
| | Structural injuries related to thoracotomy | Neurologic (phrenic and recurrent laryngeal nerves), thoracic duct, spinal cord; bronchopleural fistula, tracheobronchial disruption |
| | Surgical complications | Cardiac herniation, tension pneumothorax, bleeding, torsion of residual lobe, wound infection |
| | Cardiopulmonary complications | Supraventricular dysrhythmias, acute cor pulmonale, atelectasis, pneumonia, PE |
| **Pain management** | Spinal opioids – epidural or intrathecal<br>Parenteral opioids (iv, im, continuous iv, PCA [see Appendix]).<br>Intercostal blocks<br>Interpleural analgesia<br>Epidural local anesthetics<br>Cryoanalgesia<br>Transcutaneous nerve stimulation | Effective analgesia is essential for patient to cough, deep breathe and ambulate early. Thoracic epidural is often recommended, but lumbar route is as effective and safer. Intraop, administer a single bolus of hydromorphone (1.0-1.5 mg) in 10 ml NS. In immediate postop period, 0.2-0.3 mg/kg of hydromorphone infused through epidural. Fentanyl 40-100 $\mu$g bolus in 10 ml NS for breakthrough pain. |
| **Tests** | CXR, ABG and others as indicated. | |

**References**


1. Sabiston DC Jr, Spencer FC: *Surgery of the Chest*, 5th edition, Vol II. WB Saunders Co, Philadelphia: 1990.
2. Baue AE, ed: *Glenn's Thoracic and Cardiovascular Surgery*, 5th edition, Volume II. Geha AS, Hammond GL, Laks H, Naunheim KS, co-eds. Appleton & Lange, Norwalk, CT: 1991.
3. Capan LM, Turndorf H, Chandrakant P, et al: Optimization of arterial oxygenation during one-lung anesthesia. *Anesth Analg* 1980; 59(11):847-51.

4. Brodsky JB, Mark JBD: A simple technique for accurate placement of double-lumen endobronchial tubes. *Anesth Rev* 1983; 10:26-30.
5. Shulman M, Sandler AN, Bradley JW, et al: Postthoracotomy pain and pulmonary function following epidural and systemic morphine. *Anesthesiology* 1984: 61(5):569-75.
6. Benumof JL: One-lung ventilation and hypoxic pulmonary vasoconstriction: implications for anesthetic management. *Anesth Analg* 1985; 64(8):821-33.
7. Brodsky JB, Chaplan SR, Brose WG, Mark JBD: Continuous epidural hydromorphone for postthoracotomy pain relief. *Ann Thorac Surg* 1990: 50(6):888-93.

# WEDGE RESECTION OF LUNG LESION

## SURGICAL CONSIDERATIONS

**Description: Wedge resection** (removal of a mass and 1 cm margins in a manner that does not remove an entire anatomical pulmonary segment) may be carried out for a number of reasons. A known or suspected cancer may be removed by this limited resection. There is general agreement that this is an appropriate operation for patients with limited pulmonary reserve who are unable to withstand lobectomy. Wedge resection also is used for resection of single- or multiple-metastatic lesions from various primary neoplasms. A single metastasis may be removed through a limited thoracotomy incision. At the other extreme, **sternotomy** may be carried out to remove bilateral lesions. Wedge resection is also indicated for diagnostic and therapeutic purposes in lesions which defy diagnosis by less invasive techniques. Incisions vary with location and number of lesions and technique employed. **Limited thoracotomy**, **standard thoracotomy**, or **median sternotomy** may be used under different circumstances. **Stapling** (Fig 5-2), **clamp and suture** technique, or **excision and suture** technique may be used for lesions in different locations. Chest tubes are used for postop drainage.

**Usual preop diagnosis**: Metastatic tumor to the lungs; occasionally primary lung cancer; unknown pulmonary lesion

### SUMMARY OF PROCEDURE

| | |
|---|---|
| **Position** | Lateral or supine |
| **Incision** | Limited and related to location of solitary lesion; sternotomy for bilateral lesions |
| **Special instrumentation** | DLT |
| **Surgical time** | < 1 - 3 hrs, depending on number of lesions |
| **EBL** | < 500 cc |
| **Postop care** | ICU; careful attention to pulmonary toilet, chest tube output |
| **Mortality** | Minimal |
| **Morbidity** | Air leaks<br>Cardiac dysrhythmias |
| **Procedure code** | 32500 (wedge resection); 32095 (biopsy) |
| **Pain Score** | 2-6 |

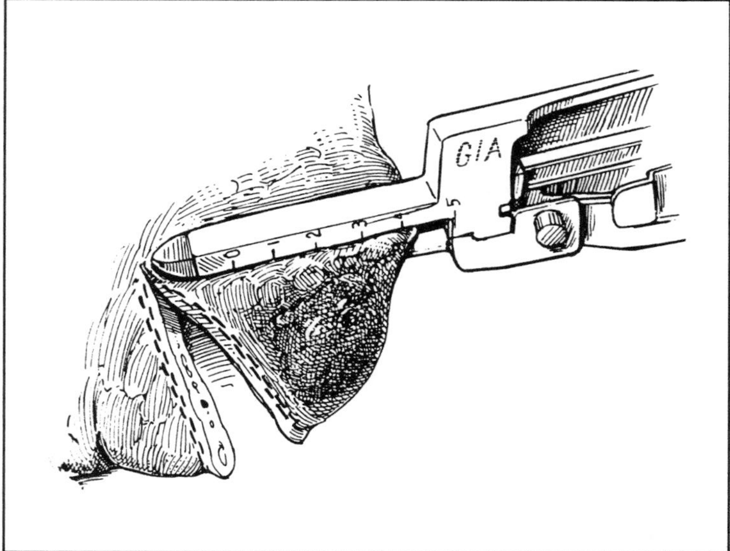


**Figure 5-2.** Stapler used to perform wedge incision. (Reproduced with permission from *Johnson's Surgery of the Chest*, 5th edition. Year Book Medical Pub: 1985.

### PATIENT POPULATION CHARACTERISTICS

**Age range** 30s-60s most common
**Male:Female** 1:1
**Incidence** Common thoracic procedure
**Etiology** Variable – neoplasm or inflammatory disease

---

## ANESTHETIC CONSIDERATIONS

### PREOPERATIVE

**Respiratory** PFTs similar to open thoracotomy. Further evaluation directed toward an underlying disease (e.g., immunocompromised patient for open-lung Bx, patient with metastatic lesions, etc.).
**Tests:** PFTs (see "Pulmonary Resection"); CXR; if chest CT available, look for airway obstruction that could interfere with DLT placement; Hct; ABG.

**Cardiovascular** **Tests:** ECG – look for evidence of RV hypertrophy, conduction problems and prior ischemia.

**Neurological** Hx of previous back surgery, peripheral neuropathy. Examine lumbar area for skin lesions, infection, deformities. Avoid placement of epidural catheter in patient with neurologic problems.

**Musculoskeletal** Patients with lung cancer may have myasthenic (Eaton-Lambert) syndrome with increased sensitivity to non-depolarizing muscle relaxants. Monitor relaxation with peripheral nerve stimulator.

**Hematologic** Patients are often anemic from primary disease. Consider preop blood transfusion.
**Tests:** Hct

**Laboratory** Other tests as indicated from H&P.

**Premedication** Midazolam 1-2 mg/iv if patient anxious. When epidural opioids are planned, avoid opioid or sedative premedication which can potentiate postop respiratory effects of spinal opioids.

### INTRAOPERATIVE

**Anesthetic technique:** GETA, often combined with epidural. Consider DLT if OLV needed.

**Induction** Thiopental 3-5 mg/kg iv, succinylcholine 1 mg/kg, or vecuronium 0.1 mg/kg for tracheal intubation.

**Maintenance** Balanced technique: $O_2$, isoflurane and iv opioids, usually fentanyl. $N_2O$ used during two-lung ventilation but discontinued during OLV. Epidural catheter seldom used because pain from limited incision is easily treated by conventional analgesic therapy. If epidural used, follow same guidelines as for open thoracotomy (opioid dosage may be reduced).

**Emergence** Extubate in OR, transfer in head-up position to PACU or ICU breathing $O_2$ by mask.

**Blood and fluid requirements** IV: 18 g x 1
NS/LR @ 2 cc/kg/hr

**Monitoring** Standard monitors (see Appendix).
± Arterial line
Arterial line needed occasionally.

**Positioning** Lateral decubitus, or supine, with wedge under back on operated side.
✓ and pad pressure points.
✓ eyes.

**Ventilation** ETT; DLT or BB rarely needed; TV (12-15 cc/kg/hr) during two-lung and OLV.

### POSTOPERATIVE

**Complications** Atelectasis
Pneumonia
Fluid overload

| | | |
|---|---|---|
| **Pain management** | Parenteral opioids (iv, im, continuous iv, PCA [see Appendix]).<br>Intercostal blocks<br>Interpleural analgesia | Bolus of bupivacaine 0.25%, 0.5 ml/kg/hr, followed by continuous infusion of 0.2 ml/kg/hr). |

**References**


1. Sabiston DC Jr, Spencer FC: *Surgery of the Chest*, 5th edition, Vol II. WB Saunders Co, Philadelphia: 1990.
2. Baue AE, ed: *Glenn's Thoracic and Cardiovascular Surgery*, 5th edition, Volume II. Geha AS, Hammond GL, Laks H, Naunheim KS, co-eds. Appleton & Lange, Norwalk, CT: 1991.
3. Mitchell RL: The lateral limited thoracotomy incision: standard for pulmonary operations. *J Thorac Cardiovasc Surg* 1990; 99(4):590-5.


# CHEST-WALL RESECTION

## SURGICAL CONSIDERATIONS

**Description:** Removal of portions of the thoracic cage may be required under several circumstances. Perhaps the most common indication is lung cancer which has invaded the chest wall. Other indications include primary tumors of the chest wall and areas of radiation necrosis. If the tumor or other disease process involves the skin, an appropriate area of skin – sometimes as much as 4 or 5 cm around the tumor – must be resected along with the specimen. Underlying subcutaneous tissue and muscle should always be resected in continuity; however, the tumor itself must not be exposed. Wide skin flaps are frequently necessary as well. Resection of larger areas of the chest wall may require extensive reconstruction. Limited resection (1-5 cm segments of 1-3 ribs) generally requires limited chest-wall reconstruction (including the use of plastic mesh replacement with or without methylmethacrylate, rib grafts, and muscle or myocutaneous flaps). Extensive reconstruction of the chest wall (procedures that are often complex and time-consuming) is usually carried out in conjunction with plastic surgeons. Removal of anterolateral or anterior portions of the chest wall, particularly resections that include the sternum, are associated with greater postop instability than are resections of posterior portions of the chest wall, which are protected by the back muscles and scapula. Thus, anterior resections may require more extensive reconstruction with wide preparation and draping.

**Usual preop diagnosis**: Lung cancer with chest-wall attachment; primary tumor of the chest wall (bone, cartilage or soft tissue); radiation necrosis

### SUMMARY OF PROCEDURE

| | |
|---|---|
| **Position** | Supine or lateral |
| **Incision** | Over mass to be resected |
| **Special instrumentation** | Bone instruments; Marlex® (or other) mesh; methylmethacrylate |
| **Surgical time** | 1 - 8 hrs |
| **Closing considerations** | May require help of plastic surgeon in extensive cases. |
| **EBL** | 100-2000 cc |
| **Postop care** | PACU or ICU; some patients require temporary ventilatory support. |
| **Mortality** | < 5% |
| **Morbidity** | Paradoxical chest wall-motion (less in posterior resections)<br>Pneumothorax<br>Wound complications |
| **Procedure code** | 19260 (including chest wall); 21559 (soft tissue only) |
| **Pain score** | 3-8 |

### PATIENT POPULATION CHARACTERISTICS

| | |
|---|---|
| **Age range** | Adults of all ages, rarely children |
| **Male:Female** | 1:1 |
| **Incidence** | Relatively rare |
| **Etiology** | Unknown |
| **Associated conditions** | Lung cancer<br>Metastatic disease |

## ANESTHETIC CONSIDERATIONS

See Anesthetic Considerations following "Repair of Pectus Excavatum or Carinatum" (below).

**References**

1. Sabiston DC Jr, Spencer FC: *Surgery of the Chest*, 5th edition, Vol II. WB Saunders Co, Philadelphia: 1990.
2. Baue AE, ed: *Glenn's Thoracic and Cardiovascular Surgery*, 5th edition, Volume II. Geha AS, Hammond GL, Laks H, Naunheim KS, co-eds. Appleton & Lange, Norwalk, CT: 1991.

# REPAIR OF PECTUS EXCAVATUM OR CARINATUM

## SURGICAL CONSIDERATIONS

**Description:** Standard bony and cartilaginous repair of a pectus excavatum (funnel chest) or carinatum (pigeon breast) is usually elective surgery to improve contour and body image. There is no documentation that these repairs have any positive effect on cardiopulmonary function, although some surgeons feel that it can be more than a cosmetic procedure. To repair pectus excavatum, enough pairs of costal cartilages – usually 4-6 – must be removed to be able to mobilize and elevate the sternum. Depending on the severity of the defect and patient's age, fixation of the sternum in the corrected position may be necessary. Repair of pectus carinatum is somewhat more varied because the defects are more varied; however, removal of cartilages and correction of the position of the sternum are still the mainstays of treatment.

A midline incision provides the most satisfactory access to the cartilages and sternum. For cosmetic reasons, however, it may be important to use a curvilinear transverse incision, particularly in females. This incision requires extensive mobilization of subcutaneous and muscle flaps. The wound complication rate is somewhat greater after transverse incisions. The costal cartilages are moved by subperichondrial dissection. This may be tedious and time-consuming, especially since 4 or 5, or even more, pairs of cartilages need to be removed. The elevation of the sternum is usually fairly straightforward, and is usually accompanied by a transverse sternal osteotomy. Intercostal muscle bundles may be left attached to the sternum or may be detached and reattached for better positioning of the sternum. Sternal support normally is not used in infants, but may be used in older children. The most common method of support is the use of a transverse metal strut resting on the ribs, but beneath the sternum. This is removed at a later date. The final position of the sternum is easier to predict following repair of pectus carinatum than following repair of pectus excavatum. Because of the negative intrathoracic pressure it is easier to hold the sternum down than up. Ideally, patients for repair of pectus excavatum are just under school age. Satisfactory repair, however, may be carried out at almost any time during childhood. As full growth is attained, results tend to be less favorable. Pectus carinatum generally has its onset during adolescence, and it is well to let the patient complete his or her growth spurt prior to undertaking repair. In certain circumstances, particularly in teenage girls and patients who do not engage in strenuous sports, subcutaneous, custom-made implants may be placed to improve body contour without necessitating major bony and cartilaginous repairs. These are usually carried out by plastic surgeons.

**Usual preop diagnosis**: Pectus excavatum or carinatum

## SUMMARY OF PROCEDURE

| | |
|---|---|
| **Position** | Supine |
| **Incision** | Transverse or vertical |
| **Special instrumentation** | Bone instruments; sometimes metal struts or wires for reconstruction |
| **Antibiotics** | Cefazolin 1 gm iv q 8 hrs x 36-48 hrs |
| **Surgical time** | 2 - 3 hrs |
| **Closing considerations** | Pleural and wound drainage common |
| **EBL** | 100 - 500 cc |
| **Postop care** | ICU |
| **Mortality** | Minimal |
| **Morbidity** | Pneumothorax: 5-10%<br>Paradoxical chest wall motion → hypoventilation/atelectasis |
| **Procedure code** | 21740 |
| **Pain score** | 4-5 |

## PATIENT POPULATION CHARACTERISTICS

| | |
|---|---|
| **Age range** | Usually children 5-10 yrs; sometimes teenagers; rarely adults |
| **Male:Female** | 1:1 |
| **Incidence** | Unusual |
| **Etiology** | Unknown |
| **Associated conditions** | Marfan syndrome |

# ANESTHETIC CONSIDERATIONS

**(Procedures covered: chest-wall resection; repair of pectus excavatum/carinatum)**

## PREOPERATIVE

| | |
|---|---|
| **Respiratory** | Seldom interferes with ventilation; no special studies indicated. Severe pectus deformity can be associated with restrictive pulmonary disease.<br>**Tests:** CXR; PFT, if indicated from H&P. |
| **Cardiovascular** | With severe pectus, the deformity results in right-ventricular-outflow-tract obstruction (RVOTO) with restriction of ventricular filling in the sitting position. Right heart catheterization may demonstrate low cardiac index during upright exercise.<br>**Tests:** ECG |
| **Hematologic** | **Tests:** Hct |
| **Laboratory** | Other tests as indicated from H&P. |
| **Musculoskeletal** | Chest-wall resection performed for invasive or metastatic cancer; patient may be malnourished, anemic; pectus repair of chest-wall deformity for cosmetic, orthopedic or cardiopulmonary indications; pectus deformity usually asymptomatic. |
| **Premedication** | Midazolam 1-2 mg iv if patient anxious. When epidural opioids are planned, avoid opioid or sedative premedication which can potentiate postop respiratory effects of spinal opioids. |

## INTRAOPERATIVE

**Anesthetic technique:** GETA, occasionally combined with epidural.

| | |
|---|---|
| **Induction** | Standard induction (see Appendix). If severe RVOTO, high-dose opioid/$O_2$ technique (e.g., fentanyl 25 $\mu$g/kg and midazolam 0.1-0.1 mg/kg). Avoid myocardial depressants; if RVOTO very severe, consider high-dose opioid anesthetic technique. |
| **Maintenance** | Standard maintenance (see Appendix) or high-dose opioid technique (fentanyl 50-100 $\mu$g/kg) for patient with severe RVOTO. |
| **Emergence** | Extubate in OR; if high-dose opioid → ICU for later extubation. |

| | | |
|---|---|---|
| **Blood and fluid requirements** | IV: 18 ga x 1<br>LR/NS @ 1-2 ml/kg/hr | Usually minimal blood loss. Fluid restriction unnecessary since extrapulmonary operation. |
| **Monitoring** | Standard monitors (see Appendix). | |
| **Positioning** | ✓ and pad pressure points.<br>✓ eyes. | |
| **Complications** | Pneumothorax | Unintentional pleural tear can cause pneumothorax. Intraop deterioration with increased ventilatory pressure suggests pneumothorax. D/C $N_2O$. Insert chest tube immediately following operation. |

**POSTOPERATIVE**

| | | |
|---|---|---|
| **Complications** | Hypoventilation<br>Flail chest<br>Atelectasis | Although most patients do not require postop ventilatory support, with extensive chest-wall resection, patient may hypoventilate. Paradoxical chest wall movement during spontaneous ventilation with flail chest; postop atelectasis from splinting. |
| **Pain management** | Depends on site and extent of chest wall resected. Parenteral or epidural opioids. | Epidural opioids particularly useful if flail chest present – reduces need for ventilatory support. |

**References**

1. Sabiston DC Jr, Spencer FC: *Surgery of the Chest*, 5th edition, Vol II. WB Saunders Co, Philadelphia: 1990.
2. Baue AE, ed: *Glenn's Thoracic and Cardiovascular Surgery*, 5th edition, Volume II. Geha AS, Hammond GL, Laks H, Naunheim KS, co-eds. Appleton & Lange, Norwalk, CT: 1991.
3. Garcia VF, Seyfer AE, Graeber GM: Reconstruction of congenital chest-wall deformities. *Surg Clin North Am* 1989; 69(5):1103-18.
4. Ghory MJ, James FW, Mays W: Cardiac performance in children with pectus excavatum. *J Pediatr Surg* 1989; 24(8):751-55.
5. Onodera M, Fukuda S, Taga K, et al: Anesthesia for pectus excavatum. *Japanese J Anesth* 1990; 39(12):1690-93.

# THORACOPLASTY

## SURGICAL CONSIDERATIONS

**Description:** The objective of a **thoracoplasty** (removal of several ribs) is to permanently obliterate an existing pleural space or to collapse a portion of the lung. Formerly, this operation was used in the treatment of tuberculosis (TB); but, because of better drug therapy, appropriate pulmonary resection and the decrease in incidence of TB, thoracoplasty is now rare. The procedure was also used for obliterating empyema spaces and helping to close bronchopleural fistulas (BPFs). The use of **pedicled muscle flaps** (serratus anterior, pectoralis major and latissimus dorsi are the most common) or an **omental transposition** have largely replaced thoracoplasty for filling empyema spaces and encouraging closing of BPFs. These operations are less deforming and better tolerated physiologically since they do not result in paradoxical motion of the chest wall.

Thoracoplasty is accomplished by removing several ribs in a subperiosteal fashion, allowing the underlying chest wall to collapse. This collapse is aided by the normally negative intrapleural pressure. Since the periosteum is left intact, the ribs will regenerate, resulting in a permanent, bony collapse of the chest wall. If the objective of the thoracoplasty is to obliterate a relatively small space (meaning that segments of only 2-3 ribs need be removed), the procedure may be done in a single stage, with little postop physiologic impairment of respiration. If extensive thoracoplasty is necessary, however, the procedure may be done in stages to minimize postop chest-wall instability and resultant respiratory problems.

**Usual preop diagnosis**: Pulmonary TB; BPF; empyema

### SUMMARY OF PROCEDURE

| | |
|---|---|
| **Position** | Usually lateral |
| **Incision** | Along rib line |
| **Special instrumentation** | Bone instruments |
| **Unique considerations** | May be TB or fungal infection |
| **Antibiotics** | Depends on causative agent |
| **Surgical time** | 2 - 3 hrs |
| **EBL** | 500 cc or more |
| **Postop care** | ICU |
| **Mortality** | Minimal |
| **Morbidity** | Paradoxical chest-wall motion → atelectasis → hypoxemia: 10%<br>Pneumothorax: Rare |
| **Procedure code** | 32900/32905 |
| **Pain score** | 7-8 |

### PATIENT POPULATION CHARACTERISTICS

| | |
|---|---|
| **Age range** | Middle age or older adults |
| **Male:Female** | 1:1 |
| **Incidence** | Rare |

## ANESTHETIC CONSIDERATIONS

See Anesthetic Considerations following "Drainage of Empyema" (below).

References

1. Sabiston DC Jr, Spencer FC: *Surgery of the Chest*, 5th edition, Vol II. WB Saunders Co, Philadelphia: 1990.
2. Baue AE, ed: *Glenn's Thoracic and Cardiovascular Surgery*, 5th edition, Volume II. Geha AS, Hammond GL, Laks H, Naunheim KS, co-eds. Appleton & Lange, Norwalk, CT: 1991.

# DRAINAGE OF EMPYEMA

## SURGICAL CONSIDERATIONS

**Description:** Collections of pus in the pleural cavity require appropriate and adequate drainage. In the acute situation, and particularly if the fluid is thin, **tube thoracostomy** at the bedside may suffice. In other circumstances, more formal drainage in the OR environment may be required. In the acute situation, **thoracotomy** and **decortication of the pleura** may be indicated, accompanied by generous tube drainage. With chronic localized empyema, **resection of the rib, local debridement**, and **tube drainage** may suffice. On rare occasions, construction of an **Eloesser flap** may be indicated. This is a permanent, skin-lined flap which creates an opening into a chronic empyema cavity. A tongue-shaped flap is based either superiorly or inferiorly over the rib immediately above or below (as the case may be) the intended area of localized rib resection. After elevation of the flap, resection of several-centimeter segments of 1 or 2 ribs is carried out and the chronic empyema space is entered. The flap is then sutured to the underlying parietal pleura or wall of the empyema cavity and the cavity is left open for permanent drainage. A variant of this procedure, called the **Clagett**

**procedure,** is carried out for empyema (with or without bronchopleural fistula) following **pneumonectomy**, since closed drainage rarely suffices in such a situation. The principal is the same: that is, an epithelial-lined, permanent opening to achieve drainage of an empyema. In the Clagett procedure, the opening is generally made anterolaterally and dependently so that drainage is effective and the patient can handle dressing changes without assistance. Segments of 2 or 3 ribs are removed and the skin is sutured to the parietal pleura, leaving a permanent opening for drainage and irrigation. Without an underlying lung, and with a relatively fixed mediastinum, this procedure is well-tolerated physiologically.

**Usual preop diagnosis**: Non-tuberculosis empyema

### SUMMARY OF PROCEDURE

| | Eloesser or Clagett | Tube Thoracostomy |
|---|---|---|
| **Position** | Usually lateral | Lateral |
| **Incision** | Over empyema pocket for Eloesser; low anterolateral for Clagett | Lateral |
| **Special instrumentation** | None | Large tubes |
| **Unique considerations** | Patient may have BPF | Local or GA |
| **Antibiotics** | Depends on causative agent | ⇐ |
| **Surgical time** | 1 hr; occasionally more | < 1 hr |
| **Closing considerations** | Wound left open | None |
| **EBL** | 100 cc | Minimal |
| **Postop care** | PACU → room | ⇐ |
| **Mortality** | Minimal | ⇐ |
| **Morbidity** | Fluid drainage<br>Bleeding: Rare | Air leak |
| **Procedure code** | 32036 | 32035 |
| **Pain score** | 3-4 | 2-3 |

### PATIENT POPULATION CHARACTERISTICS

| | |
|---|---|
| **Age range** | Usually adults |
| **Male:Female** | 1:1 |
| **Incidence** | Decreasing |
| **Etiology** | Pneumonia<br>Esophageal leak<br>Bronchial leak<br>Lymphatic or hematogenous spread<br>Post-trauma or surgery |

## ANESTHETIC CONSIDERATIONS

**(Procedures covered: thoracoplasty; drainage of empyema)**

### PREOPERATIVE

**Respiratory**

Patients usually have pre-existing pulmonary disease. Procedure often is performed for empyema in the presence of BPF following lung resection (particularly pneumonectomy), penetrating injury to chest, or rupture of a cyst or bulla. When possible, surgeon should drain empyema under local anesthesia before induction, with patient sitting upright. If empyema loculated, complete drainage may not be possible.

**Tests:** PFTs; ABG; obtain CXR to determine efficacy of preop chest drainage; if chest CT available, look for airway obstruction that could interfere with DLT placement.

**Cardiovascular** **Tests:** No specific cardiac problems.

**Neurological** √ Hx of back surgery, peripheral neuropathy. Examine lumbar area for skin lesions, infection, deformities. Avoid placement of epidural catheter in patient with neurologic problems.

**Musculoskeletal** Patients with lung cancer may have myasthenic (Eaton-Lambert) syndrome with increased sensitivity to non-depolarizing muscle relaxants. Monitor relaxation with peripheral nerve stimulator.

**Hematologic** Transfuse patients with preop Hct < 25% (Hb level necessary to maintain adequate $O_2$ content). Obtain autologous blood during the month before surgery.
**Tests:** Hct; PT; PTT

**Laboratory** Other tests as indicated from H&P.

**Premedication** Midazolam 1-2 mg iv if patient anxious. When epidural opioids are planned, avoid opioid or sedative premedication which can potentiate postop respiratory effects of spinal opioids.

## INTRAOPERATIVE

**Anesthetic technique:** GETA; seldom use combined epidural technique.

**Induction** Consider awake tracheal intubation with sedated, spontaneously breathing patient. Rapid-sequence induction with cricoid pressure is an alternative. Intubate with DLT; isolate lungs to protect from aspiration and tension pneumothorax. Use DLT with bronchial lumen to side opposite BPF. Contamination of the healthy lung from aspiration of pus is a major concern. Large DLT provides snug fit in bronchus and limits aspiration. Pus may appear in tracheal lumen (lumen to the diseased lung); suction frequently to avoid soiling good lung.

**Maintenance** $O_2$ and isoflurane (1.0-1.5%); less required if epidural local anesthetics used. Avoid $N_2O$, especially during OLV, since hypoxemia during OLV is unpredictable; use $FiO_2$=1.0. Lidocaine (1.5% or 2%) 10-12 ml, administered via epidural every 45 min, or bupivacaine (0.5%) 10-12 ml every 1.5-2.0 hrs. Hydromorphone (1.0-1.5 mg) or morphine (5.0-7.5 mg) in 10 ml NS through epidural. Following intubation, isolate lung with DLT or BB. Chest tube is then removed while chest is prepped for operation. Ventilate only the healthy lung. Since BPF is an abnormal communication between bronchial tree and pleural cavity, if no chest tube present, conventional intubation with IPPV can produce tension pneumothorax. Keep unclamped and do not remove a functioning chest tube until lung is isolated and ventilation to diseased lung stopped. Once chest is opened, there is no chance of pneumothorax, but the large air leak through BPF may prevent satisfactory ventilation of that lung. High-frequency ventilation (HFV) is recommended by some, but studies show no benefit; in some patients the BPF is actually increased with HFV.

**Emergence** Prior to closing of the chest, lungs are inflated to 30 cm $H_2O$ pressure to re-inflate atelectatic areas and to check for significant air leaks. The surgeon will insert chest tubes to drain pleural cavity and aid lung re-expansion. Patient is extubated while still in OR. If postop ventilation is required (rare), the DLT is exchanged for an ETT. If BPF is still open, consider selective ventilation postop through DLT. Ventilate each lung separately; use smaller TVs to lung with BPF.

| | | |
|---|---|---|
| **Blood and fluid requirements** | IV: 16 - 18 ga x 1<br>Restrict iv fluids; usually administer 1000-1500 cc NS/LR ± 1 U autologous blood if available; use vasopressor (ephedrine 5-10 mg iv bolus or phenylephrine 50-100 $\mu$g iv bolus) if hypotensive. | An overhydrated patient is at increased risk of right heart failure. Use of epidural local anesthetics can cause hypotension in a volume-restricted patient; vasopressor often needed. |
| **Monitoring** | Standard monitors (see Appendix).<br>± CVP and/or PA line | It is mandatory to follow oxygenation continuously during OLV. Currently this can be done only with pulse oximetry, although continuous intra-arterial $PO_2$ monitoring may soon be commercially available. |
| **Positioning** | Axillary roll, "airplane" for upper arm; avoid hyperextending arms.<br>√ and pad pressure points.<br>√ eyes. | |

### POSTOPERATIVE

| | | |
|---|---|---|
| **Complications** | Tension pneumothorax<br>Aspiration pneumonia ("down" lung) | Functioning chest tube necessary to prevent tension pneumothorax. |
| **Pain management** | Analgesic requirements minimal. | |

**References**

1. Sabiston DC Jr, Spencer FC: *Surgery of the Chest*, 5th edition, Vol II. WB Saunders Co, Philadelphia: 1990.
2. Baue AE, ed: *Glenn's Thoracic and Cardiovascular Surgery*, 5th edition, Volume II. Geha AS, Hammond GL, Laks H, Naunheim KS, co-eds. Appleton & Lange, Norwalk, CT: 1991.
3. Benjaminsson E, Klain M: Intraoperative dual-mode independent lung ventilation of a patient with bronchopleural fistula. *Anesth Analg* 1981; 60(2):118-19.
4. Bishop MJ, Benson MS, Sato P, Pierson DJ: Comparison of high-frequency jet ventilation with conventional mechanical ventilation for bronchopleural fistula. *Anesth Analg* 1987; 66(9):833-38.
5. Langston HT: Thoracoplasty: the how and the why. *Ann Thorac Surg* 1991; 52(6):1351-53.

# RESECTION OF TRACHEA FOR STENOSIS OR TUMOR

## SURGICAL CONSIDERATIONS

**Description: Tracheal resection** with **primary anastomosis** may be carried out for tracheal stenosis or for tumor. The approach to the trachea varies, depending on the nature of the lesion, its location, and the extent of resection and reconstruction that is to be carried out. The simplest resection is of the **cervical** trachea for tracheal stenosis or localized tumor. This can be done through a cervical incision alone with primary tracheal anastomosis. Longer and/or more inferiorly located lesions may be approached through a cervical incision, combined with **sternotomy**.

When operating through a cervical incision, it is important that the dissection be carried out on the anterior and posterior surface of the trachea, leaving the vascular attachments laterally to assure good blood supply to the remaining trachea. This also minimizes the chance of injury to the recurrent laryngeal nerves. Generous amounts of trachea may be mobilized inferior to the incision by this method, so that the anastomosis may be carried out without tension. After the lesion is resected, the distal trachea is intubated across the operative field and maintained in this fashion, while the tracheal anastomosis is being done using interrupted sutures of absorbable material. The ETT, which had been inserted from above, is left in the superior portion of the trachea; and, after the anastomosis is completed, the ETT is advanced into the distal trachea, while the tube which had crossed the field is removed (Fig 5-3). After the anastomosis is completed and the wound closed, it is important that tension be avoided on the suture line. Some surgeons prefer to put a suture from the skin of the chin to the anterior chest in order to hold the neck in flexion for a few days. Others use a plaster jacket for the same purpose.

For tumors of the mid-trachea, a **right thoracotomy** approach, either alone or combined with sternotomy, may be necessary. For particularly complex tracheal tumors requiring carinal resection and complex reconstruction, a transverse, or clam shell, incision may be necessary. All tracheal resections require excellent communication and cooperation between surgeon and anesthesiologist. Special anesthetic techniques, including intubation of the distal trachea across the surgical field, jet ventilation, etc., may be necessary. Rarely, CPB will be indicated for a complex tracheal resection and reconstruction.

**Usual preop diagnosis**: Tracheal stenosis or tumor (adenoid cystic carcinoma or squamous cell carcinoma most common)

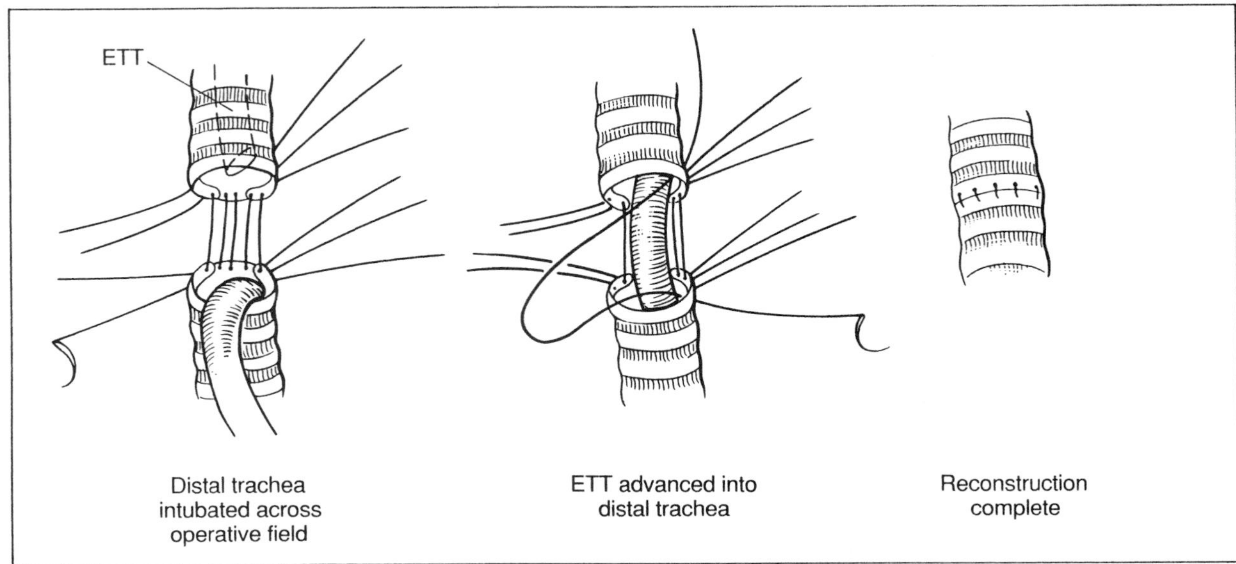


**Figure 5-3.** Stages of tracheal reconstruction. Note ETT in distal trachea. (Reproduced with permission from Grillo HC: *Current Problems in Surgery*. Year Book Medical Publishers: 1970.)

### SUMMARY OF PROCEDURE

| | Cervical Approach | Sternotomy | Right Thoracotomy |
|---|---|---|---|
| **Position** | Supine | ⇐ | Left lateral decubitus |
| **Incision** | Transverse low cervical | Cervical plus sternotomy | Right thoracotomy |
| **Surgical time** | 3 hrs | 3 - 4 hrs | 4 hrs |
| **Closing considerations** | Neck flexion (chin stitch) | ⇐ | ⇐ |
| **EBL** | 200 cc | 350 cc | 350-500 cc |
| **Postop care** | ICU | ⇐ | ⇐ |
| **Mortality** | < 5% | 5% | ⇐ |
| **Morbidity** | Retained secretions<br>Dehiscence<br>Recurrent stenosis<br>Recurrent/superior laryngeal nerve injury<br>Granuloma | ⇐ | ⇐ |
| **Procedure code** | 31780/31785 | 31781/31786 | ⇐ |
| **Pain score** | 3-4 | 5-6 | 7-9 |

### PATIENT POPULATION CHARACTERISTICS

| | |
|---|---|
| **Age range** | Wide variation |
| **Male:Female** | 1:1 |
| **Incidence** | Rare |
| **Etiology** | Stenosis usually 2° to intubation or injury<br>Tumor 2° smoking |

## ANESTHETIC CONSIDERATIONS

### PREOPERATIVE

**Respiratory** Initial presentation may involve Sx of airway obstruction which may be misdiagnosed as asthma, hemoptysis or pneumonitis. A careful evaluation of the airway is usually preceded by bronchoscopy. Lesion should be identified by site and size. Using this information, estimate what

| | | |
|---|---|---|
| | size ETT will easily pass lesion site. | |
| | **Tests:** PFTs; flow/volume loops; CT scan to determine extent of tracheal obstruction. | |
| **Laboratory** | Other tests as indicated from H&P. | |
| **Premedication** | Patients with stridor or critical airway lesions should not receive preop sedation. It is probably best to avoid sedation in all patients. | |

## INTRAOPERATIVE

**Anesthetic technique:** GETA

| | | |
|---|---|---|
| **Induction** | Be prepared for airway emergency. Surgeon must be present and prepared for emergency rigid bronchoscopy and/or to perform tracheostomy below lesion. Mask inhalational induction with spontaneous ventilation; avoid iv drugs that could depress ventilation. Avoid muscle relaxants; if necessary, consider small doses of succinylcholine. Halothane/$O_2$ is preferred for smooth induction with depression of cough reflex; avoid $N_2O$. High concentrations of halothane may be necessary. Helium has been recommended to decrease resistance to flow past the obstruction; however, helium is not usually available.<br>Have a variety of laryngeal blades and uncut ETTs of all sizes, including thin (5 mm) tubes. If ETT passes beyond lesion, can begin IPPV. If ETT cannot be passed, spontaneous ventilation with 100% $O_2$ and halothane is required. For carinal resections, use armored ETTs, which can be placed by surgeon directly into each bronchus during resection. An armored tube is preferable because it is constantly being removed while the surgeon works; also, there is less kinking, so less chance to obstruct. | |
| **Maintenance** | Standard maintenance (see Appendix). $FiO_2$ = 1.0 during apneic oxygenation; continuous monitoring with pulse oximetry mandatory. Consider HFV through a small-diameter catheter if ETT interferes with operation. HFV will require iv anesthesia since inhalational agents cannot be delivered predictably; CPB can be used (rare). | |
| **Emergence** | Early extubation; presence of ETT and IPPV can disrupt fresh suture line. Remove ETT as soon as patient is awake enough to protect airway, but before bucking and coughing occur. | |
| **Blood and fluid requirements** | IV: 18 ga x 1 (left arm)<br>NS/LR @ 3 ml/kg/hr | |
| **Monitoring** | Standard monitors (see Appendix). | Left radial artery cannulation permits uninterrupted monitoring of BP during periods of innominate artery compression. Placement of iv in left arm allows unimpeded infusion. Right extremity pulse oximetry will help detect innominate artery occlusion (which otherwise could lead to stroke.) |
| **Positioning** | √ and pad pressure points.<br>√ eyes. | |
| **Airway management** | ETT replaced with sterile ETT and circuit intraop. | Once the trachea is divided, the surgeon places a sterile ETT in the distal trachea. The original ETT is withdrawn above the surgical site. The surgeon attaches a sterile anesthesia circuit to distal ETT for ventilation. Then, the surgeon places a suture through the distal tip of the original ETT. Prior to re-anastomosis of trachea, the distal trachea is suctioned to remove accumulated blood and secretions. After a posterior suture line is completed, the original ETT is pulled through the trachea and the distal tube (which is below the resection) is removed. Reattach and ventilate patient through original ETT. |
| **Complications** | Tracheal edema | Corticosteroids (dexamethasone 6-8 mg iv) to reduce tracheal edema. |
| | Injury to neck | Any structure in the neck can be damaged, including superior and recurrent laryngeal nerves, trachea and thoracic duct. |

### POSTOPERATIVE

| | | |
|---|---|---|
| **Complications** | Tracheal disruption | Neck swelling, subcutaneous emphysema, and inability to ventilate, indicate loss of air-tight anastomosis. Immediate re-exploration of neck is essential. |
| | Recurrent laryngeal nerve injury | Bilateral (occasionally unilateral) laryngeal nerve damage may result in airway obstruction, necessitating reintubation. Mask ventilation may be ineffective. |
| **Position** | Keep head flexed to reduce tension on tracheal suture line. | |
| **Pain management** | Parenteral opioids (see Appendix) once patient is fully awake. | |

**References**

1. Sabiston DC Jr, Spencer FC: *Surgery of the Chest*, 5th edition, Vol II. WB Saunders Co, Philadelphia: 1990.
2. Baue AE, ed: *Glenn's Thoracic and Cardiovascular Surgery*, 5th edition, Volume II. Geha AS, Hammond GL, Laks H, Naunheim KS, co-eds. Appleton & Lange, Norwalk, CT: 1991.
3. Young-Beyer P, Wilson RS: Anesthetic management for tracheal resection and reconstruction. *J Cardiothoracic Anesth* 1988; 2(6):821-35.
4. Grillo HC, Mathisen DJ: Surgical management of tracheal strictures. *Surg Clin North Am* 1988; 68(3):511-24.

# EXCISION OF MEDIASTINAL TUMOR

## SURGICAL CONSIDERATIONS

**Description:** Tumors in the anterior mediastinum are usually removed through a **median sternotomy**, while tumors in the middle and posterior mediastinum are usually removed through a **lateral thoracotomy**. Some cysts or small tumors may be excised using **video-thoracoscopy** (see "Video-Thoracoscopy," below). Mediastinal tumors that are well-encapsulated are generally removed in a straightforward fashion. If anterior mediastinal tumors are not well-encapsulated and are attached to pericardium or lung on either side, appropriate portions of these attached structures may be removed in continuity with the tumor. If there is attachment to phrenic nerves on either side, one nerve may be sacrificed if necessary to remove the tumor completely. In patients with anterior mediastinal tumors, invasion of the major vascular structures, particularly the aorta and arch vessels, presents an even greater problem. Posterior mediastinal tumors are usually benign. Even so, they may be densely adherent to the posterior chest wall structures. On occasion, dissection can result in injury to an intercostal vessel. Mediastinal tumors sometimes cause tracheal compression and special anesthetic techniques may be necessary to safely secure the airway. Close communication between the surgeon and anesthesiologist is essential.

**Usual preop diagnosis**: Thymoma; teratodermoid; ganglioneuroma; lymphoma; schwannoma

### SUMMARY OF PROCEDURE

| | |
|---|---|
| **Position** | Supine or lateral |
| **Incision** | Median sternotomy or lateral thoracotomy |
| **Special instrumentation** | Sternal or rib retractors |
| **Surgical time** | ≤ 2 hrs |
| **EBL** | < 500 cc |
| **Postop care** | Frequently ICU |
| **Mortality** | Minimal |
| **Morbidity** | Bleeding |
| **Procedure code** | 39220/39200 |
| **Pain score** | 5-8 |

## PATIENT POPULATION CHARACTERISTICS

| | | | | |
|---|---|---|---|---|
| **Age range** | All ages | | | |
| **Male:Female** | 1:1 | | | |
| **Associated conditions** | Anterior mediastinum:<br>Thymoma<br>Teratoma<br>Pericardial cyst<br>Lymphoma<br>Parasternal (Morgagni) hernia<br>Lipoma | Superior mediastinum:<br>Goiter<br>Aneurysm<br>Parathyroid tumor<br>Esophageal tumor<br>Angiomatous tumor | Middle mediastinum:<br>Lymphoma<br>Lymph node inflammation<br>Bronchogenic tumor<br>Bronchogenic cyst | Posterior mediastinum:<br>Neurogenic tumor<br>Aneurysm (enteric cyst)<br>Esophageal tumor<br>Bronchogenic tumor |

## ANESTHETIC CONSIDERATIONS

See Anesthetic Considerations following "Mediastinoscopy" (below).

**References**

1. Sabiston DC Jr, Spencer FC: *Surgery of the Chest*, 5th edition, Vol II. WB Saunders Co, Philadelphia: 1990.
2. Baue AE, ed: *Glenn's Thoracic and Cardiovascular Surgery*, 5th edition, Volume II. Geha AS, Hammond GL, Laks H, Naunheim KS, co-eds. Appleton & Lange, Norwalk, CT: 1991.

# MEDIASTINOSCOPY

## SURGICAL CONSIDERATIONS

**Description:** **Mediastinoscopy** is performed by passing a short endoscope into the upper mediastinum through a small transverse incision just above the sternal notch (Fig 5-4). This procedure is used to biopsy mediastinal lymph nodes and masses as far down as the carina and upper mainstem bronchi. Blunt dissection is carried out in the pretracheal fascial plane. Nodes anterior to the trachea and in the right pretracheal region are readily accessible to biopsy by this technique (Fig 5-5); nodes on the left side are not so accessible. Occasionally, one can biopsy subcarinal nodes by this technique. The proximity of major vascular structures (Fig 5-6) leads to the potential for massive hemorrhage.

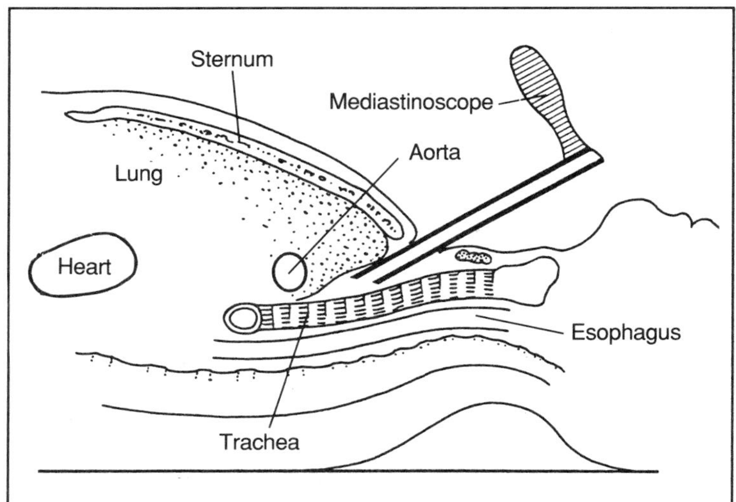


**Figure 5-4.** Insertion of mediastinoscope. (Reproduced with permission from Hurt R, Bates M: *Essentials of Thoracic Surgery*. Butterworths: 1986.)

**Variant procedure or approaches:** For nodes on the left side of the mediastinum, an **anterior mediastinotomy (Chamberlain procedure)**, usually in the second interspace, may be carried out instead of mediastinoscopy. tive being safe biopsy of the target node or mass. A tube is left during closure; it may be removed after closure of the chest or left overnight.

**Usual preop diagnosis:** Carcinoma of the lung with enlarged mediastinal nodes; mediastinal node enlargement 2° lymphoma, thymoma and others

## SUMMARY OF PROCEDURE

| | |
|---|---|
| **Position** | Supine |
| **Incision** | For mediastinoscopy, suprasternal; usually left 2nd interspace for anterior mediastinotomy. |
| **Special instrumentation** | Mediastinoscope for mediastinoscopy only; none for anterior mediastinotomy |
| **Surgical time** | ≤ 1 hr |
| **EBL** | Minimal (but risk of significant blood loss if major vascular injury occurs. |
| **Postop care** | PACU → room |
| **Mortality** | < 1% |
| **Morbidity** | Bleeding<br>Pneumothorax: Rare<br>Vocal cord paralysis: Rare<br>Esophageal perforation: Rare<br>Pleural tear: Rare<br>Tracheal laceration: Rare |
| **Procedure code** | 39400 (mediastinoscopy)<br>32905 (anterior mediastinotomy) |
| **Pain score** | 2 (mediastinoscopy); 2-3 (anterior mediastinotomy) |

## PATIENT POPULATION CHARACTERISTICS

| | |
|---|---|
| **Age range** | Adults, usually > 50 yrs |
| **Male:Female** | Male > female |
| **Incidence** | Frequently part of evaluation for patients with lung cancer |
| **Associated conditions** | Lung cancer<br>Lymphoma |

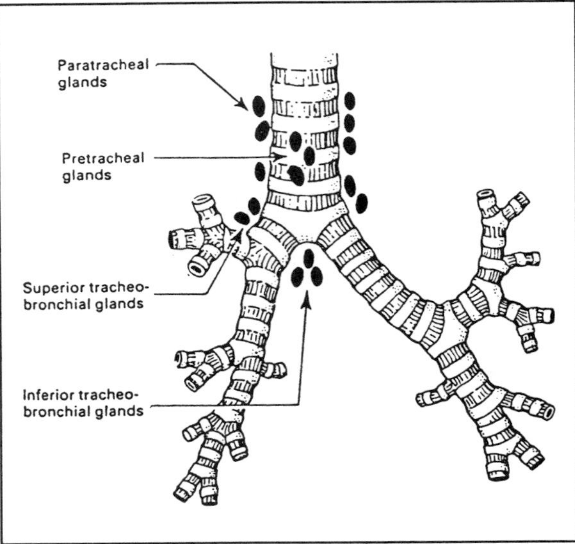


**Figure 5-5.** Common lymph node sites accessible to mediastinoscope biopsy. (Reproduced with permission from Hurt R, Bates M: *Essentials of Thoracic Surgery.* Butterworths: 1986.)

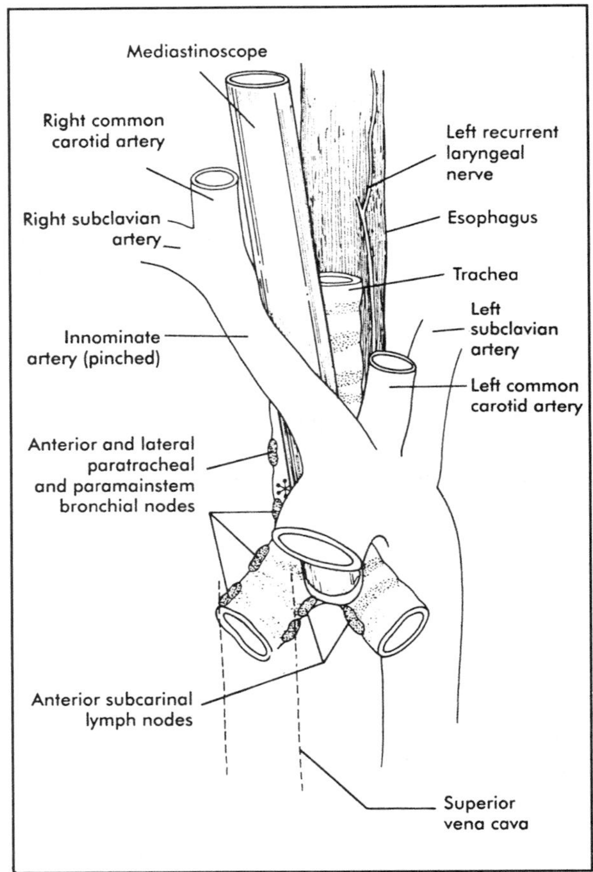


**Figure 5-6.** Relationship of mediastinoscope to trachea and great vessels. (Reproduced with permission from Petty C: Right radial artery pressure during mediastinoscopy. *Anesth Analg* 1979; 58:428. Modified in Rogers MC: *Principals & Practices of Anesthesiology.* Mosby-Year Book, St Louis:1993.)

## ANESTHETIC CONSIDERATIONS

### PREOPERATIVE

Mediastinoscopy is performed to ascertain extrapulmonary spread of pulmonary tumors, diagnose anterior mediastinal masses (neurogenic tumors, cysts, lymphomas, thymomas, parathyroid and substernal thyroid tissue). This technique also may be used for the placement of electrodes for atrial pacing of the heart. If a thoracic aneurysm is present or SVC is obstructed, mediastinoscopy is contraindicated. Anatomy is distorted and vessels can be punctured inadvertently by the mediastinoscope.

**Respiratory** — Question patient with anterior mediastinal mass about ability to lie supine; change in position may cause superior caval obstruction or cardiac and airway compression by mediastinal mass (may be apparent only following induction or on emergence from anesthesia). If significant airway compression or SVC obstruction is present, consider preop radiation or chemotherapy.
**Tests:** If airway compression is present, obtain PFTs with flow/volume loops in upright and supine positions (Fig 5-7 shows flow volume loop). Order CT scan to determine airway distortion or compression and anatomic involvement with other intrathoracic structures.

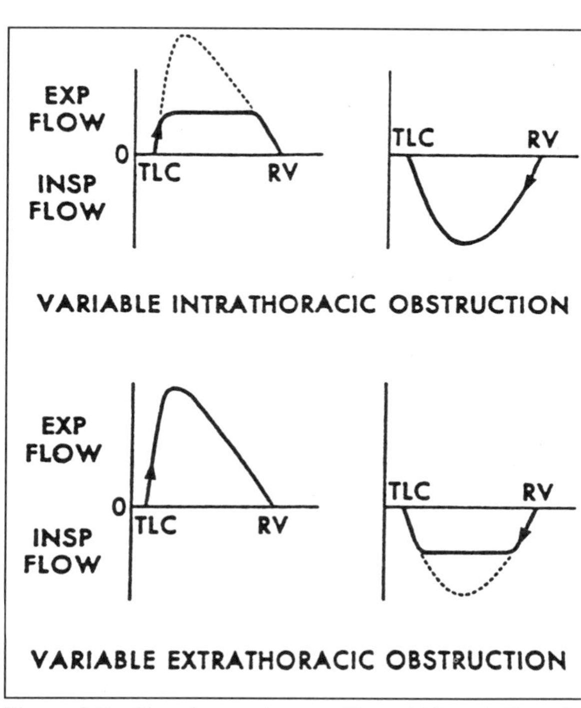


**Figure 5-7.** Flow loop volume: with variable extrathoracic lesion, the alteration in the flow volume loop is seen by flow limitation and a plateau on inspiration. The reverse occurs with variable intrathoracic lesions. (Reproduced with permission from Acręs J, Kryger MH: Clinical significance of pulmonary function tests. *Chest.* 1981; 80:207-11.)

**Cardiovascular** — Aortic angiogram if thoracic aneurysm is present.
**Tests:** As indicated by H&P.

**Musculoskeletal** — Patients with lung cancer may have myasthenic (Eaton-Lambert) syndrome with increased sensitivity to non-depolarizing muscle relaxants. Monitor relaxation with peripheral nerve stimulator.

**Neurologic** — Patient may have ↑ICP if SVC is obstructed. Obtain neurology cosultation.

**Laboratory** — Others tests as indicated from H&P.

**Premedication** — Midazolam 1-2 mg iv; meperidine 1 mg/kg iv immediately preop.

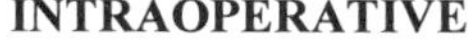

### INTRAOPERATIVE

**Anesthetic technique:** GETA

**Induction** — Consider awake FOB intubation or use short-acting muscle relaxant. Complete or partial airway obstruction by anterior mediastinal mass can be due to changes in lung and chest-wall mechanics associated with changes in the patient's position (sitting to supine during procedure) or to muscle relaxation. A surgeon familiar with rigid bronchoscopy should be in room ready to bypass obstruction.

**Maintenance** — $O_2$ (100%) and isoflurane (1-1.5%). Avoid $N_2O$, especially during OLV. Short-acting muscle relaxant and narcotics as required.

**Emergence** — Extubation in OR

**Blood and fluid requirements** — IV: 18 ga x 1
NS/LR @ 1-2 ml/kg/hr

Have blood for transfusion available in OR prior to surgery. With venous bleeding, fluids given through an iv in upper limb may enter mediastinum through a tear

| | | |
|---|---|---|
| | | in the vein. A large-bore iv cannula should then be placed in lower limb for fluid and blood transfusions. |
| **Monitoring** | Standard monitors (see Appendix).<br>Blood in OR | BP cuff on left arm; radial artery line and pulse oximeter on right. Mass or mediastinoscope can compress innominate artery, causing reduction in right-radial pulse and right-arm BP. If only right-arm BP is measured, patients may be treated inappropriately for "hypotension." Suspect great vessel compression if right-arm pressure is lower than left, or if right-arm BP disappears in the presence of a normal ECG. Arterial compression can compromise cerebrovascular perfusion → cerebral ischemia stroke. |
| **Positioning** | Head-up position<br>✓ and pad pressure points.<br>✓ eyes. | In patients with an anterior mediastinal mass, the head-up position reduces mass compression effect on airway and vascular structures. Patients with SVC obstruction, if placed in head-down position with IPPV (further impedes venous return of thoracic cavity), are at ↑risk of airway edema and airway obstruction following extubation. |
| **Complications** | Bleeding | Surgical tamponade through mediastinoscope may be indicated. For major hemorrhage, emergency thoracotomy or median sternotomy may be required to stop bleeding. |
| | Air embolism | Can occur from laceration of mediastinal vein.<br>Head elevation increases risk of embolism, particularly if patient breathes spontaneously. |
| | Airway rupture or obstruction | Monitor $ETCO_2$ and $ETN_2$.<br>Vagally mediated reflex bradycardia from compression of the trachea or great vessels. |
| | Tracheal collapse | Acute obstruction may require rigid bronchoscope to reopen airway. |

### POSTOPERATIVE

| | | |
|---|---|---|
| **Complications** | Pneumothorax (see previous section).<br>Recurrent laryngeal nerve damage<br>Bleeding | Bilateral laryngeal nerve damage may result in airway obstruction, necessitating reintubation. Mask ventilation may be ineffective. |
| **Pain management** | Parenteral opioids (see Appendix). | |
| **Tests** | CXR on all patients to R/O pneumothorax. (See Postoperative Complications for "Thoracoscopy.") | |


**References**

1. Sabiston DC Jr, Spencer FC: *Surgery of the Chest*, 5th edition, Vol II. WB Saunders Co, Philadelphia: 1990.
2. Baue AE, ed: *Glenn's Thoracic and Cardiovascular Surgery*, 5th edition, Volume II. Geha AS, Hammond GL, Laks H, Naunheim KS, co-eds. Appleton & Lange, Norwalk, CT: 1991.
3. Barash PG, Tsai B, Kitahata LM: Acute tracheal collapse following mediastinoscopy. *Anesthesiology* 1976; 44(1):67-8.
4. Petty C: Right radial artery pressure during mediastinoscopy. *Anesth Analg* 1979; 58(5):428-30.
5. Vaughan RS: Anesthesia for mediastinoscopy. *Anaesthesia* 1978; 33(2):195-98.
4. Neuman GG, Weingarten AE, Abramowitz RM, et al: The anesthetic management of the patient with an anterior mediastinal mass. *Anesthesiology* 1984; 60(2):144-47.
6. Vueghs PJ, Schurink GA, Vaes L, Langemeyer JS: Anesthesia in repeat mediastinoscopy: a retrospective study of 101 patients. *J Cardiothorac Vasc Anesth* 1992; 6(2):193-95.

# BRONCHOSCOPY – FLEXIBLE AND RIGID

## SURGICAL CONSIDERATIONS

**Description:** Most **flexible fiber optic bronchoscopy (FOB)** is done under topical anesthesia and does not require the services of an anesthesiologist. When flexible FOB precedes other surgery, it is usually carried out in an anesthetized patient through the ETT, using a special adaptor. **Rigid bronchoscopy**, alone or in combination with other procedures such as **mediastinoscopy** or **thoracotomy**, however, is usually done under GA. Ventilation during rigid bronchoscopy under GA may be carried out using a special adaptor (Racine) or a Sander's attachment (see Anesthetic Considerations, below). **Laser bronchoscopy** may be carried out using flexible or rigid bronchoscopes. $FiO_2$ of 0.4 or less is necessary when laser is in use.

**Usual preop diagnosis**: Carcinoma of the lung, primary or recurrent; hemoptysis; obstruction; foreign body; benign tumor

### SUMMARY OF PROCEDURE

| | Fiber Optic Bronchoscopy | Rigid Bronchoscopy | Laser Bronchoscopy |
|---|---|---|---|
| **Position** | Supine | ⇐ | ⇐ |
| **Special instrumentation** | FOB and instrument | Rigid bronchoscope and instrument | Nd:YAG laser and bronchoscope |
| **Unique considerations** | None | ⇐ | Keep $FiO_2 \leq 0.4$ during use of laser |
| **Surgical time** | < 30 min | ⇐ | 1 hr |
| **EBL** | Minimal | ⇐ | ⇐ |
| **Postop care** | PACU → room | ⇐ | ⇐ |
| **Mortality** | Minimal | ⇐ | 5% |
| **Morbidity** | Barotrauma | ⇐ | ⇐ |
| | Airway obstruction | ⇐ | Airway fire |
| | Pneumothorax | ⇐ | Hemorrhage |
| | | Tooth damage | Perforation |
| | | Tracheal laceration | |
| | | Pneumomediastinum | |
| | | Esophageal perforation | |
| **Procedure code** | 31622/31625 | ⇐ | 31641 |
| **Pain score** | 1 | 1 | 1 |

### PATIENT POPULATION CHARACTERISTICS

| | |
|---|---|
| **Age range** | Usually adults > 50 |
| **Male:Female** | 1:1 |
| **Associated conditions** | Lung cancer<br>Airway obstruction |

## ANESTHETIC CONSIDERATIONS

### PREOPERATIVE

**Respiratory** H&P to focus on underlying condition. Evaluate for acute and chronic pulmonary problems by H&P and lab and radiologic studies.

**Tests:** ABG (indicated if patient has Hx of heavy tobacco use, has SOB at rest or has poor exercise tolerance); PFT; CXR. Hypoxemia ($PaO_2 < 70$ mmHg) and/or hypercapnia ($PaCO_2 > 45$ mmHg) indicate significant respiratory impairment and predict increased risk.

**Cardiovascular** Many patients have Hx of cardiac disease. Cardiology consultation should be obtained for acute change in cardiac status or for patient with poorly controlled chronic disease.

**Tests:** ECG; others as indicated from H&P.

**Musculoskeletal** Patients with lung cancer may have myasthenic (Eaton-Lambert) syndrome with increased sensitivity to non-depolarizing muscle relaxants. Monitor relaxation with peripheral nerve stimulator.

**Hematologic** Blood crossmatch not necessary unless high risk of hemorrhage from Bx. (Check with surgeon.) Adequate $O_2$-carrying capacity important.

**Tests:** Hb/Hct

**Laboratory** Other tests as indicated from H&P.

**Premedication** Anti-sialagogue (prefer glycopyrrolate 0.2 mg iv, no central anticholinergic effects); atropine or scopolamine also can be used. Light sedation with midazolam 1-2 mg iv and/or fentanyl, 50-100 $\mu$g iv. Avoid heavy sedation that might impair postop ventilation.

## INTRAOPERATIVE

**Flexible bronchoscopy:** Anesthetic technique for flexible FOB requires sedation or GA. Anxious patients and those with respiratory compromise may not tolerate sedation for awake FOB; and patients with Hx of gastric reflux or aspiration are not candidates for awake FOB.

**Sedation with topical anesthesia** Sedate patient as necessary to ensure comfort and cooperation (midazolam 1-2 mg iv and/or fentanyl 50-100 $\mu$g iv. Spray palate, pharynx, larynx, vocal cords and trachea with lidocaine (4%), using nebulizer, or have patient gargle viscous lidocaine (4%).

**Transtracheal local anesthesia:** pass needle through cricothyroid membrane, aspirate air into syringe, and then inject lidocaine (2%), 2 ml. Remove needle quickly since injection causes cough (spreads the anesthetic). Perform superior laryngeal nerve blocks. Insert needle anterior to superior cornu of thyroid cartilage. After resistance is felt, aspirate gently, then inject lidocaine (2%) 2 ml; repeat on other side. Alternatively, hold base of tongue forward and, using Krause's forceps, place pledgets soaked in local anesthetic in each pyriform fossa to block the internal branch of superior laryngeal nerve. Patient can hold a suction catheter in the mouth to remove oral secretions and waste anesthetic gasses. A special face mask (Patil-Syracuse) incorporates a diaphragm through which the FOB can pass while patient breathes $FiO_2$=1. Use a special oral airway (Ovassapian) to guide FOB over back of tongue into trachea to prevent damage to FOB by teeth. Limit amount of suctioning by surgeon since suctioning through FOB decreases $FiO_2$ and FRC, $\rightarrow \downarrow PaO_2$.

**General anesthesia:** Almost any anesthetic technique is acceptable. A large ETT has less resistance to air flow; minimum size is 8 mm for adult FOB. If patient requires ETT < 8 mm, use a pediatric FOB. FOB through ETT causes PEEP effect, which can lead to hypotension in hypovolemic patient.

**Rigid bronchoscopy:** Anesthetic technique utilizing rigid bronchoscopy provides superior visualization and improved suctioning, and allows introduction of Bx forceps. Requires GA.

**Induction** Pre-oxygenate to completely de-nitrogenate patient. Use only small amount of iv opioids since postop analgesic requirements are minimal; postop respiratory depression should be avoided. Thiopental 3-5 mg/kg, succinylcholine 1 mg/kg or mivacurium 0.2 mg/kg.

**Maintenance** Isoflurane and 100% $O_2$; succinylcholine drip (1 gm/250 cc NS, titrated to effect; be aware of onset of phase II block at doses > 5-6 mg/kg). Short-acting, non-depolarizing agents (atracurium, vecuronium or mivacurium) also can be used. Manual IPPV through side-arm of rigid bronchoscope. High flow (up to 20 L/min) to compensate for leak. Hyperventilate patient in preparation for periods of apnea. Ventilation must be interrupted whenever surgeon removes eyepiece to suction or Bx. Manually ventilate to compensate for compliance changes that occur when bronchoscope is in trachea (ventilating both lungs) and when it is in bronchus (ventilating one lung). $O_2$ flush is used to compensate for leak; bypasses anesthetic vaporizer. Frequent flushing lowers anesthetic concentration. **Sanders Injection System** – jet ventilation using Venturi effect – is an alternative. Uninterrupted ventilation is possible since the presence of eyepiece is not necessary for ventilation. Fewer interruptions may shorten length of procedure. Requires iv anesthesia (e.g., propofol @ 100-200 $\mu$g/kg/min), since high fresh-gas flow makes inhalational anesthetic concentrations unpredictable. Entrainment of air results in variable $O_2$ at distal tip. If total thoracic compliance is low, adequacy of ventilation is difficult to evaluate; patient easily hypoventilated. The greater need for muscle relaxation to move chest wall increases risk of residual weakness immediately postop.

**Emergence** Can be "stormy." Patient may cough violently to clear secretions and blood. Reintubate with ETT after rigid bronchoscopy. Patient must be fully awake before extubation, with no residual neuromuscular blockade. A smooth emergence may be facilitated by early suctioning of the airway, use of an anti-sialagogue and lidocaine (1 mg/kg iv) to decrease airway sensitivity. The sitting position improves breathing and clearance of secretions. Continue supplemental $O_2$.

| | | |
|---|---|---|
| **Blood and fluid requirements** | Blood usually not required.<br>IV: 18 ga x 1<br>NS/LR @ 2 cc/kg/hr | Transfusion unnecessary unless complicated by massive hemorrhage; be prepared for emergency thoracotomy. Usually restrict iv fluids to avoid fluid overload. |
| **Monitoring** | Standard monitors (see Appendix). | Note: $ETCO_2$ not accurate during rigid bronchoscopy because of dilution effect at sample port. |
| **Positioning** | ✓ and pad pressure points.<br>✓ eyes.<br>Shoulder roll for rigid bronchoscopy | |
| **Complications** | Hypoxemia | Monitor pulse oximetry continuously. If patient hypoxemic, surgeon must withdraw bronchoscope into trachea. If problem persists, remove bronchoscope and ventilate by mask or ETT. |
| | Hypercapnia | Common, due to hypoventilation. Ventricular dysrhythmias due to respiratory acidosis and "light" anesthesia. Treat by hyperventilation (increased rate) which lowers $CO_2$ and deepens inhalational anesthesia; iv lidocaine for dysrhythmias. |
| | Bleeding | Requires frequent suctioning. For major hemorrhage, place uncut ETT down healthy bronchus and ventilate good lung. May require thoracotomy using DLT or bronchial blocker (BB) to isolate and/or tamponade bleeding site. |

## POSTOPERATIVE

| | | |
|---|---|---|
| **Complications** | Hypoventilation<br>Dental damage<br>Airway trauma<br>Pneumothorax<br>Hemorrhage<br>Risk of aspiration | Incomplete reversal of muscle relaxants or opioid overdosage can cause hypoventilation. Obtain ABG if patient has difficulty breathing or is overly sedated. Be prepared to reintubate patient. |
| | Airway obstruction (bronchospasm, bleeding, dislodged tumor, foreign body) | If nerve blocks used to depress gag reflex, no eating or drinking for several hrs post-bronchoscopy. |
| **Pain management** | Minimal pain; easily treated with iv opioids. | |
| **Tests** | CXR | Obtain CXR in recovery room to check for atelectasis, pneumothorax, mediastinal emphysema. |

**References**

1. Sabiston DC Jr, Spencer FC: *Surgery of the Chest*, 5th edition, Vol II. WB Saunders Co, Philadelphia: 1990.
2. Baue AE, ed: *Glenn's Thoracic and Cardiovascular Surgery*, 5th edition, Volume II. Geha AS, Hammond GL, Laks H, Naunheim KS, co-eds. Appleton & Lange, Norwalk, CT: 1991.
3. Fraioli RL, Sheffer LA, Steffenson JL: Pulmonary and cardiovascular effects of apneic oxygenation in man. *Anesthesiology* 1973; 39(6):588-96.
4. Graham DR, Hay JG, Clague J, et al: Comparison of three different methods used to achieve local anesthesia for fiber optic bronchoscopy. *Chest* 1992; 102(3):704-7.
5. Charlton GA, Burns, AM, Jellicoe J, et al: Anaesthesia for diagnostic rigid bronchoscopy: sequential midazolam/flumazenil compared to intermittent thiopentone. *J Cardiothorac Anesth* 1989; 3(5 Suppl 1):26-8.

# ANESTHETIC CONSIDERATIONS FOR LASER RESECTION

## PREOPERATIVE

Typically, these patients present with a long Hx of smoking and consequent pulmonary dysfunction, complicated by an airway mass (endobronchial, carinal or tracheal) causing respiratory distress.

**Respiratory** It is important to define the exact location and magnitude of any tracheal mass, in order to estimate an appropriate size for the ETT and the likelihood of obstruction on induction. CXR and CT scan should be studied. PFTs and flow volume loops may help to characterize the lesion.
**Tests:** PFTs; ABGs; CXR; CT scan (to determine site of airway obstruction)

**Musculoskeletal** Although there may be no clinically detectable muscle weakness, some of these patients will have Eaton-Lambert syndrome → ↑ sensitivity to muscle relaxants.

**Hematologic** Transfuse patients with preop Hct < 25% (or < 30% if CAD present).
**Tests:** Hct

**Laboratory** Other tests as indicated from H&P.

**Premedication** Minimal; avoid respiratory depressants.

## INTRAOPERATIVE

**Anesthetic technique:** GETA or local anesthesia with heavy sedation. Unexpected patient movement may be disastrous. Nd:YAG laser can be transmitted through a flexible quartz monofilament passed through either a rigid bronchoscope or FOB. The rigid bronchoscope provides improved visibility and better debris retrieval. It also maintains the airway with less chance of fire since metal is non-ignitable (it can reflect the laser beam, however, causing tissue damage), although manual ventilation through the side-arm may be more difficult. FOB is used with local anesthesia or through ETT under GA.

**Induction** **Without airway obstruction:** Standard induction (see Appendix).
**With airway obstruction:** Awake FOB may precede intubation in order to determine the feasibility of tracheal intubation. In patients with less severe obstruction, an inhalation induction with spontaneous ventilation may be appropriate. Avoid muscle relaxants until the airway has been secured. For FOB resections, a large, red rubber ETT is preferred as it is less flammable, and less combustible toxic products are released if ignited than if a plastic ETT is ignited. Special "laser ETTs" are not needed since Nd:YAG laser is fired distal to the tip of the ETT.

**Maintenance** Use isoflurane, air ($N_2$) and $O_2$ mixture. Keep $FiO_2 < 0.4$. Avoid $N_2O$, which supports combustion. Short-acting, non-depolarizing relaxant or succinylcholine infusion should be used since it is essential that the operating field be stationary to avoid damage to tissue from a misdirected laser beam. If the patient becomes hypoxemic, ventilate the lungs with higher $FiO_2$ and ask the surgeon to stop.

**Emergence** Following rigid bronchoscopy, the patient usually is reintubated until awake and breathing well and protective airway reflexes have returned. Patient should be recovered in the sitting position.

| | | |
|---|---|---|
| **Blood and fluid requirements** | IV: 14-16 ga x 1-2<br>NS/LR @ 1-2 ml/kg/hr | Can be "stormy" – bleeding and secretion clearance a problem. There is a potential for massive blood loss following inadvertent perforation of a major blood vessel. |
| **Monitoring** | Standard monitors (see Appendix). | Continuous pulse oximetry essential; monitor $ETCO_2$ to assess adequacy of ventilation. Keep alveolar $O_2 < 40\%$. |
| **Positioning** | ✓ and pad pressure points.<br>✓ eyes. | |
| **Complications** | Airway obstruction | From tumor, blood, tissue debris, etc. |
| | Hypoxemia/hypercarbia | From inadequate ventilation. |
| | Bleeding | Can be massive from perforation of blood vessel by laser. Apply topical epinephrine following laser photocoagulation to control bleeding. |
| | Perforation of tracheobronchial tree | Pneumothorax, pneumomediastinum and cardiac arrest. |
| | Airway fire | Rx: stop ventilation, remove $O_2$ source, extubate trachea to decrease inhalation of toxic products. Suction all debris from airway. Ventilate patient by mask, then re-intubate. Prior to extubation, perform bronchoscopy to re-evaluate airway damage and suction debris. |

### POSTOPERATIVE

| | | |
|---|---|---|
| **Complications** | Airway edema | Only the surface of the affected tissue is visibly changed; there may be underlying edema formation. Patient may require emergency reintubation if airway obstruction due to edema occurs. Steroids usually given (dexamethasone 6-8 mg iv). Complications such as hemorrhage or obstruction can be delayed up to 48 hrs. |
| **Pain management** | Minimal pain; rarely requires analgesics | |
| **Tests** | Continuous pulse oximetry monitoring. Frequent ABGs. | |

**References**

1. Sabiston DC Jr, Spencer FC: *Surgery of the Chest*, 5th edition, Vol II. WB Saunders Co, Philadelphia: 1990.
2. Baue AE, ed: *Glenn's Thoracic and Cardiovascular Surgery*, 5th edition, Volume II. Geha AS, Hammond GL, Laks H, Naunheim KS, co-eds. Appleton & Lange, Norwalk, CT: 1991.
3. McCaughan JS Jr, Barabash RD, Penn GM, Glavan BJ: Nd:YAG laser and photodynamic therapy for esophageal and endobronchial tumors under general and local anesthesia. Effects on arterial blood gas levels. *Chest* 1990; 98(6):1374-78.
4. Chan AL, Tharratt RS, Siefkin AD, et al: Nd:YAG laser bronchoscopy. Rigid or fiber optic mode? *Chest* 1990; 98(2):271-75.
5. Vanderschueren RG, Westermann CJ: Complications of endobronchial neodymium:YAG (Nd:YAG) laser application. *Lung* 1990; 168 Suppl:1089-94.
6. Warner ME, Warner MA, Leonard PF: Anesthesia for Neodymium:YAG (Nd:YAG) laser resection of major airway obstructing tumors. *Anesthesiology* 1984; 60(3):230-32.
7. Blomquist S, Algotsson L, Karlsson SE: Anaesthesia for resection of tumours in the trachea and central bronchi using the Nd:YAG-laser technique. *Acta Anaesthiol Scand* 1990; 34(6):506-10.

# VIDEO-THORACOSCOPY

## SURGICAL CONSIDERATIONS

**Description:** While thoracoscopy itself is not new, **video-thoracoscopy** is a relatively new technique which is rapidly gaining popularity. Video-thoracoscopy is most often used for assessment of pleural processes of unknown etiology, such as pleural effusion that has defied diagnosis. Its use is accepted for treatment of spontaneous pneumothorax due to apical blebs, for biopsy of peripheral infiltrates or nodules, and for drainage of pleural effusions and other fluid collections. Accessible, small lung cancers may be removed using the videoscope. **Heller myotomy** and **upper dorsal sympathectomy** can be done using video-thoracoscopy. Less well-accepted procedures using video capabilities include **lobectomy**, **pneumonectomy** and **esophagectomy**. Use of a DLT to provide collapse of the ipsilateral lung is mandatory, since satisfactory visualization of the pleural cavity is impossible without this collapse of the lung. The patient is usually in the lateral position. Several small incisions are used, usually 3; sometimes 4 or more. The video-thoracoscope is placed through the first incision and the pleural cavity is inspected. Other small incisions are then made for insertion of instruments. The position of the video-thoracoscope and instruments may be interchanged, depending on the location of the problem.

**Usual preop diagnosis**: Pleural disease (e.g, effusions); recurrent empyema; recurrent pneumothorax; localized lung masses, achalasia, pulmonary infiltrates

### SUMMARY OF PROCEDURE

| | |
|---|---|
| **Position** | Lateral |
| **Incision** | Usually 3 small incisions (portals) |
| **Special instrumentation** | Video thoracoscope with thoracoscopy instruments |
| **Unique considerations** | DLT required |
| **Surgical time** | 1 - 3 hrs |
| **Closing considerations** | Chest tube placed |

| | |
|---|---|
| **EBL** | Minimal, although there is a risk for major bleeding |
| **Postop care** | Chest tube |
| **Mortality** | Minimal |
| **Morbidity** | Major vascular injury: Rare |
| **Procedure code** | Depends on procedure carried out |
| **Pain score** | 2-3 |

### PATIENT POPULATION CHARACTERISTICS

| | |
|---|---|
| **Age range** | All age groups |
| **Male:Female** | 1:1 |
| **Associated conditions** | Pleural effusions<br>Lung mass<br>Pneumothorax |

---

## ANESTHETIC CONSIDERATIONS

### PREOPERATIVE

Procedure for diagnosis of pleural disease, drainage of effusions, chemical pleurodesis, open-lung biopsy. Video thoracoscopy is also used for wedge resections (see Anesthetic Considerations for "Wedge Resection of Lung Lesion" (above). H&P exam directed at underlying disease. Preop lab tests depend on indications for thoracoscopy. If for respiratory disease, may require PFTs, ABG, etc. If for metastatic disease, preop studies determined by underlying primary disease.

### INTRAOPERATIVE

**Anesthetic technique:** Either regional or GETA.

**Regional anesthesia:** The incision site is infiltrated with local anesthetics, and intercostal nerve blocks are performed at the level of incision and at several levels above and below incision. When surgeon enters chest, air enters pleural cavity, causing partial pneumothorax. Patient usually tolerates this. Thoracoscope in chest-wall incision prevents complete lung collapse.

**General anesthesia:** The patient is intubated with DLT to selectively collapse operated lung. Anesthetic choice optional, but $FiO_2 = 1$ during OLV. GA allows IPPV with complete re-expansion of lung without pain, if pleurodesis performed.

| | | |
|---|---|---|
| **Induction** | Standard induction (see Appendix). | |
| **Maintenance** | $O_2$ (100%) and isoflurane (1-1.5%). Avoid $N_2O$, especially during OLV. Short-acting muscle relaxant and narcotics as required. | |
| **Emergence** | Extubation in OR | |
| **Blood and fluid requirements** | IV: 18 ga x 1<br>NS/LR @ 2 cc/kg/hr | |
| **Monitoring** | Standard monitors (see Appendix). | |
| **Positioning** | ✓ and pad pressure points.<br>✓ eyes. | |
| **Complications** | Air leak from lung | Air leak obvious on re-expansion of lung. |
| | Bleeding | Excessive blood drainage via chest tube; falling Hct |
| | Injury to intrathoracic structures | |

### POSTOPERATIVE

| | | |
|---|---|---|
| **Complications** | Tension pneumothorax | In the absence of chest tube, air leak can lead to pneumothorax (rare). This may manifest as wheezing, hyperresonance, decreased chest-wall movement, dyspnea, |

| | |
|---|---|
| | subcutaneous emphysema, tracheal shift, dysrhythmias, cardiovascular collapse, ↓$PO_2$ and ↓$SaO_2$.<br>CXR diagnostic. Requires immediate decompression of tension pneumothorax with large-bore iv cannula through chest wall, followed by chest tube and continuous suction. |
| **Pain management** | Small incision<br>Analgesic requirements |
| **Tests** | CXR postop |


**References**

1. Sabiston DC Jr, Spencer FC: *Surgery of the Chest*, 5th edition, Vol II. WB Saunders Co, Philadelphia: 1990.
2. Baue AE, ed: *Glenn's Thoracic and Cardiovascular Surgery*, 5th edition, Volume II. Geha AS, Hammond GL, Laks H, Naunheim KS, co-eds. Appleton & Lange, Norwalk, CT: 1991.
3. Rusch VW, Mountain C: Thoracoscopy under regional anesthesia for the diagnosis and management of pleural disease. *Am J Surg* 1987; 154(3):274-78.
4. Oakes DD, Sherck JP, Brodsky JB, Mark JBD; Therapeutic thoracoscopy. *J Thorac Cardiovasc Surg* 1984; 87(2):269-73.
5. Landreneau RJ, Hazelrigg SR, Ferson PF, et al: Thoracoscopic resection of 85 pulmonary lesions. *Ann Thorac Surg* 1992; 54(3):415-19.
6. Miller, DL, Allen MS, Trastek VF, et al: Videothorascopic wedge excision of the lung. *Ann of Thorac Surg* 1992; 54(3): 410-14.


# THYMECTOMY

## SURGICAL CONSIDERATIONS

**Description: Thymectomy** for myasthenia gravis is usually carried out through a median sternotomy incision. In these circumstances, the thymus may be grossly normal. The thymus is an H-shaped organ with long inferior tails heading toward the diaphragm and smaller superior ones extending up into the neck. The only major vascular structure usually encountered is the thymic vein which enters the left brachiocephalic vein as it crosses anterior to the arterial structures in the anterior mediastinum. The thymus gland is anterior to all of this. Dissection is generally started inferiorly, and it is important to remove the entire thymus gland, particularly in patients with myasthenia gravis. This may involve entry into one or both pleural cavities. The dissection is carried superiorly anterior to the left brachiocephalic vein and into the neck, removing the superior tails as well. Some surgeons prefer the **cervical approach** for thymectomy in myasthenia gravis. All agree that the cervical approach is not suitable if the patient has a thymoma (with or without myasthenia gravis).

**Usual preop diagnosis**: Myasthenia gravis; thymoma

### SUMMARY OF PROCEDURE

| | Sternotomy | Cervical Approach |
|---|---|---|
| **Position** | Supine | ⇐ |
| **Incision** | Median sternotomy | Suprasternal |
| **Special instrumentation** | None | Special sternal retractor |
| **Surgical time** | 1 - 2 hrs | ⇐ |
| **EBL** | < 500 cc | ⇐ |
| **Postop care** | ICU – special attention to muscle strength related to respiratory function. | ⇐ |

| | Sternotomy | Cervical Approach |
|---|---|---|
| **Mortality** | < 5% | ⇐ |
| **Morbidity** | Infection<br>Pneumothorax<br>Hemothorax | ⇐ |
| **Procedure code** | 60520 | ⇐ |
| **Pain score** | 5-7 | 2 |

### PATIENT POPULATION CHARACTERISTICS

| | |
|---|---|
| **Age range** | Usually young adults |
| **Male:Female** | Females > males |
| **Incidence** | Infrequent |
| **Etiology** | Unknown |
| **Associated conditions** | Myasthenia gravis<br>Benign or malignant thymoma |

---

## ANESTHETIC CONSIDERATIONS

### PREOPERATIVE

**Respiratory** Obtain preop PFTs; patient may have marked reduction in VC 2° muscle weakness; establish baseline spirometry values.
**Tests:** PFTs

**Neurological** Review neurological assessment. Patients often exhibit diplopia, ptosis, and easy fatiguability of muscles. Difficulties with swallowing and speaking are common. Review tests (EMGs, Tensilon® test) done by neurologist to evaluate the adequacy of drug therapy (steroids, anticholinesterases). 10-50% of the patients with thymomas will have myasthenia gravis and >85% of myasthenics will have thymus abnormalities.

**Musculoskeletal** Determine adequacy of anticholinesterase medication. Evaluate hand strength, inspiratory efforts, and PFTs. Note that an excess of anticholinesterase agents can cause weakness indistinguishable from myasthenia.

**Laboratory** Other tests as indicated from H&P.

**Premedication** Avoid premedication; for the anxious patient, give a small dose of midazolam (1-2 mg); avoid opioids or any other sedatives that may depress ventilation. Controversy exists as to whether to continue anticholinesterase immediately preop since postop drug requirements are markedly reduced. If patient is on steroids, give hydrocortisone (100 mg iv bolus) prior to induction, then q 8 hrs x 24 hrs.

### INTRAOPERATIVE

**Anesthetic technique:** GETA, combined with epidural if transsternal thymectomy.

**Induction** Mask inhalational induction to avoid muscle relaxants entirely; or iv thiopental 2-4 mg/kg induction without muscle relaxants; small dose of succinylcholine (0.5 mg/kg) can be used to facilitate intubation (see below).

**Maintenance** Standard maintenance (see Appendix). Patients with myasthenia gravis have increased sensitivity to non-depolarizing muscle relaxants, which usually are not required (especially during cervical thymectomy). If relaxants are needed, titrate small amounts of drug, using a peripheral nerve stimulator to maintain single twitch. Atracurium is useful since it is rapidly eliminated; intubation dose (0.1-0.2 mg/kg iv). Alternatively, succinylcholine 0.5 mg/kg iv can be used. Patients on anticholinesterase therapy may have increased tolerance to succinylcholine. Avoid drugs with neuromuscular blocking effects (anti-dysrhythmics, diuretics, aminoglycosides). If the patient has normal ventilatory function, then spontaneous ventilation during cervical thymectomy may be appropriate. Patients undergoing sternotomy, and any patient with decreased pulmonary reserve, require mechanical ventilation.

| | | |
|---|---|---|
| **Emergence** | Extubate when fully awake; usually immediate postop ventilation is not necessary. Whether intubated or not, monitor patient for pulmonary function using inspiratory effort meter (PIP) and spirometry (TV). Avoid residual pharmacologic neuromuscular blockade which will lead to hypoventilation and increase risk of gastric aspiration if protective airway reflexes are inadequate. | |
| **Blood and fluid requirements** | IV: 18 ga x 1<br>NS/LR @ 1-2 ml/kg/hr | |
| **Monitoring** | Standard monitors (see Appendix). | Avoid muscle relaxants if possible; if not, use neuromuscular twitch monitor. |
| **Positioning** | ✓ and pad pressure points.<br>✓ eyes. | |

**POSTOPERATIVE**

| | | |
|---|---|---|
| **Complications** | Pneumothorax | Pleura can be entered; if so, chest tube needed. (For Dx and Rx, see "Thoracoscopy.") |
| **Pain management** | Parenteral opioids (see Appendix).<br>Epidural opioids (see Appendix). | Avoid respiratory depression; parenteral opioids for cervical incision, epidural opioids for median sternotomy. |
| **Drug management** | Usually decreased anticholinesterase requirement in the immediate postop period. | Begin anticholinesterase drugs at half preop dose. Consider "cholinergic" crisis. Sx include increased salivation, sweating, abdominal cramps, urinary frequency, fasciculations and weakness from anticholinesterase overdosage. If patient experiences increasing weakness with drug therapy, intubation and ventilation may be necessary. |
| **Tests** | Tensilon® | Neurologists can perform Tensilon® test to determine if patient has adequate anticholinesterase therapy. Determine muscle strength postop (grip strength and sustained head lift). |


**References**

1. Sabiston DC Jr, Spencer FC: *Surgery of the Chest*, 5th edition, Vol II. WB Saunders Co, Philadelphia: 1990.
2. Baue AE, ed: *Glenn's Thoracic and Cardiovascular Surgery*, 5th edition, Volume II. Geha AS, Hammond GL, Laks H, Naunheim KS, co-eds. Appleton & Lange, Norwalk, CT: 1991.
3. Smith CE, Donati F, Bevan DR: Cumulative dose-response curves for atracurium in patients with myasthenia gravis. *Can J Anaesth* 1989; 36(4):402-6.
4. Burgess FW, Wilcosky B Jr: Thoracic epidural anesthesia for transsternal thymectomy in myasthenia gravis. *Anesth Analg* 1989; 69(4):529-31.
5. Kirsch JR, Diringer MN, Borel CO, et al: Preoperative lumbar epidural morphine improves postoperative analgesia and ventilatory function after transsternal thymectomy in patients with myasthenia gravis. *Crit Care Med* 1991; 19(12):1474-79.
6. Baraka A: Anaesthesia and myasthenia gravis. *Can J Anaesth* 1992; 39:476-86.


# EXCISION OF BLEBS OR BULLAE

## SURGICAL CONSIDERATIONS

**Description:** Pulmonary blebs or bullae requiring surgical treatment may vary from small, apical blebs – most usually seen in young people with spontaneous pneumothorax – to expanding, giant bullae causing respiratory distress. The small blebs can be excised through **video-thoracoscopy** (see previous section), although some surgeons still prefer an open technique for this procedure. Giant bullae are generally removed by **open thoracotomy**, although these lesions also may be excised by video-thoracoscopic techniques. Our preference is for **stapling** across the base and excising the lesion. **Clamp and suture** techniques may be used as well. It is important to ensure an air-tight closure if possible. Particularly in patients with giant bullae and emphysema, prolonged air leaks may occur postop, and these can be very debilitating. Patients undergoing operation for giant bullae frequently have limited pulmonary reserve and present formidable operative risks. Since the operation is planned to improve their pulmonary function, however, these patients frequently do well following operation. Pleural abrasion or **pleurectomy** may accompany the excision of blebs or bullae. The blebs in young patients with recurrent spontaneous pneumothorax are usually located at the apex of the upper lobe. Bullae in patients with emphysema are usually in the upper lobe but may be anywhere in the lung. Preop localization by CT scan is usually sufficient. If a thoracotomy is done, the approach is usually lateral.

**Usual preop diagnosis**: Spontaneous pneumothorax 2° ruptured blebs; giant bullae causing respiratory distress

### SUMMARY OF PROCEDURE

| | |
|---|---|
| **Position** | Usually lateral |
| **Incision** | Axillary |
| **Special instrumentation** | Staplers |
| **Surgical time** | 1 - 3 hrs |
| **EBL** | < 500 |
| **Postop care** | PACU → room; ICU for giant bullae |
| **Mortality** | Minimal |
| **Morbidity** | Air leak: 20% or more in giant bullae |
| **Procedure code** | 32141 |
| **Pain score** | 5-7 |

### PATIENT POPULATION CHARACTERISTICS

| | |
|---|---|
| **Age range** | Young adults (blebs/small bullae); elderly (large bullae) |
| **Male:Female** | Males more frequent |
| **Incidence** | Not uncommon |
| **Etiology** | Smoking for emphysema |
| **Associated conditions** | Spontaneous pneumothorax<br>Emphysema<br>Long smoking Hx<br>α-antitrypsin deficiency |

---

## ANESTHETIC CONSIDERATIONS

### PREOPERATIVE

| | |
|---|---|
| **Respiratory** | Cysts may be bronchogenic, post-infective, infantile or emphysematous. Bullae usually result from destruction of alveolar tissue; they represent end-stage emphysematous disease associated with severe COPD. Patient may have incapacitating dyspnea. With blebs, elicit Hx of repeat pneumothoraces. Obtain PFTs and ABG for baseline. Patient may have little pulmonary reserve. $CO_2$ retention may be present.<br>**Tests:** CXR; presence of pneumothorax; if chest CT available, look for airway obstruction that could interfere with DLT placement and also bilateral disease; Hct; ABG. |
| **Cardiovascular** | **Tests:** ECG |
| **Neurological** | ✓ Hx for previous back surgery, peripheral neuropathy. Examine lumbar area for skin lesions, infection, deformities. Avoid placement of epidural catheter in patient with neurologic problems. |
| **Hematologic** | Transfuse patient with preop Hct < 25%. T&C 2-4 U of blood or obtain 1-3 U of autologous blood during the month before surgery.<br>**Tests:** Hct |
| **Laboratory** | Other tests as indicated from H&P. |
| **Premedication** | Midazolam 1-2 mg iv if patient anxious. When epidural opioids are planned, avoid opioid or sedative premedication which can potentiate postop respiratory effects of spinal opioids. |

## INTRAOPERATIVE

**Anesthetic technique:** GETA – may be combined with epidural.

**Induction** Awake intubation or GA with patient breathing spontaneously. Intubate with DLT. If muscle relaxants are used to facilitate tracheal intubation, patient will need IPPV. If cyst or bleb ruptures, a tension pneumothorax can result on the operated side or on the opposite side if bilateral disease is present.

**Maintenance** IPPV with small TVs until chest is opened. Inhalational anesthesia supplemented with epidural, local anesthetics or iv opioids. Avoid $N_2O$ at all times since bullae may be filled with air.

**Emergence** Re-expand lung under direct vision to check for major air leaks. Extubate patient early. Post-bullectomy, unlike other thoracotomy, patients have greater functional lung tissue than preop.

| | | |
|---|---|---|
| **Blood and fluid requirements** | IV: 16 ga x 1<br>NS/RL @ 1-2 ml/kg/hr<br>Restrict iv fluids.<br>Use vasopressor (ephedrine 5-10 mg iv bolus or phenylephrine 50-100 μmg iv bolus) if hypotensive. | An overhydrated patient is at increased risk of right heart failure. Use of epidural local anesthetics can cause hypotension in a volume-restricted patient; vasopressor often needed. |
| **Monitoring** | Standard monitors (see Appendix).<br>± CVP line<br>± PA line | Optional CVP and/or PA line for patients with co-existing cardiac disease. |
| **Positioning** | ✓ and pad pressure points.<br>✓ eyes.<br>Axillary roll; "airplane" for upper arm. | |
| **Ventilation** | DLT or BB needed to separate the lungs. | Allows IPPV of the "good" lung. Use gentle IPPV with smaller, more frequent TVs than during routine thoracotomy. Inspiratory pressure should not exceed 10 cm $H_2O$ to reduce likelihood of rupture of bullae in opposite lung. Treat intraop hypoxemia with CPAP to up lung. In extreme cases consider CPB (rare). |
| **Complications** | Tension pneumothorax | Can occur on either side during induction, only on non-operated side after chest is open, and again on either side postop. Presents with increased ventilatory pressure, progressive tracheal deviation, wheezing, cardiovascular collapse. CXR to rule out tension pneumothorax. Treatment: insertion of chest tube. |

## POSTOPERATIVE

| | | |
|---|---|---|
| **Complications** | Hypoventilation<br>Dental damage<br>Airway trauma<br>Pneumothorax<br>Hemorrhage<br>Risk of aspiration | Incomplete reversal of muscle relaxants or opioid overdosage can cause hypoventilation. Obtain ABG if patient has difficulty breathing or is overly sedated. Be prepared to reintubate patient. |
| | Airway obstruction (bronchospasm, bleeding, dislodged tumor, foreign body) | If nerve blocks used to depress gag reflex, no eating or drinking for several hrs post-bronchoscopy. |
| **Pain management** | Epidural opioids (see Appendix).<br>Parenteral opioids (see Appendix). | Parenteral opioids are adequate if procedure performed through a thoracoscope. |
| **Tests** | Ventilate operated lung with PIP = 30 cm $H_2O$ to observe for air leaks. | |

## References


1. Sabiston DC Jr, Spencer FC: *Surgery of the Chest*, 5th edition, Vol II. WB Saunders Co, Philadelphia: 1990.
2. Baue AE, ed: *Glenn's Thoracic and Cardiovascular Surgery*, 5th edition, Volume II. Geha AS, Hammond GL, Laks H, Naunheim KS, co-eds. Appleton & Lange, Norwalk, CT: 1991.
3. Normandale JP, Feneck RO: Bullous cystic lung disease. Its anesthetic management using high frequency jet ventilation. *Anaesthesia* 1985; 40(12):1182-85.
4. Benumof JL: Sequential one-lung ventilation for bilateral bullectomy. *Anesthesiology* 1987; 67(2):268-72.
5. Connolly JE, Wilson A: The current status of surgery for bullous emphysema. *J Thorac and Cardiovasc Surg* 1989; 97(3):351-61.
6. Ohta M, Nakahara K, Yasumitsu T, et al: Prediction of postoperative performance status in patients with giant bulla. *Chest* 1992; 101(3): 668-73.


## General References


1. Kaplan JA, ed: *Thoracic Anesthesia.* Churchill-Livingstone, New York: 1991.
2. Brodsky JB, ed: Thoracic anesthesia. In *Problems in Anesthesia.* JB Lippincott, Philadelphia: 1990.
3. Marshall BE, Longnecker DE, Fairley HB, eds: *Anesthesia for Thoracic Procedures.* Blackwell Scientific, Boston: 1988.
4. Benumof JL: *Anesthesia for Thoracic Surgery.* WB Saunders, Philadelphia: 1987.

**Surgeons**

**R. Scott Mitchell, MD** *(Cardiac, Vascular Surgery)*
**Norman E. Shumway, MD, PhD** *(Cardiac Surgery)*
**James I. Lin Fann, MD** *(Vascular Surgery)*
**Bruce A. Reitz, MD** *(Heart/Lung Transplantation)*

# 6. CARDIOVASCULAR SURGERY

**Anesthesiologists**

**Gordon R. Haddow, MB, ChB, FFA(SA)** *(Cardiac, Vascular Surgery)*
**Kristi L. Peterson, MD** *(Vascular Surgery)*
**Lawrence Siegel, MD** *(Heart/Lung Transplantation)*

**Surgeons**

**R. Scott Mitchell, MD**
**Norman E. Shumway, MD, PhD**

# 6.1 CARDIAC SURGERY

**Anesthesiologist**

**Gordon R. Haddow, MB ChB, FFA(SA)**

# CARDIOPULMONARY BYPASS

## SURGICAL CONSIDERATIONS

The development of cardiopulmonary bypass (CPB) technology has allowed the repair of many congenital and acquired lesions of the heart and great vessels. Designed to replace cardiac and pulmonary functions, full CPB requires a blood pump and oxygenator. The pump may be of the roller-head or centrifugal variety, with the latter producing less trauma to formed blood elements. The oxygenator may bubble gases ($O_2$ and $CO_2$) through a blood-filled reservoir (bubble oxygenator), or allow $O_2$ and $CO_2$ to diffuse through a thin membrane into the surrounding blood (membrane oxygenator). Utilization of any blood pump requires at least partial heparinization (ACT >180 sec), and introduction of an oxygenator mandates full heparinization (ACT >400 sec).

**Full CPB** typically drains systemic venous return via the right atrium into a venous reservoir, from which the blood is pumped through an oxygenator and then returned to the aorta or femoral artery, completely bypassing the heart and lungs (Fig 6.1-1). **Partial CPB** usually supports only a portion of the body — typically the infradiaphragmatic portion — and may use the patient's lungs as an oxygenator (left atrium → femoral artery), or a mechanical oxygenator (femoral vein → femoral artery). Full CPB is utilized during a sternotomy for work on the heart, ascending aorta, and transverse arch. Partial CPB, in which some systemic venous blood returns to the heart and is ejected into the aorta, is usually employed for work on the descending or thoracoabdominal aorta. Heparin-coated components, which may partially or totally eliminate the necessity for any heparin, may soon become clinically available.

After exposure of the relevant organs (heart or descending thoracic aorta), and after heparinization, venous and arterial cannulae must be placed intraluminally. **Cannulation of the heart** usually involves venous drainage from the right atrium, with either two cannulae inserted through the atrium into the SVC and IVC (bicaval), or via a larger, dual-stage cannula draining the right atria and IVC. Bicaval cannulation reduces venous return (and rewarming) to the heart, and allows caval snares to be placed so that the right atrium can be opened without introducing air into the venous return. Occasionally, atrial manipulation for cannulation can depress cardiac output, with resultant hypotension. This usually can be reversed with volume replacement. Aortic cannulation ususally is not associated with any physiologic pertur-

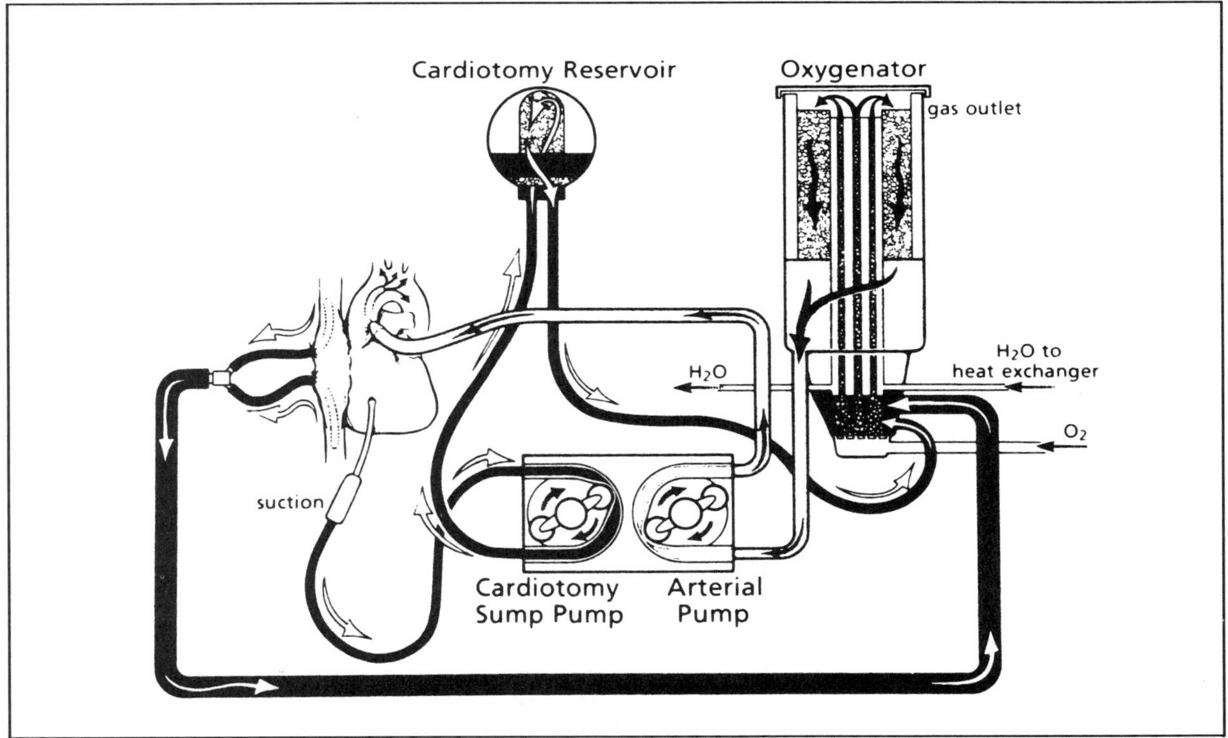


**Figure 6.1-1.** Schematic representation of the CPB circuit. (Reproduced with permission from Hardy JD: *Hardy's Textbook of Surgery*, 2nd edition. JB Lippincott: 1988.)

bation, although HTN must be avoided to minimize aortic complications. Once the cannulae are in place and connections made to the bypass circuit, CPB may be instituted electively. Most cardiac operations are conducted under mild hypothermia (28°C), unless profound hypothermic circulatory arrest is to be utilized. In that case, a target temperature of 18°C is desirable. For operations on the descending thoracic aorta, normothermia is maintained.

**Cessation of CPB** is accomplished by gradually decreasing pump flows, allowing for right heart filling, and gradually replenishing the circulating blood volume. Pulmonary and coronary vasodilation are mandatory during this phase, as there appears to be heightened vasoreactivity after periods of ischemia and hypothermia. For periods of cardiac arrest, during which the heart is deprived of its arterial blood supply, the metabolic demands of the myocardium must be minimized. This is usually accomplished by achieving diastolic arrest with a hyperkalemic cardioplegic solution, and also by lowering myocardial temperature to < 15°C. Frequent reinfusions of cardioplegia maintain hypothermia, prevent lactic acid accumulation, and deliver some minimally available dissolved $O_2$.

The **physiologic response to CPB** is complex, and is associated with a massive catecholamine release which resolves after its cessation. Subsequent changes include abnormal bleeding tendencies, increased capillary permeability, leukocytosis, renal dysfunction and impairment of the immune response. Hemodilution, non-pulsatile flow, hypothermia, exposure of formed elements to non-endothelial surfaces, complement activation, protein denaturation, cascading effects within the coagulation and fibrinolytic system, and activation of the kallikrein-bradykinin cascade, all contribute to this unphysiologic state, and account for much of the morbidity and mortality after CPB.

Many physiologic variables are now controlled by the anesthesiologist, perfusionist and surgeon, including systemic flow and perfusion pressure, arterial $O_2$ and $CO_2$, temperature and Hct. Other physiologic parameters follow either directly or indirectly. Thus, physiologic monitoring for the anesthesiologist and perfusionist include, at a minimum, arterial pressure, CVP, ABG determination (preferably on-line during CPB), cardiac output, UO and ECG. Constant communication among surgeons, perfusionist and anesthesiologist is mandatory for a smooth operation.

**Secondary effects of CPB** demand some special considerations during the final stages of the procedure and chest closure. Adverse effects on coagulation have already been mentioned, and vigorous attention to maintenance and replacement of coagulation factors is essential. The capillary leak phenomenon results in interstitial myocardial and pulmonary edema. Decreased myocardial performance and compliance mandate an increased preload, especially during the physical act of chest closure, where a transient rise in intramediastinal pressure may depress systemic venous return. Similarly, decreased pulmonary compliance and gas exchange mandate vigilance over inspiratory pressures and lung volumes during chest closure, as mediastinal volume is physically decreased.

---

# ANESTHETIC CONSIDERATIONS FOR CARDIOPULMONARY BYPASS (CPB)

This segment is not meant to be a definitive text on cardiopulmonary bypass, but rather a guide to the anesthetic management of bypass. Communication among surgeons, anesthesiologists and pump technicians is of vital importance in carrying out this procedure.

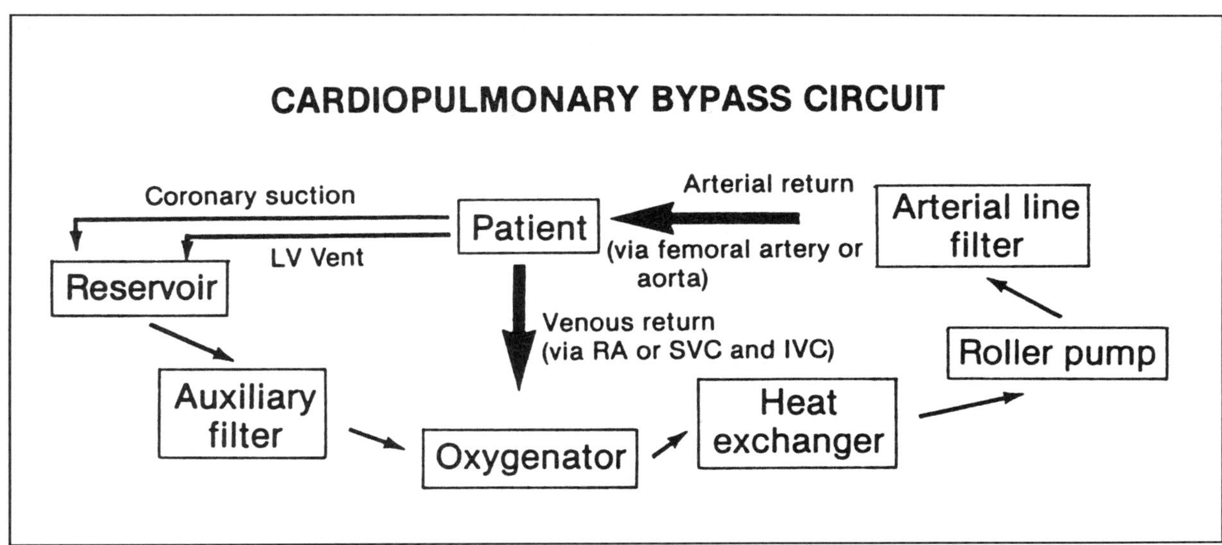


**Figure 6.1-2.** CPB circuit. (Reproduced with permission from Tinker JH: Technical aspects of cardiopulmonary bypass. In Thomas SJ, ed: *Manual of Cardiac Anesthesia*, 2nd edition. Churchill Livingstone: 1993.)

## PREPARATION FOR BYPASS

**Pre-bypass/ anticoagulation** ✓ baseline ACT (normal = 90-130 sec). Heparin (3 mg[~300 U]/kg) is administered via a central vein (✓ back-bleeding to verify intravascular position) or by the surgeon directly into the atrium (preferred). ✓ ACT 3 min after heparin. It is essential to ensure adequate anticoagulation (ACT >400 sec).

**Aortic cannulation** Control MAP to ~70 mmHg for cannulation to ensure that the aortotomy does not extend. If needed, vasodilators may be used. The arterial line should be inspected for air bubbles.

**Venous cannulation** Venous cannulation may be associated with atrial dysrhythmias. Blood loss can be excessive.

**Pupils** Assess pupil symmetry for later comparison.

## TRANSITION ONTO CPB

**Stop ventilation**

**Withdraw PA catheter** Commencing bypass is a dangerous period for the patient as a result of the many hemodynamic changes that occur. D/C ventilation once there is no pulmonary blood flow. Withdraw PA catheter 4-5 cm.

**Stop infusions** Stop iv drugs and reduce iv fluid infusions to TKO.

**Anticoagulation** ACT should be checked after 5 min on CPB to ensure anticoagulation (ACT >400 sec).

**Oxygenation** Verify oxygenation by checking arterial inflow color, in-line sensors and by ABG within 5 min of beginning CPB.

**Flow** ✓ for adequate venous drainage (CVP falls to a low level). Ensure adequate arterial inflow. Initial pressures may be very low, but will usually increase.

**Anesthesia** Anesthetics (e.g., fentanyl and midazolam) may be needed. A repeat dose (e.g., 10 mg pancuronium) should be given to prevent movement or shivering (which increases $O_2$ requirements).

**Pupils** Assess pupils. Unilateral dilation may indicate arterial inflow into the innominate artery (unilateral carotid perfusion).

## BYPASS PERIOD

**Anticoagulation** ACT levels should be checked regularly (q 20-30 min) and kept at >400. Add heparin (5,000-10,000 U), if needed.

**Pressure/flow** There is controversy about safe flows and pressures. Generally, flows of 1.2-3 $L/m^2/min$ are used, with pressures of 30-80 mmHg. A MAP of 50-60 mmHg is probably best for cerebral perfusion and does not result in excessive non-coronary blood flow.

**Acid-base status** Alpha-stat (ABG measured and interpreted at 37° regardless of actual patient temperature) regulation of acid-base status is preferred because of maintenance of normal cerebral flow and autoregulation on CPB.

**Hct/Electrolytes** Generally, Hct will fall to ~20, which is acceptable in most patients. Hypokalemia is common and should be corrected. A $K^+$ >4.5 mEq/L is desirable.

**UO** Keep UO >1 ml/kg/hr. If needed, mannitol and/or furosemide should be given (assuming pump flow is adequate).

**Temperature** During bypass the temperature is usually maintained at ~28°C.

## TERMINATION OF BYPASS

**Rewarming** Prior to discontinuing CPB, the patient should have a core temperature of at least 36.5°C.

**Anesthesia/relaxation** Patient awareness may be a problem during rewarming. D/C volatile agents and give benzodiazepine (5-10 mg) ± a narcotic to prevent awareness. In addition, a muscle relaxant should also be given.

**Acid-base/electrolytes/Hct** ✓ electrolyte, acid-base status and Hct. Correct acidosis. $K^+$ 4.5-5.5, normal ionized $Ca^{++}$, and Hct ≥ 20 should be assured.

**Air maneuvers** Air maneuvers (to remove intracardiac and intra-aortic air) are carried out when the heart is opened. Ventilation is commenced once there is pulmonary blood flow and will aid in the evacuation of air. Pleural fluid should be removed.

## WEANING FROM BYPASS

**Prior to weaning** Prior to weaning from CPB, the aortic cross-clamp should have been off for 30 min to allow rewarming and reperfusion of the heart. Defibrillation is often needed and pacing may be required. Normal sinus rhythm (NSR) or A-V pacing is preferred. Vasoactive drugs should be available. Once normal temperature, ventilation, cardiac rhythm and reperfusion are established, bypass may be terminated. The heart is gradually volume-loaded (transfused from oxygenator) to adequate filling pressures and bypass flow slowly decreased over 15-45 sec until it is off. Return to bypass in the event of progressive cardiac distension or dysfunction. Assess CO, BP and adjust vascular resistance as necessary. Inotropic agents are often required at this stage.

**Reversal of anticoagulation** Once patient is off CPB, anticoagulation must be reversed with protamine (1-1.3 mg/100 U), administered slowly over 10-30 min, since rapid administration is associated with ↓BP. (Treat with α-agonists and volume.) Other reactions include pulmonary HTN and true allergic reactions. ✓ ACT to ensure that it has returned to control (90-130 sec).

**BP management** Vasoactive support is often needed in the post-bypass period – the need varying with surgical procedure, disease process and underlying cardiac function. In general, SBP should be limited to 120 mmHg to avoid stress on the aortotomy site.

## COAGULATION AND CPB

**General** Bleeding is common post-CPB and may be considerable. Both preop and intraop factors contribute to this. A knowledge of these factors and the tests involved will aid with the management of these patients.

**Preop factors** Hx of previous bleeding during surgery is important. Many drugs may contribute to bleeding: ASA/NSAIDs (platelet dysfunction), anticoagulants (heparin, Coumadin®) and fibrinolytic agents. These should be stopped preop, if possible, or their action reversed. Other pathological processes (e.g., liver failure/congestion, renal failure or hemophilia) also play a role. Preop testing is important and should include PT, PTT, platelet count and bleeding time, as a minimum.

**Intraop factors** CPB is associated with ↓platelet count and function. Circulating clotting factors are decreased and fibrinolysis occurs.

Continued on page 6...

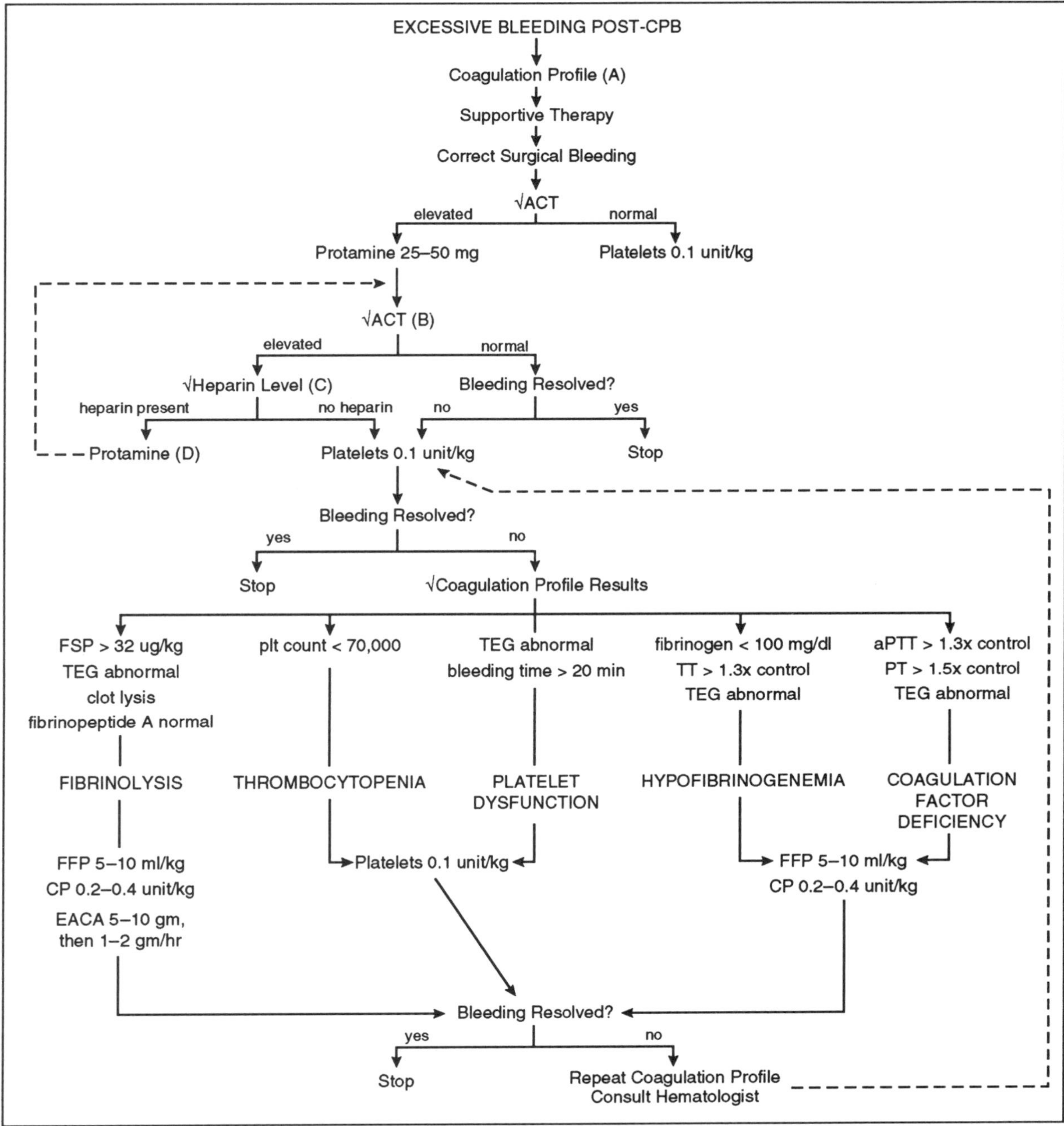


**Figure 6.1-3.** An algorithm for the treatment of patients bleeding excessively after CPB: (A) Commonly includes platelet count, PT, aPTT, TT, fibrinogen level, FSPs. Template bleeding time or TEG is desirable if available and feasible. (B) Heparin level may be checked at this step. (C) Most commonly by *in vitro* whole blood protamine titration (manual or automated); alternatively, by protamine-corrected TT. (D) Protamine dose determined by measured heparin level. Disseminated intravascular coagulation (DIC) is a rare cause of post-CPB hemorrhage and therefore is not included in the outline of coagulation profile results and treatment of post-CPB hemostatic abnormalities shown in the lower portion of the figure. It would be suspected on the occurrence of hypofibrinogenemia, thrombocytopenia, and elevated fibrinopeptides, in association with increased FSPs, clot lysis, or a TEG characteristic of fibrinolysis. The treatment of DIC includes identification and arrest of the inciting cause and coagulant replacement with FFP, CP, and platelets. EACA should not be administered to the patient with DIC and secondary fibrinolysis because of the risk of intravascular thrombosis.
ACT = activated coagulation time; aPTT = activated partial thromboplastin time; CP = cryoprecipitate; EACA = epsilon-aminocaproic acid; FFP = fresh frozen plasma; FSP = fibrin(ogen) split products; plt count = platelet count, PT = prothrombin time; TEG = thromboelastogram; TT = thrombin time. (Reproduced with permission from Hensley FA Jr, Martin DE: *The Practice of Cardiac Anesthesia*. Little, Brown: 1990.)

**Post-CPB bleeding**

The common causes of post-CPB bleeding are: surgical, inadequate heparin reversal, ↓number of platelets and platelet dysfunction, ↓clotting factors, fibrinolysis, DIC, excessive BP. Surgical causes and inadequate heparin reversal (✓ ACT) should be ruled out. If no surgical cause is found and ACT is normal, platelets (10 U) should be infused. PT, PTT, platelet count, TT, reptilase time, fibrinogen and FSP should be checked. The TEG may prove very useful. (See Fig 7.11-4 and Table 7.11-1 in "Liver/Kidney Transplantation" in the "General Surgery" section.)

---

**References**


1. DiNardo JA: Management of cardiopulmonary bypass. In *Anesthesia for Cardiac Surgery*. DiNardo JA, Schwartz MJ, eds. Appleton & Lange, Norwalk CT: 1990, Ch 9, 217-52.
2. Ream AK: Cardiopulmonary bypass. In *Acute Cardiovascular Management*. Ream AK, Fogdall RP, eds. JB Lippincott, Philadelphia: 1982, Ch 15, 456-80.
3. Fogdall RP: The post-bypass period. In *Acute Cardiovascular Management*. Ream AK, Fogdall RP, eds. JB Lippincott, Philadelphia: 1982, Ch 15, 456-80.
4. Larach DR: Anesthetic management during cardiopulmonary bypass. In *The Practice of Cardiac Anesthesia*. Hensley FA, Martin DE, eds. Little, Brown, Boston: 1990, Ch 7, 223-51.
5. Romanoff ME, Larach DR: Weaning from cardiopulmonary bypass. In *The Practice of Cardiac Anesthesia*. Hensley FA, Martin DE, eds. Little, Brown, Boston: 1990, Ch 8, 252-66.
6. Campbell FW, Jobes DR, Ellison N: Coagulation management during and after cardiopulmonary bypass. In *The Practice of Cardiac Anesthesia*. Hensley FA, Martin DE, eds. Little, Brown, Boston: 1990, Ch 18, 546-83.
7. Ellison N: Coagulation evaluation and management. In *Acute Cardiovascular Management*. Ream AK, Fogdall RP, eds. JB Lippincott, Philadelphia: 1982, Ch 24, 773-805.

# CORONARY ARTERY BYPASS DISEASE GRAFT SURGERY

## SURGICAL CONSIDERATIONS

**Description**: Coronary artery bypass grafting (CABG) is the most frequently performed cardiac operation (Fig 6.1-4). Since the discovery that coronary thrombosis is the causative event for MI, many schemes have been devised to augment the restricted coronary blood flow, including collateral pericardial blood to epicardial arteries and implantation of the internal mammary artery with unligated side-branches into the LV muscle. With the discovery by Favalaro that saphenous veins can be anastomosed to the epicardial coronary arteries, a new era of myocardial revascularization began. Basically, the technique involves bypass to a narrowed or occluded epicardial coronary greater than 1 mm in diameter with a small-diameter conduit (usually reversed saphenous vein or internal mammary artery) distal to the narrowed segment, with the proximal arterial inflow source being the ascending aorta. The mammary artery may be mobilized from the chest wall, leaving its proximal origin with the subclavian artery intact (pedicled graft), or the mammary may be transected and its proximal end anastomosed to the aorta or saphenous vein as a "free mammary graft."

The heart is approached through a median sternotomy, with the patient supported on full CPB (see separate section on CPB). Although various operative strategies may be used, the most common regimen is for all distal (epicardial) anastomoses to be performed during a single period of aortic cross-clamping and cardiac arrest. During that period of induced asystole, myocardial protection is achieved by hypothermia and occasional reperfusion via antegrade or retrograde cardioplegia. Cardiac standstill and a bloodless field are mandatory to allow these very demanding small-diameter anastomoses to be constructed with no obstruction to flow in a minimal amount of time. The cross-clamp is then removed and the heart allowed to resume beating. A partially occluding aortic cross-clamp can then be applied to allow construction of the proximal aortic anastomoses. After a sufficient period of resuscitation, the patient is weaned from CPB, and decannulation, heparin reversal and chest closure are allowed to proceed as previously noted.

The choice of conduit depends on availability and durability. Historically, the saphenous vein was the first small vessel conduit with acceptable patencies, but with prolonged experience it appears that 50% of vein grafts will be significantly diseased or occluded at 10 yrs. The internal mammary artery appears to have superior long-term performance, with approximately 90% 10-year patency rates. Other arterial conduits, such as the left gastroepiploic artery, superficial epigastric artery and the radial artery are being investigated as to their long- and short-term durability. Typical target arteries include the distal right coronary and its major terminal branch, the posterior descending artery. From the left circulation, the left anterior descending (LAD), with its diagonal and septal branches, is the most important, having been

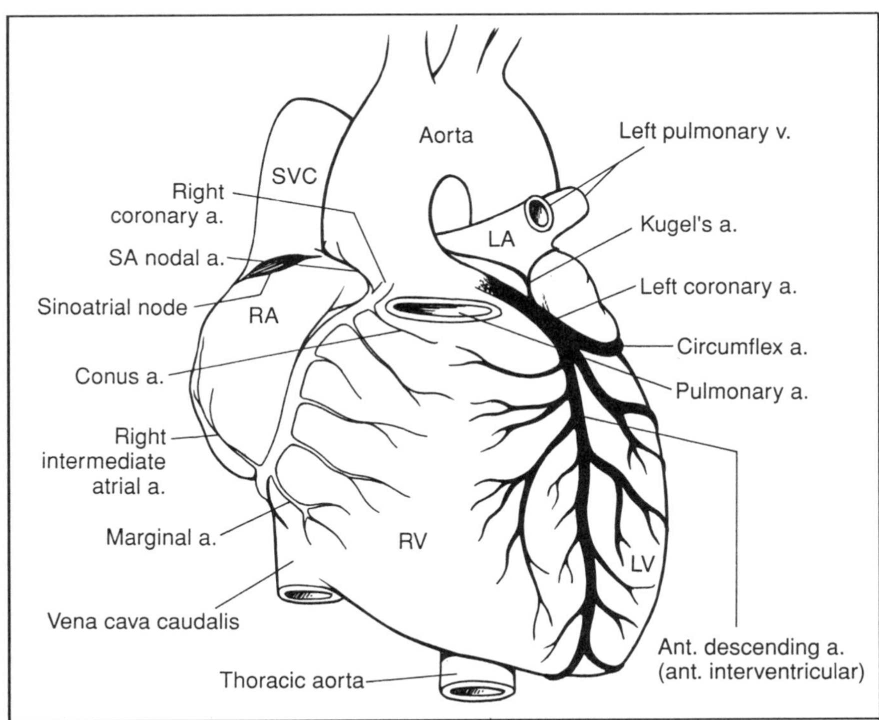


**Figure 6.1-4.** Coronary artery circulation – anterior view. (Reproduced with permission from Edwards EA, Malone PD, Collins JJ Jr: *Operative Anatomy of the Thorax*. Lea & Febiger, Philadelphia: 1972.)

estimated to supply blood to 60% of the left ventricle. The left circumflex coronary artery courses in the posterior atrioventricular groove, and is not easily accessible for bypass, which is usually performed to its obtuse marginal or posterolateral branches.

In a randomized study on coronary artery surgery, (CASS)[1], coronary bypass was noted to be superior to medical management for relief of angina, and to prolong life in patients with left main CAD, and in patients with 3-vessel disease and impaired LV function. Other patients may receive bypass for intractable angina refractory to medical management.

**Usual preop diagnosis**: CAD with Class 3 or 4 angina (angina with minimal exertion or at rest)

### SUMMARY OF PROCEDURE

| | |
|---|---|
| **Position** | Supine |
| **Incision** | Median sternotomy with legs prepped for saphenous vein harvest |
| **Special instrumentation** | Complete hemodynamic monitoring |
| **Unique considerations** | Avoidance of cardiac ischemia |
| **Antibiotics** | Cefamandole 1 gm iv at induction |
| **Surgical time** | 3.5 - 4.5 hrs |
| **Closing considerations** | Prevention of coagulopathy; maintenance of preload |
| **EBL** | 500-600 cc |
| **Postop care** | ICU: 1-3 d, intubated |
| **Mortality** | 2-4% |
| **Morbidity** | Overall: 3-6%<br>MI: 3-6%<br>Pneumonia: 5%<br>CVA: 1-2% |
| **Procedure code** | 33510-33516 (CABG); 33533-33536 (combined arterial-venous arterial); 33517-33523 (venous) |
| **Pain score** | 7-8 |

### PATIENT POPULATION CHARACTERISTICS

| | |
|---|---|
| **Age range** | 60-80 yrs (mean = 74 yrs) |
| **Male:Female** | 2:1 |
| **Incidence** | Common |
| **Etiology** | Coronary atherosclerosis |
| **Associated conditions** | LV failure<br>Pulmonary HTN<br>Ischemic mitral regurgitation<br>Diabetes mellitus<br>Obstructive pulmonary disease |

---

## ANESTHETIC CONSIDERATIONS

**(Procedures covered: coronary artery bypass disease graft surgery; left ventricular aneurysmectomy)**

### PREOPERATIVE

History, examination and tests will divide these patients broadly into two groups: (1) high-risk, characterized by poor LV function (cardiac failure; EF < 40%; LVEDP >18 mmHg; CI < 2.0 L/mm/m$^2$; ventricular dyskinesias; 3-vessel disease; occlusion of left main or left main equivalent; valvular disease; recent MI; ventricular aneurysm; VSD; MI in progress; and old age); and (2) low-risk, characterized by good LV function. The type of monitoring chosen will depend on which group the patient is in.

**Respiratory** Hx of smoking or COPD; patient should be encouraged to stop smoking at least 2 wks prior to surgery. Treat COPD and optimize therapy prior to surgery.
**Tests:** CXR; PFTs; as indicated by H&P.

**Cardiovascular** In the preop assessment, the following factors will affect patient management and surgical outcome:
-Hx of angina (stable, unstable at rest, and precipitating factors).
-The patient's exercise tolerance will provide a clue to LV functions and surgical outcome.
-The presence of CHF (Sx: SOB, PND, orthopnea, DOE, pulmonary edema, JVD, 3rd-heart sound).
-Recent (< 6 mo) MI, dysrhythmias, HTN, vascular disease (particularly carotid stenosis, aortic disease).
-Valvular disease (particularly mitral regurgitation [MR] or aortic stenosis [AS]) or the presence of a VSD or LV aneurysm may portend increased risk of perioperative complications.
**Tests:** 12-lead ECG: ✓ ischemia (area involved), LVH, previous MI, dysrhythmias. Exercise stress testing: ✓ effort tolerance, area of ischemia, maximal HR and BP before ischemia occurs, dysrhythmias. Thallium scan: ✓ component of reversible ischemia. ECHO (may be combined with stress ECHO): ✓ LV function, wall motion abnormalities, valvular disease, VSD. Cardiac catheterization: ✓ extent and location of disease, LV function, valvular pathology, VSD, LVEDP, LV aneurysm.

**Post-infarction VSD** The development of a post-infarction VSD is associated with high operative morbidity and mortality because of the difficulty in repairing the lesion due to friable tissue, difficulty in obtaining hemostasis, emergent nature of the condition and possible pulmonary edema. These patients effectively have poor LV function and should be considered as high risk. They often require support, including IABP, during induction, pre-bypass and post-bypass.

**LV aneurysm** LV aneurysm is usually a late complication of infarction; however, it can occur early, when it is usually associated with cardiac rupture (and high mortality). These patients usually have poor myocardial function and should be anesthetized with full monitoring, including PA catheterization. Post-bypass, the LV cavity is reduced in size and compliance. To ensure an adequate CO, maintain adequate preload, a higher than normal HR (A-V pacing if needed) and sinus rhythm, and consider the use of inotropes. LV aneurysms are often associated with dysrhythmias and may require cardiac mapping (see "Cardiac Mapping and Ablation Procedures," below). Hemostasis is often difficult to obtain, and adequate iv access is a necessity. Treatment usually entails the use of blood and blood products.

**Emergency revascularization** Emergency revascularization occurs in the setting of acute MI, often with acute LV failure or after failed PTCA, where the patient may be stable, suffering acute ischemia and hemodynamically unstable, or even in full cardiac arrest. Factors to consider in these cases are: full stomach (and the need for rapid-sequence induction in the face of ischemia); the prior use of fibrinolytic agents (with increased risk of hemorrhage); need for inotropes; anti-anginals; IABP; and dysrhythmias. These patients have a higher morbidity and mortality. In patients who have received fibrinolytic agents, consider the post-bypass use of antifibrinolytic agents (e.g., aminocaproic acid).

**Neurological** Previous stroke or carotid artery disease Hx/Sx should be documented and evaluated.

**Endocrine** Diabetes is common and perioperative control of blood glucose is important.
**Tests:** Blood glucose

**Renal** ✓ baseline renal function, as CPB places these patients at risk for renal failure.
**Tests:** Creatinine; BUN; electrolytes (particularly $K^+$)

**Hematologic** Patients are often on ASA or dipyridamole therapy, which may lead to increased intraop hemorrhage. These agents should be stopped 5-10 d before surgery, if possible. Some patients may be on anticoagulants (usually heparin in the immediate preop period). Heparin should be stopped 2-4 hrs preop; however, in some patients, heparin infusion is continued into the OR. Other patients may have received fibrinolytic agents which put them at increased risk for intraop hemorrhage.
**Tests:** Bleeding time; PT; PTT; platelet count

**Laboratory** Hb/Hct; other tests as indicated from H&P. T&C 8 U PRBCs.

**Premedication** Patients should be instructed to continue all medications (e.g., nitrates, β-blockers; $Ca^{++}$ antagonists, anti-dysrhythmics and anti-hypertensives) prior to surgery, with the exception of diuretics on the day of surgery. Allaying anxiety may decrease the incidence of perioperative ischemia and help with the pre-induction placement of lines. Typical preop sedation includes diazepam (10 mg po) or lorazepam (1-2 mg po) the night before and again 1-2 hrs before arrival in the OR, with the addition of morphine (0.1 mg/kg im) and scopolamine (0.3 mg im). Severely compromised patients will require less premedication.

## INTRAOPERATIVE

**Anesthetic technique:** GETA

**Induction** Generally, a high-dose narcotic technique (e.g., fentanyl 20-100 μg/kg or sufentanil 5-20 μg/kg), supplemented by etomidate (0.1-0.3 mg/kg) or midazolam (50-350 μg/kg), is appropriate. As with all cardiac cases, the speed of induction and total drug dose depends on the patient's cardiac function and pathology. Muscle relaxation may be obtained using pancuronium (0.1 mg/kg), given slowly to avoid tachycardia, or vecuronium (possibility of bradycardia, especially if the patient is β-blocked). It is important to avoid the sympathetic response to laryngoscopy. The use of high-dose narcotics, esmolol (100-500 μg/kg over 1 min, followed by 40-100 μg/kg/min infusion), SNP (0.5-3 μg/kg/min), lidocaine (1-2 mg/kg) or a combination of these agents, may decrease or ablate this response. NTG (0.5-2 μg/kg/min) also may be used during induction if evidence of ischemia occurs.

**Maintenance** Usually high-dose narcotic (total: fentanyl 50-100 μg/kg or sufentanil 10-20 μg/kg) with midazolam (50-350 μg/kg) for amnesia. Those patients with good LV function may benefit from the decreased myocardial $O_2$ demand associated with the use of volatile agents (2° contractility). $N_2O$ is generally avoided.

**Emergence** Transported to ICU, sedated, intubated and ventilated.

**Blood and fluid requirements**
IV: 14 ga x 1-2
NS/LR @ 6-8 ml/kg/hr
UO 0.5-1 ml/kg/hr
Warm all fluids.
Humidify gasses.

**Monitoring**

Standard monitors (see Appendix). — Standard and invasive monitors placed prior to induction.

Arterial line — ✓ BP in both arms. Right radial preferred if left internal mammary artery (LIMA) graft, because retraction of the sternum may compress the left subclavian.

CVP or PA catheter — In the low-risk/good LV function group, CVP is adequate; high-risk/poor LV function, a PA catheter is useful for hemodynamic monitoring, weaning from bypass and vasoactive therapy. Some groups use routine PA catheterization for all patients undergoing CABG surgery.

ECG — 5-lead monitoring II and $V_5$ (or area most at risk for ischemia).

TEE — Will reflect regional wall motion abnormalities, papillary muscle dysfunction and mitral regurgitation (MR).

**Myocardial $O_2$ Balance**

Supply – Coronary blood flow:
- Perfusion pressure (DP-LVEDP)
- Diastolic filling time (HR)
- Blood viscosity (optimal Hct=30)
- Coronary vasoconstriction:
  - -Spasm
  - -$PaCO_2$ (hypocapnia → constriction)
  - -α-sympathetic activity

Supply – $O_2$ delivery:
- $O_2$ sat
- Hct
- Oxyhemoglobin dissociation curve

Demand – $O_2$ consumption
- BP (afterload)
- Ventricular volume (preload)
- Wall thickness (↓subendocardial perfusion)
- HR
- Contractility

The balance of myocardial $O_2$ supply vs demand is important in the management of these patients. The goal of anesthesia is to ensure that this balance remains in equilibrium and that no ischemia occurs, or, if it does, that it is treated promptly. Those patients with poor LV function or complicated disease will benefit from maintenance of contractility (avoid volatile agents) and a high $FiO_2$. Whereas those with good LV function may benefit from the mild cardiac depression (↓demand associated with the addition of low-dose volatile agents). Certain events are associated with increased risk of intraop ischemia: intubation, incision, sternotomy, cannulation, tachycardia, ↑BP or ↓BP, ventricular fibrillation or distension, inadequate cardioplegia, emboli, spasm or inadequate revascularization. Care should be taken to avoid these complications and to ablate responses to stimuli.

| | | |
|---|---|---|
| **Detection of ischemia** | ECG | ST segment depression or elevation or a new T-wave alteration may suggest ischemia. Monitoring 2 leads – one lateral (e.g., $V_5$) and one inferior (e.g., II) give the best detection rate. |
| | PA catheter | Elevations of PCWP may be indicative of ischemia. A new V-wave on the PCWP trace is a better sign of possible ischemia (papillary muscle dysfunction). |
| | TEE | The appearance of a new regional wall motion abnormality is the most sensitive indication of ischemia, but it requires expert interpretation and constant monitoring. |
| **Treatment of ischemia** | Caused by tachycardia:<br>Esmolol (100-500 μg/kg)<br>↑anesthesia<br>Verapamil (2.5-10 mg iv)<br>Caused by ↑BP:<br>NTG (0.5-4 μg/kg/min)<br>↑anesthesia<br>Caused by ↓BP:<br>Phenylephrine (0.5-0.75 mg/kg/min)<br>↑preload<br>Caused by ↓↓HR:<br>A-V pacing | While avoidance of ischemia is the goal, when it does occur it should be treated aggressively. Treatment may include inotropic support (e.g., dopamine 1-5 μg/kg/min or dobutamine 0.5-30 μg/kg/min). If LV failure persists despite other therapy, an IABP may be inserted. |
| **Positioning** | ✓ and pad pressure points.<br>✓ eyes. | |

## POSTOPERATIVE

| | | |
|---|---|---|
| **Complications** | Infarction<br>Ischemia<br>Tamponade<br>Dysrhythmias<br>Cardiac failure<br>Coagulopathy<br>Hemorrhage | Ventilate patient 24-48 hrs. Postop control of ischemia is important since hemodynamic instability may be associated with inadequate pain relief, awakening and ventilation. |
| **Pain management** | Parenteral opioids for pain relief<br>Benzodiazepine for sedation | |
| **Tests** | ECG<br>CPK<br>CXR<br>Electrolytes<br>ABG<br>Coagulation profiles | |

**References**


1. Rogers WJ, Coggin CJ, Green B, et al: 10-year followup of quality of life in patients randomized to receive medical treatment or coronary artery bypass graft surgery. *Circulation* 1990; 82(5):1647-58.
2. O'Connor JP, Wynands JE: Anesthesia for myocardial revascularization. In *Cardiac Anesthesia*, 2nd edition. Kaplan JA, ed. WB Saunders Co, Philadelphia: 1987, Ch 15, 551-88.
3. Hourow JC, Hensley FA, Merin RG: Anesthetic management for myocardial revascularization. In *The Practice of Cardiac Anesthesia*. Hensley FA, Martin DE, eds. Little, Brown & Co, Boston: 1990, Ch 11, 325-49.

# LEFT VENTRICULAR ANEURYSMECTOMY

## SURGICAL CONSIDERATIONS

**Description**: Extensive MI may result in large areas of myocardial necrosis, with subsequent aneurysm formation. LV failure may ensue as a result of continuous LV dilatation or mitral insufficiency 2° annular dilatation or involvement of papillary muscles. Indications for this surgery include worsening CHF and increased dysrhythmias. Typically, apical dilatation with maintenance of basilar myocardial contractility allows for aneurysm resection and preservation of both myocardial contractility and chamber size to produce an adequate cardiac output. Operation is commenced in the usual manner, establishing CPB (see separate section on CPB), cross-clamping the aorta, establishing myocardial protection, and then assessing the left ventricle. A thinned, dilated ventricular segment with full-thickness scar formation, can be resected, and ventricular continuity restored with improvement of ventricular geometry and myocardial energy demands. Coronary bypass can be performed during this same period. Then air is removed from the left side of the heart, the cross-clamp removed and coronary perfusion re-established. After a sufficient period of resuscitation and return of vigorous contractility, bypass is discontinued, not infrequently with the assistance of intra-aortic balloon pump (IABP) to augment forward output. Decannulation, protamine administration and closure proceed as described in CPB, above.

**Usual preop diagnosis**: LV aneurysm with CHF

### SUMMARY OF PROCEDURE

| | |
|---|---|
| **Position** | Supine |
| **Incision** | Median sternotomy; ± leg incision for saphenous vein harvest if coronary bypass is planned. |
| **Unique considerations** | Preparations (ECG leads) should be made for pre- or postop IABP or assist device (LVAD) |
| **Antibiotics** | Cefamandole 1 gm iv at induction |
| **Surgical time** | Aortic cross-clamp: 40 - 100 min<br>CPB: 70 - 130 min<br>Total: 3 - 4 hrs |
| **EBL** | 300-400 cc |
| **Postop care** | ICU x 1-3 d, intubated; usually requires inotropic support ± mechanical support (LVAD, IABP). |
| **Mortality** | 5-7% |
| **Morbidity** | Overall: 8-10%<br>Requirement for IABP: 10%<br>Respiratory insufficiency: 5%<br>CVA: 2-3% |
| **Procedure code** | 33542 |
| **Pain score** | 7-10 |

### PATIENT POPULATION CHARACTERISTICS

| | |
|---|---|
| **Age range** | 50-70 yrs |
| **Male:Female** | 3:1 |
| **Incidence** | Uncommon |
| **Etiology** | Usually the end result of MI 2° CAD |
| **Associated conditions** | Mitral insufficiency<br>Pulmonary HTN<br>CAD |

## ANESTHETIC CONSIDERATIONS

See Anesthetic Considerations following "Coronary Artery Bypass Disease Graft Surgery" (above).

**References**

1. Mills NL, Everson CT, Hockmuth DR: Technical advances in the treatment of left ventricular aneurysm. *Ann Thor Surg* 1993; 55:792-800.

# AORTIC VALVE REPLACEMENT

## SURGICAL CONSIDERATIONS

**Description:** Disease of the aortic valve may present as valvular stenosis, insufficiency, or a combination of the two. Valvular disease most commonly occurs as a result of rheumatic disease, but may also occur 2° calcific degeneration (aortic sclerosis) in the elderly. Congenitally bicuspid valves and endocarditis account for most of the remainder. Repair of the aortic valve is rarely possible, and most conditions require valve replacement. The three most commonly used **prostheses** are: porcine bioprostheses, especially in the older patient; mechanical prostheses, with the necessity for lifelong anticoagulation; and cryo-preserved homografts, which unfortunately are expensive and in short supply. The operation, on full CPB, is usually performed through a median sternotomy. After routine bicaval and aortic cannulation, the patient is taken onto full CPB. Left heart drainage is accomplished through a pulmonary artery vent, a left atrial vent usually inserted through the right superior pulmonary vein, or via a LV vent inserted through the LV apex. Because of the LV hypertrophy, myocardial protection is of utmost importance. Stanford favors hyperkalemic, hypothermic cardioplegic arrest, augmented by topical cooling either with a continuous infusion of cold saline into the pericardial well or with a cooling jacket. Cardioplegic administration can be achieved either antegrade into the coronary ostia or retrograde via the coronary sinus. Myocardial temperature is monitored continuously.

After the heart is arrested, the aorta is opened to expose the aortic valve. The rheumatic, stenotic valve, including aortic annulus, is frequently heavily calcified, and all calcium must be debrided to allow the prosthetic valve to be securely seated. This is frequently a tedious and time-consuming procedure, but one which then allows the remainder of the procedure to proceed in a timely fashion. After excision of the valve leaflet and debridement of the annulus, assuring that no particulate debris embolizes into the ventricle or coronary arteries, the annulus is measured to assure a proper match between prosthetic valve and annulus and an appropriate valve prosthesis is selected. Interrupted sutures are then placed through the annulus for its entire circumference, then passed through the sewing ring of the prosthesis. The prosthesis is then lowered into the annulus and securely tied in place. Proper sizing and positioning are mandatory to prevent perivalve leaks or impingement on the coronary ostia. Systemic rewarming is initiated during the final stages of the valve implantation and the LV allowed to fill during aortic closure. With the patient in the head-down position, all remaining air is vented from the left heart and aorta, and the cross-clamp removed to allow myocardial perfusion. The heart is allowed to recover from this period of ischemia, and after sufficient resuscitation, with continuous venting of air from the aorta, the patient is weaned from CPB. Vasodilators are almost always utilized, as there appears to be excessive vasospasm present in both the coronary and pulmonary circulations after hypothermia. Decannulation and heparin reversal with protamine are then accomplished in the routine manner.

**Usual preop diagnosis:** Severe aortic stenosis with syncope, chest pain or CHF; aortic insufficiency with CHF

### SUMMARY OF PROCEDURE

| | Valve Replacement with Prosthesis | Homograft Valve Replacement |
|---|---|---|
| **Position** | Supine | ⇐ |
| **Incision** | Median sternotomy | ⇐ |
| **Special instrumentation** | TEE; hemodynamic monitoring; CPB | TEE or surface ECHO |
| **Unique considerations** | ECHO assessment of valve function and regional wall motion intraop | ECHO assessment of annular size and intraop evaluation of valve function after implantation |
| **Antibiotics** | Cefamandole 1 gm iv at incision | ⇐ |
| **Surgical time** | Aortic cross-clamp: 45 min | 60 min |
| | CPB: 90 min | 105 min |
| | Total: 3 hrs | ⇐ |
| **EBL** | 300 - 400 cc | ⇐ |
| **Postop care** | ICU x 1-3 d, intubated; hypertrophied, noncompliant LV requiring high preload. | ⇐ |
| **Mortality** | 5-8% | ⇐ |
| **Morbidity** | Pneumonia: 5-10% | ⇐ |
| | Neurological sequela: transient: 3-7%; CVA: 1-2%; permanent: 1-2% | |
| | Infection: 1% | |

| | | |
|---|---|---|
| **Procedure code** | 33405 | ⇐ |
| **Pain score** | 7-10 | 7-10 |

### PATIENT POPULATION CHARACTERISTICS

**Age range** Bicuspid valves: 50-60 yrs; rheumatic: 55-80 yrs (mean = 58 ± 13 yrs)

**Male:Female** 3:1

**Incidence** 70-100 cases/yr in tertiary care center

**Etiology** Post-rheumatic: Majority of patients
Aortic sclerosis
Progressive stenosis of a bicuspid aortic valve
Endocarditis

**Associated conditions** Post-stenotic dilatation of the ascending aorta (may require separate surgical attention)
Rheumatic mitral valvular involvement
CAD
CHF

---

## ANESTHETIC CONSIDERATIONS

### PREOPERATIVE

**Respiratory** Respiratory compromise may occur 2° pulmonary congestion (LV failure) and pleural effusion. An effusion, if significant, should be drained prior to surgery as it may impair oxygenation and, with IPPV, may impair venous return → ↓CO + ↓myocardial perfusion.
**Tests:** CXR

**Cardiovascular** **Aortic stenosis (AS):** Sx are those of angina pectoris (if at rest may indicate concurrent CAD), syncope and CHF (indicates severe disease with 2-yr life expectancy). The ejection murmur of AS is best heard at the 2nd right interspace. ECG shows LVH. Important points in the preop investigations include:
-Aortic orifice size – moderate AS = 0.7-0.9 $cm^2$; critical AS = < 0.5 $cm^2$ (normal = 2.6-3.5 $cm^2$)
-Aortic valvular gradient – severe = > 70 mmHg
-Ejection fraction (EF) – ↓EF indicates evidence of LV failure (normal = >0.6).
-Coronary angiography – associated CAD often demonstrated.
AS → ↑LV work (↑pressure load) → LV concentric hypertrophy → ↓LV diastolic function + ↑risk for ischemia ($MVO_2$ + $O_2$ supply):
-Reliance on atrial "kick" – important to maintain normal sinus rhythm (NSR).
-Sensitivity to changes in SVR: ↓SVR → ↓↓BP → ↓myocardial perfusion + ↓CO → ↓↓↓BP
-Sensitivity to volume changes – hypovolemia → ↓pre-load → ↓↓CO
-Sensitivity to rate changes – tachycardia → ↓ejection time → ↓myocardial perfusion
-↑LV wall tension + ↑duration of systole → ↑$MVO_2$
-↑LVEDP + ↑wall thickness and tension + ↓diastolic aortic pressure → ↓$O_2$ supply
**Aortic regurgitation (AR):** Sx include DOE, orthopnea, PND, palpitations and, less frequently, angina. Exercise tolerance may remain reasonably good, even with severe AR. Acute AR is very poorly tolerated. The pandiastolic murmur of AR is loudest over the sternum and left lower sternal border.
AR → chronic LV volume overload → LV eccentric hypertrophy → massive cardiomegaly → LV failure (CHF) → ↑LVEDP → ↑PA pressure and pulmonary congestion.
-Possibility of ischemia: ↑$MVO_2$ and ↓supply (↓diastolic pressure, ↑HR)
-Sensitivity to rate changes – ↓HR → ↑AR + ↓CO
-Sensitivity to changes in SVR – ↑SVR → ↑regurgitation + ↓CO.
**Tests:** ECG: ✓ hypertrophy, LV strain, ischemia, rhythm. ECHO: ✓ LV function, valve area, regurgitant fraction. Angiography: ✓ LV function, right heart pressure, CAD, valve area, regurgitant fraction.

**Hepatic** CHF may result in passive liver congestion with decrease in liver function and possible coagulopathy.
**Tests:** LFTs; PT; PTT

**Neurological** Syncopal episodes may have resulted in neurologic deficits. These should be well-documented.

**Renal** Pre-renal failure is often associated with AR 2° ↓CO.
**Tests:** BUN; creatinine, creatinine clearance; electrolytes

**Hematologic** **Tests:** Hb/Hct; clotting profile to investigate abnormalities. T&C for 8 U PRBCs.

**Laboratory** ✓ digitalis level and electrolytes; other tests as indicated from H&P.

**Premedication** Beware of over-sedation in patients with AS where ↓BP could be detrimental. Light premedication with an anxiolytic is usually sufficient. Digitalis and diuretics should be continued.

## INTRAOPERATIVE

**Anesthetic technique:** GETA

**Induction** **Aortic stenosis (AS):** Typically, $O_2$ with high-dose narcotic (e.g., fentanyl 20-100 μg/kg). Avoid sufentanil in AS because of ↓BP. Etomidate (0.1-0.3 mg/kg), midazolam (50-350 μg/kg) may be used to supplement the above. Paralysis with vecuronium or pancuronium (0.1 mg/kg, depending on desired HR. Induction is a critical period. CPB and surgeons should be available and ready to proceed. Danger is hypotension with a cycle of ischemia, further hypotension and more ischemia. Hypotension should be treated aggressively with fluid and α-adrenergic agonists (phenylephrine 50-100 μg iv bolus, infusion 0.1-0.75 μg/kg/min). Critical AS patients may benefit from the use of phenylephrine as an infusion during induction and pre-bypass. The avoidance of hypotension is even more critical in the presence of CAD. Drugs causing tachycardia should be avoided. Atrial fibrillation (AF) or SVT should be treated with cardioversion. β-blockers and other negative inotropes are generally contraindicated. Ventricular irritability should be treated early as ventricular fibrillation may be refractory to defibrillation. Beware of vasodilators, including NTG.
**Aortic Regurgitation (AR):** Again, $O_2$ with high-dose narcotic (e.g., fentanyl 20-100 μg/kg or sufentanil 6-10 μg/kg). Etomidate (0.1-0.3 mg/kg) or benzodiazepines (e.g., midazolam 50-350 μg/kg) may be used to supplement the opiates. Muscle relaxation with pancuronium (0.1 mg/kg). These patients benefit from fluid augmentation, high normal HR (90 bpm) with afterload reduction (e.g., SNP 0.25-2 μg/kg/min) to improve forward flow.

**Maintenance** High-dose narcotic (e.g., fentanyl 50-100 μg/kg). Low-dose volatile agent/air/$O_2$. Relaxant. (See Anesthetic Considerations for "Cardiopulmonary Bypass."

The following table summarizes the goals of intraop management:

| | AS | AR |
|---|---|---|
| LV preload | ↑ | Normal to ↑ |
| Heart rate | Normal to Slow ↓ | Modest ↑ |
| Rhythm | NSR | NSR |
| Contractility | Maintain | Maintain |
| SVR | Modest ↑ | ↓ |
| PVR | Maintain | Maintain |

**Post-Bypass** **Aortic stenosis (AS):** Post-bypass, patients may be hyperdynamic and require vasodilators for HTN, although inotropes also may be needed. Because of the hypertrophied, non-compliant ventricle, filling pressure may be higher than normally required.
**Aortic regurgitation (AR):** In the immediate post-bypass period, patients with AR may require inotropic support (e.g., dopamine 3-10 μg/kg/min, dobutamine 5-10 μg/kg/min, epinephrine 25-100 ng/kg/min) is often needed. Maintain LV filling. Other supportive measures (e.g., IABP) may be necessary.

**Emergence** Transport to ICU sedated, intubated and ventilated.

**Blood and fluid requirements**
IV: 14 ga x 1-2
NS/LR @ 6-8 ml/kg/hr
UO 0.5-1 ml/kg/hr
Warm all fluids.
Humidify gasses.
8 U blood cross-match

| | | |
|---|---|---|
| **Monitoring** | Standard monitors (see Appendix).<br>Arterial line<br>CVP line<br>PA catheter<br>ECG<br>TEE<br>Urinary catheter | Standard and invasive monitors should be placed prior to induction.<br>CVP may underestimate left-side pressures. In acute AR, PCWP may underestimate true LVEDP.<br>$V_5$ lead should be monitored for ischemia.<br>TEE may be useful to estimate LV filling and regional wall motion abnormalities. |
| **Positioning** | ✓ and pad pressure points.<br>✓ eyes. | |

### POSTOPERATIVE

| | | |
|---|---|---|
| **Complications** | Hemorrhage<br>Tamponade<br>Cardiac failure<br>Dysrhythmias<br>Ischemia | Postop ventilation is usually required for 24 hrs. Inotropic and vasodilator therapy is usually continued into the postop period, and then weaned. |
| **Pain management** | Parenteral opioids for pain relief<br>Benzodiazepine for sedation | |
| **Tests** | ECG<br>CXR<br>Electrolytes<br>Coagulation profile<br>HCT | |

**References**

1. Scott WC, Miller DC, Haverich A, Dawkins K, Mitchell RS, Jamieson SW, Oyer PE, Stinson EB, Baldwin JC, Shumway NE: Determinants of operative mortality for patients undergoing aortic valve replacement. Discriminant analysis of 1,479 operations. *J Thorac Cardiovasc Surg* 1985; 89(3):400-13.
2. Jackson JM, Thomas SJ: Valvular heart disease. In *Cardiac Anesthesia*, 2nd edition. Kaplan JA, ed. WB Saunders Co, Philadelphia: 1987, Ch 16, 596-614.
3. Moore RA, Martin DE: Anesthetic management for the treatment of valvular heart disease. In *The Practice of Cardiac Anesthesia.* Hensley FA Jr, Martin DE, eds. Little, Brown and Co, Boston: 1990, 350-85.

# MITRAL VALVE REPAIR OR REPLACEMENT

## SURGICAL CONSIDERATIONS

**Description**: Mitral valve repair or replacement is utilized typically for the correction of post-rheumatic mitral valvular stenosis or insufficiency, as well as mitral valve prolapse, degenerative mitral insufficiency, or repair after endocarditis. For mitral regurgitation 2° posterior leaflet abnormalities (myxomatous degeneration, torn chordae) or pure annular dilatation, most valves can be repaired. For severe rheumatic calcific mitral stenosis, mitral valve replacement with preservation of subannular structures may be necessary.

The technique of mitral valve repair or replacement is similar regardless of the mitral valve pathology. After aortic and bicaval venous cannulation, CPB (see separate section on CPB) is established, and the left heart vented through the PA. After cross-clamping the aorta, diastolic arrest is accomplished with cardioplegia administered via the aortic root, augmented with topical cooling with either continuous pericardial saline infusion or a cooling jacket. Exposure is accomplished via a vertical incision in the left atrium just posterior to atrial septum. If the left atrium is not large enough, access may be gained via an incision in the right atrium, and then incising the atrial septum, with caval snares in place to prevent air entry into the venous cannulae.

After suitable exposure, the atrium, atrial appendage and mitral valve are carefully inspected, and a decision is made to repair or replace the valve. Repair of regurgitant valves caused primarily by posterior leaflet problems is usually possible. Similarly, annular dilatation 2° LV enlargement is also usually possible by means of a ring annuloplasty. Regurgitation 2° anterior leaflet abnormalities are more problematic, requiring significant expertise, and may be less durable. Pre- and postop evaluation is greatly facilitated by use of TEE. Valve replacement can be performed after excising the valve leaflets; or, the leaflets may be preserved in an attempt to keep the benefits of the subvalvar apparatus to global ventricular performance. After appropriate excision and debridement, the annulus is rimmed with interrupted sutures which are passed through the sewing ring of the valve prosthesis. The prosthesis is carefully positioned, and the sutures tied. After filling both the LV and atrium with blood, the atrium is closed, air evacuated from the left heart, and the cross-clamp removed to allow coronary perfusion. After a satisfactory period of resuscitation, and after all air has been evacuated from the circulation, CPB may be discontinued, usually with the assistance of vasodilator agents. TEE may be utilized at this stage to assess adequacy of mitral valve repair.

**Variant procedure or approaches**: **Mitral commissurotomy** may be done closed (e.g., during pregnancy).

**Usual preop diagnosis**: Class 3 or 4 CHF 2° mitral insufficiency or mitral stenosis

## SUMMARY OF PROCEDURE

| | Mitral Valve Replacement/Repair | Closed Commissurotomy |
|---|---|---|
| **Position** | Supine | Right lateral decubitus |
| **Incision** | Median sternotomy | Left lateral thoracotomy |
| **Special instrumentation** | TEE and epicardial ECHO to assess valve function and regional wall motion; CPB | Performed without CPB. |
| **Unique considerations** | Special loading conditions may be used to estimate the amount of mitral regurgitation, which is frequently afterload-dependent. | ⇐ |
| **Antibiotics** | Cefamandole 1 gm iv | ⇐ |
| **Surgical time** | Aortic cross-clamp: 45 - 150 min<br>CPB: 90 - 200 min<br>Total: 3 - 4 hrs | Total: 2 hrs |
| **EBL** | 300-400 cc | 200-400 cc |
| **Postop care** | ICU x 1-3 d, intubated; vasodilator therapy for reversal of pulmonary HTN and afterload reduction | ⇐ |
| **Mortality** | 5-8% | < 5% |
| **Morbidity** | Pneumonia: 10-15% | ⇐ |
| | CNS complications: | |
| | Transient neurologic dysfunction: 5-10% | ⇐ |
| | CVA: 1-2% | ⇐ |
| | Infection: < 1% | ⇐ |
| **Procedure code** | 33425 (mitral valve repair)<br>33430 (mitral valve replacement) | 33420 |
| **Pain score** | 7-10 | 7-10 |

## PATIENT POPULATION CHARACTERISTICS

| | | |
|---|---|---|
| **Age range** | 40-75 yrs | 20-40 yrs |
| **Male:Female** | 1:1 | Almost exclusively pregnant females |
| **Etiology** | Post-rheumatic: Majority of cases | ⇐ |
| | Increased aging | ⇐ |
| | Myxomatous degeneration | ⇐ |
| | Ischemic etiologies: Increasing | ⇐ |
| **Associated conditions** | Aortic valvular involvement with rheumatic disease, CAD, pulmonary HTN and tricuspid regurgitation. | ⇐ |

## ANESTHETIC CONSIDERATIONS

### PREOPERATIVE

**Respiratory** Pulmonary congestion, edema, pleural effusions may be present, with an overall restrictive lung pattern. Pleural effusions should be drained prior to surgery if significant (↓oxygenation, ↓venous return with IPPV). ↑LA volume may compress the left recurrent laryngeal nerve → left vocal cord paralysis (Ortner's syndrome).
**Tests:** CXR; PFTs, if indicated

**Cardiovascular** **Mitral Stenosis (MS):** Sx include exertional dyspnea and fatigue, progressing to pulmonary edema, atrial fibrillation (AF) and hemoptysis. Embolic events occur in 15% of patients. The openi ıg snap and diastolic murmur of MS are best heard between apex and left sternal border. The ECG may show AF or wide-notched P-waves. It is important to grade the severity of MS by symptomatology and valve area: mild = 1.5-2 $cm^2$; moderate = 1-1.5 $cm^2$; and severe = < 1.0 $cm^2$ (normal = 4-6 $cm^2$). AF is often the factor precipitating deterioration in these patients. Because of the decreased LV filling, these patients are sensitive to:
-Loss of atrial "kick" – maintain NSR.
-Volume changes – keep full.
-Rate changes – avoid ↑HR → ↓diastolic filling time → ↓CO
Pathophysiology:
-MS → ↓LVH filling → ↓CO
-MS → ↑LA pressure → pulmonary edema + ↑PA pressure → ↑PVR → RV failure + TR + left shift of iv septum → ↓CO → ↑LA pressure → ↑LA volume →AF and thrombi.

**Mitral Regurgitation (MR):** May be acute (MI/endocarditis) or chronic (often associated with MS). Chronic Sx include: palpitations, DOE, PND, fatigue and orthopnea. Acute MR may lead to sudden ↓↓CO and pulmonary edema. MR can be classified as mild (< 30% regurgitant fraction [RF]), moderate (30-60% RF); or severe (>60% RF). The pansystolic murmur is loudest at the apex. The ECG may show LA and LV overload. MR patients are sensitive to:
-Changes in SVR: ↑SVR → ↑RF → ↓CO + ↓BP
↓SVR → ↓RF → ↑CO + ↑BP
-Change in HR – ↓HR → acute LA volume overload.
Mild ↑HR → ↑CO
Pathophysiology:
-Acute MR → ↑↑LA pressure → ↓CO + ↓BP → ↑HR + ↑contractility → ↑$O_2$ demand
→ ↑LV diastolic volume → ↑LVEDP → ↑$O_2$ demand
-Chronic MR → ↑LA volume + AF → pulmonary edema → RV failure.
→ LV volume overload → LVH → ↓CO + LV failure.
**Tests:** ECG: ✓ LVH, left and right atrial enlargement, rhythm. ECHO: ✓ RF, valve pressure gradients, LV function, valve pressure gradient and area.

**Neurological** The large left atrium and AF may result in thrombus formation, with the possibility of embolism. Neurological deficits should be documented.

**Gastrointestinal** Hepatic congestion may → decreased function, which may be reflected in coagulation problems.
**Tests:** LFTs; PT; PTT

**Renal** ↓CO may lead to renal failure.
**Tests:** BUN; creatinine; electrolytes

**Hematologic** Because of the potential for thromboembolism, these patients may be on anticoagulants, which may be given up to the day before surgery. In the case of Coumadin®, anticoagulant effects can be reversed by the use of FFP and vitamin K.
**Tests:** PT; PTT

**Laboratory** T&C for 8-10 U PRBCs. Hb/Hct; coagulation profile; other tests as indicated from H&P.

**Premedication** Premedication with an anxiolytic (e.g., lorazepam 1-2 mg po, midazolam 0.05-0.2 mg/kg im) or an analgesic (e.g., morphine 0.1-0.2 mg/kg), or a combination of these agents may be used, depending on patient status.

### INTRAOPERATIVE

**Anesthetic technique:** GETA

**Induction** Typically, high-dose narcotic (fentanyl 20-100 μg/kg or sufentanil 5-20 μg/kg), supplemental midazolam (50-350 μg/kg) or etomidate (0.1-0.3 mg/kg). Use pancuronium (MR) or vecuronium (MS) (0.1 mg/kg), depending on the desired HR to facillitate intubation.

**Mitral stenosis:** Hypotension should be treated with fluid, but beware of precipitating pulmonary edema. Occasionally phenylephrine may be needed to maintain SVR. Tachycardia should be avoided and if it occurs should be treated (↑anesthesia, esmolol if ventricular function is preserved). Sinus rhythm should be maintained. New onset atrial flutter/AF should be treated with defibrillation. Avoid factors that may increase PVR ($N_2O$, acidosis, hypoxia, hypercarbia).
**Mitral regurgitation (MR):** Maintain or augment preload, depending on response to fluid load. Inotropic agents may be useful to maintain contractility. Afterload reduction will improve forward flow. Generally SNP (0.5-4 μg/kg/m) is used, but NTG (0.5-4 μg/kg/m) may be more appropriate in patients with ischemia-induced regurgitation. Avoid ↑ PVR caused by $N_2O$, acidosis, hypoxia or hypercarbia. IABP may be useful perioperatively in those patients with acute MR due to MI (↓afterload, ↑coronary perfusion pressure).

**Maintenance**

High-dose narcotic, (total: fentanyl 50-100 μg/kg, or sufentanil 15-20 μg/kg), with benzodiazepine (e.g., midazolam 50-350 μg/kg) for amnesia, occasionally low-dose isoflurane, $O_2$/Air.

The following table summarizes the goals of intraop management:

| Parameter | Mitral Stenosis | Mitral Regurgitation |
|---|---|---|
| LV preload | Normal to ↑ | Normal → ↑ |
| Heart Rate | ↓ | ↑ |
| Rhythm | NSR | NSR |
| Contractility | Maintain | Maintain |
| SVR | Normal | ↓ |
| PVR | Avoid ↑ | Avoid ↑ |

**Post-bypass**

Although patients with MS generally do well after valve replacement, inotropes (e.g., dopamine, dobutamine) are occasionally necessary. This is especially true late in the disease when cardiomyopathy may be present.

**Emergence**

Transport to ICU, intubated and ventilated.

**Blood and fluid requirements**

IV: 14 ga x 1-2
NS/LR @ 6-8 ml/kg/hr
Maintain UO 0.5-1 ml/kg/hr
Warm all fluids.
Humidify gasses.

**Monitoring**

Standard monitors (see Appendix).
Arterial line
CVP line
PA catheter
Urinary catheter

Standard and invasive monitoring should be placed prior to induction. Care should be exercised with PA catheter insertion because the dilated PA may be susceptible to rupture with the catheter. In MS, PCWP may overestimate LV filling pressure because of stenosis.

TEE

TEE may help in volume management, regional wall motion abnormalities (post-acute MI) and in assessing the success of mitral valve repair. Occasionally the use of a valve ring during repair may cause systolic anterior motion of the valve leaflet, with resultant regurgitation, as seen on ECHO.

**Positioning**

√ and pad pressure points.
√ eyes.

## POSTOPERATIVE

**Complications**

Hemorrhage
Tamponade
Cardiac failure
Dysrhythmias
Conduction defects
Atrioventricular disruption

Postop ventilation 24-48 hrs. Inotropic support or vasodilator therapy may be needed. IABP for mitral incompetence, especially in the presence of acute MR as a result of infarction.

| | |
|---|---|
| **Pain management** | Parenteral opioids for pain relief<br>Benzodiazepine for sedation |
| **Tests** | ECG<br>CXR<br>ABG<br>Coagulation profile<br>Electrolytes |

**References**


1. Cobanoglu A, Grunkenmeier GL, Aru GM, McKinley CL, Starr A: Mitral replacement: clinical experience with a ball-valve prosthesis; twenty-five years later. *Ann Surg* 1985; 202(3):376-83.
2. Scott WC, Miller DC, Haverich A, Mitchell RS, Oyer PE, Stinson EB, Jamieson SW, Baldwin JC, Shumway NE: Operative risk of mitral valve replacement: Discriminant analysis of 1329 procedures. *Circulation* 1985; 72(3P+2):II-108-19.
3. Galloway AC, Colvin SB, Baumann FB, et al: A comparison of mitral valve reconstruction with mitral valve replacement: intermediate-term results. *Ann Thorac Surg* 1989; 47:655-62.
4. Jackson JM, Thomas SJ: Valvular Heart Disease. in *Cardiac Anesthesia*, 2nd edition. Kaplan JA, ed. WB Saunders Co, Philadelphia: 1987, Ch 16, 614-23.
5. Moore RA, Martin DE: Anesthetic Management for the Treatment of Valvular Heart Disease. In *The Practice of Cardiac Anesthesia*. Hensley FA, Martin DE, eds. Little, Brown and Co, Boston: 1990, 350-85.


# TRICUSPID VALVE REPAIR

## SURGICAL CONSIDERATIONS

**Description**: Insufficiency of the tricuspid valve is almost always due to left-side valvular disease, with tricuspid annular dilatation and resultant valvular insufficiency usually 2° pulmonary HTN. Some congenital conditions (Ebstein's deformity) may persist into early adulthood, when replacement is usually necessary. Tricuspid repair is normally possible in the absence of primary involvement of tricuspid leaflets. The procedure is usually accomplished on CPB (see separate section on CPB), either with the heart fibrillating or during a brief period of aortic cross-clamping and diastolic arrest. After instituting CPB and snaring the venous cannulae to prevent air entry into the pump circuit, the tricuspid valve is exposed through an incision in the right atrium. In the absence of leaflet involvement by the rheumatic process, repair usually can be accomplished by a simple **annuloplasty**. After atrial closure, evacuation of air and myocardial resuscitation, the patient is weaned from CPB with vasodilator agents. Temporary pacing wires are usually inserted and passed to the anesthesiologist in case inadvertent injury to the AV node or His bundle cause complete heart block.

**Variant procedure or approaches**: Tricuspid **valve replacement**

**Usual preop diagnosis**: Tricuspid regurgitation, 2° annular dilatation 2° pulmonary HTN and left-side failure

### SUMMARY OF PROCEDURE

| | |
|---|---|
| **Position** | Supine |
| **Incision** | Median sternotomy |
| **Special instrumentation** | Intraop ECHO; hemodynamic monitoring; CPB |
| **Antibiotics** | Cefamandole 1 gm iv at induction |
| **Surgical time** | Aortic cross-clamp: 30 - 40 min<br>CPB: 70 - 80 min<br>Total: 3 - 4 hrs |
| **EBL** | 400-800 cc (Long-standing tricuspid regurgitation may result in impaired hepatic production of coagulation factors.) |
| **Postop care** | ICU x 1-3 d, intubated; vasodilator therapy for pulmonary HTN |
| **Mortality** | 2-3% |

**Morbidity** Third-degree heart block: 10%; RV: 2-3%
**Procedure code** 33452, 33465
**Pain score** 7-10

### PATIENT POPULATION CHARACTERISTICS

**Age range** 50-75 yrs
**Male:Female** 1:1
**Incidence** Rare
**Etiology** Rheumatic
Congenital (Ebstein's)

**Associated conditions** Rheumatic involvement of left-side valves with pulmonary HTN

---

## ANESTHETIC CONSIDERATIONS

### PREOPERATIVE

**Cardiovascular** Tricuspid regurgitation (TR) is usually well-tolerated and Sx (↓CO) may go unnoticed, masked by Sx associated with left-side valvular disease and pulmonary HTN. Occasionally TR is 2° endocarditis and raises the suspicion of iv drug abuse. TR may be caused by pulmonary HTN → ↑RV afterload → RV dilation, ↑RV wall tension → dilation of tricuspid valve annulus and TR.
Pathophysiology:
-TR → ↓CO 2° ↑RV size → shift of the intraventricular septum to the left → ↓LV size, ↓LV compliance → LV underloading due to ↓LV size and ↓RV stroke volume.
-TR → atrial fibrillation (AF) 2° ↑right atrial size. In isolated insufficiency, the ↑ in right atrial pressure may result in shunting across a patent foramen ovale (PFO), leading to paradoxical embolization with potentially disastrous consequences.
**Tests:** ECG: ✓AF. ECHO: ✓relative chamber size, contractility, PFO, valve lesions. Cardiac catheterization: ✓ contractility, cardiac output, pulmonary pressures and their response to vasodilators, other valvular pathology.

**Respiratory** Pulmonary HTN (>25 mmHg mean pressure), pulmonary edema and effusions may be present.
**Tests:** CXR: ✓ pulmonary edema, pleural effusion.

**Renal** Chronic venous congestion may lead to pre-renal failure.
**Tests:** BUN; creatinine; electrolytes

**Hepatic** Hepatic congestion may lead to impaired synthetic function, particularly coagulation factors.
**Tests:** PT; PTT.

**Hematologic** **Tests:** Hb/Hct; other tests as indicated from H&P and symptoms. Consider viral testing (HIV, hepatitis in isolated tricuspid endocarditis or in iv drug abusers). T&C 8 U PRBCs.

**Laboratory** Other tests as indicated from H&P.

**Premedication** Standard premedication (see Appendix) is usually appropriate.

### INTRAOPERATIVE

**Anesthetic technique:** GETA

**Induction** Typically, $O_2$ and high-dose narcotic (fentanyl 20-100 μg/kg or sufentanil 10-20 μg/kg) with etomidate (0.1-0.3 mg/kg) or midazolam (50-150 μg/kg). Muscle relaxation is obtained with a non-depolarizing agent (e.g., pancuronium 0.1 mg/kg, vecuronium 0.1 mg/kg).

**Maintenance** The choice of narcotic/benzodiazepine/$O_2$ or volatile agent and $O_2$ will be determined by the underlying lesion and ventricular function. Avoid $N_2O$ (pulmonary HTN). Low-dose isoflurane may be used. Benzodiazepines (e.g., midazolam 50-300 μg/kg, diazepam 0.3-0.5 mg/kg) may be used for amnesia. Exact choice of agents for maintenance depends on underlying lesion, ventricular function and co-existing disease. Management goals of TR are often those of co-existing valvular problems. The general principles, however, are: (1) Adequate preload (↓preload ↓RV stroke volume). (2) HR: normal-to-increased. (3) Contractility: normal. May require inotropic support for ↑PVR, anesthetic myocardial depression or IPPV. (4) PVR: normal or decrease (high PVR ↓RV stroke volume). (5) SVR: little effect unless it affects left-side pathology.

**Emergence** To ICU intubated and ventilated x 24-48 hrs.

| | | |
|---|---|---|
| **Blood and fluid requirements** | IV: 14 ga x 1-2<br>NS/LR @ 6-8 ml/kg/hr<br>UO 0.5-1 ml/kg/hr<br>Warm all fluids.<br>Humidify gasses.<br>8-10 U PRBC cross-match | Because of the possibility of PFO and R→L shunt, ensure that all venous lines are clear of air. |
| **Monitoring** | Standard monitors (see Appendix).<br>Arterial line<br>CVP or PA catheter<br>Urinary catheter | Standard and invasive monitoring should be placed prior to induction.<br>CVP may be a poor indicator of RV or LV filling. PA catheter may be helpful in the management of fluid balance, cardiac output and management of pulmonary HTN, but may be difficult to place and will require removal while valve or annular ring is placed. |
| | TEE | Because RV distention may affect LV filling and stroke volume, TEE may be useful in judging filling and relative LV size. |
| **Pulmonary HTN** | ↑PVR can result from:<br>↓$PaO_2$<br>↑$PaCO_2$<br>↓pH<br>$N_2O$<br>α-agonists | In TR, the control of PVR is important because ↑PVR may result in ↓CO. Hypoxia, hypercarbia, acidosis, $N_2O$ or α-agonists may increase PVR. PVR may be reduced with hypocarbia, inotropic support with dobutamine (5-10 μg/kg/min), isoproterenol (10-50 ng/kg/m) or amrinone (loading 0.75 mg/kg, infusion 2-20 μg/kg/min) and by using pulmonary vasodilators – NTG (1-4 μg/kg/min), SNP (0.5-4 μg/kg/min), prostaglandin $E_1$ (0.05-0.4 μg/kg/min), or NO (inhaled to effect – experimental at this stage). |
| **Positioning** | ✓ and pad pressure points.<br>✓ eyes. | |
| **Complications** | Coagulopathy<br>Hemorrhage<br>RV failure | Coagulopathy 2° prolonged bypass time for multiple valve replacements.<br>RV failure 2° ↑PVR (previously, RV decompressed by tricuspid incompetence). Rx includes inotropes dobutamine (5-10 μg/kg/min), isoproterenol (25-100 ng/kg/min), amrinone (loading 0.75 mg/kg, infusion 2-20 μg/kg/min), epinephrine (25-100 ng/kg/min), avoidance of factors causing ↑PVR, and the use of pulmonary vasodilators. |

## POSTOPERATIVE

| | | |
|---|---|---|
| **Complications** | Hemorrhage<br>Coagulopathy<br>Dysrhythmias<br>RV failure<br>Infection<br>Renal impairment | Inotropic support and pulmonary vasodilators will need to be continued. Avoid those factors which ↑PVR. |
| **Pain management** | Parenteral opioids for pain relief<br>Benzodiazepine for sedation | |
| **Tests** | ECG<br>Coagulation profile<br>Renal panel: BUN, creatinine<br>ABG<br>Electrolytes | |

**References**

1. Jackson JM, Thomas SJ: Valvular heart disease. In *Cardiac Anesthesia*, 2nd edition. Kaplan JA, ed. WB Saunders Co, Philadelphia: 1987, Ch 16, 589-634.
2. Moore RA, Martin DE: Anesthetic management for the treatment of valvular heart disease. In *The Practice of Cardiac Anesthesia*. Hensley FA Jr, Martin DE, eds. Little, Brown and Co, Boston: 1990, Ch 12, 350-86.

# SEPTAL MYECTOMY/MYOTOMY

## SURGICAL CONSIDERATIONS

**Description:** Patients with asymmetric septal hypertrophy usually present with symptoms 2° LV outflow tract obstruction, increased diastolic dysfunction and stiffness, or a combination of the two, manifested as syncope, CHF or severe chest pain. The systolic hemodynamic abnormality is caused by anterior leaflet of the mitral valve being drawn into the LV outflow tract, and abutting the asymmetrically hypertrophied intraventricular septum, narrowing the LV outflow track, and producing a large intracavitary gradient. Additionally, severe mitral insufficiency may result. The most common surgical procedure for asymmetric septal hypertrophy is **septal myectomy/myotomy**. After institution of CPB, aortic cross-clamping and cardioplegic arrest, the aorta is opened, and visualization of the subvalvar ventricular septum attained. Bimanual palpation, as well as TEE visualization, can localize the asymmetric hypertrophy. Using the right coronary orifice as a landmark, the ventricular septum is longitudinally incised with two parallel incisions approximately 1 cm apart, with care being taken to avoid injury of the papillary muscle or mitral valve chordae. A trough of the hypertrophied septum is then excised, alleviating the LV outflow tract obstruction. Removal of a portion of the asymmetrically hypertrophied myopathic septum also usually reduces the systolic anterior motion (SAM) of the anterior mitral leaflet, reduces the intracavitary gradient and mitral regurgitation. Infrequently, mitral valve replacement may be necessary for persistent mitral regurgitation.

**Usual preop diagnosis**: Asymmetric septal hypertrophy with CHF, chest pain, and/or syncope

### SUMMARY OF PROCEDURE

| | |
|---|---|
| **Position** | Supine |
| **Incision** | Median sternotomy |
| **Special instrumentation** | TEE; hemodynamic monitoring; CPB |
| **Unique considerations** | Because of LV hypertrophy, maintenance of adequate preload is essential. Afterload must also be maintained to prevent LV outflow tract obstruction (LVOTO). |
| **Antibiotics** | Cefamandole 1 gm iv at induction |
| **Surgical time** | 2.5 hrs |
| **EBL** | 150 cc |
| **Postop care** | ICU, intubated on ventilator 24-36 hrs |
| **Mortality** | 3-4% |
| **Morbidity** | Complete heart block: 5%<br>Persistent mitral regurgitation: 5%<br>New aortic insufficiency: 2-5%<br>CVA: < 1%<br>VSD: < 1% |
| **Procedure code** | 33416 |
| **Pain score** | 6-10 |

### PATIENT POPULATION CHARACTERISTICS

| | |
|---|---|
| **Age range** | 20-80 yrs (mean = 45 yrs) |
| **Male:Female** | 1:1 |
| **Incidence** | 10/yr at Stanford University Medical Center |
| **Etiology** | Asymmetric septal hypertrophy |

# ANESTHETIC CONSIDERATIONS

## PREOPERATIVE

**Respiratory** Affected only 2° to cardiac failure.

**Cardiovascular** Patients with idiopathic hypertrophic subaortic stenosis (IHSS) often present with Sx of syncope, angina pectoris (CAD), CHF and palpitations. The main feature of IHSS is dynamic LV outflow tract obstruction (LVOTO) 2° to septal hypertrophy and a possible venturi effect which draws the anterior mitral valve leaflet into the outflow tract. LVOTO → ↑LV hypertrophy → ↓compliance and ↓diastolic function → ↑LVEDP, making diastolic filling dependent on preload and atrial contraction. Obstruction is worsened by decreased preload or afterload, increased contractility or HR. IHSS also results in ↑$MVO_2$ and ↓coronary perfusion, especially to the septum and subendocardium, which increases the risk of ischemia. Hypertrophy occurs throughout the whole myocardium and may lead to further dysfunction. Mitral regurgitation (MR), caused by a venturi suction effect, is often present and is exacerbated by the same conditions that increase LVOTO. (Note that ↓ afterload → ↑MR, unlike the usual [non-venturi-suction] form of MR.) Patients are often on β-blockers or $Ca^{++}$ antagonists. These should be continued to day of surgery.

**Tests:** ECG: ✓ Q-waves (indicative of septal hypertrophy); short PR interval with slurred QRS complex; supraventricular tachycardia; LV hypertrophy.

ECHO: ✓ septal hypertrophy; MR; LV hypertrophy, myocardial dysfunction.

Cardiac catheterization: ✓ LVOT pressure gradient which may increase with provocation (e.g., Valsalva maneuver); obliteration of the LV cavity; MR; CAD.

**Neurological** Document syncope and any neurological deficits that may have arisen.

**Laboratory** Hb/Hct; electrolytes; other tests as indicated from H&P.

**Premedication** Avoid activation of the sympathetic nervous system since this will cause ↑HR and ↑inotropy → ↓CO + ↓BP. Thus, adequate anxiolysis is essential and can be obtained by premedication with a benzodiazepine (e.g., midazolam 0.05-0.2 mg/kg im, lorazepam 1-2 mg po or diazepam 5-10 mg po). Avoid ↓SVR, and maintain β-blockade and $Ca^{++}$ channel blocker therapy.

## INTRAOPERATIVE

**Anesthetic technique:** GETA

**Induction** Typically, high-dose narcotic (fentanyl 20-100 μg/kg; avoid sufentanil due to vasodilation) supplemented by etomidate (0.1-0.3 mg/kg), midazolam (50-350 μg/kg) or thiopental (2-4 mg/kg). Ketamine should be avoided due to the activation of the sympathetic nervous system. Introduction of a volatile agent prior to intubation may be helpful. Vecuronium (0.1 mg/kg) for muscle relaxation. Use pancuronium with caution (tachycardia) and avoid d-tubocurarine (hypotension).

**Maintenance** $O_2$ and narcotic (fentanyl 50-100 μg/kg) + volatile agent – most commonly, halothane because of decreased contractility and preservation of SVR; however, halothane may lead to loss of normal sinus rhythm (NSR). Isoflurane is relatively contraindicated (↓SVR). Midazolam (50-350 μg/kg) can be used for amnesia. The cornerstone of anesthesia for IHSS is to avoid factors which will increase LVOTO: (1) ↓preload; (2) ↓afterload; (3) ↑contractility; (4) loss of NSR; and (5) ↑HR.

**Emergence** To ICU intubated and ventilated x 24-48 hrs.

**Blood and fluid requirements**
IV: 14 ga x 1-2
NS/LR @ 6-8 ml/kg/hr
Maintain UO 0.5-1 ml/hr
Warm fluids.
Humidify gasses.

**Monitoring**
Standard monitors (see Appendix).
Arterial line
PA catheter
TEE
Urinary catheter

Standard and invasive monitors should be placed prior to induction. A PA catheter is useful for assessment of LV filling (keep high normal PCWP) and for monitoring SVR (normal-to-high). A pacing or pace port PA catheter may be useful for conduction problems occurring postop. TEE is useful to judge LV filling, LV contractility, LVOTO, MR and VSD.

| | | |
|---|---|---|
| **Intraoperative problems** | ↓Preload | Rx: volume, phenylephrine |
| | ↓Afterload | Rx: phenylephrine |
| | ↑Contractility | Rx: esmolol, halothane |
| | ↑HR | Rx: esmolol |
| | Loss of NSR | Rx: cardioversion, verapamil |
| | Complete heart block | Patients should have reliable means of pacing, if necessary, including temporary ventricular leads. |
| | VSD | The septum may be damaged, resulting in a VSD (diagnosed by TEE). If present, it should be repaired. |
| **Position** | √ and pad pressure points.<br>√ eyes. | |

## POSTOPERATIVE

| | | |
|---|---|---|
| **Complications** | Hemorrhage | Dx: from chest tube drainage. Rx with blood and factors as needed. √ coagulation status. May require re-exploration. |
| | Complete heart block | Postop ventilation 24-36 hrs. Pacing should be available. Occasionally, inotropes of vasodilators required. β-blockers and $Ca^{++}$ antagonists usually discontinued. |
| | Late VSD | Late VSD, indicated by development of a murmur, will require repair. |
| | Tamponade | Dx: by rising filling pressure, equalization of CVP and PADP, ↓CO, ↓UO and by ECHO. Rx: re-exploration and drainage. |
| **Pain management** | Parenteral opioids for pain relief<br>Benzodiazepine for sedation | |
| **Tests** | ECG: √ conduction problems<br>ABG<br>ECHO: √ LVOTO; VSD<br>Coagulation profile<br>Electrolytes | |


**References**

1. Morrow AG, Reitz BA, Epstein SE, Henry WL, Conkle DM, Itscoitz SB, Redwood DR: Operative treatment in hypertrophic subaortic stenosis. Techniques, and the results of pre- and postoperative assessment in 83 patients. *Circulation* 1975; 52(1):88-102.
2. Maron BJ, Bonow RO, Cannon RO III, Leon MB, Epstein SE: Hypertrophic cardiomyopathy. Interrelations of clinical manifestations, pathophysiology, and therapy. *N Engl J Med* 1987; 316(13):780-89; 316(14):844-52.
3. Reich DL, Brooks III JL, Kaplan JA: Uncommon Cardiac Diseases. In *Anesthesia and Uncommon Diseases*, 3rd edition, Chap 8. Katz J, Benumof JL, Kadis LB, eds. WB Saunders Co, Philadelphia: 1990, Ch 8, 341-43.
4. Jackson JM, Thomas SJ: Valvular Heart Disease. In *Cardiac Anesthesia*, 2nd edition. Kaplan JA, ed. WB Saunders Co, Philadelphia: 1987, Ch 16, 589-634.
5. Hilgenberg JC: Cardiomyopathies. In *Anesthesia and Co-existing Disease*, 2nd edition. Stoelting RK, Dierdorf SF, eds. Churchill Livingstone, New York: 1988., Ch 8, 129-33.

# CARDIAC MAPPING AND ABLATION PROCEDURES

## SURGICAL CONSIDERATIONS

**Description**: Cardiac dysrhythmias may occur 2° abnormal or accessory conduction pathways in the heart. Electrophysiologic testing can localize these abnormal pathways, evaluate their suppressibility by dysrhythmic medications, and even ablate, with radiofrequency, certain localized pathways. Surgical ablation is possible for those pathways not amenable to catheter-directed radiofrequency ablation. For polymorphic dysrhythmias not amenable to ablation or pharmacologic suppression, automatic implantable cardiac defibrillators (AICD) can be highly effective by delivering a depolarizing shock after detecting the dysrhythmia. The evaluation decision tree proceeds as follows: monomorphic ventricular tachycardia (VT) → pharmacologic suppression; if unsuccessful, mapping with catheter or surgical ablation. Polymorphic VT → pharmacologic suppression, if unsuccessful, mapping and catheter ablation, if still unsuccessful → AICD.

Surgical ablation is performed on CPB (see section on CPB). After routine cannulation and implantation of electrophysiologic leads, an attempt is made to induce VT. If successful, and the patient remains stable, electrophysiologic mapping is performed. Avoidance of anti-dysrhythmics is important at this stage. If the patient is hemodynamically unstable, CPB is begun, and the mapping procedure completed. Once complete, the heart is arrested, and during hypothermic cardiac arrest, the dysrhythmogenic focus is excised or cryoblated. For polymorphic VT, an AICD is usually implanted. Initially, this was performed through a left anterior thoracotomy, but some lead systems have progressed so that only subcutaneous patches, a superior caval electrode, and RV pacing leads are necessary, as is an incision for the defibrillator. Defibrillator testing requires multiple episodes of VT or ventricular fibrillation (VF) with rescue "shocks," which may produce some cardiac instability. For polymorphic dysrhythmias not amenable to ablation or pharmacologic suppression, implantable automatic defibrillators can be highly effective in delivering a depolarizing shock after detecting the dysrhythmia.

**Usual preop diagnosis**: Supra-ventricular tachycardia (SVT); ventricular tachycardia or fibrillation; Wolff-Parkinson-White (WPW) syndrome; Lown-Ganong-Levine (LGL) syndrome

### SUMMARY OF PROCEDURE

| | Mapping and/or Ablation | Automatic Defibrillator |
|---|---|---|
| **Position** | Supine | Supine, with slight elevation of left chest |
| **Incision** | Median sternotomy | Central venous access (left subclavian vein) with either pericardial defibrillator patches, placed through an anterior thoracotomy, or subcutaneous patches. |
| **Special instrumentation** | Electrophysiologic instrumentation; defibrillator patches on skin; CPB | External defibrillator; DLT to allow collapse of left lung; defibrillator patches/paddles on skin |
| **Unique considerations** | Avoid anti-dysrhythmic agents during induction, if possible. | None |
| **Antibiotics** | Cefamandole 1 gm iv at induction | ⇐ |
| **Surgical time** | Aortic cross-clamp: 30 - 60 min<br>CPB: 70 - 150 min<br>Total: 3 - 4 hrs | Total: 2 - 3 hrs (no CPB) |
| **EBL** | 300-400 cc | < 100 cc |
| **Postop care** | ICU x 2 d; ECG monitoring x 7 d | ICU x 1 d; ECG monitoring x 7 d |
| **Mortality** | 5-15% (highly dependent on mechanism of dysrhythmia. If aberrant pathway (WPW), 1-2%; if 2° LV aneurysm with ischemic dysfunction, 5-15%) | 1-2% |
| **Morbidity** | Overall: 10%<br>Recurrent VT/VF: 20-30%<br>MI: 2-5% | Respiratory complications: 2-5%<br>CVA: 1%<br>2% |
| **Procedure code** | 93325 | 33222, 33245, 33246 |
| **Pain score** | 6-10 | 5-10 |

### PATIENT POPULATION CHARACTERISTICS

**Age range** 30-70 yrs in general
WPW and other anatomical pathways: 2-50 yrs
Acquired dysrhythmias from ischemic damage: 50-75 yrs

**Male:Female** 2:1

**Incidence** Rare

**Etiology** SVT, usually 2° congenital bypass tracts
VT and VF, usually 2° ischemia-induced changes such as LV aneurysm formation or an irritable peri-infarct zone

---

## ANESTHETIC CONSIDERATIONS

### PREOPERATIVE

Patients may be divided into two populations based on symptomatology, associated pathology and probable outcome: (1) **Superventricular dysrhythmias**: e.g., Wolff-Parkinson-White. These patients are usually young and otherwise healthy. May be associated with Ebstein's anomaly (tricuspid valve defect → RV failure), mitral valve disease or CAD. Low perioperative mortality (1%). (2) **Ventricular dysrhythmias**: usually older patients with significant ventricular dysfunction (EF 10-35%) and other pathologies such as CAD or cardiac failure. Procedure is often accompanied by LV aneurysmectomy or myocardial revascularization (see "Coronary Artery Bypass Graft Surgery," above). Mortality is 15% for mapping/ablation, but much less for AICD implantation.

**Respiratory** May have associated pulmonary disease 2° smoking.
**Tests:** CXR; PFT as indicated from H&P.

**Cardiovascular** 1) **Supraventricular dysrhythmias**: Occasionally associated disease as above. Look for precipitating factors in the dysrhythmia and any methods that have been used to terminate the dysrhythmia. Usually drug therapy is terminated prior to surgery to make the dysrhythmia inducible. Note type of drugs used, especially those used to terminate a dysrhythmia.
2) **Ventricular dysrhythmias**: Inquire about any methods that have been used to terminate the dysrhythmia. Look for associated conditions – CAD, CHF, cardiomyopathy, LV aneurysm, HTN, mitral insufficiency, diabetes. Generally these patients will have poor LV function with increased sensitivity to myocardial depressants. It is important to note that these patients may be on combinations of anti-dysrhythmics. Many of these drugs have significant negative inotropic effects. Of special note is amiodarone, which has been associated with intractable bradydysrhythmias, refractory vasodilation and difficulty in weaning from CPB.
3) **AICD**: AICD patients are left on full medication as it is usually impossible to wean them from anti-dysrhythmic medications before surgery.
**Tests:** ECG: ✓ dysrhythmia, ischemia. Electrophysiologic report: ✓ type of dysrhythmia, means of termination – pharmacologic or electrical. ECHO: ✓ ventricular function, wall motion abnormalities, valvular problems. Cardiac angiography: ✓ ventricular function, CAD, valvular disease, LV aneurysm.

**Renal** Patients with poor ventricular function may have associated renal compromise. Electrolyte abnormalities ($K^+$, $Mg^{++}$) may be associated with increased cardiac irritability and should be corrected preop.
**Tests:** BUN; creatinine; electrolytes

**Hematologic** Hb/Hct; T&C for 8 U (AICD patients are not T&C'd)

**Laboratory** Other tests as indicated from H&P.

**Premedication** Typically, a benzodiazepine (e.g., lorazepam 1-2 mg po, midazolam 0.05-0.2 mg/kg im), morphine (0.1-0.2 mg/kg), or a combination, depending on LV function.

### INTRAOPERATIVE

**Anesthetic technique:** GETA

**Induction** Exact type of induction depends on the planned surgery, need for CPB, ventricular function and whether prolonged (12+ hr) postop ventilation will be necessary. For patients with supraventricular dysrhythmias and good LV function, early extubation in the ICU can be planned. For these patients, induction with thiopental (2-4 mg/kg) or etomidate (0.1-0.3 mg/kg), with low-to-moderate dose narcotic (e.g., fentanyl 5-20 μg/kg) and muscle relaxation with vecuronium (0.1 mg/kg) is often used. For patients with poor ventricular function, a high-dose narcotic (e.g., fentanyl 20-100 μg/kg), 100% $O_2$ and muscle relaxation with vecuronium (0.1 mg/kg) is appropriate. Many patients for AICD implantation may be extubated at the end of the procedure; therefore, a low-dose narcotic (e.g., fentanyl 3-10 μg/kg), plus etomidate (0.1-0.3 mg/kg), is often used. Muscle relaxation with vecuronium (0.1 mg/kg) is satisfactory.

**Maintenance**

Maintenance of anesthesia for **superventricular dysrhythmias:** Generally, mapping is done prior to bypass, but after cannulation. If the focus is left-side, cardioplegia is used after mapping; but right-side foci are usually done with normothermic bypass and a beating heart. This has relevance in the increased heparin requirements (↑metabolism), so that frequent ACTs should be performed. If rapid cardiac rates are induced, myocardial $O_2$ demand will be high. Ensure amnesia with a benzodiazepine (e.g., midazolam 50-350 μg/kg).

Maintenance of anesthesia for **ventricular dysrhythmias:** These foci are usually left-side and 2° to CAD. Both epicardial and endocardial mapping are often needed and are carried out under normothermic bypass. The same consideration of increased heparin requirement and ↑$MVO_2$ during induced ventricular tachycardia apply. In addition, the ventricle may be open while the aorta is not cross-clamped. It is important that the aortic valve remain closed during this period to prevent air entering the aorta. Adequate aortic pressure is important and may be obtained with a phenylephrine infusion (0.15-0.75 μg/kg iv). During the procedure, ventricular tissue may be excised, and this, together with the already compromised ventricle, may result in difficulty in terminating CPB. Inotropes and IABP may be required. Coagulopathies, particularly 2° low platelets, may occur during prolonged normothermic bypass. Ensure amnesia with a benzodiazepine (e.g., midazolam 50-350 μg/kg).

Maintenance for **AICD:** AICD devices have leads for sensing rate and for delivering a 10-30 J shock to prevent sustained ventricular fibrillation joules. These may be placed via a small anterior thoracotomy or via a transvenous route. Verification of placement involves the induction of ventricular fibrillation or tachycardia and the testing of the device's capability in converting this to NSR. External defibrillation should be available at all times, as should anti-dysrhythmics. While the device is tested, the patient should be ventilated with 100% $O_2$. Multiple testing cycles can result in depressed LV function and inotropes may be needed.

**Emergence**

AICD patients are often extubated at the end of surgery, especially if a transvenous approach is used. If, however, multiple test shocks are needed or the heart displays evidence of injury (need for inotropes, ST segment abnormalities), then extubation may need to be deferred to ICU. Generally, with supraventricular and ventricular dysrhythmia patients (where sternotomy is performed), emergence is deferred to ICU. Electrophysiologic testing is usually repeated a few wks after surgery.

**Blood and fluid requirements**

IV: 14 ga x 1-2
NS/LR @ 6-8 ml/kg/min
UO 0.5-1 ml/kg
Warm all fluids.
Humidify gasses.

**Monitoring**

Standard monitors (see Appendix).
Arterial line
CVP line
PA catheter
Urinary catheter

A CVP or PA catheter may be placed according to LV function. Generally, in all cases, a PA sheath should be used. If a PA catheter is chosen it should be advanced when the chest is open and access to the heart is available because of the potential for inducing dysrhythmias. These lines may be placed with the aid of local anesthesia (lidocaine) prior to induction of GA.

External defibrillation pads

Because anti-dysrhythmics may affect the mapping procedure, they should be avoided whenever possible. Defibrillation or cardioversion is the treatment of choice. For this, external pads and internal paddles are essential.

| | | |
|---|---|---|
| **Monitoring, continued** | TEE | TEE is useful to assess LV function before and after mapping, ablation and AICD testing. |
| | Temperature | Normothermia should be maintained, since decreased temperature may affect conduction in aberrant pathways and, thus, the mapping procedure. |
| **Positioning** | Roll under shoulders for median sternotomy and under left chest for AICD.<br>✓ and pad pressure points.<br>✓ eyes. | |

**POSTOPERATIVE**

| | | |
|---|---|---|
| **Complications** | Recurrent dysrhythmias<br>Hemorrhage<br>Coagulopathy<br>Ischemia | The AICD is switched off or left on, depending on whether the patient is going to the ICU or the ward. Defibrillation should always be available. |
| **Pain management** | Parenteral opioids for pain relief<br>Benzodiazepine for sedation | |
| **Tests** | CXR: ✓ line placement, pneumothorax<br>ECG: ✓ ischemia dysrhythmias<br>Electrophysiologic testing<br>Coagulation profile<br>Electrolytes | |

**References**


1. Cox JL: Anatomic-electrophysiologic basis for the surgical treatment of refractory ischemic ventricular tachycardia. *Ann Surg* 1983; 198(2):119-29.
2. Cox JL, Gallagher JJ, Cain ME: Experience with 118 consecutive patients undergoing surgery for the Wolff-Parkinson-White syndrome. *J Thorac Cardiovasc Surg* 1985; 90(4):490-501.
3. Stull MW, Luck JC, Martin DE: Anesthesia for patients with electrophysiologic disorders. In *The Practice of Cardiac Anesthesia*. Hensley FA Jr, Martin DE, eds. Little, Brown and Co, Boston: 1990, Ch 16, 493-524.
4. Feinberg BI: Anesthesia and Electrophysiologic Procedures. In *Cardiac Anesthesia*, 2nd edition. Kaplan JA, ed. WB Saunders Co, Philadelphia: 1987, Ch 19, 751-84.


# PACEMAKER INSERTION

## SURGICAL CONSIDERATIONS

**Description**: Pacemaker insertion may be required for relief of abnormalities of the conduction system. A transvenous pacemaker lead may be placed via the subclavian vein, through the tricuspid valve into the right ventricle (single-chamber pacing); or two leads may be placed, one into the right atrium and the other into the right ventricle (dual-chamber pacing). Typically, 2nd- or 3rd-degree heart block is the diagnostic indication, although sick sinus syndrome and other abnormalities also may be found. Access to the subclavian veins is usually attained percutaneously, although a cut-down may be used to expose the cephalic vein in the deltopectoral groove. Passage of a guide wire into the right ventricle may cause frequent premature ventricular beats which usually subside spontaneously with repositioning of the guide wire or lead. After ventricular and/or atrial lead placement, the pacing lead will have to be tested for sensing threshold, pacing threshold, depolarization amplitude and lead resistance. After satisfactory placement of the pacing leads, the actual pacemaker generator unit is connected and then placed in a subcutaneous pocket at the site of percutaneous lead placement.

**Usual preop diagnosis**: Abnormalities of S-A nodal function (SSS) or A-V nodal function (heart block)

## SUMMARY OF PROCEDURE

| | |
|---|---|
| **Position** | Supine |
| **Incision** | Left subclavicular; mostly percutaneous |
| **Special instrumentation** | Fluoroscopy with fluoro-table |
| **Unique considerations** | Patient usually awake with mild sedation |
| **Antibiotics** | Cefamandole 1 gm iv at induction |
| **Surgical time** | 1 hr |
| **EBL** | Minimal |
| **Postop care** | PACU → CCU; ECG monitoring x 2-4 hrs; chest radiograph to document lead configuration. |
| **Mortality** | 0-1% |
| **Morbidity** | Lead displacement: 1-2%<br>Pneumothorax: 1-2% |
| **Procedure code** | 33200, 33201, 33206, 33218 |
| **Pain score** | 2 |

## PATIENT POPULATION CHARACTERISTICS

| | |
|---|---|
| **Age range** | 50-80 yrs |
| **Male:Female** | 2:1 |
| **Incidence** | Infrequent |
| **Etiology** | CAD<br>Cardiac valve repair/replacement |
| **Associated conditions** | Complete heart block with syncope<br>Sick sinus syndrome<br>Paroxysmal tachycardia<br>SVTs |

---

# ANESTHETIC CONSIDERATIONS

## PREOPERATIVE

The indications for permanent pacemaker insertion are usually bradydysrhythmias (e.g., 3rd-degree heart block, sinus node dysfunction, etc.) or, less commonly, tachycardia (e.g., atrial flutter not responsive to medical therapy). There are many different types of pacemakers, which are classified according to the chamber paced, chamber sensed, response to sensing, programmability and anti-tachyrhythmia functions. The anesthesiologist should be aware of the type of pacemaker to be implanted and the means for external control.

| | |
|---|---|
| **Cardiovascular** | Evaluate patient for associated disease, including CAD (~50%), HTN (~20%), cardiomyopathy, CHF, valvular defect, and for any symptoms or recent changes related to the conduction problems (syncope, CHF). It is important to know the reason for pacemaker implantation and the patient's escape rhythm. These patients are often on anti-dysrythmics, diuretics, cardiac glycosides and a variety of other cardiovascular agents, which should be continued up to the day of surgery.<br>**Tests:** Exercise tolerance by Hx; ECG: ✓ rate, ischemic changes, rhythm; other tests as indicated by H&P; ✓ serum digoxin and other anti-dysrhythmic levels. |
| **Pacemaker** | If a permanent pacemaker is already in place, its type and present functional state should be assessed. (Sx of problems include chest pain, palpitations, syncope and weakness.) If no permanent pacemaker, a temporary transvenous pacemaker should be placed prior to surgery, except in unusual circumstances.<br>**Tests:** ECG: ✓ Valsalva maneuver or carotid sinus massage – may slow the heart sufficiently to allow the permanent pacemaker to fire and allow assessment of function. A rate lower than the set rate may indicate battery failure. CXR: ✓ lead continuity. |
| **Hematologic** | Hct or Hb |
| **Laboratory** | ✓ $K^+$ level, which can affect pacing threshold, lead to loss of pacemaker capture if low, or ventricular tachycardia, if high. Other tests as indicated from H&P. |
| **Premedication** | Standard premedication (see Appendix). |

## INTRAOPERATIVE

**Anesthetic technique:** Permanent pacemakers are commonly placed via the transvenous route, requiring only local anesthesia and MAC with sedation. For epicardial pacemaker placement, GETA is required. These patients should be transported to OR monitored. Care is taken to avoid dislodging temporary pacing electrodes. The function of the temporary pacemaker should be checked prior to induction.

**General anesthesia:**

| | | |
|---|---|---|
| **Induction** | Usually anesthesia can be induced with STP (3-5 mg/kg) or etomidate (0.2-0.3 mg/kg), in combination with an opiate (e.g., fentanyl 1-2 μg/kg) to attenuate the response to intubation. Vecuronium or pancuronium (0.1 mg/kg) will provide adequate muscle relaxation. | |
| **Maintenance** | Standard maintenance (see Appendix). Avoid excessive hyperventilation (→ ↓$K^+$) and use volatile agents with caution, as they may increase A-V conduction time. | |
| **Emergence** | Generally, patient is extubated at the end of the case. | |
| **Blood and Fluid requirements** | Minimal fluid requirements<br>IV: 16 ga x 1<br>NS/LR @ 4-6 ml/kg/hr | |
| **Monitoring** | Standard monitors (see Appendix).<br>Urinary catheter | Rarely, arterial line if patient disease indicates. |
| **Electrocautery interference** | Minimize by:<br>-Using bipolar cautery, if possible.<br>-Grounding pad on leg.<br>-Limiting cautery output.<br>-Limiting cautery use. | The use of electrocautery may interfere with pacemaker function and result in dysrhythmias or failure of the pacemaker. Monitor ECG and pulse (since electrical activity does not mean cardiac output) for interference. Have a magnet available to convert the pacemaker to asynchronous mode (check that this is possible and will not change the programming of the pacemaker. |
| **Complications** | Dysrhythmias<br>Air embolism<br>Cardiac tamponade<br>Hemo/pneumothorax<br>Hemorrhage | Availability of temporary pacing is important because complete heart block or dislodgement of leads may occur. In addition, pharmacologic agents (atropine, 0.5-2 mg; isoproterenol 10-100 ng/kg/min) to increase HR should be available . |

## POSTOPERATIVE

| | |
|---|---|
| **Complications** | Dislodging of electrodes<br>Dysrhythmias<br>Pneumothorax<br>Tamponade |
| **Pain management** | Parenteral opioids for pain relief<br>Benzodiazepine for sedation |
| **Tests** | ECG<br>CXR<br>Electrolytes |

**References**


1. Simon AB: Perioperative management of the pacemaker patient. *Anesthesiology* 1977; 46(2):127-31.
2. Zaidan JR: Pacemakers. *Anesthesiology* 1984; 60(4):319-34.

# PERICARDIECTOMY

## SURGICAL CONSIDERATIONS

**Description:** Constrictive pericarditis, either acute or chronic, interferes with ventricular filling, reducing stroke volume and depressing the cardiac index. Although there are many possible etiologies (infectious, nephrogenic, post-radiation), the diagnosis remains unknown for a majority of patients. Typically, patients present with a progressive history of breathlessness, fatiguability, or peripheral or abdominal swelling, often months to years after the inciting event. The diagnosis may be confirmed by cardiac catheterization, with equalization of end diastolic pressures, although volume loading may be necessary to demonstrate this in the patient under medical management. The differentiation between constrictive pericardial disease and restrictive myocardial disease may be difficult, and may coexist in a single patient. Once this diagnosis has been confirmed, surgical **pericardiectomy** should be undertaken, since the outlook without surgical relief is one of gradual, but persistent deterioration. Although surgical mortality remains in the 10-15% range, long-term relief for survivors is good. Since these patients are usually significantly hemodynamically compromised, intensive monitoring is indicated. Approach may be through a median sternotomy or left anterolateral thoracotomy. Removal of both visceral and parietal pericardium is essential for relief, but dense adhesions of these layers to underlying muscle may make this dissection very difficult, tedious and bloody, especially if the visceral pericardium and epicardium are involved in the constrictive process. CPB (see separate section on CPB) may be utilized for hemodynamic instability, but it obviously increases bleeding complications. Complete excision from both ventricular surfaces is mandatory. Most perioperative difficulties evolve from cardiac failure.

**Variant procedure or approaches**: A limited **pericardial window**, draining fluid into the left hemithorax, may relieve tamponade, but will be of no benefit for a true constrictive process.

**Usual preop diagnosis**: Constrictive pericarditis

### SUMMARY OF PROCEDURE

| | Median Sternotomy | Anterolateral Thoracotomy |
|---|---|---|
| **Position** | Supine | Supine, with elevation of left hemithorax |
| **Incision** | Midline | Fifth interspace |
| **Special instrumentation** | TEE; full hemodynamic monitoring; CPB standby | ⇐ |
| **Antibiotics** | Cefamandole 1 gm iv at induction | ⇐ |
| **Surgical time** | 2 - 5 hrs, depending on tenacity of visceral peel | ⇐ |
| **Closing considerations** | Avoid volume overload and cardiac distention. Chronically depressed hearts may require inotropic or mechanical support (i.e., IABP) postop. | ⇐ |
| **EBL** | 100-500 cc | ⇐ |
| **Postop care** | ICU; intubated x 4-6 hrs. Hemodynamic monitoring. Low cardiac output state may persist postop. | ⇐ |
| **Mortality** | 5-15%,[5] predominantly from cardiac failure | ⇐ |
| **Morbidity** | Persistent CHF: 5%<br>Transient phrenic nerve dysfunction: < 1% | ⇐ |
| **Procedure code** | 33100 | ⇐ |
| **Pain score** | 7-10 | 7-10 |

### PATIENT POPULATION CHARACTERISTICS

| | |
|---|---|
| **Age range** | 10-80 yrs (median = 45 yrs)[6] |
| **Male:Female** | 2:1 |
| **Incidence** | 3-4 patients/yr at tertiary referral center |
| **Etiology** | Majority unknown. Infectious, radiation, prior cardiac operation, rheumatic pericarditis, amyloid deposition |
| **Associated conditions** | Restrictive myocardial diseases |

# ANESTHETIC CONSIDERATIONS

## PREOPERATIVE

Pericardiectomy is most commonly performed for patients with constrictive pericarditis, while pericardial window procedures are used for patients with cardiac tamponade.

**Respiratory** Restrictive disease may be present due to fibrosis (e.g., post-TB) or pleural effusions. This may impair oxygenation and, if the effusions are significant, may ↓venous return on institution of IPPV, resulting in rapid decompensation (↓CO). Drain prior to surgery.

**Tests:** CXR: ✓ active disease, fibrosis, effusions, pericardial calcification; ABG; PFT: as indicated by CXR and Sx, and if time permits.

**Cardiovascular** Of importance is the presence or absence of a pericardial effusion. A large effusion which develops slowly (chronic pericarditis) may cause little or no Sx. Conversely, a small and rapidly forming effusion may lead to cardiac tamponade. While the cardiovascular signs for both tamponade and constriction are similar (pulsus paradoxus, venous HTN, exaggerated venous pulsations, hypotension, tachycardia), it is important to differentiate between them as it may affect intraop management. Constrictive pericarditis can be differentiated from cardiac tamponade by ECHO, by pulsus paradoxus (frequent with tamponade; rare with constrictive pericarditis). Kussmaul's sign (distention of the jugular veins on inspiration) is rare with tamponade and common with constrictive pericarditis. Electrical alternans is present with tamponade and absent in constrictive pericarditis. Examination of the RV pressure wave form is unchanged in tamponade, but shows a dip and prominent Y descent in constrictive pericarditis.

Anesthetic management is influenced by the planned procedure, the underlying process (constriction or tamponade) and its severity. Clues to severity are the physical symptoms and the degree of tachycardia, hypotension and the filling pressure. (While it is not possible to give exact figures, a HR of >100 bpm, systolic BP < 100 mmHg and a filling pressure > 15 mmHg are probably significant.) In addition, it is important to assess concurrent cardiac problems: cardiomyopathy, CAD or valvular disease (especially in constrictive disease associated with TB, radiation therapy or in rheumatoid diseases such as lupus).

**Tests:** ECG: ✓ low-voltage complexes, electrical alternans. ECHO: ✓ pericardial effusion, calcification of pericardium, valvular lesions, myocardial function.

**Gastrointestinal** Chronic hepatic congestion may lead to decreased synthetic function (↓procoagulants). Development of ascites may result in ↑intra-abdominal pressure. Because of this and the fact that these are sometimes emergency procedures, consider possible full stomach.

**Tests:** LFTs; PT; PTT

**Renal** Renal failure may cause pericarditis and, conversely, pericarditis may cause renal failure (2° pre-renal factors: ↑venous pressure, ↓perfusion pressure). This may affect the choice of drugs used for anesthesia that depend on renal clearance (particularly muscle relaxants).

**Tests:** BUN; creatinine, creatinine clearance; electrolytes

**Hematologic** Some renal or hepatic conditions may be associated with coagulation disorders. These include both procoagulant and platelet problems. If possible, any coagulopathy should be corrected prior to surgery with FFP, platelets or both. Consult with a hematologist if necessary.

**Tests:** Hb/Hct; PT; PTT; platelet count; bleeding time

**Laboratory** Other tests as indicated from H&P.

**Premedication** Little or no premedication may be indicated. Otherwise, a benzodiazepine may be used (e.g., midazolam 0.05-0.2 mg/kg im). Consider full-stomach precautions – $H_2$-antagonists (e.g., ranitidine 50 mg iv), metoclopramide (10 mg iv), antacids (e.g., Na citrate 0.3 M 30 ml po).

## INTRAOPERATIVE

**Anesthetic technique:** GETA. Consider pericardiocentesis or pericardial window under local anesthesia prior to induction, as drainage of even a small amount of fluid may dramatically improve the patient's status. The considerable manipulation of the heart, extensive dissection, blood loss, dysrhythmias and unrelieved tamponade make pericardiectomy cases a challenge.

**Induction** Typically, ketamine 1-2 mg/kg or etomidate 0.2-0.3 mg/kg ± narcotic (fentanyl 2-30 μg/kg), depending on patient status. Consider maintaining spontaneous ventilation in tamponade patients until drained, as institution of IPPV may result in rapid decompensation and cardiac arrest due to ↓↓venous return. Otherwise, succinylcholine (1 mg/kg) with cricoid pressure (full stomach) or pancuronium (0.1 mg/kg) for muscle relaxation.

| | | |
|---|---|---|
| **Maintenance** | Narcotic (fentanyl 20-100 μg/kg), low-dose volatile agent, midazolam (50-350 μg/kg), or a combination of these agents in 100% $O_2$. CO is dependent on maintaining a high preload to ensure adequate cardiac filling, avoiding and treating bradycardia and preserving myocardial contractility. The use of inotropes (dobutamine, isoproterenol or epinephrine) may be necessary. Alpha-agonists should be avoided but, on occasion, may be needed to increase coronary perfusion. These anesthetic considerations apply to both tamponade and constrictive disease. | |
| **Emergence** | In general, plan for extubation in the OR in the case of pericardial window and transport to ICU for postop ventilation following pericardiectomy. | |
| **Blood and fluid requirements** | IV: 14 ga (or 7 Fr) x 1-2<br>UO: 0.5-1 ml/kg/hr<br>Warm fluids and humidify gasses.<br>T&C 8 U for pericardiectomy. | During pericardiectomy, anticipate rapid blood loss (a major cause of mortality). For this reason, CPB should be available on standby for all pericardiectomy procedures. |
| **Monitoring** | Standard monitors (see Appendix) .<br>Arterial line<br>CVP line<br>PA catheter<br>TEE<br>Urinary catheter | All monitors should be place prior to induction. PA catheters aid the management of filling pressures, CO and afterload. TEE may be useful to gauge filling volume and degree of relief of pericardial constriction. |
| **Complications** | Cardiac tamponade<br>Dysrhythmias | Intrathoracic pressure associated with IPPV may produce a ↓↓CO in these patients (because of ↓venous return). Spontaneous ventilation, therefore, is preferred until the tamponade is drained. |
| | Hemorrhage<br>Coagulopathy<br>Heart failure | Hemorrhage is not usually a problem unless penetrating trauma is the cause of the tamponade.<br>Once constriction is relieved, myocardial function does not return to normal quickly. Inotropes are often needed. Due to extensive dissection and hemorrhage, coagulopathies may develop and should be treated aggressively. |
| **Positioning** | √ and pad pressure points.<br>√ eyes. | |

## POSTOPERATIVE

| | | |
|---|---|---|
| **Complications** | Hemorrhage<br>Coagulopathy<br>Ventricular hypofunction<br>Dysrhythmias<br>Ischemia | Following pericardial window surgery, patients improve with the relief of the tamponade. Post pericardiectomy patients, however, may have a continuation of intraop dysrhythmias and myocardial depression. Inotropes (e.g., dopamine 5-10 μg/kg/min) may be needed for 24-48 hrs. Normal cardiac function can take 4-6 wks to return. Postop ventilation for 24-48 hrs. |
| **Pain management** | Parenteral opioids for pain relief<br>Benzodiazepine for sedation | |
| **Tests** | ECG<br>CXR<br>ABG<br>Coagulation profile<br>Electrolytes | |


**References**

1. McCaughan BC, Schaff HV, Piehler JM, Danielson GK, Orszulak TA, Puga JR, Connolly DC, McGoon DC: Early and late results of pericardiectomy for constrictive pericarditis. *J Thorac Cardiovasc Surg* 1985; 89:340.
2. Lake CL: Anesthesia and pericardial disease. Anesth Analg 1983; 62(4):431-43.
3. Reich DL, Brooks JL, Kaplan JA: Uncommon cardiac disease. In *Anesthesia and Uncommon Diseases*, 3rd edition. Katz J, Benumof JL, Kadis LB, eds. WB Saunders Co, Philadelphia: 1990, Ch 8, 356-61.
4. Legler DC: Uncommon diseases and cardiac anesthesia. In *Cardiac Anesthesia*, 2nd edition. Kaplan JA, ed. WB Saunders Co, Philadelphia: 1987, Ch 20, 804-12.

**Surgeons**

**James I. Lin Fann, MD**
**R. Scott Mitchell, MD**

# 6.2 VASCULAR SURGERY

**Anesthesiologists**

**Kristi L. Peterson, MD**
**Gordon R. Haddow, MB, ChB, FFA(SA)**

# CAROTID ENDARTERECTOMY

## SURGICAL CONSIDERATIONS

**Description:** Carotid endarterectomy (CEA) is one of the most commonly performed vascular surgery procedures in the U.S. Because of presumed microemboli from stenotic/ulcerated plaques at the carotid bifurcation, CEA has been championed as an effective procedure to reduce the risk of subsequent stroke. Recently, the NASCET trial has determined, in a prospective, randomized, blinded trial, that CEA is more effective than medical therapy for symptomatic patients with internal carotid artery narrowings between 60-90%[1] Symptoms are usually hemispheric (contralateral, upper or lower extremity paresis or numbness) or retinal (unilateral monocular blindness). Symptoms may be transient (TIA, or reversible ischemic neurological deficit [RIND]) or permanent (CVA). The status of surgical intervention for asymptomatic carotid stenosis remains equivocal. Currently, many surgeons would recommend prophylactic CEA only for asymptomatic carotid stenosis greater than 85%. Although some surgeons routinely prefer local anesthesia, most prefer GA with careful hemodynamic monitoring because of the frequent concomitant CAD.

The carotid artery is approached through an oblique neck incision along the anterior border of the sternocleidomastoid muscle. After division of the common facial vein, the carotid sheath is opened and the carotid artery is exposed, avoiding injury to the phrenic, vagus, ansa hypoglossi and hypoglossal nerves. After controlling the internal, external and common carotid arteries, heparin is administered, and the internal, external and common carotid arteries are clamped sequentially. An indwelling shunt may be utilized, at the discretion of the surgeon. An endarterectomy plane is established proximally, and developed distally into both the external and internal branches, with establishment of a fine tapered end point. After removal of all thrombus, loose smooth muscle fibers, and endothelium, the arteriotomy is closed, with or without a patch, the artery flushed and flow restored. The incision is then closed, after meticulous hemostasis has been assured.

**Usual preop diagnosis:** Carotid artery disease

### SUMMARY OF PROCEDURE

| | |
|---|---|
| **Position** | Supine, with neck extended and turned away from the side of the lesion. |
| **Incision** | Anterior to sternocleidomastoid from earlobe to base of neck, or curvilinear in a skin crease over the carotid bifurcation. |
| **Special instrumentation** | Complete hemodynamic monitors; EEG monitors; ± shunt |
| **Unique considerations** | Capability to measure stump pressure may be needed. This can be accomplished by a high-pressure arterial line being passed off the field to a pressure transducer. During carotid cross-clamping, it is imperative that there be no intraop hypotension. An in-dwelling shunt may be utilized to restore carotid perfusion during CEA. Heparin 10,000 U 5 min prior to cross-clamping, and protamine 50 mg after restoration of flow. |
| **Antibiotics** | Cefamandole 1 gm iv at induction of anesthesia |
| **Surgical time** | Carotid cross-clamp: 30 min; total operating time: 90 min |
| **Closing considerations** | In order to assess the patient's neurologic status, it is best to be able to awaken and extubate the patient at the conclusion of the procedure. Avoidance of HTN is also critical during this period, since the endarterectomy tissues are thin and friable. |
| **EBL** | 100-200 cc |
| **Postop care** | ICU x 12-24 hrs; BP control; cardiac monitoring |
| **Mortality** | 1% |
| **Morbidity** | MI: Major cause of postop mortality<br>Cranial nerve injury (recurrent and superior laryngeal nerves): 39%<br>Restenosis<br>Asymptomatic: 9-12%<br>Symptomatic: < 3%<br>Neurologic complications: < 2%<br>Hemorrhage: 1%<br>False aneurysm: < 0.5% |
| **Procedure code** | 35301 |
| **Pain score** | 3-10 |

### PATIENT POPULATION CHARACTERISTICS

| | |
|---|---|
| **Age range** | 55-80 yrs |
| **Male:Female** | 3:1 |
| **Incidence** | Second most common vascular surgical procedure (after AAA repair) |
| **Etiology** | Arteriosclerosis<br>Fibro-muscular dysplasia |
| **Associated conditions** | Significant CAD coexists with carotid artery disease in at least 30% of patients, necessitating careful cardiac and hemodynamic monitoring. |

## ANESTHETIC CONSIDERATIONS

See Anesthetic Considerations for "Carotid Thromboendarterectomy" in "Other Neurosurgery" section.

**References**

1. NASCET Collaborators: *N Eng J Med* 1991; 325:445-53.

# REPAIR OF THORACIC AORTIC ANEURYSMS

## SURGICAL CONSIDERATIONS

**Description**: Repairs of aneurysms of the ascending, transverse arch and descending thoracic aorta are performed to repair expanding or leaking aneurysms or prophylactically to prevent rupture. Patients with Sx of rapid expansion or aneurysm leaking[1] may require urgent repair. Each surgical type – ascending, arch and descending – is considered separately as follows. Aneurysms of the **ascending aorta** may arise 2° the degenerative changes of atherosclerosis (exacerbated by old age, HTN, tobacco use), from inborn errors of metabolism (Marfan syndrome), or from post-stenotic dilatation and continued expansion of a chronic dissection. Diseases of the entire aorta, including the sinuses of Valsalva, as in Marfan syndrome and annuloaortic ectasia, require replacement of the entire aorta with a composite, valved conduit, while acquired diseases usually allow replacement of the aorta distal to the sinotubular ridge. Repair of the ascending aorta is usually accomplished on full CPB with an aortic cross-clamp placed just proximal to the innominate artery, and arterial inflow through the femoral artery. The aneurysmal ascending aorta is replaced with a Dacron® tube graft from the sinotubular ridge to the innominate artery. Dilatation of the sinuses of Valsalva mandates replacement with a valved conduit sewn proximally to the aortic annulus and distally to the aorta at the innominate, with coronary ostia re-implanted in the side of the tube graft.

Aneurysms of the **aortic arch** are the least common of the thoracic aorta. Because of the need for concomitant replacement of the arch vessels, however, they are the most complex to repair. Total CPB is utilized, and cerebral protection is accomplished either by CPB perfusion of one or all cerebral vessels, or by profound hypothermic circulatory arrest at 15-18° C. Repair can originate from the aortic annulus and extend distally to the mid-descending thoracic aorta at the level of the carina. Routine caval cannulation is accomplished via a median sternotomy, and arterial access is gained via the femoral artery. If circulatory arrest is to be used, the patient is cooled to 15-18°C, the heart is arrested and, with no distal cross-clamp, distal anastomosis is accomplished, followed by implantation of the head vessels attached to an island of aorta. Perfusion is then reinstituted, the graft clamped proximal to the innominate artery, and the proximal anastomosis performed, while the patient is being rewarmed. Alternatively, if one elects to perfuse the cerebral vessels, the innominate and left carotid arteries can be individually cannulated and perfused via a "Y" connection from the femoral arterial perfusion line. The necessity for profound hypothermic circulatory arrest is thus avoided. After completion of the distal aortic, arch vessel island, and proximal aortic anastomoses, weaning from CPB and subsequent steps proceed in a routine fashion.

Repair of aneurysms of the **descending thoracic aorta** is usually performed for symptomatic and leaking aneurysms, enlarging aneurysms, and aneurysms of sufficient size to warrant prophylactic repair. **Aneurysmorrhaphy** is accomplished through a left posterolateral thoracotomy on partial CPB. After entry into the left thorax, venous drainage for CPB may be obtained from the PA or the femoral vein; and arterial return is via the femoral artery. If partial bypass without an oxygenator is elected, thus minimizing the amount of heparin necessary, venous access can be gained via the pulmonary veins or left atrium, and arterial return via the femoral artery or distal thoracic aorta. After institution of bypass, the aorta is cross-clamped above and below the aneurysm, the aorta divided, a tube graft interposed, and clamps removed. The patient is weaned from bypass, and the operation is terminated in the routine fashion.

**Usual preop diagnosis**: Enlarging or symptomatic aortic aneurysm

## SUMMARY OF PROCEDURE

| | Ascending Aorta | Transverse Arch | Descending Aorta |
|---|---|---|---|
| **Position** | Supine | ⇐ | Lateral decubitus with left side up |
| **Incision** | Median sternotomy | ⇐ | Left posterolateral thoracotomy with access to femoral artery and vein |
| **Special instrumentation** | CPB, if used. | Complete hemodynamic monitors; CPB | ⇐ + DLT; lower extremity BP monitor |
| **Unique considerations** | Routine CPB hemodynamic monitoring | If profound hypothermic arrest is utilized, neuro-protective adjuncts, including local hypothermia, barbiturates and steroids, should be used. | One-lung ventilation (OLV); partial CPB |
| **Antibiotics** | Cefamandole 1 gm iv | ⇐ | ⇐ |
| **Surgical time** | Aortic cross-clamp: 40 - 120 min<br>CPB: 70 - 150 min<br>Total: 2.5 - 5 hrs | Aortic cross-clamp: 75 - 120 min<br>Circulatory arrest: 30 - 45 min<br>CPB: 3 - 4.5 hrs<br>Total: 4 - 6 hrs | Aortic cross-clamp: 25 - 45 min<br>CPB: 30 - 60 min<br>Total: 2.5 - 4.5 hrs |
| **Closing considerations** | Aggressive management of coagulopathy, if a long pump run is necessary. | Aggressive management of coagulopathy | Replacement of DLT with single-lumen tube |
| **EBL** | 300-400 cc | 400-700 cc | 200-300 cc |
| **Postop care** | ICU, intubated 5-20 hrs, depending on preop condition. | ICU, intubated 24-48 hrs. | ICU, intubated 5-25 hrs. |
| **Mortality** | 5-10% | 10-15%[3] | ⇐ |
| **Morbidity** | Renal failure: 5-10%[2] | – | 10-15% |
| | CVA: 4-6% | 2-5% | 2-4% |
| | Respiratory insufficiency: 3-5% | 10% | 10-15% |
| | MI: 2-5% | ⇐ | 2-4% |
| **Procedure code** | 33860 | 33870 | 33875 |
| **Pain score** | 7-10 | 7-10 | 9-10 |

## PATIENT POPULATION CHARACTERISTICS

| | | | |
|---|---|---|---|
| **Age range** | 23-80 yrs (mean = 55 yrs) | 50-75 yrs | 34-79 yrs (mean = 65 yrs) |
| **Male:Female** | 3:1 | 2:1 | 2.5:1 |
| **Incidence** | 15-20/yr at tertiary center | 10-15/yr at tertiary center | 10-20/yr at tertiary center |
| **Etiology** | Degenerative disease | ⇐ | ⇐ |
| | Atherosclerotic disease | ⇐ | ⇐ |
| | | Chronic dissections | ⇐ |
| **Associated conditions** | CHF: 50%<br>Angina: 30%<br>HTN: 30%<br>COPD: 15% | Aortic valve disease: 30%<br>COPD: 20%<br>CAD: 15% | HTN: 65%<br>CAD: 50%<br>COPD: 30%<br>CHF: 10% |

## ANESTHETIC CONSIDERATIONS

### PREOPERATIVE

In contrast with thoracic aortic dissections, Sx of thoracic aortic aneurysms may be of a more chronic nature. A ruptured or leaking aneurysm, however, may have a more precipitous presentation. Patients may be asymptomatic; however, most will have coexisting CAD, PVD, and/or cardiovascular disease.

**Cardiovascular** — **Arch and ascending aneurysms** (60-70% of aneurysms): commonly associated with HTN, syphilis, cystic medial necrosis or connective tissue disorder (e.g., Marfan syndrome, atherosclorosis). CHF may occur 2° to dilation of the aortic annulus and aortic incompetence. Aneurysmal compression or intrinsic disease of the coronary arteries may result in myocardial ischemia.
**Descending** (30%): usually associated with HTN, cystic medial necrosis, Marfan syndrome, atherosclorosis.
**Tests:** ECG: ✓ for LVH, ischemia. ECHO: ✓ for valvular disease, size and extent of aneurysm, LV function. Angiography: ✓ exact extent of aneurysm (allows planning of procedure and sites for arterial monitoring), coronary artery anatomy and degree of occlusion.

**Respiratory** — Recurrent laryngeal nerve palsy may lead to hoarseness (ascending/arch aneurysms). Stridor or dyspnea may be present 2° tracheal or bronchial compression. Hemoptysis or a hemorrhagic pleural effusion suggest aneurysmal leakage or rupture. The implications include the possibility of compromised oxygenation, risk of massive hemorrhage on thoracotomy, increased intrathoracic pressure and consequent decreased venous return (especially when IPPV is instituted).
**Tests:** CXR: ✓ for widened mediastinum, distortion of trachea and left main bronchus (because it may affect the placement of DLT); others as indicated from H&P.

**Neurologic** — Any deficit should be well-documented as neurologic sequelae frequently occur after surgery.

**Renal** — Renal problems may occur 2° to AR and heart failure, HTN, or involvement of renal arteries in the aneurysm.
**Tests:** BUN; creatinine, creatinine clearance; electrolytes

**Gastrointestinal** — Descending aneurysms that involve the coeliac or superior mesenteric arteries may result in bowel ischemia.
**Tests:** ABG: ✓ persistent metabolic acidosis. Abdominal x-ray: ✓ ileus.

**Hematological** — If time permits, consider autologous blood donation; pre-existing coagulopathy increases risk of the procedure.
**Tests:** PT; PTT; bleeding time; Hct/Hb

**Laboratory** — Syphilis serology; others as indicated from H&P.

**Premedication** — Pain and anxiety may significantly contribute to HTN and should be treated (e.g., morphine 0.1 mg/kg im ± midazolam 0.025-0.1 mg/kg iv or 0.05-0.2 mg/kg im); but avoid obtundation. Since many of these patients present emergently, consider full-stomach precautions – $H_2$ antagonists (e.g., ranitidine 50 mg iv), metoclopramide (10 mg iv), antacids (e.g., Na citrate 0.3 M 30 cc po).

### INTRAOPERATIVE

**Anesthetic technique:** The anesthetic management of patients with aortic dissections and aortic aneurysms are similar in many respects. For intraop and postop management of these conditions, see Anesthetic Considerations for "Repair of Thoracic Aortic Dissections."

**References**


1. Skeehan TM; Cooper JR Jr: Anesthetic management for thoracic aneurysms and dissections. In *The Practice of Cardiac Anesthesia*. Hensley FA Jr, Martin DE, eds. Little, Brown and Co, Boston: 1990, Ch 15, 461-92.
2. Roseberg JN, Shine T, Nugent M: Thoracic aortic disease. In *Cardiac Anesthesia,* 2nd edition. Kaplan JA, ed. WB Saunders Co, Philadelphia: 1987, Ch 18, 725-50.
3. Pressler BA, McNamara JJ: Thoracic aortic aneurysm. Natural history and treatment. *J Thorac Cardiovasc Surg* 1980; 79:489-98.
4. Moreno-Cabral CE, Miller DC, Mitchell RS, Stinson EB, Oyer PE, Jamieson SW, Shumway NE: Degenerative and atherosclerotic aneurysms of the thoracic aorta. *J Thor Cardiovasc Surg* 1984; 88:1020-32.
5. Galloway AC, Colvin SB, Mendola CL, Hurwitz JB, Baumann FG, Harris LJ, Culliford AT, Grossi EA, Spencer FC: Ten-year operative experience with 165 aneurysms of the ascending aorta and aortic arch. *Circ* 1989; 80(Suppl 1):I-249-56.
6. Crawford ES, Snyder DM: Treatment of aneurysms of the aortic arch. *J Thorac Cardiovasc Surg* 1983; 85:237-46.

# REPAIR OF ACUTE AORTIC DISSECTIONS AND DISSECTING ANEURYSMS

## SURGICAL CONSIDERATIONS

**Description**: Repair of acute aortic dissection is performed to prevent life-threatening complications such as hemorrhage, tamponade and heart failure secondary to acute aortic valvular insufficiency, and to redirect flow into the true lumen. Emergent repair of acute ascending dissections is generally accepted therapy to prevent rupture of the aortic root with exsanguination or pericardial tamponade. Mortality for acute ascending dissection is estimated at 1% per hour, for the first 48 hours. The management of descending thoracic aortic dissections remains controversial, but surgical intervention probably should be recommended only for younger patients, patients with uncontrolled pain or evidence for continued expansion or extravasation, and those with branch-vessel compromise.

Ascending dissections typically produce sharp, tearing retrosternal pain that penetrates straight through to the subscapular area. The presentation, however, is so frequently variable that for any patient in extremis, especially with migratory pain or vacillating findings, and even asymptomatic patients with valvular aortic regurgitation, should be considered for the diagnosis. With a suggestive history, a new murmur, or a pulse deficit, an enlarged mediastinal shadow on chest radiography should prompt further diagnostic efforts. CT scanning, MRI and aortography may all be diagnostic, but no diagnostic modality has 100% sensitivity. Recently, TEE has enjoyed popularity for it appears highly sensitive in detecting a mobile intimal flap in the ascending or descending aorta. In addition, TEE can provide useful information regarding aortic regurgitation, periaortic hematoma and flow within a false channel. It is usually available at the bedside, or in the emergency ward, and does not subject the patient to a contrast load.

Once diagnosed, these patients are transported immediately to the OR. Through a median sternotomy, venous access is gained via the right atrium, and arterial inflow is supplied through a femoral artery. CPB is established, the patient cooled to 18°C, and circulatory support discontinued. During a period of profound circulatory arrest, the ascending aorta is opened, and the tear localized. The repair is carried distally into the arch, if the entire dissection can be resected, and the distal aortic layers are re-approximated with a Teflon® felt strip supporting the medial and advential layers. The distal graft anastomosis is then completed, the graft clamped, the bypass pump restarted and systemic warming commenced. Proximally, the aortic root is reconstructed, again using Teflon® felt layers to support the medial and adventitial layers, and re-suspend the aortic valve, which can be salvaged in approximately 85% of cases. The heart is then cleared of air, and the cross-clamp removed to allow reperfusion of the coronary circulation. After a sufficient period of resuscitation, the patient is weaned from CPB. Aggressive management of an acquired coagulopathy is not unusual prior to chest closure.

Repair of dissections involving the descending thoracic aorta is accomplished through a left thoracotomy utilizing partial CPB. Venous drainage is usually via the femoral vein, although the PA or pulmonary vein may be used. Arterial access is via the femoral artery. After institution of CPB, the dissected aorta above and below the most damaged area is cross-clamped and the aorta transected. After oversewing patent intercostal arteries, the medial and adventitial layers are buttressed with Teflon® felt, and an interposition Dacron® graft is sewn into place. After evacuation of air, clamps are removed, and the patient weaned from CPB. Heparin reversal, decannulation and closure are accomplished in the usual manner.

**Usual preop diagnosis**: Acute dissection of the ascending aorta (see Fig 6.2-1 for types of dissection).

**SUMMARY OF PROCEDURE**

| | Ascending Aorta | Descending Aorta |
|---|---|---|
| **Position** | Supine | Lateral decubitus, left side up |
| **Incision** | Median sternotomy | Left lateral thoracotomy |
| **Unique considerations** | Full hemodynamic monitoring, with provisions for circulatory arrest, topical hypothermia, barbiturates and steroids; TEE | DLT |
| **Antibiotics** | Cefazolin 1 gm iv | ⇐ |
| **Surgical time** | Cross-clamp: 30 - 50 min | 30 - 60 min |
| | Circulatory arrest: 20 - 30 min | – |
| | CPB: 60 - 100 min | 35 - 60 min |
| | Total: 3 - 5 hrs | ⇐ |

| | | |
|---|---|---|
| **Closing considerations** | Aggressive management of coagulopathy, which frequently develops consumption of platelets. | Replace DLT with single-lumen ETT. |
| **EBL** | 400 - 800 cc | 600-800 cc |
| **Postop care** | ICU: 1 - 2 d, intubated | ⇐ |
| **Mortality** | 10-25% | ⇐ |
| **Morbidity** | Bleeding: 3-8%<br>Respiratory insufficiency: 2-5%<br>CVA: 2-4% | Paraplegia: 5%<br>CVA: 1-2%<br>MI: 1-2% |
| **Procedure code** | 33860 | 33875 |
| **Pain score** | 7-10 | 9-10 |

## PATIENT POPULATION CHARACTERISTICS

| | |
|---|---|
| **Age range** | 40-70 yrs |
| **Male:Female** | 3:2 |
| **Incidence** | 10/100,000 |
| **Etiology** | Degenerative aortic disease |
| **Associated conditions** | HTN<br>Secondary aortic regurgitation<br>Bicuspid aortic valve<br>Marfan syndrome |

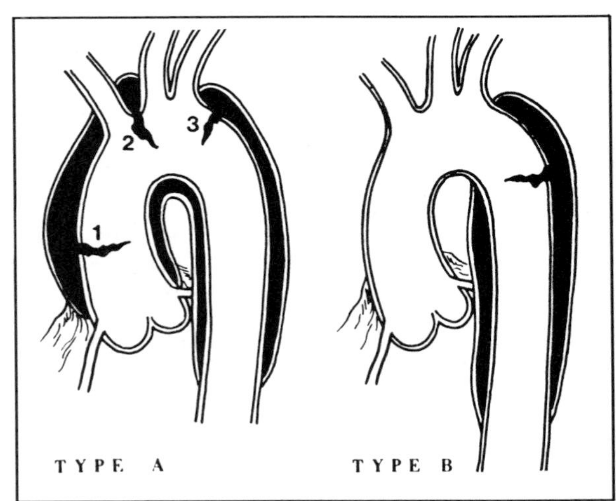


**Figure 6.2-1.** Types of dissections: Type A = ascending aortic dissection; Type B = descending aortic aneurysm. (Reproduced with permission from Miller DC, Stinson EB, et al: Aortic dissections. *J Thorac Cardiovasc Surg* 1979; 78:367.)

---

# ANESTHETIC CONSIDERATIONS

## PREOPERATIVE

Sx are usually of sudden onset and depend on the site of dissection and specific organ involvement. Aortic dissections are divided into 2 types, depending on the site of initial dissection: **Type A** – ascending and arch aorta, and **Type B** – descending aorta. Initial treatment involves the use of anti-hypertensive medications (e.g., SNP) to control BP and β-blockers (e.g., esmolol) to ↓contractility. Type A dissections usually require urgent surgery.

| | |
|---|---|
| **Respiratory** | ✓ for recurrent laryngeal nerve palsy with chronic aneurysmal dilation. Tracheal and left main bronchus compression → difficult intubation, atelectasis; hemoptysis 2° rupture into lung; hemothorax → compromised oxygenation, ↑intrathoracic pressure → ↓ venous return, especially with IPPV.<br>**Tests:** CXR: ✓ for widened mediastinum, tracheal or left main bronchus compression and distortion (affects DLT placement), atelectasis, pleural effusion (or hemothorax 2° rupture). |
| **Cardiovascular** | Aortic dissections may be associated with chronic HTN, cystic medial necrosis or other connective tissue disorder (e.g., Marfan syndrome) and trauma. Dissection may result in cardiac tamponade, acute aortic valve incompetence, acute cardiac failure, angina, MI or rupture of the aorta. Dissection of major arteries may result in ↓ or absent peripheral pulses which may affect the placement sites for intra-arterial monitoring and central venous access. Pain and anxiety may result in HTN, while rupture or leakage may result in hypotension and shock.<br>**Tests:** ECG: ✓ for Sx of LVH, ischemia or infarction, low voltage (tamponade). ECHO: ✓ for site of dissection, valvular competence, LV function, pericardial effusion or tamponade. Angiography: ✓ for site of dissection (Type A or B), valvular function, involvement of coronary and other major arteries, sites of rupture, LV function. CT scan: ✓ site and extent of dissection. |
| **Neurological** | Deficits are not uncommon, especially with Type B dissections where the blood supply to the spinal cord may be jeopardized. Document carefully. |

| | |
|---|---|
| **Renal** | Renal failure 2° renal artery involvement in dissection, shock or cardiac failure. UO should be closely monitored during initial medical therapy.<br>**Tests:** UO; BUN; creatinine; electrolytes |
| **Gastrointestinal** | Compromised blood supply to the bowel or liver may result in ischemia → metabolic acidosis and ↓liver function.<br>**Tests:** ABG: ✓ persistent metabolic acidosis; LFTs |
| **Hematologic** | Coagulopathy may be present 2° massive hemorrhage or liver involvement, and can increase risk of the surgery.<br>**Tests:** PT; PTT; bleeding time; Hct/Hb |
| **Laboratory** | Other tests as indicated from H&P. |
| **Premedication** | Since many of these patients present emergently, consider full-stomach precautions: $H_2$-antagonists (ranitidine 50 mg iv), metoclopramide (10 mg iv), antacids (Na citrate 0.3 M 30 cc po). Alleviate anxiety and pain, which may worsen HTN, but avoid obtundation (e.g., morphine 0.1 mg/kg im, ± midazolam 0.025-0.1 mg/kg iv or 0.05-0.2 mg/kg im). |

## INTRAOPERATIVE

**Anesthetic technique:** GETA. Pre-induction control of BP and contractility (NTG or SNP to SBP = 105-115 and esmolol to HR = 60-80) is important in preventing extension of the dissection or rupture of the aneurysm. Fluid resuscitation may be necessary prior to induction. If present, cardiac tamponade should be relieved by pericardiocentesis.

| | |
|---|---|
| **Induction** | Control of hypertensive response to laryngoscopy is important and may be accomplished with high-dose narcotic (fentanyl 20-100 μg/kg or sufentanil 5-20 μg/kg) with etomidate (0.1-0.3 mg/kg) or midazolam (50-350 μg/kg) and esmolol (100-500 μg/kg over 1 min, followed by 50-100 μg/kg/min infusion). SNP (0.5-3 μg/kg/min) and/or pretreatment with lidocaine (1.5 mg/kg) also may be required to further control the hypertensive response to laryngoscopy. Avoid ketamine because of its hypertensive effect. Muscle relaxation may be obtained using vecuronium or pancuronium (0.1 mg/kg). Remember the possibility of a full stomach in this patient population. Hence a modified rapid-sequence induction (cricoid pressure with manual ventilation and non-depolarizing muscle relaxant) may achieve the two goals of relatively rapid induction and intubation and tight control of BP. Usually a left DLT is used in patients with descending lesions to improve surgical access; however, it may be difficult to place due to aneurysmal compression of the trachea and left mainstem bronchus, and it is associated with a small risk of aneurysmal rupture. For these reasons, a right DLT may be preferred. FOB is useful to verify ET placement. |
| **Maintenance** | $O_2$/narcotic/benzodiazepine: low-dose volatile agent may be used to control BP (MAP = 60-80), although infusion of vasopressors, vasodilators or inotropes may be necessary. Control HR (< 80; anesthesia, esmolol), and contractility (β-blockade or inotropes, depending on circumstances. Benzodiazepines may be used for amnesia (midazolam 50-350 μg/kg; diazepam 0.3-0.5 mg/kg). Most type A aneurysms and ascending/arch aneurysms require hypothermic CPB (see Anesthetic Considerations for "Cardiopulmonary Bypass" section). Intraop anesthetic considerations are governed primarily by the site of the aortic pathology. These considerations are discussed below. |
| **Emergence** | Transported to ICU, sedated, intubated and ventilated x 24-48 hrs. Following repairs of the descending aorta (thoracotomy incision), weaning from ventilator may be aided by epidural narcotics after documentation of normal spinal cord function and coagulation. |

| | | |
|---|---|---|
| **Blood and fluid requirements** | Anticipate large blood loss.<br>IV: 14 ga - 7 Fr x 2<br>NS/LR @ 6-8 ml/kg/hr<br>Warm all fluids.<br>Humidify gasses.<br>Cross-match 8-10 U of blood.<br>UO 0.5-1 cc/kg/hr | In Type A dissections and arch aneurysms, if possible, avoid iv placement in the left arm or left IJ/subclavian veins because of the possibility of innominate vein ligation. Mannitol (0.5-1 gm/kg iv) should be given if renal perfusion is compromised by dissection or before cross-clamping. Consider normovolemic hemodilution if the patient is stable and the Hct >35. |
| **Monitoring** | Standard monitors (see Appendix).<br>Arterial line<br>PA catheter<br>Urinary catheter | Arterial line site is dependent on the type of surgery and the location of the lesion. Because the right subclavian artery may be compromised in patients with ascending lesions, the left radial or femoral arteries may need to be used. Aortic arch lesions may involve the vascular supply to both upper extremities, hence, femoral artery catheterization may be necessary. In ascending lesions, |

| | | |
|---|---|---|
| **Monitoring, continued** | | two artery lines may be required – right radial (above clamp pressure) and left femoral (below clamp pressure). Consult with surgeon as to best site. |
| | TEE | TEE is useful to assess cardiac function, regional wall motion abnormalities, valvular pathology, aortic valvular repair (if required as part of a Type A repair). Probe passage may increase compression of the trachea, impeding ventilation. Caution should be used in the presence of aneurysmal compression of the esophagus. |
| | Temperature | Monitor both core (rectal/bladder) and nasopharyngeal/ tympanic membrane temperature (as indicative of brain temperature) – important in deep hypothermic arrest. |
| | EEG (arch/ascending lesions) | EEG may help in assessing effectiveness of cerebral protection (silent EEG) or adequacy of cerebral perfusion. |
| | SSEPs (descending lesions) | SSEPs may detect posterior spinal perfusion problems, but cannot detect anterior cord dysfunction or predict postop paraplegia. Both EEG and SSEP may require expert help to set up, monitor and interpret. |
| **Complications** | Hemorrhage<br>Coagulopathy | Both are common. Hemorrhage should be treated with crystalloid, colloid or blood, as indicated. |
| **Ascending lesions** | CPB<br>Aortic regurgitation<br>Coronary arteries | Usual site of cannulation for CPB is the femoral artery. Aortic valve replacement may be necessary. Patients may have myocardial ischemia 2° coronary artery occlusion; may require CABG or re-implantation of vessels. |
| | Deep hypothermic arrest | Cerebral protective measures and selective perfusion of cerebral vessels may be required. (See below.) |
| **Arch lesions** | CPB<br>Deep hypothermic arrest | Usual site of cannulation for CPB is femoral artery. Cerebral protection relies on hypothermia (15-18°C) and drugs (methylprednisolone [Solu-Medrol®] 1 gm, mannitol 0.5-1 gm/kg, STP 30 mg/kg) to reduce $CMRO_2$ and neuronal injury. The head is surface cooled (protect eyes and ears from cold injury). Monitor EEG to ensure absence of brain electrical activity. Monitor tympanic membrane or nasopharyngeal temperatures as an indication of brain temperature. Avoid hyperglycemia and maintain normal pH and $PaCO_2$ when measured at 37°C (alpha stat). Maintain muscle relaxation. |
| **Descending lesions** | Pre-cross-clamping | Mannitol (0.5-1 gm/kg) should be given prior to clamp application to provide renal protection, even if a shunt is placed. Hypothermia (32-34°C) may protect spinal cord. |
| | Shunt | A heparin-bonded shunt may be used from the aortic arch to the femoral artery to provide distal perfusion. |
| | Partial bypass | Partial CPB may be used to provide distal perfusion. In this arrangement, the heart perfuses the head and upper extremities, while CPB is used to perfuse and oxygenate the lower body. Venous drainage is from the femoral vein, PA or left atrium and returned via the femoral artery. Distal and proximal pressures are altered by controlling cardiac filling, pump flow and vasodilators. |
| | Cross-clamping | Application of clamp may → acute HTN with ischemia and LV failure. This may be controlled by partial bypass, shunting or use of vasodilators (SNP 0.5-4 μg/kg/min, NTG 0.5-4 μg/kg/min). During cross-clamping, monitor UO and √metabolic acidosis (renal or bowel ischemia) with serial ABGs. Cross-clamp time should be < 30 min to reduce incidence of paraplegia. |

| | | |
|---|---|---|
| **Descending lesions, continued** | Unclamping | Unclamping may result in severe hypotension and myocardial depression. Hypovolemia, acidosis, vasodilator factors and reactive hyperemia have been implicated as the cause. Prior to unclamping, ensure adequate volume status (PCWP 2-5 mmHg above patient's normal); treat acidosis; have vasopressors available, and the clamp should be released slowly over 1-2 min. Use of partial bypass or a shunt to ensure distal perfusion will mitigate unclamping shock. |
| **Positioning** | Arch and ascending: supine, shoulder roll. ✓ and pad pressure points. Descending: lateral decubitus, axillary roll, pillow between knees. ✓ pressure points, eyes. | |

## POSTOPERATIVE

| | | |
|---|---|---|
| **Complications** | Myocardial ischemia, failure<br>Dysrhythmias<br>Hemorrhage<br>Coagulopathy<br>Renal failure<br>Bowel ischemia<br>Respiratory failure | A DLT may be required in lesions of the descending aorta, if hemorrhage continues from left lung; otherwise, the tube may be replaced at the end of procedure by a single-lumen ETT. BP should be controlled to MAP 60-80 and HR < 100 to decrease the likelihood of repeat dissection or graft dehiscence. |
| | Paraplegia | Anterior spinal artery syndrome |
| **Pain management** | Parenteral opioids for pain relief<br>Benzodiazepines for sedation | |
| **Tests** | ECG: ischemia, infarction, dysrhythmias.<br>CXR: line and ETT placement, pulmonary contusion.<br>Coagulation profile<br>Renal: BUN; creatinine<br>ABG: Respiratory, gut ischemia<br>CT Scan: CNS or spinal neurologic deficits<br>Electrolytes | |


**References**

1. Miller DC, Mitchell RS, Oyer PE, Stinson EB, Jamieson SW, Shumway NE: Independent determinants of operatality for patients with aortic dissections. *Circ* 1984; 70(Suppl I):I-153-64.
2. Skeehan TM, Cooper CR: Anesthetic management for thoracic aneurysms and dissections: in *The Practice of Cardiac Anesthesia* Hensley FA, Martin DE, eds. Little, Brown and Company, Boston: 1990, Ch 15.
3. Roseberg JN, Shine T, Nugent M: Thoracic aortic disease: in *Cardiac Anesthesia*, 2nd edition. Kaplan JA, ed. WB Saunders Co, Philadelphia: 1987, Ch 18, 725-50.
4. Wickey GS, Hickey PR: Brain protection during cardiac surgery. In *The Practice of Cardiac Anesthesia.* Hensley FA Jr, Martin DE, eds. Little, Brown and Co: 1990, Ch 24, 710-27.
5. Hickey PR; Anderson NP: Deep hypothermic circulatory arrest: a review of pathophysiology and clinical experience as a basis for anesthetic management. *J Cardiothorac Anesth* 1987; 1(2):137-55.

# REPAIR OF ANEURYSMS OF THE THORACOABDOMINAL AORTA

## SURGICAL CONSIDERATIONS

**Description:** Aneurysms of the thoracoabdominal aorta may occur because of degenerative aortic disease (atherosclerosis), as a consequence of hereditary disorders of metabolism (Marfan syndrome), or as a sequela of chronic aortic dissections. These aneurysms are classified as to extent: Group I consists of aneurysms that involve most of the descending thoracic and upper abdominal aorta. Group II involves most of the descending thoracic aorta and most or all of the abdominal aorta. Group III involves the distal thoracic and varying segments of the abdominal aorta. Group IV involves most or all of the abdominal aorta, including the origins of the visceral vessels.

Repair of these aneurysms is an extensive, difficult and demanding procedure, as blood flow to the entire body below the neck is interrupted, with resultant renal and visceral ischemia. Additionally, the blood supply to the spinal cord may arise from lumbar and/or intercostal vessels in the affected aortic segment, producing critical cord ischemia during cross-clamping and postop paraplegia.

Almost all thoracoabdominal aneurysm repairs are performed through a thoracoabdominal incision using the **inclusion technique** as advocated by **Crawford**, et al.[1] After opening the chest, the incision is extended across the costal cartilage onto the abdomen. The diaphragm is radially incised to the aortic hiatus, and the retroperitoneal dissection plane established anterior to the psoas musculature. All intra-abdominal contents, as well as the left kidney, are reflected anteriorly. Only proximal aortic control is established. After minimal heparinization, single-lung anesthesia is established to allow collapse of the left lung, the proximal aorta at the aneurysm neck is cross-clamped, and the aneurysm incised. Back-bleeding from patent intercostals, mesenteric and renal vessels can be controlled by balloon catheters; and aggressive blood salvage with autotransfusion devices is mandatory. The repair entails suturing a tube graft proximally to the divided aorta, and then sewing islands of aortic tissue containing intercostal visceral vessels onto appropriate size holes in the side of the tube graft to allow reperfusion of important intercostal, celiac axis, superior mesenteric, renal arteries and, finally, the distal aorta or iliac arteries. Since there is obligate visceral ischemia during the period of cross-clamping (which must be limited to less than 60-75 minutes), the operation must proceed expeditiously.

Alternatively, in an effort to afford both spinal cord and visceral protection through hypothermia, the operation may be performed on CPB during a period of profound hypothermic circulatory arrest, but with marked exacerbation of hemorrhagic complications.

After aortic cross-clamping, the aneurysm is opened and the repair performed from within the aneurysm, sewing on-lay patches of the intercostal, mesenteric and renal vessels to openings created in the tube graft. This no-clamp technique allows reasonable management of these very extensive aneurysms, but results in an obligatory and ongoing blood loss through back-bleeding of visceral vessels until the anastomoses are complete.

**Usual preop diagnosis:** Expanding, painful or large thoracoabdominal aneurysm

### SUMMARY OF PROCEDURE

| | |
|---|---|
| **Position** | Right lateral decubitus; hips rotated posteriorly to 45° and left arm draped forward over an airplane sling. Axillary roll placed. |
| **Incision** | Posterolateral thoracotomy incision, in appropriate interspace, extended across the costal margin to midline, then extended inferiorly as a midline abdominal incision. The incision is one of the largest incisions in surgery, necessitated by the absolute need for exposure in this difficult area, and is, unfortunately, associated with a lot of postop pain. |
| **Special instrumentation** | DLT; CPB; NG tube |
| **Unique considerations** | OLV with collapse of left lung necessary for most cases. Cold LR may be injected into renal or visceral arteries for organ preservation. Alternatively, operation can be performed under profound hypothermic circulatory arrest for spinal cord protection in patients with chronic dissections. Cell savers and rapid-infusion devices used to augment red-cell salvage and rapid-transfusion requirements. Frequently, operation is performed with only proximal cross-clamping; so there may be an obligate ongoing blood loss from visceral arterial orifices, as well as from distal aorta and iliac arteries. |
| **Antibiotics** | Cefamandole 1 gm iv |

**Surgical time** 6 hrs. Proximal aortic cross-clamping until completion of visceral revascularization may extend to 60 min. Longer cross-clamp times may be anticipated in patients with chronic aortic dissections for which profound hypothermic circulatory arrest is frequently utilized.

**Closing considerations** OR → ICU, intubated x 24-48 hrs.

**EBL** Ongoing back-bleeding from visceral and iliac vessels results in substantial volume loss during cross-clamping, approaching 5-7 L. Most red-cell volume may be salvaged and returned through a RBC salvage system.

**Postop care** ICU, intubated and ventilated x 24-72 hrs. Re-warming, hemodynamic monitoring and volume resuscitation are often required in ICU.

| | Aneurysm Group: | Group I | Group II | Group III | Group IV |
|---|---|---|---|---|---|
| **Mortality** | | – | 10-25% | – | 5% |
| **Morbidity** | Paraplegia | – | 25% | – | 2% |
| | Other neurological complications | – | 1% | – | – |
| | Renal insufficiency | – | 2-5% | – | – |
| | Respiratory failure | – | 10% | – | – |
| | Graft infection | – | 1-6% | – | – |
| | MI | – | – | – | – |
| | Graft failure | – | Rare | – | – |
| | Graft thrombosis | – | – | – | – |
| | False aneurysm | – | – | – | – |
| | Embolization | – | – | – | – |
| | Bowel ischemia | – | 2-10% | – | – |
| | Impotence | Rare | ⇐ | ⇐ | ⇐ |
| | Ureteral injury | Rare | ⇐ | ⇐ | ⇐ |

**Procedure code** 33877

**Pain score** 6-10

### PATIENT POPULATION CHARACTERISTICS

**Age range** Non-Marfan: 55-75 yrs
Marfan: 35-55 yrs

**Male:Female** 3:1

**Incidence** < 5 cases/yr in most hospitals, except major referral centers

**Etiology** Predominantly atherosclerotic. Patients with Marfan syndrome may present with a progressive dilatation of a chronic dissection.

**Associated conditions** HTN: 75%
CAD: 30%
Obstructive pulmonary disease: 30%
Renal insufficiency: 15%

---

## ANESTHETIC CONSIDERATIONS

### PREOPERATIVE

**Respiratory** Chronic pulmonary disease is associated with postop morbidity. Preop preparation with bronchodilators, cessation of smoking, incentive spirometry and chest physiotherapy may decrease the risk of postop problems.

**Tests:** CXR: ✓ for distortion of the left mainstem bronchus which may affect placement of the DLT. May need PFTs, ABG to determine severity of pulmonary disease.

**Cardiovascular** CAD is the most frequent cause of perioperative and late death in elective thoracoabdominal aortic aneurysm repair. It is commonly associated with HTN.

**Tests:** ECG –✓ for LVH and ischemia.

| | |
|---|---|
| **Neurological** | Increased risk of spinal cord ischemia with cross-clamping of the aorta; therefore, any preop neurologic deficits should be well-documented. The use of deep hypothermic circulatory arrest may be used in patients with chronic aortic dissections. |
| **Renal** | Preop renal dysfunction increases the potential for postop renal problems. Aneurysmal involvement of the renal arteries may also occur.<br>**Tests:** BUN; creatinine, creatinine clearance |
| **Gastrointestinal** | Aneurysmal involvement of the inferior mesenteric and superior mesenteric arteries may cause visceral ischemia.<br>**Tests:** Abdominal x-ray (ileus); ABG (metabolic acidosis) |
| **Hematologic** | Pre-existing coagulopathy increases risk. Many patients have been on ASA preop. Excessive alcohol use is associated with anemia, thrombocytopenia and low production of vitamin K-dependent factors. Rarely, a DIC process may occur within the lumen of the aneurysm.<br>**Tests:** PT; PTT; bleeding time; platelet count; Hct |
| **Laboratory** | UA; electrolytes; radiologic assessment of aneurysm (ultrasonography, computerized tomography and arteriography) |
| **Premedication** | Anxiety and pain may contribute to HTN and risk of aneurysmal rupture. Morphine 0.1 mg/kg im and midazolam 0.07 mg/kg im. Full-stomach precautions for emergent procedures (e.g., metoclopramide 10 mg iv, ranitidine 50 mg iv, Na citrate 30 cc po). |

## INTRAOPERATIVE

**Anesthetic technique:** GETA. The goals of anesthesia for this procedure are to: (1) preserve myocardial, renal, pulmonary, CNS and visceral organ function; (2) maintain adequate intravascular volume so that cardiac output is not impaired; and (3) control BP so that the transmural pressure across the aneurysm does not increase, thereby increasing the risk of rupture. Provide good perfusion of other organs. CPB is used to accomplish deep hypothermic circulatory arrest. The rationale for this use is controversial. Deep hypothermic cardiac arrest (DHCA) may confer spinal cord protection and is usually reserved for patients with chronic dissections. CPB may also be used for distal perfusion of organs and afterload protection of the left ventricle. Partial CPB is usually reserved for suprarenal or supraceliac aneurysms in order to perfuse bowel and kidneys. (See Anesthetic Considerations for "Cardiopulmonary Bypass" and "Repair of Thoracic Aortic Dissections" for more discussion on CPB and DHCA.)

| | |
|---|---|
| **Induction** | Prevent hypertensive response to laryngoscopy with high-dose narcotic technique (fentanyl 10-50 μg/kg or sufentanil 5-15 μg/kg) and the use of benzodiazepine (midazolam 50-300 μg/kg) or etomidate (0.1-0.3 mg/kg). Esmolol 100-500 μg/kg over 1 min, NTP 0.5-3 μg/kg, or lidocaine administered either by topical spray or an iv dose of 1.5 mg/kg will also decrease the cardiovascular response to intubation. Muscle relaxation for intubation may be achieved with vecuronium (beware of ↓HR) or pancuronium (0.1 mg/kg). Etomidate is useful in unstable patients for emergent repair following rupture or ongoing dissection. A modified rapid-sequence induction may be necessary in emergent cases. A DLT is mandatory for this procedure; however, it may be difficult to position due to distorted anatomy. FOB may be helpful to position DLT. |
| **Maintenance** | $O_2$/air/narcotic, ± low-dose volatile agent. Benzodiazepines may be used for amnesia (e.g., midazolam 50-300 μg/kg, diazepam 0.3-0.5 mg/kg). In hemodynamically unstable patients, scopolamine (400 μg) provides amnesia. Maintain cardiac output and control of BP at preop levels. These patients may have increased hemodynamic variability on cross-clamping aorta, 2° bleeding and coexisting disease. Keeping the patient warm may be difficult due to large incision and visceral exposure. |
| **Emergence** | Deferred to ICU. Postop ventilation 24-72 hrs. DLT may need to be maintained postop 2° to facial, oral, and airway edema. |

| | | |
|---|---|---|
| **Blood and fluid requirements** | Anticipate large blood loss.<br>IV: 14 ga x 2 or 7.0 Fr x 2<br>Rapid infuser<br>Cell saver<br>PRBCs cross-match 8-10 U.<br>Warm fluids and humidify gasses.<br>Maintain UO 0.5-1 ml/kg/hr. | Large incision and visceral exposure requires administration of large volumes of fluid. Consider use of mannitol furosamide, ACE inhibitors or low-dose dopamine 1-3 μg/kg/ min if concerned about renal function and UO. |
| **Monitoring** | Standard monitors (see Appendix).<br>PA catheter<br>ST segment analysis | ✓ for increases in PA pressures and PCWP, decrease in CO, TEE wall motion abnormalities and changes in EF. Consult with surgeon regarding placement of cross-clamp |

| | | |
|---|---|---|
| **Monitoring, continued** | Arterial line<br>UO<br>± EEG<br>SSEP<br>TEE<br>Bladder temperature | so arterial line will not be affected. TEE is a good monitor for ventricular filling and myocardial ischemia. Monitor core temperature (rectal, bladder). Nasopharyngeal or tympanic membrane temperature (indicative of brain temperature) is monitored for circulatory arrest cases. EEG, SSEPs may be useful in assessment of cerebral protection and spinal cord perfusion problems. |
| **Cross-clamping** | Clamping | Application of cross-clamp at supraceliac level probably produces the greatest hemodynamic stress experienced by surgical patients. Application of the clamp may result in HTN and ischemia. Preload, afterload and HR can be controlled with SNP (0.25-5 μg/kg/min) and esmolol (100-500 μg/kg/min) infusions. |
| | Unclamping | Ensure adequate volume; replace blood loss. Just before removal of the cross-clamp, filling volumes are allowed to rise gradually, avoiding the occurrence of myocardial ischemia. Dilators are discontinued. Hypotension may occur with removal of cross-clamp 2° hypovolemia, reactive hyperemia, acidosis or myocardial dysfunction. If necessary, surgeon can reclamp or occlude the aorta. |
| **Positioning** | Right axillary roll<br>√ and pad pressure points.<br>√ eyes. | Right lateral decubitus with hips rotated posteriorly. Left arm placed in airplane sling or supported by pillows. |
| **Complications** | Myocardial ischemia<br>HTN<br>Coagulopathy<br>Hemorrhage<br>Hemostasis<br>Hypothermia<br>Other organ ischemia | Coagulopathy due to dilutional and consumptive processes.<br><br>Hypothermia may exacerbate coagulopathy, cause dysrhythmias and depress cardiac contractility. |

## POSTOPERATIVE

| | | |
|---|---|---|
| **Complications** | Myocardial ischemia<br>Neurologic deficits 2° cerebral or spinal cord ischemia<br>Renal failure<br>Respiratory failure | BP should be closely controlled postop to decrease bleeding from graft site and raw surfaces. |
| **Pain management** | Epidural narcotics (see Appendix). | Epidural is placed only after normal neurologic and coagulation status is determined. |
| **Tests** | CXR line placement and ETT placement<br>Coagulation profile<br>ABG analysis | |

**References**

1. Crawford ES, Crawford JL, Safi HJ, Coselli JS, Hess KR, Brooks B, Norton HJ, Glaeser DH: Thoracoabdominal aortic aneurysms: Preoperative and intraoperative factors determining immediate and long-term results of operations in 605 patients. *J Vasc Surg* 1986; 3(3):389-404.
2. Crawford ES, Walker HSJ III, Solen SA, Normann NA: Graft replacement of aneurysm in descending thoracic aorta: results without bypass or shunting. *Surgery* 1981; 89: 73-85.
3. Roizen MF, Beaupre PN, Alpert RA, et al: Monitoring with two-dimensional transesophageal echocardiography. Comparison of myocardial function in patients undergoing supracelias, suprarenal-infraceliac, or infrarenal aortic occlusion. *J Vasc Surg* 1984; 1:300-5.
4. Bailin MT, Davison KJ: Amnesia for abdominal aortic reconstruction: One approach at Massachusetts General Hospital. In *Anesthesia for Vascular Surgery*. Churchill Livingstone, New York: 1990, Ch 12.

# SURGERY OF THE ABDOMINAL AORTA

## SURGICAL CONSIDERATIONS

**Description**: Operations on the abdominal aorta are generally performed for aneurysmal or occlusive diseases. Although aortic aneurysms may involve the supra-renal aorta, the majority are infra-renal in origin, and may extend into the iliac arteries (Fig 6.2-2). Most (>95%) are asymptomatic, and are discovered incidentally during investigation of another medical problem. Because of the associated increased risk for rupture as the aneurysm increases in size, most vascular surgeons recommend prophylactic repair for aneurysms >5 cm in cross-section dimension. Repair also is indicated for painful aneurysms, those that have been associated with atheroembolism, and when there is documented recent increase in size, or evidence of leak or rupture. CAD coexists in 30-40% of these patients, and should be assessed preop.

The operative repair may be either transperitoneal or retroperitoneal. After exposure of the abdominal aorta from the level of the renal vein distally to the iliac arteries, the aorta is cross-clamped, distally at first to prevent atheroembolism, and then proximally. Graft origin is usually from the infra-renal aorta, but may arise from the infra-mesenteric aorta or even the supra-celiac aorta. Graft termination may be to the distal aorta above the bifurcation (tube graft), to the common or external iliac arteries (Y graft), or the femoral arteries. Immediately prior to cross-clamping, vasodilators are increased to reduce afterload, which is significantly increased with application of the aortic cross-clamp. The aorta is then incised, lumbar vessels oversewn, and the aorta transected to allow an interposition graft to be sewn into place. The retroperitoneal approach has many advocates, as it may require less volume intraop, may be associated with less temperature loss, and may result in a shorter period of postop adynamic ileus. In a randomized, prospective study, however, no significant difference could be detected between these two approaches as regards blood loss or postop recovery time.

Aorto-iliac occlusive disease can be a significant cause of lower extremity arterial insufficiency. Although the operative approach may be similar to that for aneurysmal disease, there exists a significant difference intraop in that there are not such profound changes associated with aortic clamping, since there is already some element of increased afterload 2° the occlusive disease. Nevertheless, hemodynamic monitoring is mandatory to allow for rapid volume shifts, and to assure adequate preload and sufficient afterload reduction, especially during the period of aortic cross-clamping.

**Variant procedure or approaches:** In the rare patient with COPD severe enough to preclude weaning from the ventilator postop, extra-anatomic grafts (e.g., axillo-femoral, ilio-femoral and femoral-femoral bypass) can be constructed under local anesthesia.

**Usual preop diagnosis**: Abdominal aortic aneurysm (AAA); severe aorto-iliac stenosis sufficient to cause debilitating buttock, thigh or calf claudication; isolated-inflow (aorto-iliac) disease (rarely the sole cause for ischemic symptoms at rest or for tissue loss, except as a result of embolic complications)

### SUMMARY OF PROCEDURE

| | **Transperitoneal Approach** | **Retroperitoneal Approach** |
|---|---|---|
| **Position** | Supine | Supine with mild elevation of left flank |
| **Incision** | Midline abdominal | Left subcostal, left oblique, along 10th rib toward umbilicus |
| **Special instrumentation** | Self-retaining retractor; TEE | ⇐ |
| **Unique considerations** | Will need pharmacologic manipulation to decrease afterload or increase preload coincident with clamping or unclamping of aorta. | ⇐ (The retroperitoneal approach is not used for emergency cases.) |
| **Antibiotics** | Cefamandole 1 gm iv | ⇐ |
| **Surgical time** | 3 - 5 hrs | ⇐ |
| **EBL** | 500 cc | ⇐ |
| **Postop care** | ICU 8-16 hrs, intubated. Requires aggressive volume administration to allow for 3rd-space loss in 1st 12 hrs postop. Patient comfort and respiratory management markedly improved by epidural catheter for postop analgesia. Careful cardiac monitoring. | ⇐ |

| | Transperitoneal Approach | Retroperitoneal Approach |
|---|---|---|
| **Mortality** | 2-5% elective; 50% emergent | ⇐ |
| **Morbidity** | MI: 10-15% (3% fatal) | ⇐ |
| | Respiratory insufficiency/pneumonia: 5-10% | |
| | Lower extremity ischemia: 2-5% | |
| | Renal insufficiency: 2-5% | |
| | Bowel complications: 3-4% | |
| | Hemorrhage: 2-4% | |
| | CVA: < 1% | |
| | Infection: < 1% | |
| | Paraplegia: < 0.4% | |
| **Procedure code** | 35001-35103 (aneurysm) | ⇐ |
| **Pain score** | 8-10 | 7-10 |

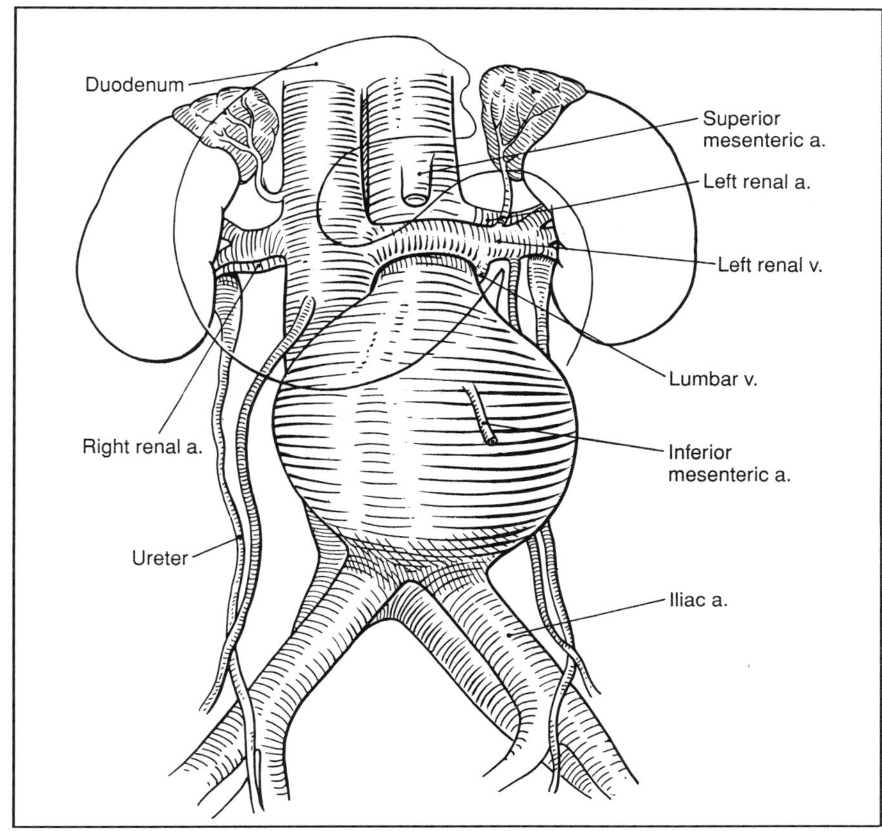


**Figure 6.2-2.** Aneurysm of the abdominal aorta. (Reproduced with permission from Calne R, Pollard SG: *Operative Surgery*. Gower Medical Pub: 1992.)

## PATIENT POPULATION CHARACTERISTICS

| | |
|---|---|
| **Age range** | 55 yrs + |
| **Male:Female** | 4:1 |
| **Incidence** | 3% of males >55 yrs; >5% of patients >50 yrs in a general cardiology clinic[1,2] |
| **Etiology** | Atherosclerosis |
| | Marfan syndrome |
| | Ehlers-Danlos syndrome |
| | Dissection |
| | Infection, including syphilis |
| **Associated conditions** | CAD |
| | Obstructive pulmonary disease |
| | Cerebrovascular disease |
| | Renal insufficiency |

## ANESTHETIC CONSIDERATIONS

### PREOPERATIVE

**Respiratory** Many patients have COPD and a long Hx of smoking. Preop preparation including bronchodilators, cessation of smoking, incentive spirometry and chest physiotherapy will decrease the risk of postop complications.

**Tests:** CXR. May need PFTs and ABG to determine severity of pulmonary disease.

**Cardiovascular** CAD is the most common cause of morbidity and mortality in this patient population. HTN increases risk of aneurysmal rupture; hence, preop control of BP is essential. ✓ BP in both arms to determine placement of arterial line intraop (arterial line should be placed in arm with higher BP).

**Tests:** Radiologic assessment of aneurysm using ultrasonography, computerized tomography, arteriography and MRI. ECG: ✓ for evidence of ischemia, infarction and LVH.

**Renal** Chronic renal insufficiency occurs frequently in this patient population 2° HTN, diabetes mellitus and atherosclerotic renovascular disease. Hypovolemia 2° radiographic dye studies and bowel prep → renal failure.

**Tests:** BUN, creatinine; creatinine clearance; electrolytes; U/A

**Hematologic** Preop coagulation disorders should be corrected. Many patients are on ASA, which should be discontinued 7 d preop. Alcohol abuse can be associated with anemia, thrombocytopenia and decreased vitamin K-dependent factors. Preop autologous blood donation decreases transfusion risks.

**Tests:** PT; PTT; bleeding time; Hct; CBC

**Laboratory** Other tests as indicated from H&P.

**Premedication** Anxiety and pain may cause HTN and increase risk of aneurysmal rupture. Sedatives and analgesics should be used as indicated (see Appendix). Full-stomach precautions for emergent procedures (see Appendix).

### INTRAOPERATIVE

**Anesthetic technique:** GETA, combination of epidural and GA. The goals of anesthesia are to: (1) preserve myocardial, renal, pulmonary and CNS perfusion; (2) maintain adequate intravascular volume and cardiac output; (3) anticipate the surgical maneuvers that will affect BP and blood volume; and (4) control BP to minimize risk of rupture while ensuring perfusion of other organs.

**Induction** Undesirable cardiovascular responses may be minimized by using a high-dose narcotic technique (e.g., fentanyl 10-50 μg/kg or sufentanil 5-15 μg/kg) if the patient is to remain intubated postop. This can be used in conjunction with a benzodiazepine (midazolam 50-300 μg/kg). If it is planned to extubate the patient postop, anesthesia should be induced using less narcotic (e.g., fentanyl 5 μg/kg) in conjunction with STP (2-4 mg/kg) or etomidate (0.2-0.4 mg/kg). If an epidural will be used for postop pain relief, no further iv doses of narcotic should be given intraop. Patients with an epidural typically receive 10 cc of 2% lidocaine or 10 cc of 0.5% bupivacaine intraop. A sensory block is obtained and induction is begun. Muscle relaxants are chosen to minimize tachycardia or hypotension (e.g., vecuronium 0.1 mg/kg). If there is a hemodynamic response to oral airway insertion, tracheal lidocaine or further anesthetic is given before gentle laryngoscopy and intubation. Etomidate is useful for induction in hemodynamically unstable patients. Full-stomach precautions may be necessary.

**Maintenance** $O_2$/air/narcotic and volatile agent. $N_2O$ can be used, but it may cause bowel distention. Combining epidural and GA offers good abdominal relaxation. Patients receiving epidural local anesthesia may require phenylephrine to treat ↓BP 2° sympathetic blockade. Epidural catheter placement before systemic anticoagulation is a safe technique. Narcotic epidural analgesia should be given within an hour of skin incision if morphine 3-8 mg is used. If hydromorphone (0.5-0.8 mg) is given epidurally, it is given within an hour of abdominal closure. Patient may become hypothermic 2° large incision with visceral exposure and prolonged operation.

**Emergence** Patients who have had uneventful surgery, especially utilizing a retroperitoneal approach, are frequently extubated in the OR, or shortly after arrival in the ICU. Patients with severe cardiac or pulmonary disease generally are mechanically ventilated for 24-48 hours. Prevention of HTN and tachycardia during emergence may require titration of ß-adrenergic-blocking drugs (e.g., esmolol 50-300 μg/kg/min) and/or vasodilators (e.g., SNP 0.25-5.0 μg/kg/min) or NTG (0.25-5.0 μg/kg/min). It is important to assure full reversal from neuromuscular blockade.

| | | |
|---|---|---|
| **Blood and fluid requirements** | Major blood loss<br>IV: 14 ga (or 7.0 Fr) x 2<br>4 U PRBC<br>UO 0.5-1 ml/kg/hr<br>Warm all fluids.<br>Humidify all gasses. | Use of rapid infusion and blood-salvaging devices helpful. Consider acute normovolemic hemodilution. Hemorrhage should be treated with crystalloid, colloid or blood as appropriate. |
| **Monitoring** | Standard monitors (see Appendix). | Monitor for cardiac ischemia. Automated ST segment analysis is useful. |
| | CVP line | The measurement of CVP may be sufficient in patients with good ventricular function and exercise tolerance. |
| | PA catheter | In patients with recent MI, Hx of CHF, Hx of unstable angina, multi system disease or in those presenting emergently (without the benefit of a complete workup), however, a PA catheter is appropriate.. |
| | TEE | TEE is invaluable for assessing cardiac changes 2° cross-clamping and unclamping the aorta. |
| | Arterial line<br>Urinary catheter | The arterial line is generally placed in the radial artery of the arm having the higher BP (if difference exists). |
| **Cross-clamping** | ↑↑ Afterload – HTN<br>↓ Preload<br>↑ Filling pressures<br>± ↓ Spinal cord perfusion<br>± ↓ Renal perfusion<br>↓ Perfusion to viscera below the clamp | Application of aortic cross-clamp causes HTN proximal to the clamp. In a healthy heart, this is well-tolerated with minimal increase in filling pressure. In hearts with poor ventricular function, filling pressures generally rise. Control of preload, afterload and HR can be accomplished with vasodilators and ß-blockers. Negative inotropic agents, like ß-blockers and inhalational anesthetics are used cautiously. Occlusion of infrarenal aorta decreases renal blood flow. Ensure adequate intravascular volume and CO. Consider use of mannitol, furosemide or low dose of dopamine 1-3 mg/kg/min to maintain UO. |
| **Aortic unclamping** | ↓↓ Afterload<br>Volume loading<br>Lactate washout<br>± Phenylephrine | Immediately before unclamping, D/C dilators and negative inotropic agents. Gradually increase filling pressures (volume loading) to avoid myocardial ischemia. ↓↓BP may occur with removal of cross-clamp 2° to hypovolemia, reactive hyperemia or myocardial dysfunction. Reperfusion of lower limbs and washout of lactate does not usually require use of $HCO_3$. Patients with an epidural sympathetic block often require phenylephrine support during unclamping. The surgeon can reclamp or occlude the aorta, if ↓↓BP persists. |
| **Positioning** | √ and pad pressure points.<br>√ eyes. | |
| **Complications** | Myocardial ischemia<br>HTN<br>Hemorrhage<br>Coagulopathy<br>Hypothermia<br>Organ ischemia | Hypothermia may cause dysrhythmias, depress contractility and exacerbate coagulopathy. |

## POSTOPERATIVE

| | |
|---|---|
| **Complications** | Myocardial ischemia<br>Renal failure<br>Respiratory failure |
| **Pain management** | Epidural narcotics (see Appendix). |

| | | |
|---|---|---|
| **Tests** | CXR to ✓ line and ETT placement<br>ABG<br>Coagulation profile<br>BUN; creatinine | BP should be closely controlled postop to decrease bleeding from graft site and raw surfaces. |


**References**

1. Darling RC, Messina CR, Brewster DC, Ottinger LW: Autopsy study of unoperated abdominal aortic aneurysms. The case for early resection. *Circulation* 1977; 56(3 Suppl):II-161-64.
2. Taylor LM Jr, Porter JM: Basic data related to clinical decision-making in abdominal aortic aneurysms. *Ann Vasc Surg* 1987; 1(4):502-4.
3. Story RJ, Wylie EJ: Surgical management of arterial lesions of the thoracoabdominal aorta. *Am J Surg* 1972; 126:157-64.
4. Dunn E, Prager RL, Fry W, Kirsh MM: The effect of abdominal aortic cross-clamping on myocardial function. *J Surg Res* 1977; 22:463-68.
5. Gooding JM, Archie JP Jr, McDowell H: Hemodynamic response to infrarenal aortic cross-clamping in patients with and without coronary artery disease. *Crit Care Med* 1980; 8:382-85.
6. Falk JL, Rackow EC, Blumenberg R, et al: Hemodynamic and metabolic effects of abdominal aortic cross-clamping. *Am J Surg* 1981; 142:174-77.
7. Foster JH, Bolasny BL, Gobbel WG Jr, Scott HW Jr: Comparative study of elective resection and expectant treatment of abdominal aortic aneurysm. *Surg Gynecol Obstet* 1969; 129:1-9.


# INFRAINGUINAL ARTERIAL BYPASS

## SURGICAL CONSIDERATIONS

**Description**: Due to the limited durability of distal bypass procedures, bypass to the infrainguinal arteries is indicated only for salvage of the severely ischemic lower extremity, as manifest by gangrene, ischemic ulceration or ischemic rest pain. Less frequently, it is used to alleviate functional ischemia of claudication, or leg discomfort with exercise. Its use is predicated on the pre-existence of adequate inflow to the level of the groin or femoral artery. Other necessary components include an adequate target vessel, preferably in continuity with runoff into the plantar arch of the foot, and an adequate conduit, preferably autologous saphenous vein. Long-term patency rates of non-autologous conduits to the below-knee arteries is distinctly inferior to that of saphenous vein, and should be avoided whenever possible. This population, almost by definition, includes patients with diabetes mellitus, CAD and cerebrovascular disease, all of which must be assessed preop.

The operative repair usually involves incisions at the groin distal bypass sites to expose the donor and recipient arteries, and to harvest leg or arm venous conduit. The operative approaches are rather similar. An unobstructed inflow source – usually the common femoral, superficial femoral or deep femoral artery – is exposed in the groin. The target distal artery, usually at the level of the knee or below, can be approached through a medial incision. More distally, the peroneal and anterior tibial arteries can be approached laterally at the mid-tibial level. At the level of the malleolus, both the dorsalis pedis and posterior tibial arteries can be revascularized. After control of donor and recipient vessels, an anatomic tunnel is created, and the bypass conduit (saphenous vein, prosthetic graft) passed through its length. After administration of 10,000 U of heparin, the distal anastomosis is constructed first, followed by the proximal anastomosis. A completion arteriogram confirms unobstructed flow. Heparin is then partially reversed, meticulous hemostasis obtained, and the wounds closed.

Although conventional wisdom has held that the anesthetic and operative risks for these patients undergoing distal reconstructions are low, recent data have shown little difference in postop morbidity and mortality when compared with patients undergoing a major inflow procedure within the abdomen.[1]

**Usual preop diagnosis**: Severe peripheral vascular disease; CAD; diabetes mellitus; HTN; obstructive PA disease. (These are almost ubiquitous co-morbidities.)

### SUMMARY OF PROCEDURE

| | |
|---|---|
| **Position** | Supine |
| **Incision** | Groin, medial knee, ± distal leg incisions; + incision to harvest venous conduit |
| **Antibiotics** | Cefamandole 1 gm iv at induction of anesthesia |
| **Surgical time** | 2 - 5 hrs |
| **Closing considerations** | Optimization of coagulation status |
| **EBL** | 200-300 cc |
| **Postop care** | Possible ICU x 24 hrs; careful monitoring is mandatory as patients are at risk for myocardial ischemia. |
| **Mortality** | 2-4%[2] |
| **Morbidity** | MI: 5-12%<br>Respiratory insufficiency: 5%<br>Infection: 2-5%<br>Amputation: 2-4%<br>CVA: < 1% |
| **Procedure code** | 35556 (fem-pop); 35558 (fem-fem) - vein graft<br>35656 (fem-pop); 35661 (fem-fem) - prosthetic graft |
| **Pain score** | 4-6 |

### PATIENT POPULATION CHARACTERISTICS

| | |
|---|---|
| **Age range** | >55 yrs (mean age = >70 yrs) |
| **Male:Female** | 4:1 |
| **Incidence** | Claudication fairly common in elderly; however, 75% will remain untreated, but stable, over 2-5 yrs, with < 5% requiring amputation. |
| **Etiology** | Arteriosclerosis (primarily)<br>Chronic embolic disease (rare)<br>Vasculitis<br>Popliteal artery entrapment<br>Cystic adventitial disease of popliteal artery |
| **Associated conditions** | CAD<br>Cerebrovascular disease<br>Diabetes mellitus<br>HTN<br>Obstructive pulmonary disease |

## ANESTHETIC CONSIDERATIONS

**(Procedures covered: infrainguinal arterial bypass; lumbar and upper extremity sympathectomy; thrombectomy or vein excision)**

### PREOPERATIVE

Patients presenting for peripheral vascular surgery may suffer from major systemic diseases, including CAD, HTN and diabetes. Three types of occlusive vascular disease have been described: Type 1 – isolated to the aortic and iliac bifurcations; is not associated with CAD. Type 2 – diffuse pattern involving coronary and cerebral circulations, associated with a higher incidence of diabetes and HTN. Type 3 – involves small vessels, especially of the lower limbs and is associated with higher postop morbidity and mortality.

| | |
|---|---|
| **Respiratory** | Vascular patients frequently have Hx of smoking and COPD. Preop evaluation of pulmonary function helps to determine whether regional vs GA is appropriate, while providing baseline values for postop comparison.<br>**Tests:** CXR; PFTs; ABG |
| **Cardiovascular** | Vascular surgery of the lower extremities is often associated with ↑morbidity and mortality 2° ↑incidence of CAD and HTN in this patient population.<br>**Tests:** ECG – ✓ for LVH and ischemia; other tests as indicated from H&P. |

**Neurological** Increased incidence of cerebrovascular disease. Careful neurological assessment is necessary to document existing deficits.

**Endocrine** Increased incidence of diabetes, which may be associated with peripheral and autonomic neuropathies (silent MI, labile BP) and delayed gastric emptying. Insulin requirements for most diabetic patients can be managed by administering one half the usual a.m. dose of insulin once a dextrose-containing iv (e.g., D5LR) has been established. Frequent blood glucose measurements should be made perioperatively.

**Renal** There is a higher incidence of renal artery disease and renal insufficiency in this patient population.
**Tests:** BUN; creatinine; creatinine clearance; electrolytes; UA

**Hematologic** Many patients presenting for this surgery are taking anticoagulant/antiplatelet medications. Inquire as to bleeding or bruising tendency.
**Tests:** Hct; PT; PTT; platelets

**Laboratory** As indicated from H&P.

**Premedication** Continue usual medications up to time of surgery. Anxiety can contribute to HTN and tachycardia. Premedicate conservatively (midazolam 5 mg im) for elderly patients. If ischemic pain is present, a narcotic such as morphine (3-7 mg im) can be given. Avoid im administration in patients on anticoagulant therapy.

## INTRAOPERATIVE

**Anesthetic technique:** Either regional anesthesia or GETA may be used. For infrainguinal arterial bypass, there is no evidence that either regional or GA is superior for promoting graft survival. To date, no study has shown a difference in patient mortality between these anesthetic techniques. **Lumbar sympathectomy** may be accomplished with a regional or GA. **Upper extremity sympathectomy** is done transthoracically (axillary and anterior approach) and a DLT helps facilitate the surgery. A DLT is not necessary for the supraclavicular approach. (See "Thoracic Anesthesia" section for discussion of DLT management.) For **thrombectomy**, GETA with IPPV may reduce the risk of pulmonary emboli.

**General anesthesia:**

**Induction** Hemodynamic stability is important; therefore, a slow, gradual induction is carried out. Preoxygenation is followed by smooth iv induction using small, incremental doses of fentanyl (1-2 $\mu$g/kg), then STP is given in divided doses (50-75 mg at a time) until the patient is asleep. A full dose of muscle relaxant is given and ventilation is controlled. Muscle relaxation is not necessary during the procedure, but muscle relaxant is given to facilitate intubation. The muscle relaxant is chosen to avoid undesirable effects on HR. Alternatively, if the LV function is poor, and the depressant effects of STP cannot be tolerated, a high-dose narcotic technique (e.g., fentanyl 10-50 $\mu$g/kg) is appropriate.

**Maintenance** Standard maintenance (see Appendix). If high-dose narcotic technique is used, benzodiazepines are given for amnesia. Continued muscle relaxation is unnecessary. These surgical procedures are associated with minimal hemodynamic instability.

**Emergence** Tracheal extubation should be based on standard criteria, such as adequacy of ventilation, return of airway reflexes and reversal of muscle relaxation. Control of BP is accomplished with vasodilators (e.g., NTG 0.1-4.0 $\mu$g/kg/min or SNP 0.25-5.0 $\mu$g/kg/min). Esmolol can be given in incremental doses of 10 mg or by infusion (50-200 $\mu$g/kg/min).

**Regional anesthesia:** Patients presenting for regional anesthesia must have a normal coagulation profile; also, they cannot be on heparin, urokinase or streptokinase. The important goals in regional anesthesia are to achieve hemodynamic stability while establishing an adequate block. An epidural or spinal catheter is frequently used to infuse a gradual onset and to prevent an excessively high block. Hemodynamic stability can be improved by infusing 500-1000 cc of crystalloid before performing the block. The patient may be placed in the lateral decubitus position (with operative side down), which may provide a denser and more prolonged block on that side. Achieving a T8-T10 level is optimal. Over-zealous hydration may → CHF in this patient population, when the vasodilation 2° regional sympathectomy dissipates. The use of regional anesthesia in patients receiving intraop anticoagulation is controversial. We feel it is a relatively safe procedure and have not had a complication with this technique. If blood is aspirated after placement of an epidural, we remove the catheter and then replace it at a different interspace. Patients on ASA should have a normal bleeding time and patients on mini-dose heparin should have a normal PTT before use of regional anesthesia.

**Spinal** — **One-shot spinal:** 1% hyperbaric tetracaine (6-10 mg) or 0.75% bupivacaine (10-15 mg). Add epinephrine 0.2 mg (generally increases duration of block about 50%) or phenylephrine 5 mg (generally increases duration of block about 100%). Do not add vasoconstrictor if patient is diabetic.

**Continuous spinal:** A 20-ga catheter is placed via an 18-ga Tuohy needle. 0.5% hyperbaric tetracaine or 0.75% bupivacaine is titrated to desired anesthetic level (T10-T8). Catheters should be re-dosed every 60-80 min or as soon as BP trends upward. The risk of spinal headache is very low with continuous spinals.

**Epidural** — Lidocaine 2% with 1:200,000 epinephrine or 0.5% bupivacaine is used. Titrate to desired anesthetic level (T10-T8).

| | | |
|---|---|---|
| **Blood and fluid requirements** | Minimal-to-moderate blood loss<br>IV: 14 or 16 ga x 1<br>Warm fluids.<br>Humidify gasses.<br>Maintain UO 0.5-1 ml/kg. | |
| **Monitoring** | Standard monitors (see Appendix).<br>ST-segment analysis<br>Arterial line | An arterial line is most often used in patients with severe cardiopulmonary disease, in brittle diabetics, or for patients undergoing upper extremity sympathectomy (transthoracic approach and DLT). Blood sampling for ABGs, electrolytes, glucose and Hct is facilitated by the use of an arterial line. |
| | ± CVP/PA catheters | CVP and PA catheters are not routinely used because large changes in intravascular volumes are uncommon. Patients with poor LV function, recent MI or severe valvular disease may need PA monitoring. |
| **Positioning** | ✓ and pad pressure points.<br>✓ eyes. | Diabetic patients may be at risk of skin ischemia due to poor positioning or inadequate padding of limbs, etc. |
| **Complications** | HTN<br>Ischemia<br>Hypothermia<br>Hemorrhage<br>Pneumothorax | Pneumothorax may occur with supraclavicular approach to sympathectomy. |

## POSTOPERATIVE

| | | |
|---|---|---|
| **Complications** | CHF<br>Hypothermia<br>Graft occlusion<br>Pneumothorax | Infrainguinal bypass: Avoid over-hydration; when epidural sympathectomy fades, these patients are at increased risk for CHF. Maintain normovolemia so that peripheral vasoconstriction (which may limit outflow to the graft) does not occur. Hypothermia causes vasoconstriction and also may limit outflow to the graft. |
| **Pain management** | Epidural/spinal opiates (see Appendix).<br>PCA | Epidural (or spinal) catheter may be used for postop analgesia (see Appendix). |
| **Tests** | CXR if central line placed<br>Hct | |

**References**


1. Krupski WC, Layug EL, Reilly LM, Rapp JH, Mangano DT: Comparison of cardiac morbidity between aortic and infrainguinal operations. Study of Perioperative Ischemia (SPI) Research Group. *J Vasc Surg* 1992; 15(2):354-65.
2. Veith FJ, Gupta SK, Samson RH, et al: Progress in limb salvage by reconstructive arterial surgery combined with new or improved adjunctive procedures. *Ann Surg* 1981; 194:386-401.
3. McKenzie PJ, Wishart HY, Dewar KM, Gray I, Smith G: Comparison of the effects of spinal anaesthesia and general anaesthesia on postoperative oxygenation and perioperative mortality. *Br J Anaesth* 1980; 52(1):49-54.

4. Covino BG: *Reasons to preferentially select regional anesthesia.* IARS Review Course Lectures, 60th Congress. International Anesthesia Research Society, Cleveland: 1986, 61-5.
5. Carli F, Gabrielczyk M, Clark MM, Aber VR: An investigation of factors affecting postoperative rewarming of adult patients. *Anaesthesia* 1986; 41(4):363-69.
6. Damask MC, Weissman C, Barth A, et al: General vs epidural – which is the better anesthetic technique for femoral-popliteal bypass surgery?. *Anaesth Analg* 1986; 65:539.
7. Cousins MJ, Wright CJ: Graft; muscle, skin blood flow after epidural block in vascular surgical procedures. *Surg Gynecol Obstet* 1971; 133(1):59-64.
8. Terry HJ, Allan JS, Taylor GW: The effect of adding lumbar sympathectomy to reconstructive arterial surgery in the lower limb. *Br J Surg* 1970; 57(1):51-5.
9. Murphy TM: Spinal, epidural and caudal anesthesia. In *Anesthesia*, Vol 2, 2nd edition. Miller RD, ed. Churchill Livingstone, New York: 1986, 1061-1111.
10. Vaughan MS, Vaughan RW, Cork RC: Postoperative hypothermia in adults: relationship of age, anesthesia, and shivering to rewarming. *Anesth Analg* 1981; 60(10):746-51.
11. Park WY, Balingit BE, MacNamara TE: Effects of patient age, pH of cerebrospinal fluid, and vasopressors on onset and duration of spinal anesthesia. *Anesth Analg* 1975; 54(4):455-58.
12. Concepciono M, Maddi R, Francis D, Rocco AG, Murray E, Covino BG: Vasoconstrictors in spinal anesthesia with tetracaine – a comparison of epinephrine and phenylephrine. *Anesth Analg* 1984; 63(2):134-38.
13. Rao TL, El-Etr AA: Anticoagulation following placement of epidural and subarachnoid catheters: an evaluation of neurologic sequelae. *Anesthesiology* 1981; 55(6):618-20.
14. Varkey GP, Brindle GF: Peridural anaesthesia and anti-coagulant therapy. *Can Anaesth Soc J* 1974; 21(1):106-9.
15. Denny N, Masters R, Pearson D, Rend J, Sihota M, Selander D: Postdural puncture headache after continuous spinal anesthesia. *Anesth Analg* 1987; 66(8):791-94.
16. Harris JP, May J: Upper extremity sympathectomy. In *Vascular Surgery*, 3rd edition. Rutherford RB, ed. WB Saunders Co, Philadelphia: 1989, 190-897.
17. Collin GJ, Rich HM, Clagett GP: Clinical results of lumbar sympathectomy. *Am Surgery* 1981; 47:31-35.
18. Dalessandri KM, Carson SN, Tillman P, et al: Effect of lumbar sympathectomy in distal arterial obstruction. *Arch Surgery* 1983; 118:1157-60.

# LUMBAR SYMPATHECTOMY

## SURGICAL CONSIDERATIONS

**Description**: The role of **lumbar sympathectomy** is not well-defined.[1,2] The procedure is used selectively in patients with causalgia, inoperable lower limb ischemia with rest pain or toe gangrene, symptomatic vasospastic disorders (e.g., Raynaud's phenomenon, frostbite), and sometimes as an adjunct to distal revascularization procedures.[1-3] Causalgia responds well to lumbar sympathectomy, especially if performed early in the clinical course. There may be some benefit of the procedure in 50-60% of patients with rest pain or ischemic ulceration.[4] Sympathectomy may increase collateral blood flow and local skin blood flow.[5] Scleroderma with impending "minor" amputation may benefit from sympathectomy with improved wound healing.[2] Sympathetic denervation involves the division of preganglionic fibers along their segmental origins and resection of corresponding relay ganglia.[1] For most clinical indications, L2 and L3 **ganglionectomy** sufficiently sympathectomizes the lower extremity.

The **anterolateral retroperitoneal approach (Flowthow)** is most commonly performed because of the adequate exposure and a relatively well-tolerated incision.[1] For this approach, an oblique incision is made through the abdominal musculature, extending from the lateral border of the rectus abdominus to the anterior axillary line. Cephalad and caudad blunt dissection is performed between the transversalis fascia and peritoneum. The dissection is continued in a retroperitoneal fashion. The psoas muscle is identified, with care being taken to leave the ureter and gonadal vessels attached to overlying peritoneum. The sympathetic chain is identified between the psoas muscle and the vertebra (medial to psoas and overlying the transverse process of lumbar vertebra). The sympathetic chain is dissected free from surrounding tissue, clipped proximally and distally, and resected. On the left side, the sympathetic chain is lateral to the abdominal aorta; on the right, the sympathetic chain is beneath the IVC. Hemostasis is achieved and abdominal wall closed in layers.

A **posterior approach** (**Royle**) is used less often because of significant postop paraspinous muscle spasms. In this approach, a transverse lumbar incision is made. The paraspinous muscles are partially divided and retracted to expose the vertebra. The sympathetic chain is identified and resected as described. The anterior/transperitoneal approach is performed in conjunction with an abdominal aortic or intraperitoneal procedure. Dissection is carried to the psoas muscle; the retroperitoneum is entered and the sympathetic chain is isolated in the groove between the psoas and the vertebra. The sympathetic chain is clipped proximally and distally and resected. **Adson's anterior transperitoneal** approach is used when combined with an abdominal aortic or other intraperitoneal procedure.

**Usual preop diagnosis**: Causalgia; inoperable arterial occlusive disease with limb-threatening ischemia causing rest pain, ulceration or superficial digital gangrene; symptomatic vasospastic disorders (e.g., Raynaud's phenomenon or frostbite)

### SUMMARY OF PROCEDURE

| | Anterolateral Retroperitoneal | Posterior | Anterior Transperitoneal |
|---|---|---|---|
| **Position** | Supine (flank slightly raised); widen distance between costal margin and iliac crest. | Prone | Supine |
| **Incision** | Oblique (lateral edge of rectus to ribs at anterior axillary line) | Posterior transverse over mid-lumbar region | Transverse or midline abdominal |
| **Special instrumentation** | Self-retaining retractor | ⇐ | ⇐ |
| **Unique considerations** | May use frozen section to confirm specimen. | ⇐ | ⇐ |
| **Antibiotics** | None | ⇐ | None, per se, depending on associated procedure |
| **Surgical time** | 2 - 3 hrs | 3 hrs | 4 hrs |
| **Closing considerations** | Flex table to facilitate abdominal wall closure; occasionally drain is placed. | ⇐ | ⇐ |
| **EBL** | 50-100 cc (unless complicated) | 50-100 cc | ⇐ |
| **Postop care** | PACU → ward. (May require cardiac and hemodynamic monitoring in high-risk patients, or if combined with distal revascularization. | ⇐ | ⇐ |
| **Mortality**[3-5] | Minimal | ⇐ | ⇐ |
| **Morbidity** | Postsympathectomy neuralgia: 50% | ~50% | ⇐ |
| | Sexual derangement – retrograde ejaculation (usually bilateral L1 sympathectomy): 25-50% | ~25-50% | ⇐ |
| | Wound hematoma: 10% | ~10% | ⇐ |
| | Wound infection: 1-3% | ~1-3% | ⇐ |
| | | Paraspinous muscle spasms | |
| **Procedure code** | 64818 | ⇐ | ⇐ |
| **Pain score** | 5 | 5 | 5 (related to primary procedure) |

### PATIENT POPULATION CHARACTERISTICS

| | |
|---|---|
| **Age range** | 38-91 yrs; younger patients with vasospastic disease; older patients with peripheral vascular disease |
| **Male:Female** | 2:1 |

**Incidence** Unknown. Approximately 30 cases/yr at SUMC, mainly for inoperable lower extremity ischemia or as an adjunct to revascularization procedures.

**Etiology** Peripheral vascular disease (rest pain and tissue loss)
Vasospastic disorders
Causalgia

**Associated conditions** Peripheral vascular disease: Rare
Vasospastic disorders: Rare

## ANESTHETIC CONSIDERATIONS

See Anesthetic Considerations following "Infrainguinal Arterial Bypass" (above).

**References**

1. Shannon FL, Rutherford RB: Lumbar sympathectomy: Indications and technique. In *Vascular Surgery*, 3rd edition. Rutherford RB, ed. WB Saunders Co, Philadelphia: 1989, 764-73.
2. Boltax RS: Lumbar sympathectomy: a place in clinical medicine. *Conn Med* 1989; 53(12):716-17.
3. AbuRahma AF, Robinson PA: Clinical parameters for predicting response to lumbar sympathectomy in patients with severe lower limb ischemia. *J Cardiovasc Surg* 1990; 31(1):101-6.
4. Repelaer van Driel OJ, van Bockel JH, van Schilfgaarde R: Lumbar sympathectomy for severe lower limb ischaemia: results and analysis of factors influencing the outcome. *J Cardiovasc Surg* 1988, 29(3):310-14.
5. Norman PE, House AK: The early use of operative lumbar sympathectomy in peripheral vascular disease. *J Cardiovasc Surg* 1988; 29(6):717-22.

# UPPER EXTREMITY SYMPATHECTOMY

## SURGICAL CONSIDERATIONS

**Description**: **Upper extremity sympathectomy** is the surgical treatment for hyperhidrosis, reflex sympathetic dystrophy, post-traumatic pain syndromes and certain vasospastic disorders affecting the hands and digits.[1-3] Palmar hyperhidrosis is especially responsive to surgical sympathectomy.[2] The results achieved with sympathectomy for upper extremity ischemic and post-traumatic pain syndromes are less favorable. It is recommended that T2 and T3 ganglia be excised and the stellate ganglion spared. Manipulation of the stellate ganglion is associated with increased incidence of Horner's syndrome.[2] The **supraclavicular approach** was introduced in 1935[3] and is still used commonly. The **axillary, extrapleural approach** of **Atkins** was designed to provide an anatomic approach to the sympathetic chain. **Roos**' modification of the Atkins technique includes an extrapleural approach to the sympathetic chain after resection of the first rib. This is very useful for identifying the exact level of the sympathetic chain, and is associated with less postop pain because rib retraction is unnecessary. The **anterior thoracic approach** involves a limited thoracotomy through the third interspace, which provides excellent exposure. It is, however, associated with the morbidity and mortality of a thoracotomy. Part of the sympathetic chain below the stellate ganglion may be excised more readily via this approach. All of these methods have intrinsic advantages and disadvantages, but only the supraclavicular and axillary methods are used widely. Newer techniques, such as **CT-guided phenol sympathetic block** and **trans-thorascopic sympathectomy**, have been developed and may yield comparable short- and long-term results.[2,4]

**Usual preop diagnosis**: Hyperhidrosis; ischemia; post-traumatic pain syndromes; vasospastic disorders; various forms of arteritis

### SUMMARY OF PROCEDURE

| | Supraclavicular | Axillary Transthoracic Or Extrapleural | Anterior Transthoracic |
|---|---|---|---|
| **Position** | Supine | Lateral decubitus (arm supported to avoid brachial plexus traction) | Supine (slight lateral decubitus) |
| **Incision** | Above medial 1/3 of clavicle | For **transthoracic:** transverse lower axilla (enter thorax at 2nd or 3rd interspace); for **extrapleural:** transverse axillary (resect 1st rib) | Anterior thoracotomy (enter thorax at 3rd interspace and divide 3rd-costal cartilage) |
| **Special instrumentation** | DLT | ⇐ | ⇐ |
| **Antibiotics** | None | ⇐ | ⇐ |
| **Surgical time** | 3 - 4 hrs | ⇐ | ⇐ |
| **Closing considerations** | May need drain. | Chest tube placed and connected to water seal for transthoracic approach. | Chest tube placed and connected to water seal. |
| **EBL** | 100-200 cc | ⇐ | ⇐ |
| **Postop care** | PACU → ward | ⇐ | ⇐ |
| **Mortality** | Minimal | ⇐ | ⇐ |
| **Morbidity** | Post-sympathectomy neuralgia: Common | ⇐ | ⇐ |
| | Pleurotomy: 10% | – | – |
| | Pleural effusion: 7% | ~7% | ⇐ |
| | Gustatory sweating: 6% | ~6% | ⇐ |
| | Horner's syndrome: 4% | ~4% | ⇐ |
| | Pneumonia: 3% | ~3% | ⇐ |
| | Atelectasis: 2% | ~2% | ⇐ |
| | Phrenic nerve injury: 2% | – | – |
| | Pneumomediastinum: 2% | – | – |
| | Subclavian artery injury: 2% | – | – |
| | Lymphocele: 1% | – | – |
| | Wound hematoma: 1% | – | – |
| | Chylous fistula: Rare | ⇐ | – |
| | Winged scapula: Rare | ⇐ | – |
| **Procedure code** | 64804 | 64802 | 64809 |
| **Pain score** | 4 | 5 | 5 |

### PATIENT POPULATION CHARACTERISTICS

| | |
|---|---|
| **Age range** | 11-45 yrs |
| **Male:Female** | 1:1 |
| **Incidence** | Hyperhidrosis ≤ 1% of the population (palmar hyperhidrosis in 0.15-0.25%) |
| **Etiology** | Hyperhidrosis: strong family Hx<br>Vasospasm and arteritides: Idiopathic<br>Ischemia: Peripheral vascular disease, trauma, autoimmune disease |
| **Associated conditions** | Peripheral vascular disease<br>Trauma<br>Autoimmune disease |

## ANESTHETIC CONSIDERATIONS

See Anesthetic Considerations following "Infrainguinal Arterial Bypass" (above).

**References**

1. Harris JP, May J. Upper extremity sympathectomy. In *Vascular Surgery*, 3rd edition. Rutherford RB, ed. WB Saunders Co, Philadelphia: 1989, 890-97.
2. Hashmonai M, Kopelman D, Kein O, Schein M: Upper thoracic sympathectomy for primary palmar hyperhidrosis: long-term follow-up. *Br J Surg* 1992; 79(3):268-71.
3. Moran KT, Brady MP: Surgical management of primary hyperhidrosis. *Br J Surg* 1991; 78(3):279-83.
4. Pace RF, Brown PM, Gutelius JR: Thorascopic transthoracic dorsal sympathectomy. *Can J Surg* 1992; 35(5):509-11.


# VENOUS SURGERY – THROMBECTOMY OR VEIN EXCISION

## SURGICAL CONSIDERATIONS

**Description**: Standard therapy for acute DVT consists of anti-coagulation, bed rest and elevation of the extremity.[1,8] Surgical thrombectomy for acute iliofemoral DVT remains controversial. **Venous thrombectomy** is recommended for patients with threatened limb loss or venous gangrene caused by massive DVT associated with high compartment pressures and arterial insufficiency (phlegmasia cerulea dolens).[1,8] Venous thrombectomy requires exposure of the femoral vein via a groin cutdown. The common femoral vein is isolated (located medial or posteromedial to the femoral artery) and controlled proximally and distally. The patient is given iv heparin at this stage, if not already heparinized. A transverse venotomy is followed by extraction of the thrombus, using forceps and Fogarty embolectomy catheters. Distal thrombi are expressed through the same incision with the aid of an Esmarch bandage placed on the extremity.[1] After complete removal of the thrombus, the venotomy is closed with nonabsorbable sutures and flow through the femoral vein re-established. The femoral incision is closed in layers. A plastic/Silastic® drain may or may not be used. The best results of thrombectomy are obtained in young patients with the first episode of proximal (iliofemoral) thrombosis.

Nonsuppurative thrombophlebitis of the superficial veins may develop due to local trauma, prolonged inactivity, fungal infection or the use of oral contraceptives.[1] Suppurative thrombophlebitis may occur as a complication of iv line placement or iv drug abuse. Underlying varicose veins may predispose to thrombophlebitis. Migratory superficial thrombophlebitis may be associated with chronic ischemia of the extremities in Buerger's disease, or it may develop in patients with a malignancy.[1] Conservative management with hot compresses, nonsteroidal anti-inflammatory medications, and elevation of the extremity is effective in most cases. Rarely, **excision** of the acutely thrombosed greater saphenous vein is indicated to prevent progression of thrombosis to the saphenofemoral junction and into the deep venous system.[1] Vein excision is simply approached by a longitudinal incision directly over the affected vein. The phlebitic vein is dissected from the surrounding tissue, ligated proximally and distally, and removed. The surrounding fibrotic tissue is debrided gently. The wound is irrigated and packed open with moist gauze. Suppurative phlebitis is treated with iv antibiotics and complete excision of the involved vein segment through multiple small incisions.

**Usual preop diagnosis**: Lower limb venous thrombosis threatening viability; femoral thrombosis < 10 d; iliac thrombosis < 3 wks; floating thrombi at hip level; acute deep or superficial venous thrombosis; suppurative thrombophlebitis

### SUMMARY OF PROCEDURE

| | Thrombectomy | Vein Excision |
|---|---|---|
| **Position** | Supine | ⇐ |
| **Incision** | Ipsilateral longitudinal or oblique groin incision | Multiple small incisions along the course of vein to be excised |
| **Special instrumentation** | Fogarty embolectomy catheters; RBC salvage system | None |
| **Unique considerations** | IPPV during thrombectomy may decrease chance of PE 2° ↓venous return → more complete extraction of the thrombus. | None |

| | Thrombectomy | Vein Excision |
|---|---|---|
| **Antibiotics** | None, unless the patient has a septic thrombus (antibiotic is dependent on blood culture) | Dependent on culture of aspirate. Usually a septic patient is on broad-spectrum antibiotics (guided by culture). |
| **Surgical time** | 2 - 3 hrs | 1 - 3 hrs |
| **Closing considerations** | None | Wound packed open for drainage |
| **EBL** | 50-250 cc | ⇐ |
| **Postop care** | PACU → ward; ICU in high-risk patients; heparin administered before and after procedure, followed by Coumadin® for 1-6 mo.[8] | PACU → ward; support stockings |
| **Mortality** | Minimal (depending on underlying illness) | Minimal |
| **Morbidity** | Post-thrombotic syndrome: < 10-44%[8]<br>Venous stasis<br>Non-pitting edema<br>Brawny induration<br>Aching pain | Minimal |
| **Procedure code** | 34421 | 35860 |
| **Pain score** | 3 | 2 |

### PATIENT POPULATION CHARACTERISTICS

**Age range** Young adult-elderly

**Male:Female** 1:2

**Incidence** 6-7 million in U.S. have adverse effects from chronic venous stasis[3]; 500,000 have complications of leg ulceration

**Etiology**
Chronic primary varicose veins
Defective venous valves
Impaired pumping action of muscles in leg
Previous iliofemoral thrombophlebitis
Obstruction of venous return

**Associated conditions**
Multifactoral:
- Varicose veins
- Underlying malignancy
- Altered coagulation status (hypercoagulability – acquired or congenital)
- Hx of DVT/thrombophlebitis

## ANESTHETIC CONSIDERATIONS

See Anesthetic Considerations following "Infrainguinal Arterial Bypass" (above).

**References**


1. Gloviczki P, Merrell SW: Surgical treatment of venous disease. *Cardiovasc Clin* 1992; 22(3):81-100.
2. Johnson G Jr: The management of venous disorders: Introduction and general considerations. In *Vascular Surgery*, 3rd edition. Rutherford RB, ed. WB Saunders Co, Philadelphia: 1989, 1480-82.
3. Lofgren KA: Surgical management of chronic venous insufficiency. *Acta Chir Scand Suppl* 1988; 544:62-8.
4. O'Donnell TF Jr: Clinical diagnosis and classification of chronic venous insufficiency. In *Vascular Surgery*, 3rd edition. Rutherford RB, ed. WB Saunders Co, Philadelphia: 1989, 1504-12.
5. Burnham SJ: Varicose veins: Patient selection and treatment. In *Vascular Surgery*, 3rd edition. Rutherford RB, ed. WB Saunders Co, Philadelphia: 1989, 1512-17.
6. Large J: Surgical treatment of saphenous varices, with preservation of the main great saphenous trunk. *J Vasc Surg* 1985; 2(6):886-91.
7. Friedell ML, Samson RH, Cohen MJ, Simmons GT, Rollins DL, Mawyer L, Semrow CM. High ligation of the greater saphenous vein for treatment of lower extremity varicosities: the fate of the vein and therapeutic results. *Ann Vasc Surg* 1992; 6(1):5-8.
8. Lord RS, Chen FC, et al: Surgical treatment of acute deep venous thrombosis. *World J Surg* 1990; 14(5):694-702.
9. Sottiurai VS: Surgical correction of recurrent venous ulcer. *J Cardiovasc Surg* 1991; 32(1):104-9.
10. Bergan JJ, Yao JS, et al. Surgical treatment of venous obstruction and insufficiency. *J Vasc Surg* 1986; 3(1):174-81.

# SURGERY FOR PORTAL HYPERTENSION

## SURGICAL CONSIDERATIONS

**Description:** Alcoholic liver disease is the major cause of portal HTN. End-stage liver disease with cirrhosis is the 10th leading cause of death in the U.S. (exceeding 23,000/year). 15-20% of patients with portal HTN have variceal hemorrhage during the first year of diagnosis (additional 5-10 % incidence of bleeding per year), and the initial episode of variceal hemorrhage is associated with 50% mortality. Portal HTN (>15 mmHg) develops when splanchnic venous flow to the right heart becomes impeded.[1-6] Medical and surgical therapeutic interventions are directed not at portal HTN per se, but at its complications, notably bleeding esophageal varices. Intractable ascites and hypersplenism are less common indications for operative therapy. Presinusoidal portal HTN, unlike sinusoidal or post-sinusoidal obstruction, is not associated with severe hepatocellular disease; thus, the prognosis for patients with presinusoidal block is better than those with sinusoidal or postsinusoidal disease. Shunt procedures can be classified as **total shunts** (decompression of the portal venous system) or **selective shunts** (decompression of only the varix-bearing area).[2,4,7]

There are two general types of total shunt procedures.[2,8] The **end-to-side portacaval shunt** (Fig 6.2-3A) is technically simpler and may be more appropriate in emergency situations. It is associated with immediate control of hemorrhage in the majority of cases. The portacaval shunt, however, does eliminate portal perfusion of the liver and does not decompress the hepatic sinusoids. Alternatively, the **functional side-to-side shunt** (Fig 6.2-3B) allows decompression of hepatic sinusoids and may preserve some degree of portal perfusion of the liver. Also, it is more effective in controlling ascites. Variations of the side-to-side shunt include: **portacaval**, **splenorenal**, **mesocaval (Clatworthy)**, and **portarenal** (rarely used).

For the **end-to-end** and **side-to-side portacaval shunts**, the approach is via an extended right subcostal incision. **Cholecystectomy** usually is not performed because of likelihood of profuse bleeding from the liver bed. The hepatoduodenal ligament is identified, and the portal vein is exposed from the hilum of the liver to the pancreas. The gastroduodenal and right gastric branches may be divided to provide additional exposure of the portal vein. The IVC is exposed by incising the peritoneum just beneath the hepatic triad. Proximal and distal control of the portal vein is achieved; a side-biting clamp is placed on the IVC. In order to perform an **end-to-side portacaval shunt**, the portal vein is divided and oversewn proximally; the end-to-side anastomosis is performed from the portal vein to the IVC. The alternative is to perform a side-to-side anastomosis of the portal vein to the IVC without division of the portal vein.

The **proximal splenorenal shunt** is approached through a left thoracoabdominal or transabdominal incision. The spleen is isolated and removed, and the distal splenic vein is mobilized from the distal pancreatic bed. The left renal vein is exposed and controlled. The distal splenic vein is then anastomosed in an end-to-side fashion to the mid renal vein. The **mesocaval shunt** is indicated in cases of ascites, periportal fibrosis, portal vein thrombosis and Budd-Chiari syndrome.[5] The mesocaval shunt (Fig 6.2-3C) is approached through a vertical midline incision. The colon is retracted cephalad and the superior mesenteric vein (SMV) is identified at the root of the mesentery. A length of the SMV is isolated and encircled. A **Kocher maneuver** (mobilization of the duodenum) is performed and the IVC is exposed anteriorly and laterally. A side-biting clamp partially occludes the IVC and a 14-20 mm Dacron® graft is anastomosed in an end-to-side fashion to the IVC. The graft is clamped and the side-biting clamp removed from the IVC, thereby restoring flow via the IVC. The SMV is clamped and an end-to-side anastomosis created from the graft to the SMV. Flow is thus re-established from the SMV through the graft to the IVC.

Selective shunts are designed to decompress esophageal varices, while some portal perfusion of the liver is maintained.[4,9,10] The hallmark example of this approach is the **distal splenorenal shunt (Warren)** (Fig 6.2-3D), which is seldom used in emergency situations. The principal feature of this shunt is disconnection of the splenic and superior mesenteric venous drainage systems. The distal splenorenal shunt is approached through a left chevron or extended left subcostal incision. The lesser sac is entered after division of the gastroepiploic vessels and mobilization of the splenic flexure of the colon. The stomach is retracted cephalad and the peritoneum overlying the inferior aspect of the pancreas incised. The splenic vein is identified and controlled proximally and distally. The inferior mesenteric vein is divided. The splenic vein is divided proximally and the proximal stump oversewn. Then the splenic vein is mobilized from the pancreatic bed. The left renal vein is identified and 5-7 cm of the vein is isolated. The splenic vein is anastomosed in an end-to-side fashion to the renal vein. The coronary vein is ligated close to its origin. The distal splenorenal shunt decompresses the stomach, distal esophagus and spleen and controls variceal hemorrhage in 85% of patients.[9]

**Variant procedure or approaches**: **Total shunt** (e.g., portacaval, proximal splenorenal, mesocaval); **selective shunt** (e.g., Warren); **non-shunt procedures** (e.g., **Sugiura**, **Hassab**, and **esophageal transection with stapling)**

**Usual preop diagnosis**: Bleeding esophageal varices (as a result of portal HTN); ascites; hypersplenism

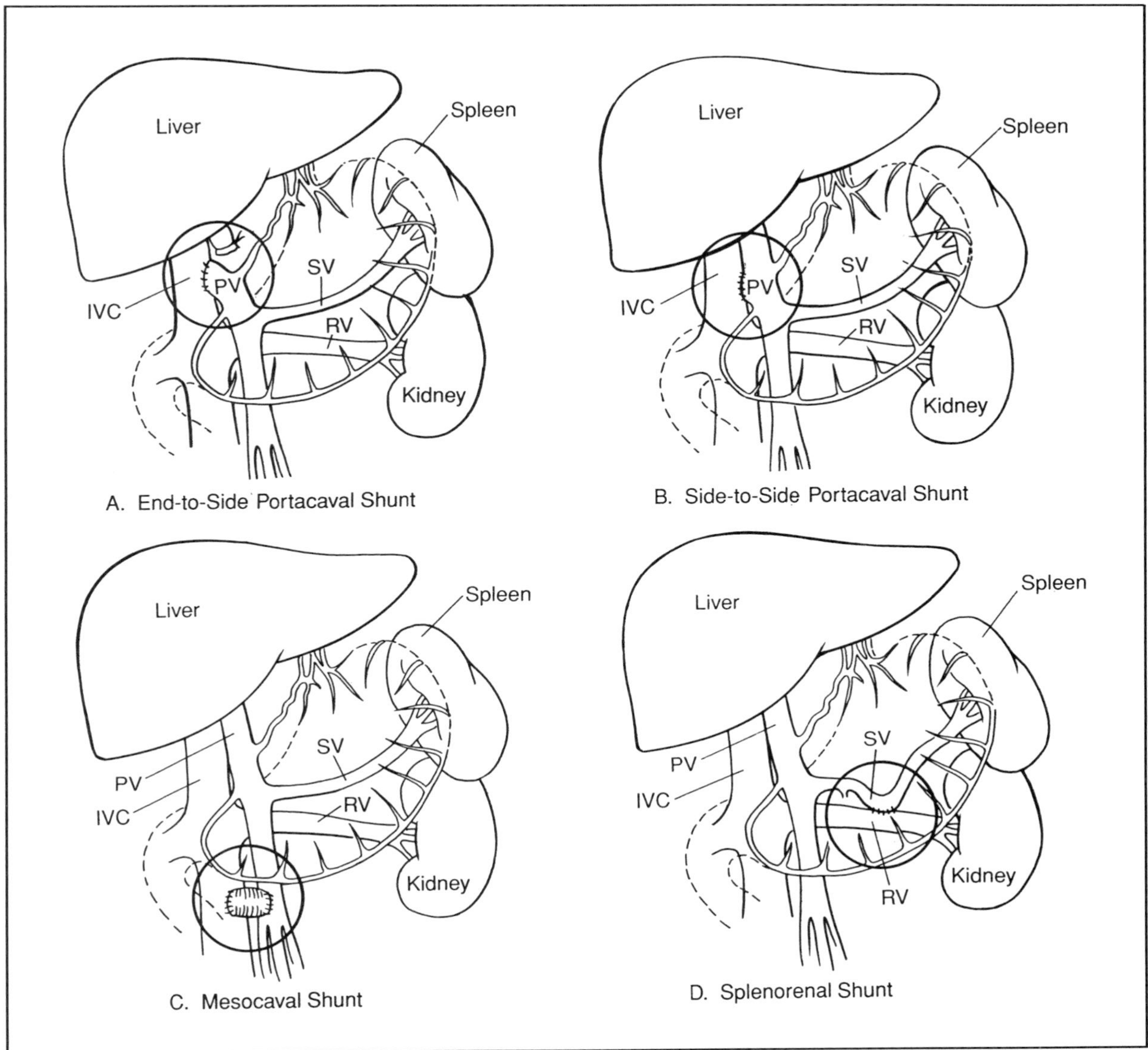


**Figure 6.2-3.** Types of shunt: (A) End-to-side portacaval; (B) side-to-side portacaval; (C) mesocaval shunt; (D) splenorenal. (Reproduced with permission from Hardy JD: *Hardy's Textbook of Surgery*, 2nd edition. JB Lippincott, 1988.)

## SUMMARY OF PROCEDURES (TOTAL AND SELECTIVE SHUNTS)

| | Portacaval | Proximal Splenorenal | Mesocaval | Distal Splenorenal (Warren) |
|---|---|---|---|---|
| **Position** | Supine | Supine ± left flank elevated | Supine | Supine, left side elevated slightly |
| **Incision** | Extended right subcostal – may be lengthened or converted to left thoracoabdominal | Left thoracoabdominal or left subcostal, or vertical midline | Vertical midline abdominal | Left chevron or left subcostal with midline extension |
| **Special instrumentation** | Self-retaining retractor | ⇐ | ⇐ | ⇐ |
| **Unique considerations** | May need FFP; consider cell-saver. | ⇐ | ⇐ | ⇐ |

| | Portacaval | Proximal Splenorenal | Mesocaval | Distal Splenorenal |
|---|---|---|---|---|
| **Antibiotics** | Cefazolin 1 gm iv | ⇐ | ⇐ | ⇐ |
| **Surgical time** | 4 - 6 hrs | ⇐ | ⇐ | ⇐ |
| **Closing considerations** | None | ⇐ | ⇐ | ⇐ |
| **EBL** | 1000-2000 cc | ⇐ | ⇐ | ⇐ |
| **Postop care** | Patient → ICU; careful fluid management; consider Na restriction; may require PA catheter. | ⇐ | ⇐ | ⇐ |
| **Mortality**[1,2,3,5,7,8,9,17,18] | Emergency: 38%<br>Elective: 3%<br>Child's A: 0-15%<br>Child's B: 1-43%<br>Child's C: 6-58% | 5-10% | ⇐ | 1-16% |
| **Morbidity**[1,5,7,8,15] | Late liver failure: 50% | ~50% | ⇐ | – |
| | Encephalopathy: 32%<br>Child's A: 8%<br>Child's B: 20%<br>Child's C: 30% | ~32% | ⇐ | 5-47% (overall)<br>5% at 2 yrs<br>12% at 3-6 yrs<br>27% at 10 yrs |
| | Early rebleeding: 0-19% | ~0-19% | ⇐ | Loss of selectivity: 60% (@ 2 yrs) |
| | Shunt thrombosis: 1-10% | 20% | 9-30% | Recurrent variceal hemorrhage (shunt occlusion): 3-19% |
| | Pancreatitis: – | – | –<br>Duodenal obstruction<br>Erosion through bowel wall | Portal vein thrombosis: 4-10% |
| **Procedure code** | 37140 | 37180 | 37160 | 37181 |
| **Pain score** | 6 | 6 | 6 | 6 |

Note: In addition to the shunt procedure itself, other factors that determine postop morbidity and mortality include: severity of hepatocellular disease, degree of hepatic reserve, and urgency of the procedure. Although the specific numbers may vary, several comparative series have shown no difference in operative mortality rate or long-term survival rate among the various shunt procedures.[2-4,7]

## NON-SHUNT PROCEDURES

**Non-shunt procedures** are designed to devascularize the esophagogastric region, thus eliminating acute variceal hemorrhage.[11] Procedures of this type include: **portazygous disconnection**; **splenectomy**; **coronary vein ligation**; and **transesophageal** or **transgastric varix ligation**.

The **Sugiura** operation, approached via abdominal and thoracic incisions, includes esophageal transection and devascularization, splenectomy and pyloromyotomy.[12] This procedure is usually performed in two operative stages, with the second stage sometimes delayed. The **Hassab** procedure involves devascularization of the upper half of the stomach and splenectomy, thus effectively disconnecting the esophageal varices.[11,13] This operation has been reserved in some centers for the failures of sclerotherapy. Finally, **esophageal transection**, using a stapling device, disconnects the varices in the lower esophagus. This is accomplished by placing a row of staples at the esophagus just above the esophagogastric junction.[3,11,14-16] Because portal perfusion of the liver is maintained after the non-shunt procedures, hepatic function is preserved.[5]

## SUMMARY OF NON-SHUNT PROCEDURES

| | Sugiura (2 Stages) | Hassab | Esophageal Transection with Stapling |
|---|---|---|---|
| **Position** | Supine, left side elevated | Supine | ⇐ |
| **Incision** | Abdominal stage: midline; thoracic stage: left thoracotomy | Vertical midline | ⇐ |
| **Special instrumentation** | Self-retaining retractor | ⇐ | ⇐ |
| **Unique considerations** | None | ⇐ | ⇐ |
| **Antibiotics** | Cefazolin 1 gm iv | ⇐ | ⇐ |
| **Surgical time** | 4 - 6 hrs for both stages | 4 hrs | ⇐ |
| **EBL** | 1000-2000 cc | ⇐ | ⇐ |
| **Postop care** | ICU; careful hemodynamic monitoring; PA catheterization | ⇐ | ⇐ |
| **Mortality**[5,12-15,19] | Overall: 5-14% | | 10-83% |
| | Emergent: 14% (≤ 60%) | 12-38% | |
| | Elective: 3% | 10% | |
| **Morbidity**[1,5,12-15,19] | Recurrent hemorrhage: 2-50% | 7% | 0-50% |
| | Esophagopleural leak: 6% | – | 3% |
| | Encephalopathy: 3% | 1-25% | 33% |
| | Ascites: 2% | 4% | 11% |
| | Wound infection: 2% | – | 11% |
| **Procedure code** | 43401 | ⇐ | ⇐ |
| **Pain score** | 6 | 5 | 5 |

## PATIENT POPULATION CHARACTERISTICS[8,14,17,19]

**Age range** 11-72 yrs (mean age = 48 yrs); depending on etiology: pediatric (e.g., congenital hepatic fibrosis) to adult (e.g., alcoholic liver disease)

**Male:Female** 2-8:1

**Incidence** Rare

**Etiology**
Alcoholic liver disease (alcoholic hepatitis, chronic alcoholism, cirrhosis)
Postnecrotic cirrhosis
Portal vein thrombosis
Splenic vein occlusion
Hematologic diseases
Hepatic vein occlusion
Schistosomiasis
Congenital hepatic fibrosis
Sarcoidosis
Sinusoidal occlusion (vitamin A toxicity, Gaucher's disease)
Veno-occlusive disease

**Associated conditions**
Alcohol dependency
Cirrhosis/liver failure
Poor nutritional status
Coagulopathy
Encephalopathy

## ANESTHETIC CONSIDERATIONS

**(Procedures covered: shunt and non-shunt procedures for portal hypertension surgery)**

### PREOPERATIVE

**Respiratory** Hypoxemia may be present 2° ascites, V/Q mismatch, ↑R → L pulmonary shunting, atelectasis, pulmonary infections and ↓pulmonary diffusing capacity.
**Tests:** ABG; PFTs, as indicated; CXR

**Cardiovascular** Patients presenting with portal HTN often have a hyperdynamic circulatory state with ↑plasma volume, ↑CO and ↓SVR with a decreased ability to ↑SVR or ↑HR in response to stimuli. Ventricular performance may be abnormal (CHF) especially in patients with alcoholic liver disease. Ascites → ↑intrathoracic pressure, ↓FRC, ↓venous return and ↓CO. Older patients in this population usually have CAD.
**Tests:** ECG. If LV function in question, ECHO or angiography.

**Hepatic** The physical manifestations of hepatic disease include palmar erythema, caput medusae, spider angiomas and gynecomastia. Albumin and other products of liver synthesis (e.g., coagulation factors) may be decreased. Encephalopathy may be present as a result of impaired ammonia metabolism.
**Tests:** Bilirubin; albumin; PT; SGOT; SGPT; ammonia; alk pos

**Gastrointestinal** Portal HTN eventually results in esophageal and gastric varices. Patients may present emergently with profuse GI bleeding. Ascites occurs in approximately 80% of patients with portal HTN and splenomegaly is invariably present. As a result of elevated intra-abdominal pressure from ascites, and slow gastric emptying, a rapid-sequence induction with full-stomach precautions will be necessary.

**Renal** Portal HTN → ↓GFR and ↓renal blood flow → renal failure.
**Tests:** UA; creatinine clearance as indicated from H&P

**Hematologic** These patients are often anemic as a result of poor nutrition, malabsorption, and intestinal tract blood loss. Hypersplenism may be present (platelet count < 50,000 and WBC < 2,000). Synthesis of all coagulation factors is decreased except factor VIII and fibrinogen. A low-grade DIC may be present. Cross-match for 8-10 U PRBC.
**Tests:** CBC; platelet count; bleeding time; PT; PTT; DIC screen

**Pharmacologic** The liver is the major site of drug biotransformation; however, the effects of hepatic dysfunction on drug elimination and disposition are inconsistent.

**Laboratory** These patients may have significant electrolyte disturbances (e.g., ↓↓$Na^+$, ↓$K^+$).
**Tests:** Electrolytes and others as indicated from H&P.

**Premedication** If premedication is appropriate, small doses of anxiolytic such as midazolam (0.5-1 mg iv) are preferable. Avoid im medications in patients with possible coagulopathy. Full-stomach precautions are necessary. Metoclopramide (10 mg iv) and ranitidine (50 mg iv) may be given 60 min before surgery.

### INTRAOPERATIVE

**Anesthetic technique:** GETA. Preservation of intravascular volume and myocardial stability can be a challenge in these patients.

**Induction** Rapid-sequence induction with STP (3-5 mg/kg) and succinylcholine (1-2 mg/kg) should be used. Replace blood loss and ensure normovolemia before induction (if possible). Etomidate (0.2 mg/kg) or ketamine (1 mg/kg) may be preferable for induction in hemodynamically unstable patients.

**Maintenance** High-dose narcotic technique with fentanyl (50-100 μg/kg) or sufentanil (10-15 μg/kg) and low-dose isoflurane. Midazolam (0.1-0.2 mg/kg) is often given in conjunction with the narcotic to ensure amnesia during times of hemodynamic instability when isoflurane cannot be tolerated. $N_2O$ is avoided to prevent bowel distention. Muscle relaxation is needed (e.g., vecuronium 0.1 mg/kg or less, titrated using a nerve stimulator).
**NB:** After drainage of ascitic fluid there may be a precipitous drop in BP requiring rapid volume replacement ± vasopressor.

**Emergence** Generally deferred to ICU due to large fluid shifts and transfusion requirements. Patients who have undergone uneventful and nonemergent surgery may be candidates for extubation.

| | | |
|---|---|---|
| **Blood and fluid requirements** | IV: 14 ga x 2 or 7.0 Fr x 2<br>Anticipate large blood loss.<br>Rapid infuser<br>RBC salvage device<br>8-10 U PRBC<br>Warm all fluids.<br>Humidify all gasses.<br>Warming blanket<br>Bair-Hugger®-type warmer | FFP, platelets and cryo should be available to treat coagulopathy. |
| **Monitoring** | Standard monitors (see Appendix).<br>Arterial line<br>CVP or PA catheter<br>UO | Arterial and central pressure monitoring are essential.<br>A PA catheter is useful in this setting because most patients are cirrhotic and may have excessive blood loss and large fluid shifts.<br>In these procedures, prevention of hypothermia is important. UO is measured and is helpful as a monitor of renal perfusion. Mannitol (0.25-1 gm/kg iv) may be needed to maintain UO.<br>In patients with large varices, avoid esophageal placement of temperature probes or stethoscopes. |
| | ABGs | Serial ABGs to determine adequacy of ventilation and normal acid base status should be done.<br>Hct, coagulation slides and $Ca^{++}$ should be measured following replacement of large blood volumes. |
| | Electrolytes<br>Blood glucose | Electrolytes and glucose also should be monitored. Glucose metabolism in liver disease may be impaired → ↓glucose. |
| **Positioning** | ✓ and pad pressure points.<br>✓ eyes. | |
| **Complications** | Coagulopathy<br>Hemorrhage<br>Hypothermia | |

## POSTOPERATIVE

| | | |
|---|---|---|
| **Complications** | Coagulopathy<br>Hypothermia<br>Encephalopathy<br>Renal failure | |
| **Pain management** | PCA (see Appendix).<br>Parenteral opiates | |
| **Tests** | CXR: line placement<br>Hct<br>Electrolytes<br>Glucose | DIC screen, if continued bleeding. |


**References**

1. Johansen K, Helton WS: Portal hypertension and bleeding esophageal varices. *Ann Vasc Surg* 1992; 6(6):553-61.
2. Smith GW, Cameron JL, Malt RA, Turcotte JG: Total portosystemic shunts. In *Vascular Surg*ery, 3rd edition. Rutherford RB, ed. WB Saunders Co, Philadelphia: 1989, 1155-72.
3. Smith GW: The surgical management of portal hypertension. In *Vascular Surgery*, 3rd edition. Rutherford RB, ed. WB Saunders Co, Philadelphia: 1989, 1116-22.
4. Van Stiegmann G: Selective shunts. In *Vascular Surgery*, 3rd edition. Rutherford RB, ed. WB Saunders Co, Philadelphia: 1989, 1173-82.
5. Collini FJ, Brener B: Portal hypertension. *Surg Gynecol Obstet* 1990; 170(2):177-92.
6. Rikkers LF: New concepts of pathophysiology and treatment of portal hypertension. *Surgery* 1990; 107(5):481-88.

7. Langer B, Taylor BR, Greig PD: Selective or total shunts for variceal bleeding. *Am J Surg* 1990; 160(1):75-9.
8. Levine BA, Sirinek KR:The portacaval shunt. Is it still indicated? *Surg Clin North Am* 1990; 70(2):361-78.
9. Henderson JM: The distal splenoral shunt. *Surg Clin North Am* 1990; 70(2):405-23.
10. Henderson JM, Millikan WJ Jr, Galloway JR: The Emory perspective of the distal splenorenal shunt in 1990. *Am J Surg* 1990; 160(1):54-9.
11. Terblanche J: Emergency management of variceal hemorrhage. In *Vascular Surgery*, 3rd edition. Rutherford RB, ed. WB Saunders Co, Philadelphia: 1989, 1136-45.
12. Orozco H, Mercado MA, Takahashi T, Hernandez-Ortiz J, Capellan JF, Garcia-Tsao G: Elective treatment of bleeding varices with the Sugiura operation over 10 years. *Am J Surg* 1992; 163(6):585-89.
13. Hassab MA: Nonshunt operations in portal hypertension without cirrhosis. *Surg Gynecol Obstet* 1970; 131(4):648-54.
14. Huizinga WK, Angorn IB, Baker LW: Esophageal transection versus injection sclerotherapy in the management of bleeding esophageal varices in patients at high risk. *Surg Gynecol Obstet* 1985; 160(6):539-46.
15. Hoffmann J: Stapler transection of the oesophagus for bleeding oesophageal varices. *Scand J Gastroenterol* 1983; 18(6):707-11.
16. Takasaki T, Kobayashi S, Muto H, Suzuki S, Harada M, Nakayama K: Transabdominal esophageal transection by using a suture device in cases of esophageal varices. *Int Surg* 1977; 62(8):426-28.
17. Smith GW: Use of hemodynamic selection criteria in the management of cirrhotic patients with portal hypertension. *Ann Surg* 1974; 179(5):782-90.
18. Turcotte JG, Lambert MJ III: Variceal hemorrhage, hepatic cirrhosis, and portacaval shunts. *Surgery* 1973; 73(6):810-17.
19. Bothe A: Portal hypertension: Nonshunting procedures. In *Current Surgical Therapy*, 4th edition. Cameron JL, ed. Mosby Year Book, St Louis: 1992, 302-5.
20. Smith GW: The Surgical management of portal hypertension. In *Vascular Surgery*, 3rd edition. WB Saunders Co, Philadelphia: 1989, 1116-22.
21. Turcolte: Variceal hemorrhage, hepatic cirrhosis and portocaval shunts. *Surgery* 1973; 73:810-17.
22. Haberer Jp, Schoeffler P, Couderc E, Duraldestin P: Fentanyl pharmacokinetics in anesthetized patients with cirrhosis. *Br J Anaesth* 1982; 54:1267.
23. Gelman S, Fowler KC, Smith: Liver circulation and function during isoflurane and halothane anesthesia. *Anesthesiology* 1984; 6:726.

# ARTERIOVENOUS ACCESS FOR HEMODIALYSIS

## SURGICAL CONSIDERATIONS

**Description: Peripheral subcutaneous arteriovenous (AV) fistula**, or **prosthetic graft**, is the current procedure of choice for patients requiring permanent hemodialysis access.[1-3] The blood flow in the autogenous AV fistula increases with time, and the resulting vein wall thickening prevents venous tears and infiltration during dialysis.

The standard AV fistula is usually constructed by anastomosing the cephalic vein to the radial artery at the wrist level (**Brescia-Cimino** fistula). Other locations include the "snuff box," or antebrachium. Vascular access using vascular substitutes or prosthetic grafts is performed when there is a lack of suitable veins in patients who have had failed access procedures, peripheral vein sclerosis, or severe arterial disease involving the upper extremity. Forearm grafts are constructed as a direct communication between the radial or ulnar artery and the antecubital or brachial vein, or as a "loop" between the brachial artery and these veins. Similarly, an access can be constructed in the upper arm as a communication between the brachial artery above the elbow and the basilic or axillary vein in a straight fashion.[1] The polytetrafluoroethylene (Teflon®) graft has become the mainstay for hemodialysis access in patients who are not candidates for Brescia-Cimino fistula placement. These grafts are associated with a primary patency rate of 50-60% at 2-3 years.[2,3]

**Variant procedure or approaches: Forearm AV fistula** (Brescia-Cimino fistula), **loop or straight shunt** using vascular substitute in forearm, and **upper arm straight shunt**

**Usual preop diagnosis:** End-stage renal failure requiring hemodialysis

## SUMMARY OF PROCEDURE

| | Forearm AV Fistula | Forearm Loop or Straight Graft | Upper Arm Straight Graft |
|---|---|---|---|
| **Position** | Supine, arm abducted | ⇐ | ⇐ |
| **Incision** | Longitudinal or transverse at wrist or "snuff box" | Transverse at antecubital fossa and/or at wrist; counterincision in forearm | Transverse or longitudinal in upper arm |
| **Special instrumentation** | Arm/hand table (for arm abduction); Doppler flow probe may be used. | ⇐ | ⇐ |
| **Unique considerations** | Local anesthesia; consider brachial plexus block (increased incidence of hematoma); heparinization | ⇐ | ⇐ |
| **Antibiotics** | None | Vancomycin 1 gm iv | ⇐ |
| **Surgical time** | 1 - 2 hrs | ⇐ | ⇐ |
| **Closing considerations** | Use of Doppler to ✓ shunt patency | ⇐ | ⇐ |
| **EBL** | 25-50 cc | 25-100 cc | ⇐ |
| **Postop care** | Hemodynamic monitoring for poor-risk patients; can be done as outpatient. | ⇐ | ⇐ |
| **Mortality**[1-3] | Minimal, depending on associated risk factors | ⇐ | ⇐ |
| **Morbidity**[1-3] | Thrombosis: 20% | 8-32% | ~8-32% |
| | Technical failure: 10-15% | ⇐ | ⇐ |
| | Arterial steal: Rare | Similar | ⇐ |
| | Cardiac failure: Rare | Similar | ⇐ |
| | Infection: Rare | 10% | ⇐ |
| | No-venous-outflow: Rare | 6% | ~6% |
| | Seroma: Rare | ⇐ | ⇐ |
| | Venous aneurysm: Rare | ⇐ | ⇐ |
| | Venous HTN: Rare | Similar | ⇐ |
| **Procedure code** | 36820 | 36830 | ⇐ |
| **Pain score** | 1 | 2 | 2 |

## PATIENT POPULATION CHARACTERISTICS

| | |
|---|---|
| **Age range** | Pediatric and adult population (mean age = 56 yrs in one series) |
| **Male:Female** | 1:1 |
| **Incidence** | Hemodialysis access is one of the most commonly performed procedures by vascular surgeons. |
| **Etiology** | Glomerulonephritis<br>Diabetes<br>HTN<br>Pyelonephritis |
| **Associated conditions** | Diabetes mellitus<br>Peripheral vascular disease/CAD |

## ANESTHETIC CONSIDERATIONS

See Anesthetic Considerations following "Permanent Vascular Access" (below).

**References**

1. Haimov M: Circulatory access for hemodialysis. In *Vascular Surgery*, 3rd edition. Rutherford RB, ed. WB Saunders Co, Philadelphia: 1989, 1073-85.
2. Hill SL, Donato AT: Complications of dialysis access: a six-year study. *Am J Surg* 1991; 162(3):265-67.
3. Schuman ES, Gross GF, Hayes JF, Standage BA: Long-term patency of polytetrafluoroethylene graft fistulas. *Am J Surg* 1988; 155(5):644-46.

# PERMANENT VASCULAR ACCESS

## SURGICAL CONSIDERATIONS

**Description**: Silastic® or plastic catheters are placed in patients who require venous access for chronic antibiotic therapy, TPN, chemotherapy or hemodialysis.[1-6] **Hickman**, **Broviac** and **Groshong catheters** are made of silicone rubber or plastic with a cuff near the skin exit site. In theory, these cuffs serve as barriers to infection. Access is generally achieved via subclavian, IJ or femoral vein puncture. These catheters are available in various sizes and in single- or double-lumen configurations. Larger diameter (13 Fr) Hickman or Permacath® DL catheters have been introduced for hemodialysis.[1-3] **Mediport® and Portacath® devices** have a metallic or plastic reservoir connected to the catheters and are intended for complete subcutaneous implantation. These catheters are used in chronically ill patients, particularly those requiring chemotherapy. The implantable access ports have been associated with improved patient comfort and reduced infection rates.[4] Long-term catheter survival is limited by infection. Removal and replacement of the catheter is the only way to eradicate the infection.

**Variant procedure or approaches**: Two major distinctions: Hickman/Broviac catheters (no reservoir) vs Mediport®/Portacath® catheters (subcutaneous with reservoir). Subclavian, IJ or femoral vein puncture, depending on vein status, previous operations and patient comfort.

**Usual preop diagnosis**: Chronic antibiotic therapy; TPN; chemotherapy; end-stage renal failure

### SUMMARY OF PROCEDURE

| | Hickman/Broviac/Groshong | Mediport®/Portacath® |
|---|---|---|
| **Position** | Supine, slight Trendelenburg | ⇐ |
| **Incision** | Puncture site (subclavian, IJ or femoral vein); subcutaneous tunnel for passage of catheter. Alternative: cephalic or IJ vein cutdown to achieve access.[7] | Puncture site (subclavian, IJ or femoral vein); subcutaneous pocket for port. Alternative: cephalic or IJ vein cutdown to achieve access.[7] |
| **Special instrumentation** | Image intensifier or fluoroscope | ⇐ |
| **Unique considerations** | Local anesthesia; may need iv sedation; monitor for ectopy during placement. | ⇐ |
| **Antibiotics** | Usually none; consider cefazolin 1 gm iv. | ⇐ |
| **Surgical time** | 30 - 90 min | 45 - 90 min |
| **EBL** | 10-25 cc | 25-50 cc |
| **Postop care** | CXR in recovery room; may be outpatient. | ⇐ |
| **Mortality**[1,2] | Minimal | ⇐ |
| **Morbidity**[1-4,6] | Catheter thrombosis: 25% | 4% |
| | Skin exit site infection: 13% | – |
| | Poor flow: 10-13% | ~10-13% |
| | Catheter sepsis: 5-8% | 2% |
| | Arterial puncture: 6% | ~6% |
| | Local bleeding: 5% | – |
| | SVC thrombosis: 5% | ~5% |

| | | |
|---|---|---|
| **Morbidity, continued** | Catheter displacement: 3% | ~3% |
| | Subclavian thrombosis: 2% | ~2% |
| | Pneumothorax 1-2% | ~1-2% |
| | Failed attempt: 1% | ~1% |
| | Infection: 3-5/1000 cath days | – |
| | | Pocket hematoma: 2% |
| | | Pocket infection: 3% |
| | | Catheter leakage: 1% |
| **Procedure code** | 36533 | ⇐ |
| **Pain score** | 1 | 2 |

### PATIENT POPULATION CHARACTERISTICS

| | |
|---|---|
| **Age range** | Pediatrics and adults, 8-80 yrs |
| **Male:Female** | 1:1 |
| **Incidence** | Depending on underlying disease |
| **Etiology** | Access for chemotherapy<br>Infections<br>Hemodialysis<br>Chronic TPN |
| **Associated conditions** | Malignancy<br>Chronic illness/infection<br>Renal failure |

---

## ANESTHETIC CONSIDERATIONS FOR VASCULAR ACCESS

**(Procedures covered: vascular access; arteriovenous access for hemodialysis)**

### PREOPERATIVE

The patient populations presenting for vascular access surgery are extremely diverse. Patients requiring vascular access for chemotherapy, TPN and chronic antibiotic therapy frequently can be done with MAC (see Appendix). Also presenting for these procedures are end-stage renal failure patients who need arteriovenous access for hemodialysis (generally involving the upper extremity). These patients return to the OR frequently for revising or replacing of fistulas. They are often ASA III & IV patients who may require GA or an upper extremity block. Anesthetic considerations for the chronic renal patient are discussed below.

| | |
|---|---|
| **Respiratory** | Pulmonary edema may be present from fluid overload. CHF and uremic pleuritis can occur. Pneumonias occur more frequently in these patients due to depressed immune systems. Hemodialysis contributes to hypoxemia due to V/Q mismatch and hypoventilation.<br>**Tests:** CXR; ABG. Consider PFTs. |
| **Cardiovascular** | Often have HTN related to hypervolemia and a disorder of the renin-antiogensin system. May have LVH 2° to HTN. Cardiomyopathy, pericarditis and pericardial effusion occur with uremia. Hypervolemia and hypoalbuminemia can contribute to CHF. Uremic patients often have defective aortic and carotid body reflex arcs. Ejection murmurs are common.<br>**Tests:** ECG; others as indicated from H&P. |
| **Renal** | A comprehensive preop evaluation should include an assessment of renal function and adequacy of recent dialysis therapy. Ascertaining the patient's usual and recent weights is useful. Dialysis is usually advisable shortly before anesthesia and surgery. The symptoms of uremia (Plt dysfunction, electrolyte/fluid abnormalities, CNS and GI disturbances) improve with dialysis. If a transfusion is needed, it is best done during dialysis so intravascular volume can be controlled.<br>**Tests:** Serum BUN; creatinine. If patient produces urine, consider creatinine clearance, UA. |
| **Hematologic-coagulation** | Chronic anemia with Hct ranging from 15-21 g/dL. Normochromic, normocytic anemia present due to bone marrow depression, lack of erythropoietin, nutritional deficiency and diminished red-cell survival time. Patients adjust to chronic anemia through ↑CO and ↑1,3 DPG levels. Accumulation of waste products inhibit Plt function. Defects do occur in the coagulation cascade, but PT and PTT are usually normal.<br>**Tests:** CBC; Plt; PT; PTT; bleeding time |

| | |
|---|---|
| **Gastrointestinal** | Uremic patients commonly have hiccups, anorexia, N&V and diarrhea. They are very prone to developing GI bleeds. Renal failure causes ↓gastric emptying. Premedication with metoclopramide (10 mg po) and ranitidine (150 mg po) will ↓gastric volume and pH. |
| **Nervous system** | CNS Sx of uremia range from malaise to seizures to coma. Fatigue and intellectual impairment commonly occur. Peripheral and autonomic neuropathies exist. Peripheral neuropathy presents as itching and paresthesias of the lower extremities. Autonomic dysfunction can cause postural hypotension. Document deficits carefully. |
| **Endocrine** | Diabetes frequently may be the cause of renal failure, with its attendant problems. **Tests:** Glucose |
| **Immune system** | Often depressed. Patients prone to sepsis. Hepatitis B and HIV infections from blood products may exist. |
| **Metabolic and biochemical** | Accumulation of potassium, urea, parathyroid hormone (hypercalcemia), magnesium, aluminum (neurotoxicity), acid metabolites and phosphate occurs. Knowing hyperkalemia exists is of importance because of the potential for fatal cardiac dysrhythmias. Shift of the oxyhemoglobin curve to the right occurs due to the metabolic acidosis and increased 2,3 DPG (improves tissue oxygenation). Hyponatremia is a common electrolyte disturbance in chronic renal failure. |
| **Premedication** | If warranted, it is best to use light premedication with sedatives or opioids due to the possibility of exaggerated effects. (See Appendix.) |

## INTRAOPERATIVE

**Anesthetic technique:** GA, upper extremity block or MAC.

**Regional anesthesia:** May be advantageous due to decreased number of drug effects. See section on upper extremity blocks (see Anesthetic Considerations following "Dorsal Stabilization and Extensor Synovectomy of the Rheumatoid Wrist"). If the patient was very recently dialyzed, there may be a residual heparin effect. Regional anesthesia is contraindicated if coagulopathy is present.

**General anesthesia:** The duration of action and elimination of many anesthetic drugs is altered in the patient with renal failure.

| | |
|---|---|
| **Induction** | Renal failure reduces protein binding; therefore, highly protein-bound drugs may produce prolonged and exaggerated effects. Acidemia increases the proportion of agent existing in the nonionized, unbound state, which increases its availability to effector sites (e.g., brain). In addition, renal failure patients require a lower dose of STP for induction due to the increased permeability of the blood-brain barrier 2° uremia. Because ketamine and benzodiazepines are less heavily protein-bound than barbiturates, the induction dose does not need to be decreased as much. Ketamine may exaggerate pre-existing HTN. Succinylcholine is not associated with greater than normal increases in potassium in renal-failure patients. It should be avoided, however, if the $K^+$ >5.5 mEq/L. Repeated doses of succinylcholine do not prolong muscle relaxation, since serum cholinesterase levels are normal in renal failure. Non-depolarizing muscle relaxants such as pancuronium and d-tubocurarine have delayed excretion and increased duration of action. Atracurium elimination is not significantly affected in renal failure. Similarly, vecuronium does not have a significantly increased duration of action. |
| **Maintenance** | Inhalation anesthesia offers the advantage of not being renally eliminated. Biotransformation may produce some inorganic fluoride (nephrotoxin); however, this is not an issue in dialysis patients. There is less fluoride released with halothane than isoflurane, but because of myocardial depression with halothane, isoflurane may be a better choice of inhalation anesthesia. Opioids can produce an increased magnitude and duration of effect. Increased accumulation of morphine glucuronides → prolonged respiratory depression. An accumulated metabolite of meperidine (normeperidine) can cause seizures. Fentanyl is a good choice, due to its rapid tissue redistribution. |
| **Emergence** | Prolonged effect of anticholinesterases (e.g., neostigmine and edrophonium) effectively offsets prolongation of blockade. Other factors affecting reversal of non-depolarizers should be taken into account. These include acid-base status, depth of blockade, temperature and use of drugs such as diuretics or antibiotics, which can potentiate blockade. |

| | | |
|---|---|---|
| **Blood and fluid requirements** | IV: 18-20 ga x 1<br>NS @ 1-2 cc/kg/hr | IV access may be difficult; avoid iv placement in operated arm. Minimize fluids in renal-failure patients. |
| **Monitoring** | Standard monitors (see Appendix). | Avoid BP cuff placement on operated arm. |

| | | |
|---|---|---|
| **Positioning** | √ and pad pressure points.<br>√ eyes. | |
| **Complications** | Local anesthetic toxicity | See section on axillary blocks in Appendix. |

### POSTOPERATIVE

| | | |
|---|---|---|
| **Complications** | Nerve damage<br>Hematoma | These are rare complications of brachial plexus blocks. |
| **Pain management** | PO analgesics | |

**References**


1. Gibson SP, Mosquera D: Five years' experience with the Quinton Permcath for vascular access. *Nephrol Dial Transplant* 1991; 6(4):269-74.
2. Wisborg T, Flaatten H, Koller ME: Percutaneous placement of permanent central venous catheters: experience with 200 catheters. *Acta Anaesthesiol Scand* 1991; 35(1):49-51.
3. Donnelly PK, Hoenich NA, Lennard TW, Proud G, Taylor RM: Surgical management of long-term central venous access in uraemic patients. *Nephrol Dial Transplant* 1988; 3(1):57-65.
4. Franceschi D, Specht MA, Farrell C: Implantable venous access device. *J Cardiovasc Surg* 1989; 30(1):124-29.
5. Silberman H, Berne TV, Escandon R: Prospective evaluation of a double-lumen subclavian dialysis catheter for acute vascular access. *Am Surg* 1992; 58:443-45.
6. Bour ES, Weaver AS, Yang HC, Gifford RR: Experience with the double lumen Silastic catheter for hemoaccess. *Surg Gynecol Obstet* 1990; 171(1): 33-9.
7. Chuter T, Starker PM: Placement of Hickman-Broviac catheters in the cephalic vein. *Surg Gynecol Obstet* 1988; 166(2):163-64.
8. Kaufman BS, Contreras J: Preanesthetic assessment of the patient with renal disease. *Anesth Clin North Am* 1990; 8:677.
9. Ghoneim MM, Pandya H: Plasma protein binding of thiopental in patients with impaired renal or hepatic function. *Anesthesiology* 1975; 42:545.
10. Don HF, Dieppa RA, Taylor P: Narcotic analgesics in anuric patients. *Anesthesiology* 1975; 42:745.
11. Bastron RD: Anesthetic considerations for patients with end-stage renal disease. In *Refresher Course in Anesthesiology*. Barash PG, eds. JB Lippincott, Philadelphia: 1985, 13.
12. Gibson TP: Renal disease and drug metabolism: an overview. *Am J Kidney Dis* 1986; 8:17.
13. Mazze RI, Calverley RK, Smith NT: Inorganic fluoride nephrotoxicity: prolonged enflurane and halothane anesthesia in volunteers. *Anesthesiology* 1977; 46:1265.


# VENOUS SURGERY – VEIN STRIPPING AND PERFORATOR LIGATION

## SURGICAL CONSIDERATIONS

**Description**: Chronic venous insufficiency results from static blood flow in the deep, superficial and perforating veins of the lower extremity.[3] Clinical manifestations include pathologic changes in the skin and subcutaneous tissues, such as pigmentation, dermatitis, induration and ulceration around the lower portion of the leg.[1,3] The condition is most commonly caused by defective venous valves, and less often by obstruction to the venous return or impaired pumping action of the muscles in the leg.[3] The disorder is sometimes the residual of previous iliofemoral thrombophlebitis. Varicose veins of the primary type, particularly those of long duration, are a common cause of chronic venous insufficiency of milder degrees.[3] Most symptoms respond well to conservative management, which includes compression stockings, elevation of the extremity and topical treatment of ulcerations. Failure of medical management is an indication for surgical intervention. Split-thickness skin grafting is indicated for large ulcers to accelerate healing and shorten hospitalization time.[1,3] **Ligation of perforators** is best performed when the ulcer has completely healed. The classic approach of **Linton** is rarely used today. If the quality of the skin overlying the perforators prevents a direct approach, **subfascial ligation** of the perforators may be performed through a short, posterior midline incision.[9] The incompetent greater or lesser saphenous veins are resected only if patency of the deep system is confirmed. Venous ulcers recur in 30% of patients after surgical therapy, and ulcerations persist for prolonged period in 15% of patients.[1] Adjunctive procedures include: **valvuloplasty**, **vein transposition** and **venous valve transplant**.[9,10]

**Usual preop diagnosis**: Chronic deep venous insufficiency

### SUMMARY OF PROCEDURE

| | |
|---|---|
| **Position** | Supine |
| **Incision** | **Vein stripping:** longitudinal or oblique groin incision and transverse incision at medial malleolus; transverse incision over posterior lower leg for lesser saphenous vein stripping. **Perforator ligation:** longitudinal incision along medial aspect of tibia to posterior medial malleolus. |
| **Special instrumentation** | Vein stripper |
| **Antibiotics** | If patient has an associated venous ulcer, preop antibiotics should be based on culture results; cefazolin 1 gm iv generally, if culture results are not available. |
| **Surgical time** | 3 hrs |
| **Closing considerations** | None |
| **EBL** | 50-250 cc |
| **Postop care** | PACU → ward; anti-embolism stockings and SCDs |
| **Mortality** | Minimal |
| **Morbidity**[3,9] | Persistence of non-healing ulcer: 20-53% |
| **Procedure code** | 37700 |
| **Pain score** | 3 |

### PATIENT POPULATION CHARACTERISTICS

| | |
|---|---|
| **Age range** | Young adult-elderly (generally older adults, although present in younger patients as well). |
| **Male:Female** | 1:2 |
| **Incidence** | 6-7 million people in U.S. have adverse effects from chronic venous stasis;[3] 500,000 have complications of leg ulceration. |
| **Etiology** | Chronic primary varicose veins<br>Defective venous valves<br>Impaired pumping action of muscles in leg<br>Previous iliofemoral thrombophlebitis<br>Obstruction of venous return |
| **Associated conditions** | Varicose veins<br>History of DVT/thrombophlebitis |

## ANESTHETIC CONSIDERATIONS

See Anesthetic Considerations following "Venous Surgery – Varicose Vein Stripping" (below).

**References**

See references for "Venous Surgery – Thrombectomy or Vein Excision."

# VENOUS SURGERY — VARICOSE VEIN STRIPPING

## SURGICAL CONSIDERATIONS

**Description**: In patients with primary varicose veins, no definite cause has been identified, although age, female sex, pregnancy, obesity and positive family history are predisposing factors.[1,2] The causes of secondary varicosity include incompetence or obstruction of the deep veins as a result of previous DVT, tumor, trauma or congenital or acquired arteriovenous fistulas.[1] Usual indications for operative therapy include aching, swelling, heaviness, cramps, itching, cosmesis, stasis dermatitis, pigmentation, burning and ulcers.[1-5] Surgical treatment is contraindicated in: pregnant patients; elderly patients who are considered high risk; and patients with arterial insufficiency of the lower extremities, lymphedema, skin infection or coagulopathy.[1,3]

There are two principal approaches: the **stab avulsion technique** and **high ligation and stripping**.[5,6] With **stab avulsion**, the varicosities are marked preop. Small transverse or longitudinal incisions are made directly over these varicosities, which are dissected from the surrounding subcutaneous tissue (with undermining of the skin) and bluntly removed or avulsed. Firm pressure over the region being operated on will achieve hemostasis. After removal of all marked varicosities, sterile dressings are placed and a compression bandage wrapped around the affected leg. The patient is instructed to keep the leg elevated as much as possible while convalescing at home. The chief advantage of the stab avulsion technique is preservation of the saphenous vein when it is not directly involved with varicosities.

If there is valvular incompetence of the saphenous vein, the treatment of choice is **stripping (avulsion)** of the incompetent portion of the greater and lesser saphenous veins, together with avulsion of the superficial varicose veins of the thigh and calf.[1] **High ligation and stripping** refers to the removal of the greater saphenous vein from the level of medial malleolus to the saphenofemoral junction. A small transverse incision is made at the level of the ankle and the saphenous vein is dissected free. A longitudinal or oblique incision at the groin permits isolation of the saphenous vein at the saphenofemoral junction. The greater saphenous vein is ligated proximally and distally. After a **venotomy**, a plastic or metallic vein stripper is passed and the vein is removed or stripped in a distal-to-proximal fashion. Sterile dressings are applied, followed by a compressive dressing.

If all varicose veins are removed and the incompetent segment of the saphenous vein is stripped, 85% of the patients will have good-to-excellent results at late follow-up.[1] These procedures can be performed with regional or GA.

**Usual preop diagnosis**: Varicose veins; symptoms of venous insufficiency; cosmetic considerations

### SUMMARY OF PROCEDURE

| | Stab Avulsion Technique | High Ligation and Stripping |
|---|---|---|
| **Position** | Supine | ⇐ |
| **Incision** | Varicosities marked preop; short stab incisions made and veins avulsed with small forceps. | Varicosities marked preop; small transverse incision over saphenous vein proximal to medial malleolus; proximal saphenous vein exposed via groin incisions and stripper passed. |
| **Special instrumentation** | None | Vein stripper |
| **Unique considerations** | May be facilitated by tourniquet. | ⇐ |
| **Antibiotics** | None | ⇐ |
| **Surgical time** | 2 - 3 hrs | ⇐ |
| **Closing considerations** | Leg compressed with elastic wrap | ⇐ |
| **EBL** | 50-250 cc | 50-150 cc |
| **Postop care** | PACU → ward; support stockings | ⇐ + Elevate foot of bed 10°; short periods of ambulation |
| **Mortality** | Minimal | ⇐ |
| **Morbidity**[6,7] | Recurrence: < 10% | ⇐ |
| | Hematoma: Rare | ⇐ |
| | Infection: Rare | ⇐ |
| | Postop DVT: Rare | 5% |
| | Nerve injury: Rare | ⇐ |

| | Stab Avulsion Technique | High Ligation and Stripping |
|---|---|---|
| **Morbidity, continued** | Lymph fistula: Rare | ⇐ |
| | Femoral artery injury: Nil | Very rare |
| **Procedure code** | 37720/37730 | ⇐ |
| **Pain score** | 2 | 2 |

### PATIENT POPULATION CHARACTERISTICS

**Age range** Wide range, young adult-elderly (average = 48 yrs)

**Male:Female** 1:3

**Incidence** 24,000,000 in U.S.

**Etiology** Primary varicose veins: no definite cause (predisposing factors include age, female sex, pregnancy, obesity and positive family Hx)
Secondary varicose veins: incompetence or obstruction of the deep veins from DVT, tumor, trauma or high venous pressures due to congenital or acquired arteriovenous fistulas

**Associated conditions** Older age
Pregnancy
Obesity
DVT
Tumor
Trauma

---

## ANESTHETIC CONSIDERATIONS

**(Procedures covered: varicose vein stripping; vein stripping and perforator ligation)**

### PREOPERATIVE

Patients presenting for varicose vein surgery are a generally healthy patient population (ASA I & II). Preop considerations and tests, therefore, should be guided by the H&P.

**Hematologic** If regional anesthesia planned, check patient's coagulation status.
**Tests:** Platelet count; CBC with differential; PT; PTT; bleeding time (if on ASA, NSAIDs or dipyridamole (Persantine®)

**Laboratory** UA; other tests as indicated from H&P.

**Premedication** If necessary, standard premedication (see Appendix).

### INTRAOPERATIVE

**Anesthetic technique:** General, regional or local anesthesia ± sedation are all appropriate anesthetic techniques. Choice depends on factors such as extent of surgery, patient physical status and patient and surgeon preference.

**Regional anesthesia:**

**Spinal** Single-shot vs continuous: Patient in sitting or lateral decubitus position (operative site down) for placement of hyperbaric subarachnoid block. Doses of local anesthetics are as follows for T10-T12 level: 5% lidocaine in 7.5% dextrose 50-75 mg; 0.75% bupivacaine in 8% dextrose 7-10 mg; 0.5% tetracaine in 5% dextrose 10-12 mg. For continuous spinal, titrate local anesthetic to desired surgical level (T12). Large doses of hyperbaric local anesthetic should be avoided as they can cause postop cauda equina syndrome.

**Epidural** Patient in sitting or lateral decubitus position for placement of epidural catheter. After locating the epidural space, administer a test dose (e.g., 3 ml of 1.5% lidocaine with 1:200,000 epinephrine) to elucidate whether the catheter is subarachnoid or intravascular. Titrate local anesthetic until desired surgical level is obtained (3-5 ml at a time) usually < 15 ml.

**Local** Requires gentle surgical technique. Surgical field block, plus ilioinguinal and iliohypogastric nerve blocks using 0.5% bupivacaine with 1:200,000 epinephrine. Usually done by surgeon.

**General anesthesia:**

| | |
|---|---|
| **Induction** | Mask/LMA vs ETT: Standard induction (see Appendix). Mask GA (or LMA) may be suitable for many patients. |
| **Maintenance** | Standard maintenance (see Appendix). |
| **Emergence** | No special considerations. |
| **Blood and fluid requirements** | Minimal blood loss<br>IV: 18 ga x 1<br>NS/LR @ 5-8 cc/kg/hr |
| **Monitoring** | Standard monitors (see Appendix). |
| **Positioning** | √and pad pressure points.<br>√eyes. |

## POSTOPERATIVE

| | | |
|---|---|---|
| **Complications** | Cauda equina syndrome | The diagnosis of cauda equina syndrome (urinary and fecal incontinence, paresis of lower extremities, perineal hyperethesias) should be sought in the postop period in patients who have received large doses of intrathecal local anesthetic during continuous spinal techniques. Check patients for bowel or bladder dysfunction and perineal sensory deficits. If present, consider a neurology consultation and continue follow-up of the patient's neurologic dysfunction. |
| | Urinary retention common with regional anesthesia | Patients with urinary retention may require intermittent catheterization until urinary function resumes. |
| **Pain management** | PO analgesics:<br>Acetaminophen and codeine (Tylenol® #3 1-2 tab q 4-6 hrs)<br>Oxycodone and acetaminophen (Percocet® 1 tab q 6 hrs) | Regional anesthesia should provide sufficient analgesia postop. |

**References**

See references for "Venous Surgery – Thrombectomy or Vein Excision."

1. Johnson G: The management of venous disorders: introduction and general considerations. In *Vascular Surgery*, 3rd edition. Rutherford RB, ed. WB Saunders Co, Philadelphia: 1989, 190-897.
2. Glorickzki P, Merrell SW: Surgical treatment of venous disease. *Cardiovasc Clin* 1992; 22(3):81-100.
3. Coon WW: Epidemiology of venous thromboembolism. *Am Surg* 1977; 186:149.
4. Harlan JM, Harker LA: Hemostasis, thrombosis and thromboembolic disorders. *Med Clin North Am* 1981; 65:855.

**Surgeon**

**Bruce A. Reitz, MD**

## 6.3 HEART/LUNG TRANSPLANTATION

**Anesthesiologist**

**Lawrence Siegel, MD**

# SURGERY FOR HEART TRANSPLANTATION

## SURGICAL CONSIDERATIONS

**Description:** Although heart transplantation has been practiced since 1967, it has had its greatest expansion since the early 1980s with the introduction of cyclosporine immunosuppression. Currently, there are approximately 150 transplant centers and 2,200 heart transplant procedures performed yearly in the U.S. Indications for heart transplantation range from hypoplastic left heart syndrome in the neonate to cardiomyopathy and ischemic heart disease in the adult. Recipients usually have end-stage heart disease manifested by CHF and a prognosis of less than 1-year survival. Many patients are on inotropic drugs or on some type of additional mechanical assist, such as the use of an intra-aortic balloon pump (IABP) or an implanted LV assist device. Current immunosuppressive protocols consist of a combination of cyclosporine with prednisone and azathioprine. Immunosuppression begins either immediately preop or perioperatively and will continue throughout the life of the patient. Current 1-year survival averages 85% in most centers, with 5-year survival of > 60%.

Following median sternotomy, the pericardium is opened, with care being taken to preserve the phrenic nerve. The aorta and vena cava are cannulated, the aorta is cross-clamped and caval tapes (tourniquets to prevent VAE) are applied. The aorta and PA are then transected. This is followed by an incision through the atria, and the recipient heart is removed. The donor heart is prepared by opening the left atrium through the pulmonary veins, separating the aorta and PA. The donor heart is attached by a long continuous suture line around the left atrium, followed by similar suture line around the right atrium. Next, the PA and aorta are anastomosed to their respective recipient vessels. Multiple de-airing maneuvers are followed by aortic unclamping and rewarming and resuscitation of the heart. Normal sinus rhythm (NSR) is established and CPB discontinued. Heparin is reversed, hemostasis is secured, and the chest is closed in a routine manner.

**Neonatal heart transplantation** differs in that the PA is cannulated if the ductus arteriosus is patent. Reconstruction of the aortic arch in the patient with hypoplastic left heart syndrome requires CPB with deep hypothermia (< 18°C) and circulatory arrest. The heart is then excised and the transverse aortic arch is opened beyond the ductus arteriosus to minimize risk of late coarctation. The donor heart is prepared with special attention to trimming the transverse aortic tissue for subsequent reconstruction. The left and right atrium, PA and aorta are sutured in place. The new ascending aorta and right atrium are cannulated and CPB with rewarming is reinstituted. Chest closure is routine.

**Usual preop diagnosis:** Cardiomyopathy; CAD with ischemic cardiomyopathy; CHD (e.g., hypoplastic left heart syndrome or anomalous left coronary artery); end-stage valvular heart disease

### SUMMARY OF PROCEDURE

| | Adult Heart Transplant | Neonate Heart Transplant |
|---|---|---|
| **Position** | Supine | ⇐ |
| **Incision** | Median sternotomy | ⇐ |
| **Special instrumentation** | Ascending aortic, SVC and IVC cannulae | Ascending aortic and right atrial cannulae |
| **Unique considerations** | Due to complete excision of the heart, use of a PA catheter is usually not feasible. | Deep hypothermia with circulatory arrest |
| **Antibiotics** | Erythromycin 500 mg + cefamandole 1 gm iv | Erythromycin 5-10 mg/kg + cefamandole 10-30 mg/kg iv |
| **Surgical time** | Cross-clamp: 45 - 60 min<br>Surgery: 3 - 4 hrs | Circulatory arrest: 45 - 60 min<br>Surgery: 3 - 4 hrs |
| **Closing considerations** | Temporary AV pacing wires are usually placed. A PA catheter may be advanced, especially if there are concerns about residual pulmonary HTN and donor right heart function. An isoproterenol infusion is started intraop to keep HR = 100-110, and to help improve right heart function and ↓PVR. | Temporary ventricular pacing wire is usually placed. Temporary transthoracic left atrial line may be placed. Extensive aortic suture line requires avoidance of postop hypertensive episodes. |
| **EBL** | 500-1500 cc | 50-100 cc |
| **Postop care** | Cardiac ICU: 1-2 d of assisted ventilation; 2-3 d stay. | Pediatric ICU x 1-2 d of assisted ventilation; 4-5 d stay, with attention to pulmonary care. |

| | | |
|---|---|---|
| **Mortality** | < 5% | ⇐ |
| **Morbidity** | Early acute rejection episodes from 10-21 d: 50%<br>Infection, particularly pulmonary: 10%<br>Pulmonary HTN with right heart dysfunction: < 10%<br>Dysrhythmias with nodal rhythms: 5%<br>Bleeding: 2-4%<br>Hyperacute rejection: Rare (< 1%)<br>Intra-coronary air emboli | Respiratory problems: 20%<br>Infection: 10%<br>Pulmonary vasospasm with right heart dysfunction: < 10%<br>Bleeding: 2-4% |
| **Procedure code** | 33945 | ⇐ |
| **Pain score** | 8-10 | 8-10 |

### PATIENT POPULATION CHARACTERISTICS

| | | |
|---|---|---|
| **Age range** | 18-65 yrs (average 45-50 yrs) | 1 d-2 mo |
| **Male:Female** | 7:3 | 1:1 |
| **Incidence** | 2200/yr (U.S.) | Rare |
| **Etiology** | Cardiomyopathy: 50%<br>CAD with multiple previous infarcts: 48%<br>Others: 2% | No apparent correlation with any specific genetic disorder.<br>Cardiomyopathy: 49%<br>CHD: 42%<br>Other: 7% |
| **Associated conditions** | CHF | Other congenital anomalies |

---

## ANESTHETIC CONSIDERATIONS

### PREOPERATIVE

Patients scheduled for heart transplantation are terminally ill, typically with CHF, which has a mortality of >50% in 2 yrs. (Studies have shown that patients with severe CHF have a rapid mortality of 50% in 6 mo.) The progression of cardiovascular disease is usually well-documented in these patients. A history of recent exacerbation of cardiac dysfunction should be sought and all data should be interpreted in light of interval changes.

**Respiratory** The presence of pulmonary HTN and elevated pulmonary vascular resistance (PVR) may be disclosed by catheterization. The severity of the abnormality and the responsiveness to specific vasodilators must be determined.

**Tests:** Right heart catheterization

**Cardiovascular** Indicators to consider include: hemodynamic status; LV ejection fraction (EF) (mortality is rapid in patients with EF < 10% and is worse for patients with EF of 10-20%, as compared with those with EF >20%); myocardial structure and morphology, symptoms and functional capacity; neuroendocrine status; serum sodium; and dysrhythmia. Unfortunately, while these measures show trends with mortality, they are not individually strong enough to predict a particular patient's course. Low $O_2$ consumption (< 10%) is associated with poor survival. Normal $O_2$ consumption is 40 ml/kg/min. In practice, however, this measure is too severe, as many patients awaiting heart transplantation have $O_2$ consumption of 20 ml/kg/min. Dysrhythmia is a major cause of death, and electrophysiology studies of these patients may not be helpful because dysrhythmia tends to be non-inducible in them. This phenomenon frustrates efforts to select and test anti-dysrhythmic drug therapy. The effectiveness of past anti-dysrhythmic therapy should be reviewed.

**Tests:** ECG; cardiac catheterization; ECHO

**Hematologic** Hepatic dysfunction may result from some component of RV failure and may reduce synthetic function. Patients with dilated cardiomyopathy or previous cardiac surgery are frequently treated with anti-coagulants to reduce the risk of thrombus formation, although the efficacy of this therapy has not been studied. Mild hepatic dysfunction and chronic anticoagulation may contribute to postop bleeding. The anticoagulant effect of warfarin should be reversed with FFP.

**Tests:** Hct; PT; PTT; fibrin; platelets

**Endocrine** Neuroendocrine abnormalities are often present in severe CHF cases. The cardiomyopathy produces low cardiac output → compensatory sympathetic activation and renin-angiotensin activity. The result is excessive vasoconstriction with salt and $H_2O$ retention, which further impair myocardial performance. Markedly worse survival is seen in CHF patients with serum sodium < 130. This may indicate the importance of neuroendocrine pathophysiology, or may simply be evidence of the severity of the CHF. It may also simply indicate that patients with more severe CHF are treated with more diuretics. When patients are treated with an angiotensin-converting enzyme inhibitor such as enalapril, the serum sodium is normalized and survival chances are improved because of the slowing of the progression of CHF, not from alteration in the incidence of sudden death.

**Tests:** Electrolytes; creatinine

**Laboratory** Evidence of renal and hepatic dysfunction should be sought by H&P and lab studies. Hypokalemia is generally not treated in view of the potassium in the graft.

**Premedication** Although anxious, these patients are usually well-informed and psychologically prepared to undergo heart transplantation. They respond well to the reassurance of the preop visit, and pharmacologic premedication usuallly is not necessary. $O_2$ therapy should commence prior to transport of the patient to the OR. Reassuring the family of a patient who suffers from rapidly progressive cardiac dysfunction also is valuable. The patient may be at increased risk for pulmonary aspiration of gastric contents because of the unscheduled nature of the transplant surgery, and use of oral cyclosporine immediately preop may be appropriate. Ranitidine (50 mg) and metoclopramide (10 mg) may be administered iv, which is most efficiently accomplished in the OR.

## INTRAOPERATIVE

**Anesthetic technique:** GETA. After the patient is placed on operating table, $O_2$ and non-invasive monitors are applied. Dyspnea (a complication of the supine position) can be treated by raising the back of the table. As infection is a much-feared complication in the immunosupressed transplant patient, aseptic technique is extremely important. Airway equipment is pre-sterilized, and a disposable circle system and bacterial filters are used. Aseptic technique is used in inserting and securing all vascular catheters. The anesthesia machine should be equipped with a supply of air to control the $FiO_2$.

**Induction** A CVP catheter is usually inserted prior to induction of anesthesia. Anesthesia is not induced until the team harvesting the graft reports that the donor heart appears to be normal. The patient is denitrogenated ($FiO_2$=1.0), and cricoid pressure is applied just before induction.

Induction agents include fentanyl (5-20 μg/kg) or sufentanil (1-4 μg/kg). Etomidate (0.1-0.2 mg/kg) is useful in permitting rapid control of the airway and for assuring lack of patient awareness. Midazolam also may be used. Vecuronium (0.15 mg/kg), pancuronium (0.1 mg/kg), or a combination of these two agents should be administered immediately to permit airway control.

Care must be taken to avoid bradycardia, which often results in low cardiac output in these patients. Immediate control of the airway is crucial, as hypercarbia and hypoxia must be avoided. Narcotic-induced chest-wall rigidity can be avoided by gradual and incremental dosing.

The patient can be expected to have a low cardiac output, resulting in a delayed induction of anesthesia which must be anticipated to avoid anesthetic overdosage. Low cardiac output and volume-contracted condition make patient initially very sensitive to anesthetics. High preload is often necessary, and iv fluid is often administered to compensate for the vasodilating effect of anesthetic-mediated sympatholysis. Inotropic support may be necessary when induction is poorly tolerated.

Patient should be ventilated by mask, and cricoid pressure released only after the airway has been secured with a cuffed ETT. The usual aids for managing the unexpectedly difficult airways should be readily available. Antibiotics are administered, and additional monitors (urinary catheter with thermistor, nasopharyngeal temperature probe, TEE or esophageal stethoscope) are set up. If there is a delay in the anticipated arrival of the graft, the donor should be covered and kept warm and skin prep should be delayed. Additional narcotics should be administered only in immediate anticipation of the commencement of surgery.

**Maintenance** Typical cumulative anesthetic doses for the entire intraop course are: fentanyl 50 μg/kg or sufentanil 10-15 μg/kg; midazolam 0.2 mg/kg; vecuronium 0.3 mg/kg or pancuronium 0.2 mg/kg; scopolamine 0.07 mg/kg.

**Termination of CPB**

Junctional rhythm is common in the denervated transplanted heart. Isoproterenol 10-75 ng/kg/min is used to achieve a HR of 100-120 bpm. Isoproterenol is also useful in providing inotropic support and pulmonary vasodilation (see below). When sinus rhythm is achieved, it is common to observe 2 P-waves. The original atrial tissue produces non-conducting P-waves. Responses mediated by vagal tone will be observed in the rate of the original atrial tissue and have no clinical importance beyond the ease with which the ECG is interpreted. Atropine and neostigmine do not affect HR. HTN does not produce reflex bradycardia. The graft atrium produces normally conducted P-waves.

The graft-conductive tissue contains adrenergic receptors and responds normally to norepinephrine, epinephrine and isoproterenol.

Inotropic support with dopamine (2-10 μg/kg/min), isoproterenol and epinephrine (20-100 ng/kg/min) may be necessary, especially if pulmonary circulation promotes RV failure. A PA catheter may be helpful in guiding the use of inotropes and vasodilators.

TEE and RV EF catheters are also used at times. RV failure may be produced by the presence of air in the RCA. Visual inspection may demonstrate this problem, and one should wait for the passage of the air and the resolution of ischemia before terminating CPB.

SNP (0.2-2.0 μg/kg/min) is used for afterload reduction. Prostaglandin $E_1$ ($PGE_1$) (20-100 ng/kg/min) and NTG (0.2-2.0 μg/kg/min) may be used for pulmonary vasodilation, especially if a preop catheterization study demonstrates responsiveness of the pulmonary circulation. Isoproterenol infusion (2-20 μg/kg/min) may provide appropriate pulmonary vasodilation, chronotropy and inotropy. IV fluid and vasodilators must be given with particular care, as the flow produced by the denervated heart is quite sensitive to preload.

**Post-bypass hemorrhage**

Post-bypass bleeding is a common problem brought on by the preop use of anticoagulants, the depressed synthetic function of the liver in chronic heart failure, and the trauma of CPB. Following administration of protamine, infusion of platelets, FFP and RBCs may be necessary. Cryoprecipitate is occasionally needed, especially for patients with previous chest surgery. The use of aprotinin, epsilon amino caproic acid (EACA) or tranexamic acid may be appropriate in some cases.

**Immuno-suppression**

Methylprednisolone 500 mg is given after bypass is terminated.

**Diuresis**

There may be little urine production, especially if patient received high-dose diuretics preop. Cyclosporine may exacerbate renal dysfunction. Mannitol and furosemide may be needed to induce diuresis.

**Transport**

A sterile, disposable Jackson-Rees system is used in transporting the patient to the ICU.

**Blood and fluid requirements**

Possible severe bleeding
IV: 14-16 ga x 1-2
NS/LR @ 4-6 cc/kg/hr

Bleeding is often a major problem after termination of CPB. A second catheter is inserted in patients with previous chest surgery.

**Monitoring**

Standard monitors (see Appendix).
Arterial line
CVP/PA catheter
UO

If the transplant patient is very dyspneic in the supine position, or if the initial time estimate for the arrival of the graft is substantially in error, it may be advantageous to insert the CVP catheter immediately following induction. A 20-ga catheter is placed percutaneously in a radial artery; a triple-lumen catheter is used for those patients who do not have significant pulmonary HTN. An 8.5 Fr introducer is used for patients with elevated pulmonary vascular resistance in anticipation that a PA catheter may be necessary to manage right heart failure following the transplantation. The left IJ vein is the preferred site of cannulation, which leaves the right IJ unscarred for repeated endomyocardial Bx of the transplanted heart.

**Positioning**

✓ and pad pressure points.
✓ eyes.
Arms padded at sides
Chest roll

## POSTOPERATIVE

| | | |
|---|---|---|
| **Complications** | RV dysfunction | RV failure may occur in patients with pulmonary HTN and high RV afterload. |
| | Pulmonary HTN | Maneuvers which exacerbate pulmonary HTN should be avoided. These include: hypoxia, hypercarbia, acidosis and extremes of lung volume. Efforts to treat pulmonary HTN with vasodilator therapy may be complicated by impaired V/Q matching with hypoxemia and by systemic hypotension producing poor right coronary perfusion and RV ischemia. Inotropic support of the RV may be necessary. Isoproterenol infusion (2-20 $\mu$g/kg/min) is attractive because it combines inotropy, pulmonary vasodilation and chronotropy. |
| | Oliguria<br>Drug side effects:<br>- Cyclosporine: HTN, nephrotoxicity, hepatotoxicity<br>- Corticosteroids: glucose intolerance, HTN, obesity, hyperlipidemia, aseptic necrosis of hip, bowel perforation, infection<br>- Azathioprine: anemia, thrombocytopenia, leukopenia, hepatotoxicity | Pre-existing impairment may lead to chronic low output state. Other renal problems may be related to cyclosporine toxicity, diuretic toxicity or CPB. Rx by optimizing hemodynamics: consider reduction or elimination of nehprotoxins; and consider continuing use of diuretics. Cyclosporine nephrotoxicity occurs in most patients. A functional toxicity with ↓GFR occurs at low dose and is reversible. Tubular toxicity with morphologic changes occurs at high doses and is generally clinically unimportant and reversible. The most serious damage is vascular interstitial toxicity, which occurs over months at high doses and is not reversible. |
| **Pain management** | PCA (see Appendix) after weaning from mechanical ventilation. | |
| **Tests** | Creatinine, Hct | |

**References**


1. Baumgartner WA, Reitz BA, Achuff SA, eds: *Heart and Heart-Lung Transplantation.* WB Saunders Co, Philadelphia: 1990.
2. Cirella VN, Pantuck CB, Lee YJ, Pantuck EJ: Effects of cyclosporine on anesthetic action. *Anesth Analg* 1987; 66(8):703-6.
3. Grebenik CR, Robinson PN: Cardiac transplantation at Harefield. A review from the anaesthetist's standpoint. *Anaesthesia* 1985; 40(2):131-40.
4. Cannon DS, Rider AK, Stinson EB, Harrison DC: Electrophysiologic studies in the denervated transplanted human heart. II. Response to norepinephrine, isoproterenol and propranolol. *Am J Cardiol* 1975; 36(7):859-66.
5. Govier AV: Anesthesia and cardiac transplantation. In *Anesthesia and the Heart Patient.* Estafanous FG, ed. Butterworths, Boston: 1989, 99-107.
6. Demas K, Wyner J, Mihm FG, Samuels S: Anesthesia for heart transplantation. A retrospective study and review. *Br J Anaesth* 1986; 58(12):1357-64.
7. Kormos RL, Thompson M, Hardesty RL, et al: Utility of preoperative right heart catheterization data as a predictor of survival after heart transplantation. *J Heart Transplant* 1986; 5:391.
8. Schulte-Sasse Y, Hess W, Tarnow J: Pulmonary vascular response to nitrous oxide in patients with normal and high pulmonary vascular resistance. *Anesthesiology* 1982; 57(1):9-13.
9. Massie BM, Conway M: Survival of patients with congestive heart failure: past, present, and future prospects. *Circulation* 1987; 75(5 P+2):IV11-9.
10. Keogh AM, Freund J, Baron DW, Hickie JB: Timing of cardiac transplantation in idiopathic dilated cardiomyopathy. *Am J Cardiol* 1988; 61(6):418-22.
11. Lee WH, Packer M: Prognostic importance of serum sodium concentration and its modification by converting-enzyme inhibition in patients with severe chronic heart failure. *Circulation* 1986; 73(2):257-67.
12. The CONSENSUS Trial Study Group: Effects of Enalapril on mortality in severe congestive heart failure. Results of the Cooperative North Scandinavian Enalapril Survival Study. *N Engl J Med* 1987; 316(23):1429-35.
13. Costard A, Hill I, Schroeder J, Fowler M: Response to nitroprusside-Predictor of early post transplant mortality. *J Am Coll Cardiol* 1989; 14:62A.
14. Kriett JM, Kaye MP: The Registry of the International Society for Heart and Lung Transplantation: eighth official report – 1991. *J Heart Lung Transplant* 1991; 10(4):491-98.
15. Waterman PM, Bjerke R: Rapid-sequence induction technique in patients with severe ventricular dysfunction. *J Cardiothorac Anesth* 1988; 2:602-6.

16. Ryffel B, Foxwell BM, Gee A, Greiner B, Woerly G, Mihatsch MJ: Cyclosporine – relationship of side effects to mode of action. *Transplantation* 1988; 46(2 Suppl):90S-96S.
17. Starling RC, Cody RJ: Cardiac transplant hypertension. *Am J Cardiol* 1990; 65(1):106-11.
18. Propst J, Siegel L, Feeley T: Aprotinin reduces transfusions during repeat sternotomy for heart transplantation. *Anesthesia Analgesia* 1993; 76(25):5337.
19. Ream AK, Fowles RE, Jamieson S: Cardiac transplantation. In *Cardiac Anesthesia*, 2nd edition. Kaplan JA, ed. WB Saunders Co, Philadelphia: 1987, 881-91.

# SURGERY FOR LUNG AND HEART/LUNG TRANSPLANTATION

## SURGICAL CONSIDERATIONS

**Description:** With the availability of cyclosporine, the ability to successfully transplant the heart and both lungs was proven in monkeys and then successfully applied in a patient in March of 1981. Subsequently, single-lung transplantation was successfully performed in 1984 and an *en bloc*, double-lung transplant in 1986. Clinical lung transplantation of these various types has increased markedly in the last few years, and, currently, approximately 700 single-lung transplants, 200 bilateral lung transplants, and 60 heart-lung transplants are performed in the U.S. each year.

Current indications for heart-lung transplantation are primarily those of combined heart and lung disease, including Eisenmenger's syndrome due to a congenital heart defect with irreversible pulmonary HTN. Certain types of diffuse lung disease, such as cystic fibrosis and primary pulmonary HTN without significant heart failure, are also treated in some centers by heart-lung transplantation. Recipients for single-lung transplant usually have end-stage pulmonary disease without significant sepsis. This includes patients with interstitial fibrosis, emphysema, and lymphangioleiomyomatosis. Some patients with pulmonary vascular disease, such as primary pulmonary HTN or pulmonary HTN associated with an ASD, have undergone single-lung transplantation with or without cardiac repair. Bilateral lung transplantation is now performed usually as a sequential single-lung transplant, with the major indications being septic lung disease, such as cystic fibrosis, chronic bronchiectasis, severe bullous emphysema, or pulmonary vascular disease with or without cardiac repair. Current immunosuppressive protocols consist of a combination of cyclosporine with prednisone and azathioprine, with or without early induction therapy, using a cytolytic agent such as antithymocyte globulin. Immunosuppression may begin preop and continue throughout the life of the patient. Current one-year survival averages between 60% and 70% for the various types of lung transplants.

**Heart-lung transplants** are usually performed through a median sternotomy, although occasionally bilateral, transsternal thoracotomy has been employed. **Single-lung transplants** (usually left side) and **bilateral sequential lung transplants** use a lateral thoracotomy or transsternal bilateral thoracotomy. Single- and double-lung transplants are greatly facilitated with single-lung (one-lung) ventilation (OLV), which is essential for the procedures. If this type of ventilation is not feasible, a bronchial-blocker must be inserted through the operative field during pneumonectomy and re-implantation. CPB is routinely used for heart-lung transplantation, and is used for either single- or bilateral-lung transplantation, depending on the stability of the patient during OLV and/or clamping of the PA. Patients with severe pulmonary HTN undergoing single- or double-lung transplantation will almost always require CPB to reduce PA pressure during clamping. For combined transplants, the recipient heart is removed as for standard heart transplantation (see "Surgery for Heart Transplantation"). A portion of the PA near the ligamentum arteriosum, however, is left intact in order to preserve the recurrent laryngeal nerve. Next, each recipient lung is excised and the trachea is transected above the carina. For single-lung transplant, usually the left recipient lung is excised, leaving a bronchial stump and vascular pedicles for the PA and veins (left atrium). For bilateral lung transplants, both recipient lungs are removed, the trachea transected just above the carina, and the main PA and left atrium prepared for subsequent anastomosis.

**Implantation of the grafts** involves a tracheal anastomosis, aortic and right atrial anastomosis for heart-lung transplants, and a bronchial anastomosis with PA and pulmonary venous anastomosis for single-lung transplantation. **Bilateral sequential lung transplants** are performed as if they were single-lung transplants. CPB requires heparinization and protamine reversal. Prior to closure, extensive exploration for potential bleeding sites within the posterior mediastinum is carried out with placement of right and left pleural and mediastinal drainage. Thoracotomies are closed in standard fashion with routine chest tube drainage.

**Usual preop diagnosis**: End-stage heart and lung disease, such as Eisenmenger's syndrome; cystic fibrosis; primary pulmonary HTN; emphysema; bronchiectasis; lymphangioleiomyomatosis; interstitial pulmonary fibrosis; sarcoidosis; and other unusual forms of lung disease

## SUMMARY OF PROCEDURE

| | Heart-Lung Transplant | Single-Lung Transplant | Bilateral Lung Transplant |
|---|---|---|---|
| **Position** | Supine | Lateral thoracotomy | Supine |
| **Incision** | Median sternotomy, usual; bilateral anterior thoracotomy, occasionally | Posterolateral thoracotomy | Transsternal bilateral thoracotomy |
| **Special instrumentation** | Ascending aortic, SVC and IVC cannulae | Occasional need for a bronchial-blocker to be inserted through the operative field. | Occasional cannulation, as noted for heart-lung Tx, occasional need for bronchial-blocker. |
| **Unique considerations** | CPB. If recipient has had previous thoracotomies, collaterals in the mediastinum may be troublesome. Some patients with cystic fibrosis have severe bilateral scarring, requiring extensive dissection in order to remove the recipient lung. | ± CPB. Patient may become severely hypoxic or hypercarbic during OLV, requiring need for CPB. During right thoracotomy, cannulation can be performed through the thorax, but left thoracotomy may require femoral artery and vena cannulation. | CPB. Thoracotomy is usually performed on left side first, with implantation of the lung on this side, followed by completion of the right-side thoracotomy and right-lung transplantation. If patient becomes unstable, cannulation in the thorax is usually possible to facilitate transplantation. |
| **Antibiotics** | Continue specific antibiotic regime. Coverage for pseudomonas is suggested in patients with cystic fibrosis. | Cefazolin 1 gm iv | ⇐ with appropriate coverage for pseudomonas in patients with cystic fibrosis. |
| **Surgical time** | 4 - 5 hrs | 2 - 3 hrs | 5 - 6 hrs |
| **Closing considerations** | Temporary pacing wire applied and isoproterenol infusion is usually started intraop to keep HR between 100-110, as with a cardiac transplant. | Ventilation with as low an $FiO_2$ as possible to maintain a $PO_2$ >90. Minimize MAP and iv fluid. | ⇐ |
| **EBL** | 500-2000 cc | < 500 cc (more if CPB is used) | 500-2000 cc |
| **Postop care** | Cardiac ICU: 3-7 d; 1-2 d assisted ventilation | ⇐ | ⇐ |
| **Mortality** | 10-15% | 10% | 10-15% |
| **Morbidity** | Early acute rejection episodes from 10-21 d: 75% | – | – |
| | Infection, particularly pulmonary: 30-40% | ⇐ | ⇐ |
| | Pulmonary interstitial edema: 20% | Bleeding: 2-4% | ⇐ |
| | | Bronchial leak or stenosis: 2-4% | ⇐ |
| | Return for bleeding: 4-6% | | |
| | Hyperacute rejection: Rare | | |
| **Procedure code** | 33935 | 33999 | ⇐ |
| **Pain score** | 8-10 | 8-10 | 8-10 |

## PATIENT POPULATION CHARACTERISTICS

| | | | |
|---|---|---|---|
| **Age range** | 3 mo - 55 yrs (average 30-40 yrs) | 1 yr - 65 yrs | 1 yr - 65 yrs |
| **Male:Female** | 1:1 | ⇐ | ⇐ |

| | Heart-Lung Transplant | Single-Lung Transplant | Bilateral Lung Transplant |
|---|---|---|---|
| **Incidence** | 60/yr (U.S.)<br>200/yr (worldwide) | 600/yr (U.S.)<br>1000/yr (worldwide) | 200/yr (U.S.)<br>400/yr (worldwide) |
| **Etiology** | Eisenmenger's syndrome<br>CHD<br>Cystic fibrosis<br>Pulmonary vascular disease<br>Other lung diseases | Acquired chronic lung disease<br>Pulmonary vascular disease | Cystic fibrosis<br>Interstitial fibrosis<br>Emphysema |
| **Associated conditions** | Severe cyanosis and polycythemia<br>Diabetes in patients with cystic fibrosis<br>Sinus infections in patients with cystic fibrosis | Right heart dysfunction<br>Pulmonary valve insufficiency and tricuspid valve insufficiency | Diabetes<br>Sinus infections in patients with cystic fibrosis |

## ANESTHETIC CONSIDERATIONS FOR HEART-LUNG TRANSPLANTATION

### PREOPERATIVE

Patients scheduled for heart-lung transplantation are terminally ill, although they may still be able to maintain limited activity. Indications include primary pulmonary HTN, Eisenmenger's syndrome, cystic fibrosis and combined cardiac and pulmonary disease. The standard pre-anesthetic evaluation is supplemented with considerations particular to these patients. The progression of disease is usually well-documented.

**Respiratory** Patients with severe pulmonary HTN (80/60 mmHg) have enlarged pulmonary arteries. Vocal cord dysfunction (Sx: hoarseness, inability to phonate "e") may occur when the left recurrent laryngeal nerve is stretched by an enlarged PA, making these patients at increased risk for pulmonary aspiration. Appropriate precautions to avoid aspiration should be taken (see Induction, below).
**Tests:** ABG; cardiac catheterization

**Cardiovascular** Hx of recent exacerbation of symptoms should be sought and cardiac catheterization data interpreted in light of interval changes. The severity of pulmonary HTN and the responsiveness to specific vasodilators during catheterization should be reviewed.
**Tests:** ECG; cardiac catheterization; ECHO

**Neurological** R → L intracardiac shunting may be present in patients with pulmonary HTN, and Hx of embolic episodes should be sought. Extra care should be used to avoid injection of even small quantities of intravenous air.

**Hematologic** The medication schedule should be verified with particular attention to the recent use of anticoagulants.
**Tests:** Hct; PTT; PT; platelet count; fibrinogen

**Laboratory** Evidence of renal and hepatic dysfunction should be sought by H&P and lab studies. Hypokalemia is generally not treated because the heart-lung graft is preserved with potassium and implantation will reverse hypokalemia.

**Premedication** Although anxious, these patients are usually well-informed and psychologically prepared. They respond well to the reassurance of the preop visit and pharmacologic premedication usually is not necessary. $O_2$ therapy should commence prior to transport of patient to the OR. Patient may be at increased risk for pulmonary aspiration of gastric contents because of the unscheduled nature of the surgery, the use of oral cyclosporine immediately preop, and the presence of recurrent laryngeal nerve damage. Ranitidine (50 mg) and metoclopramide (10 mg) may be administered iv preop.

### INTRAOPERATIVE

**Anesthetic technique:** GETA. Infection is a much-feared complication in the immunosupressed transplant patient; thus, aseptic technique is important. Airway equipment is pre-sterilized. A disposable circle system and bacterial filters are used. Aseptic technique is used in inserting and securing all vascular catheters. The anesthesia machine should be equipped with a supply of air to permit control of the $FiO_2$. Anesthesia is not induced until the team harvesting the graft reports that it appears to be normal to direct inspection.

**Induction**

Once in OR, the patient should be placed on the operating table and $O_2$ and non-invasive monitors applied. A patient who is dyspneic in the supine position may be treated by raising the back of the table. Cricoid pressure must be used when the patient is at risk for aspiration of gastric contents. A major goal of anesthetic induction is the avoidance of further increases in pulmonary vascular resistance (PVR) by guarding against respiratory acidosis, hypoxia, $N_2O$, light anesthesia and extremes of lung volume. When hemodynamically tolerated, fentanyl (30 $\mu$g/kg) is useful in blunting the pulmonary vascular response to intubation.

Etomidate (0.1-0.2 mg/kg) may be used when hypotension limits administration of narcotics. Vecuronium (0.15 mg/kg), pancuronium (0.1 mg/kg), or a combination of the 2, should be administered early to permit rapid airway control. Midazolam and scopolamine produce amnesia. $N_2O$ is not used because it exacerbates pulmonary HTN, reduces $FiO_2$ and expands intravascular air bubbles. Patient should be ventilated by mask, and cricoid pressure released only after the airway has been secured with a cuffed ETT. Excessive pressure of the cuff on the trachea should be avoided. An ETT of internal diameter of 8.0 mm will facilitate FOB postop.

**Maintenance**

Typical total anesthetic doses for the entire intraop course are: fentanyl 50 $\mu$g/kg or sufentanil 10-15 $\mu$g/kg; midazolam 0.2 mg/kg; vecuronium 0.3 mg/kg or pancuronium 0.2 mg/kg; scopolamine 0.07 mg/kg.

**Termination of CPB**

After tracheal anastomosis is completed, lungs are ventilated with $FiO_2 = 0.21$ at 5 bpm and a TV of 6 ml/kg. When bladder temperature reaches 36°C, ventilation is increased to 10 breaths/min and TV of 12 ml/kg. TV should be adjusted to eliminate atelectasis and to achieve a peak inflation pressure of 25-30 cm $H_2O$ with the chest open. The $FiO_2$ is increased to 0.4 and may be altered in response to pulse oximetry and blood gas data. $FiO_2$ is limited in the hope of curtailing free radical injury. PEEP may be used to enhance oxygenation and is adjusted with an appreciation of the effect of lung volume on PVR. Hypoxemia must be avoided. Hyperkalemia may be treated with calcium (10 $\mu$g/kg), glucose (50 gm), insulin (10 U) and diuresis.

Junctional rhythm is common in the denervated transplanted heart. Isoproterenol (10-75 mg/kg/min) is used to achieve a HR of 100-120 beats/min.

When sinus rhythm is achieved, it is common to see 2 P-waves. The residual atrial tissue produces non-conducting P-waves. Responses mediated by vagal tone will be seen in the rate of the original atrial tissue and have no clinical importance beyond the ease with which the ECG is interpreted.

Atropine and neostigmine do not affect HR.

HTN does not produce reflex bradycardia.

The graft atrium produces normally conducted P-waves. The graft-conductive tissue contains adrenergic receptors and responds normally to norepinephrine, epinephrine and isoproterenol.

The cardiac output of the denervated heart is quite sensitive to preload; thus, iv fluid and vasodilators must be given with particular care.

SNP is used for afterload reduction. $PGE_1$ (20-100 ng/kg/min), isoproterenol and NTG (0.2-2.0 $\mu$g/kg/min) also may be used for pulmonary vasodilation.

Inotropic support with dopamine (2-10 $\mu$g/kg/min), isoproterenol and epinephrine (20-100 ng/kg/min) may be necessary, especially if pulmonary HTN and RV failure occur.

**Immuno-suppression**

Methylprednisolone 500 mg is given after bypass is terminated.

**Diuresis**

There may be little urine production, especially if patient received high-dose diuretics preop. Cyclosporine may exacerbate renal dysfunction. Mannitol and furosemide may be needed to induce diuresis.

**Transport**

A sterile, disposable Jackson-Rees system is used in transporting the patient to the ICU.

| | | |
|---|---|---|
| **Blood and fluid requirements** | Anticipate large blood loss.<br>IV: 14-16 ga x 2 | Bleeding is often a major problem after termination of CPB. Patients with intracardiac defects are at increased risk for cerebral embolic events. Care must be taken to remove all air bubbles from intravascular lines. |
| **Control of blood loss** | Post-bypass bleeding is a common problem. | Post-bypass bleeding is exacerbated by preop use of anticoagulants, depressed synthetic liver function, trauma of CPB; and/or previous chest therapy. |
| | Coagulation therapy necessary. | Coagulation therapy may include: protamine (30 $\mu$g/kg); platelets; FFP; RBCs; EACA (70-400 $\mu$g/kg); DDAVP; aprotinin. |

| | | |
|---|---|---|
| | Possible severe bleeding | Severe bleeding prompts further therapy: cryoprecipitate; Factor IX concentrate. |
| **Monitoring** | Standard monitors (see Appendix).<br>Arterial line<br>CVP/PA catheter<br>UO | If patient is very dyspneic in the supine position, or if the initial time estimate for the arrival of the graft is substantially in error, it may be advantageous to insert the CVP catheter following anesthetic induction. An introducer permits the rapid insertion of a PA catheter when necessary. The left IJ vein is the preferred site of cannulation, leaving the right IJ unscarred for repeated endomyocardial biopsies of the transplanted heart. |

## POSTOPERATIVE

| | | |
|---|---|---|
| **Complications** | Oliguria | There may be little urine production, especially if patient received high-dose diuretics preop. Cyclosporine may exacerbate renal dysfunction. Diuresis may be induced with mannitol and furosemide. |
| | Pulmonary edema | Pulmonary edema may be problematic, given the lack of lymphatic drainage. Diuresis and restriction of iv fluid may help. |
| | RV dysfunction | RV failure may occur in patients with pulmonary HTN and high RV afterload. |
| | Pulmonary HTN | Maneuvers which exacerbate pulmonary HTN should be avoided. These include: hypoxia, hypercarbia, acidosis and extremes of lung volume. Efforts to treat pulmonary HTN with vasodilator therapy may be complicated by impaired V/Q matching with hypoxemia and by systemic hypotension producing poor right coronary perfusion and RV ischemia. Inotropic support of the RV may be necessary. Isoproterenol is attractive because it combines inotropy, pulmonary vasodilation and chronotropy. |
| | Rejection<br>Infection | Monitor rejection Sx with transvenous endomyocardial Bx and transbronchial Bx. |
| | Drug side effects:<br>-Cyclosporine: HTN, nephrotoxicity, hepatotoxicity<br>-Corticosteroids: glucose intolerance, HTN, obesity, hyperlipidemia, aseptic necrosis of hip, bowel perforation, infection<br>-Azathioprine: anemia, thrombocytopenia, leukopenia, hepatotoxicity | Cyclosporine nephrotoxicity occurs in most patients. A functional toxicity with reduced GFR occurs at low dose and is reversible. Tubular toxicity with morphologic changes occurs at high doses and generally is clinically unimportant and reversible. The most serious damage is vascular interstitial toxicity, which occurs over months at high doses and is not reversible. |
| **Pain management** | PCA (see Appendix). | |

### References


1. Baumgartner WA, Reitz BA, Achuff SA, eds: *Heart and Heart-Lung Transplantation.* WB Saunders Co, Philadelphia: 1990.
2. Sale JP, Patel D, Duncan B, Waters JH: Anaesthesia for combined heart and lung transplantation. *Anaesthesia* 1987; 42(3):249-58.
3. Reitz BA, Wallwork JL, Hunt SA, Pennock JL, Billingham ME, Oyer PE, Stinson EB, Shumway NE: Heart-lung transplantation: successful therapy for patients with pulmonary vascular disease. *N Engl J Med* 1982; 306(10):557-64.
4. Schulte-Sasse U, Hess W, Tarnow J: Pulmonary vascular responses to nitrous oxide in patients with normal and high pulmonary vascular resistance. *Anesthesiology* 1982; 57(1):9-13.
5. Pearl RG, Rosenthal MH: Anesthetic management of patients with pulmonary hypertension. *Problems in Anesthesia* 1987; 1:448-62.
6. Cirella VN, Pantuck CB, Lee YJ, Pantuck EJ: Effects of cyclosporine on anesthetic action. *Anesth Analg* 1987; 66(8):703-6.
7. Pucci A, Forbes RD, Berry GJ, Rowan RA, Billingham ME: Accelerated post-transplant coronary arteriosclerosis in combined heart-lung transplantation. *Transplant Proc* 1991; 23(1P+2):1228-29.

8. Scott JP, Sharples L, Mullins P, Aravot DJ, Stewart S, Otulana BA, Higenbottom TW, Wallwork J: Further studies on the natural history of obliterative bronchiolitis following heart-lung transplantation. *Transplant Proc* 1991; 23(1P+2):1201-2.
9. Theodore J, Robin ED, Morris AJ, Burke CM, Jamieson SW, Van Kessel A, Stinson EB, Shumway NE: Augmented ventilatory response to exercise in pulmonary hypertension. *Chest* 1986; 89(1):39-44.
10. Theodore J, Morris AJ, Burke CM, Glanville AR, Van Kessel A, Baldwin JC, Stinson EB, Shumway NE, Robin ED: Cardiopulmonary function at maximum tolerable constant work rate exercise following human heart-lung transplantation. *Chest* 1987; 92(3):433-39.
11. Starnes VA, Theodore J, Oyer PE, Billingham ME, Sibley RK, Berry G, Shumway NE, Stinson EB: Evaluation of heart-lung transplant recipients with prospective, serial transbronchial biopsies and pulmonary function studies. *J Thorac Cardiovasc Surg* 1989; 98(5P+1):683-90.
12. Ryffel B, Foxwell BM, Gee A, Greiner B, Woerly G, Mihatsch MJ: Cyclosporine – relationship of side effects to mode of action. *Transplantation* 1988; 46(2 Suppl):90S-96S.

---

## ANESTHETIC CONSIDERATIONS FOR LUNG TRANSPLANTATION

### PREOPERATIVE

The patient presenting for lung transplantation typically has end-stage pulmonary fibrosis or emphysema, although other diseases, such as pulmonary HTN, also may be treated by single-lung transplantation. Double-lung transplantation can be used to treat cystic fibrosis and bronchiectasis. The progression of the disease is usually well-documented; however, Hx of recent exacerbation of symptoms should be sought.

**Respiratory** Assess the patient's ability to undergo one-lung ventilation (OLV) by review of the ventilation-perfusion scan. If little perfusion of the non-operative lung is present, anticipate the need for CPB.[7] The extent of the restrictive lung disease and diffusion abnormality must be assessed preop. For example, room-air $PaO_2$ < 45 mmHg predicts the need for CPB.

**Tests:** PFT; V/Q scan; ABG

**Airway** Patients with severe pulmonary HTN (80/60 mmHg) have enlarged pulmonary arteries. Vocal cord dysfunction (Sx: hoarseness, inability to phonate "e") may occur when the left recurrent laryngeal nerve is stretched by an enlarged PA, making these patients at increased risk for pulmonary aspiration; therefore, appropriate precautions to avoid aspiration should be taken (see Induction, below).

**Cardiovascular** Evidence of RV dysfunction with tricuspid regurgitation should be sought by physical exam, ECHO and cardiac catheterization. RV ejection fraction (EF) may be estimated with radionuclide ventriculography (normal EF = >50%). Pulmonary HTN is considered to be severe and may produce RV failure when pressure is >2/3rds of systemic arterial pressure. Note response to specific vasodilators recorded during catheterization.

**Tests:** Preview cardiac catheterization data; ECG; mean PAP >40 mmHg and PVR >5 mmHg/min/L may predict the need for partial CPB.

**Neurological** R → L intracardiac shunting may be present in patients with pulmonary HTN, and Hx of embolic episodes should be sought. Extra care should be used to avoid injection of even small quantities of intravenous air.

**Musculoskeletal** Chronic cachexia precludes the procedure.

**Hematologic** Polycythemia 2° chronic hypoxemia is common. Autologous blood is indicated in OR, after induction of anesthesia.

**Tests:** Hct

**Laboratory** Other tests as indicated from H&P.

**Premedication** Patients awaiting lung transplantation are generally well-informed about the planned perioperative course. These patients respond well to the reassurance of the preop visit, and pharmacologic premedication is usually not necessary. $O_2$ therapy, with the usual home $O_2$ regimen, should commence prior to transport to the OR. Patient may be at ↑ risk for pulmonary aspiration of gastric contents because of the unscheduled nature of the surgery, the use of oral cyclosporin immediately prior to surgery and the presence of recurrent laryngeal nerve damage. Ranitidine (50 mg) and metoclopramide (10 mg) may be administered iv prior to surgery.

## INTRAOPERATIVE

**Anesthetic technique:** GETA. Infection is a much-feared complication in the immunosuppressed transplant patient; thus, aseptic technique is important. Airway equipment is pre-sterilized. A disposable circle system and bacterial filters are used. Aseptic technique is used in inserting and securing all vascular catheters.

**Induction** Typically, fentanyl 30 mg/kg (incremental doses) after invasive monitors placed, ± etomidate 0.1-0.2 mg/kg when rapid control of the airway is desirable; vecuronium 0.15 mg/kg or pancuronium 0.1 mg/kg (avoid succinylcholine 2° ↓HR); midazolam 0.1 mg/kg or scopolamine 0.005 mg/kg for amnesia. Cricoid pressure must be used when the patient is at risk for aspiration because of the unscheduled nature of the surgery, use of preop oral cyclosporin and possible vocal cord dysfunction associated with stretch injury of the recurrent laryngeal nerve. Avoid further increases in pulmonary vascular resistance (PVR) by guarding against hypoxemia, acidosis, hypercarbia, light anesthesia and extremes of lung volume.

**Maintenance** Typically, narcotic/$O_2$/air/± isoflurane (in absence of hypoxemia and right heart failure). Typical total anesthetic doses for the entire intraop course: fentanyl 50-75 μg/kg or sufentanil 10-15 μg/kg, midazolam 0.2 mg/kg, vecuronium 0.3 mg/kg, or pancuronium 0.2 mg/kg or pipecuronium 0.2 mg/kg, scopolamine 0.07 mg/kg.

**Emergence** Prior to closure of the chest, lungs are inflated to 35 cm $H_2O$, in order to re-inflate atelectatic areas and check adequacy of bronchial closure. At the conclusion of surgery, both lumens of the DLT should be aspirated and the tube replaced with a single-lumen 8.0 mm (ID) ETT. The patient is transported to the ICU intubated and ventilated.

**Blood and fluid requirements**

IV: 14 or 16 ga x 1-2
NS/LR @ 4 ml/kg/hr]

Patients with intracardiac defects are at increased risk for cerebral embolic events; take care to remove all air bubbles from intravascular lines.

**Monitoring**

Standard monitors (see Appendix).
Arterial line
PA catheter
Urinary catheter with thermistor

ECG leads should be covered with tape to insure that electrical contact is not degraded by prep solution or blood. An 8.5 Fr introducer and a thermodilution PA catheter are inserted prior to induction of anesthesia. Mixed venous oximetry may be desirable during OLV, and with partial CPB. RV EF measurement may be useful. The catheter should be advanced into the main PA. Be careful of air embolization during catheter insertion. Patients who are profoundly dyspneic (high negative intrathoracic pressure) are at high risk for venous air embolism; consider inserting the catheter after GA and IPPV have been instituted. Oxygenation must be watched closely. Blood gases are sampled at 10-min intervals.

TEE

TEE is useful for evaluating RV function.

**One-lung ventilation (OLV)**

DLT: 41 Fr (men); 39 Fr (women)
Use large VT (12-15 ml/kg) during regular and OLV.

A disposable DLT is inserted in the left mainstem bronchus to permit surgical access. Verification of tube position by auscultation may be difficult due to the severity of the lung disease. FOB is used to verify proper tube placement. Positioning of the bronchial cuff in the proximal left mainstem bronchus does not interfere with surgical access to the bronchus. The position of the DLT should be verified after the patient is moved to the lateral position. Progressive deterioration of oxygenation should be treated before frank hypoxemia develops. Finally, verify ventilation and proper functioning of the tube, then eliminate volatile anesthetic or vasodilators which may blunt hypoxic pulmonary vasoconstriction. Apply $O_2$ with CPAP at 5 cm $H_2O$ to the non-dependent lung. Further adjustment of CPAP may enhance oxygenation. The non-dependent lung may be re-inflated with $O_2$ if necessary to achieve adequate oxygenation. If adequate oxygenation cannot be achieved, CPB should be initiated.

| | | |
|---|---|---|
| **PA clamping** | Improve V/Q mismatch.<br>Improve oxygenation.<br>PAP ↑↑ → RVF | Clamping of the PA will improve V/Q mismatch and oxygenation; however, severe pulmonary HTN and right heart failure may develop. Vasodilators, such as NTG (0.2-2 $\mu$g/kg/min), SNP (0.2-10 $\mu$g/kg/min) or $PGE_1$ (20-100 ng/kg/min), should be used to treat pulmonary HTN and reduce RV afterload; however, care must be taken to avoid systemic hypotension. Inotropic support for the RV may be necessary (dopamine [2-10 $\mu$g/kg/min] or epinephrine [20-100 ng/kg/min]). The right atrial pressure should be monitored for evidence of tricuspid regurgitation associated with RV dilation. |
| **PA unclamping** | PIP: 20-25 mm $H_2O$<br>$O_2$ sat: 95-100%<br>PEEP: 5-10 mmHg | Temporary unclamping of the PA may be necessary to allow further pharmacologic therapy. If right heart failure cannot be controlled pharmacologically, CPB should be initiated. The PA should not be unclamped until ventilation is possible to the transplanted lung. Perfusion without oxygenation of the transplanted lung would produce profound shunt and hypoxemia. TV should be adjusted to eliminate atelectasis and to achieve a PIP of 20-25 cm $H_2O$ with the chest open. The $FiO_2$ (0.35) is limited in the hope of curtailing free radical injury. PEEP may be used to enhance oxygenation. |
| **Positioning** | For single-lung:<br>Supine → lateral decubitus<br>Axillary roll<br>Airplane splint<br>Avoid hyperextension (>90°)<br>For double-lung:<br>Supine with arms above head for bilateral subcostal incision.<br>√ and pad pressure points.<br>√ eyes. | Verify proper endobronchial location after moving to the lateral position.<br><br>Difficult access to airway after patient positioned. |

## POSTOPERATIVE

| | | |
|---|---|---|
| **Complications** | Pulmonary edema<br>Infection: bacterial, viral, fungal or protozoan<br>Side effects of immunosuppressive agents:<br>-Cyclosporine: hepatotoxicity, HTN nephrotoxicity, seizures<br>-Corticosteroids: HTN, osteoporosis, glucose intolerance, hyperlipidemia<br>-Azathioprine: anemia, thrombocytopenia, leukopenia | Pulmonary edema may be problematic given the lack of lymphatic drainage. Diuresis and restriction of iv fluid may help. Mannitol and furosemide can be used to induce diuresis.<br>Immunosuppression drugs typically include: cyclosporin, azathioprine and corticosteroids. Polyclonal antilymphocyte globulin or monoclonal antilymphocyte antibodies also may be used. |
| **Pain management** | Epidural narcotics (see Appendix).<br>Parenteral narcotics (see Appendix). | Postop analgesia may be provided by infusion of narcotics through an epidural catheter. If CPB is used, the insertion of the epidural catheter should be delayed until normal coagulation function is documented in the ICU. |

**References**

1. Siegel LC: Selection of anesthetic agent for thoracic surgery. In *Problems in Anesthesia*, Vol 4. Brodsky JB, ed. JB Lippincott, Philadelphia: 1990, 249-63.

2. Siegel LC, Brodsky JB: Choice of anesthetic agents for intrathoracic surgery. In *Thoracic Anesthesia*, 2nd edition. Kaplan JA, ed. Churchill Livingstone, New York: 1991.
3. Conacher ID, McNally B, Choudhry AK, McGregor CGA: Anaesthesia for isolated lung transplantation. *Br J Anaesth* 1988; 60(5):588-91.
4. Conacher ID: Isolated lung transplantation: a review of problems and guide to anaesthesia. *Br J Anaesth* 1988; 61(4):468-74.
5. Benumof JL. Partridge BL, Salvatierra C, Keating J: Margin of safety in positioning modern double-lumen endotracheal tubes. *Anesthesiology* 1987; 67(5):729-38.
6. Capan LM, Turndorf H, Chandrankant P, et al: Optimization of arterial oxygenation during one-lung anesthesia. *Anesth Analg* 1980; 59(1):847-51.
7. Hurford WE, Kolker AC, Strauss W: The use of ventilation/perfusion lung scans to predict oxygenation during one-lung anesthesia. *Anesthesiology* 1987; 67(5):841-44.
8. Eishi K, Takazawa A, Nagatsu M, Hirata K, et al: Pulmonary flow-resistance relationships in allografts after single lung transplantation in dogs. *J Thorac Cardiovasc Surg* 1989; 97(1):24-9.
9. Scherer RW, Vigfusson G, Hultsch E, et al: Prostaglandin F2a improves oxygen tension and reduces venous admixture during one-lung ventilation in anesthetized paralyzed dogs. *Anesthesiology* 1985; 62(1):23-8.
10. Thomas BJ, Siegel LC: Anesthetic and postoperative management of single-lung transplantation. *J Cardiothoracic Vasc Anesth* 1991; 5(3):266-67.
11. DeMajo WAP: Anesthetic technique for single lung transplantation. In *The transplantation and replacement of thoracic organs*. Cooper DKC, Novitsky D, eds. Kluwer Academic Publishers, Boston: 1990.
12. The Toronto Lung Transplant Group: Experience with single-lung transplantation for pulmonary fibrosis. *JAMA* 1988; 259(15):2258-62.
13. Maurer JR, Winton TL, Patterson GA, Williams TR: Single-lung transplantation for pulmonary vascular disease. *Transplant Proc* 1991; 23(1 P+2):1211-12.
14. Kramer MR, Marshall SE, McDougall IR, Kloneck A, Starnes VA, Lewiston NJ, Theodore J: The distribution of ventilation and perfusion after single-lung transplantation in patients with pulmonary fibrosis and pulmonary hypertension. *Transplant Proc* 1991; 23(1 P+2):1215-16.
15. Marshall SE, Lewiston NJ, Kramer MR, Sibley RK, Berry G, Rich JB, Theodore J, Starnes VA: Prospective analysis of serial pulmonary function studies and transbronchial biopsies in single-lung transplant recipients. *Transplantat Proc* 1991; 23(1 P+2):1217-19.
16. Williams EL, Jellish WS, Modica PA, Eng CC, Tempelhoff R: Capnography in a patient after single lung transplantation. *Anesthesiology* 1991; 74(3):621-22.
17. Colley PS, Cheney FW: Sodium nitroprusside increases Qs/Qt in dogs with regional atelectasis. *Anesthesiology* 1977; 47(4):388.
18. Carere R, Patterson GA, Liu P, Williams T, Maurer J, Grossman R: Right and left ventricular performance after single and double lung transplantation. The Toronto Lung Transplant Group. *J Thorac Cardiovasc Surg* 1991; 102(1):115-23.
19. Sekela ME, Noon GP, Holland VA, Lawrence EC: Differential perfusion: potential complication of femoral-femoral bypass during single lung transplantation. *J Heart Lung Transplant* 1991; 10(2):322-24.
20. Demajo WAP: Pulmonary transplantation. In *Thoracic Anesthesia*, 2nd edition. Kaplan J, ed. Churchill Livingstone, New York: 1991, 555-62.

## 7. GENERAL SURGERY

### Surgeons

**Harry A. Oberhelman, MD, FACS** *(Esophageal, Intestinal, Hepatic, Pancreatic, Peritoneal, Endocrine Surgery)*
**Mark A. Vierra, MD** *(Stomach, Biliary Tract Surgery)*
**James M. Stone, MD** *(Colorectal Surgery)*
**Stefanie S. Jeffrey, MD, FACS** *(Breast Surgery)*
**Edward J. Alfrey, MD** *(Liver/Kidney Transplantation)*
**Donald C. Dafoe, MD** *(Liver/Kidney Transplantation)*
**Velerig Selivanov, MD** (Trauma Surgery)

### Anesthesiologists

**Steven K. Howard, MD** *(Esophageal, Stomach, Intestinal, Colorectal, Hepatic Biliary, Pancreatic, Peritoneal, Breast, Endocrine Surgery)*
**Gordon R. Haddow, MB, ChB, FFA(SA)** *(Liver/Kidney Transplantation)*
**Price Stover, MD** *(Liver/Kidney Transplantation)*
**Linda Foppiano, MD** *(Trauma Surgery)*

**Surgeon**

**Harry A. Oberhelman, MD, FACS**

## 7.1 ESOPHAGEAL SURGERY

**Anesthesiologist**

**Steven K. Howard, MD**

# ESOPHAGEAL DIVERTICULECTOMY

## SURGICAL CONSIDERATIONS

**Description:** Diverticula of the esophagus may be of congenital or acquired origin. The most common sites are **hypopharyngeal (Zenker's)**, just above the cricopharyngeal sphincter, and in the **epiphrenic** area just above the distal high-pressure zone. The usual treatment consists of excision of the diverticulum, combined with a cricopharyngeal myotomy or a lower esophagomyotomy (Fig 7.1-2). Care must be taken not to enter the esophageal lumen. If this occurs, the mucosal tear is approximated with fine cat-gut or Dexon® sutures. The **hypopharyngeal diverticulum** is approached through either side of the neck. The upper esophagus is exposed by retracting the sternocleidomastoid muscle and carotid sheath laterally and the thyroid gland medially. The diverticulum is located in the prevertebral space. Care is taken not to injure the recurrent laryngeal nerve. Following excision of the diverticulum, a **myotomy** is performed, starting on the upper esophagus and curving across the cricopharyngeal muscle near the neck of the diverticulum. The epiphrenic diverticulum is approached through the left chest and the dissection started at the pulmonary hilum. Care is taken not to injure the vagus nerves as the esophagus is mobilized downward. The diverticulum is freed from the right pleura and posterior mediastinum. Once the diverticulum has been freed, an **esophagomyotomy** is performed on the side opposite the diverticulum. The diverticulum is then excised, leaving a cuff of the neck to suture the mucosa carefully. The muscle layer is then approximated over the mucosal closure.

**Variant procedure or approaches:** The hypopharyngeal diverticulum is approached through either side of the neck, while the epiphrenic diverticulum is approached via a left thoracotomy.

**Usual preop diagnosis:** Esophageal diverticulum

### SUMMARY OF PROCEDURE

| | Hypopharyngeal | Epiphrenic |
|---|---|---|
| **Position** | Supine | Right lateral decubitus |
| **Incision** | Left or right cervical | Left thoracotomy |
| **Special instrumentation** | None | Chest retractor |
| **Unique considerations** | Care not to injure recurrent laryngeal nerve | 10 cm myotomy |
| **Antibiotics** | Cefotetan 1 gm preop | ⇐ |
| **Surgical time** | 1 - 2 hrs | ⇐ |
| **Closing considerations** | Inspect for perforation | ⇐ |
| **EBL** | 50-100 ml | 100-200 ml |
| **Postop care** | PACU | ICU x 1-2 d |
| **Mortality** | < 1% | ⇐ |
| **Morbidity** | Recurrent nerve paralysis: < 5%<br>Temporary phonetic problems: < 5%<br>Esophageal stricture: < 3%<br>Esophageal fistula: < 2% | Atelectasis: 5-10%<br>Esophageal stricture: < 5%<br>Esophagal perforation: < 2% |
| **Procedure code** | 43130 | 43135 |
| **Pain score** | 6-7 | 7-9 |

### PATIENT POPULATION CHARACTERISTICS

| | |
|---|---|
| **Age range** | 38-92 yrs (50% of patients >70 yrs) |
| **Male:Female** | 1:1 |
| **Incidence** | Uncommon |
| **Etiology** | Uncoordinated cricoesophageal muscle and lower esophageal sphincter: 100%<br>Weakness of esophageal wall: 100% |
| **Associated conditions** | Cachexia: 25-30%<br>Hiatus hernia with or without reflux: 25%<br>Chronic pulmonary infection: 15-20% |

# ESOPHAGOSTOMY

## SURGICAL CONSIDERATIONS

**Description**: Esophagostomy is performed to divert oral secretions away from the esophagus to a stoma pouch in certain types of esophageal perforation. In addition, it may be utilized for feeding purposes when the patient cannot swallow due to obstructive lesions of the pharynx. Through a left cervical incision, the sternocleidomastoid muscle and carotid sheath are retracted laterally and the thyroid medially, exposing the cervical esophagus (Fig 7.1-1). The esophagus is mobilized, with care being taken not to injure the recurrent laryngeal nerve. The esophagus is brought to the skin surface as a loop or end stoma and sutured to the skin with absorbable sutures.

**Variant procedure or approaches**: The procedure is usually performed via a left cervical approach; the right side is an alternative.

**Usual preop diagnosis**: Esophageal perforation; nasopharyngeal cancer; esophageal atresia

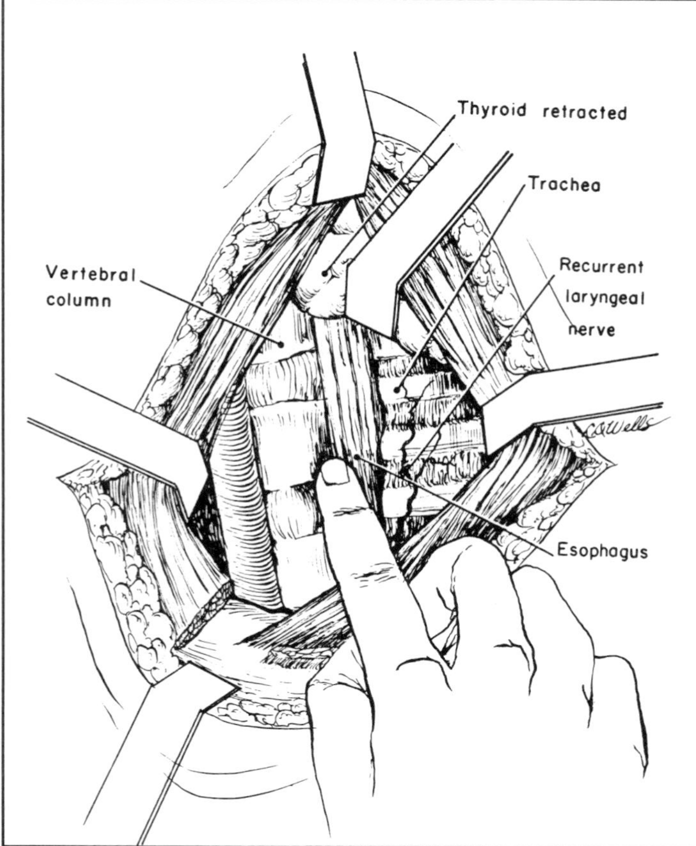


**Figure 7.1-1.** Surgical anatomy for cervical esophagostomy. (Reproduced with permission from Nora PF, ed: *Operative Surgery Principles and Techniques*. WB Saunders Co: 1990.)

### SUMMARY OF PROCEDURE

| | |
|---|---|
| **Position** | Supine, with head rotated to right |
| **Incision** | Cervical |
| **Antibiotics** | Cefotetan 1 gm 30 min preop |
| **Surgical time** | 45 mins |
| **EBL** | 25-50 ml |
| **Postop care** | Stoma pouch to collect saliva; PACU → room |
| **Mortality** | < 0.1% |
| **Morbidity** | Skin irritation: 15-20%<br>Saliva leakage: 5-10%<br>Wound infection: < 5% |
| **Procedure code** | 43352 |
| **Pain score** | 5-7 |

### PATIENT POPULATION CHARACTERISTICS

| | |
|---|---|
| **Age range** | Variable – 20-60 yrs |
| **Male:Female** | 1:1 |
| **Incidence** | Not uncommon |
| **Etiology** | Surgically created |
| **Associated conditions** | Esophageal perforation or atresia: 50%<br>Pharyngeal cancer: 50% |

## ANESTHETIC CONSIDERATIONS

See "Anesthetic Considerations for Esophageal Surgery" following "Esophagectomy," at the end of this section.

**References**

1. Urskel HC Jr, et al: Improved management of esophageal perforation: exclusion and division in continuity. *Ann Surg* 1974; 179:587.

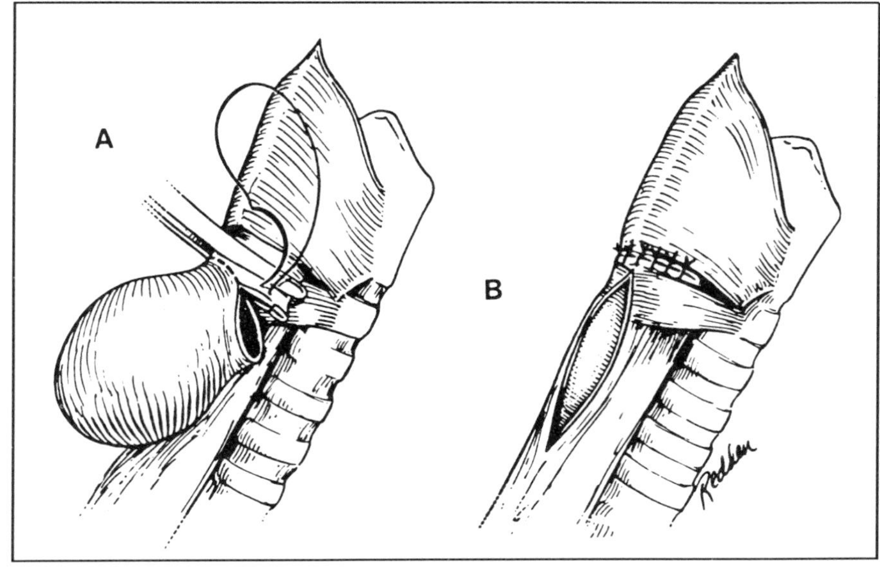


**Figure 7.1-2.** Esophageal diverticulectomy: (A) Excision of Zenker's diverticulum; (B) Division of the cricopharyngeus (myotomy) reduces the chance of recurrence or postop dysphagia. (Reproduced with permission from Hardy JD: *Hardy's Textbook of Surgery*, 2nd edition. JB Lippincott: 1988.)

## ANESTHETIC CONSIDERATIONS

See "Anesthetic Considerations for Esophageal Surgery" following "Esophagectomy," at the end of this section.

**References**

1. Little AG, Ferguson MK, Skinner DB: *Diseases of the Esophagus*, Vol. II, Benign Diseases. Futura Publishing, New York: 1990.

# CLOSURE OF ESOPHAGEAL PERFORATION

## SURGICAL CONSIDERATIONS

**Description**: Esophageal perforation may be spontaneous, instrumental, traumatic, or 2° intrinsic esophageal disease. Spontaneous perforations commonly occur in the lower third of the esophagus. Instrumental perforations may occur at any level, but are most common just above the cardia and in the cervical esophagus. The level of traumatic perforation depends on the location of the penetrating wound. Symptoms of esophageal perforation at the cricopharyngeal sphincter include neck pain, fever and crepitations in the substernal and neck areas. Perforation in the mediastinum may result in hydropneumothorax, mediastinitis, fever and substernal pain. Cervical perforations are managed with antibiotics and drainage in the cervical area. Therapy for thoracic esophageal perforation generally requires drainage of the pleural cavity and antibiotics. Open thoracotomy with closure of the perforation and an onlay patch of pleura may be indicated, depending on the size of the perforation and the patient's condition.

**Variant procedure or approaches**: Cervical or right thoracic drainage are indicated when the perforation occurs in the neck or high in the mediastinum.

**Usual preop diagnosis**: Esophageal perforation

## SUMMARY OF PROCEDURE

| | Left Thoracotomy | Cervical or Thoracic Drainage |
|---|---|---|
| **Position** | Left lateral decubitus | Supine or right lateral decubitus |
| **Incision** | Left thoracotomy | Cervical or right chest |
| **Antibiotics** | Cefotetan 2 gm iv | ⇐ |
| **Surgical time** | 2 hrs | 1 hr |
| **Closing considerations** | Chest drain | Cervical or thoracic drain |
| **EBL** | 100-200 ml | 50-100 ml |
| **Postop care** | Chest tube to suction; PACU → room | ⇐ |
| **Mortality** | 5-10% | 2-5% |
| **Morbidity** | Pneumonia: 5-10% | – |
| | Esophageal leak: 2-5% | 10% |
| | Pericarditis: 1-3% | |
| **Procedure code** | 43415 | 32020, 43410 |
| **Pain score** | 8-10 | 8-10 |

## PATIENT POPULATION CHARACTERISTICS

| | |
|---|---|
| **Age range** | Variable – 20-80 yrs |
| **Male:Female** | 1:1 |
| **Incidence** | 1 in 8,000 admissions |
| **Etiology** | Instrumental (endoscopy, dilatation, intubation)<br>Traumatic (penetrating, foreign body, caustic agents)<br>Intrinsic disease (carcinoma, peptic ulceration)<br>Spontaneous |
| **Associated conditions** | Esophageal stricture: 75%<br>Cancer: 25% |

# ANESTHETIC CONSIDERATIONS

See "Anesthetic Considerations for Esophageal Surgery" following "Esophagectomy," at the end of this section.

**References**

1. Orringer MB: The Mediastinum. In *Operative Surgery*, 3rd edition. Nora PF, ed. WB Saunders Co, Philadelphia: 1990, 370-73.

# ESOPHAGOMYOTOMY

## SURGICAL CONSIDERATIONS

**Description**: Esophagomyotomy is performed for achalasia and other motility disorders to facilitate esophageal emptying into the stomach. It consists of incising the muscular layer of the distal esophagus and continuing down across the gastroesophageal junction for at least 1 cm (Heller).[1] The muscle is dissected back from the mucosa so that roughly 180° is exposed (Fig 7.1-3). The distal esophagus is mobilized either from below the diaphragm or via a left thoracic approach. Care is taken not to injure the vagus nerve.

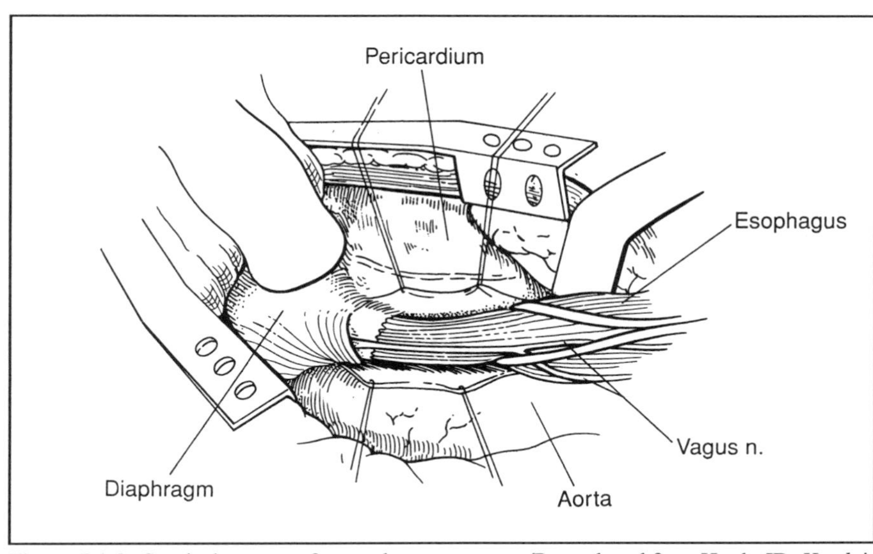


**Figure 7.1-3.** Surgical anatomy for esophagomyotomy. (Reproduced from Hardy JD: *Hardy's Textbook of Surgery*, 2nd edition. JB Lippincott: 1988.)

When approached from the abdomen, the esophagus is exposed by incising the gastroesophageal ligament. The distal esophagus is mobilized and pulled downward to perform the myotomy.

**Variant procedure or approaches**: The procedure is usually performed through a left thoracotomy, but some surgeons prefer a **transabdominal approach**.

**Usual preop diagnosis**: Achalasia

### SUMMARY OF PROCEDURE

| | Thoracic Approach | Abdominal Approach |
|---|---|---|
| **Position** | Right lateral decubitus | Supine |
| **Incision** | Left thoracotomy in 6th interspace | Midline upper abdomen |
| **Special instrumentation** | Chest retractor | Denier retractor |
| **Unique considerations** | Care should be taken to avoid extending gastric myotomy too far to prevent esophageal reflux. | ⇐ |
| **Antibiotics** | Cefotetan 1-2 gm 30 min preop | ⇐ |
| **Surgical time** | 1 - 2 hrs | ⇐ |
| **Closing considerations** | √ for perforation. Consider fundoplication to prevent esophageal reflux.[2] | ⇐ |
| **EBL** | 150-200 ml | 100-150 ml |
| **Postop care** | ICU x 1-2 d | PACU → room |
| **Mortality** | $< 0.5\%$ | ⇐ |
| **Morbidity** | Esophagitis: $\leq 20\%$ | ⇐ |
| | Transient dysphagia/reflux: 5% | ⇐ |
| | Esophageal leak: 1-2% | ⇐ |
| **Procedure code** | 43331 | 43330 |
| **Pain score** | 7-9 | 6-8 |

### PATIENT POPULATION CHARACTERISTICS

| | |
|---|---|
| **Age range** | 30-50 yrs |
| **Male:Female** | 1:1 |
| **Incidence** | 0.6/100,000 |
| **Etiology** | Neuromuscular disorder of unknown etiology often characterized by absence of ganglion cells of Auerbach's plexus: 100% |
| **Associated conditions** | Predisposition to development of carcinoma: 1-20%<br>Pulmonary complications 2° aspiration: 5-10% |

## ANESTHETIC CONSIDERATIONS

See "Anesthetic Considerations for Esophageal Surgery" following "Esophagectomy," at the end of this section.

**References**

1. Ellis FH Jr, Crozier RE, Watkins E Jr: Operation for esophageal achalasia. Results of esophagomyotomy without an antireflex. *J Thorac Cardiovasc Surg* 1984; 88(3):344-51.
2. Belsey R: Functional disease of the esophagus. *J Thorac Cardiovasc Surg* 1966; 52(2):164-88.

# ESOPHAGOGASTRIC FUNDOPLASTY

## SURGICAL CONSIDERATIONS

**Description**: Esophagogastric fundoplasty represents a variety of operations designed to prevent esophageal reflux by wrapping the fundus of the stomach around a 3-4 cm segment of the lower esophagus. This fundal wrapping acts to reinforce the lower esophageal sphincter. Surgery may be performed transabdominally or transthoracically, depending on surgeon's preference. The most commonly employed is the **Nissen fundoplication**, utilizing both the anterior and posterior walls of the stomach. They are sutured together around the lower esophagus with non-absorbable sutures (Fig 7.1-4A). This is accomplished by incising the gastro-splenic ligament and ligating 3 or 4 short gastric vessels. Care must be taken not to injure the spleen or vagus nerves during the repair.

**Variant procedure or approaches**: Modifications of the Nissen fundoplication include the **Hill procedure**, in which the gastroesophageal junction is sutured to the median arcuate ligament of the diaphragm or to the pre-aortic fascia (Fig 7.1-4B). Another modification is the **Belsey Mark IV** repair, in which there is a 240° semi-fundoplication between the stomach and esophagus (Fig 7.1-5.) making it easier for the patient to overcome the resistance of the wrap. There are proponents of each repair, although the Nissen fundoplication remains the procedure most widely used.

**Usual preop diagnosis**: Sliding hiatus (hiatal) hernia or free reflux

### SUMMARY OF PROCEDURE

| | Nissen Fundoplication | Hill Procedure[1] | Belsey Mark IV[2] |
|---|---|---|---|
| **Position** | Supine | ⇐ | Right lateral decubitus |
| **Incision** | Midline abdominal | ⇐ | Left posterolateral thoracotomy |
| **Special instrumentation** | #40-50 Hurst dilators; NG tube | NG tube | Chest retractor; NG tube |
| **Unique considerations** | Fundoplication should be loose; parietal cell vagotomy performed if peptic ulcer disease present. | ⇐ | ⇐ |

| | Nissen Fundoplication | Hill Procedure | Belsey Mark IV |
|---|---|---|---|
| **Antibiotics** | Cefotetan 1-2 gm 30 min preop | ⇐ | ⇐ |
| **Surgical time** | 1 - 2 hrs | ⇐ | ⇐ |
| **Closing considerations** | Inspect spleen for bleeding | ⇐ | ⇐ |
| **EBL** | 100-150 ml | ⇐ | 100-200 ml |
| **Postop care** | PACU → room | ⇐ | ICU x 1-2 d |
| **Mortality** | < 0.5% | ⇐ | ⇐ |
| **Morbidity** | Recurrent hernia: 20% | ⇐ | ⇐ |
| | Gas-bloat syndrome: 10-20% | < 5% | ⇐ |
| | Temporary dysphagia: 5-10% | 5% | 2% |
| | Gastric fistula: < 2% | ⇐ | ⇐ |
| **Procedure code** | 43324 | ⇐ | ⇐ |
| **Pain score** | 6-8 | 7-8 | 7-9 |

### PATIENT POPULATION CHARACTERISTICS

| | |
|---|---|
| **Age range** | 46-60 yrs |
| **Male:Female** | 1:2 |
| **Incidence** | Not uncommon |
| **Etiology** | Esophagogastric reflux: 100%<br>Esophageal hiatus hernia: 80-90% |
| **Associated conditions** | Diverticulosis of colon: 30-35%<br>Cholelithiasis: 25-30% |

## ANESTHETIC CONSIDERATIONS

See "Anesthetic Considerations for Esophageal Surgery" following "Esophagectomy," at the end of this section.

**References**

1. Hill LD: Progress in the surgical management of hiatal hernia. *World J Surg* 1977; 1(4):425-36.
2. Belsey R: Mark IV repair of hiatal hernia by the transthoracic approach. *World J Surg* 1977; 1(4):475-81.

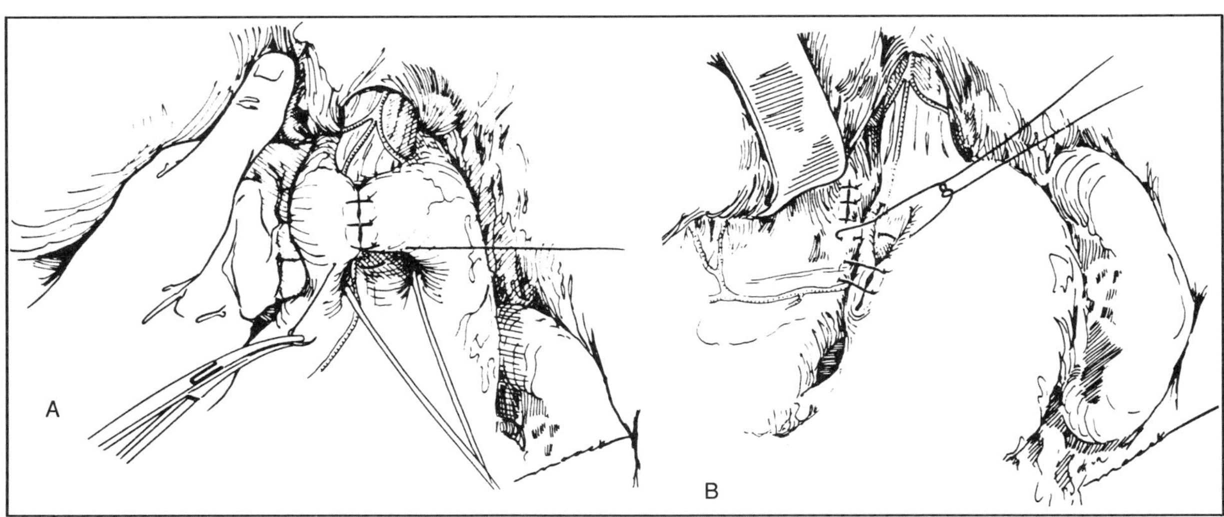


**Figure 7.1-4.** (A) Nissen fundoplication may be performed via either the transabdominal or transthoracic approach; (B) Hill repair is performed through the abdomen. (Reproduced with permission from Hardy JD: *Hardy's Textbook of Surgery*, 2nd edition. JB Lippincott: 1988.)

# ESOPHAGECTOMY

## SURGICAL CONSIDERATIONS

**Description:** Esophagectomy is commonly performed for malignant disease of the middle and lower thirds of the esophagus. It may also be indicated for Barrett's esophagus (peptic ulcer of lower esophagus ± stricture) and for peptic strictures that fail dilatation. Lesions in the lower third are usually approached via a left thoracoabdominal incision, while middle-third lesions are best approached via the abdomen and right chest (**Ivor Lewis**). Resections of the eso-

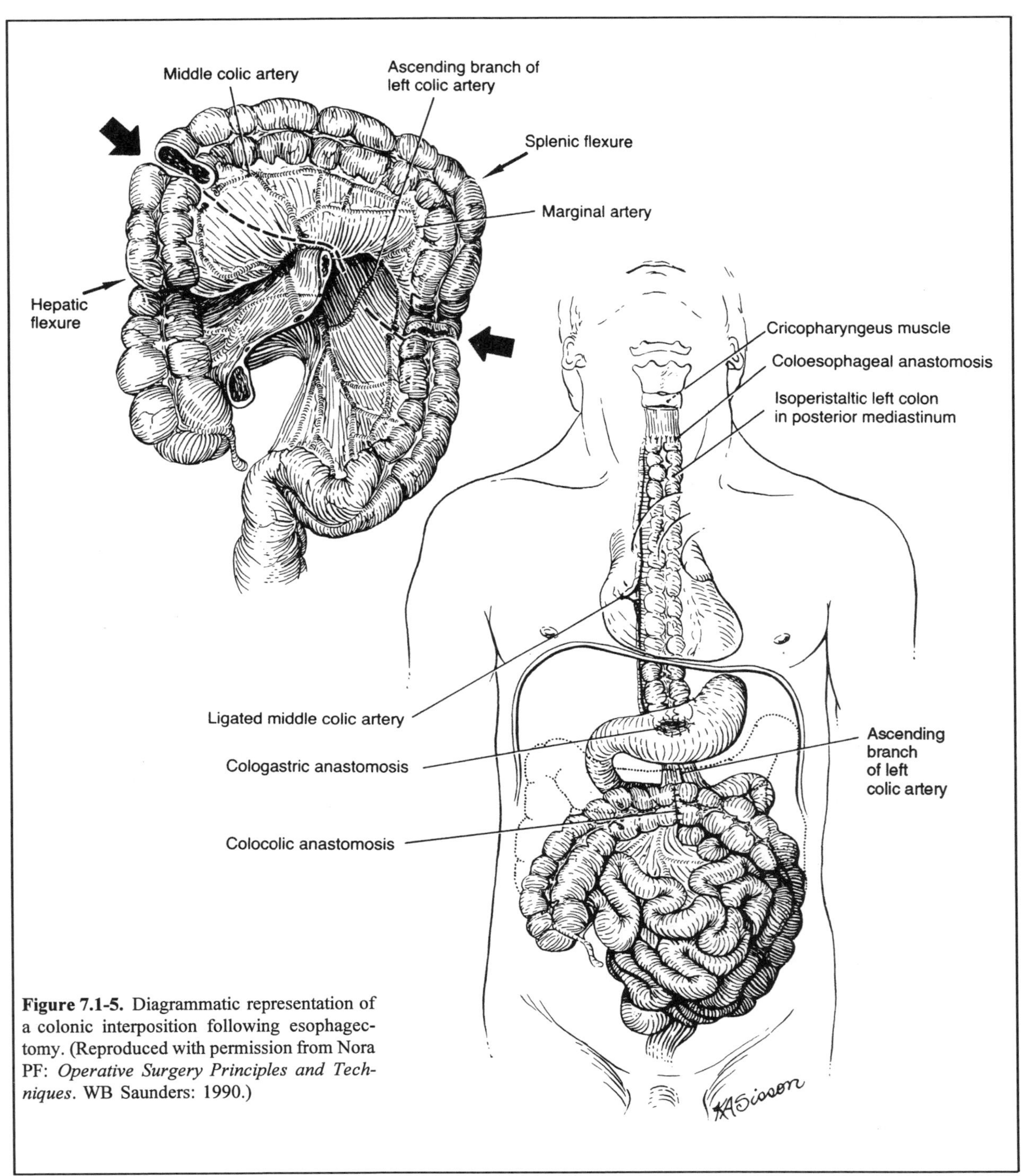


**Figure 7.1-5.** Diagrammatic representation of a colonic interposition following esophagectomy. (Reproduced with permission from Nora PF: *Operative Surgery Principles and Techniques*. WB Saunders: 1990.)

phagogastric junction for malignant disease are best performed through a left thoracoabdominal approach, in which a portion of the proximal stomach is removed, along with a coeliac node dissection.

The esophagus is removed *en bloc*, along with its pleural coverings, the adjacent lymph nodes, subcarinal lymph nodes and the thoracic duct. The azygos vein is divided and a segment removed where it courses close to the wall of the esophagus. Mobilization of the stomach is achieved by dividing the short gastric vessels to the spleen and the left gastric artery. The celiac axis is cleaned free of all lymph nodes and the gastric-colic ligament incised. Following the **Kocher maneuver** (reflecting duodenum) and a **Ramstedt-Fredet** or **Heineke-Mikulicz pyloroplasty**, the stomach is pulled into the chest and anastomosed to the proximal cut end of the esophagus. This is usually done with an EEA stapling instrument.

**Variant procedure or approaches: Orringer** introduced the so-called "**blind esophagectomy**" done via the abdomen and neck by blunt dissection. This is useful primarily for benign esophageal lesions or malignant lesions of the pharynx and larynx where the pharynx and/or upper esophagus require resection.

**Total esophagectomy** may be done via an abdominal and right thoracotomy approach with colonic interposition and anastomosis in the neck (Fig 7.1-5). Either the right or left side of the colon can be mobilized for interposition. Both depend on the middle colic artery and the marginal artery of the colon for their vascular supply. When the proximal portion of the right colon is utilized, the interposed segment of bowel is isoperistaltic, but when the left colon is brought up, the segment is antiperistaltic. Although the colonic interposition is said to function primarily as a conduit for food, it is found that the isoperistaltic colonic segment functions better. In either case, the colonic segment is connected to the body of the stomach after suturing the esophageal-colonic anastomosis.

**Usual preop diagnosis:** Carcinoma of esophagus or gastroesophageal junction; Barrett's esophagus; benign strictures

**SUMMARY OF PROCEDURE**

| | Esophagectomy | Blind Esophagectomy | Esophago-gastrectomy | Total Esophagec-tomy + Colonic Interposition |
|---|---|---|---|---|
| **Position** | Supine and left lateral decubitus | Supine | Left lateral decubitus | Supine and right lateral decubitus |
| **Incision** | Midline abdominal + right or left chest and/or cervical incisions | Cervical and midline abdominal | Thoracoabdominal across costal margin | Midline + right thoracic and cervical |
| **Special instrumentation** | Chest retractor ± EEA stapler | Denier retractor | Chest retractor ± EEA stapler | Chest retractor |
| **Unique considerations** | DLT | None | DLT | ⇐ |
| **Antibiotics** | Cefotetan 2 gm pre-op | ⇐ | ⇐ | ⇐ |
| **Surgical time** | 3 - 4 hrs | 4 - 5 hrs | 3 - 4 hrs | 5 - 6 hrs |
| **Closing considerations** | Lung expansion | Pneumothorax | Lung expansion | Vascular integrity of colonic interposition |
| **EBL** | 200-300 ml | 500-600 ml | 200-300 ml | 500-600 ml |
| **Postop care** | ICU x 1-2 d | ⇐ | ⇐ | ICU x 2-3 d |
| **Mortality** | 5-10% | ⇐ | ⇐ | 10% |
| **Morbidity** | Respiratory complications: 15-20% | ⇐ | ⇐ | ⇐ |
| | Anastomotic leakage: < 5% | 5-10% | < 5% | 10% |
| | Anastomotic stricture: < 5% | ⇐ | ⇐ | 10% |
| | Wound infection: < 5% | ⇐ | ⇐ | ⇐ |
| **Procedure code** | 43110 | ⇐ | 43120 | 43110 |
| **Pain score** | 7-9 | 6-8 | 7-9 | 7-9 |

### PATIENT POPULATION CHARACTERISTICS

| | |
|---|---|
| **Age range** | 40-80 yrs |
| **Male:Female** | 2:1 for carcinoma |
| **Incidence** | 1-2% of malignant disease |
| **Etiology** | Alcohol and tobacco<br>Dietary factors - hot foods<br>Lye burns |
| **Associated conditions** | Barrett's esophagus<br>Hiatus hernia<br>Reflux esophagitis<br>Radiation esophagitis<br>Caustic burns |

---

## ANESTHETIC CONSIDERATIONS FOR ESOPHAGEAL SURGERY

**(Procedures covered: esophagostomy; treatment of esophageal diverticulectomy; closure of esophageal perforation; esophagomyotomy; esophagogastric fundoplasty; esophagectomy)**

### PREOPERATIVE

**Respiratory** A history of gastric reflux suggests the possibility of recurrent aspiration pneumonia: ↓pulmonary reserve and ↑risk of regurgitation/aspiration during anesthetic induction. (See Premedication, below.) If thoracic approach is planned, patient should be evaluated to insure that OLV can be tolerated (see below).

Determine if patient has been exposed to bleomycin, which may cause pulmonary toxicity (above a total dose of 300 U/m$^2$); toxicity may be made worse by high concentrations of $O_2$. Many patients with esophageal cancer have a long history of smoking, with consequent respiratory impairment.

**Tests:** PFTs ($FEV_1$, FVC), ABG can be helpful in predicting likelihood of perioperative pulmonary complications and probability that patient may require postop mechanical ventilation. (Patients with baseline hypoxemia/hypercarbia on room air ABG will have a higher likelihood of postop complications and need for postop ventilatory support. Severe restrictive or obstructive lung disease will also increase the chance of pulmonary morbidity in the perioperative period) A-P, lateral CXR.

**Cardiovascular** Patient may be hypovolemic and malnourished from dysphagia or anorexia. Chemotherapeutic drugs (daunorubicin, adriamycin) may cause cardiomyopathies. Often seen if total dose is >550 mg/m$^2$. Chronic alcohol abuse may also produce a toxic cardiomyopathy. CHF, if present, may be refractory to treatment; however, preop optimization of cardiac status is essential. (Consider cardiac consultation.)

**Tests:** If cardiomyopathy suspected, ECHO or MUGA scan will provide data on ejection fraction. ECG, to rule out myocardial ischemia as cause of pain/heartburn.

**Hematologic** Encourage preop autologous blood donation.

**Tests:** CBC with differential; coagulation profile (PT/PTT)

**Laboratory** UA; electrolytes; glucose; creatinine; BUN; bilirubin; transaminases; alkaline phosphatase; albumin. Other tests as indicated from H&P.

**Premedication** Midazolam (0.07-0.08 mg/kg im). Morphine (0.08-0.15 mg/kg im). Consider $H_2$-antagonists, metoclopramide (10 mg iv 1 hr preop), and Na citrate (30 cc po 30 min preop).

### INTRAOPERATIVE

**Anesthetic technique:** GETA (with or without epidural for postop analgesia). If postop epidural analgesia is planned, placement and testing of the catheter prior to anesthetic induction is helpful. (This is accomplished by injecting 5-7 cc of 1% lidocaine via the epidural catheter, and eliciting a segmental block.) If a thoracic or abdominothoracic approach is performed, placement of a DLT is indicated, as one-lung anesthesia provides excellent surgical exposure. (For additional discussion, see Anesthetic Considerations in "Lobectomy and Pneumonectomy" in "Thoracic Surgery" section.)

**Induction** Patients with esophageal disease are often at risk for pulmonary aspiration; therefore, the trachea should be intubated with the patient awake or after rapid-sequence induction with cricoid pressure. Awake intubation: (1) Blind nasal: topical vasoconstrictor to nose (1% phenylephrine or 4% cocaine on cotton-tipped applicators). Advance ETT until at laryngeal inlet; when patient inspires, advance ETT into trachea. Manipulation of ETT or head may be necessary for successful placement. (2) **Fiber optic intubation**: topical oropharyngeal anesthesia with 10% lidocaine spray. Transtracheal administration of 4% lidocaine (2 cc) with 23 ga needle. ETT is guided into trachea under visualization with the fiber optic bronchoscope (see FOL in "Anesthetic Considerations for Thoracolumbar Procedures" in "Neurosurgery" section). If patient is clinically hypovolemic, restore intravascular volume prior to induction and titrate induction dose of sedative/hypnotic agents.

**Maintenance** Standard maintenance (see Appendix), without $N_2O$. Alternatively, a combined technique may be used. A local anesthetic (1.5-2% lidocaine with 1:200,000 epinephrine 12-15 ml q 60 min) can be injected into an epidural catheter to provide both anesthesia and optimal surgical exposure (contracted bowel and profound muscle relaxation). Be prepared to treat hypotension with fluid and vasopressors. GA is administered to supplement regional anesthesia and for amnesia. Systemic sedatives (droperidol, opiates, benzodiazepines, etc.) should be minimized during epidural opiate administration as they increase the likelihood of postop respiratory depression. If epidural opiates are used for postop analgesia, a loading dose (e.g., hydromorphone 1.0-1.5 mg) should be administered at least 1 hr before conclusion of surgery.

**Emergence** The decision to extubate at the end of surgery depends on patient's underlying cardiopulmonary status and the extent of the surgical procedure. Patient should be hemodynamically stable, warm, alert, cooperative, and fully reversed from any muscle relaxants prior to extubation. Patients who require postop ventilation should have the DLT changed to a single-lumen ETT prior to transport to ICU. Weaning from mechanical ventilation should begin when patient is awake and cooperative, able to protect the airway, and have adequate return of pulmonary function (as measured by VC of $\geq$15 cc/kg, MIF-25 cm $H_2O$, respiratory rate < 25 and ABG which approaches preop baseline).

| | | |
|---|---|---|
| **Blood and fluid requirements** | IV: 14-16 ga x 1<br>NS/LR @ 8-12 cc/kg/hr<br>Fluid warmer | T&C for 4 U PRBC. Platelets, FFP and cryoprecipitate (if required) should be administered according to lab tests (platelet count, PT, PTT, DIC screen, thromboelastography [TEG]). |
| **Monitoring** | Standard monitors (see Appendix).<br>Urinary catheter<br>Arterial line | Plus others as indicated by patient's status. Attempt to prevent hypothermia during long operations. Consider heated humidifier, warming blanket, warming room temperature, keeping patient covered until ready for prep, etc. |
| **Positioning** | If lateral decubitus position, axillary roll, airplane arm holder.<br>✓ pressure points, including ears, eyes and genitals.<br>✓ radial pulses to ensure correct placement of axillary roll (if misplaced, will compromise distal pulses). | Problems that can arise include: brachial plexus injuries, damage to soft tissues, ears, eyes, genitals from malpositioning. |
| **Complications** | Hypoxemia | Hypoxemia during OLV may result from malposition of DLT $\rightarrow$ $\downarrow$vent. Rx: ✓ position and adjust. 100% $FiO_2$, PEEP to ventilated lung, CPAP to non-ventilated lung, return to double-lung ventilation. Temporary clamping of the PA may be necessary to $\uparrow O_2$ saturation. |

## POSTOPERATIVE

| | | |
|---|---|---|
| **Complications** | Atelectasis<br>Aspiration<br>Hemorrhage | For atelectasis or aspiration, recover the patient in the Fowles position<br>For hemorrhage, ✓ coags; replace factors as necessary. |

| | | |
|---|---|---|
| **Complications, continued** | Pneumothorax<br>Hemothorax | Dx for pneumothorax and hemothorax: wheezing, coughing, ↓$PO_2$, ↑$PCO_2$. Confirm by CXR. Rx: chest tube drainage as necessary. In emergency (e.g., tension pneumothorax) use needle aspiration. Supportive Rx: $O_2$, vasopressors, volume, ± ETT and IPPV. |
| | Hypoxemia<br>Hypoventilation | For hypoxemia and hypoventilation, adequate analgesia, supplemental $O_2$. |
| | Recurrent laryngeal nerve injury | For laryngeal nerve injury, indirect visualization of vocal cords; patient usually will be hoarse. |
| | Esophageal anastomotic leak<br>Pain | Surgical repair for esophageal anastomotic leak |
| **Pain management** | Epidural analgesia: hydromorphone (0.8-1.5 mg load; 0.2-0.3 mg/hr infusion)<br>PCA (see Appendix). | Patient should recover in ICU or hospital ward that is accustomed to treating side effects of epidural opiates (e.g., respiratory depression, breakthrough pain, nausea, pruritus). |
| **Tests** | CBC; ABG; CXR (rule out pneumothorax, atelectasis) | |

**References**


1. Orringer MB, Orringer JS: Esophagectomy without thoracotomy: a dangerous operation? *J Thorac Cardiovasc Surg* 1983; 85(1):72-80.
2. Belsey R: Reconstruction of the esophagus with left colon. *J Thorac Cardiovasc Surg* 1965; 49:33-55.
3. Eisenkraft JB, Cohen E, Kaplan JA: Anesthesia for Thoracic Surgery. In *Clinical Anesthesia.* Barash, PG, Cullen BF, Stoelting RK eds. JB Lippincott Co, Philadelphia: 1989, 918.
4. Patterson GA, Cooper JD: Complications of thoracotomy. In *Anesthesia for Thoracic Procedures.* Marshall BE, Longnecker DE, Fairley HB, eds. Blackwell Scientific Publications, Boston: 1988, 559-79.

**Surgeon**

**Mark A. Vierra, MD**

# 7.2 STOMACH SURGERY

**Anesthesiologist**

**Steven K. Howard, MD**

# GASTRIC RESECTIONS

## SURGICAL CONSIDERATIONS

**Description: Total gastrectomy** is performed most commonly for gastric cancer, and may include **omentectomy**, **lymph node dissection**, and/or **splenectomy**, depending on the extent of the tumor, condition of the patient, and surgeon's preference. Occasionally it is performed for uncontrollable symptoms due to Zollinger-Ellison syndrome. Rarely, this procedure may be used for control of hemorrhage from diffuse gastritis. Even more rarely, patients with intractable post-gastrectomy symptoms may eventually require total gastrectomy.

In a gastric resection, the abdomen is entered through an upper midline incision and the lateral segment of the left lobe of the liver is retracted to the patient's right, exposing the esophagogastric junction. The omentum is taken off of the colon and the spleen is delivered; then the splenic vessels are divided, leaving the spleen attached to the stomach by the short gastric vessels. The vessels to the stomach are individually ligated and divided; then the duodenum is divided just distal to the pylorus. The stomach is divided at or near the esophagogastric junction. The jejunum is divided just beyond the Ligament of Trietz, and the distal end is brought up through a hole in the mesentery of the colon and anastomosed to the esophagus. The duodenum is closed with either sutures or staples. Intestinal continuity is established by anastomosing the end of the proximal limb of the jejunum to a Roux limb of jejunum, approximately 60 cm distal to the anastomosis with the esophagus. A drain is then placed. Occasionally, following total gastrectomy, the surgeon may choose to create a jejunal reservoir to simulate a stomach. This does not add appreciably to the duration, difficulty or morbidity of the operation, but its efficacy is not widely accepted. A nasogastric tube is advanced across the esophagojejunal anastomosis and the abdomen is closed. Total gastrectomy has traditionally been associated with a morbidity and mortality out of proportion to the operation's apparent magnitude. This is most likely a consequence of the patient's underlying condition, which often includes advanced malignancy and, almost invariably, some degree of malnutrition.

**Variant procedure or approaches:** Exposure for a **hemigastrectomy** is similar to, but less extensive than that required for a total gastrectomy. The abdomen is entered through an upper midline or right subcostal incision, but the lateral segment of the left lobe of the liver is simply retracted superiorly. If the resection is performed for cancer, an **omentectomy** may still be performed; however, it would be unusual to intentionally perform a **splenectomy**. The blood supply to the distal stomach is divided, and the duodenum is divided just beyond the pylorus. The body of the stomach is divided, using either clamps and sutures or staples, at a level appropriate for the pathology. If the resection is for cancer, an adequate proximal margin will dictate the proximal line of resection; if for a benign gastric ulcer, approximately half of the distal stomach is resected (preferably excising the ulcer itself). Reconstruction may be either to the duodenum (**Billroth I**), loop of jejunum (**Billroth II**) (Fig 7.2-1), or to a **Roux-en-Y loop of jejunum**. The anastomoses may be stapled or sewn; then the abdomen is closed.

**Usual preop diagnosis**: Total gastrectomy: gastric malignancy; Zollinger-Ellison syndrome; hemorrhage 2° diffuse gastritis. Hemigastrectomy: gastric cancer; gastric ulcers

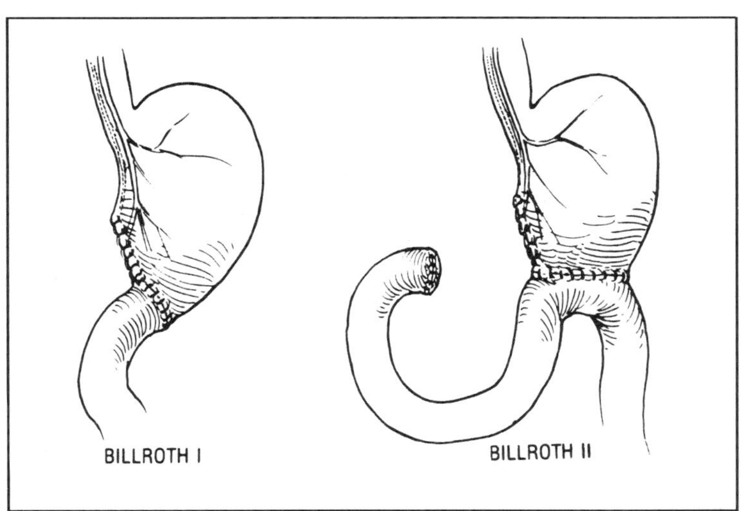


**Figure 7.2-1.** Anatomy of duodenostomy (Billroth I) and gastrojejunostomy (Billroth II). (Reproduced with permission from Hardy JD: *Hardy's Textbook of Surgery*, 2nd edition. JB Lippincott: 1988.)

### SUMMARY OF PROCEDURE

| | Total Gastrectomy | Hemigastrectomy |
|---|---|---|
| **Position** | Supine | ⇐ |
| **Incision** | Upper midline or bilateral subcostal | Upper midline or right subcostal |
| **Special instrumentation** | Upper hand or other self-retaining costal retractor | Upper hand or other costal retractor |
| **Antibiotics** | ± Cefazolin 1 gm iv | ⇐ |
| **Surgical time** | 2 - 4 hrs | 1.5 - 2 hrs |
| **Closing considerations** | Muscle relaxation required; NG suction | ⇐ |
| **EBL** | 500+ cc, with potential for significantly more. | 100-500 cc |
| **Postop care** | PACU | ⇐ |
| **Mortality** | 0-22% | 0-1.8% (may be >10% if emergency) |
| **Morbidity** | Pulmonary complications: 15%<br>Re-operation: 0-5%<br>Esophagojejunal leak<br>Sepsis<br>Late anastomotic stricture<br>Cardiac complications | Anastomotic leak<br>Wound infection<br>Cardiopulmonary complications |
| **Procedure code** | 43620 | 43630 |
| **Pain score** | 7-8 | 7-8 |

### PATIENT POPULATION CHARACTERISTICS

| | |
|---|---|
| **Age range** | Mostly elderly |
| **Male:Female** | Male predominance |
| **Incidence** | Declining, due to declining incidence of gastric cancer and gastric ulcer, and medical treatment for Zollinger-Ellison syndrome |
| **Etiology** | Gastric cancer and ulcer associated with:<br>Advanced age<br>Alcohol and tobacco use<br>Geographic location |
| **Associated conditions** | Weight loss: Common<br>Anemia: Common<br>Malnutrition: Common<br>Zollinger-Ellison syndrome: Rare (Avoid $H_2$-antagonists prop, if intraop gastric pH monitoring is planned by surgeon.) |

## ANESTHETIC CONSIDERATIONS

See Anesthetic Considerations following "Operations for Peptic Ulcer Disease" (below).

**References**

1. Heberer G, Teichmann RK, Kramlin HJ, Gunther B: Results of gastric resection for carcinoma of the stomach: the European experience. *World J Surg* 1988; 12(3):374-81.
2. Dent DM, Madden MB, Price SK: Randomized comparison of R1 and R2 gastrectomy for gastric carcinoma. *Br J Surg* 1988; 75(2):110-12.
3. Longmire WP Jr: Gastric carcinoma: is radical gastrectomy worthwhile? *Ann R Coll Surg Engl* 1980; 62(1):25-30.
4. Herrington LL Jr: Vagotomy and antrectomy. In *Surgery of the Stomach, Duodenum and Small Intestine*, 2nd edition. Scott HW Jr, Sawyers JL, eds. Blackwell Scientific Publications, Boston: 1992, 524-39.

# OVERSEW GASTRIC OR DUODENAL PERFORATION

## SURGICAL CONSIDERATIONS

**Description:** These operations are usually emergencies, and patients usually have peritonitis at presentation. Closure of the perforation alone, as opposed to performance of a definitive ulcer operation, is performed based on the surgeon's assessment of the patient's ability to tolerate a more extensive operation and the risk of recurrent ulceration.

In the younger patient with duodenal perforation (and where there is no delay in the diagnosis), a **highly selective vagotomy** may be added to closure of the perforation. Stomach or duodenum perforation is almost always a consequence of peptic ulcer disease, although on rare occasion, it may be caused by penetrating trauma. While perforation of the duodenum is almost never a consequence of malignant ulceration, perforation of the stomach due to malignant ulceration must always be considered. For this reason, the preferred treatment of a perforated gastric ulcer includes **resection**. If the general condition of the patient is poor or local inflammation is present, a biopsy of the ulcer, followed by closure, may be prudent. Biopsy of a perforated duodenal ulcer, on the other hand, is seldom necessary. In patients who are not systemically ill at the time of operation and who do not have severe peritonitis, some surgeons prefer to do a definitive ulcer operation such as a **vagotomy and pyloroplasty** or **highly selective vagotomy** at the time of closure of the perforation. Under other circumstances, closure of the perforation alone may be appropriate.

For closure of perforations, an upper midline incision is usually used, although a right subcostal incision may be appropriate. The liver is retracted superiorly and the area of perforation identified. A nasogastric tube will have been placed preop and should remain on suction throughout the case to minimize ongoing leakage from the perforation area. Perforation of the stomach may be handled either by resection (see "Gastric Resections," above), or by biopsy and simple suture closure. Perforation of the duodenum is usually repaired by simple suture of the site. Omentum is often used to buttress the area of closure of the stomach or duodenum. Closed suction drains are placed near the area of perforation and the abdomen is irrigated. Abdominal closure is routine, and the skin may be closed either primarily or packed open, depending on surgeon's preference.

**Variant procedure or approaches:** In certain patients, **nonoperative management** of perforated ulcer may be appropriate. In general, this has a relatively high likelihood of success in otherwise healthy patients with sealed duodenal perforation, but is much less reliable in frailer patients. While this may be a reasonable approach in some patients, there is no data to suggest that it is safer than traditional operative treatment.

**Usual preop diagnosis:** Perforated peptic ulcer

### SUMMARY OF PROCEDURE

| | |
|---|---|
| **Position** | Supine |
| **Incision** | Midline |
| **Special instrumentation** | Costal retractor |
| **Unique considerations** | Patients usually have peritonitis. |
| **Antibiotics** | ± Cefazolin 1 gm iv |
| **Surgical time** | 1 hr |
| **Closing considerations** | Muscle relaxation required for closure; NG suction |
| **EBL** | Minimal |
| **Postop care** | PACU |
| **Mortality** | 5-15%, largely dependent on patient population |
| **Morbidity** | Pneumonia<br>Intra-abdominal abscess<br>Wound infection<br>Reperforation |
| **Procedure code** | 43840 (gastrorrhaphy, suture of perforated duodenal or gastric ulcer, wound or injury) |
| **Pain score** | 7 |

### PATIENT POPULATION CHARACTERISTICS

| | |
|---|---|
| **Age range** | Adult, increasingly elderly, especially women |
| **Male:Female** | Previous heavy male predominance still exists for duodenal ulcer, but large increase in incidence in gastric perforation in women >65. |
| **Incidence** | Fairly common. Stable incidence, but with change in distribution, especially more elderly women. |
| **Etiology** | Peptic ulcer disease<br>Non-steroidal medications<br>Malignancy, if gastric |
| **Associated conditions** | Malignancy (if perforation is gastric)<br>Non-steroidal medications<br>Steroid use, especially during pulse therapy<br>Other risk factors for PUD (e.g., alcoholism, smoking, etc.) |

## ANESTHETIC CONSIDERATIONS

See Anesthetic Considerations following "Operations for Peptic Ulcer Disease" (below).

**References**

1. Hennessy E: Perforated peptic ulcer: mortality and morbidity in 603 cases. *Aust NZ J Surg* 1969; 38(3):243-52.
2. Jick SS, Perera DR, Walker AM, Jick H: Non-steroidal anti-inflammatory drugs and hospital admission for perforated peptic ulcer. *Lancet* 1987; 2(8555):380-82.
3. Hugh TB: Perforated peptic ulcers. In *Maingot's Abdominal Operations*, 9th edition. Schwartz SI, Ellis H, eds. Appleton & Lange, Norwalk, CT: 1989, 627-645.
4. Sawyers JL: Acute perforation of peptic ulcer. In *Surgery of the Stomach, Duodenum and Small Intestine*. Scott HW Jr, Sawyers JL, eds. Blackwell Scientific Publications, Boston: 1992, 566-72.

# OPERATIONS FOR PEPTIC ULCER DISEASE

## SURGICAL CONSIDERATIONS

**Description:** Gastric ulcers are commonly associated with advanced age, and patients often have other medical problems, particularly cardiovascular and pulmonary. Currently there is a trend toward more emergency operations for bleeding gastric ulcers, particularly in elderly women and perhaps related to increasing use of non-steroidal medications. All operations for peptic ulcer disease require exposure of the upper abdomen, and may be performed using either an upper midline or a long, right subcostal incision. The choice of surgical procedure depends on a number of considerations, including whether it is performed as an emergency or electively; the reason for performing the procedure (common factors include bleeding, perforation, intractability or gastric outlet obstruction); duration of symptoms; condition of the patient; and experience of the surgeon.

**Vagotomy and antrectomy (V&A):** This is the most extensive of the operations performed for peptic ulcer disease, and is generally reserved for low-risk patients with significant intractable symptoms. The esophageal hiatus is exposed either by taking down the lateral segment of the left lobe of the liver and reflecting it to the patient's right, or by retracting this segment of the liver superiorly to gain exposure. The phrenoesophageal ligament is divided and the anterior and posterior vagus nerves (there may be more than one of each involved) are identified by feel. Division of all vagal trunks at the esophageal hiatus is performed, and specimens of the nerves are sent for pathology. The blood supply to the antrum is then divided, usually by dividing the right gastric and gastroepiploic vessels first. The gastro-

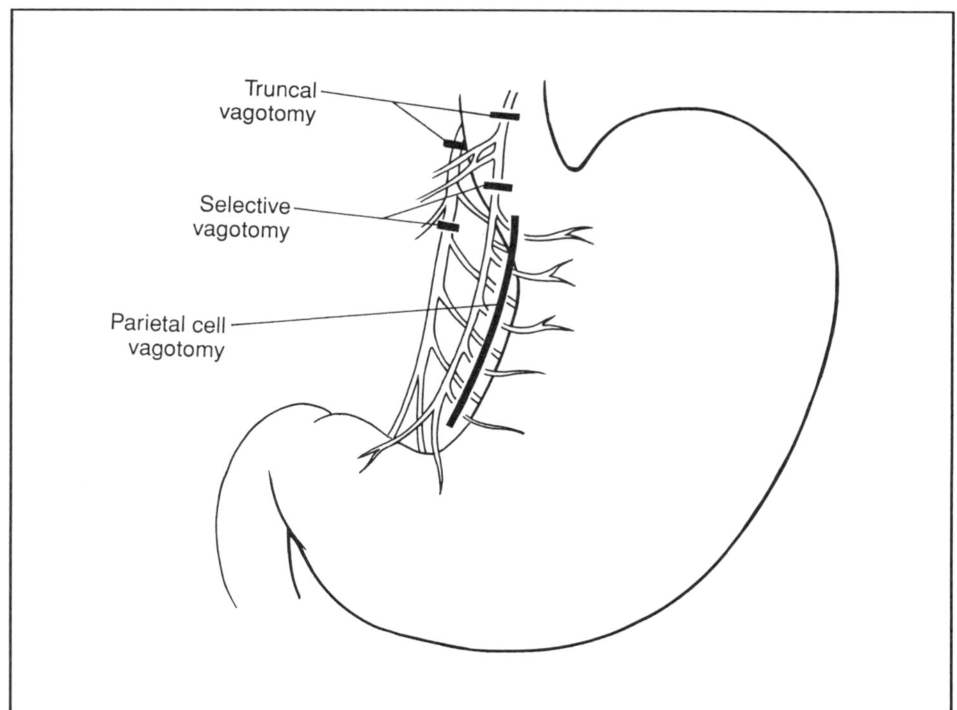


**Figure 7.2-2.** Types of vagotomy. Heavy lines incicate where vagal trunks are cut.

hepatic ligament is divided and the stomach elevated off of its attachments to the transverse colon. The gastric antrum is resected, leaving the duodenum just beyond the pylorus and dividing the stomach just above the junction of the body with the antrum. Reconstruction may be as a **Billroth I** (stomach-to-duodenum) or **Billroth II** (stomach-to-jejunal loop) (Fig 7.2-1). The anastomosis may be stapled or hand-sewn. Drains are not commonly used if a Billroth I is performed, but may be used in Billroth II because of the concern for a leak from the duodenal stump.

**Vagotomy and pyloroplasty (V&P)**: This is the most commonly performed operation for peptic ulcer disease in the U.S. and is especially common for emergency operations. It is generally accepted to be simpler and safer to perform than V&A, but not as effective at preventing recurrence of ulcer disease. The abdominal incision and exposure of the hiatus to perform a vagotomy is the same as for vagotomy and pyloroplasty. After division of both vagal trunks (Fig 7.2-2), a longitudinal incision is made through the pylorus. The incision is then sutured together transversely, completing the pyloroplasty.

**Parietal cell vagotomy (PCV):** This operation requires even more meticulous exposure of the esophageal hiatus than that needed for a truncal vagotomy. The hiatus is exposed as above, and the main vagal trunks supplying the stomach are identified, but not divided. The stomach is retracted downward, and it is often helpful to divide a portion of the gastrocolic omentum to facilitate grasping the stomach. Branches supplying the body of the stomach (Fig 7.2-2), however, are individually divided and ligated with fine ligatures. Because the nerve fibers run with the blood vessels to the stomach, this necessarily involves division of the blood supply to the proximal lesser curvature of the stomach. This dissection is carried to the region of the "crow's foot" of the stomach, which is preserved. By denervating only the acid-producing portion of the stomach, while preserving innervation to the antrum, gastric acidity is diminished without significantly impairing gastric motility or emptying. A pyloroplasty is, therefore, not necessary. The operation is relatively tedious compared to the other procedures, and is usually performed electively or, rarely, urgently if there is a recent perforation and minimal soilage. It can be recommended only for duodenal ulcer disease, not gastric ulcer. Side-effects of this operation are generally less than with other ulcer operations.

**Variant procedure or approaches**: At the time of this writing, there have been several attempts to perform vagotomy, particularly PCV or vagotomy and pyloroplasty, **laparoscopically**. There is not enough experience to date, however, to describe its usefulness.

**Usual preop diagnosis**: V&P: complications of duodenal ulcer disease (bleeding, perforation and gastric outlet obstruction). V&A: duodenal and prepyloric ulcer disease. PCV: isolated duodenal ulcer disease; recent perforation and minimal peritoneal soilage

## SUMMARY OF PROCEDURE

| | V&P | V&A | PCV |
|---|---|---|---|
| **Position** | Supine | ⇐ | ⇐ |
| **Incision** | Midline or long subcostal | ⇐ | Midline |
| **Special instrumentation** | Costal margin retractor | ⇐ | ⇐ |
| **Antibiotics** | ± Cefazolin 1 gm iv | ⇐ | ⇐ |
| **Surgical time** | 1 - 2 hrs | 1.5 - 3 hrs | 1.5 - 2.5 hrs |
| **Closing considerations** | Muscle relaxation required for closure; NG suction | ⇐ | ⇐ |
| **EBL** | < 250 cc; greater for emergency surgeries | 250-500 cc | < 250 cc |
| **Postop care** | PACU | ⇐ | ⇐ |
| **Mortality** | 0-2% (most series include emergencies) | 0-1.6% (most series do not include emergencies) | 0-0.4% |
| **Morbidity** | Dumping and diarrhea: 6-20% | 17-27% | – |
| | Recurrence: 4.9-12.3% | 0-2% | 5-15% (39.3-5%) |
| | | | Impaired gastric emptying: 0.3% |
| | | | Necrosis, lesser curve: < 0.3% |
| | | | PE: rare |
| **Procedure code** | 43630 (hemigastrectomy or distal subtotal gastrectomy)<br>43640<br>43640-22 (special difficulty if laparoscopic) | 43635<br>43635-22 (special difficulty if laparoscopic) | 43641 (PCV or HSV)<br>43641-22 (special difficulty if laparoscopic) |
| **Pain score** | 6 | 6 | 6 |

## PATIENT POPULATION CHARACTERISTICS

| | |
|---|---|
| **Age range** | Adults |
| **Male:Female** | Male > female |
| **Incidence** | Declining |
| **Etiology** | Acid hypersecretion<br>Abnormal mucosal permeability and repair mechanisms<br>Helicobacter pylori |
| **Associated conditions** | Gastrinoma: Rare<br>Hyperparathyroidism: Rare |

---

# ANESTHETIC CONSIDERATIONS

**(Procedures covered: gastric resections; oversew gastric/duodenal perforation; operations for peptic ulcer disease; duodenotomy)**

## PREOPERATIVE

Patients presenting for gastric surgery generally comprise 2 groups: (1) those presenting for emergency surgery following GI bleeding or perforation, and (2) those presenting with gastric carcinoma or elective treatment of peptic ulcer disease. Patients in the first group are often hemodynamically unstable and require rapid preop assessment and appropriate fluid therapy. It is prudent to consider full-stomach precautions in both patient groups.

**Respiratory** Patients with GI bleeding are prone to aspiration of blood and gastric contents. If this has occurred, patient may have significant respiratory insufficiency (in urgent need of tracheal intubation for "protection" of airway).

**Cardiovascular** Hypovolemia may be severe due to N&V, diarrhea, poor po intake or GI blood loss. Sx include ↓skin turgor, ↑HR, ↓BP, ↓UO. Correct hypovolemia prior to inducing anesthesia.
**Tests:** Orthostatic vital signs; ECG

**Renal** GI fluid loss can lead to renal and electrolyte abnormalities.
**Tests:** Electrolytes; BUN; creatinine; glucose; UA

**Hematologic** Polycythemia 2° GI fluid loss may be present; patients with GI bleeding will likely be anemic and may have a coagulopathy.
**Tests:** CBC with platelets; PT; PTT

**Laboratory** Bilirubin; transaminases; alkaline phosphatase; albumin; calcium

**Premedication** Standard premedication (see Appendix) for elective procedures. Consider $H_2$-antagonist, metoclopramide (10 mg iv 1 hr preop), and Na citrate (30 cc po 15-30 min preop).

## INTRAOPERATIVE

**Anesthetic technique:** GETA ± epidural for postop analgesia. If postop epidural analgesia is planned, placement of catheter prior to anesthetic induction is helpful to establish correct placement in the epidural space (accomplished by injecting 5-7 cc of 1% lidocaine via the epidural catheter, eliciting a segmental block).

**Induction** The patient with gastric disease or upper GI bleeding is often at risk for pulmonary aspiration, and the trachea should be intubated with the patient awake or after rapid-sequence induction with cricoid pressure. (See "Rapid-Sequence Induction" in Appendix.) If patient is clinically hypovolemic, restore intravascular volume (colloid, crystalloid or blood) prior to induction, and titrate induction dose of sedative/hypnotic agents.

**Maintenance** Standard maintenance (see Appendix) without $N_2O$. **Combined epidural/light GA**: Local anesthetic (1.5-2% lidocaine with 1:200,000 epinephrine (12-15 cc q 60 min) can be injected into the epidural catheter to provide both anesthesia and optimal surgical exposure (contracted bowel and profound muscle relaxation). Be prepared to treat hypotension with fluid and vasopressors. GA is administered to supplement regional anesthesia and for amnesia. Systemic sedatives (droperidol, opiates, benzodiazepines, etc.) should be minimized during epidural opiate administration as they increase the likelihood of postop respiratory depression. Treat hypotension with fluid and vasopressors. If epidural opiates are used for postop analgesia, a loading dose (e.g., hydromorphone 1.0 mg) should be administered at least 1 hr before the conclusion of surgery.

**Emergence** The decision to extubate at the end of surgery depends on the patient's underlying cardiopulmonary status and extent of the surgical procedure. Patient should be hemodynamically stable, warm, alert, cooperative and fully reversed from any muscle relaxants prior to extubation. Continued intubation and mechanical ventilation may be required if the patient is unable to protect the airway, or has not had adequate return of pulmonary function (as measured by VC of 15 cc/kg, MIF of -25 cm $H_2O$, RR < 25 and ABGs which approach patient's baseline).

**Blood and fluid requirements** Anticipate large third-space losses.
IV: 14-16 ga x 1
Fluid warmer

T&C for 4 U PRBC. Platelets, FFP and cryoprecipitate should be administered according to lab tests (platelet count, PT, PTT, DIC screen, thromboelastography).

**Monitoring** Standard monitors (see Appendix)
UO
ABG
± CVP catheter

+ Others as indicated by patient's status. Try to prevent hypothermia during long operations. Consider heated humidifier, warming blanket, warming room temperature, keeping patient covered until ready for prep, etc.

**Positioning** ✓ and pad pressure points.
✓ eyes.

**Complications** Acute hemorrhage
Hypoxemia 2° abdominal packs
↓FRC

## POSTOPERATIVE

**Complications** Atelectasis
Hemorrhage
Ileus
Hypothermia

**Pain management** Epidural analgesics (see Appendix).
PCA (see Appendix).

**Tests** CXR if CVP placed perioperatively.

**References**


1. Goligher JC, Pulvertaft CN: Comparison of different operations. In *After Vagotomy*. Williams JA, Cox AG, eds. Butterworths, London: 1969, 83-118.
2. Jordan PH Jr, Condon RE: A prospective evaluation of vagotomy-pyloroplasty and vagotomy-antrectomy for treatment of duodenal ulcer. *Ann Surg* 1970; 72(4):547-63.
3. Goligher JC, Pulvertaft CN, De Dombal FT, Congers JH, Duthie HL, Fether DB, Latchmore AJ, Shoesmith JH, Smiddy FG, Willson-Pepper J: Five to eight-year results of Leeds-York controlled trial of elective surgery for duodenal ulcer. *Br Med J* 1968; 2(608):781-87.
4. Thompson JC, Wiener I: Evaluation of surgical treatment for duodenal ulcer: short- and long-term effects. *Clin Gastroenterol* 1984; 13(2):569-600.
5. Johnston D: Duodenal and gastric ulcer. In *Maingot's Abdominal Operations*, 9th edition. Schwartz SI, Ellis H, eds. Appleton & Lange, Norwalk, CT: 1989, 599-625.
6. Hoffmann J, Jensen HE, Christiansen J, Olesen A, Loud FB, Hauch O: Prospective controlled vagotomy trial for duodenal ulcer. Results after 11-15 years. *Ann Surg* 1989; 209(1):40-5.
7. Moreno GE, Narbona AB, Charo DT, Figueroa AJ: Proximal gastric vagotomy. A prospective study of 829 patients with four-year follow-up. *Acta Chir Scand* 1983; 149(1):69-76.
8. Gorey TF, Lennon F, Heffernan SJ: Highly selective vagotomy in duodenal ulceration and its complications. A 12-year review. *Ann Surg* 1984; 200(2):181-84.
9. Clark CG, Fresini H, Aranjo JG, Boulos PB: Proximal gastric vagotomy or truncal vagotomy and drainage for chronic duodenal ulcer? *Br J Surg* 1986; 73(4):298-300.
10. Herrington L, Sawyers JL: Complications following gastric operations. In *Maingot's Abdominal Operations*, 9th edition. Schwartz SI, Ellis H, eds. Appleton & Lange, Norwalk, CT: 1989, 701-30.
11. Johnston D: Vagotomy. In *Maingot's Abdominal Operations*, 9th edition. Schwartz SI, Ellis H, eds. Appleton & Lange, Norwalk, CT: 1989, 647-65.


# OPERATIONS FOR MORBID OBESITY

## SURGICAL CONSIDERATIONS

**Description:** Procedures devised to promote weight loss are of two fundamental types: (1) **gastric partitioning procedures**, which work by decreasing the size of the gastric pouch, thereby limiting the amount of food that can be consumed at one time; and (2) **malabsorptive procedures**, which work by bypassing most of the small bowel and creating a state of chronic malabsorption. Of these two general types of procedures, the partitioning procedures are generally less effective at promoting weight loss than are the malabsorptive procedures, but are much more popular because they are associated with far fewer serious side-effects.

The partitioning procedure most commonly used today is the **vertical banded gastroplasty (VBG)**. The abdomen is entered through an upper midline incision and the esophagogastric junction is exposed either by retracting the liver superiorly or by taking down the ligamentous attachments of the lateral segment of the left lobe of the liver and retracting this down and to the patient's right. The vessels to the lesser curvature are taken down for a short distance near the esophagogastric junction and the posterior attachments of the stomach are taken down. A large bougie is passed by the anesthesiologist into the stomach and an EEA circular stapler is used to create a hole in the stomach adjacent to the bougie near the esophagogastric junction. Through this, a special stapler with thick, strong staples is passed and is fired up along the esophagus, creating a pouch of approximately 30 cc in volume. This leaves an outlet to the remainder of the stomach of only 1-2 cm, which is reinforced with a bond of mesh. A nasogastric tube is placed through the gastroplasty into the distal stomach and the abdomen is closed without drains.

Less commonly used is the **gastroplasty with Roux-en-Y gastroenterostomy**. Exposure is similar to that for a VBG. The upper stomach is mobilized and two rows of staples are used to partition the stomach into a small proximal and large distal pouch. A Roux segment of jejunum is then anastomosed to the small proximal pouch to provide drainage of it. A nasogastric tube is placed and the abdomen is closed without drains.

**Variant procedure or approaches**: An alternative to these procedures is the **jejunoileal bypass (JI)**, in which the proximal jejunum is anastomosed to the terminal ileum. Exposure may be through a short, mid-abdominal or right, transverse incision and is generally less than is needed for a gastroplasty. The proximal jejunum is anastomosed to the terminal ileum, creating a chronic state of malabsorption. A nasogastric tube is placed and the abdomen is closed without drains.

**Usual preop diagnosis**: Morbid obesity (100 lbs above ideal body weight or 100% over ideal body weight), generally in combination with some medical condition felt to be worsened by the obesity (e.g., osteoarthritis, diabetes, respiratory insufficiency, CHF)

**SUMMARY OF PROCEDURE**

| | **Gastroplasty** | **JI Bypass** |
|---|---|---|
| **Position** | Supine | ⇐ |
| **Incision** | Midline | ⇐ |
| **Special instrumentation** | Large OR tables; heavy-duty retractors; special stapling devices | ⇐ (except no need for special staplers) |
| **Unique considerations** | Prophylactic cholecystectomy often advocated. Pneumatic compression boots may not be large enough; subcutaneous heparin used commonly. | ⇐ |
| **Antibiotics** | ± Cefazolin 1 gm iv | ⇐ |
| **Surgical time** | 2 - 3 hrs | ~1.5 - 3 hrs |
| **Closing considerations** | Anticipate 1+ hr closure time; NG suction | ⇐ |
| **EBL** | < 500 cc | ⇐ |
| **Postop care** | Postop ventilation may be necessary; DVT precautions | ⇐ |
| **Mortality** | 0.5-1.6% | ⇐ |
| **Morbidity** | PE: 1-1.6% | ⇐ |
| | Wound infection: 4-8% | ⇐ |
| | Anastomotic leak: 3% | ⇐ |
| | Dehiscence: 1.6% | ⇐ |
| **Procedure code** | 43842 (VBG) | 43844 (gastric bypass other than Roux-en-Y gastroenterostomy for morbid obesity); 43846 (gastric bypass with Roux-en-Y gastroenterostomy for morbid obesity) |
| **Pain score** | 7 | 5-6 |

**PATIENT POPULATION CHARACTERISTICS**

| | |
|---|---|
| **Age range** | Adult |
| **Male:Female** | ~1:1 |
| **Incidence** | Rare |
| **Etiology** | Multifactorial |
| **Associated conditions** | Respiratory insufficiency<br>$CO_2$ retention<br>CHF<br>Diabetes<br>Unusually high risk of DVT and PE |

# ANESTHETIC CONSIDERATIONS

## PREOPERATIVE

Morbid obesity is variably defined (>100 pounds over ideal body weight or 2 times ideal body weight), and may be associated with increased perioperative mortality and morbidity. Obstructive sleep apnea (OSA) is common in the morbidly obese patient.

**Respiratory** Increased $O_2$ consumption and $CO_2$ production (e.g., increased basal metabolic rate). Decreased chest wall compliance (↓20-60%), normal lung compliance. Reduced ERV and FRC, so that tidal breathing may fall within the range of closing capacity → V/Q abnormalities. Supine position decreases FRC further → worsening hypoxemia. Increased minute ventilation is required to remain normocarbic. There is a normal response to $CO_2$ unless patient develops the obesity hypoventilation ("Pickwickian") syndrome (↑$PaCO_2$, ↓$PaO_2$, loss of hypercarbic drive, sleep apnea, hypersomnolence, polycythemia, pulmonary HTN, CHF). Tracheal intubation often is difficult in this patient population.

**Tests:** CXR; PFTs (FVC, $FEV_1$, $MMEF_{25-75}$ ± bronchodilators; room-air ABG)

**Cardiovascular** Blood volume and CO increase with rising weight. HTN is very common (use correct size BP cuff). LV dysfunction may be present; patient unable to increase CO or tolerate ↑blood volume. Pulmonary HTN may be present in OSA. Obesity is a risk factor for CAD and sudden death. Anticipate problems with vascular access.

**Tests:** ECG; others as indicated from H&P. (Patient with SOB may require MUGA scan and ECHO for LV function, as SOB can have a cardiac or pulmonary etiology.

**Endocrine** Glucose intolerance and diabetes mellitus (DM) common.

**Tests:** Fasting glucose

**Hepatic** Liver function is often abnormal and drug metabolism may be significantly affected. Combined with altered pharmacokinetics, many drugs (e.g., midazolam and vecuronium) may have unpredictably prolonged action.

**Gastrointestinal** Increased intra-abdominal pressure, gastric volume and acidity, with an increased incidence of hiatal hernia, make this patient population at risk for pulmonary aspiration of gastric contents.

**Musculoskeletal** Higher incidence of airway problems in obese patients. Careful airway examination is paramount. These patients are excellent candidates for fiber optic intubation. Establish availability of OR table large enough to accommodate morbidly obese patient.

**Hematologic** Polycythemia may occur 2° chronic hypoxemia

**Tests:** CBC

**Laboratory** Other tests as indicated from H&P.

**Premedication** Sedatives are best given either orally or iv in monitored environment. The sleep apneic patient may be especially sensitive to sedatives and narcotic drugs. Intramuscular medications can be erroneously injected into adipose tissues. Consider anti-cholinergics if performing awake fiber optic intubation (glycopyrrolate 0.2 mg iv 30 min preop). Take full-stomach precautions: metoclopramide (10 mg iv 60 min preop); $H_2$-antagonist (ranitidine 5 mg iv); non-particulate antacid (3 M Na citrate) 30 cc, 15 min prior to induction.

## INTRAOPERATIVE

**Anesthetic technique:** GETA ± epidural for postop analgesia.

**Induction** Patient at risk for aspiration of gastric contents, and should be intubated either awake (see Appendix) or after rapid-sequence induction with cricoid pressure. Err on the side of caution (awake intubation) as the incidence of difficult mask ventilation and intubation is high in obese patients. Following successful intubation and induction of anesthesia, a NG tube should be placed and the stomach contents suctioned. Lipophilic drugs (STP) will have a greater volume of distribution, than others, and dosage increases might have to be made. If using combined anesthetic approach, placement of an epidural catheter should be accomplished, with the patient in the sitting position. A bilateral sensory block (using 5-7 cc 1.5% lidocaine) prior to induction will help confirm correct placement of the catheter within the epidural space. Verification of placement is particularly important in this population since regional anesthesia in the obese patient is technically more difficult.

| | | |
|---|---|---|
| **Maintenance** | Standard maintenance (see Appendix). $N_2O$ can be used if bowel distention is not a concern for surgical exposure/closure. Obese patients metabolize volatile anesthetics to a greater extent than their non-obese counterparts. Thus, isoflurane or desflurane may be the volatile anesthetic of choice.<br>**Combined epidural/GA:** Local anesthetic (1.5-2% lidocaine with 1:200,000 epinephrine 8-12 $\mu$l q 60 min) can be injected incrementally into the epidural catheter to provide both anesthesia and optimal surgical exposure (contracted bowel and profound muscle relaxation). The dose of local anesthetic administered via the epidural catheter should be decreased to 75% of normal dose. Be prepared to treat hypotension with fluid and vasopressors (ephedrine 5-10 mg iv, phenylephrine 50-100 $\mu$g iv). GA is administered to supplement regional anesthesia and for amnesia. Sedative drugs (droperidol, opiates, benzodiazepines, etc.) should be minimized in the presence of epidural opiates, as they increase the likelihood of postop respiratory depression. If epidural opiates are used for postop analgesia, a loading dose (e.g., hydromorphone 1.0 mg) should be administered 1-2 hrs before conclusion of surgery. | |
| **Emergence** | Elective ICU admission for postop care should be considered. The decision to extubate at the end of surgery depends on patient's underlying cardiopulmonary status and the extent of the surgical procedure. Patients should be hemodynamically stable, warm, alert, cooperative and fully reversed from any muscle relaxants prior to extubation. | |
| **Blood and fluid requirements** | Anticipate large fluid loss.<br>IV: 14-16 ga x 1-2<br>NS/LR @ 10-15 cc/kg/hr<br>Warm all fluids.<br>Humidify gasses. | Guide fluid management by UO, filling pressure. T&C for 2 U PRBCs. |
| **Monitoring** | Standard monitors (see Appendix).<br>UO | Invasive monitoring as clinically indicated. |
| **Positioning** | ✓ and pad pressure points.<br>✓ eyes.<br>Supine position = ↓FRC<br>Avoid Trendelenburg. | Supine positioning decreases lung volumes, which may increase V/Q abnormality, resulting in hypoxemia. This is exacerbated by use of the Trendelenburg position, which usually is not well-tolerated by morbidly obese patients. |
| **Complications** | Hypoxemia 2° ↓FRC | |

## POSTOPERATIVE

| | | |
|---|---|---|
| **Complications** | Hypoxemia<br>Hypercarbia<br>DVT<br>PE<br>Atelectasis | Recover patient in sitting position to improve ventilatory mechanics. Give supplemental $O_2$. |
| **Pain management** | Epidural analgesia: hydromorphone (0.8-1.5 mg load, 0.2-0.3 mg/hr infusion)<br>PCA (see Appendix). | Patient should be recovered in ICU or hospital ward accustomed to treating side effects of epidural opiates (e.g., respiratory depression, breakthrough pain, nausea, pruritus). |
| **Tests** | ABG<br>CXR | Others as clinically indicated. |

**References**


1. Griffen W Jr: In *Surgical Management of Morbid Obesity*. Griffen WO Jr, Printen KJ, eds. Marcel Dekker, New York: 1987, 27-45.
2. Lechner GW, Callender AK: Subtotal gastric exclusion and gastric partitioning: a randomized prospective comparison of one hundred patients. *Surgery* 1981; 90(4):637-44.
3. Linner JH: Comparative effectiveness of gastric bypass and gastroplasty: a clinical study. *Arch Surg* 1982; 117(5):695-700.
4. Flickinger DG, Pories WJ: Gastric bypass and other gastric restrictive procedures for morbid obesity. In *Surgery of the Stomach, Duodenum, and Small Intestine*, 2nd edition. Scott HW, Sawyers JL, eds. Blackwell Scientific Publications, Boston: 1992, 638-52.

5. Gastrointestinal surgery for severe obesity: Proceedings of a National Institutes of Health Consensus Development Conference. March 25-27, 1991, Bethesda, MD. *Am J Clin Nut* Feb 1992; 55(2 Suppl):487S-619S.
6. Buckley FP: Anesthesia and obesity and gastrointestinal disorders. In *Clinical Anesthesia.* Barash PG, Cullen BF, Stoelting RK, eds. JB Lippincott, Philadelphia: 1989, 1117-31.
7. Buckley FP, Robinson NB, Simonowitz DA, Dellinger EP: Anaesthesia in the morbidly obese. A comparison of anaesthetic and analgesic regimens for upper abdominal surgery. *Anaesthesia* 1983; 38(9):840-51.
8. Rawal N, Sjostrand V, Christofferson E, et al: Comparison of intramuscular and epidural morphine for postoperative analgesia in the grossly obese. Influence on postoperative ambulation and pulmonary function. *Anesth Analg* 1986; 63:583.
9. Buckley FP: Anesthetizing the morbidly obese patient. *ASA Annual Refresher Course Lectures* 1992; 163:1-6.
10. Fox GS, Whalley DG, Bevan DR: Anaesthesia for the morbidly obese. Experience with 110 patients. *Br J Anaesth* 1981; 53(8):811-16.

# GASTROSTOMY

## SURGICAL CONSIDERATIONS

**Description:** A gastrostomy is a tube placed through the abdominal wall directly into the stomach. Such tubes can be used for gastric decompression or for feeding, and they may be permanent or temporary. Patients undergoing gastrostomy placement often have neurologic impairment which compromises their ability to handle oral secretions and increases their risk of aspiration. **Percutaneous gastrostomy**, in contrast to the other techniques, is most commonly performed using intravenous sedation and local anesthesia.

**Variant procedure or approaches**: The traditional **Stamm gastrostomy** is most commonly placed at the time of a laparotomy performed for another purpose, or may be performed through a separate, small laparotomy incision in patients in whom endoscopic placement is not possible for technical reasons. The incision may be upper midline or transverse directly over the stomach. The anterior wall of the stomach is identified and two pursestring sutures are placed in the stomach around the site at which the tube will enter. The gastrostomy tube is introduced through the abdominal wall directly over the intended site of entry into the stomach. A small hole is made in the stomach in the center of the pursestring sutures, the tube is introduced into the stomach, and the pursestrings are tied securely around the tube. The wound is then closed. General anesthesia is usually preferred, but the operation may be performed under local anesthesia in thin patients.

The **Janeway gastrostomy** is a technical modification, also requiring performance of a laparotomy. The greater curvature of the stomach is identified and a stapler placed across a portion of this, creating a tube that arises from the main body of the stomach. The staple line may be oversewn and then the end of the tube is brought through the abdominal wall and matured to the skin as a small stoma. This allows for permanent access to the stomach with removal of the tube between feedings, and is useful in patients with long-term dependence on gastrostomy access. The Janeway gastrostomy is rarely used, though young patients with neurologic impairment who are expected to need lifetime gastrostomy feeding are good candidates.

In **percutaneous (endoscopic) gastrostomy**, the stomach is intubated endoscopically and the gastric and abdominal walls punctured under endoscopic guidance. The gastrostomy tube is introduced through the mouth and passed through the stomach and abdominal wall from inside out. In most centers this has become the most common technique of gastrostomy placement due to its simplicity and because, in most patients, it can be performed under local anesthesia with MAC. Previous gastric operations may make endoscopic placement difficult or dangerous, as may some obstructing lesions of the esophagus or pharynx.

**Usual preop diagnosis**: Temporary gastrostomies are often used after major abdominal surgery as an alternative to NG suction. Percutaneous gastrostomies are often placed in patients with advanced malignancy and intestinal obstruction or inadequate oral intake, and in patients with neurologic impairment and difficulty eating.

## SUMMARY OF PROCEDURE

| | Stamm | Janeway | Percutaneous |
|---|---|---|---|
| **Position** | Supine | ⇐ | ⇐ |
| **Incision** | Midline or transverse | ⇐ | Puncture |
| **Special instrumentation** | None | ⇐ | Endoscope, percutaneous gastrostomy kit |
| **Antibiotics** | ± Cefazolin 1 gm iv | ⇐ | ⇐ |
| **Surgical time** | 45 min | 1 hr | 0.5 - 1 hr |
| **Closing considerations** | Muscle relaxation for closure | ⇐ | None |
| **EBL** | Minimal | ⇐ | ⇐ |
| **Mortality** | Minimal | ⇐ | ⇐ |
| **Morbidity** | Wound infection: 2.1-9% | ⇐ | – |
| | Hemorrhage: 0.9-1.1% | ⇐ | ⇐ |
| | Aspiration pneumonia: 2.2% | ⇐ | 1.6% |
| | Failure to function: 2.2% | ⇐ | – |
| **Procedure code** | 43830 | 43832 | 43750 |
| **Pain score** | 4-5 | 5 | 1-2 |

## PATIENT POPULATION CHARACTERISTICS

| | |
|---|---|
| **Age range** | All ages, though with peaks in infancy and the elderly |
| **Male:Female** | ~1:1 |
| **Incidence** | Common |
| **Etiology** | (See Preop Diagnosis, above.) |
| **Associated conditions** | Gastrostomy placed at the time of laparotomy when NG drainage is anticipated for a prolonged period<br>For feeding in the neurologically impaired or in those with complex upper digestive difficulties<br>Advanced malignancy (for either feeding or palliative decompression) |

# ANESTHETIC CONSIDERATIONS

See "Anesthetic Considerations for Ostomy Procedures" in "Intestinal Surgery" section.


**References**

1. Gauderer MW, Stellato TA: Gastrostomies: evolution, techniques, indications and complications. *Curr Probl Surg* 1986; 23(9):657-719.
2. Grant JP: Comparison of percutaneous endoscopic gastrostomy with Stamm gastrostomy. *Ann Surg* 1988; 207(5):598-603.
3. Shellito PC, Malt RA: Tube gastrostomy. *Ann Surg* 1985; 201(2):180-85.
4. Webster MW Jr, Carey LC, Ravitch MM: The permanent gastrostomy: use of the gastrointestinal anastomotic stapler. *Arch Surg* 1975; 110(5):658-60.

**Surgeon**

**Harry A. Oberhelman, MD, FACS**

## 7.3 INTESTINAL SURGERY

**Anesthesiologist**

**Steven K. Howard, MD**

# DUODENOTOMY

## SURGICAL CONSIDERATIONS

**Description:** A duodenotomy is performed to ligate a bleeding vessel at the base of a duodenal ulcer or to perform some procedure on the ampulla of Vater. It is important to be familiar with the anatomy of the proximal duodenum in relation to the major and minor pancreatic duct orifices. The duodenotomy may be made longitudinally or transversely, depending on the surgeon's preference. A transverse opening allows one to close the duodenotomy without tension, however, it must be placed very accurately for the purpose of exposure. Bleeding vessels at the base of an ulcer must be secured with suture ligatures. Care must be taken to avoid perforating the duodenum when performing a sphincterotomy.

**Usual preop diagnosis:** Duodenal ulcer; impacted common duct stone

### SUMMARY OF PROCEDURE

| | |
|---|---|
| **Position** | Supine |
| **Incision** | Midline abdominal or subcostal |
| **Unique considerations** | Magnifying glasses if operation involves lesser pancreatic sphincter |
| **Antibiotics** | Cefotetan 2 gm preop |
| **Surgical time** | 1 - 2 hrs |
| **Closing considerations** | Secure closure of duodenum |
| **EBL** | Minimal |
| **Postop care** | NG decompression |
| **Mortality** | < 0.5% |
| **Morbidity** | Duodenal leak: < 5%<br>Postop pancreatitis: < 3% |
| **Procedure code** | 44010 |
| **Pain score** | 6-8 |

### PATIENT POPULATION CHARACTERISTICS

| | |
|---|---|
| **Age range** | Any age |
| **Male:Female** | 1:1 |
| **Incidence** | Not uncommon |
| **Etiology** | Duodenal ulcer<br>Impacted common duct stone |
| **Associated conditions** | Bleeding duodenal ulcer: 50-60%<br>Chronic pancreatitis: 20-25%<br>Impacted common duct stones: 10-15% |

## ANESTHETIC CONSIDERATIONS

See Anesthetic Considerations following "Operations for Peptic Ulcer Disease" in "Stomach Surgery" section.

**References**

1. Nora PF: *Operative Surgery: Principles and Techniques*, 3rd edition. WB Saunders Co, Philadelphia: 1990.

# APPENDECTOMY

## SURGICAL CONSIDERATIONS

**Description:** Appendectomy is performed for appendicitis or suspected appendicitis. The negative laparotomy rate has been reduced by the judicious use of ultrasonography, laparoscopy and barium enema. Through a RLQ (McBurney) or right paramedian incision, the cecum is exposed and pulled into the wound (Fig 7.3-1). The appendix is then delivered through the wound, and the mesoappendix is clamped, cut and ligated. The appendix is removed by crushing and ligating, and then transecting the base. The appendiceal stump may be invaginated into the wall of the cecum or left alone. In some instances it may be easier to divide the base of the appendix before delivering the appendix into the wound. The wound should be left open and soft drains used in cases of perforated appendix. In children, the appendix may be inverted and allowed to slough off internally. Recently, appendectomy has been performed via the laparoscope. Following insufflation of the peritoneal cavity, the appendix is mobilized and the mesoappendix and appendix divided using the gastrointestinal anastomosis (GIA) stapler. The appendix is delivered through the umbilical port (camera port).

**Usual preop diagnosis:** Appendicitis

### SUMMARY OF PROCEDURE

| | |
|---|---|
| **Position** | Supine |
| **Incision** | RLQ (McBurney's[1]) or right paramedian |
| **Unique considerations** | Variation in stump closure; NG tube if prolonged ileus is expected. |
| **Antibiotics** | Cefotetan 1 gm preop |
| **Surgical time** | 1 hr |
| **Closing considerations** | Skin wound should not be closed when appendix has perforated. Drain in presence of well-defined abscess cavity. |
| **EBL** | < 75 ml |
| **Postop care** | Wound care when left open |
| **Mortality** | Perforation: 2%<br>Non-perforation: < 0.1 |
| **Morbidity** | Pelvic, subphrenic, or intra-abdominal abscess (perforation): 20%<br>Wound abscess: < 5%<br>Fecal fistula: < 1%<br>Wound hematoma: < 0.5%<br>Ileus: Variable |
| **Procedure code** | 44950 |
| **Pain score** | 5-7 |

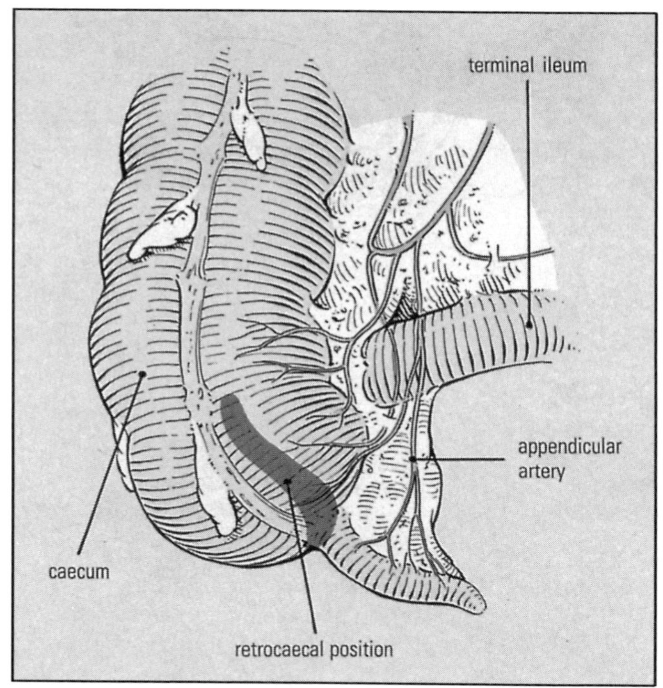


**Figure 7.3-1.** Relevant anatomy for appendectomy. (Reproduced with permission from Calne R, Pollard SG: *Operative Surgery.* Gower Medical Pub: 1992.)

### PATIENT POPULATION CHARACTERISTICS

| | |
|---|---|
| **Age range** | Any age |
| **Male:Female** | 1:1 |
| **Incidence** | 1/15 persons |
| **Etiology** | Obstruction[2]: 80-90%<br>Fecaliths: 75%<br>Carcinoid tumors: < 5% |
| **Associated conditions** | None |

# ANESTHETIC CONSIDERATIONS

**(Procedures covered: appendectomy; excision of Meckel's diverticulectomy)**

## PREOPERATIVE

| | |
|---|---|
| **Respiratory** | Respiratory impairment can occur 2° acute abdominal pain and splinting. Tachypnea and hyperpnea can be heralding Sx of appendiceal perforation and sepsis. Patients with acute appendicitis should be treated as if they have a full stomach. Consider administration of metoclopramide (10 mg iv) and $H_2$ blocker (ranitidine 50 mg iv), as well as Na citrate 0.3 M 30 cc po.<br>**Tests:** ABG; CXR, if clinically indicated. |
| **Cardiovascular** | May be dehydrated from fever, emesis and decreased oral intake. Assess volume status with vital signs in the supine and standing positions (if possible) and hydrate adequately prior to proceeding with anesthetic induction.<br>**Tests:** ECG, if indicated from H&P. |
| **Gastrointestinal** | Patient typically has abdominal pain with N&V. Muscular resistance to abdominal palpation of the abdominal wall frequently parallels the severity of the inflammatory process. With spreading peritoneal irritation (as with perforation), patient will develop abdominal distension and paralytic ileus.<br>**Tests:** Electrolytes |
| **Hematologic** | Moderate leukocytosis (10,000-18,000) with moderate left shift. Hemoconcentration is probable, if patient is dehydrated.<br>**Tests:** CBC |
| **Laboratory** | UA; others as indicated from H&P. |
| **Premedication** | Opiate premedication (morphine 0.08-0.15 mg/kg im) is indicated after patient is scheduled for surgery. If surgical intervention is still in question, administration of opiates may mask Sx of appendicitis. |

## INTRAOPERATIVE

**Anesthetic technique:** GETA, with rapid-sequence iv induction, followed by ET intubation. (If systemic sepsis absent, hydration adequate, patient cooperative, and high abdominal exploration unlikely, then regional anesthetic can be considered.)

| | | |
|---|---|---|
| **Induction** | STP 3-5 mg/kg + succinylcholine 1-1.5 mg/kg iv in rapid sequence, with assistant holding cricoid pressure until successful placement of ETT is confirmed. Restore intravascular volume prior to anesthetic induction if patient is clinically hypovolemic. | |
| **Maintenance** | Standard maintenance (see Appendix), without $N_2O$. | |
| **Emergence** | The patient should be extubated awake after return of airway reflexes. | |
| **Blood and fluid requirements** | IV: 16-18 ga x 1<br>NS/LR @ 5-8 cc/kg/hr | |
| **Monitoring** | Standard monitors (see Appendix). | |
| **Positioning** | ✓ and pad pressure points.<br>✓ eyes. | Others, as indicated by patients's status. |
| **Complications** | Sepsis | |

## POSTOPERATIVE

| | | |
|---|---|---|
| **Complications** | Sepsis (possible with appendiceal rupture) | Adequate Abx coverage. |
| | Paralytic ileus | Time |
| | Atelectasis | Adequate pain control, incentive spirometry, early ambulation |
| **Pain management** | PCA (see Appendix). | |
| **Tests** | As indicated clinically | |

**References**


1. McBurney C: Experience with early operative interference in cases of disease of the vermiform appendix. *NY Med J* 1889; 50:676-84.
2. Van Zwalenburg C: The relation of mechanical distention to the etiology of appendicitis. *Ann Surg* 1905; 41:437-50.
3. Cook CE: Anesthesia for abdominal surgery. In *Clinical Anesthesia Procedures of the Massachusetts General Hospital*, 3rd edition. Firestone LL, Lebowitz PW, Cook CE, eds. Little, Brown, Boston: 1988, 271-86.


# MECKEL'S DIVERTICULECTOMY

## SURGICAL CONSIDERATIONS

**Description:** Meckel's diverticulum is a true congenital diverticulum, usually arising within two feet of the ileocecal valve. It was first described by Meckel[1] in 1809. Excision of a Meckel's diverticulum is indicated for bleeding, obstruction, perforation, inflammation, intussusception, and when there is a palpable mass near the base of the diverticulum. Ectopic mucosa is present in roughly 50% of symptomatic patients, with gastric mucosa the most frequent.[2] After entering the peritoneal cavity, the distal ileum, along with the diverticulum, is delivered into the wound. The diverticulum is excised and the wound closed in two layers. Following excision of the diverticulum, care must be taken not to narrow the bowel lumen during closure.

**Usual preop diagnosis:** Meckel's diverticulum; "left-side appendicitis"

### SUMMARY OF PROCEDURE

| | |
|---|---|
| **Position** | Supine |
| **Incision** | Midline abdominal or RLQ (McBurney's) |
| **Antibiotics** | Cefotetan 1-2 gm preop |
| **Surgical time** | 1 hr |
| **EBL** | < 100 ml |
| **Mortality** | < 0.5% |
| **Morbidity** | Wound infection: 5%<br>Pulmonary complication: < 5%<br>Anastomotic leak: < 1% |
| **Procedure code** | 44800 |
| **Pain score** | 6-8 |

### PATIENT POPULATION CHARACTERISTICS

| | |
|---|---|
| **Age range** | < 40 yrs |
| **Male:Female** | 3:1 |
| **Incidence** | 1-2% |
| **Etiology** | Congenital |
| **Associated conditions** | None |

## ANESTHETIC CONSIDERATIONS

See Anesthetic Considerations following "Appendectomy" (above).

**References**


1. Meckel JF: Ulcer die divertikel an darmkanal. *Arch Physiol* 1809; 9:421-53.
2. Söderlund S. Meckel's diverticulum. A clinical and histologic study. *Acta Chir Scand* 1959 (Suppl 248); 13-233.

# ENTEROSTOMY

## SURGICAL CONSIDERATIONS

**Description:** **Enterostomy** is performed for stenting the small intestine with a long tube, for feeding purposes, for bypassing small or large bowel obstructions, and following total proctocolectomy. An intestinal tube is either purse-stringed into the small bowel and brought through the abdominal wall, or the intestine itself is brought to the exterior and fashioned into a stoma. Different tubes are used for feeding, according to surgeon's preference. After purse-stringing the tube in the bowel, the seromuscular layer of the jejunum is sutured over the tube for a distance of 3-4 cm before exiting through the abdominal wall. The **Brooke ileostomy** is created by bringing a two-inch segment of ileum through an abdominal wall stab wound. The ileum is folded back on itself and sutured to the skin edge or dermis (Fig 7.3-2). Some surgeons secure the ileum to the underlying peritoneum, but this is not necessary.

**Variant procedure or approaches:** There are various intestinal or drainage tubes that may be inserted into the bowel, depending on the function required. For example, certain tubes are used for feeding, while others may be used for drainage or decompression.

**Usual preop diagnosis:** Intestinal obstruction due to extensive adhesions; following removal of the large intestine (including the rectum); for enteral feedings.

### SUMMARY OF PROCEDURE

| | Enterostomy | Feeding Jejunostomy | Ileostomy |
|---|---|---|---|
| **Position** | Supine | ⇐ | ⇐ |
| **Incision** | Midline abdominal | ⇐ | ⇐ |
| **Antibiotics** | Cefotetan 1-2 gm preop | ⇐ | ⇐ |
| **Surgical time** | 1 - 1.5 hrs | ⇐ | ⇐ |
| **Closing considerations** | Securing tube to abdominal wall | ⇐ | Viable stoma |
| **EBL** | < 100 ml | ⇐ | ⇐ |
| **Postop care** | Tube irrigation | ⇐ | Stoma care |
| **Mortality** | < 0.5% | ⇐ | ⇐ |
| **Morbidity** | Ileus: 60-70% | ⇐ | ⇐ |
| | Wound infection: < 5% | ⇐ | ⇐ |
| | | | Stoma necrosis: < 2% |
| **Procedure code** | 44300 | ⇐ | 44310 |
| **Pain score** | 5-6 | 5-6 | 5-6 |

### PATIENT POPULATION CHARACTERISTICS

| | |
|---|---|
| **Age range** | 20-65 yrs |
| **Male:Female** | 1:1 |
| **Incidence** | Common |
| **Etiology** | Intestinal obstruction: 60-70%<br>Diseases resulting in total proctocolectomy: 10-15%<br>Inability to eat: 5-10% |
| **Associated conditions** | Inflammatory bowel disease<br>Intestinal adhesions<br>Inability to eat orally |

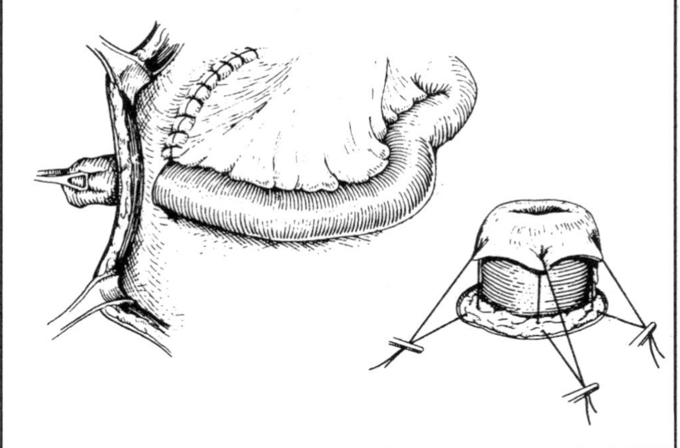

**Figure 7.3-2.** Brooke ileostomy. (Reproduced with permission from Hardy JD: *Rhoad's Textbook of Surgery*, 5th edition. JB Lippincott: 1977.)

## ANESTHETIC CONSIDERATIONS FOR OSTOMY PROCEDURES

**(Procedures covered: enterostomy; ileostomy; gastrostomy; gastrojejunostomy)**

### PREOPERATIVE

This patient population is very diverse and includes those with inflammatory bowel disease, cancer or post-CVA, and those presenting following trauma. Thus, the patient population ranges from the otherwise healthy to the critically ill. Many of these patients will have abnormal protective airway reflexes and are at risk of aspiration of gastric contents.

**Respiratory** Patients may have abnormal laryngeal reflexes and difficulty swallowing, making them prone to aspiration of gastric contents and associated pneumonitis; decreased pulmonary reserve and hypoxemia can be seen in patients with pulmonary infections.
**Tests:** PA, lateral CXR to rule out pneumonia. Consider ABG.

**Cardiovascular** Patients are likely to be hypovolemic 2° chronically poor po intake and malnutrition.
**Tests:** ECG; orthostatic vital signs

**Neurological** Patients often sick and debilitated (e.g., post-CVA).

**Laboratory** CBC with differential; coagulation profile (PT; PTT); UA; electrolytes; glucose; creatinine; BUN; bilirubin; transaminases; alkaline phosphatase; albumin; calcium; others as indicated from H&P.

**Premedication** Depends on patient status. Titrate small doses of benzodiazepines (midazolam 0.25-0.5 mg iv) or opiate (fentanyl 25-50 μg iv). Consider $H_2$-antagonists and metoclopramide (10 mg iv 60 min preop).

### INTRAOPERATIVE

**Anesthetic technique:** MAC with local anesthesia to area of incision for gastrostomy; otherwise, GA is appropriate for ostomy procedures.

**Induction** Patient may be at risk for pulmonary aspiration. If GA is planned, the trachea should be intubated while patient is awake or after rapid-sequence induction with cricoid pressure. If patient is hypovolemic, volume status should be restored before induction, and doses of sedative/hypnotic should be titrated to effect.

**Maintenance** **MAC:** Titration of sedatives (midazolam 0.25-1 mg iv) and analgesics (fentanyl 25-50 μg iv).
**GA:** Standard maintenance (see Appendix).

**Emergence** Trachea should be extubated after return of protective laryngeal reflexes, if patient at risk for aspiration of gastric contents.

**Blood and fluid requirements** Minimal blood loss
IV: 16-18 ga x 1
NS/LR @ 5-8 cc/kg/hr

**Monitoring** Standard monitors (see Appendix). Others as clinically indicated.

**Positioning** √ and pad pressure points.
√ eyes.

### POSTOPERATIVE

**Complications** Atelectasis
Aspiration
Hypoxemia
Hypercarbia

**Pain management** PCA (see Appendix)

#### References

1. Brooke BN: The management of an ileostomy, including its complications. *Lancet* 1952; 2:102-4.

# CONTINENT ILEOSTOMY POUCH (KOCK)

## SURGICAL CONSIDERATIONS

**Description:** A **Kock pouch**[1] consists of an internal reservoir fashioned from the distal ileum and an intussuscepted nipple valve used to provide continence. Approximately 45 cm of small bowel are required for construction of the pouch and valve. After suturing two limbs of the ileum together over a distance of 15 cm, the distal segment is intussuscepted over itself to form the nipple valve. The pouch is then sutured closed and mounted beneath the abdominal wall stoma site (Fig 7.3-3). The stoma is made flush with the skin for cosmetic reasons and left intubated for 1 month with a special plastic catheter. The pouch requires catheterization for evacuation of its contents 3-4 times a day. The continent ileostomy reservoir has been modified by **Barnett**[2] to include the construction of an isoperistaltic valve with an intestinal collar around its base to prevent deintussusception and valve prolapse. These procedures are typically performed as part of or following **bowel resection**.

**Usual preop diagnosis:** Inflammatory bowel disease; familial polyposis or malfunctioning ileostomies

### SUMMARY OF PROCEDURE (KOCK OR BARNETT POUCH)

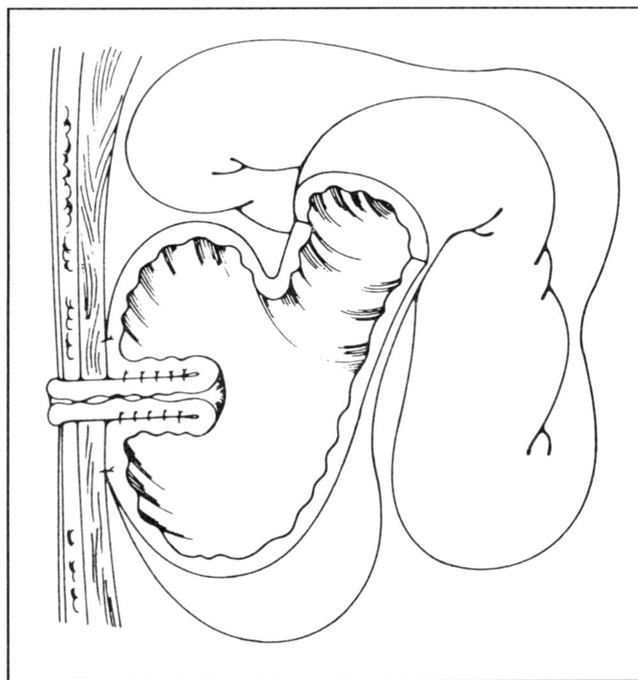

**Figure 7.3-3.** Continent ileostomy or Kock pouch. (Reproduced with permission from Hardy JD: *Hardy's Textbook of Surgery*, 2nd edition. JB Lippincott: 1988.)

| | |
|---|---|
| **Position** | Supine |
| **Incision** | Midline abdominal |
| **Special instrumentation** | GIA or TA staplers |
| **Antibiotics** | Usual bowel prep with antibiotics; cefotetan 2 gm preop |
| **Surgical time** | 2 - 3 hrs |
| **Closing considerations** | Valve vascularity |
| **EBL** | 200-300 ml |
| **Postop care** | Maintain pouch decompression |
| **Mortality** | < 1% |
| **Morbidity** | Intestinal ileus: 5%<br>Wound infection: < 5%<br>Intestinal obstruction: 2-3%<br>Pouch fistula: 1-3%<br>Valve necrosis: < 0.5% |
| **Procedure code** | 44316 |
| **Pain score** | 6-8 |

### PATIENT POPULATION CHARACTERISTICS

| | |
|---|---|
| **Age range** | 18-80 yrs |
| **Male:Female** | 1:1 |
| **Incidence** | Common |
| **Etiology** | Ileostomy: 50%<br>Proctocolectomy: 5% |
| **Associated conditions** | Extracolonic inflammatory bowel manifestations: 10% |

## ANESTHETIC CONSIDERATIONS

See Anesthetic Considerations following "Enterostomy" (above).

**References**


1. Kock NG: Intra-abdominal "reservoir" in patients with permanent ileostomy. Preliminary observations on a procedure resulting in fecal "continence" in five ileostomy patients. *Arch Surg* 1969; 99(2):223-31.
2. Barnett WO: Modified techniques for improving the continent ileostomy. *Am Surg* 1984; 50(2):66-9.

# SMALL BOWEL RESECTION WITH ANASTOMOSIS

## SURGICAL CONSIDERATIONS

**Description:** Resection of the small bowel is performed for a number of diseases (listed below). After entering the peritoneal cavity, the involved small bowel is delivered into the wound and the lesion resected between bowel clamps (Fig 7.3-4). Varying amounts of mesentery are included, depending on the diagnosis. More extensive resections indicated for malignant disease include regional lymph nodes. Re-anastomosis may be accomplished by various suturing techniques or stapling. The peritoneal cavity may be accessed through vertical or transverse incisions. Operative techniques include **open end-to-end, closed end-to-end, side-to-side**, or **stapled, functional end-to-end anastomoses**.

**Usual preop diagnosis:** Intestinal obstruction, complicated by intestinal gangrene due to adhesions, internal hernia, volvulus, intussusception, mesenteric vascular occlusion, Crohn's disease, radiation enteritis, intestinal fistulae, small bowel tumors, and trauma.[1]

### SUMMARY OF PROCEDURE

| | |
|---|---|
| **Position** | Supine |
| **Incision** | Vertical or transverse |
| **Unique considerations** | Adequate fluid resuscitation; NG tube |
| **Antibiotics** | Cefotetan 1-2 gm preop |
| **Surgical time** | 1 - 3 hrs |
| **EBL** | 50-100 cc |
| **Postop care** | NG or long intestinal tube decompression |
| **Mortality** | Varies according to etiology: 1-5% |
| **Morbidity** | Atelectasis: < 10%<br>Intestinal ileus: < 10%<br>Wound infection: < 5%<br>Intestinal leak, fistula: < 3% |
| **Procedure code** | 44120 |
| **Pain score** | 7-9 |

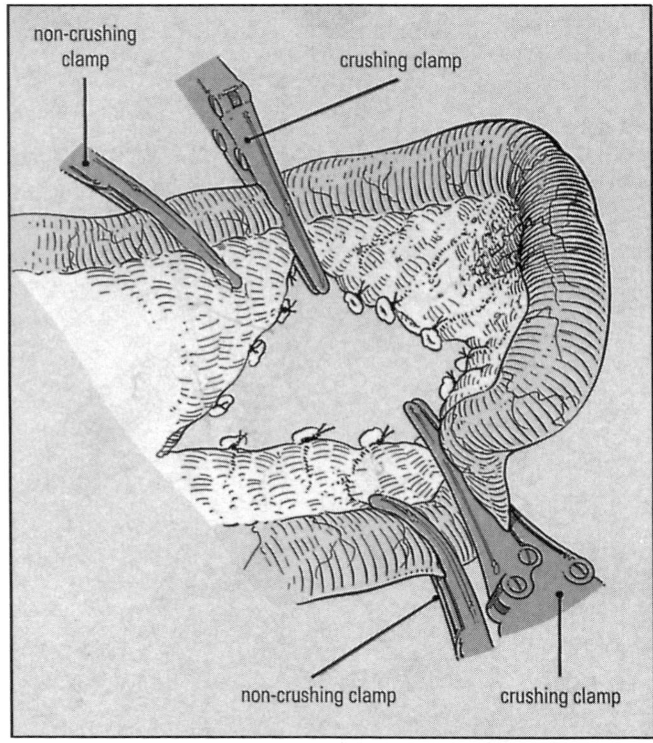


**Figure 7.3-4.** Application of bowel clamps. (Reproduced with permission from Calne R, Pollard SG. *Operative Surgery*. Gower Medical Pub: 1992.)

### PATIENT POPULATION CHARACTERISTICS

| | |
|---|---|
| **Age range** | 20-70 yrs |
| **Male:Female** | 1:1 |
| **Incidence** | Common |
| **Etiology** | Interference with blood supply (obstruction, strangulated hernia, volvulus, mesenteric thrombosis)<br>Trauma<br>Tumors<br>Crohn's disease |
| **Associated conditions** | Multiple, depending on etiology (see Preop Diagnosis). |

## ANESTHETIC CONSIDERATIONS

See Anesthetic Considerations following "Closure of Enteric Fistulae" (below).

**References**

1. Zollinger RM Jr, Zollinger RM: *Atlas of Surgical Operations*, 6th edition. Macmillan, New York: 1988.

# ENTEROLYSIS

## SURGICAL CONSIDERATIONS

**Description:** Enterolysis consists of separating loops of bowel adhesed to other loops or the abdominal wall by sharp dissection, and excising adhesive bands. Care must be taken to avoid producing enterotomies. In recurrent cases of intestinal obstruction, small bowel plication or intraluminal tube stenting may be utilized. Plication is achieved by suturing the bowel or its mesentery so that the small bowel is aligned in an orderly manner without kinks. This also can be accomplished by threading a long, intra-abdominal tube orally down through the small intestine.[1] This has the effect of holding the bowel in a non-obstructed position while new adhesions form.

**Usual preop diagnosis:** Intra-abdominal adhesions

### SUMMARY OF PROCEDURE

| | |
|---|---|
| **Position** | Supine |
| **Incision** | Midline abdominal |
| **Special instrumentation** | Sometimes a long intestinal tube is used for decompression and fixation of bowel loop. |
| **Unique considerations** | Bowel decompression |
| **Antibiotics** | Cefotetan 1-2 gm preop |
| **Surgical time** | 1 - 4 hrs |
| **Closing considerations** | Adequate decompression to permit wound closure |
| **EBL** | 150-500 cc |
| **Postop care** | PACU; continued intestinal decompression 4-7 d |
| **Mortality** | 1-3% |
| **Morbidity** | Wound abscess: 15-20%<br>Prolonged ileus: 10-20%<br>Fistula formation: < 10%<br>Pulmonary complications: 5-10%<br>Recurrent intestinal obstruction: 5-8% |
| **Procedure code** | 44005 |
| **Pain score** | 5-7 |

### PATIENT POPULATION CHARACTERISTICS

| | |
|---|---|
| **Age range** | Any age |
| **Male:Female** | 1:1 |
| **Incidence** | Common |
| **Etiology** | Previous intra-abdominal operative procedure: >90%<br>Malignant tumors: 15-20%<br>Hernias: 10-15%<br>Volvulus: 5-10%<br>Inflammatory bowel disease: 5%<br>Gallstone ileus: < 5%<br>Intussusception: < 5% |

## ANESTHETIC CONSIDERATIONS

See Anesthetic Considerations following "Closure of Enteric Fistulae" (below).

**References**

1. Close MB, Christensen NM: Transmesenteric small bowel plication or intraluminal tube stenting. Indications and contraindications. *Am J Surg* 1979; 138(1):89-96.

# CLOSURE OF ENTERIC FISTULAE

## SURGICAL CONSIDERATIONS

**Description:** Enteric fistulae may occur between the bowel and abdominal wall (enterocutaneous), between loops of the intestine (enteroenteric or enterocoelic), or between the bowel and bladder or vagina (enterovesical or enterovaginal). Surgical repair is usually reserved for fistulae to the abdominal wall, bladder and vagina, and consists of excising the fistula and repairing the bowel and the other organ separately. Most fistulae are characterized by the adherence of the two visceral organs with a communication between their lumens.

The organs involved are separated by blunt-sharp dissection and repaired locally after excision of the indurated margins of the defect. In the case of both the small and large intestine, it may be necessary to resect a segment of bowel with the defect and to perform an end-to-end anastomosis. If the repair sites involved lie close together, it is important to interpose tissue, such as the omentum, between the viscera to minimize chance of recurrence. Occasionally a fistula may be bypassed rather than surgically resected.

**Usual preop diagnosis:** Enteric fistula

### SUMMARY OF PROCEDURE

| | |
|---|---|
| **Position** | Supine |
| **Incision** | Midline abdominal |
| **Unique considerations** | Preop nutritional support and fistula wound care |
| **Antibiotics** | Cefotetan 2 gm preop |
| **Surgical time** | 1 - 4 hrs |
| **Closing considerations** | Separation of repairs by interposition of omentum and other tissue |
| **EBL** | 50-300 cc |
| **Postop care** | NG decompression until bowel function returns; TPN support |
| **Mortality** | 0-5% |
| **Morbidity** | Ileus: 60-70%<br>Pulmonary complications: 10%<br>Recurrent fistula: 5-10%<br>Wound infection: 5-10% |
| **Procedure code** | 44640 (closure of intestinal cutaneous fistula)<br>44641 (closure of enterovesical fistula with bowel or resection)<br>44660 (closure of enterovesical fistula with intestinal or bladder resection) |
| **Pain score** | 6-8 |

### PATIENT POPULATION CHARACTERISTICS

| | |
|---|---|
| **Age range** | Any age |
| **Male:Female** | 1:1 |
| **Incidence** | Common |
| **Etiology** | Anastomotic leaks: 60-70%<br>Carcinoma: 10-15%<br>Crohn's disease: 5-10%<br>Iatrogenic bowel injury: 5-10%<br>Perforative diverticulitis: 5-10%<br>Radiation enteritis: 5%<br>Foreign body perforation: < 5% |
| **Associated conditions** | Malnutrition: 30%<br>Inflammatory bowel disease: 25%<br>Cancer: 15% |

# ANESTHETIC CONSIDERATIONS FOR INTESTINAL AND PERITONEAL PROCEDURES

**(Procedures covered: exploratory laparotomy; small bowel resection; enterolysis; closure of enteric fistulae; excision of intra-abdominal tumor; drainage of subdiaphragmatic abscess)**

## PREOPERATIVE

Patients requiring exploratory laparotomy are often at risk for aspiration of gastric contents. Precautions to prevent this are necessary to help assure safe patient outcome.

**Respiratory** — Respiratory insufficiency can be present due to intra-abdominal pathology; ↓FRC → ↑A-a gradient and arterial hypoxemia; diaphragmatic impairment and splinting → ↑respiratory insufficiency.
**Tests:** CXR; consider ABG.

**Cardiovascular** — Patient is likely to be critically ill and should be evaluated for presence of hypovolemia (hypotension, tachycardia) and should receive adequate volume replacement before anesthetic induction.
**Tests:** ECG; orthostatic vital signs

**Musculoskeletal** — Abdominal rigidity may be present; abdominal pain is common.

**Gastrointestinal** — Diarrhea, vomiting and prolonged npo status can lead to electrolyte abnormalities.
**Tests:** Electrolytes; glucose

**Renal** — Renal insufficiency/failure may be present, especially in elderly and/or chronically ill patients, and in those who are hypovolemic.
**Tests:** BUN; creatinine; electrolytes; routine UA

**Laboratory** — CBC with differential; platelet count; PT; PTT

**Premedication** — Standard premedication (see Appendix). Consider $H_2$-antagonists (e.g., ranitidine 50 mg iv 1 hr preop), metoclopramide (10 mg iv 1 hr preop) and Na citrate (30 cc po < 30 min preop).

## INTRAOPERATIVE

**Anesthetic technique:** GETA ± epidural for postop analgesia. If postop epidural analgesia is planned, placement of catheter prior to anesthetic induction is helpful to establish correct placement in the epidural space (accomplished by injecting 5-7 cc of 1% lidocaine via the epidural catheter, eliciting a segmental block).

**Induction** — The patient with abdominal pathology is often at risk for pulmonary aspiration and the trachea should be intubated with patient awake or after rapid-sequence iv induction with cricoid pressure. (See Standard Induction Techniques in Appendix.) If patient is clinically hypovolemic, restore intravascular volume (colloid, crystalloid or blood) prior to induction and titrate induction dose of sedative/hypnotic agents.

**Maintenance** — **Balanced anesthesia** without $N_2O$. (See "Standard Maintenance Techniques" in Appendix.) Complete muscle relaxation should be assured.
**Combined epidural and light general anesthetic:** Local anesthetic (1.5-2% lidocaine with 1:200,000 epinephrine 12-15 cc q 60 min) can be injected into the epidural catheter to provide both anesthesia and optimal surgical exposure (contracted bowel and profound muscle relaxation). Be prepared to treat hypotension with fluid and vasopressors. GA is administered to supplement regional anesthesia and for amnesia. If epidural opiates are used for postop analgesia, a loading dose (e.g., hydromorphone 1.0 mg) should be administered at least 1 hr before the conclusion of surgery. Systemic sedatives (droperidol, opiates, benzodiazepines, etc.) should be minimized during this type of anesthetic as they increase the likelihood of postop respiratory depression. An NG tube should be placed and kept on intermittent suction.

**Emergence** — The decision to extubate at the end of surgery depends on the patient's underlying cardiopulmonary status and the extent of the surgical procedure. Patients should be hemodynamically stable, warm, alert, cooperative, and fully reversed from any muscle relaxants prior to extubation. If the above criteria are not met, patient should remain intubated and transported to ICU for further care.

**Blood and fluid requirements** — IV: 14-16 ga x 1-2
T&C for 4 U RBCs.
NS/LR @ 10-15 cc/kg/hr
Fluid warmer

Platelets, FFP and cryoprecipitate should be administered according to lab tests (platelet count, PT, PTT, DIC screen, thromboelastography).

| | | |
|---|---|---|
| **Monitoring** | Standard monitors (see Appendix).<br>UO<br>± Arterial line<br>± CVP/PA catheter | Invasive monitors, as indicated by patient's status. Prevent hypothermia during long operations. Consider heated humidifier, warming blanket, warm room temperature, keeping patient covered until ready for prep, etc. |
| **Positioning** | ✓ and pad pressure points.<br>✓ eyes. | |
| **Complications** | Hemorrhage<br>Sepsis | Acute septic shock may require PA catheter and aggressive hemodynamic support. |

**POSTOPERATIVE**

| | | |
|---|---|---|
| **Complications** | Sepsis<br>Hemodynamic instability<br>Atelectasis<br>Hypoxemia<br>Hemorrhage<br>Ileus | Pulmonary function abnormalities may persist for 1 wk postop (↓vital capacity and ↓FRC) |
| **Pain management** | Epidural analgesia (see Appendix).<br>PCA (see Appendix). | Patient should be recovered in ICU or ward accustomed to treating the side-effects of epidural opiates (e.g., respiratory depression, breakthrough pain, nausea, pruritus). |
| **Tests** | CBC; CXR (if central line placed); electrolytes; glucose | Others as directed by intraop course. |

**References**


1. Aguirre A, Fischer JE, Welch CE: The role of surgery and hyperalimentation in the therapy of gastrointestinal-cutaneous fistulae. *Ann Surg* 1974; 180(4):393-401.
2. Merritt WT: Anesthesia for gastrointestinal surgery. In *Principles and Practice of Anesthesiology*. Rogers MC, Tinker JH, Covino BG, Longnecker DE, eds. Mosby-Year Book, Inc, St. Louis: 1993, 1967-89.

**Surgeon**

**James M. Stone, MD**

# 7.4 COLORECTAL SURGERY

**Anesthesiologist**

**Steven K. Howard, MD**

# PARTIAL COLECTOMY WITH ANASTOMOSIS

## SURGICAL CONSIDERATIONS

**Description:** This procedure is used for resection of any portion of the abdominal colon with primary anastomosis (Fig 7.4-1). The most common types of partial colectomy are: **total abdominal colectomy**, **right hemicolectomy**, **sigmoid colectomy** and **left hemicolectomy**. Occasionally, **cecectomy** or **short segmental resections** are performed. Most patients presenting for elective colectomy undergo preop bowel preparation that consists of mechanical cleaning of the colon, and administration of preop oral antibiotics. As a result of the bowel prep, patients are frequently hypovolemic and hypokalemic when they come to the OR.

**Partial colectomy** may be performed via midline or transverse abdominal incisions, depending on the underlying disease, portion of colon to be resected and surgeon's preference. In general, midline incisions are preferred when: a high-lying splenic flexure must be mobilized; inflammatory bowel disease is present; the extent of colon resection is not known preop; and/or combined hepatic resection is anticipated. Transverse incisions are commonly used for right hemicolectomy or sigmoid colectomy. The anastomosis may be hand-sewn or stapled; in the abdominal colon, there is no clear advantage to either anastomic technique. The modified lithotomy position – thighs abducted and extended, knees flexed and legs supported by stirrups (Allen universal, Lloyd-Davies) – is useful when intraop lower endoscopy is planned, and when an anastomosis to the distal sigmoid or rectum is anticipated (e.g., sigmoid resection for diverticular disease). In this position, a stapling device may be passed through the anus to perform the anastomosis. Ureteral stents may be placed prior to laparotomy when an inflammatory mass is present in the pelvis (sigmoid diverticulitis, ileocolic or sigmoid Crohn's disease), when there has been prior irradiation of the operative field and when a bulky or recurrent pelvic cancer is resected.

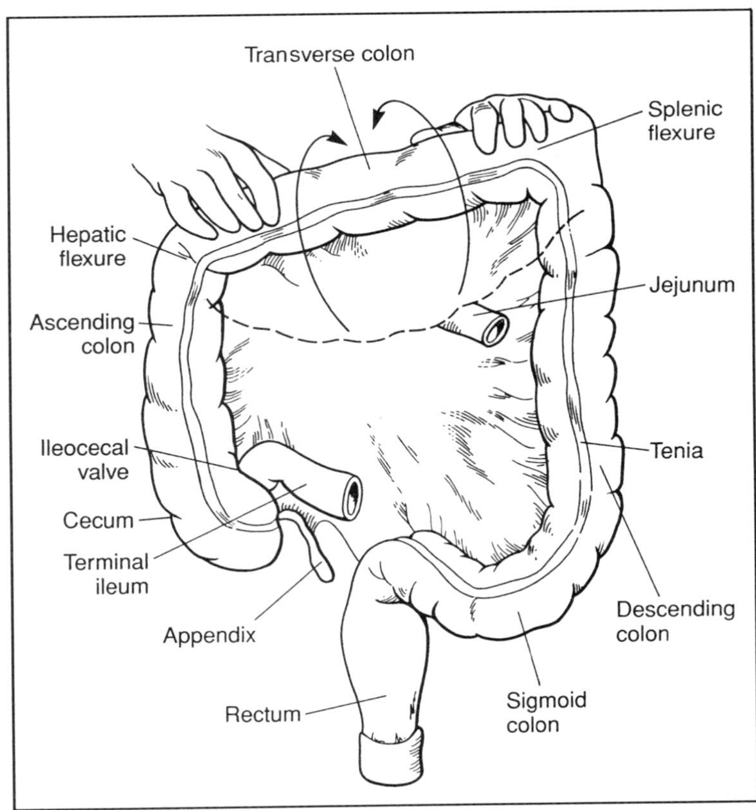


**Figure 7.4-1.** Anatomy of the colon. (Reproduced with permission from Hardy JD: *Hardy's Textbook of Surgery*, 2nd edition. JB Lippincott: 1988.)

The sequence of steps in partial colectomy is the same for all parts of the colon. The first step is mobilization, performed along the line of Toldt (separating the retroperitoneum from the peritoneum) for the right, left and sigmoid colon, and among the greater omentum for the transverse colon. Proximal and distal sites for resection are selected and the intervening mesentery is taken between clamps. Finally, the bowel is transected and an anastomosis is effected. During mobilization of the pelvic colon, care must be exercised to identify and preserve the ureter. During mobilization of the hepatic flexure, care is taken not to injure the duodenum.

Creation of a **colostomy** may be desirable in patients who are hemodynamically unstable, or when local conditions such as inflammation, carcinomatosis, ischemia or unprepped bowel are present. The distal end of the resected colon may be brought through the skin as a mucous fistula, or it may be oversewn and placed within the peritoneal cavity.

**Usual preop diagnosis:** Colon cancer; diverticular disease; Crohn's disease; ulcerative colitis; trauma; ischemic colitis; lower GI hemorrhage; intractable constipation; colon volvulus

## SUMMARY OF PROCEDURE

| | |
|---|---|
| **Position** | Supine or modified lithotomy |
| **Incision** | Transverse or vertical midline |
| **Unique considerations** | Bowel prep, or underlying disease may result in dehydration, electrolyte abnormalities or anemia. |
| **Antibiotics** | Cefotetan 1 gm iv |
| **Surgical time** | 1 - 3 hrs |
| **Closing considerations** | Colostomy or ileostomy matured after wound is closed (requires 10 - 20 min). |
| **EBL** | 100-300 cc (500-2000 cc if splenic injury, loss of major vascular pedicle or repeat operation for cancer, Crohn's disease) |
| **Postop care** | ICU for underlying disease; NG tube for distention or vomiting. Avoid use of long-lasting anticholinergics (e.g., Phenergan®). |
| **Mortality** | 0.5-2% (mostly related to underlying disease) |
| **Morbidity** | SBO: 5-10%<br>Wound infection: 4-10%<br>For anastomosis-anastomotic leak: 2-4%<br>Wound dehiscence: 1-2%<br>Bleeding: 1%<br>Splenic injury: 1% |
| **Procedure code** | 44140 (with anastomosis); 44141 (with colostomy); 44144 (with mucofistula) |
| **Pain score** | 8 |

## PATIENT POPULATION CHARACTERISTICS

| | Crohn's Disease | Colon cancer | Trauma | Diverticula |
|---|---|---|---|---|
| **Age range** | 2nd-4th decade | 5th-7th decade | 2nd-4th decades | >40 yrs |
| **Male:Female** | 1:1 | 1.3:1 | 3:1 | 1:1 |
| **Incidence** | 1-6/100,000 | 30/100,000 | 1-2/100,000 | 10/100,000 |
| **Etiology** | Unknown | Genetic: 5% | Trauma | Western: low-fiber diet |
| **Associated conditions** | Malnutrition<br>Anemia<br>Intra-abdominal sepsis<br>Intestinal fistulae<br>Perianal disease<br>Nephrolithiasis<br>Sclerosing and ankylosing spondylitis | Iron deficiency<br>Colonic obstruction<br>Colonic perforation | Liver fracture<br>Spleen fracture<br>Rib fracture<br>Closed-head injury<br>Penetration of viscera adjacent to colon injury | Hemorrhoids<br>Chronic constipation |

# ANESTHETIC CONSIDERATIONS

See Anesthetic Considerations following "Stoma Closure and Repair Surgeries" (below).

**References**


1. Benn PL, Wolff BG, Ilstrup DM: Level of anastomosis and recurrent colonic diverticulitis. *Am J Surg* 1986; 151(1):269-71.
2. Corman ML, Veidenheimer MC, Coller JA: Colorectal carcinoma: a decade of experience at the Lahey Clinic. *Dis Colon Rectum* 1979; 22(7):477-79.
3. Lock MR, Fazio VW, Farmer RG, Jagelman DG, Lavery IC, Weakly FL: Proximal recurrence and the fate of the rectum following incisional surgery for Crohn's disease of the large bowel. *Ann Surg* 1981; 194(6):754-60.
4. Flint LM, Vitale GC, Richardson JD, Polk HC Jr: The injured colon: relationships of management to complications. *Ann Surg* 1981; 193(5):619-23.

# REPAIR OF CECAL OR SIGMOID VOLVULUS

## SURGICAL CONSIDERATIONS

**Description:** Cecal volvulus occurs only in people with an abnormally mobile right colon. It accounts for 30-40% of colon volvulus in the U.S. Patients characteristically present with symptoms of intestinal obstruction, dehydration and a "coffee-bean" deformity arising from the RLQ seen on a plain abdominal radiograph. If there is clinical evidence of bowel necrosis, the patient must be taken directly to the OR for resection of nonviable bowel. In the case of cecal volvulus, a primary anastomosis usually can be performed but, with sigmoid volvulus, a colostomy normally is created. On occasion, a contrast enema is required to confirm the diagnosis. The treatment consists of correction of fluid and electrolyte disturbances, NG tube decompression, as well as detorsion and fixation of the colon. A related condition known as cecal bascule, is said to exist when a mobile cecum folds in an anterior direction on top of a fixed ascending colon. The treatment for cecal bascule is identical to that of cecal volvulus.

Cecal volvulus may be treated by **resection** of the right colon, **detorsion and cecopexy**, or **detorsion and tube cecostomy**. **Right hemicolectomy** for cecal volvulus is performed in a similar manner to the way it is performed for any other condition. In cecal (or sigmoid) volvulus with ischemia, an attempt should be made to ligate the vascular supply to the colon prior to detorsion. This is done to avoid a sudden washout of the toxic byproducts of ischemia and bacterial overgrowth into the circulation. The intent of **cecopexy** is to re-create the normal situation of short, non-mobile peritoneal attachments to the right colon. Cecopexy is performed by suturing the colon to the parietal peritoneum in the right gutter. Some authors have advocated creating a flap of parietal peritoneum from the hepatic flexure to the cecum along the right gutter. The flap is lifted and the right colon is placed under the flap and against the denuded area of retroperitoneum. The flap is sutured to the anterior wall of the right colon with serosal sutures. Presumably, dense adhesions from the deperitonealized gutter will further fix the colon in place. The advantage of cecopexy is that there is no need to open the colon; the disadvantages are that the greatly distended cecum is not decompressed, and that the fixation often fails and recurrent volvulus ensues. **Tube cecostomy**, on the other hand, allows decompression of the cecum, and provides a more secure point of fixation. Tube cecostomy is performed by placing a pursestring suture in the anterior wall of the cecum, opening the cecum through the center of the pursestring, and placing a large (>32 Fr) mushroom catheter in the cecum. The tube exits the abdominal wall through a stab wound separate from the incision. The disadvantages are that leakage and irritation around the tube invariably occur, and that the colon must be opened.

Sigmoid volvulus occurs in people with abnormally elongated sigmoid colons, along with narrowly-based mesenteric attachments. It accounts for 60-70% of colon volvulus in the U.S. The majority of patients will come from chronic nursing facilities and are usually elderly or on chronic neuropsychiatric medications. Most cases of sigmoid volvulus can be reduced with a rigid proctoscope or a flexible sigmoidoscope. After detorsion (reduction), a bowel prep can be performed, followed by definitive surgery.

If a bowel prep can be performed, sigmoid volvulus is treated by **resection** of the redundant sigmoid with a **colorectal anastomosis**. This resection is performed in the typical fashion, with attention given to early ligation of the vascular supply. If a bowel prep cannot be performed, or if the patient is already completely dependent on nursing care for bowel function or is so frail that an absolutely minimal operation must be done, a sigmoid colostomy can be very simply created at the most redundant part of the sigmoid colon. If there is a question about the viability of the colon, the nonviable colon is resected, the distal sigmoid colon is oversewn and dropped into the pelvis (**Hartmann's procedure**), and the proximal end of the sigmoid is exteriorized as an end colostomy. Operative detorsion alone should not be performed because the recurrence rate is prohibitively high.

**Usual preop diagnosis:** Cecal volvulus; sigmoid volvulus

### SUMMARY OF PROCEDURE

| | Cecopexy | Tube Cecostomy | Sigmoid Resection, Anastomosis |
|---|---|---|---|
| **Position** | Supine | ⇐ | Supine or modified lithotomy |
| **Incision** | Transverse RLQ or lower midline | ⇐ | Transverse LLQ or lower midline |
| **Special instrumentation** | None | Large (>32 Fr) drainage tubes; mushroom; Depezzar or Foley catheters | Surgical staplers |

| | Cecopexy | Tube Cecostomy | Sigmoid |
|---|---|---|---|
| **Unique considerations** | Detorsion may result in hypotension, wheezing, or other manifestations of the sudden influx of the byproducts of ischemia and bacterial overgrowth into the circulation. | ⇐ | ⇐ |
| **Antibiotics** | Cefotetan 1 gm iv | ⇐ | ⇐ |
| **Surgical time** | 60 min | ⇐ | 60 - 90 min |
| **Closing considerations** | Abdomen will be distended; vital capacity may be limited by closure | None | ⇐ |
| **EBL** | < 200 ml | ⇐ | 200-400 ml |
| **Postop care** | Watch for respiratory compromise from distension | Irrigate with cecostomy tube with 30 ml saline TID | None |
| **Mortality** | 30% (gangrenous cecum); 5-10% (viable cecum) | ⇐ | 60-80% (gangrenous sigmoid); 5-15% (viable sigmoid) |
| **Morbidity** | Recurrent volvulus: 20% | 5%<br>Tube irritation and fecal soilage: 80-100% | Anastomotic leaks: 5-10%<br>PE: 2-5%<br>MI: 2-4% |
| **Procedure code** | 44050 | 44300 | 44140 |
| **Pain score** | 8 | 8 | 8 |

### PATIENT POPULATION CHARACTERISTICS

| | Cecal Volvulus | Sigmoid Volvulus |
|---|---|---|
| **Age range** | Peak in 7th-8th decade | ⇐ |
| **Male:Female** | 1:2 | 1:1 |
| **Incidence** | ≤ 60 yrs old: 0.45/100,000<br>> 60 yrs old: 5.6/100,000 | ⇐<br>> 60 yrs old: 8.8/100,000 |
| **Etiology** | Lack of fixation of the right colon | Elongated sigmoid colon with short mesenteric attachment |
| **Associated conditions** | Dehydration | Chronic constipation<br>Mental retardation<br>Neuropsychiatric conditions |

---

## ANESTHETIC CONSIDERATIONS

See Anesthetic Considerations following "Stoma Closure and Repair Surgeries" (below).

# STOMA CLOSURE AND REPAIR SURGERIES

## SURGICAL CONSIDERATIONS

**Description:** The intestine may be exteriorized as a loop, divided loop or end stoma. With an end stoma, the defunctionalized bowel distal to the stoma may also be exteriorized as a mucous fistula, dropped back into the abdomen as a **Hartmann's procedure**, or totally resected as in a **proctectomy**. With loop stomas, both the afferent and efferent ends of bowel exit the abdominal wall through the same opening; therefore, these stomas may be closed (anastomosed) with a circumstomal incision. The closure of an end stoma with mucous fistula or Hartmann's procedure requires a formal **laparotomy**.

The most frequent indications for stomal revision are stomal stenosis, stomal retraction, parastomal hernia, parastomal fistula, and poorly sited stomas. Many cases of stomal stenosis and retraction may be corrected with local operations through circumstomal incisions. A formal abdominal incision is generally required for the correction of parastomal hernia, which frequently requires re-siting the stoma. The repair of peristomal fistula, which generally requires resection of the involved bowel, also requires a formal laparotomy. On occasion, a stoma may be re-sited or diseased bowel may be resected through a parastomal incision. These patients frequently receive a bowel prep and, as a result, are frequently hypovolemic and hypokalemic when they come to the OR.

**Closure of a loop stoma** is performed through a circular incision, placed just outside the mucocutaneous junction of the stoma and the skin. The proximal and distal ends of the bowel are separated from the subcutaneous tissue, the anterior fascia, and then the posterior fascia. The bowel is cleaned of adherent skin and the previously opened antimesenteric border of the bowel is simply closed with sutures. Alternatively, the previously exteriorized portion of bowel is resected, and the two ends are anastomosed with either sutures or staples. On rare occasion, it is necessary to extend the incision transversely through the abdominal wall to safely effect an anastomosis. The fascia is closed in the standard fashion. The time-honored practice of leaving the skin and subcutaneous tissues open has been challenged by many surgeons.

**Closure of an end stoma** with a mucous fistula generally requires a midline abdominal incision. After entering the peritoneal cavity, the functioning stoma and mucous fistula are identified and then freed from their attachment to the abdominal wall via circumstomal incisions. Intervening structures are moved out of the way and an anastomosis is created via sutured or stapled technique. The procedure is nearly identical for closure of a stoma with a long, defunctionalized, intraperitoneal Hartmann's procedure (resection of a diseased portion of colon with proximal colostomy and distal stump closure). On occasion, retrograde passage of a flexible endoscope via the rectum helps to identify the Hartmann's limb (distal stump). When the defunctionalized limb consists of only the pelvic rectum, it is frequently helpful to pass a rigid proctoscope into the rectum to help identify the distal end. It is only necessary to clean enough of the rectal wall to accommodate the head of an EEA stapler. The stapler is passed per rectum with the sharp trocar retracted inside the stapler. When the abdominal surgeon confirms proper placement of the stapler by feeling the outline of the staple-containing ring throughout the rectal wall, the perineal operator advances the trocar through the rectal wall. The abdominal operator then removes the trocar and locks the anvil (pursestringed within the proximal bowel) to the stapler shaft. The perineal operator closes and fires the stapler, while the abdominal operator holds the adjacent viscera out of the way. The anastomosis is tested by infusing air into the rectum after filling the pelvis with NS.

In **paracolostomy hernia** repair, the abdomen may be entered via a midline or a transverse parastomal incision. The stoma is freed from the abdominal wall and the hernia is repaired via direct suture approximation of the fascial edges or placement of a prosthetic mesh. Although most surgeons prefer to move the stoma to a fresh location, some have advocated simply closing the fascia around the stoma or placing the stoma via a hole cut through a piece of prosthetic mesh used to bridge the hernia gap. Since colostomy closure is at best a clean-contaminated case, the risk of periprosthetic infection is very real.

Simple closure of the internal opening of a parastomal fistula is rarely successful; in nearly all situations resection of the diseased bowel will be done and either an anastomosis will be performed or the resected end will be used to form a new stoma. The external fistula track(s) will be unroofed or excised. This creates an open wound adjacent to the stoma and may impair bag fit to the point that re-siting the stoma is necessary.

**Usual preop diagnosis:** Stomal stenosis, retraction, parastomal hernia, fistula

## SUMMARY OF PROCEDURE

| | Closure of Loop Stoma | Closure of End Stoma | Repair of Parastomal Hernia |
|---|---|---|---|
| **Position** | Supine | Supine or modified lithotomy* | Supine |
| **Incision** | Circumstomal | Midline or transverse abdominal | Midline or circumstomal |
| **Special instrumentation** | Anastomotic staplers | Endoscope for closure of Hartmann's procedure | Prosthetic mesh |
| **Antibiotics** | ** | ** | ** |
| **Surgical time** | 60 - 90 min | 1 - 3 hrs | ⇐ |
| **Closing considerations** | Requires only a few fascial staples; skin may be left open | None | Stoma matured after abdomen closed |
| **EBL** | < 100 ml | 100-500 ml | < 100 ml |
| **Mortality** | 1% | 2-4% | 1% |
| **Morbidity** | Anastomotic leak | ⇐ | Recurrent hernia |
| | SBO | ⇐ | Peristomal infection |
| | Wound infection | ⇐ | Stomal ischemia |
| **Procedure code** | 44620 | 44625 | 44346 |
| **Pain score** | 5 | 8 | 6 |

* The modified lithotomy position is used for closure of a Hartmann's procedure when an endoscope or stapling device may need to be passed through the anus.

** Bowel prep consists of mechanical cleaning of the colon, accomplished with cathartics or lavage solutions, as well as oral antibiotics. A commonly used regimen is: neomycin 1 gm po and erythromycin base 1 gm po, given at 1 pm, 2 pm, and 10 pm on the night before surgery. An intravenous 2nd generation cephalosporin may be given at the time of induction.

## PATIENT POPULATION CHARACTERISTICS

| | |
|---|---|
| **Age range** | Variable |
| **Male:Female** | 1:1 |
| **Incidence** | Not uncommon |
| **Etiology** | Protection or avoiding an insecure anastomosis |
| | Traumatic injuries to the colon |
| | Complete colonic obstruction |
| | Colonic infections such as diverticulitis |
| | Inflammatory processes such as Crohn's disease or ulcerative colitis |
| | After emergency resection for ischemic colitis |
| **Associated conditions** | Multiple trauma |
| | Inflammatory bowel disease |
| | Colon cancer |
| | Gut ischemia |

---

# ANESTHETIC CONSIDERATIONS FOR LARGE BOWEL SURGERY

**(Procedures covered: partial colectomy with anastomosis; repair of cecal or sigmoid volvulus; stoma closure and repair surgeries)**

## PREOPERATIVE

Patients presenting for this group of surgical procedures have in common an increased risk for pulmonary aspiration. In addition, patients with bowel obstruction, particularly of the small intestine, must be treated urgently as the obstruction may rapidly progress to bowel necrosis, perforation and septic shock.

| | |
|---|---|
| **Respiratory** | Respiratory insufficiency 2° acute abdominal process (e.g., pain, splinting, sepsis, metabolic acidosis) and bowel distention limiting diaphragmatic excursion (↓TV, ↓FRC)<br>**Tests:** CXR; consider ABG. |
| **Cardiovascular** | Hemodynamic instability 2° sepsis or pain (tachycardia, labile BP). Hypovolemia due to fever, poor po intake, vomiting, diarrhea. Restoring intravascular volume and hemodynamic stability are goals prior to induction of anesthesia.<br>**Tests:** Orthostatic vital signs; ECG |
| **Renal** | Electrolyte abnormalities common.<br>**Tests:** Electrolytes; glucose; BUN; creatinine |
| **Gastrointestinal** | An NG tube should be in place and the stomach emptied before induction of anesthesia. |
| **Musculoskeletal** | Abdominal musculature may be rigid due to acute abdominal process. |
| **Hematologic** | Hemoconcentration due to GI fluid loss; anemia due to acute GI bleeding.<br>**Tests:** CBC with platelets; PT; PTT |
| **Laboratory** | Other tests as indicated from H&P. |
| **Premedication** | Light standard premedication (see Appendix) is usually appropriate. For aspiration prophylaxis, ranitidine 50 mg iv 1 hr before induction, followed by Na citrate (30 cc, 3 M, po) immediately before induction, will significantly decrease the acidity of gastric contents. Metoclopramide is contraindicated in patients with bowel obstruction or perforation. |

## INTRAOPERATIVE

**Anesthetic technique:** GETA ± epidural for postop analgesia. If postop epidural analgesia is planned, placement of catheter prior to anesthetic induction is helpful to establish correct placement in the epidural space (accomplished by injecting 5-7 cc of 1% lidocaine via the epidural catheter, eliciting a segmental block).

| | |
|---|---|
| **Induction** | The patient with an acute abdominal process is at risk for pulmonary aspiration; trachea should be intubated with patient awake or after rapid-sequence induction with cricoid pressure (see Appendix.) If patient is clinically hypovolemic, restore intravascular volume (colloid, crystalloid or blood) prior to induction, and titrate induction dose of sedative/hypnotic agents. |
| **Maintenance** | Standard maintenance (see Appendix) without $N_2O$. **Combined epidural/GA:** local anesthetic (1.5-2% lidocaine with 1:200,000 epinephrine (12-15 cc q 60 min) can be injected into the epidural catheter to provide both anesthesia and optimal surgical exposure (contracted bowel and profound muscle relaxation). Be prepared to treat hypotension with fluid and vasopressors. GA is administered to supplement regional anesthesia and for amnesia. If epidural opiates are used for postop analgesia, a loading dose (e.g., hydromorphone 1.0 mg) should be administered at least 1 hr before conclusion of surgery. Systemic sedatives (droperidol, opiates, benzodiazepines, etc.) should be minimized during epidural opiate administration as they increase the likelihood of postop respiratory depression. |
| **Emergence** | The decision to extubate at the end of surgery depends on the patient's underlying cardiopulmonary status and extent of surgical procedure. Patient should be hemodynamically stable, warm, alert, cooperative and fully reversed from any muscle relaxants prior to extubation, and have adequate return of pulmonary function (as measured by VC of 15 cc/kg, MIF of -25 cm $H_2O$, RR < 25 and ABG which approaches patient's baseline). |

| | | |
|---|---|---|
| **Blood and fluid requirements** | Anticipate large third-space losses.<br>IV: 14-16 ga x 1<br>NS/LR @ 10-15 cc/kg/hr<br>Fluid warmer<br>T&C for 4 U PRBCs. | Platelets, FFP and cryoprecipitate should be administered according to lab tests (platelet count, PT, PTT, DIC screen, thromboelastography). |
| **Monitoring** | Standard monitors (see Appendix).<br>UO<br>± Arterial line<br>± CVP | Invasive monitoring, as indicated by patient's status. Prevent hypothermia during long operations. Consider heated humidifier, warming blanket, warming room temperature, keeping patient covered until ready for preop, etc. |
| **Positioning** | ✓ and pad pressure points.<br>✓ eyes. | |
| **Complications** | Septic shock | Hemodynamic instability 2° hemorrhage, sepsis. |

### POSTOPERATIVE

| | | |
|---|---|---|
| **Complications** | Hypoxemia<br>Hemodynamic instability<br>Sepsis | Hypoxemia may be 2° atelectasis. |
| **Pain management** | Epidural analgesia (see Appendix)<br>PCA (see Appendix) | |
| **Tests** | CBC; CXR (if central line placed); electrolytes; glucose | |

#### References

1. Condon RE, Wittmann DH: The use of antibiotics in general surgery. *Curr Prob Surg* 1991; 28(12):801-949.

# TOTAL PROCTOCOLECTOMY

## SURGICAL CONSIDERATIONS

**Description:** Total proctocolectomy involves excision of the entire colon, rectum and anus (Fig 7.4-2). The end of the ileum may be fashioned into an **end ileostomy (Brooke ileostomy)**, **continent ileostomy (Koch pouch)** or an **ileoanal pouch**. Most patients request the ileoanal pouch procedure to avoid the need for a stoma. The bacterial load of the colon is greatly diminished by mechanical cleaning, which may be accomplished by cathartics or non-absorbed, lavage solutions. As a result of this bowel prep, patients are frequently hypokalemic and hypovolemic. Oral antibiotics are also given the night before surgery to further diminish the bacterial load. Neomycin 1 gm and erythromycin base 1 gm taken at 1 pm, 2 pm, and 11 pm on the day before surgery are commonly used. Many other regimens of absorbed and/or non-absorbed antibiotics, however, are equally effective. The efficacy of parenteral broad spectrum antibiotics, given at the time of induction, has not been established, although it is widely practiced.

**Total proctocolectomy** is performed through a midline incision. In the setting of ulcerative colitis, the small bowel is inspected for Crohn's disease or evidence of an unexpected colon cancer. In the setting of familial adenomatous polyposis (FAP), a search is made for unexpected intestinal cancers, metastases or desmoid tumors. The right colon is mobilized first and then the small bowel mesentery is mobilized to allow for creation of an ileostomy. The transverse colon may be mobilized by separating it from the greater omentum, or the greater omentum may be resected along with the specimen. The descending colon is mobilized, and the splenic flexure is taken down from both the transverse and descending colon sides. The sigmoid colon is then mobilized to the level of the sacral promontory. At this time, the ileum is transected at the ileocecal valve and the vascular supply to the colon is divided between clamps. Unless a malignancy is present, the mesentery may be taken at a convenient level near the bowel wall. At the level of the sacral promontory, the superior rectal artery and vein are divided between clamps. The dissection continues close to the rectal wall to avoid injury to the presacral sympathetic and the pelvic parasympathetic nerves. This diminishes the chances of postop impotence or retrograde ejaculation.

When the dissection reaches the pelvic floor, the perineal phase of the operation begins. A circumferential incision is made at the anal verge, and the intersphincteric space is identified. The dissection proceeds cephalad in the intersphincteric plane until the abdominal dissection is encountered and the specimen is removed. The abdomen and perineum are irrigated and a presacral drain is brought out of a stab wound adjacent to the perineal incision. The levator, external sphincter muscles, and skin are closed in layers. (If a second operating team is available, time may be saved by performing the perineal dissection while the abdominal colon is being mobilized.) A circular incision is made over an ileostomy site (which was marked preop) and a muscle-splitting incision is carried through the rectus fascia and muscle. The terminal ileum is mobilized and cleaned of its mesentery sufficiently to allow 5 cm to project above the skin when it is led through the stoma site. With the stoma projecting through the abdominal wall, the midline fascia and skin are closed. Retention sutures may be used in malnourished patients, as well as those taking chronic, high-dose corticosteroids. After the skin is closed, an everting, **Brooke ileostomy** is performed.

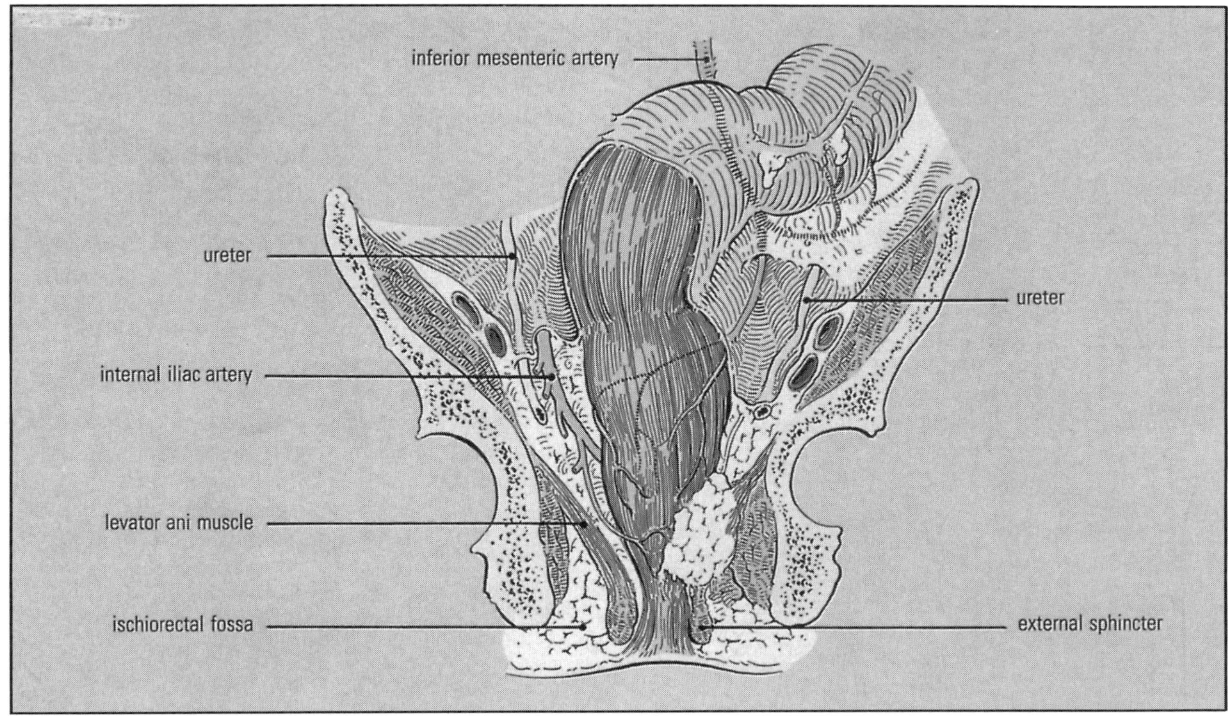


**Figure 7.4-2.** Relevant anatomy for proctocolectomy, colectomy. (Reproduced with permission from Calne R, Pollard SG: *Operative Surgery*. Gower Medical Pub: 1992.)

**Variant procedure or approaches:** With the **continent ileostomy procedure**, removal of the colon, rectum and anus is unchanged from above. The terminal ileum is used to create an intra-abdominal reservoir as well as a sphincter mechanism (nipple valve). This is accomplished by sewing two loops of ileum together to form a pouch. A nipple valve is formed by intussuscepting ileum into itself and the pouch. The walls of the adjacent intussuscepted ileum are fixed together with several rows of staples. The patient does not wear an ileostomy appliance because stool collects in the ileal reservoir. The reservoir is emptied 3 to 4 times/day by passing a catheter through the nipple valve.

With the **ileoanal pouch procedure**, the anus and sphincter mechanism are preserved. A short segment of the distal rectal muscle tube is also preserved after the mucosa has been surgically removed. A reservoir (pouch), made from the terminal ileum, is anastomosed to the top of the anus. A temporary ileostomy is commonly performed at the same time. After the ileoanal pouch procedure, patients have 5-7 bowel movements in a 24-hour period. The ileoanal pouch procedure is contraindicated in patients with Crohn's disease, or anal incontinence. Obesity, advanced age, and severe underlying medical problems are relative contraindications. These operations may be performed more rapidly by two teams working simultaneously in the abdomen and perineum.

**Usual preop diagnosis:** Ulcerative colitis; familial adenomatous polyposis; Crohn's colitis

## SUMMARY OF PROCEDURE

| | **Total Proctocolectomy With End Ileostomy** | **Total Proctocolectomy With Continent Ileostomy** | **Total Colectomy, Mucosal Proctectomy, Ileoanal Pouch** |
|---|---|---|---|
| **Position** | Modified lithotomy | ⇐ | ⇐ |
| **Incision** | Long midline | ⇐ | ⇐ |
| **Special instrumentation** | 2-table setup (separate abdominal and perineal instruments); deep pelvic instruments | 2-table setup; long, non-cutting linear staplers; Koch catheters; deep pelvic instruments | 2-table setup; anal retractors; spinal needle; 1:200,000 epinephrine; deep pelvic instruments |

| | Total Proctocolectomy With End Ileostomy | Total Proctocolectomy With Continent Ileostomy | Colectomy, Proctectomy, Ileoanal Pouch |
|---|---|---|---|
| **Unique considerations** | Patients frequently on chronic high-dose corticosteroids. | ⇐ | ⇐ + Epinephrine solutions injected under the rectal mucosa to facilitate dissection and reduce bleeding. |
| **Antibiotics** | Cefotetan 1 gm iv | ⇐ | ⇐ |
| **Surgical time** | 3 - 4 hrs | 3 - 7 hrs | ⇐ |
| **Closing considerations** | Ileostomy completed after skin closed (15-30 min). | None | Temporary ileostomy commonly used, completed after skin closure. |
| **EBL** | 300-1000 ml (most blood loss during pelvic and perineal dissections. | ⇐ | ⇐ |
| **Postop care** | Transient inability to void common. | Maintain patency of catheter draining pouch; transient inability to void common. | Small bowel mesentery lengthened by dissection around duodenum. This frequently necessitates use of postop NG tube. Transient inability to void common. |
| **Mortality** | 2-5% (older patients and those with underlying medical problems) | 0-2% | ⇐ |
| **Morbidity** | Dyspareunia: 30% | ⇐ | 5-10% |
| | Stoma complications: 20% | – | – |
| | SBO: 10-15% | ⇐ | ⇐ |
| | Impotence: 2-4% | ⇐ | ⇐ |
| | | Nipple valve failure: 20-50% | – |
| | | Persistent perineal wound: 30% | – |
| | | Pouchitis: 20-30% | ⇐ |
| | | Intra-abdominal sepsis: 5% | – |
| | | Pouch incontinence: 5% | – |
| | | | Nocturnal incontinence: 20% |
| | | | Poor function: 5% |
| | | | Pelvic sepsis: 0-4% |
| **Procedure code** | 44155 | 44156 | 44153 |
| **Pain score** | 8 | 8 | 8 |

## PATIENT POPULATION CHARACTERISTICS

| | Ulcerative colitis | Familial adenomatous polyposis |
|---|---|---|
| **Age range** | 3rd-5th decade | 2nd-4th decade |
| **Male:Female** | 1:1 | ⇐ |
| **Incidence** | 6-10/100,000 | 100-150 cases/yr |
| **Etiology** | Unknown | Genetic |
| **Associated conditions** | Cushing's syndrome<br>Anemia<br>Malnutrition<br>Colorectal cancer<br>Sclerosing cholangitis | Colorectal cancer<br>Desmoid tumors<br>Adenomas or cancers of the duodenum and small intestine<br>Brain tumors (Turcot's syndrome)<br>Adrenal adenomas<br>Osteomas |

## ANESTHETIC CONSIDERATIONS

See Anesthetic Considerations following "Operations for Rectal Incontinence" (below).

**References**

1. Francois Y, Dozois RR, Kelly KA, Beart RW Jr, Wolff BG, Pemberton JH, Ilstrup DM: Small intestinal obstruction complicating ileal pouch-anal anastomosis. *Ann Surg* 1989; 209(1):46-50.
2. Metcalf AM, Dozois RR, Kelly KA: Sexual function in women after proctocolectomy. *Ann Surg* 1986; 204(6):624-7.
3. Wexner SD, Wong WD, Rothenberger DA, Goldberg SM: The ileoanal reservoir. *Am J Surg* 1990; 159(1):178-85.
4. Jarvinen HJ, Makitie A, Sivula A: Long-term results of continent ileostomy. *Int J Colorectal Dis* 1986; 1(1):40-3.
5. Kelly KA, Pemberton JH, Wolff BG, Dozois RR: Ileal pouch-anal anastomosis. *Curr Prob Surg* 1992; 29(2):57-131.
6. Condon RE, Wittmann DH: The use of antibiotics in general surgery. *Curr Prob Surg* 1991; 28(2):801-949.

# OPERATIONS FOR RECTAL PROLAPSE

## SURGICAL CONSIDERATIONS

**Description:** Rectal prolapse (procidentia) is intussusception of the full thickness of the rectal wall beyond the anal canal. It must be distinguished from rectal mucosal prolapse, caused by elongation of the mucosal attachments to the underlying sphincter muscle, and internal intussusception, where the upper rectum folds into the lower rectum, but does not descend into the sphincter mechanism. Rectal mucosal prolapse is treated as part of the spectrum of hemorrhoidal disease, and internal intussusception rarely benefits from surgery. Procidentia is frequently associated with anal incontinence. The surgical approaches to procidentia are determined by patient age, concurrent medical disease, sphincter function, and the amount of prolapsed tissue.

Surgical treatment of procidentia may be undertaken through an abdominal or a perineal approach. The **abdominal approaches** have a lower recurrence rate and, because they do not diminish the capacity of the rectal reservoir, are generally preferable for maintaining fecal continence. The primary abdominal approach is **rectopexy**, in which the rectum is mobilized in the posterior plane from the sacral promontory to the levator muscles. The rectum is then pulled cephalad and sutured to the presacral fascia with multiple non-absorbable sutures. Many surgeons routinely perform **sigmoid resection** along with rectopexy. They contend that removal of the redundant sigmoid further diminishes the chance of late recurrence and may improve constipation; and that it avoids the possibility of sigmoid volvulus. (Pulling the rectum up creates a long sigmoid colon on a short mesenteric base, the anatomic condition necessary for volvulus.) The rectum may also be suspended by use of a sling attached to the rectum and secured to the presacral fascia. A number of approaches have been described, the most popular being the **Ripstein procedure**. **Sling procedures** have equivalent recurrence rates but higher complication rates. They also require that mobilization of the rectum along the presacral plane is carried to the level of the levators. A band of Marlex™ mesh is sewn to the presacral fascia below the level of the sacral promontory, upward traction is placed on the rectum and several interrupted sutures are placed from the rectum to the mesh.

When patients are deemed too feeble to undergo laparotomy, prolapse may be repaired via a **perineal approach**. The most common of these is **perineal rectosigmoidectomy** (or **Altmeir procedure**). The prolapsed rectum is withdrawn through the anal canal to its full extent, and a circumcision is made in the outer tube of the prolapsed bowel just distal to the dentate line. This exposes the inner tube of prolapsed bowel, along with its mesentery, which is transected at the level of the anal verge. A primary anastomosis is made between the cut ends of the inner and outer bowel. Prior to anastomosis, the levator muscles are often approximated in the midline in an effort to aid continence. When the volume of prolapsed tissue is small, the **Delorme procedure** is often performed. During this procedure, the mucosa is stripped off the prolapsed rectum, and the prolapsed rectal muscle is foreshortened by plication until it resides above the sphincters.

**Usual preop diagnosis:** Full-thickness rectal prolapse (procidentia)

## SUMMARY OF PROCEDURE

| | Rectopexy | Rectopexy with Sigmoid Resection | Perineal Recto-sigmoidectomy | Delorme Procedure |
|---|---|---|---|---|
| **Position** | Supine, modified lithotomy; deep Trendelenburg | ⇐ | Prone jackknife; lithotomy | ⇐ |
| **Incision** | Low transverse; low midline | ⇐ | No external incision | ⇐ |
| **Special instrumentation** | Deep pelvic instruments; teflon mesh if sling planned; sterile titanium thumbtacks (for bleeding from presacral venous plexus) | Deep pelvic instruments; sterile titanium thumbtacks (useful for bleeding from presacral venous plexus) | Hip-roll for jackknife position; anastomosis may be created with EEA™ stapler. | Hip-roll for jackknife position |
| **Unique considerations** | Presacral venous plexus bleeding may occur in procedures for recurrence; bowel prep may cause dehydration or hypokalemia. | ⇐ | Epinephrine solutions may be used to diminish bleeding; bowel prep may cause dehydration or hypokalemia. | ⇐ |
| **Antibiotics** | Cefotetan 1 gm iv | ⇐ | ⇐ | ⇐ |
| **Surgical time** | 1 - 2 hrs | 1 - 3 hrs | ⇐ | 1.5 - 2 hrs |
| **EBL** | < 100 cc; more if re-operation | 100-300 cc; more if re-operation | 100-200 cc | 100 cc |
| **Postop care** | No rectal probes or medications | ⇐ | ⇐ | ⇐ |
| **Mortality** | 0-2% | 0-4% | 1-4% | 0-1% |
| **Morbidity** | Rectal stricture (with sling): 5-10% | – | – | – |
| | Recurrent prolapse: 2-8% | 2-5% | 20-40% | 5-10% |
| | Pelvic infection: 5% | Anastomotic leak: 2-4% | – | – |
| **Procedure code** | 45540 | 45550 | 45130 | 45541 |
| **Pain score** | 7 | 7 | 2 | 2 |

## PATIENT POPULATION CHARACTERISTICS

| | |
|---|---|
| **Age range** | Women: peak incidence in 6th-7th decade; men: evenly distributed through age range |
| **Male:Female** | 1:4 |
| **Incidence** | Unknown |
| **Etiology** | Decreased pelvic muscular support<br>Congenital deficiency of rectal support<br>Pudendal neuropathy<br>Chronic constipation and straining<br>Multiparity<br>Myelomeningocele<br>Spina bifida<br>Cystic fibrosis (children)<br>Acute parasitic diarrheal illness (children) |
| **Associated conditions** | Fecal incontinence<br>Urinary stress incontinence<br>Rectocele<br>Cystocele |

## ANESTHETIC CONSIDERATIONS

See Anesthetic Considerations following "Operations for Rectal Incontinence" (below).

**References**

1. Watts JD, Rothenberger DA, Buls JG, Goldberg SM, Nivajvongs S: The management of procidentia. 30 years' experience. *Dis Colon Rectum* 1985; 28:(2)96-102.
2. Gordon PH, Hoexter B: Complications of the Ripstein procedure. *Dis Colon Rectum* 1978; 21(4):277-80.
3. Wassef R, Rothenberger DA, Goldbgerg SM: Rectal Prolapse. *Curr Prob Surg* 1986; 23(6):397-451.
4. Freidman R, Muggia-Sulam M, Freund HR: Experience with the one-stage perineal repair of rectal prolapse. *Dis Colon Rectum* 1983; 26(2):789-91.

# RESECTION OF RECTAL LESIONS

## SURGICAL CONSIDERATIONS

**Description:** Many lesions within the distal two-thirds of the rectum can be excised through a **transanal approach**. Most benign lesions are amenable to a local transanal approach, and the application of local excision is increasing in the treatment of favorable, early-stage adenocarcinomas of the rectum. The most common benign tumors treated by local excision are adenomas. Lesions such as carcinoid tumor, endometrioma and solitary rectal ulcer also may be locally excised. **Transanal excision** of benign lesions may be performed in the submucosal plane, while suspected malignancies are excised by removing the entire thickness of the rectal wall. A full antibiotic and mechanical bowel prep is given preop. Transanal excision is usually performed in the prone jackknife position, although the lithotomy position may be used when the lesion is located on the posterior rectal wall. A local anal block, usually 0.25% marcaine, with 1:200,000 epinephrine, is performed to relax the sphincter mechanism and minimize sphincter injury, aid in hemostasis and diminish postop pain. A short bivalve anoscope is inserted into the anal canal. Stay sutures are placed adjacent to the area of resection, and the lesion is pulled into the operative field. On occasion, lesions may be prolapsed all the way through the anus and excised outside of the body. If prolapse is not possible, the dissection starts at the distal end of the lesion and proceeds proximally. The proctotomy incision is enlarged on each side of the lesion in 1-2 cm increments; after each increment, the previous incision is closed with full-thickness, absorbable sutures. These sutures are then grasped and used for further traction. When the specimen is removed, a few final sutures are needed to close the proximal-most incision. When large tumors are resected, **rigid proctoscopy** is performed to confirm preservation of an adequate lumen.

**Variant procedure or approaches:** The **transsacral (Kraske)[1] approach** to rectal tumors offers wider exposure than the transanal approach, but is more painful and has a substantially greater likelihood of complications (wound infection, fecal fistula, incontinence). A transsacral approach is advantageous when the lesion is located behind the rectum (retrorectal tumors), and when resection of the lower sacrum or coccyx is anticipated. Transsacral resection is generally performed in the prone jackknife position. An incision is made from the posterior commissure of the anus to the base of the sacrum. The sphincter muscles are spared, but the levator muscles are divided to expose the posterior wall of the rectum. The coccyx may be disarticulated and removed at this point to improve exposure without adding to operative morbidity. It is also possible to remove the lower sacral segments through this approach, but increasing morbidity accrues as the sacral nerve roots are sacrificed. The posterior wall of the rectum is opened and the lesion, along with a full-thickness disc of rectal wall, is excised. If the lesion is on the anterior wall, two proctotomy incisions are necessary. The proctotomy incisions are closed in one or two layers with standard anastomotic techniques. The levator muscles are reapproximated and the skin is closed. Some surgeons place a drain within the retrorectal space prior to closing. The transsacral approach may be combined with an abdominal approach (abdominal-transsacral resection) in some cases of low rectal cancer.

The **transsphincteric (Mason)[2] approach** to rectal lesions also gives wider exposure than does the transanal approach, but at the expense of a substantially greater risk of fecal incontinence. Transsphincteric excision is performed with the patient in the prone jackknife position. An incision is made at the posterior commissure of the anus and is extended along the lateral border of the coccyx and sacrum. The external sphincter, internal sphincter and levator ani muscles are sequentially transsected in the posterior midline. As each muscle is cut, the cut edges are tagged with sutures to facilitate accurate reapproximation. The rectal wall is incised and the lesion is excised. The proctotomy incision is closed via standard anastomotic suturing techniques, and the individual components of the sphincter muscle are reapproximated with interrupted sutures. The overlying skin is closed in a standard fashion.

**Usual preop diagnosis:** Villous adenoma; tubular adenoma; adenocarcinoma; carcinoid tumor; endometrioma; solitary rectal ulcer; retrorectal tumors (in decreasing frequency)

### SUMMARY OF PROCEDURE

| | Transanal Excision | Transsacral Excision | Transsphincteric Excision |
|---|---|---|---|
| **Position** | Prone jackknife or lithotomy | Prone jackknife | ⇐ |
| **Incision** | Intrarectal | Anus-to-lateral sacral wall | ⇐ |
| **Special instrumentation** | Rigid proctoscope; headlight and/or fiber optic retractors; Foley catheter | Gigli or power saw if sacral resection contemplated; headlight and/or fiber optic retractors; Foley catheter | Headlight and/or fiber optic retractors; Foley catheter |
| **Unique considerations** | Bowel prep may result in dehydration and hypokalemia | ⇐ | ⇐ |
| **Antibiotics** | Cefotetan 1 gm iv | ⇐ | ⇐ |
| **Surgical time** | 15 - 120 min | 1 - 2 hrs | ⇐ |
| **EBL** | < 100 ml | < 100 ml (500 ml if sacral resection) | < 100 ml |
| **Postop care** | No rectal temperatures, suppositories, or enemas | ⇐ | ⇐ |
| **Mortality**[1,3,4,5] | 0-2% | ⇐ | ⇐ |
| **Morbidity**[1,3,4,5] | Tumor recurrence: 5-50% | 50% | 5-50% |
| | Urinary retention: 10-20% | ⇐ | ⇐ |
| | Bleeding: 2-5% | ⇐ | ⇐ |
| | Pelvic sepsis: 0-4% | ⇐ | ⇐ |
| | Ureteral injury: < 1% (minimized by use of Foley) | ⇐ | ⇐ |
| | | Fecal fistula: 10-30% | – |
| | | Fecal incontinence: 5-10% | 10-40% |
| **Procedure code** | 45170 | 45160 | 45170 |
| **Pain score** | 3 | 7 | 7 |

### PATIENT POPULATION CHARACTERISTICS

| | |
|---|---|
| **Age range** | Rectal adenomas – 5th-7th decades; rectal adenocarcinoma – 6th-9th decades; endometrioma – 2nd-4th decades; solitary rectal ulcer syndrome – 4th-8th decades; carcinoid tumors – 5th-8th decades |
| **Male:Female** | 1:1 |
| **Incidence** | Varies with disease; not uncommon |
| **Etiology** | Varies with disease |
| **Associated conditions** | Pre-existing anorectal pathology, such as fecal incontinence, may require concurrent treatment |

## ANESTHETIC CONSIDERATIONS

See Anesthetic Considerations following "Operations for Rectal Incontinence" (below).

**References**

1. Allgöwer M, Dürig M, Hochstetter A, Huber A: The parasacral sphincter-splitting approach to the rectum. *World J Surg* 1982; 6(5):539-48.
2. Mason AY: Surgical access to the rectum — a transsphincteric exposure. *Proc R Soc Med* 1970; 63(Suppl)91-4.

3. Localio SA, Eng K, Gouge TH, Ranson JH: Abdominosacral resection for carcinoma of the midrectum: ten years' experience. *Ann Surg* 1978; 188(4):475-80.
4. Biggers OR, Beart RW Jr, Ilstrup DM: Local excision of rectal cancer. *Dis Colon Rectum* 1986; 29(6):374-77.
5. Hager TH, Gall FP, Hermanek P: Local excision of cancer of the rectum. *Dis Colon Rectum* 1983; 26(3)149-51.
6. Corman ML: *Colon and Rectal Surgery*, 2nd edition. JB Lippincott Co, Philadelphia: 1989.
7. Condon RE, Wittmann DH: The use of antibiotics in general surgery. *Curr Prob Surg* 1991; 28(12):801-949.


# ANAL FISTULOTOMY/FISTULECTOMY

## SURGICAL CONSIDERATIONS

**Description:** The great majority of perianal fistulae arise as a result of infection within the anal glands located at the dentate line (cryptoglandular fistula). Fistulae may also arise as the result of trauma, Crohn's disease, inflammatory processes within the peritoneal cavity, neoplasms or as a consequence of radiation therapy. The ultimate treatment of fistula-in-ano is determined by the etiology and the anatomic course of the fistula. The principle behind treatment of cryptoglandular fistulae is to excise the offending gland, and lay open or excise all infected tissue. Fistulae that track above the majority of the sphincter mechanism must be treated by procedures that either do not cut the overlying sphincter, cut the sphincter and repair it, or cut the sphincter very gradually (seton, see below). A fistula may be treated at the time of drainage of a perianal abscess or as a separate, elective operation. The route of a fistula tract is best determined by exploration at the time of operation. While local anesthesia is acceptable for simple fistulas with known routes, many fistula operations require regional or general anesthesia because the ultimate route and depth of the fistula will not be known. Special consideration is given to fistulae that arise in the setting of Crohn's disease. Poor wound healing, the likelihood of recurrent or multiple fistulae, and the premium on sphincter function in patients with chronic diarrhea, dictates that only the most superficial fistulae can be laid open. The primary goal is palliation; specifically, to drain abscesses and prevent their recurrence. This is often accomplished by placing a Silastic® seton (a ligature placed around the sphincter muscles) around the fistula tract, and leaving it in place indefinitely. In the absence of active Crohn's disease in the rectum, attempts at fistula cure may be undertaken.

**Variant procedure or approaches:** **Fistulotomy** involves cutting all tissues superficial to a fistula so that the fistula tract is brought to the skin level. The opened, fibrotic fistula wall is often sewn to the skin edge (marsupialized). **Fistulectomy** involves excision of the entire fistula tract. When conventional fistulotomy would cause incontinence, a **seton** may be used. The seton may be gradually tightened to transect the sphincter over a matter of weeks. Setons also may be placed loosely and left in place for several weeks with the intention of creating enough local fibrosis that the sphincter will not separate when it is cut at a second operation. Other approaches that may be used to avoid fecal incontinence are **complete fistulotomy with immediate reconstruction** of the sphincter and fistulectomy with closure of the internal opening by an **endorectal advancement flap** technique.

**Usual preop diagnosis:** Fistula-in-ano

**SUMMARY OF PROCEDURE**

| | Fistulotomy or Fistulectomy | Fistulotomy with Seton | Endorectal Advancement Flap |
|---|---|---|---|
| **Position** | Prone jackknife; occasionally lithotomy | ⇐ | Prone jackknife |
| **Incision** | Perianal | ⇐ | ⇐ |
| **Antibiotics** | Cefotetan 1 gm iv | ⇐ | ⇐ |
| **Surgical time** | 15 - 60 min | ⇐ | 60 - 90 min |
| **EBL** | < 50 ml | ⇐ | ⇐ |
| **Mortality** | Minimal | ⇐ | ⇐ |

| | Fistulotomy or Fistulectomy | Fistulotomy with Seton | Advancement Flap |
|---|---|---|---|
| **Morbidity** | Fecal incontinence: 0-30%<br>Non-healing, or recurrent fistula: 5% | 10-30%<br>10-20%. (This procedure used only in complex fistulae, so complication rate appears higher.) | 0-10%<br>10-40%. (This procedure used only in complex fistulae, so complication rate appears higher.) |
| **Procedure code** | 46270, 46275, 46280 | 46275, 46280, 46285 | 46280 |
| **Pain score** | 6 | 6 | 6 |

### PATIENT POPULATION CHARACTERISTICS

| | |
|---|---|
| **Age range** | 2nd-7th decades |
| **Male:Female** | 2:1 |
| **Incidence** | Common |
| **Etiology** | Infection within the anal glands located at the dentate line (cryptoglandular fistula)<br>Trauma<br>Crohn's disease<br>Inflammatory processes within the peritoneal cavity<br>Neoplasms<br>Consequence of radiation therapy |
| **Associated conditions** | See above. |

## ANESTHETIC CONSIDERATIONS

See Anesthetic Considerations following "Operations for Rectal Incontinence" (below).

**References**


1. Parks AG, Gordon PH, Hardcastle JD: A classification of fistula-in-ano. *Br J Surg* 1976; 63(1):1-12.
2. Fazio VW: Complex anal fistulae. *Gastroenterol Clin North Am* 1987; 16(1):93-114.
3. Stone JM, Goldberg SM: The endorectal advancement flap procedure. *Int J Colorectal Dis* 1990; 5(4)232-35.


# HEMORRHOIDECTOMY

## SURGICAL CONSIDERATIONS

**Description:** Hemorrhoids are normally occurring vascular tissues, located in discrete aggregations known as hemorrhoidal cushions, within the distal rectum and anus. They are thought to play a role in the fine control of enteric continence, and are only treated if they cause a symptom that persists after conservative therapy. Hemorrhoids may cause bleeding, prolapse, mucous drainage, itching or pain (when thrombosed). The primary pathophysiologic event in the development of symptomatic hemorrhoids is thought to be mucosal prolapse caused by degeneration of the fibroelastic tissue that tethers the vascular cushions and overlying mucosa to the submucosa. All modern treatments for hemorrhoidal disease diminish prolapse by fixing the mucosa to the submucosa with scar tissue. Hemorrhoids are classified as internal, when they arise above the dentate line, or external, when they arise from below. Internal hemorrhoids are further classified by the degree of prolapse: I – protrude into lumen; II – prolapse and spontaneously reduce; III – prolapse and require manual reduction; IV – prolapsed and incarcerated. The most common symptom from external hemorrhoids is pain caused by acute thrombosis. The surgical treatment involves excision of the thrombosed hemorrhoid, usually under local anesthetic, in the office. Internal hemorrhoids may be treated by non-excisional or excisional techniques. Non-excisional techniques are generally used in the office or outpatient clinic. They do not require an anesthetic because their use is limited to the insensate tissues above the dentate line. Examples of non-excisional treatments are **rubber-band ligation**, **infrared coagulation**, **sclerotherapy** and **cryotherapy**.

**Surgical hemorrhoidectomy** may be performed in the lithotomy or prone jackknife position. An operating anoscope is placed in the anal canal and a hemorrhoid column is grasped and tented up into the lumen. An incision is started at the anal verge and a plane is developed deep to the hemorrhoidal tissue, and superficial to the sphincter muscles. When the internal sphincter is identified, the dissection proceeds in the avascular space along its luminal surface. The dissection is continued up into the rectum to include all redundant tissue. Lateral incisions along the redundant tissue are completed to excise the hemorrhoid. Care is taken to leave healthy bridges of mucosa between adjacent hemorrhoidal columns. Hemostasis is obtained with cautery and the mucosal defect may be closed with a running, absorbable suture. It is also acceptable to leave the mucosal wound open. The procedure is repeated over the other enlarged hemorrhoid columns, removing redundant tissue and leaving long vertical scars to prevent further mucosal prolapse.

**Variant procedure or approaches:** The **Whitehead hemorrhoidectomy** is similar, except that instead of discrete vertical incisions, the hemorrhoidal tissue is dissected off of the sphincter circumferentially, redundant tissue is excised, and the rectal mucosa is brought down to the dentate line and sewn in place. Lasers have not been shown to improve results in the treatment of hemorrhoids, and they typically increase cost. Sphincter stretch for symptomatic hemorrhoids (**Lord procedure**) should be abandoned, because of the high incidence of incontinence associated with it.

**Rubber-band ligation** requires no anesthesia because the band is placed on the insensate, distal rectal mucosa. A slotted anoscope is inserted into the anal canal and a hemorrhoid column is visualized. The most proximal area of redundant mucosa is grasped with a clamp and pulled into the barrel of the ligation gun. The trigger is pulled, forcing the rubber band onto the base of the tented-up hemorrhoid tissue. The encompassed tissue sloughs over a 4-7-day period, and a scar is formed between the mucosa and the underlying muscle.

**Usual preop diagnosis:** Symptomatic hemorrhoids; bleeding, prolapse or pain

## SUMMARY OF PROCEDURE

| | Hemorrhoidectomy | Whitehead Hemorrhoidectomy |
|---|---|---|
| **Position** | Prone jackknife, lithotomy or left lateral decubitus | ⇐ |
| **Incision** | Series of vertical incisions from anal verge to top of hemorrhoid columns | Circumferential intra-anal incision at the dentate line |
| **Special instrumentation** | Headlight or lighted anoscope; operating anoscope | ⇐ |
| **Antibiotics** | None | ⇐ |
| **Surgical time** | 45 - 90 min | ⇐ |
| **EBL** | < 100 ml | ⇐ |
| **Postop care** | Sitz baths, oral fluids, fiber supplements | ⇐ |
| **Mortality** | Rare | ⇐ |
| **Morbidity** | Urinary retention: 15-30% | ⇐ |
| | Incontinence: 1-6% | ⇐ |
| | Bleeding: 2-5% | ⇐ |
| | Stricture: 2-5% | ⇐ |
| | Infection: 1-2% | ⇐ |
| | | Mucosal ectropion: 2-20% |
| **Procedure code** | 46255, 46260, 45505 | 46255, 46260, 45505 |
| **Pain score** | 9 | 9 |

## PATIENT POPULATION CHARACTERISTICS

| | |
|---|---|
| **Age range** | Peak prevalence 45-65 yrs |
| **Male:Female** | 1:1 |
| **Incidence** | Prevalence 75/1,000 |
| **Etiology** | Low-fiber diet |
| | Genetic |
| | Pregnancy |
| **Associated conditions** | Constipation |

## ANESTHETIC CONSIDERATIONS

See Anesthetic Considerations following "Operations for Rectal Incontinence" (below).

**References**

1. Barron J: Office ligation of internal hemorrhoids. *Am J Surg* 1963; 105(4):563-70.
2. Buls JG, Goldberg SM: Modern management of hemorrhoids. *Surg Clin North Am* 1978; 58(3):469-78.
3. Burchell MC, Thow GB, Mannson RR: A "modified Whitehead" hemorrhoidectomy. *Dis Colon Rectum* 1976; 19(3):225-32.
4. Smith LE: Hemorrhoids. A review of current techniques and management. *Gastroenterol Clin North Am* 1987; 16(1)79-91.
5. Johanson JF, Sonnenberg A: The prevalence of hemorrhoids and chronic constipation. An epidemiologic study. *Gastroenterology* 1990: 98(2)380-86.

# OPERATIONS FOR RECTAL INCONTINENCE

## SURGICAL CONSIDERATIONS

**Description:** The majority of patients with rectal (enteric) incontinence will not be helped by surgery. In these patients, incontinence is caused by a combination of pudendal neuropathy and atrophy of the muscles of the pelvic floor. When an anatomic defect in the sphincter mechanism can be identified, surgery is likely to be beneficial.

**Sphincteroplasty** is performed in the prone jackknife position after a full mechanical and antibiotic bowel prep, which may leave patients hypovolemic and hypokalemic. An incision is placed at the anal verge, centered over the area of injured sphincter, and extended sufficiently around the anus to reach the retracted, cut edges of the sphincter. The anoderm and rectal mucosa are dissected off of the internal surface of the sphincter. The external surface of the sphincter mechanism is then dissected free to the level of the pelvic diaphragm. Care must be taken not to injure the inferior hemorrhoidal nerves during dissection around the posterior-lateral sphincter. The fibrotic portion linking the two ends of sphincter is cut, and the ends are overlapped and secured in place with two layers of interrupted horizontal mattress sutures. In women with obstetric injuries, the transverse perineal muscles are reapproximated. The anoderm is pulled down and re-secured to the skin at the anal verge. The remainder of the skin is closed as completely as possible.

**Variant procedure or approaches:** The surgical options for patients without anatomic defects in their sphincters are generally unsuccessful. The **posterior anoplasty of Parks** was designed to passively enhance continence by increasing the normally occurring angle between the rectum and the anal canal, and to increase the mechanical efficiency of weak sphincter muscle by shortening the fiber length. Lack of efficacy has limited its use, although some surgeons still perform the Parks procedure in the setting of continued incontinence after abdominal repair of rectal prolapse. The operation is performed in the prone jackknife position after a standard bowel prep. A hemispherical incision is placed at the level of the intersphincteric groove over the posterior half of the anus. The plane between the internal and external anal sphincters is identified and developed proximally to above the puborectalis muscle. The puborectalis fibers are "reefed," or pulled together, as far as possible with nonabsorbable suture. The external sphincter is plicated together in the midline with a series of nonabsorbable sutures that start at the deep external sphincter and progress to the subcutaneous sphincter. Skin is closed with absorbable sutures.

The **Thiersch operation (pinch graft)** has poor efficacy and a high complication rate and should be considered only as a procedure of last resort in patients with symptomatic rectal prolapse or fecal incontinence. As originally described, the anal canal was encircled with a silver wire which served as a passive obstacle to prolapse or defecation. In more recent years, an elastic sheet of Dacron®-impregnated Silastic® mesh has been used. Two small incisions are made on opposite sides of the anal verge. A pathway around the anal canal is created by blunt dissection and a 1.5 cm-wide piece of mesh is led around the anal canal. The ends of the mesh are overlapped in one of the incisions and either sutured or stapled together at an appropriate level of tension. The wounds are irrigated with antibiotic solution and the incisions are closed.

**Usual preop diagnosis:** Rectal (enteric) incontinence

## SUMMARY OF PROCEDURE

| | Overlapping Sphincteroplasty | Parks Postanal Repair | Modified Thiersch Procedure |
|---|---|---|---|
| **Position** | Prone jackknife | ⇐ | Prone jackknife or lithotomy |
| **Incision** | Circumanal | ⇐ | 2 small incisions lateral to the anus |
| **Special instrumentation** | Headlight | ⇐ | Headlight; Silastic® mesh |
| **Unique considerations** | Urinary catheter preop | ⇐ | None |
| **Antibiotics** | Standard bowel prep | ⇐ | Standard bowel prep, cefotetan 1 gm iv at induction; antibiotic in irrigation fluid |
| **Surgical time** | 1 - 2 hrs | 1 hr | 30 - 45 min |
| **EBL** | < 100 ml | ⇐ | ⇐ |
| **Postop care** | Early: Sitz baths, "medical colostomy"* | ⇐ | ⇐ |
| | Late: fiber supplement, stool softener | ⇐ | ⇐ |
| **Mortality** | Rare | ⇐ | ⇐ |
| **Morbidity** | Unimproved incontinence: 20% | 60-80% | 20% |
| | Improved, but minor incontinence: 30% | | Erosion of prosthesis: 30-60% |
| | Prolonged wound healing: 20% | | Obstructed defecation: 20-40% |
| | Infection: 1-2% | | |
| **Procedure code** | 46750 | 46761 | 15050 |
| **Pain score** | 8 | 7 | 6 |

* "Medical colostomy" is performed to prevent patients from having bowel movements for several days after the procedure. It involves a clear liquid diet and around-the-clock codeine pills for their constipating effect. This regimen is maintained for 3-4 d. After this period, the goal is to avoid constipation, so stool softeners and a fiber supplement are administered. Patients are instructed to take a laxative if they go more than 24 hrs without a bowel movement.

## PATIENT POPULATION CHARACTERISTICS

| | |
|---|---|
| **Age range** | Bimodal: 3rd-5th decades for obstetric injury, fistulotomy and perineal trauma; 6th-8th decades for pudendal neuropathy/pelvic floor atrophy |
| **Male:Female** | 1:4 |
| **Incidence** | Not uncommon |
| **Etiology** | Pudendal neuropathy<br>Pelvic floor atrophy<br>Obstetric injury<br>Injury during anal surgery (fistulotomy, sphincterotomy, hemorrhoidectomy)<br>Perineal trauma<br>Neurologic disease<br>Congenital anomalies |
| **Associated conditions** | Urinary incontinence<br>Chronic constipation<br>Multiparity |

## ANESTHETIC CONSIDERATIONS

**(Procedures covered: excision or repair of rectal prolapse; proctocolectomy; repair of rectal lesions, anal fistulotomy/fistulectomy; anal sphincterotomy/sphincteroplasty; hemorrhoidectomy; operations for rectal incontinence)**

### PREOPERATIVE

**Respiratory** — A careful evaluation of respiratory status is important. If patient has ↓respiratory reserve, the lithotomy position may be better tolerated than the prone or jackknife positions.
**Tests:** As indicated from H&P.

**Musculoskeletal** — Pain is likely to be present at the surgical site and should be considered when positioning patient for anesthetic induction (e.g., if patient has pain while sitting, perform regional anesthesia in the lateral decubitus position). Evaluate bony landmarks if regional anesthetic is planned.

**Hematologic** — If regional anesthesia is planned and patient is taking ASA, NSAIDs, or dipyridamole, ✓ platelet count and bleeding time.
**Tests:** CBC with differential; electrolytes; plt; bleeding time as indicated from H&P.

**Laboratory** — Other tests as indicated from H&P.

**Premedication** — Standard premedication (see Appendix).

### INTRAOPERATIVE

**Anesthetic technique:** GA, spinal or epidural techniques may be used.

**General anesthesia:**

**Induction** — **General (mask vs ETT):** Standard induction (see Appendix). Procedures done in the jackknife position may require ET intubation for airway control if a regional technique is not performed.

**Maintenance** — Standard maintenance (see Appendix).

**Emergence** — No special considerations

**Regional anesthesia:**

**Spinal** — **Single-shot vs continuous:** Patient in either sitting, lateral decubitus, prone or jackknife position for placement of a subarachnoid block. Doses of local anesthetics should be adequate to provide high lumbar level of sensory anesthesia (e.g., lidocaine 5%, 50-75 mg; tetracaine 10-14 mg; bupivacaine 8-12 mg). For continuous spinal, titrate local anesthetic to desired surgical level. Large doses of local anesthetic should be avoided as they can cause postop cauda equina syndrome.

**Epidural** — Patient in sitting or lateral decubitus position for placement of epidural catheter. A test dose (e.g., 3 cc of 1.5% lidocaine with 1:200,000 epinephrine) is administered and patient is observed for development of a subarachnoid block or symptoms of an intravascular injection. Then titrate 2% lidocaine with epinephrine (3-5 cc at a time) until desired surgical level is obtained.

**Caudal** — Patient in prone, jackknife or lateral position for placement of caudal block. After needle has been positioned properly in the caudal canal, a 3 cc test dose of 1.5% lidocaine with 1:200,000 epinephrine is injected (as above). To obtain sacral levels of anesthesia, a volume of 10 ml should be sufficient (0.25% bupivacaine or 2% lidocaine with 1:200,000 epinephrine).

| | | |
|---|---|---|
| **Blood and fluid requirements** | IV: 16-18 ga x 1<br>NS/LR @ 5-8 cc/kg/hr | Blood not likely to be required. |
| **Monitoring** | Standard monitors (see Appendix). | Others as clinically indicated. |
| **Positioning** | ✓ and pad pressure points.<br>✓ eyes. | Chest support or bolsters to optimize ventilation in the jackknife position; care in positioning the patient's extremities and genitals after turning into jackknife position. Avoid pressure on eyes and ears after turning patient. |
| **Complications** | Lithotomy position can lead to damage to peroneal nerve → foot drop. | |

## POSTOPERATIVE

| | | |
|---|---|---|
| **Complications** | Urinary retention<br>Poor wound healing<br>Atelectasis<br>Cauda equina syndrome | Catheterize until return of urinary function.<br><br>Cauda equina syndrome is characterized by varying degrees of urinary/fecal incontinence, sensory loss in the perineal area and lower extremity motor weakness. |
| **Pain management** | PCA (see Appendix).<br>Epidural analgesia (see Appendix). | PO analgesics may be suitable:<br>Acetaminophen and codeine (Tylenol® #3 1-2 tab q 4-6 hrs) or oxycodone and acetaminophen (Percocet® 1 tab q 6 hrs) |
| **Tests** | As indicated by patient status. | |

**References**

1. Parks AG. Anorectal incontinence. President's Address. *Proc Roy Soc Med* Meeting 27. 1975; 68(11):681-90.
2. Snooks SJ, Swash M, Henry MM, Setchell M: Risk factors in childbirth causing damage to the pelvic floor innervation. *Int J Colorectal Dis* 1986; 1(1):20-4.
3. Slade MS, Goldberg SM, Schottler JL: Sphincteroplasty for acquired anal incontinence. *Dis Colon Rectum* 1977: 20(1):33-5.
4. Horn HR, Schoetz DJ Jr, Coller JA, Veidenheimer MC: Sphincter repair with a silastic sling for anal incontinence and rectal procidentia. *Dis Colon Rectum* 1985; 28(11):868-72.
5. Rigler ML, Drasner K, Krejcie TC, Yelich SJ, Scholnick FT, DeFontes J, Bohner D: Cauda equina syndrome after continuous spinal anesthesia. *Anesth Analg* 1991; 72(3):275-81.
6. Dershwitz, M: Local Anesthetics. in *Clinical Anesthesia Procedures of the Massachusetts General Hospital*, 3rd edition. Firestone LL, Lebowitz PW, Cook CE eds; Little, Brown and Co, Boston: 1988,185-98.

**Surgeon**

**Harry A. Oberhelman, MD, FACS**

# 7.5 HEPATIC SURGERY

**Anesthesiologist**

**Steven K. Howard, MD**

# HEPATIC RESECTION

## SURGICAL CONSIDERATIONS

**Description:** For major lobar resections (Fig 7.5-1) the corresponding hepatic artery, portal vein and bile duct are isolated and ligated in the porta hepatis. If possible, the major hepatic vein of the involved lobe is ligated at its entry into the vena cavae.

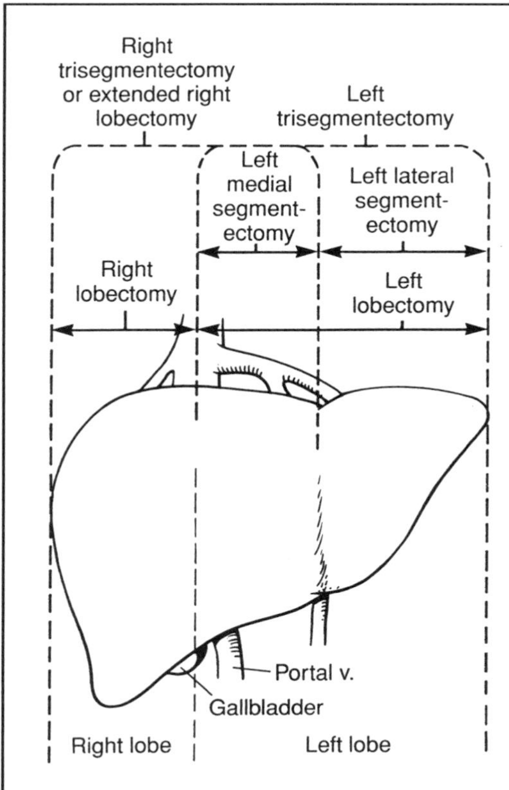


**Figure 7.5-1.** Types of liver resection. (Reproduced with permission from Hardy JD: *Hardy's Textbook of Surgery*, 2nd edition. JB Lippincott: 1988.)

Transection of the liver is done by blunt dissection utilizing the Cavitron ultrasonic suction aspirator (CUSA) and argon beam laser coagulator. During dissection through the liver substance, the visible vessels and bile ducts should be clipped or ligated. During the transection, minor-to-moderate bleeding may occur, particularly if larger veins are torn, and these must be controlled with suture ligatures. Following resection, suction drains are placed and the omentum is tacked to the cut surface of the liver for hemostasis.

As the principles and techniques of hepatic surgery have evolved, the overall mortality and morbidity have improved considerably. Since the normal liver is capable of regeneration, it is possible to resect the right or left lobe, along with a major segment of the contralateral lobe. This procedure is known as a **trisegmentectomy**. In patients afflicted with cirrhosis, the regeneration process is limited; thus, uninvolved liver should be preserved.

**Partial resection** of the liver for metastatic disease may be performed at the same time as surgical resection for the primary lesion. Although most major resections can be performed by a transabdominal approach, some surgeons prefer a thoracoabdominal approach.

**Usual preop diagnosis:** Benign and malignant primary or metastatic tumors of the liver

### SUMMARY OF PROCEDURE

| | Right/Left Lobectomy | Trisegmentectomy | Partial Resection |
|---|---|---|---|
| **Position** | Supine | ⇐ | ⇐ |
| **Incision** | Midline abdominal | ⇐ | ⇐ |
| **Special instrumentation** | Denier retractor (lifts anterior chest wall); CUSA; argon beam laser; cell saver (on occasion) | ⇐ | ⇐ |
| **Unique considerations** | Intraop ultrasound | ⇐ | ⇐ |
| **Antibiotics** | Cefotetan 2 gm preop | ⇐ | ⇐ |
| **Surgical time** | 3 - 4 hrs | 4 - 5 hrs | 1 - 2 hrs |
| **Closing considerations** | Secure adequate hemostasis | ⇐ | ⇐ |
| **EBL** | 500-2000 ml | ⇐ | 300-500 ml |
| **Postop care** | ICU x 1-3 d | ⇐ | PACU → room |

| | Right/Left Lobectomy | Trisegmentectomy | Partial Resection |
|---|---|---|---|
| **Mortality** | 3-10% | ⇐ | < 3% |
| **Morbidity** | Bile leak: 10-30% | ⇐ | ⇐ |
| | Intra-abdominal infection: 10-15% | ⇐ | 5-10% |
| | Pleural effusion: 10% | ⇐ | 5% |
| | Wound infection: 5-10% | ⇐ | 2-5% |
| | Hepatic failure: 5% | ⇐ | < 1% |
| | Postop hemorrhage: 2-3% | ⇐ | ⇐ |
| **Procedure code** | 47125 (total left lobectomy)<br>47130 (total right lobectomy | 47122 | 47120 |
| **Pain score** | 7-9 | 7-9 | 7-9 |

### PATIENT POPULATION CHARACTERISTICS

| | |
|---|---|
| **Age range** | 14-80 yrs[1] |
| **Male:Female** | 2:1 |
| **Incidence** | Primary liver cancer 4/100,000 |
| **Etiology** | Metastatic to liver from primary cancer<br>Environmental and chemical carcinogens<br>Chronic hepatitis and/or cirrhosis[2]<br>Parasitic infection (clonorchis sinensis) |
| **Associated conditions** | Chronic hepatitis<br>Cirrhosis |

## ANESTHETIC CONSIDERATIONS

See Anesthetic Considerations following "Hepatorrhaphy" (below).

**References**

1. Sitzman RJV et al: Preoperative assessment of malignant hepatic tumors. *Am J Surg* 1990; 159(1):137-42.
2. Parker GA et al: Intraoperative ultrasound of the liver affects operative decision making. *Ann Surg* 1989; 209(5):569-77.
3. Oberfield RA, Steele G Jr, Gollan JL, Sherman D: Liver cancer. *CA Cancer J Clin* 1989; July-August. 39(4):206-18.

# HEPATORRHAPHY

## SURGICAL CONSIDERATIONS

**Description**: Although most liver lacerations have stopped bleeding by the time a surgeon sees them, others require suturing or partial liver resection to control bleeding. Various techniques are available to control hemorrhage, including packing, suturing, inflow occlusion and resection. Small lacerations that have stopped bleeding require no specific therapy other than possible drainage. Lacerations that continue to bleed usually can be sutured and drained. Extensive tears of the liver that are actively bleeding may require temporary occlusion of the porta hepatis, containing the hepatic artery, portal vein and bile duct (**Pringle maneuver**) in order to excise deviated parenchyma and control bleeding with sutures, clips, coagulators, etc. Occasionally, the hepatic vein draining the involved lobe will require clamping to control back-bleeding. When the bleeding cannot be controlled, it is expedient to pack the wound, drain the abdomen and close. The pack can be removed without much risk of rebleeding within 48-72 hours.

**Usual preop diagnosis**: Trauma with CT evidence of hepatic laceration

## SUMMARY OF PROCEDURE

| | |
|---|---|
| **Position** | Supine |
| **Incision** | Midline abdominal |
| **Special instrumentation** | Denier retractor |
| **Surgical time** | 1 - 2 hrs |
| **EBL** | Variable – 300-2000 ml |
| **Mortality** | 1-2% |
| **Morbidity** | Continued bleeding: 2-3%<br>Biliary fistula<br>Perihepatic abscess<br>Intrahepatic hematoma<br>Arteroportal fistula<br>Hepatic and renal failure |
| **Procedure code** | 47350 |
| **Pain score** | 7-9 |

## PATIENT POPULATION CHARACTERISTICS

| | |
|---|---|
| **Age range** | Variable |
| **Male:Female** | 1:1 |
| **Incidence** | Rare |
| **Etiology** | Trauma (blunt vs penetrating)<br>Surgical<br>Hepatic adenomas<br>Needle biopsies of liver |
| **Associated conditions** | See Etiology, above |

---

# ANESTHETIC CONSIDERATIONS FOR HEPATIC PROCEDURES

**(Procedures covered: hepatorrhaphy; hepatic resection; other hepatic surgery)**

## PREOPERATIVE

Patients presenting for hepatic surgery may have primary or metastatic tumors from GI and other sources. Liver function may be entirely normal in these patients. Hepatocellular carcinoma is seen commonly in males >50 yrs, and is associated with chronic active hepatitis B and cirrhosis. The preop considerations listed below describe patients without cirrhosis. (See Preoperative Considerations for "Surgery for Portal Hypertension" in "Vascular Surgery" section) for evaluation of patients with cirrhosis).

| | |
|---|---|
| **Respiratory** | Respiratory function is typically normal. Tumors of the liver, however, may be metastatic from a malignancy.<br>**Tests:** CXR; others as clinically indicated. |
| **Cardiovascular** | Patients may be hypovolemic and volume status should be carefully assessed before induction of anesthesia (skin turgor, UO, orthostatic BP, HR, etc). Tumors may surround major vascular structures and impede blood flow. Consider evaluation with CT/MRI scan. |
| **Hepatic** | Liver resection can be indicated for hemangiomas, hydatid cysts and tumors. It is important to determine the size of the tumor and involvement of vascular structures preop so as to be adequately prepared for major intraop blood and fluid losses.<br>**Tests:** LFTs; albumin; ultrasound/CT/MRI |
| **Hematologic** | The liver produces all clotting factors except VIII and the degree of hepatic insufficiency determines the extent of any coagulopathy. T&C 4 U PRBCs.<br>**Tests:** CBC; PT; PTT; platelet count; others as indicated from H&P. |

**Laboratory** Tests as indicated from H&P. **NB:** For elective cases, if abnormal LFTs are present on preop labs, it is important to perform a complete medical workup. This can include reviewing old lab data, hepatitis serology and an abdominal ultrasound to rule out cholestatic causes of liver dysfunction. Surgery and anesthesia in the presence of acute hepatitis is associated with a high mortality.

**Premedication** Standard premedication (see Appendix). Consider administering vitamin K if PT is prolonged. (Beneficial results from vitamin K usually occur within 24 hrs.)

## INTRAOPERATIVE

**Anesthetic technique:** GETA ± epidural for postop analgesia. If postop epidural analgesia is planned, placement of catheter with patient in sitting position prior to anesthetic induction is helpful to establish correct placement in the epidural space (accomplished by injecting 5-7 cc of 1% lidocaine via the epidural catheter, eliciting a segmental block). The initial incision is usually right subcostal, but it may have to be extended into the right chest if surgical resection necessitates. If known beforehand, placement of a left DLT may improve surgical exposure.

**Induction** Standard induction (see Appendix). Restore intravascular volume prior to anesthetic induction. Trauma patients require awake intubation (see Appendix) or rapid-sequence induction with cricoid pressure until intubation has been confirmed. If patient is hemodynamically unstable, consider etomidate (0.2-0.4 mg/kg) or ketamine (1-3 mg/kg) in place of STP.

**Maintenance** Standard maintenance (see Appendix); $N_2O$ can be used if bowel distention is not problematic for surgical exposure/closure.

**Combined epidural/GA:** Local anesthetic (1.5-2% lidocaine with 1:200,000 epinephrine (8-12 ml q 60 min) can be injected into the epidural catheter to provide both anesthesia and optimal surgical exposure (contracted bowel and profound muscle relaxation). Be prepared to treat hypotension with fluid and vasopressors. GA is administered to supplement regional anesthesia and for amnesia. Systemic sedatives (droperidol, opiates, benzodiazepines, etc.) should be minimized during this type of anesthetic as they increase the likelihood of postop respiratory depression. If epidural opiates are used for postop analgesia, a loading dose (e.g., hydromorphone 1.0 mg) should be administered at least 1 hr before the conclusion of surgery. During surgery, maintain ventilation to avoid extremes of hypercarbia and hypocarbia.

**Emergence** For major hepatic resections, the patient will be best-cared for in an ICU. Consider keeping the patient mechanically ventilated until he/she is hemodynamically stable and ventilatory status is optimized. If surgical resection was minimal, the patient can be extubated awake after return of airway reflexes.

| | | |
|---|---|---|
| **Blood and fluid requirements** | Anticipate large blood loss.<br>IV: 14-16 ga x 2<br>NS/LR @ 10-20 cc/kg/hr<br>Fluid warmer<br>Humidify gasses.<br>Consider utilizing rapid transfusion device. | Blood loss can be significant; keep at least 2 U PRBC ahead. Lobectomies are often associated with more blood loss than wedge resections. Massive transfusions may be required and appropriate blood products should be available (e.g., 2 FFPs + 6 PLT/10 U PRBC). If procedure does not involve cancer, blood salvage devices can be utilized. |
| **Control of blood loss** | Surgical control<br>Pringle maneuver<br>Grafts<br>Sealants | Surgical control of the main blood vessels entering the hilar area (Pringle maneuver). Grafts (omental or peritoneal) or rapidly polymerizing adhesives can be applied to the raw surface of the resected segment to provide a means of hemostasis. |
| **Monitoring** | Standard monitors (see Appendix).<br>UO<br>± CVP<br>± Arterial line | Others as clinically indicated. If the extent of the resection is not known at the beginning of surgery, appropriate monitoring (CVP, arterial line, additional ivs, etc.) should be established prior to beginning resection. |
| **Positioning** | ✓ and pad pressure points.<br>✓ eyes. | |
| **Complications** | Massive hemorrhage | Ensure adequate vascular access. Consider rapid-transfusion device. |

## POSTOPERATIVE

| | | |
|---|---|---|
| **Complications** | ↓liver function<br>Hemorrhage<br>Electrolyte imbalances<br>Hypoglycemia<br>Hypothermia, shivering<br>DIC<br>Pulmonary insufficiency (atelectasis, effusion, pneumonia) | Patients with normal liver function preop may have significant postop impairment of liver function 2° loss of liver mass or surgical trauma.<br>>90% of patients will develop some form of respiratory complication. |
| **Pain management** | Epidural analgesia: (see Appendix).<br>PCA (see Appendix). | Patient should be recovered in ICU or hospital ward that is accustomed to treating the side effects of epidural opiates (e.g., respiratory depression, breakthrough pain, nausea, pruritus). |
| **Tests** | ABG; CXR; others as clinically indicated. | |


**References**

1. Feliciano DV, Jordan GL Jr, Bitondo CG, Mattox KL, Burch JM, Cruse PA: Management of 1000 consecutive cases of hepatic trauma. *Ann Surg* 1986; 204:438-45.
2. Merritt WT, Gelman S: Anesthesia for liver surgery. In *Principles and Practice of Anesthesiology*. Rogers MC, Tinker JH, Covino BG, Longnecker DE, eds. Mosby Year Book, St Louis: 1993, 1991-2034.

**Surgeon**

**Mark A. Vierra, MD**

# 7.6 BILIARY TRACT SURGERY

**Anesthesiologist**

**Steven K. Howard, MD**

# CHOLECYSTECTOMY

## SURGICAL CONSIDERATIONS

**Description:** With the advent of laparoscopic cholecystectomy, the traditional **open cholecystectomy** has become a rarity, generally reserved for gallbladders that are expected to be difficult to remove due to inflammation, previous operations and adhesions, or because of other medical problems, such as coagulopathy or cirrhosis. In most institutions, fewer than 10% of cholecystectomies will be begun as open procedures, and perhaps 5% of laparoscopic cholecystectomies will be converted to open cholecystectomies during the course of the operation due to technical difficulties, complications or unexpected findings. The open cholecystectomy of the 90s is, in general, a substantially more challenging operation, for both surgeon and anesthesiologist, than it was in previous decades.

The **open cholecystectomy** is usually performed through a right subcostal or midline incision. Upward traction is applied to the liver or gallbladder, while downward traction on the duodenum exposes the region of the cystic duct and artery and common duct. Depending on local conditions and the surgeon's preference, the gallbladder may be removed from the top down, excising the gallbladder from the liver bed and isolating the cystic duct and artery as the final stage of the operation, or the cystic duct and artery may be isolated and divided first, and the gallbladder removed retrograde from the gallbladder bed as the final step of the procedure. The anatomy of the biliary tree is quite variable, and few surgeons always remove the gallbladder in exactly the same way every time. (Fig 7.6-1 shows biliary tree anatomy.)

**Cholangiography** may be performed in either laparoscopic or open cholecystectomy and is performed at the discretion of the surgeon – some surgeons perform it in all patients and others perform it only in patients in whom there is some clinical evidence of choledocholithiasis. The cystic duct is opened and a catheter placed into the duct and secured with a ligature, tie or special cholangiogram clamp. Dye is injected into the biliary tree via the catheter and x-rays are taken. If stones are found, a common duct exploration may be performed. Alternatively, an endoscopic retrograde cholangiogram (ERCP) with stone extraction may be carried out postop. Cholangiography usually adds about 10-15 minutes to the procedure.

**Laparoscopic cholecystectomy** requires general anesthesia, just as with open cholecystectomy. It is performed under video guidance and usually involves 3-5 punctures of the abdomen. The abdomen is insufflated using a special insufflator that may deliver as much as 6-9 L of $CO_2$/minute and maintains the abdominal pressure at approximately 10-16 mmHg. After placement of the usual ports, the patient is placed in reverse Trendelenburg with the right side of the bed elevated. This helps the colon and duodenum to fall away from the gallbladder. The gallbladder is grasped and elevated and dissection of the cystic duct and artery is carried out by the surgeon, who stands on the patient's left. The cystic duct and artery are isolated, clipped and divided, and a cholangiogram may be performed. The gallbladder is then removed retrograde from the gallbladder bed, which is irrigated and suctioned dry to assure hemostasis. The patient is levelled out and the gallbladder is extracted through the umbilicus. The umbilical fascia and skin incisions are closed.

**Choledochotomy**, or **"common duct exploration,"** is the opening and exploration of the common duct for the purpose of extracting stones. The need for this may be anticipated preop or performed based on findings at operation, particularly the finding of common duct stones by cholangiography. A longitudinal incision approximately 1 cm long is made in the duct and exploration is carried out through this incision. The duct may be irrigated with NS, balloon catheters may be passed and various instruments introduced to grasp, remove or crush retained stones. The duct may be biopsied by this approach, and **choledochoscopy** – the direct visualization of the duct's interior using a small flexible scope – can be performed. Depending on the complexity of the findings, a common duct exploration can be expected to add from 30 minutes to more than an hour to the cholecystectomy. In general, the mortality of patients undergoing common duct exploration is approximately 2-5 times that of a simple cholecystectomy. This difference can be explained by the fact that patients undergoing common duct exploration tend to be older and sicker – the opening of the duct itself is not necessarily a significant physiologic insult.

In a few centers, **laparoscopic common duct exploration** is being attempted, but presently this is not a commonly performed procedure, and there has been little experience with it as yet. It is too soon to know if this procedure will become common practice. Access to the duct is usually carried out through the cystic duct by dilating the duct, rather than through a choledochotomy. The stone can be grasped and extracted with a basket introduced into the duct either under direct vision, using a small flexible choledochoscope, or under fluoroscopic guidance. There are as yet no published results that allow a prediction as to how successful this technique will be, how long it can be expected to take, or what complications might be associated with it.

**Variant procedure or approaches**: Cholecystectomy remains the mainstay of treatment for symptomatic biliary stone disease. **Nonsurgical treatment** of cholelithiasis, particularly by **oral dissolution** and/or **lithotripsy**, have very limited usefulness and are rarely used in clinical practice.

**Usual preop diagnosis**: Symptomatic cholelithiasis; acute cholecystitis; choledocholithiasis

**SUMMARY OF PROCEDURE**

| | Cholecystectomy | Laparoscopic Cholecystectomy | Cholecystectomy/ Common Duct Exploration |
|---|---|---|---|
| **Position** | Supine | Supine, reverse Trendelenburg with right side elevated | ⇐ |
| **Incision** | Right subcostal or midline | 3-5 trocar sites | Longitudinal |
| **Special instrumentation** | Costal margin retractor ± cholangiogram catheter | Laparoscopic equipment, including insufflator, video; ± x-ray or fluoroscopy for cholangiography | Choledochotomy instruments |
| **Unique considerations** | Requires intraop x-ray for cholangiogram | See Special Instrumentation, above. | May include choledochoscopy. |
| **Antibiotics** | Ampicillin, piperacillin or mezlocillin, 1-3 gm iv ± gentamicin; or cefotetan 1-2 gm iv | ⇐ | ⇐ |
| **Surgical time** | 45 - 90 min | 45 - 120 min | 1 - 2.5 hrs |
| **Closing considerations** | Muscle relaxation | ⇐ + Brief closing | Muscle relaxation |
| **EBL** | < 250 cc | Minimal | 250 cc |
| **Postop care** | PACU | ⇐ | ⇐ |
| **Mortality** | 0.7% | 0-0.1% | 0-1.5% < 60 yrs; ≤ 5% in advanced age |
| **Morbidity** | Postop bile leak: 0-9% | – | ⇐ |
| | Pancreatitis: 0-4.6% | – | 2-5% |
| | Bile duct injury: 0-0.25% | 0-0.5% | |
| | Cardiac and respiratory complications: Rare, but leading cause of death | – | |
| | Hemorrhage: Rare | – | |
| | | Conversion to open cholecystectomy: 2-5% | |
| | | Bleeding requiring transfusion: 0-0.5% | |
| | | Intestinal injury: 0-0.4% | |
| | | MI or CVA: 0-0.2% | |
| **Procedure code** | 47600 | 47605 | 47610 |
| **Pain score** | 6 | 2 | 6-7 |

**PATIENT POPULATION CHARACTERISTICS**

| | |
|---|---|
| **Age range** | Mostly adult; increases with age |
| **Male:Female** | 1:2-3 |
| **Incidence** | 600,000/yr in U.S.; 90+% performed laparoscopically. |
| **Etiology** | See Associated Conditions, below. |
| **Associated conditions** | Ileal disease<br>Cirrhosis<br>Hemolytic disorders<br>Choledocholithiasis<br>Cholangitis or active pancreatitis |

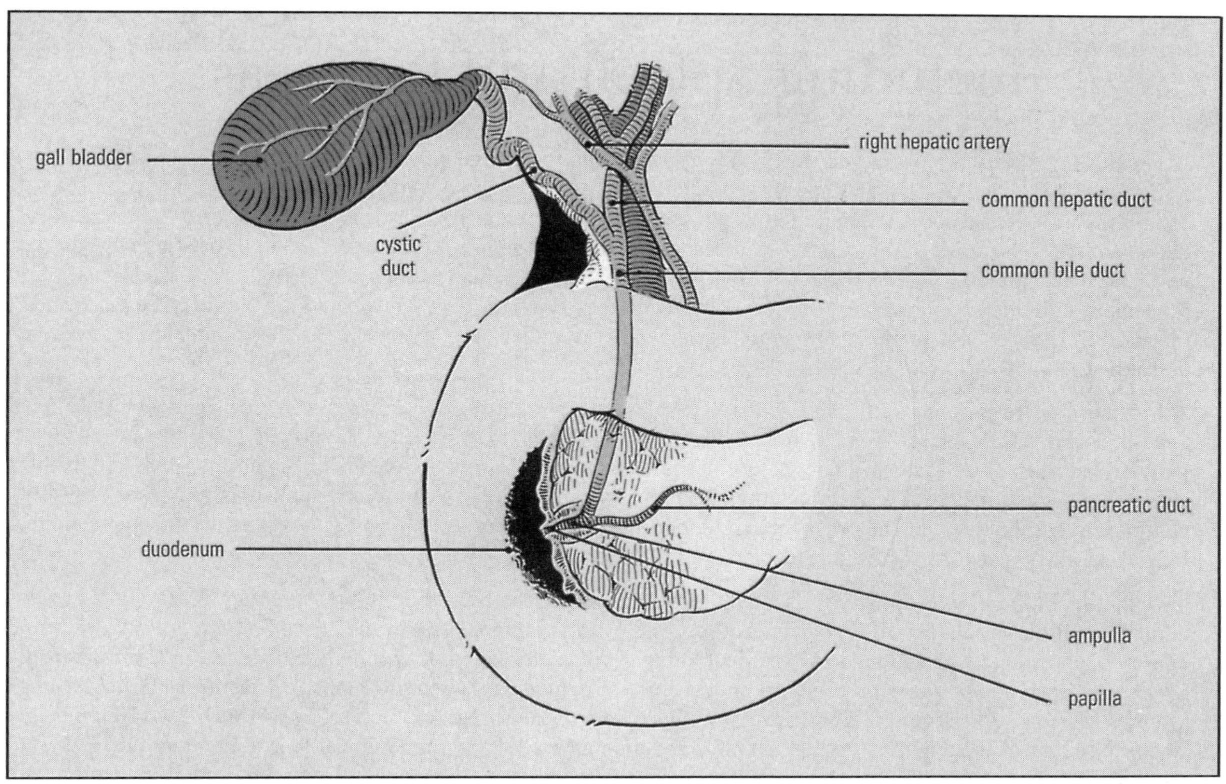


**Figure 7.6-1.** Anatomy of the biliary tree. (Reproduced with permission from Calne R, Pollard SG: *Operative Surgery*. Gower Medical Pub: 1992.)

---

## ANESTHETIC CONSIDERATIONS

See "Anesthetic Considerations for Biliary Tract Surgery," at the end of this section.

**References**

1. Brooks JR: Acute and chronic cholecystitis. In *Current Surgical Therapy*. Cameron J, ed. BC Decker, Philadelphia: 1989, Vol III, 257-62.
2. Boquist L, Bergdahl L, Andersson A: Mortality following gallbladder surgery: a study of 3,257 cholecystectomies. *Surgery* 1972; 71(4):616-24.
3. McSherry CK, Glenn F: The incidence and causes of death following surgery for nonmalignant biliary tract disease. *Ann Surg* 1980; 191(3):271-75.
4. Cuschieri A, Dubois F, Mouiel J, Mouret P, Becker H, Buess G, Trede M, Troidl H: The European experience with laparoscopic cholecystectomy. *Am J Surg* 1991; 161(3):385-87.
5. The Southern Surgeons Club: A prospective analysis of 1518 laparoscopic cholecystectomies. *New Eng J Med* 1991; 324(16):1073-78.
6. Spaw: Laparoscopic laser cholecystectomy: analysis of 500 procedures. *Surg Laparoscopy Endoscopy* 1991; 1(1):2-7.
7. Voyles CR, Petro AB, Meena AL, Haick AJ, Koury AM: A practical approach to laparoscopic cholecystectomy. *Am J Surg* 1991; 161(3):365-70.
8. Peters JH, Ellison EC, Innes JT, Liss JL, Nichols KE, Lomano JM, Roby SR, Front ME, Carey LC: Safety and efficacy of laparoscopic cholecystectomy. A prospective analysis of 100 initial patients. *Ann Surg* 1991; 213(1):3-12.
9. Zucker KA, Bailey RW, Gadacz TR, Imbembo AL: Laparoscopic guided cholecystectomy. *Am J Surg* 1991; 161(1):36-44.

# BILIARY DRAINAGE PROCEDURES

## SURGICAL CONSIDERATIONS

**Description:** Biliary drainage procedures may be performed for malignant and nonmalignant indications, and the type of drainage procedure performed depends on factors such as the nature of the biliary obstruction, the patient's overall condition and prognosis, the need for other surgical procedures and institutional expertise. **Endoscopic** and **transhepatic techniques** are increasing in use and, today, most drainage procedures of the biliary tree are performed with these techniques. There remain a significant number of patients, however, for whom a traditional surgical procedure is the most appropriate. In general, the complexity of the different operations that may be performed and the morbidity attendant to these has more to do with the indications for operation than with which procedure is performed.

All of these operations are performed, under general anesthesia, through an upper midline or right subcostal incision. Self-retaining retractors are used to retract the liver superiorly to expose the region of the porta hepatis. If the gallbladder will not be used for the bypass procedure (**cholecystojejunostomy**), then it is usually removed as the first step in the procedure (see "Cholecystectomy," above). If the patient has had previous upper right quadrant surgery, the complexity and duration of the procedure and blood loss may increase significantly. Any associated hepatic cirrhosis may make the procedure particularly demanding.

**Transduodenal sphincteroplasty** is usually performed for benign obstruction of the Ampulla of Vater or for extensive choledocholithiasis. **Endoscopic sphincterotomy** is the most commonly performed technique for opening the ampulla, and is most commonly performed by gastroenterologists outside of the OR with iv sedation. **Open sphincteroplasty** is usually reserved for patients in whom endoscopic retrograde cholangiogram (ERCP) has been unsuccessful or in whom a laparotomy is required for other reasons. For these open procedures, the second portion of duodenum is incised over the region of the ampulla, and the ampulla is cannulated. A longitudinal incision is made over the course of the ampulla and the mucosa of the ampulla is sutured to the mucosa of the duodenum with fine interrupted sutures, with care being taken not to compromise the pancreatic duct. The duodenum is closed with suture, a small closed suction drain is placed, and the wound is closed. A postop stay of five to seven days can be expected.

**Cholecystojejunostomy** is usually performed as palliation for malignant obstruction of the distal bile duct. Its advantage is that it does not require dissection of the portal triad, but the long-term results are less reliable than with the other two drainage procedures. This is partly because the gallbladder may not drain as well as the common duct, and partly because the tumor may grow to occlude the junction of the common and cystic ducts. The abdomen is opened as described above, and the region of the porta hepatis examined to assure that the cystic duct is not imminently compromised by tumor. The jejunum is then brought up to the gallbladder, usually by passing the jejunum through the transverse mesocolon. The anastomosis may be performed either to an intact loop of jejunum (**"loop cholecystojejunostomy"**) or to a Roux-en-Y loop of jejunum (**"Roux-en-Y" cholecystojejunostomy"**), and is carried out with one or two layers of sutures, depending on surgeon's preference. If a Roux-en-Y is created, a second jejuno-jejunal anastomosis must be performed.

In **choledochoduodenostomy** or **choledochojejunostomy**, an anastomosis is fashioned between the common duct and the duodenum or the common duct and Roux loop of jejunum. This is often a relatively more demanding operation than cholecystojejunostomy because it requires dissection deep in the porta hepatis to gain access to the common duct. Long-term results are more reliable, however, and these are preferred for benign disease. Exposure of the biliary tree is the same as for the above procedures. The gallbladder is always removed (if it is still present). The common duct is dissected free from the surrounding structures in the porta and an anastomosis is constructed between the common duct and the duodenum or jejunum. If the jejunum is used, it is almost always brought up as a Roux-en-Y, requiring a second jejuno-jejunal anastomosis.

**Variant procedure or approaches**: Endoscopic or transhepatic placement of temporary or permanent **biliary stents** is an increasingly common alternative to surgical drainage in patients with incurable pancreatic or biliary tract disease.

**Usual preop diagnosis**: Transduodenal sphincteroplasty: extensive choledocholithiasis, often after failed attempt at ERCP; rarely, malignant disease. Cholecystojejunostomy: malignant obstruction of distal common bile duct, usually due to pancreatic cancer. Choledochojejunostomy or choledochoduodenostomy: benign strictures of the distal bile duct; longstanding stone disease; pancreatitis; iatrogenic injury; Oriental cholangiohepatitis; after resection of some tumors of the pancreas or distal bile duct.

## SUMMARY OF PROCEDURE

| | Cholecysto-jejunostomy | Choledocho-jejunostomy | Choledocho-duodenostomy | Transduodenal sphincteroplasty |
|---|---|---|---|---|
| **Position** | Supine | ⇐ | ⇐ | ⇐ |
| **Incision** | Midline or right subcostal | ⇐ | ⇐ | ⇐ |
| **Special instrumentation** | Costal retractor | ⇐ | ⇐ | ⇐ |
| **Unique considerations** | Consider usual prep for patients with obstructive jaundice. | ⇐ | ⇐ | ⇐ |
| **Antibiotics** | Ampicillin, piperacillin or mezlocillin, 1-3 gm iv ± gentamicin; or cefotetan 1-2 gm iv | ⇐ | ⇐ | ⇐ |
| **Surgical time** | 1 hr; may be significantly greater if resection of tumor is considered. | 1.5 - 3 hrs | ⇐ | ⇐ |
| **Closing considerations** | Muscle relaxation; NG suction | ⇐ | ⇐ | ⇐ |
| **EBL** | < 250 cc (greater if tumor resection performed, or in the presence of portal HTN). | 250-500 cc (greater if tumor resection performed, or in the presence of portal HTN). | ⇐ | < 250 cc (transfusion rarely needed). |
| **Postop care** | PACU | ⇐ | ⇐ | ⇐ |
| **Mortality**[1,2,3,5,7,8] | ≤ 35% in advanced pancreatic cancer; otherwise, < 10% | ≤ 29%, with pancreatic cancer; 0.5% for benign disease | 0-5.4%[3,4,5] (usually for benign disease) | 0-7% |
| **Morbidity**[1-5,7,8] | Sepsis | ⇐ | ⇐ | – |
| | Respiratory complications | ⇐ | ⇐ | – |
| | Renal failure | ⇐ | ⇐ | – |
| | Hemorrhage | ⇐ | ⇐ | – |
| | Wound infection | ⇐ | ⇐ | – |
| | Breakdown of biliary anastomosis | ⇐ | ⇐ | Pancreatitis: Rare |
| | Thrombotic complications | ⇐ | ⇐ | Recurrent cholangitis: Rare |
| **Procedure code** | 47720(cholecystoenterostomy) 47721 (with gastroenterostomy) 47740 (Roux-en-Y cholecystoenterostomy) | 47760 (anastomosis, extrahepatic biliary ducts and GI tract) 47780 (Roux-en-Y anastomosis, extrahepatic biliary ducts and GI tract) | 47440 | 47460 (transduodenal sphincterotomy or sphincteroplasty) |
| **Pain score** | 7 | 7 | 7 | 6 |

## PATIENT POPULATION CHARACTERISTICS

| | |
|---|---|
| **Age range** | 5th-7th decade; may be younger for sphincterotomy |
| **Male:Female** | 1.1:2.1 |
| **Incidence** | Procedure-related incidence not available, but clearly declining in favor of techniques by interventional gastroenterology and radiology |
| **Etiology** | See Preop Diagnosis, above. |

**Associated conditions** Jaundiced: Very common
Fat-soluble vitamin deficiencies
Malignancy, especially pancreatic: Common
Malnutrition: Common

## ANESTHETIC CONSIDERATIONS

See "Anesthetic Considerations for Biliary Tract Surgery" at the end of this section.

**References**


1. Hines LH, Burns RP: 10 years' experience treating pancreatic and periampullary cancer. *Am Surg* 1976; 42(6):441-47.
2. Hess KW: *Surgery of the Biliary Passages and the Pancreas*. D VanNostrand Co, Princeton: 1965.
3. Baker AR, Neoptolemos JP, Carr-Locke DL, Fossard DP: Sump syndrome following choledochoduodenostomy and its endoscopic treatment. *Br J Surg* 1985; 72(6):433.
4. Birkenfeld S, Serour F, Levi S, Abulafia A, Balassiano M, Krispin M: Choledochoduodenostomy for benign and malignant biliary tract diseases. *Surgery* 1988; 103(4):408-10.
5. Sarr MG, Cameron JL: Surgical palliation of unresectable carcinoma of the pancreas. *World J Surg* 1984; 8(6):906-18.
6. Cahill CJ: Prevention of postoperative renal failure in patients with obstructive jaundice – the role of bile salts. *Br J Surg* 1983; 70(10):590.
7. Thomas CG Jr, Nicholson CP, Owen J: Effectiveness of choledochoduodenostomy and transduodenal sphincterotomy in the treatment of benign obstruction of the common duct. *Ann Surg* 1971; 173(6):845-56.
8. Ellis H: Choledocholithiasis. In *Maingot's Abdominal Operations*, 9th edition. Schwartz SI, Ellis H, eds. Appleton & Lange, Norwalk, CT: 1989, 1431-50.


# EXCISION OF BILE DUCT TUMOR

## SURGICAL CONSIDERATIONS

**Description:** Primary tumors of the extrahepatic bile ducts, including the hepatic bifurcation (Klatskin tumors) are uncommon malignancies, with the only curative treatment for them being surgical excision. Such tumors are usually classified as being proximal bile duct tumors, involving the hepatic bifurcation and above; middle bile duct tumors, involving the midportion of the common hepatic and common bile duct; and distal bile duct tumors which involve the distal bile duct, including the intrapancreatic or intraduodenal portion of the bile duct (Fig 7.6-1). The gallbladder will usually be removed in any such operation.

Distal bile duct tumors, which carry a significantly higher cure rate than either proximal bile duct or pancreatic tumors, may be treated by **pancreaticoduodenectomy**. (See "Pancreaticoduodenectomy" for discussion of this operation.)

Mid bile duct tumors are usually excised by removing a generous portion of the mid bile duct, resecting the ducts up to the hepatic bifurcation and sometimes performing a pancreaticoduodenectomy. Biliary drainage is usually established by anastomosing the proximal bile duct to a Roux loop of jejunum. For proximal bile duct tumors, most of the extrahepatic bile ducts are excised and biliary drainage is established by anastomosis of the right and left hepatic ducts to a Roux loop of jejunum. These are often technically demanding operations with the potential for major blood loss. It may be necessary to perform a major hepatic resection at the same time, and the possibility of this should always be assumed when an operation of this sort is carried out.

Surgical exposure for any of these operations is usually achieved through a long midline or transverse subcostal incision and the use of self-retaining retractors. Often, a transhepatic catheter will have been placed radiographically preop to provide relief of jaundice and to facilitate identification of the bile ducts. The liver and gallbladder are retracted superiorly while downward traction is placed on the duodenum. If the gallbladder is still in place, a cholecystectomy is performed (see "Cholecystectomy," above). For proximal bile duct tumors and mid-bile duct tumors not requiring pancreaticoduodenectomy, the bile duct is divided distally, just above the duodenum and the pancreatic portion of the bile duct is oversewn. The bile duct is then resected proximally to the level of the bifurcation of the hepatic ducts. A Roux-en-Y loop of jejunum is anastomosed to the hepatic ducts to establish biliary drainage. Drains are placed and most surgeons place a nasogastric tube for such cases.

**Variant procedure or approaches**: Endoscopic or transhepatic stenting of areas of stricture is often used as a palliative alternative to surgical excision. These are usually performed radiographically and do not require general anesthesia. They may be used as an alternative to resection or in preparation for surgery.

**Usual preop diagnosis**: Cholangiocarcinoma (common); benign strictures of the bile ducts (infrequent); sclerosing cholangitis (rare)

### SUMMARY OF PROCEDURE

| | |
|---|---|
| **Position** | Supine |
| **Incision** | Midline or subcostal |
| **Special instrumentation** | Costal retractor |
| **Unique considerations** | Many cases prove unresectable at operation. Intraop radiation therapy may be used. |
| **Antibiotics** | Ampicillin, piperacillin or mezlocillin, 1-3 gm iv, ± gentamicin; or cefotetan 1-2 gm iv |
| **Surgical time** | 3 - 8 hrs |
| **Closing considerations** | Muscle relaxation required for closure; NG suction |
| **EBL** | 500-5000 cc, depending on need for liver resection and presence of portal HTN. |
| **Postop care** | ICU postop |
| **Mortality**[1,2] | 5-10% |
| **Morbidity**[1,2] | Sepsis<br>Hemorrhage<br>Anastomotic leakage<br>Wound infection<br>Liver failure<br>PE |
| **Procedure code** | 47710 |
| **Pain score** | 7-8 |

### PATIENT POPULATION CHARACTERISTICS

| | |
|---|---|
| **Age range** | 50s-70s |
| **Male:Female** | Male >female |
| **Incidence** | 4500 cases of bile duct cancer/yr in U.S. |
| **Etiology** | Multifactorial |
| **Associated conditions** | Ulcerative colitis<br>Sclerosing cholangitis<br>Typhoid carrier state<br>Clonorchis sinensis<br>Choledochal cyst<br>Caroli's disease<br>Gallstones |

## ANESTHETIC CONSIDERATIONS

See "Anesthetic Considerations for Biliary Tract Surgery" at the end of this section.

**References**


1. Blumgart LH, Michel M: Tumours of the gallbladder and bile ducts. In *Maingot's Abdominal Operations*, 9th edition. Schwartz SI, Ellis H, eds. Appleton & Lange, Norwalk, CT: 1989, 1533-54.
2. Zinner MJ: Bile duct tumors. In *Current Surgical Therapy*, Vol III. Cameron JL, ed. BC Decker, Philadelphia: 1989, 289-91.

# CHOLEDOCHAL CYST EXCISION OR ANASTOMOSIS

## SURGICAL CONSIDERATIONS

**Description:** This rare congenital anomaly includes various types of dilatation of the biliary tree, and patients may present with cholangitis, pancreatitis or, rarely, malignancy. Although four types of cyst are commonly recognized, the vast majority consist of fusiform dilatation of much or most of the extrahepatic biliary tree. While the traditional description of choledochal cyst is that of an infant with a palpable abdominal mass and jaundice or cholangitis, this is a relatively rare presentation today. Today, many cysts are found in adults undergoing evaluation for symptoms thought to be due to gallbladder disease. These patients may present with biliary colic, pancreatitis or cholangitis. Recommended treatment consists of **excision of the cyst**, when technically safe. **Cyst-enteric bypass**, usually to a Roux loop of jejunum, is almost never performed today because of the known small, but real risk of developing malignancy in these cysts. Only in an elderly patient under unusual technical circumstances would this be appropriate.

The operation is performed through a midline or right subcostal incision. The liver is retracted superiorly and the duodenum inferiorly, exposing the biliary tree. The gallbladder is excised, along with as much of the cyst as possible. The duct is divided as distally as possible, just above the duodenum, and the cyst reflected superiorly. It is usually excised to the hepatic bifurcation, and an anastomosis is performed at this level, often between the common orifice of the right and left hepatic ducts and a Roux loop of jejunum.

Re-operative cases are not uncommon; most follow a cyst-enteric bypass. These cases may be significantly more difficult than first-time operations.

**Variant procedure or approaches**: There is an increasing tendency among gastroenterologists to perform **endoscopic sphincterotomy** in these patients, rather than to refer them for surgical resection, particularly in older patients. It remains to be seen if these patients will develop cancer in the retained cysts.

**Usual preop diagnosis**: Choledochal cyst, the most common type involving fusiform enlargement of the entire extrahepatic biliary tree

### SUMMARY OF PROCEDURE

| | |
|---|---|
| **Position** | Supine |
| **Incision** | Midline or right subcostal |
| **Special instrumentation** | Costal retractor |
| **Antibiotics** | Ampicillin, piperacillin or mezlocillin, 1-3 gm iv ± gentamicin; or cefotetan 1-2 gm iv |
| **Surgical time** | 2 - 4 hrs |
| **Closing considerations** | NG suction |
| **EBL** | 250 cc, with potentially greater blood loss in re-operations |
| **Postop care** | PACU |
| **Mortality** | Very rare |
| **Morbidity** | Anastomotic leak<br>Wound infection<br>Pulmonary complications<br>Pancreatitis |
| **Procedure code** | 47715 (excision); 47716 (bypass) |
| **Pain score** | 5-7 |

### PATIENT POPULATION CHARACTERISTICS

| | |
|---|---|
| **Age range** | Classically, 60% < 10 yrs of age, although this may be changing; also adults of all ages |
| **Male:Female** | 1:3 |
| **Incidence** | Rare in U.S.; more common in Japan |
| **Etiology** | Unclear |
| **Associated conditions** | Jaundice<br>Pancreatitis<br>Malignancy within the cyst |

# ANESTHETIC CONSIDERATIONS FOR BILIARY TRACT SURGERY

**(Procedures covered: open and laparoscopic cholecystectomy; excision of bile duct tumor; choledochal cyst excision/anastomosis; biliary drainage procedures; transduodenal sphincterotomy or sphincteroplasty)**

## PREOPERATIVE

Patients presenting for biliary tract surgery are an extremely diverse group, ranging from the otherwise healthy to the extremely ill. With the increasing popularity of laparoscopic surgery, most open cholecystectomies will be performed only on the sickest patients or when it is not possible to complete the laparoscopic procedure. These patients, therefore, generally will be sicker than those undergoing open cholecystectomy in the mid-1980s. Cirrhosis, even of a mild degree, substantially increases the risk of cholecystectomy, with hemorrhage being the greatest danger. Patients with bile duct tumors are usually jaundiced at presentation and have undergone transhepatic and/or endoscopic studies for diagnostic purposes. Often an external transhepatic biliary drain may be present and jaundice may have been relieved in this way. Rarely, a hepatic resection may be performed as part of the procedure. Prior operation or the presence of portal HTN will substantially increase the duration, complexity, and blood loss of the procedure.

**Respiratory** Pain 2° an acute abdominal process may cause splinting which, in turn, may impair respiratory function (↓FRC, hypoventilation, atelectasis). For patients undergoing laparoscopic cholecystectomy, intra-abdominal $CO_2$ insufflation may → atelectasis, ↓FRC, ↑PIP, and ↑$PaCO_2$. Studies comparing patients undergoing open vs laparoscopic cholecystectomy reveal that respiratory function is less impaired and function is recovered more quickly in patients undergoing laparoscopic cholecystectomy. Tachypnea, hyperpnea and acute respiratory alkalosis can be signs of sepsis, or due solely to pain associated with inflammation of the gall bladder.

**Cardiovascular** Patients may be dehydrated from fever, vomiting and decreased oral intake; assess hemodynamic status by evaluating BP and HR in the supine and standing positions. Fluid resuscitate if patient shows Sx of orthostatic hypotension (use 250-500 ml NS iv) until hemodynamic status improves. Patients undergoing laparoscopic cholecystectomy are prone to hemodynamic compromise 2° positioning (reverse Trendelenburg), increased intra-abdominal pressure with subsequent impairment of venous return, and unappreciated hemorrhage which is often more difficult to detect laparoscopically. Epigastric discomfort is common with biliary tract disease and can mimic symptoms of myocardial ischemia.

**Tests:** ECG and CPK isoenzymes as necessary to R/O MI; others as indicated from H&P.

**Renal** In patients with obstructive jaundice, preop administration of bile salts po may prevent renal insufficiency following surgery.[7]

**Gastrointestinal** Patients with peritonitis will exhibit guarding and may develop abdominal distention and paralytic ileus. Therefore, full-stomach precautions are warranted.

**Tests:** Bilirubin; AST (SGOT); ALT (SGPT); alkaline phosphatase; albumin

**Hematologic** Leukocytosis is often present with a moderate left shift. ✓ coags. Administer vitamin K as needed.

**Tests:** CBC, with differential and platelets; PT/PTT.

**Laboratory** Routine UA; electrolytes; glucose; creatinine; others as indicated from H&P.

**Premedication** Meperidine (1-1.5 mg/kg im) is thought to cause less sphincter of Oddi spasm than other opiates. Sphincter spasm can interfere with intraop cholangiograms and cause pain; treatment is with naloxone in 40 $\mu$g increments. Atropine (0.4-0.6 mg im or iv) or glycopyrrolate (0.2-0.3 mg im or iv) may help decrease spasm of the sphincter, and can be given in combination with the opiate. Parenteral vitamin K is indicated if PT is prolonged (10 mg/d im for 3 d). Administer $H_2$ antagonists (ranitidine 50 mg iv); metoclopramide (10 mg iv) may be given should the patient be at risk for gastric aspiration.

## INTRAOPERATIVE

**Anesthetic technique:** GETA. In patients at risk for aspiration of gastric contents, ET intubation should be accomplished either awake or following a rapid-sequence iv induction. In patients undergoing laparoscopic procedures, $CO_2$ insufflation will cause an increase in intra-abdominal pressure which will predispose to passive regurgitation of gastric contents. Hence, ET intubation is indicated. Controlled ventilation will minimize the possibility of hypercarbia from absorbed $CO_2$.

| | | |
|---|---|---|
| **Induction** | Standard induction (see Appendix) if no aspiration risk. In patients at risk of aspiration, a rapid-sequence induction should be performed (see Appendix). | |
| **Maintenance** | Standard maintenance (see Appendix). Muscle relaxants facilitate surgery and are indicated. | |
| **Emergence** | If there is a risk for aspiration of gastric contents, patient should be extubated awake after return of protective airway reflexes; otherwise, no special considerations. | |
| **Blood and fluid requirements** | Minimal blood loss<br>Possible high fluid loss<br>IV: 16-18 ga x 1<br>NS/LR @ 5-8 cc/kg/hr | Blood products usually not required. Anticipate that patient may be dehydrated and require generous iv hydration prior to anesthetic induction (e.g., 10-15 cc/kg). |
| **Monitoring** | Standard monitors (see Appendix). | Others as clinically indicated. |
| **Positioning** | √ and pad pressure points.<br>√ eyes. | A steep, reverse Trendelenburg position may be required, causing cardiorespiratory impairment. |
| **Complications** | $CO_2$ embolization<br>Subcutaneous emphysema<br>Perforation of viscus | These complications are unique to laparoscopic procedures. |

## POSTOPERATIVE

| | | |
|---|---|---|
| **Complications** | Ventilatory impairment<br>Pneumothorax<br>Atelectasis 2° surgical retraction and splinting | Monitor patients for hypoxemia in the postop period. Administer supplemental $O_2$ and consider a portable CXR to aid in the diagnosis. |
| **Pain management** | PCA: meperidine. Loading dose, 20-100 mg; incremental dose, 10 mg; lockout, 10 min. | Intercostal nerve blocks, intrapleural analgesia, or epidural analgesia are also useful techniques. Prolonged PCA meperidine is associated with ↑normeperidine → CNS disorder. |

### References


1. Crittenden SL, McKinley MJ: Choledochal cyst – clinical features and classification. *Am J Gastroenterol* 1985; 80(8):643-47.
2. Saing H, Tam PK, Le JMH, Pe-Nyun: Surgical management of choledochal cysts: a review of 60 cases. *J Pediatr Surg* 1985; 20(4):443-48.
3. Venu RP, Geenen JE, Hogan WJ, Dodds WJ, Wilson SW, Stewart ET, Soergel KH: Role of endoscopic retrograde cholangiopancreatography in the diagnosis and treatment of choledochocele. *Gastroenterology* 1984; 87(5):1144-49.
4. Nagorney DM, McIlrath DC, Adson MA: Choledochal cysts in adults: clinical management. *Surgery* 1984; 96(4):656-63.
5. Yamaguchi M: Congenital choledochal cyst: analysis of 1,433 patients in the Japanese literature. *Am J Surg* 1980; 140(5):653-57.
6. Reiestad F, Stromskag KE: Interpleural catheter in the management of postoperative pain. A preliminary report. *Reg Anes* 1986; 11:89-91.
7. Cahill CJ: Prevention of postoperative renal failure in patients with obstructive jaundice – the role of bile salts. *Br J Surg* 1983; 70(10):590.
8. Marco AP, Yeo CJ, Rock P: Anesthesia for a patient undergoing laparascopic cholecystectomy. *Anesthesiology* 1990; 73:1268-70.
9. Taylor E, Feinstein R, White PF, Soper N: Anesthesia for laparoscopic cholecystectomy. Is nitrous oxide indicated? *Anesthesiology* 1992; 76:541-43.

**Surgeon**

**Harry A. Oberhelman, MD, FACS**

# 7.7 PANCREATIC SURGERY

**Anesthesiologist**

**Steven K. Howard, MD**

# OPERATIVE DRAINAGE FOR PANCREATITIS

## SURGICAL CONSIDERATIONS

**Description**: Operative drainage for pancreatitis is usually indicated when a peripancreatic collection of fluid becomes infected. Pancreatic abscesses often develop in the lesser sac or, less often, adjacent to and along the pancreas. The infection may subsequently spread to the subphrenic spaces or into the pericolic gutters. Fistulization into adjacent organs, particularly the transverse colon, is common. Severe intra-abdominal hemorrhage from erosion into major arteries lying adjacent to the pancreas may also occur.[1] Exploration of the peritoneal cavity is performed before opening the lesser sac. Fluid or abscess collection lateral to the left and right sides of the colon should be palpated, as should the base of the transverse mesocolon and its subhepatic areas. The gastrocolic ligament is incised to approach the pancreas. There are different operative approaches, depending on location of involvement and surgeon's preference. Upper midline or transverse abdominal incisions are used most often. Posterior drainage through the bed of the 12th rib or retroperitoneal lateral approaches may be used (Fig 7.7-1).

**Usual preop diagnosis**: Pancreatitis 2° to biliary tract disease, alcoholism, idiopathic

### SUMMARY OF PROCEDURE

| | |
|---|---|
| **Position** | Supine |
| **Incision** | Midline, transverse, synchronous anterior and posterior |
| **Unique considerations** | Must perform adequate debridement of necrotic tissue and provide adequate drainage of abdomen; NG tube |
| **Antibiotics** | Cefotetan 1-2 gm 30 min preop |
| **Surgical time** | 1 - 2 hrs |
| **Closing considerations** | Adequate drainage of pancreatic bed and fluid resuscitation of patient |
| **EBL** | 300-750 ml |
| **Postop care** | Routine wound and drain care; PACU → room (occasionally ICU) |
| **Mortality** | 8-30% |
| **Morbidity** | Fistulae formation: 18-55%<br>Delayed gastric emptying: 50%<br>Unremitting sepsis: 10-30%<br>Atelectasis: 5-10%<br>Respiratory deterioration: 5%<br>Hemorrhage<br>Bowel perforations |
| **Procedure code** | 48000 |
| **Pain score** | 7-9 |

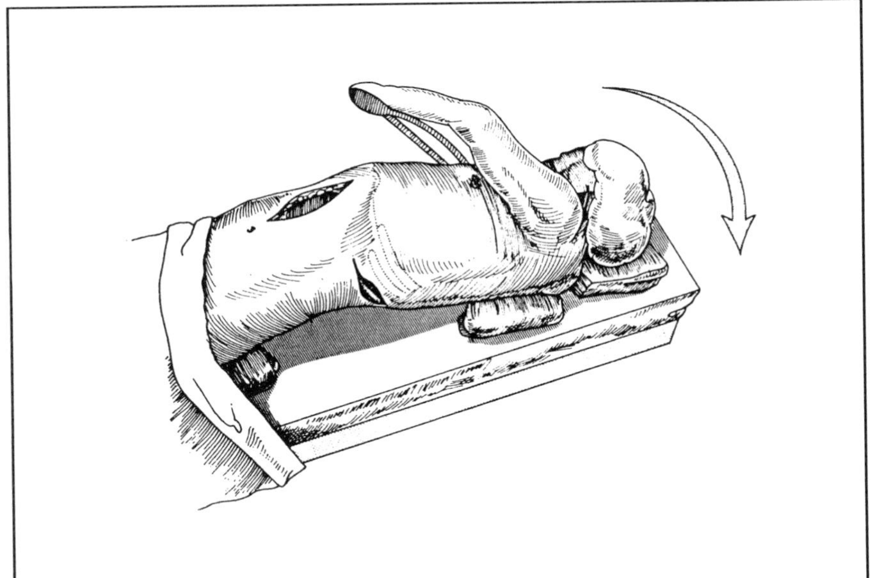

**Figure 7.7-1.** Incision for anterior and posterior drainage in pancreatitis. Note that bed or table is rotated until patient is almost supine. (Re-produced with permission from Berne TV, Donovan AJ: Synchronous anterior and posterior drainage of pancreatic abscess. *Arch Surg* 1981; 116: 527-33. Copyright 1981, American Medical Association.)

### PATIENT POPULATION CHARACTERISTICS

| | |
|---|---|
| **Age range** | 30-60 yrs |
| **Male:Female** | 1:1 |
| **Incidence** | 10-40% of patients with pancreatitis |
| **Etiology** | Alcoholism: 30-50%<br>Postop pancreatitis: 15-40%<br>Biliary tract disease: 20-30%<br>Idiopathic pancreatitis: 15-20% |
| **Associated conditions** | See Etiology, above. |

## ANESTHETIC CONSIDERATIONS

See "Anesthetic Considerations for Pancreatic Surgery" following "Whipple Resection," at the end of "Pancreatic Surgery" section.


**References**

1. Berne TV: Pancreatic abscesses. *Prob Gen Surg* 1984; 1:569-82.


# DRAINAGE OF PANCREATIC PSEUDOCYST

## SURGICAL CONSIDERATIONS

**Description**: Internal drainage of a pancreatic pseudocyst may be accomplished by anastomosing the cyst to the stomach, duodenum or other small bowel via a Roux-en-Y loop of jejunum. The procedure of choice for internal decompression depends on the location of the pseudocyst in relation to the portion of the GI tract that will provide maximal dependent drainage of the cyst. Operation is best delayed for a period of 4-6 weeks to permit maturation of the cyst wall.[1] If operation is indicated, the abdomen is entered via a midline incision. If the pseudocyst lies behind the stomach (or duodenum), it is approached anteriorly, through the posterior wall of the stomach (or duodenum). A circular portion of the posterior wall is excised, allowing entry into the cyst cavity, which is then drained. An anastomosis is created between the cyst and stomach (or duodenum) by using interrupted sutures. The anterior wall of the stomach (or duodenum) is then closed. If the cyst presents inferior to the stomach, it is anastomosed in a similar fashion to a Roux-en-Y loop of jejunum. Drains are placed appropriately. External drainage may suffice, if it is not possible to provide internal drainage. Spontaneous resolution of pancreatic pseudocyst may be expected in 20% or more of patients.[2] If infection of the pseudocyst occurs with clinical signs of sepsis, **external drainage** percutaneously under CT guidance, or operative **internal drainage** is indicated.

**Usual preop diagnosis**: Pseudocyst of pancreas 2° to acute pancreatitis

### SUMMARY OF PROCEDURE

| | Internal Drainage | External Drainage |
|---|---|---|
| **Position** | Supine | ⇐ |
| **Incision** | Midline abdominal | ⇐ |
| **Unique considerations** | Location of pseudocyst in relation to GI tract; NG tube | Accessibility for percutaneous decompression; NG tube |
| **Antibiotics** | Cefotetan 1-2 gm 30 min preop | ⇐ |
| **Surgical time** | 1 - 2 hrs | |

| | Internal Drainage | External Drainage |
|---|---|---|
| **Closing considerations** | Adequate drainage | 1 hr<br>⇐ |
| **EBL** | 100-300 mi | |
| **Postop care** | NG decompression | ⇐ |
| **Mortality**[3] | 10-12% | ⇐ |
| **Morbidity**[3] | Bleeding: 5-7% | 3-4% |
| | Recurrence: 2-3% | < 2% |
| | Sepsis: < 5% | 2-5% |
| **Procedure code** | 48520 | ⇐ |
| **Pain score** | 6-8 | 48510 |
| | | 5-7 |

### PATIENT POPULATION CHARACTERISTICS

| | |
|---|---|
| **Age range** | 15-80 yrs |
| **Male:Female** | 1:1 |
| **Incidence** | Rare |
| **Etiology** | Acute pancreatitis<br>Trauma<br>Malignancy |
| **Associated conditions** | Acute pancreatitis: 90% |

## ANESTHETIC CONSIDERATIONS

See "Anesthetic Considerations for Pancreatic Surgery" following "Whipple Resection," at the end of "Pancreatic Surgery" section.

**References**


1. Warshaw AL, Rattner DW: Timing of surgical drainage for pancreatic pseudocyst: clinical and chemical criteria. *Ann Surg* 1985; 202(6):720-24.
2. Bradley EL, Clements JL Jr, Gonzalez AC: The natural history of pancreatic pseudocysts: a unified concept of management. *Am J Surg* 1979; 137(1):135-41.
3. Grace RR, Jordan PH Jr: Unresolved problems of pancreatic pseudocysts. *Ann Surg* 1976; 184(1):16-21.


# PANCREATICO-JEJUNOSTOMY

## SURGICAL CONSIDERATIONS

**Description**: Pancreatico-jejunostomy, as advocated by **Puestow**,[1] consists of a longitudinal opening of the pancreatic duct, from the site of transection of the tail of the pancreas to a point just to the right of the mesenteric vessels. The widely opened duct is then anastomosed to a Roux-en-Y loop of jejunum (Fig 7.7-2B). This is necessary because of the multiple strictures and dilatations that occur along the duct system. Resection of the pancreatic tail and spleen are optional. Through a midline or transverse abdominal incision, the pancreas is exposed by mobilizing the duodenum (**Kocher maneuver**), exposing the head of the pancreas, and opening the lesser sac to visualize the body and tail. The pancreas is mobilized by dissecting it away from portal vein, celiac plexus and splenic vessels. Hemorrhage may complicate this stage of the surgery. The pancreatic duct may be aspirated to identify its location. A Roux-en-Y loop of jejunum is then brought up to the pancreas and anastomosed to the opened duct or pancreatic capsule. A drain is left along the anastomosis. The wound is closed in the usual fashion.

**Variant procedure or approaches**: If the obstruction of the pancreatic duct is limited to the head of the pancreas, one may merely perform a retrograde drainage; that is, anastomosing the distal transected pancreas to a Roux-en-Y loop of the jejunum (**Duval procedure** [Fig 7.7-2B]).[2]

**Usual preop diagnosis**: Chronic pancreatitis

### SUMMARY OF PROCEDURE

| | Longitudinal Pancreatico-jejunostomy (Puestow) | Caudal Pancreatico-jejunostomy (Duval) |
|---|---|---|
| **Position** | Supine | ⇐ |
| **Incision** | Midline abdominal or transverse | ⇐ |
| **Antibiotics** | Cefotetan 1-2 gm 30 min preop | ⇐ |
| **Surgical time** | 2 - 3 hrs | 1 - 2 hrs |
| **Closing considerations** | NG tube; adequate drainage | ⇐ |
| **EBL** | 300-400 ml | 100-200 ml |
| **Postop care** | NG decompression | ⇐ |
| **Mortality** | 1-4% | 2-3% |
| **Morbidity** | Failure to relieve pain: 25-50% | 25-60% |
| | Pancreatic leak: 5-10% | 5% |
| | Wound infection: 5% | ⇐ |
| **Procedure code** | 48180 | 48145 |
| **Pain score** | 6-8 | 6-8 |

### PATIENT POPULATION CHARACTERISTICS[3]

| | |
|---|---|
| **Age range** | 17-72 yrs |
| **Male:Female** | 2.5:1 |
| **Etiology** | Alcoholism<br>Biliary tract disease<br>Idiopathic<br>Trauma<br>Familial |
| **Associated conditions** | Biliary tract disease: 25-50%<br>Hyperparathyroidism: < 5% |

## ANESTHETIC CONSIDERATIONS

See "Anesthetic Considerations for Pancreatic Surgery" following "Whipple Resection," at the end of "Pancreatic Surgery" section.

**References**

1. Puestow CB, Gillesby WJ: Retrograde surgical drainage of the pancreas for chronic relapsing pancreatitis. *Arch Surgery* 1958; 76:898-907.
2. DuVal MK Jr: Caudal pancreatico-jejunostomy for chronic relapsing pancreatitis. *Ann Surg* 1954; 140(6):775-85.
3. Morrow CE, Cohen JI, Sutherland DE, Najarian JS: Chronic pancreatitis: long-term surgical results of pancreatic duct drainage, pancreatic resection, and near total pancreatectomy and islet autotransplantation. *Surgery* 1984; 96(4):608-16.

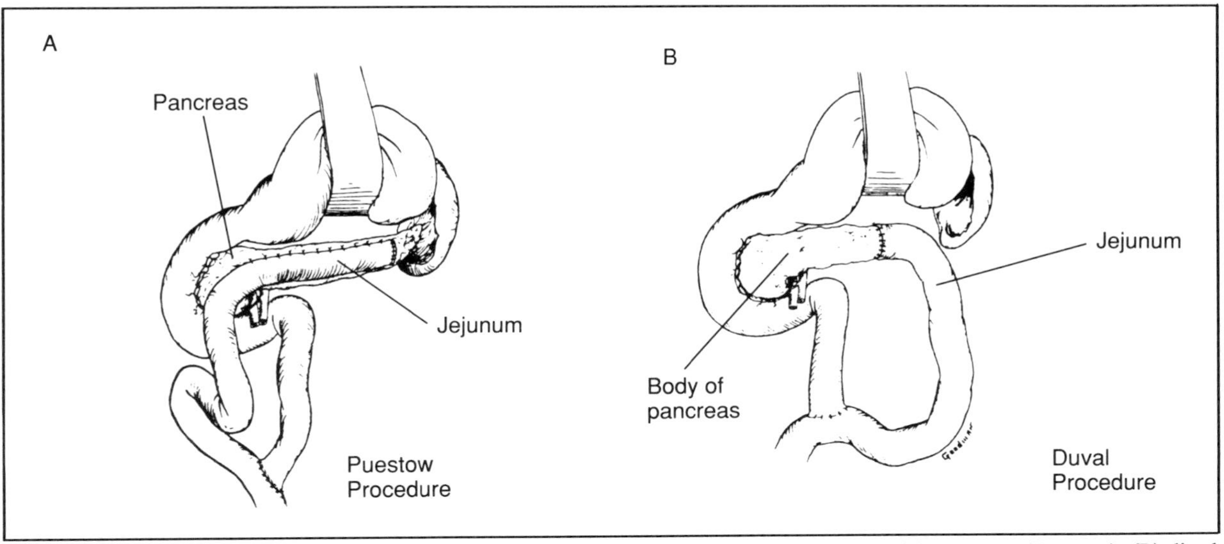


**Figure 7.7-2.** Operative management of chronic pancreatitis: (A) onlay Roux-en-Y pancreatico-jejunostomy (Puestow); (B) distal Roux-en-Y pancreatico-jejunostomy (Duval). (Reproduced with permission from Hardy JD: *Hardy's Textbook of Surgery*. JB Lippincott: 1988.)

# PANCREATECTOMY

## SURGICAL CONSIDERATIONS

**Description**: **Distal pancreatectomy** is performed for tumors in the distal half of the pancreas. The peritoneum is incised along the inferior surface of the pancreas, with care being taken to avoid tearing the middle colic vessels. Following mobilization of the spleen, the splenic artery is ligated near its origin. The gastrosplenic ligament is divided, ligating the short gastric vessels and the left gastroepiploic vessel. The inferior mesenteric vein is ligated at the inferior border of the pancreas, and the splenic vein is ligated at the proposed point of transection. The transected pancreas (Fig 7.7-3) is usually stapled and drained, although some surgeons suture the cut end and ligate the duct. The spleen may be preserved when operating for benign disease, provided the splenic vessels are ligated proximal to the splenic hilum in order to preserve collateral blood flow.

**Variant procedure or approaches**: **Subtotal pancreatectomy** usually implies resecting the pancreas from the mesenteric vessels distally, leaving the head and uncinate process intact. This procedure may be performed for tumor or chronic pancreatitis. **Child's procedure** consists of removing all of the pancreas except a rim of tissue along the lesser curvature of the duodenum; preserving the duodenum makes it unnecessary to reconstruct the bile duct. This procedure is usually reserved for patients with chronic pancreatitis.

**Usual preop diagnosis**: Carcinoma of pancreas; islet cell tumors; chronic pancreatitis

### SUMMARY OF PROCEDURE

| | Distal Pancreatectomy | Subtotal Pancreatectomy | Child's Procedure |
|---|---|---|---|
| **Position** | Supine | ⇐ | ⇐ |
| **Incision** | Midline abdominal or chevron | ⇐ | ⇐ |

| | Distal Pancreatectomy | Subtotal Pancreatectomy | Child's Procedure |
|---|---|---|---|
| **Special instrumentation** | Denier retractor | ⇐ | ⇐ |
| **Unique considerations** | NG tube | ⇐ | Preservation of vasculature of duodenum |
| **Antibiotics** | Cefotetan 1-2 gm 30 min preop | ⇐ | ⇐ |
| **Surgical time** | 2 - 3 hrs | ⇐ | 3 - 4 hrs |
| **Closing considerations** | Adequate drainage | ⇐ | ⇐ |
| **EBL** | 300-500 ml | 500-750 ml | 500-1000 ml |
| **Postop care** | NG decompression; PACU | ⇐ | ⇐ |
| **Mortality** | < 5% | ⇐ | ⇐ |
| **Morbidity** | Diabetes: 5% | ⇐ | ⇐ |
| | Wound infection: 5% | ⇐ | ⇐ |
| | Pancreatic fistula: < 5% | ⇐ | 90% |
| | Common bile duct injury | ⇐ | ⇐ |
| | Hemorrhage | ⇐ | ⇐ |
| | Duodenal necrosis | ⇐ | ⇐ |
| | Pancreatic leakage | ⇐ | ⇐ |
| | Pancreatic insufficiency | ⇐ | ⇐ |
| **Procedure code** | 48140 | 48145 | 48151 |
| **Pain score** | 6-8 | 6-8 | 6-8 |

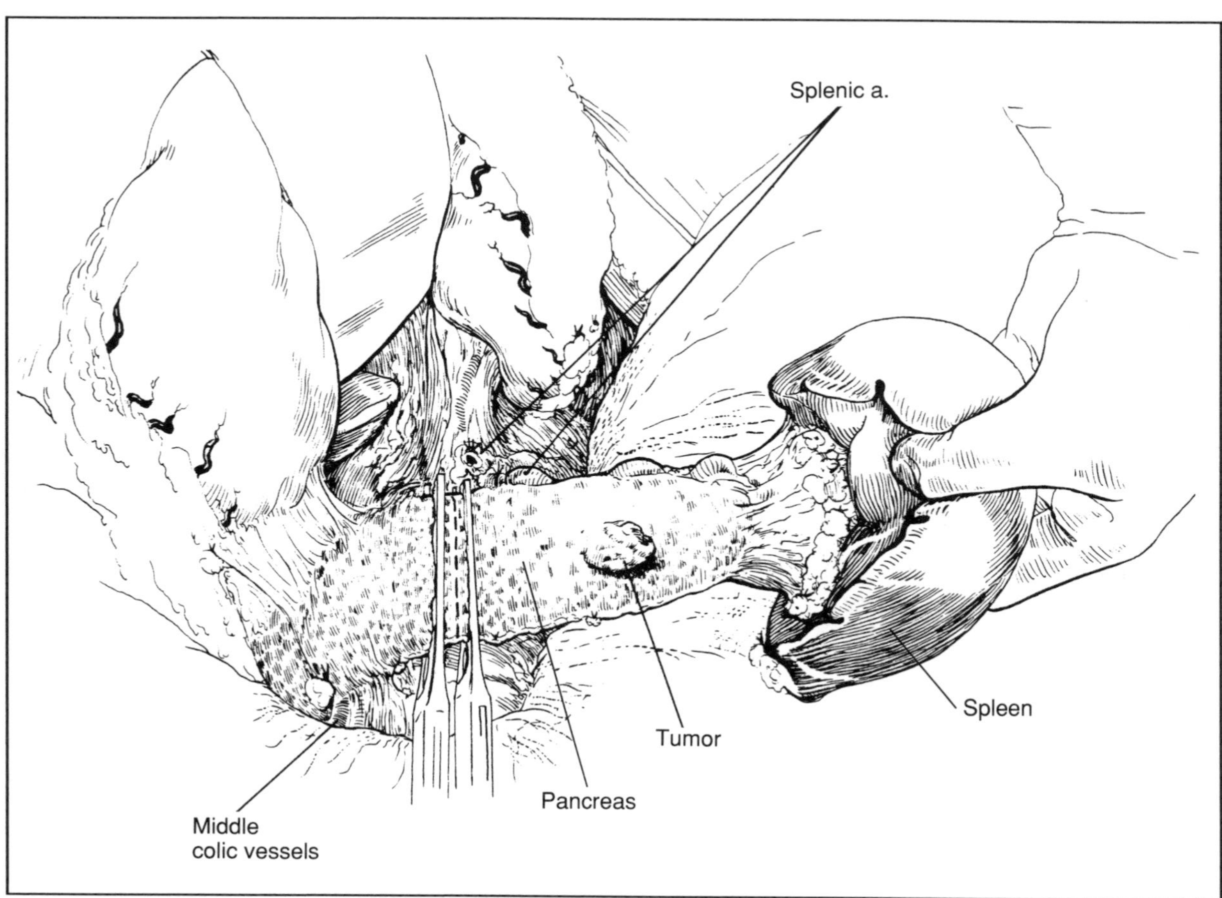


**Figure 7.7-3.** Resection of pancreatic tumor. (Reproduced with permission from Zollinger RM Jr, Zollinger RM: *Atlas of Surgical Operations*, 6th edition. Macmillan: 1988.)

## PATIENT POPULATION CHARACTERISTICS

| | |
|---|---|
| **Age range** | 30-60 yrs |
| **Male:Female** | 1:1 |
| **Incidence** | ~ 26,000/yr in U.S. |
| **Etiology** | Adenocarcinoma<br>Chronic pancreatitis<br>Islet cell tumors |
| **Associated conditions** | Alcoholism and biliary tract disease with chronic pancreatitis: 90%<br>Other endocrine disorders: 3-5% |

## ANESTHETIC CONSIDERATIONS

See "Anesthetic Considerations for Pancreatic Surgery" following "Whipple Resection," at the end of "Pancreatic Surgery" section.

References

1. Frey CF, Child CG, Fry W: Pancreatectomy for chronic pancreatitis. *Ann Surg* 1976; 184(4):403-13.

# WHIPPLE RESECTION

## SURGICAL CONSIDERATIONS

**Description:** A **Whipple resection** consists of a **pancreatoduodenectomy**, followed by an **anastomosis** of the distal pancreatic stump into the jejunum, a **choledochojejunostomy**, and a **gastrojejunostomy** (Fig 7.7-4). On entering the peritoneal cavity, one determines the resectability of the pancreatic lesion. Contraindications to resection include: involvement of the superior mesenteric vessels; infiltration by tumor into root of the mesentery; extension into the porta hepatis, with involvement of the hepatic artery; and liver metastases. If the tumor is deemed resectable, further mobilization of the head of the pancreas is performed. The common duct is transected above the cystic duct entry and the gall bladder is removed. Once the superior mesenteric vein is freed from the pancreas, the latter is transected, with care being taken not to injure the splenic vein. The stomach is transected at the antral-body junction or beyond the pylorus if uninvolved by tumor. The jejunum is transected beyond the ligament of Treitz and the

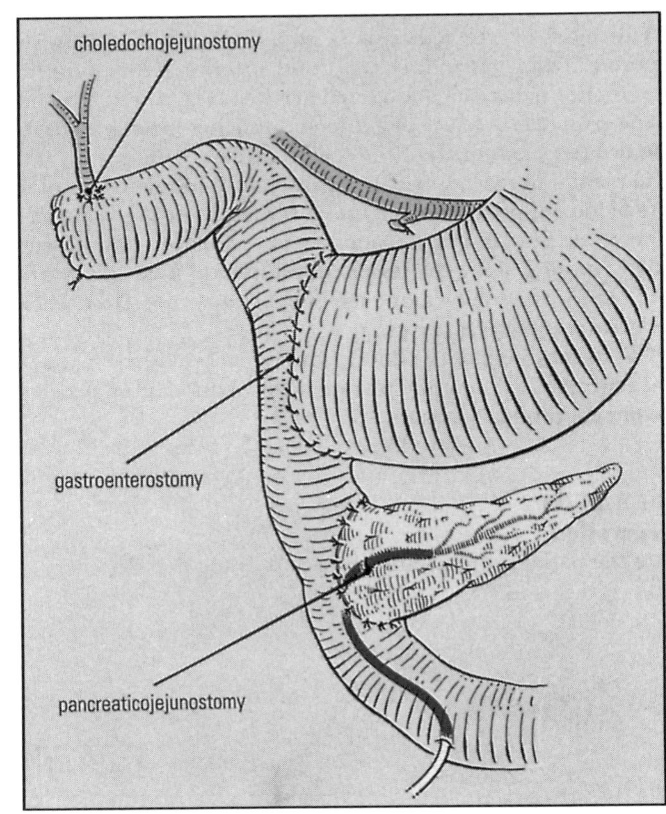


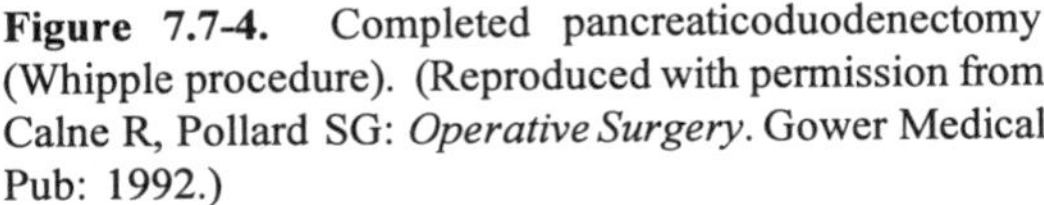
**Figure 7.7-4.** Completed pancreaticoduodenectomy (Whipple procedure). (Reproduced with permission from Calne R, Pollard SG: *Operative Surgery*. Gower Medical Pub: 1992.)

specimen removed by severing the vascular connections with the mesenteric vessels. Reconstitution is achieved by anastomosing the distal pancreatic stump, bile duct and stomach into the jejunum. Drains are placed adjacent to the pancreatic anastomosis. Some surgeons stent the latter until healing has occurred.

**Variant procedure or approaches:** There are several variants which consist of an extension of the Whipple procedure: **total pancreatectomy**; **regional pancreatectomy**, involving resection and reconstruction of the retropancreatic superior mesenteric vein and/or artery; and the pylorus-preserving **pancreatic resection**.

**Usual preop diagnosis:** Carcinoma of the pancreas; malignant cystadenomas; chronic pancreatitis

**SUMMARY OF PROCEDURE**

| | Whipple[1] | Total Pancreatectomy[2] | Regional Pancreatectomy[2] |
|---|---|---|---|
| **Position** | Supine | ⇐ | ⇐ |
| **Incision** | Midline abdominal or generous oblique | Midline abdominal or chevron | Midline abdominal or generous oblique |
| **Special instrumentation** | Denier retractor | ⇐ | ⇐ |
| **Unique considerations** | Stenting of pancreatic duct | None | Stenting of pancreatic duct |
| **Antibiotics** | Cefotetan 2 gm preop | ⇐ | ⇐ |
| **Surgical time** | 4 - 5 hrs | 4 - 6 hrs | 5 - 6 hrs |
| **Closing considerations** | Securing pancreatic stent, if used | None | Securing pancreatic stent, if used |
| **EBL** | 500-750 ml | 750-1000 ml | 750-1500 ml |
| **Postop care** | NG decompression; pancreatic decompression; PACU/ICU | NG decompression; diabetes management | ⇐ |
| **Mortality** | 8-12% | 12% | 15% |
| **Morbidity** | Delayed gastric emptying: 25% | ⇐ | < 2% |
| | Sepsis: 5-15% | 5% | 25% |
| | Hemorrhage: 5% | < 5% | 5% |
| | MI: 1-3% | ⇐ | < 5% |
| | Biliary fistula: < 2% | < 1% | < 2% |
| | Pancreatic fistula: 3-5% | NA | 3-5% |
| **Procedure code** | 48150 | 48155 | 48150 (Whipple procedure) + 37799 (resection of superior mesenteric vein) |
| **Pain score** | 7-9 | 7-9 | 7-9 |

**PATIENT POPULATION CHARACTERISTICS** (for cancer of pancreas[3])

| | |
|---|---|
| **Age range** | 50-80 yrs |
| **Male:Female** | 1:1 |
| **Incidence** | 10th most common cancer in U.S. – 28,000/yr |
| **Etiology** | Familial and genetic factors (probably most important)<br>Diabetes<br>Alcohol intake<br>Tobacco<br>Diet<br>Coffee<br>Pancreatitis |
| **Associated conditions** | See Etiology, above. |

# ANESTHETIC CONSIDERATIONS FOR PANCREATIC SURGERY

**(Procedures covered: drainage for pancreatitis; drainage of pancreatic pseudocyst; pancreatico-jejunostomy; pancreatectomy; Whipple resection)**

## PREOPERATIVE

Patients presenting for pancreatic surgery typically can be divided into three groups. (1) Those with acute pancreatitis who have failed medical treatment in the past. This group may be extremely ill, presenting for surgery during an exacerbation of pancreatitis or when the diagnosis is in doubt. (2) Patients with carcinoma of the pancreas, including hormone-secreting tumors such as insulinoma and gastrinoma (Zollinger-Ellison syndrome). (3) Patients suffering from the sequelae of chronic pancreatitis, e.g., pseudocyst or abscess.

**Respiratory** Respiratory compromise – such as pleural effusions, atelectasis and ARDS, progressing to respiratory failure – may occur in up to 50% of patients with acute pancreatitis. Postop mechanical ventilation may be needed for these patients.
**Tests:** CXR; ABG; PFT, as indicated from H&P.

**Cardiovascular** Patients with acute pancreatitis may be hypotensive and may require aggressive volume resuscitation with crystalloid and even blood prior to surgery. ECG change simulating myocardial ischemia may be seen in patients with acute pancreatitis. Severe electrolyte disturbances may be associated with acute pancreatitis and some hormone-secreting tumors of the pancreas. $\downarrow K^+$ may be severe and should be corrected preop (correction of $\downarrow Mg^{++}$ may improve $\downarrow K^+$.)
**Tests:** ECG; electrolytes; others as indicated from H&P.

**Gastrointestinal** Jaundice and abdominal pain are common presenting Sx in this group of patients. The presence of ileus or intestinal obstruction should mandate full-stomach precautions and rapid-sequence induction. Electrolyte disturbances are common with acute pancreatitis and may include hypochloremic metabolic alkalosis, $\downarrow Ca^{++}$, $\downarrow Mg^{++}$ and $\uparrow$glucose. These abnormalities should be corrected preop. Zollinger-Ellison syndrome is associated with diarrhea and severe peptic ulcer disease which may be complicated by perforation and bleeding. ViPomas are associated with massive watery diarrhea and electrolyte disturbances.
**Tests:** Electrolytes; glucose; LFTs; $CA^{++}$; amylase; others as indicated from H&P.

**Renal** Patients should be evaluated for renal insufficiency and anesthetic plan adjusted accordingly.
**Tests:** BUN; creatinine; UA; others as indicated from H&P.

**Endocrine** Many patients with acute pancreatitis may have diabetes 2° loss of pancreatic tissue. Hormone-secreting tumors of the pancreas are occasionally associated with multiple endocrine neoplasia syndromes (MEN-I, parathyroid, pancreas, pituitary and pheochromocytomas). Insulinoma is the most common hormone-secreting tumor of the pancreas and can result in hypoglycemia. Perioperative blood glucose measurements are essential.
**Tests:** Electrolytes; glucose; others as indicated from H&P (e.g., urinary VMA if pheochromocytoma suspected).

**Hematologic** Hct may be falsely elevated, due to hemoconcentration, or low, 2° hemorrhage. Coagulopathy may be present.
**Tests:** CBC with differential; platelets; PT; PTT; fibrinogen

**Laboratory** Other tests as indicated from H&P.

**Premedication** Standard premedication (see Appendix). Note: full-stomach precautions in patients with intestinal obstruction: ranitidine 50 mg iv, metoclopramide 10 mg iv 45 min preop, and 0.3 M Na citrate (30 cc po 15 min preop).

## INTRAOPERATIVE

**Anesthetic technique:** GETA ± epidural for postop analgesia. If postop epidural analgesia is planned, insertion of the catheter prior to anesthetic induction is helpful to establish correct placement in the epidural space (accomplished by injecting 5-7 cc of 1% lidocaine in order to elicit a segmental block).

**Induction** The patient with bowel obstruction or ileus is at risk for pulmonary aspiration, and rapid-sequence induction with cricoid pressure is indicated. If the patient is clinically hypovolemic, restore intravascular volume (colloid, crystalloid or blood) prior to induction and titrate induction dose of sedative/hypnotic agents. Etomidate (0.2-0.4 mg/kg iv) or ketamine (1-3 mg/kg iv) may provide less hemodynamic depression on induction of anesthesia.

| | | |
|---|---|---|
| **Maintenance** | Standard maintenance (see Appendix). Avoid $N_2O$ to minimize bowel distension. **Combined epidural/GA:** Local anesthetic (1.5-2% lidocaine with 1:200,000 epinephrine (12-15 ml q 60 min) can be injected incrementally into the epidural catheter to provide both anesthesia and optimal surgical exposure (contracted bowel and profound muscle relaxation). Be prepared to treat hypotension with fluid and vasopressors (e.g., ephedrine 5-10 mg iv). GA is administered to supplement regional anesthesia and for amnesia. Systemic sedatives (droperidol, opiates, benzodiazepines, etc.) should be minimized during this type of anesthetic as they increase the likelihood of postop respiratory depression. If epidural opiates are used for postop analgesia, a loading dose (e.g., hydromorphone 1.0 mg) should be administered 1-2 hrs before conclusion of surgery. | |
| **Emergence** | The decision to extubate at the end of surgery depends on the patient's underlying cardiopulmonary status and extent of the surgical procedure. Patients should be hemodynamically stable, warm, alert, cooperative, and fully reversed from any muscle relaxants prior to extubation. | |
| **Blood and fluid requirements** | Anticipate large fluid loss.<br>IV: 14-16 ga x 2<br>NS/LR @ 10-20 cc/kg/hr<br>Warm all fluids.<br>Humidify inhaled gasses. | Blood loss can be significant, and blood should be immediately available. Procedures tend to be long and extensive, leading to hypothermia and large 3rd-space fluid loss. If procedure does not involve cancer or infection, cell-saving devices can be utilized. Guide fluid management by UO, filling pressures, CO. |
| **Monitoring** | Standard monitors (see Appendix).<br>UO<br>Arterial line<br>± CVP or PA catheter | Most pancreatic surgery is associated with major fluid shifts and fluid loss. Invasive monitoring is usually required. In patients with cardiopulmonary compromise, a PA catheter may prove helpful for intraop fluid management. |
| **Positioning** | ✓ and pad pressure points.<br>✓ eyes. | |
| **Complications** | Hypokalemia<br>Hypovolemia | Release of pancreatic lipase → omental fat saponification → $\downarrow Ca^{++}$. Significant 3rd-space and evaporative losses contribute to hypovolemia. Major hemorrhage can occur during dissection of the pancreas from the mesenteric and portal vessels. |

### POSTOPERATIVE

| | | |
|---|---|---|
| **Complications** | Electrolyte imbalances<br>Hypovolemia<br>Hypothermia<br>Hypocalcemia<br>Hyperglycemia | Total pancreatectomy is associated with a brittle diabetes that can be very difficult to control. Subtotal resections lead to variable hyperglycemia. |
| **Pain management** | Continuous epidural analgesia (see Appendix).<br>PCA (see Appendix). | Patient should be recovered in an ICU or hospital ward that is accustomed to treating the side effects of epidural opiates (e.g., respiratory depression, breakthrough pain, nausea, pruritus). |
| **Tests** | CXR (if CVP placed); ABG; Hct. | Electrolytes; calcium; glucose; Hct; platelets – as indicated for postop management. |

**References**


1. Longmire WP Jr: Cancer of the pancreas: palliative operation, Whipple procedure, or total pancreatectomy. *World J Surg* 1984; 8(6):872-79.
2. Moossa AR, Scott MH, Lavelle-Jones M: The place of total and extended total pancreatectomy in pancreatic cancer. *World J Surg* 1984; 8(6):895-99.
3. Gordis L, Gold EB. Epidemiology of pancreatic cancer. *World J Surg* 1984; 8(6):808-21.
4. Merritt WT: Anesthesia for gastrointestinal surgery. In *Principles and Practice of Anesthesiology*. Rogers MC, Tinker JH, Covino BG, Longnecker DE, eds. Mosby-Year Book Inc, St Louis: 1993, 1967-89.

**Surgeon**

**Harry A. Oberhelman, MD, FACS**

# 7.8 PERITONEAL SURGERY

**Anesthesiologist**

**Steven K. Howard, MD**

# EXPLORATORY OR STAGING LAPAROTOMY

## SURGICAL CONSIDERATIONS

**Description: Exploratory laparotomy** is indicated primarily in patients suffering penetrating or severe abdominal blunt trauma. It is important that a thorough and systematic intra-abdominal examination be carried out to prevent missing significant injuries (e.g., ruptured duodenum, transected pancreas, etc). Any active bleeding should be controlled prior to a systematic examination. Other indications for laparotomy include certain patients with fever of undetermined origin or those in whom a specific diagnosis cannot be made, or for staging of selected patients with Hodgkin's disease. A **staging laparotomy** consists of **splenectomy**, **wedge** and **needle biopsies** of both lobes of the liver, and biopsies of the periaortic, celiac, mesenteric and porta-hepatic lymph nodes. In young women, suturing (pexing) the ovaries in the midline protects them from radiation. Indications for staging in Hodgkin's disease and lymphomas vary from institution to institution.

Basically, the procedure begins with a midline abdominal incision; then the abdomen is explored, and both needle and wedge biopsies of the liver are performed. The spleen is removed by incising the lateral peritoneal attachment and delivering the spleen into the naval. The short gastric vessels are cut and ligated and the splenic vessels exposed. These are cut individually and ligated, and the spleen is removed. Para-aortic nodes are exposed through a left para-aortic incision in the retroperitoneum, and removed for biopsy. Lymph channels are clipped to prevent lymphatic leakage. The nodes dissected extend to the inferior margin of the duodenum. It may be necessary to cross the aorta and biopsy the enlarged nodes on the right side.

**Usual preop diagnosis:** Abdominal trauma; Hodgkin's disease or other lymphomas

### SUMMARY OF PROCEDURE

| | Staging | Exploratory |
|---|---|---|
| **Position** | Supine | ⇐ |
| **Incision** | Midline abdominal | ⇐ + Transverse |
| **Special instrumentation** | Abdominal retractor | ⇐ |
| **Unique considerations** | Ovarian pexy | Careful monitoring of BP in trauma patients |
| **Antibiotics** | Cefotetan 1-2 gm preop | Cefotetan 1-2 gm iv in trauma patients |
| **Surgical time** | 1.5 - 2 hrs | Variable – 1 - 2 hrs |
| **Closing considerations** | Splenic bed hemostasis | Hemostasis |
| **EBL** | 100-200 ml | Variable – 200-500 ml |
| **Postop care** | NG decompression; PACU → room | ICU for trauma patients |
| **Mortality** | < 1% | 2-5% |
| **Morbidity** | Prolonged ileus: 10-15%<br>Pulmonary complications: 5-10%<br>Wound infection: 2-3%<br>Small bowel obstruction: 1%<br>Intraperitoneal bleeding: < 1% | ⇐ + In trauma patients:<br>Atelectasis: 5-10%<br>Wound infection: 5-10%<br>Hemorrhage: 1-3%<br>Pneumonia: < 1% |
| **Procedure code** | 49220 | 49000 |
| **Pain score** | 6-8 | 6-8 |

### PATIENT POPULATION CHARACTERISTICS

| | | |
|---|---|---|
| **Age range** | 15-60 yrs | 15-75 yrs |
| **Male:Female** | 1:1.5 | 1:1 |
| **Incidence** | Common | ⇐ |
| **Etiology** | Unknown | Trauma |
| **Associated conditions** | Hodgkin's disease: 95%<br>Lymphoma: 5% | Other visceral or vascular injuries in trauma |

# ANESTHETIC CONSIDERATIONS

## PREOPERATIVE

Typically, patients presenting for **staging laparotomy** (which usually includes splenectomy) have Hodgkin's disease or some other lymphomatous disorder. Apart from the primary disease, these patients are in reasonably good health and will not have undergone radiation or chemotherapy prior to the staging laparotomy. Patients presenting for **splenectomy** may be divided into two less healthy groups: (1) trauma patients whose management is described in "Laparotomy for trauma," and (2) a more complex group that includes myeloproliferative disorders and other varieties of hypersplenism. These two groups may present complex perioperative management problems.

**Respiratory** Patients who have splenomegaly may have a degree of left lower lobe atelectasis which should be evaluated by physical exam. Some may have been treated with bleomycin, a chemotherapeutic drug that causes pulmonary fibrosis at total doses >200 mg/m$^2$. Methotrexate and cytarabine may also cause pulmonary fibrosis. Toxic drug effects are potentiated by smoking, XRT and high $FiO_2$.

**Tests:** CXR; others as clinically indicated.

**Cardiovascular** Patients with systemic disease requiring splenectomy may be chronically ill and have decreased cardiovascular reserve. Patients who have received doxorubicin (Adriamycin®) at doses >550 mg/m$^2$, may have a dose-dependent cardiotoxicity which can be worsened by XRT. Manifestations include ↓QRS amplitude, CHF, pleural effusions and dysrhythmias.

**Tests:** ECG; ECHO or MUGA scan to determine LV function, if indicated.

**Neurological** Patients may have neurological deficits from receiving chemotherapeutic agents (e.g., vinblastine and cisplatin can cause peripheral neuropathies). Any evidence of neurologic dysfunction should be documented in the preop evaluation.

**Hematologic** Patients are likely to present with splenomegaly 2° hematologic disease (Hodgkin's disease, non-Hodgkin's lymphoma, reticulum cell sarcoma, chronic leukemia, Felty's syndrome, myeloid metaplasia, thrombotic thrombocytopenic purpura, idiopathic thrombocytopenic purpura, idiopathic autoimmune hemolytic anemia, sickle cell disease, thalassemia, hereditary elliptocytosis, hereditary spherocytosis). Cytopenias are very common.

**Tests:** CBC with differential; platelet count; bleeding time

**Hepatic** Some chemotherapeutic agents (e.g., methotrexate) may be hepatotoxic. Evaluation of LFTs should be considered in patients deemed to be at risk.

**Tests:** LFTs, if indicated from H&P.

**Renal** Some chemotherapeutic drugs (e.g., methotrexate, cisplatin) are nephrotoxic; therefore, patients exposed to such agents can present with renal insufficiency.

**Tests:** UA; electrolytes; BUN; creatinine; others as indicated from H&P.

**Laboratory** Other tests as indicated from H&P.

**Premedication** Standard premedication (see Appendix). Administer stress dose of steroids (e.g., 100 mg hydrocortisone q 8 hr on day of surgery) if patient has received them as part of chemotherapeutic regimen.

## INTRAOPERATIVE

**Anesthetic technique:** GETA ± epidural for postop analgesia. If postop epidural analgesia is planned, placement of catheter prior to anesthetic induction is helpful to establish correct placement in the epidural space (accomplished by injecting 5-7 cc of 1% lidocaine via the epidural catheter, eliciting a segmental block).

**Induction** Standard induction (see Appendix).

**Maintenance** Standard maintenance (see Appendix). **Combined epidural/GA:** Local anesthetic (1.5-2% lidocaine with 1:200,000 epinephrine (12-15 ml q 60 min) can be injected incrementally into the epidural catheter to provide both anesthesia and optimal surgical exposure (contracted bowel and profound muscle relaxation). Be prepared to treat hypotension with fluids and vasopressors (e.g., ephedrine 5-10 mg iv). GA is administered to supplement regional anesthesia and for amnesia. Systemic sedatives (droperidol, opiates, benzodiazepines, etc.) should be minimized as they increase the likelihood of postop respiratory depression. If epidural opiates are used for postop analgesia, a loading dose (e.g., hydromorphone 1.0 mg) should be administered 1-2 hrs before conclusion of surgery.

**Emergence** No special considerations

| | | |
|---|---|---|
| **Blood and fluid requirements** | IV: 14-16 ga x 1<br>NS/LR @ 10-15 cc/kg/hr<br>Fluid warmer<br>Airway humidifier | |
| **Monitoring** | Standard monitors (see Appendix). | Others as indicated by patient's status. Try to prevent hypothermia during long operations. Consider heated humidifier, warming blanket, warming room temperature, keeping patient covered until ready for prep, etc. |
| **Positioning** | ✓ and pad pressure points.<br>✓ eyes. | |
| **Complications** | Unexpected bleeding | |

**POSTOPERATIVE**

| | | |
|---|---|---|
| **Complications** | Bleeding<br>Atelectasis (usually left lower lobe) | |
| **Pain management** | Epidural analgesia<br>PCA (see Appendix). | Patient should be recovered in ICU or hospital ward that is accustomed to treating side effects of epidural opiates (e.g., respiratory depression, breakthrough pain, nausea, pruritus). |
| **Tests** | CXR, if CVP placed perioperatively; CBC and platelet count. | |


**References**

1. Rutledge R, Sheldon GF: Abdominal Trauma. In *Operative Surgery*, 3rd edition. Nora PF, ed. WB Saunders Co, Philadelphia: 1990.
2. Taylor MA, Kaplan HS, Nelsen TS: Staging laparotomy with splenectomy for Hodgkin's disease: the Stanford experience. *World J Surg* 1985; 9(3):449-60.
3. Merritt WT: Anesthesia for gastrointestinal surgery. In *Principles and Practice of Anesthesiology*. Rogers MC, Tinker JH, Covino BG, Longnecker DE, eds. Mosby Year Book, St Louis: 1993, 1967-89.
4. Rinder CS: Cancer therapy and its anesthetic implications. In *Clinical Anesthesia*. Barash PG, Cullen BF, Stoelting RK, eds. JB Lippincott, Philadelphia: 1992, 1447-64.


# SPLENECTOMY

## SURGICAL CONSIDERATIONS

**Description:** Through a midline abdominal or left subcostal incision, the spleen is mobilized by dividing the lateral peritoneal attachments while the spleen is retracted medially. (Relevant anatomy is shown in Fig 7.8-1.) Once delivered into the operative wound, the short gastric vessels are clamped, cut and ligated. The splenic artery and vein are then exposed, with care being taken not to injure the tail of the pancreas. By keeping the splenic hilum between the operator's fingers and thumb, inadvertent bleeding can be controlled easily. Accessory spleens (incidence, 15-30%) should also be looked for if the splenectomy is being done for a hematologic disorder. They are found along the cephalad and caudad edges of the pancreas behind the stomach and in the area of the gastro-hepatic ligament, greater omentum and the splenic hilum. All patients undergoing splenectomy should receive polyvalent pneumococcal vaccine either prior to operation or following surgery.

**Variant procedure or approaches:** Following trauma, efforts at splenic salvage (**splenorrhaphy**) should be made to preserve all or part of the spleen. This may be accomplished by the use of local hemostatic techniques (electrocoagulation, argon beam coagulator, Surgicel® or Gelfoam® soaked in thrombin, microfibrillar collagen, and the use of fine sutures or mattress sutures utilizing Teflon® felt pledgets).

**Usual preop diagnosis:** Staging laparotomy; trauma; immune thrombocytopenic purpura; hereditary spherocytosis; other hereditary hemolytic anemias; or a variety of myeloproliferative disorders

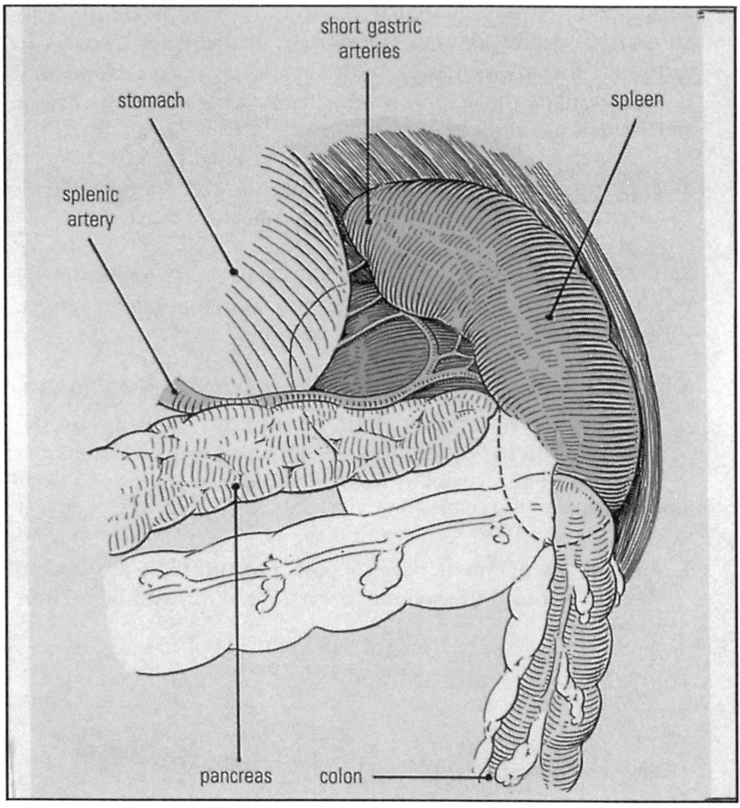


**Figure 7.8-1.** Relevant anatomy for splenectomy. (Reproduced with permission from Calne S, Pollard SG: *Operative Surgery*. Gower Medical Pub: 1992.)

**SUMMARY OF PROCEDURE**

| | Splenectomy | Splenorrhaphy |
|---|---|---|
| **Position** | Supine | ⇐ |
| **Incision** | Midline or left subcostal | ⇐ |
| **Special instrumentation** | Suitable abdominal retractors | ⇐ |
| **Unique considerations** | Potential for major blood loss during procedure; avoid splenic laceration and damage to tail of pancreas. | ⇐ |
| **Antibiotics** | Cefotetan 1 gm preop | ⇐ |
| **Surgical time** | 1 - 1.5 hrs | 1 - 2 hrs |
| **Closing considerations** | Adequate hemostasis | ⇐ |
| **EBL** | 50-100 ml | 200-500 ml |
| **Postop care** | NG decompression; PACU (non-trauma) | ⇐ |
| **Mortality** | 0-3% | ⇐ |
| **Morbidity**[1] | Thrombocytosis: 50-75% → DVT<br>Pulmonary complications: 3-23%<br>Pancreatitis and/or pancreatic fistula: 1.5-7.7%<br>Subphrenic abscess: 0-6%<br>Bleeding: 1-5%<br>Overwhelming sepsis[3]:<br>Adults: 0.3-1.8%<br>Children: ≤ 4% | ⇐ (Overall complication rate: 11.8%[2]) |
| **Procedure code** | 38100 | 38115 |
| **Pain score** | 5-7 | 5-7 |

### PATIENT POPULATION CHARACTERISTICS

| | |
|---|---|
| **Age range** | Any age |
| **Male:Female** | 1:1 |
| **Incidence** | Common |
| **Etiology** | See Preop Diagnosis, above |
| **Associated conditions** | Blood dyscrasias: 30-50%<br>Abdominal or thoracic trauma: 25%<br>Hodgkin's disease: 5-10%<br>Tumors: 5% |

## ANESTHETIC CONSIDERATIONS

See Anesthetic Considerations following "Exploratory or Staging Laparotomy" (above).

**References**

1. Pate JW, Peters TG, Andrews CR: Postsplenectomy complications. *Am Surg* 1985; 51(8):437-41.
2. Feliciano DV et al: A four-year experience with splenectomy versus splenorrhaphy. *Ann Surg* 1985; 201(5):568-75.
3. Schwartz PE et al: Postsplenectomy sepsis and mortality in adults. *JAMA* 1982; 248(18):2279-83.

# EXCISION OF INTRA-ABDOMINAL AND RETROPERITONEAL TUMORS

## SURGICAL CONSIDERATIONS

**Description**: Intra-abdominal and retroperitoneal tumors, other than those of visceral origin, consist primarily of sarcomas (liposarcoma, fibrous histiocytomas, mesenteric fibromas). They are usually approached through a long, midline incision for adequate exposure and to assess their resectability. Resection of such lesions may require excision of adjacent or involved small bowel or large intestine or other involved abdominal viscera. Care must be taken not to injure the ureters or major vessels, particularly at the root of the mesentery to the small bowel. If residual tumor remains, intraop radiation (IORT) may be indicated. In certain tumors the patient may still benefit from "tumor debulking" (removing as much tumor as possible and treating the remaining tumor with radiation and/or chemotherapy). Operative approaches are dictated by location of tumor. Although most operative approaches are transabdominal, some retroperitoneal tumors may be approached retroperitoneally via oblique incision on either side of the abdomen.

**Usual preop diagnosis**: Intra-abdominal or peritoneal tumor

### SUMMARY OF PROCEDURE

| | |
|---|---|
| **Position** | Supine |
| **Incision** | Midline abdominal |
| **Unique considerations** | Availability of blood |
| **Antibiotics** | Cefotetan 1-2 gm iv preop |
| **Surgical time** | 2 - 4 hrs |
| **Closing considerations** | Hemostasis |
| **EBL** | 300-1000 ml |

| | |
|---|---|
| **Mortality** | 1-3% |
| **Morbidity** | Respiratory problems: 5-10%<br>Wound infection: 2-4%<br>Hemorrhage: 1-3% |
| **Procedure code** | 49220 |
| **Pain score** | 8-10 |

### PATIENT POPULATION CHARACTERISTICS

| | |
|---|---|
| **Age range** | Variable, 20-75 yrs |
| **Male:Female** | 1:1 |
| **Incidence** | Common |
| **Etiology** | Unknown |
| **Associated conditions** | Partial bowel obstruction: 15-20%<br>Hydronephrosis: 10-15% |

## ANESTHETIC CONSIDERATIONS

See "Anesthetic Considerations for Other Intestinal and Peritoneal Procedures" in "Intestinal Surgery" section.

### References

1. *Color Atlas of Demonstrations in Surgical Pathology*, Vol 1. Royal College of Surgeons of Edinburgh. Williams & Wilkins: 1983, 530-43.

# DRAINAGE OF SUBPHRENIC ABSCESS

## SURGICAL CONSIDERATIONS

**Description:** Abscesses may occur in subphrenic spaces, including the right subphrenic, right subhepatic, left subphrenic, lesser sac or bare area of the liver, following peritonitis (Fig 7.8-2), abdominal surgery or trauma. It is important to know the anatomy of these spaces for making a correct diagnosis, and for treatment.

**Drainage** is accomplished by a posterior or anterior extraperitoneal approach or by a transpleural approach, depending on the location of the abscess. Lesser sac abscesses are best approached by an anterior transperitoneal route. Abscesses in the bare area of the liver are drained posteriorly. Once the abscess has been localized, the cavity is entered by finger dissection and drained. Loculations are broken up and the cavity thoroughly irrigated with NS or a suitable antibiotic solution. Appropriate drains are placed and the wound is closed in a conventional manner. Cultures are routinely obtained.

**Variant procedure or approaches:** **Percutaneous approaches** are becoming more popular as experience is gained by interventional radiologists. This technique should be reserved for unilocular collections, where sterile cavities are not penetrated, and a safe route is available.

**Usual preop diagnosis:** Subphrenic abscess

## SUMMARY OF PROCEDURE

| | Subphrenic Abscess Drainage | Percutaneous Approach |
|---|---|---|
| **Position** | Supine or lateral decubitus, right or left | ⇐ |
| **Incision** | Subcostal or oblique abdominal | None |
| **Special instrumentation** | Drainage tubes | Special catheters; CT guidance |
| **Antibiotics** | Cefotetan 1-2 gm preop | ⇐ |
| **Surgical time** | 1 hr | ⇐ |
| **EBL** | 50-100 ml | 10-25 ml |
| **Postop care** | Maintain patency of the drainage tubes | ⇐ |
| **Mortality** | < 5% | ⇐ |
| **Morbidity** | Inadequate drainage: 5-10%<br>Pulmonary complications: 5-10%<br>Bowel perforation: < 2% | ⇐ |
| **Procedure code** | 49040 | ⇐ |
| **Pain score** | 7-9 | 4-5 |

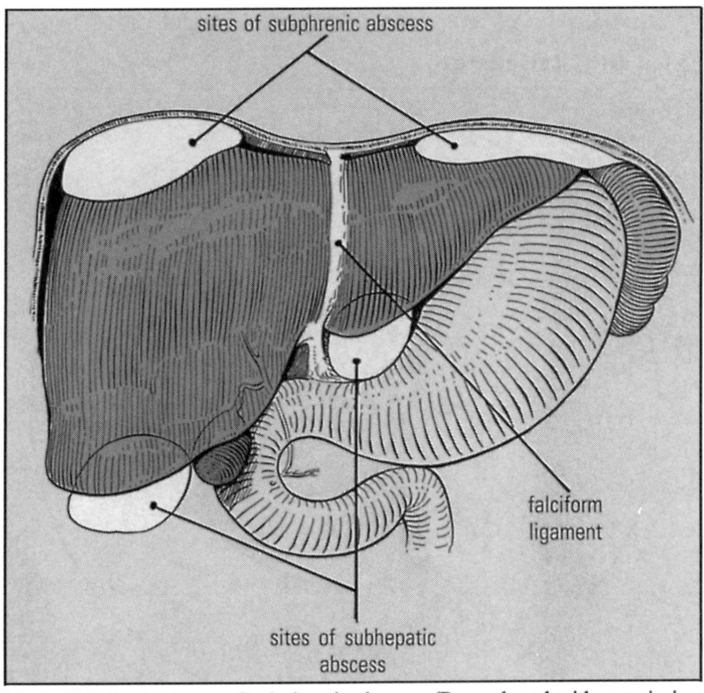

Figure 7.8-2. Anatomy of subphrenic abscess. (Reproduced with permission from Calne S, Pollard SG: *Operative Surgery*. Gower Medical Pub: 1992.)

## PATIENT POPULATION CHARACTERISTICS

| | |
|---|---|
| **Age range** | Variable, 15-80 yrs |
| **Male:Female** | 1:1 |
| **Incidence** | Common |
| **Etiology** | Postop: 70-80%<br>Peritonitis: 25-30%<br>Trauma: 5-10% |
| **Associated conditions** | See Etiology, above. |

# ANESTHETIC CONSIDERATIONS

See "Anesthetic Considerations for Other Intestinal and Peritoneal Procedures" in "Intestinal Surgery" section.

**References**

1. Nora PF: *Operative Surgery*. WB Saunders Co, Philadelphia: 1990, 466-73.

# INGUINAL HERNIORRHAPHY

## SURGICAL CONSIDERATIONS

**Description:** Groin hernias are defects in the transverse abdominis layer, where a direct hernia comes through the posterior wall of the inguinal canal and an indirect hernia comes through the internal inguinal ring. Surgical approach can be either anterior or posterior. In general, an **anterior approach** (Bassini, McVay's, Shouldice or mesh repair) is used for primary repair of an indirect or direct inguinal hernia. The **Bassini repair** consists of ligation of the hernia sac and suturing the conjoint tendon to the shelving edge of Poupart's ligament. **McVay's repair** sutures the conjoint tendon to Cooper's ligament and is usually reserved for direct inguinal hernias. **Shouldice** emphasizes the closing of the transverse fascia and transversus abdominal muscle layers. More recently, the interposing of Marlex® mesh between the conjoint tendon, the internal oblique muscle and the inguinal ligament has become popular. Other modifications are indicated in special situations.

A **posterior approach** is used by some surgeons for the repair of femoral hernias and recurrent inguinal hernias,[3] and for treating incarcerated and strangulated hernias. The **posterior preperitoneal approach** is normally performed by suturing the transversus abdominis arch on the superior aspect of the hernia defect to Cooper's ligament and the iliopubic tract on the inferior aspect of the defect.

**Usual preop diagnosis:** Groin pain or lump

### SUMMARY OF PROCEDURE

| | |
|---|---|
| **Position** | Supine |
| **Incision** | Oblique or transverse |
| **Unique considerations** | Avoid damage to nerve structure and spermatic cord. Avoid interfering with blood supply to testes. |
| **Antibiotics** | None |
| **Surgical time** | 1 - 1.5 hrs |
| **Postop care** | PACU → room |
| **EBL** | 25-50 ml |
| **Mortality** | < 0.3% |
| **Morbidity** | Wound abscess: < 3%<br>Wound hematoma: < 2% |
| **Procedure code** | 49505 |
| **Pain score** | 4-5 |

### PATIENT POPULATION CHARACTERISTICS

| | |
|---|---|
| **Age range** | 1-90 yrs |
| **Male:Female** | 85:15 |
| **Incidence** | 15/1000 |
| **Etiology** | Congenital variants<br>Reduced collagen synthesis in adults |
| **Associated conditions** | Chronic cough<br>Urinary retention<br>Chronic constipation |

## ANESTHETIC CONSIDERATIONS

See Anesthetic Considerations following "Repair of Abdominal Dehiscence" (below).

**References**

1. Barbier J, Carretier M, Richer JP: Cooper ligament repair: an update. *World J Surg* 1989; 13(5):499-505.
2. Wantz GE: The Canadian repair: Personal observation. *World J Surg* 1989; 13(5):516-21.
3. Read RC: Preperitoneal herniorrhaphy: a historical review. *World J Surg* 1989; 13(5):532-40.

# FEMORAL HERNIA REPAIR

## SURGICAL CONSIDERATIONS

**Description:** The hernia sac is exposed as it exits the preperitoneal space through the femoral canal (Fig 7.8-3). If the hernia cannot be reduced, the possibility of strangulation needs to be kept in mind. The peritoneal sac in most cases should be opened proximal to the femoral canal in order to gain control of the intestine before it reduces itself into the peritoneal cavity. If the bowel is ischemic, it may require resection. The repair consists of suturing the iliopubic tract to Cooper's ligament, taking care not to compromise the femoral vein.

**Usual preop diagnosis:** Bulging of tissues over femoral canal

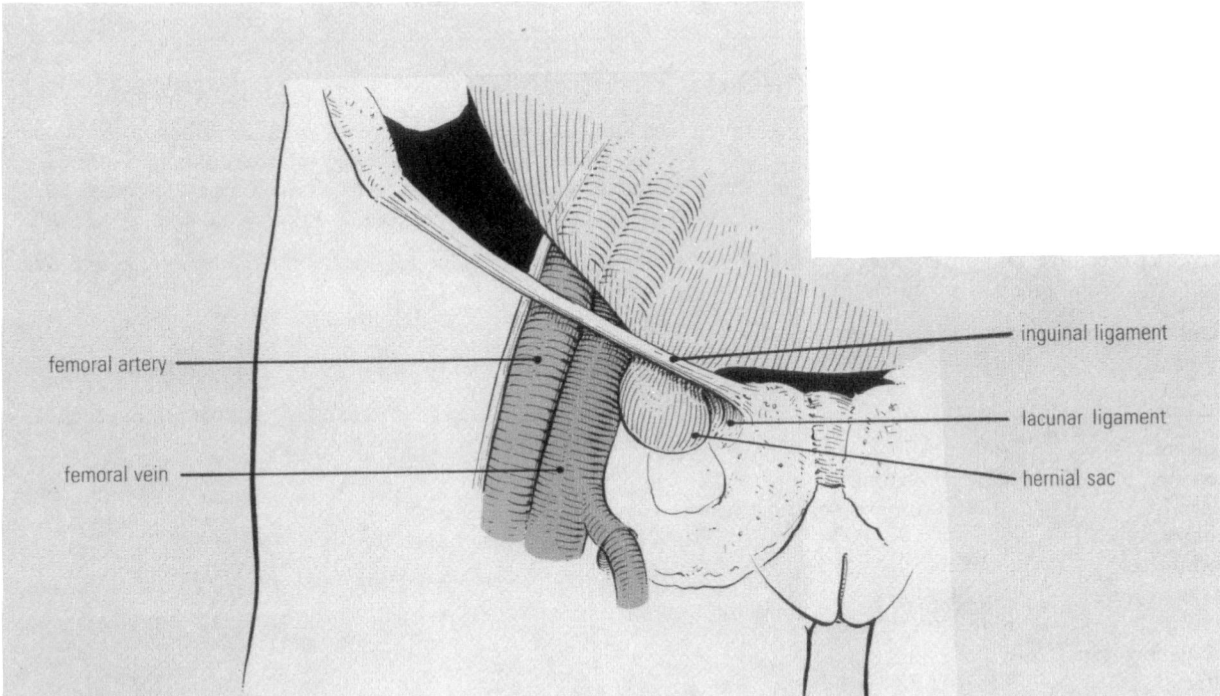


**Figure 7.8-3.** Anatomy of a femoral hernia. (Reproduced with permission from Calne R, Pollard SG: *Operative Surgery*. Gower Medical Pub: 1992.)

### SUMMARY OF PROCEDURE

| | |
|---|---|
| **Position** | Supine |
| **Incision** | Oblique |
| **Surgical time** | 1 - 1.5 hrs |
| **EBL** | 25-50 ml |
| **Postop care** | PACU → room |
| **Mortality** | < 1% (6-20% if strangulated) |
| **Morbidity** | Recurrence: 6% |
| **Procedure code** | 49550 |
| **Pain score** | 5-6 |

### PATIENT POPULATION CHARACTERISTICS

| | |
|---|---|
| **Age range** | Adults; rare in children |
| **Male:Female** | 1:3 |
| **Incidence** | 1.5% of all groin hernias |
| **Etiology** | Failure of pre-formed peritoneal sac to obliterate<br>Muscle atrophy in older age group |

## ANESTHETIC CONSIDERATIONS

See Anesthetic Considerations following "Repair of Abdominal Dehiscence" (below).

**References**

1. Bendavid R. New techniques in hernia repair. *World J Surg* 1989; 13(5):522-31.

# REPAIR OF INCISIONAL HERNIA

## SURGICAL CONSIDERATIONS

**Description**: Incisional hernias can occur after any abdominal incision, but are most common following midline incisions. Factors leading to herniation are: wound infection, trauma, inadequate suturing, and weak tissues. Following skin incision, the skin edges and subcutaneous fat are retracted and the dissection carried down to the hernia defect. The redundant hernia sac is excised and the fascia freed up on both sides of the wound. Primary closure is preferred.

**Variant procedure or approaches**: In addition to primary repair, the latter may be reinforced by an onlay mesh prosthesis, or the prosthesis may be used to fill the hernial defect.

**Usual preop diagnosis**: Incisional hernia

### SUMMARY OF PROCEDURE

| | |
|---|---|
| **Position** | Supine |
| **Incision** | Vertical or transverse |
| **Special instrumentation** | Mesh prosthesis (in some cases) |
| **Antibiotics** | Cefotetan 1-2 gm iv |
| **Surgical time** | 1 - 2 hrs |
| **Closing considerations** | Retention sutures |
| **EBL** | 100-200 ml |
| **Postop care** | NG decompression; abdominal binder; PACU → room |
| **Mortality** | < 1% |
| **Morbidity** | Ileus: 5-10%<br>Respiratory complications: 5-10%<br>Wound infection: 1-2% |
| **Procedure code** | 49560, 49560-22 (repair of incisional hernia with mesh prosthesis) |
| **Pain score** | 5-6 |

### PATIENT POPULATION CHARACTERISTICS

| | |
|---|---|
| **Age range** | 20-70 yrs |
| **Male:Female** | 1:1 |
| **Incidence** | 3-5% of midline abdominal incision |
| **Etiology** | Wound infection<br>Trauma<br>Inadequate suturing<br>Weak tissues |
| **Associated conditions** | Obesity<br>Malnutrition |

## ANESTHETIC CONSIDERATIONS

See Anesthetic Considerations following "Repair of Abdominal Dehiscence" (below).

**References**

1. Condon RE, Telford G: Anterior Abdominal Wall Hernia. In *Operative Surgery*, 3rd edition. Nora PF, ed. WB Saunders Co, Philadelphia: 1990, Ch 33.

# REPAIR OF ABDOMINAL DEHISCENCE

## SURGICAL CONSIDERATIONS

**Description:** Dehiscence implies a "splitting apart" or "bursting open" of a wound. A complete dehiscence is a separation of all layers of the abdominal wall and is often associated with an extrusion of abdominal viscera. If incomplete, the separation of fascial and muscular layers results in an incisional hernia or an obstruction of a herniated loop of intestine. The earliest sign of a wound dehiscence is the presence of a serosanguineous drainage from the wound. Minimal disruptions may be treated conservatively with occlusive dressings and an abdominal binder. Major dehiscence requires operative repair using retention sutures.

**Variant procedure or approaches:** Variations in the type of closure depend on surgeon's preference. Interrupted, non-absorbable sutures and skin bridges are often used.

**Usual preop diagnosis:** Wound dehiscence

### SUMMARY OF PROCEDURE

| | |
|---|---|
| **Position** | Supine |
| **Incision** | Closure of previous incision |
| **Unique considerations** | Adequate muscle relaxation essential |
| **Antibiotics** | Cefotetan 1-2 gm preop |
| **Surgical time** | 1 - 1.5 hrs |
| **EBL** | 50-100 ml |
| **Postop care** | Abdominal binder to relieve tension on suture line; PACU → room |
| **Mortality** | 5-10% |
| **Morbidity** | Incisional hernia: 5-10%<br>Wound infection: < 5%<br>Wound ischemia: 1-2% |
| **Procedure code** | 49900 |
| **Pain score** | 4-5 |

### PATIENT POPULATION CHARACTERISTICS

| | |
|---|---|
| **Age range** | 25-90 yrs |
| **Male:Female** | 1:1 |
| **Incidence** | 1.3% in patients < 45 yrs<br>5.4% in patients >45 yrs |
| **Etiology** | Wound infection<br>Excessive coughing or sneezing<br>Excessive abdominal distention<br>Weak tissue<br>Poor nutrition<br>Hematoma formation<br>Poor surgical technique |

| | |
|---|---|
| **Associated conditions** | Malnutrition: 25-30%<br>Ascites: 20-25%<br>Hypoproteinemia: 20%<br>Chronic anemia: 5-10%<br>Vitamin C deficiency: < 5% |

---

## ANESTHETIC CONSIDERATIONS

**Procedures covered: inguinal herniorrhaphy; femoral hernia repair; incisional hernia repair; repair of abdominal dehiscence)**

### PREOPERATIVE

Predisposing factors for hernia often include increased abdominal pressure 2° chronic cough, bladder outlet obstruction, constipation, pregnancy, vomiting and acute or chronic muscular effort. These factors should be controlled preop to avoid postop recurrence. The patient population may range from premature infants to the elderly with the possibility of multiple medical problems.

| | |
|---|---|
| **Musculoskeletal** | Pain is likely to be present in area of hernia; evaluate bony landmarks if regional anesthetic is planned. |
| **Gastrointestinal** | Hernias may become incarcerated, obstructed or strangulated, requiring emergency surgery. Fluid and electrolyte imbalance should be assumed.<br>**Tests:** Electrolytes |
| **Hematologic** | If regional anesthesia planned, check patient's coagulation status.<br>**Tests:** Platelet count; CBC with differential; PT/PTT; bleeding time (if on ASA, NSAIDs or dipyridomole [Persantine®]) |
| **Laboratory** | UA; other tests as indicated from H&P. |
| **Premedication** | If necessary, standard premedication (see Appendix). |

### INTRAOPERATIVE

**Anesthetic technique:** General, regional or local anesthesia ± sedation (MAC) are all appropriate anesthetic techniques. Choice depends on factors such as site of incision, patient physical status and preference of both patient and surgeon. GA may be preferred for incisions made above T8. Profound muscle relaxation may be necessary to facilitate exploration and repair.

**Regional anesthesia:**

| | |
|---|---|
| **Spinal** | Single-shot vs continuous: Patient in sitting or lateral decubitus position (operative site down) for placement of hyperbaric subarachnoid block. Doses of local anesthetics are as follows for T4-T6 level: 5% lidocaine in 7.5% dextrose (75-100 mg); 0.75% bupivacaine in 8.25% dextrose (10-15 mg); 0.5% tetracaine in 5% dextrose (12-18 mg). For continuous spinal, titrate local anesthetic to desired surgical level (T6). Large doses of hyperbaric local anesthetic should be avoided as they can cause postop cauda equina syndrome. |
| **Epidural** | Patient in sitting or lateral decubitus position for placement of epidural catheter. After locating the epidural space, administer a test dose (e.g., 3 ml of 1.5% lidocaine with 1:200,000 epinephrine) to elucidate whether the catheter is subarachnoid or intravascular. Titrate local anesthetic until desired surgical level is obtained (3-5 ml at a time) usually less than 20 ml. |
| **Local** | Requires gentle surgical technique. Surgical field block, plus ilioinguinal and iliohypogastric nerve blocks using 0.5% bupivacaine with 1:200,000 epinephrine. Usually done by surgeon. |

**General anesthesia:**

| | |
|---|---|
| **Induction** | Mask vs ET: Standard induction (see Appendix). Mask GA may be suitable for the patient who presents with a simple chronic hernia. If there is obstruction, incarceration or strangulation, however, a rapid-sequence induction with ET intubation is indicated. GETA also may be indicated in the patient with wound dehiscence. |

| | | |
|---|---|---|
| **Maintenance** | Standard maintenance (see Appendix). Muscle relaxants may be necessary to facilitate surgical repair. | |
| **Emergence** | Consider extubating the trachea while patient is still anesthetized to prevent coughing and straining. Patients who are at risk for pulmonary aspiration and require awake intubation or rapid-sequence induction are not candidates for deep extubation. | |
| **Blood and fluid requirements** | Minimal blood loss<br>IV: 16-18 ga x 1<br>NS/LR @ 5-8 cc/kg/hr | |
| **Monitoring** | Standard monitoring (see Appendix). | |
| **Positioning** | √and pad pressure points.<br>√eyes. | |
| **Complications** | Wound dehiscence with coughing/ straining | |

**POSTOPERATIVE**

| | | |
|---|---|---|
| **Complications** | Cauda equina syndrome | The diagnosis of cauda equina syndrome (urinary and fecal incontinence, paresis of lower extremities, perineal hyperesthesias) should be sought in the postop period in patients who have received large doses of intrathecal local anesthetic during continuous spinal techniques. √ patients for bowel or bladder dysfunction and perineal sensory deficits. If present, consider a neurology consultation and continue followup of the patient's neurologic dysfunction. |
| | Urinary retention, common with regional anesthesia | Patients with urinary retention may require intermittent catheterization until urinary function resumes. |
| **Pain management** | PO analgesics:<br>Acetaminophen and codeine (Tylenol® #3 1-2 tab q 4-6 hrs) or oxycodone and acetaminophen (Percocet® 1 tab q 6 hrs) | Surgical field block or regional anesthesia should provide sufficient analgesia postop. |

**References**


1. Hardy JD: *Critical Surgical Illness*, 2nd edition. WB Saunders Co, Philadelphia: 1980, 203-9.
2. Rigler ML, Drasner K, Krejcie TC, Yelich SJ, Scholnick FT, DeFontes J, Bohner D: Cauda equina syndrome after continuous spinal anesthesia. *Anesth Analg* 1991; 72:275-81.
3. Cousins MJ, Bridenbaugh PO, eds: *Neural Blockade Pain Management*, 2nd edition. JB Lippincott Co, Philadelphia: 1988, 685-87.

**Surgeon**

**Stefanie S. Jeffrey, MD, FACS**

# 7.9 BREAST SURGERY

**Anesthesiologist**

**Steven K. Howard, MD**

# BREAST BIOPSY

## SURGICAL CONSIDERATIONS

**Description: Breast biopsy** is the surgical removal of breast tissue for pathologic examination. Breast biopsies are done for palpable abnormalities, such as breast masses or asymmetric breast thickenings, or for non-palpable abnormalities that are seen only on mammogram. Mammographic abnormalities include microcalcifications, mammographic masses (densities) and areas of architectural distortion. With mammographic abnormalities, the breast tissue may look and feel normal at surgery and the abnormality may only be appreciated by x-ray or by microscopic examination. Therefore, the surgeon requires accurate preop localization of the abnormality to be removed. This is done under local anesthesia with mammographic guidance using a percutaneous hook-wire placed by the radiologist. The patient goes directly to the OR where the surgeon dissects along the wire and excises the abnormality marked by its hooked tip. The tissue specimen is sent for a radiograph to confirm whether the abnormality has been adequately excised. (This is known as **wire localization**, **needle localization**, or **hook-wire localization breast biopsy**.)

Breast biopsies are generally done under local anesthesia; however, the patient may require monitoring by an anesthesiologist if large amounts of intravenous sedation are anticipated, or if the patient has any medical problems. Some surgeons prefer to do breast biopsies under GA if the Bx is particularly deep in the breast, the patient is very anxious and prefers not to be awake, or the patient has submammary breast implants which may be incidentally punctured by needle injection.

**Usual preop diagnosis:** Breast mass or mammographic abnormality

### SUMMARY OF PROCEDURE

| | Breast Biopsy | Wire Localization Breast Biopsy |
|---|---|---|
| **Position** | Supine, with ipsilateral arm abducted. Table may be banked to center breast. | ⇐ |
| **Incision** | Over-breast mass or circumareolar | ⇐ + Incision may or may not incorporate skin entry site of wire. |
| **Special instrumentation** | None | Wire placed immediately preop in mammography suite. |
| **Surgical time** | 0.5 - 1 hr | 1 - 1.5 hr, depending on time it takes to get back results of specimen radiograph. |
| **Closing considerations** | Gauze bandage over wound. Some surgeons prefer patient to sit upright so breast can resume normal shape before bandaging. | ⇐ + Specimen radiograph result must be obtained prior to completion of operation. |
| **EBL** | < 25 cc | ⇐ |
| **Postop care** | PACU → home | ⇐ |
| **Mortality** | Minimal | ⇐ |
| **Morbidity** | Hematoma: < 10% | ⇐ |
| | Infection: 2-5% | ⇐ |
| | | Inability to excise mammographic abnormality: Infrequent (due to inaccurate wire placement in radiology or wire movement during patient transport or surgical prepping) |
| | | Placement or migration of the wire into the thorax or mediastinum: Very rare |
| **Procedure code** | 19120 | 19120-22 |
| **Pain score** | 2-5 | 2-5 |

### PATIENT POPULATION CHARACTERISTICS

| | | |
|---|---|---|
| **Age range** | 16-90 (usually >30 yrs) | 35-80 yrs |
| **Male:Female** | Mainly female | Only female |
| **Incidence** | Common | ⇐ |
| **Etiology** | Unknown | ⇐ |

# ANESTHETIC CONSIDERATIONS

## PREOPERATIVE

Breast masses may vary in size and depth, which will, in part, determine what type of anesthetic is most suitable for the procedure in these otherwise healthy patients. Typically, these excisional biopsies can be accomplished with sedatives and local anesthesia; however, patient wishes must be considered in the anesthetic plan. The suitability of local vs GA may be best-addressed by preop discussion with the surgical team.

| | |
|---|---|
| **Psychosocial** | Patients are likely to be very anxious concerning the possibility of breast malignancy, and should be counseled and premedicated appropriately. |
| **Laboratory** | CBC; other tests as indicated from H&P. |
| **Premedication** | Standard premedication (see Appendix) |

## INTRAOPERATIVE

**Anesthetic technique:** GA or local anesthesia ± sedation are both appropriate techniques. Choice of anesthetic technique depends on the size and depth of the suspicious lesion and the desires of the patient. Often done on an outpatient basis.

| | | |
|---|---|---|
| **MAC** | Combination of analgesics (e.g., fentanyl) and anxiolytics (e.g., midazolam), titrated to effect, are most commonly used. The surgeon may choose to add Na bicarbonate to 1% lidocaine (1:10) to reduce injection pain. The anesthesiologist may give a short-acting narcotic or a short-acting sedative hypnotic just prior to the initial injection of local anesthetic in the skin. Propofol infusion (25-75 $\mu$g/kg/min) is being used more frequently to provide a constant level of sedation. | |
| **Induction** | Standard induction (see Appendix). Mask anesthetic may be appropriate, but also may be difficult due to encroachment on the surgical field; an ETT may be required. | |
| **Maintenance** | Standard maintenance (see Appendix). Muscle relaxants are not necessary for the surgical procedure. | |
| **Emergence** | No special considerations | |
| **Blood and fluid requirements** | Minimal blood loss<br>IV: 18 ga x 1<br>NS/LR @ 3-5 cc/kg/hr | |
| **Monitoring** | Standard monitors (see Appendix)<br>Maintain verbal contact with patient if MAC. | Other monitors as clinically indicated. |
| **Positioning** | ✓ and pad pressure points.<br>✓ eyes. | |
| **Complications** | Inadequate analgesia | May have to supplement surgical field block with local anesthetic or convert to GA. |

## POSTOPERATIVE

| | |
|---|---|
| **Complications** | No specific complications anticipated |
| **Pain management** | PO analgesics (see Appendix) |
| **Tests** | As clinically indicated |

**References**

1. Bland KI, Copeland EM III, eds: *The Breast: Comprehensive Management of Benign and Malignant Diseases.* WB Saunders Co, Philadelphia: 1991.
2. Harris JR, Hellman S, Henderson IC, Kinne DW, eds: *Breast Diseases,* 2nd edition. JB Lippincott Co, Philadelphia: 1991.
3. Zelcer J, White PF: Monitored anesthesia care. In *Anesthesia,* 3rd edition. Miller RD, ed. Churchill Livingstone, New York: 1990, 1321-34.

# MASTECTOMY

## SURGICAL CONSIDERATIONS

**Description:** The treatment of breast cancer has evolved greatly in the last 30 years. The **radical mastectomy**, which removes the breast, the underlying pectoral muscles and the axillary lymph nodes, is no longer the mainstay of treatment. The two major treatment alternatives now are the **modified radical mastectomy** and **wide local excision** of the tumor (**partial mastectomy** or **lumpectomy**) with **axillary dissection**, followed by postop radiation therapy to the remaining breast tissue. Modified radical mastectomy entails removal of the breast and axillary lymph nodes, while the pectoral muscles remain in place (except when surgeons perform the **Patey procedure**, in which the pectoralis minor muscle is removed to allow a more complete dissection of the axillary lymph nodes). When a wide local excision is performed, it removes the tumor with a rim of normal surrounding tissue (i.e., surgical margins free of tumor). When a wide local excision and axillary dissection are performed at the same time, separate incisions are performed and separate instruments are generally used so that there is no cross-contamination of cancer cells between the wounds.

The axillary dissection generally removes levels I and II axillary lymph nodes: those lymph nodes that lie lateral to the edge of the pectoralis minor muscle and those that lie posterior to the pectoralis minor muscle. The level III, or highest group of axillary lymph nodes, generally cannot be reached without removing the pectoralis minor muscle. For prognostic and treatment purposes, no survival advantage can be shown in removing level III axillary lymph nodes. The disadvantages include a significant increase in postop lymphedema of the arm when these high lymph nodes are excised. As part of the axillary dissection, the surgeon preserves the thoracodorsal nerve to the latissimus dorsi muscle and the long thoracic nerve to the serratus anterior muscle, as well as the blood and nerve supply to the pectoral muscles. Preservation of the intercostobrachial nerve (sensory to the upper arm), which courses through the axillary fat pad, is optional.

A **total mastectomy** (also known as a **simple** or **complete mastectomy**) removes only the breast. There is no axillary dissection involved and it is done mainly for treatment of duct carcinoma *in situ.*

**Usual preop diagnosis:** Breast cancer; *in situ* breast cancer

### SUMMARY OF PROCEDURE

| | Modified Radical Mastectomy | Total Mastectomy (Simple Mastectomy) | Partial Mastectomy/ Axillary Lymph Node Dissection |
|---|---|---|---|
| **Position** | Supine, with ipsilateral arm abducted. Some surgeons prep arm for inclusion in the operative field. | ⇐ | ⇐ |
| **Incision** | Elliptical oblique or elliptical transverse to include nipple/ areola and previous Bx incision | ⇐ | Incision over breast mass or previous Bx site. Separate transverse incision in axilla using different instruments. |
| **Special instrumentation** | Pectoral, axillary drains usually placed prior to closure. | Pectoral drain usually placed prior to closure. | Axillary drain usually placed prior to closure. |
| **Unique considerations** | Avoid iv and BP cuff on ipsilateral arm. | ⇐ | ⇐ |
| **Surgical time** | 1.5 - 3 hrs (+ ~1 hr if immediate breast reconstruction performed) | 1 - 2 hrs (+ ~1 hr if immediate breast reconstruction performed) | 2 - 3 hrs |
| **Closing considerations** | Gauze bandage over incision site | ⇐ | ⇐ |
| **EBL** | 150-500 cc, depending on whether scalpel or electrocautery is used for breast dissection. | ⇐ | 25-100 cc |
| **Postop care** | PACU → room x 2 d | PACU → hospital x 1-2 d, or occasionally → home | ⇐ |

| | Modified Radical Mastectomy | Total Mastectomy | Partial Mastectomy/ Node Dissection |
|---|---|---|---|
| **Mortality** | Minimal | ⇐ | ⇐ |
| **Morbidity** | Lymphedema: 5-30% (depending on extent of axillary dissection) | – | Lymphedema: 5-30% (depending on extent of axillary dissection) |
| | Seroma: 25% | ⇐ | ⇐ |
| | Infection: 2-10% | ⇐ | ⇐ |
| | Flap necrosis: < 5% | ⇐ | – |
| | Hematoma: < 5% | ⇐ | < 10% |
| | Injury to axillary neurovascular structures: Rare | – | ⇐ |
| | Pneumothorax: Rare (may occur with attempts to obtain hemostasis of intercostal perforating vessels) | ⇐ | — |
| **Procedure code** | 19240 | 19180 | 19162 |
| **Pain score** | 4-8 | 4-6 | 4-8 |

### PATIENT POPULATION CHARACTERISTICS

**Age range** 20-90 yrs (generally >40 yrs)

**Incidence** Approximately 1/9 American women develop breast cancer; in 1992, 180,000 cases were diagnosed. The incidence has been increasing at a rate of 3%/yr since 1980.

**Etiology** Unknown

---

## ANESTHETIC CONSIDERATIONS

### PREOPERATIVE

Patients often have no other underlying medical problems. Some consideration, however, should be given to the anesthetic implications of metastatic spread to bone, brain, liver, lung, etc.

**Respiratory** Respiratory compromise can be present if patient has received XRT to the thorax as part of treatment. Certain chemotherapeutic drugs (e.g., bleomycin >200 mg/m$^2$) can cause pulmonary toxicity and necessitate administration of low $FiO_2$ ($\leq$ 30).

**Tests:** PA and lateral CXR (✓ for pleural effusion and rib or vertebral lesions). If patient shows any signs of respiratory compromise, obtain room air ABG. Consider PFTs (FVC, $FEV_1$, $MMEF_{25-75}$) if CXR or ABG abnormal. This will help predict pulmonary reserve and patient tolerance to GA. Patients who show signs of impaired pulmonary function might require postop care in an ICU for various reasons (e.g., mechanical ventilation, aggressive pulmonary toilet, close observation, etc.).

**Cardiovascular** Chemotherapeutic agents (e.g., doxorubicin at doses >550 mg/m$^2$) also cause cardiomyopathies. If patient was exposed to this type of drug, cardiac dysfunction may be present, and a cardiac consultation to evaluate ventricular function may be necessary.

**Tests:** ECHO or MUGA scan

**Neurological** Breast cancer often metastasizes to the CNS and can present with focal neurologic deficits, ↑ICP or altered mental status. If patient has altered mental status, full medical workup should proceed without delay; postpone surgery until cause is found. Consider neurological/neurosurgical consultation.

**Tests:** CT/MR scan should be recommended, if indicated from H&P.

**Hematologic** Patient may be anemic 2° chronic disease or chemotherapeutic agents.

**Tests:** CBC, with differential and platelet count

**Laboratory** Routine lab exam; other tests as indicated from H&P.

**Premedication** Standard premedication (see Appendix).

## INTRAOPERATIVE

**Anesthetic technique:** GA, except in the case of superficial Bx, which can be done under MAC with sedation.

**Induction** Standard induction (see Appendix)

**Maintenance** Standard maintenance (see Appendix). The use of muscle relaxants during axillary dissection should be avoided to permit surgical identification of nerves by nerve stimulator.

**Emergence** Pressure dressings are often applied with the patient anesthetized and "sitting up" at the end of the procedure. Discuss with surgeons whether or not they intend to apply this type of dressing to enable emergence to be timed appropriately.

**Blood and fluid requirements**

Minimal-to-no blood loss
IV: 16-18 ga x 1 (avoid operative side)
NS/LR @ 3-5 cc/kg/hr

**Monitoring**

Standard monitors (see Appendix)
BP cuff on arm opposite surgical site

Others as indicated by patient status.

**Positioning**

✓ and pad pressure points.
✓ eyes.

**Complications**

Pneumothorax

Deep surgical exploration may cause inadvertent entry into the patient's pleural space, causing a pneumothorax. Monitor patient for Sx of pneumothorax (e.g., ↑PIP, ↓$PaCO_2$, asymmetric breath sounds, hyperresonance to percussion over the affected side, hemodynamic instability). Dx: CXR. Rx: Chest tube, 100% $O_2$.

## POSTOPERATIVE:

**Complications**

Pneumothorax
Psychological trauma

Pneumothorax: If index of suspicion is high, maintain oxygenation (100% $FiO_2$) and ventilation; inform surgeons of the likelihood of the Dx. If patient is hemodynamically unstable (suggesting a tension pneumothorax), place a 14-ga iv catheter in the 2nd intercostal space while the surgeons set up for placement of a chest tube. If patient is hemodynamically stable and not hypoxemic, a portable CXR may aid in diagnosis.

**Pain management**

PCA (see Appendix)
PO analgesics (see Appendix)

**Tests**

Postop portable CXR, if pneumothorax is a consideration.

**Surgeon**

**Harry A. Oberhelman, MD, FACS**

## 7.10 ENDOCRINE SURGERY

**Anesthesiologist**

**Steven K. Howard, MD**

# EXCISION OF THYROGLOSSAL DUCT CYST

## SURGICAL CONSIDERATIONS

**Description**: The majority of patients with thyroglossal duct cysts are diagnosed before the age of 20. The usual presentation is a superficial midline/neck mass near hyoid bone. Following incision of the deep cervical fascia, the cyst is freed from secondary structures (Fig 7.10-1). Since the duct is in close association with the hyoid bone, the mid-portion of the bone should be excised with the cyst. The dissection is continued superiorly and posteriorly to the foramen caecum. If the duct is not entirely removed, recurrence is very likely.

**Usual preop diagnosis**: Thyroglossal duct cyst

### SUMMARY OF PROCEDURE

| | |
|---|---|
| **Position** | Supine, with neck in hyper-extended position |
| **Incision** | Transverse skin incision |
| **Surgical time** | 1 - 1.5 hrs |
| **Closing considerations** | Careful hemostasis |
| **EBL** | 25-50 ml |
| **Mortality** | < 0.1% |
| **Morbidity** | Bleeding: < 5%<br>Infection: < 5% |
| **Procedure code** | 60280 |
| **Pain score** | 5-7 |

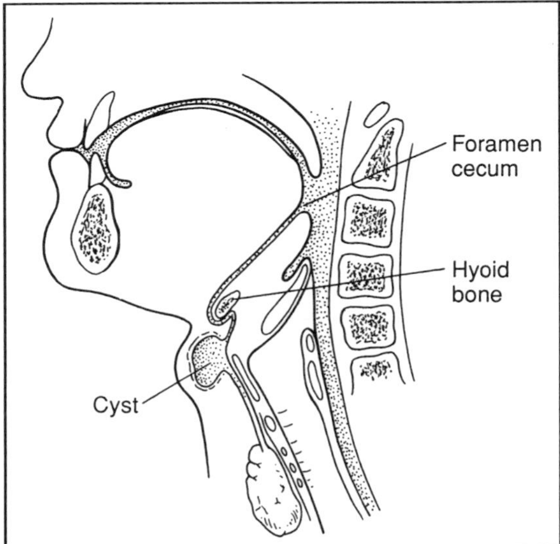


**Figure 7.10-1.** Course of thyroglossal duct, with cyst. (Reproduced with permission from Healey JE Jr: *Surgical Anatomy*, 2nd edition. BC Decker: 1990.)

### PATIENT POPULATION CHARACTERISTICS

| | |
|---|---|
| **Age range** | 10-20 yrs |
| **Male:Female** | 1:1 |
| **Incidence** | Not uncommon |
| **Etiology** | Persistence of undifferentiated epithelial cells in area of hyoid bone that later became squamous-cell epithelium or glandular tissue |

## ANESTHETIC CONSIDERATIONS

See Anesthetic Considerations following "Thyroidectomy" (below).

**References**


1. Nora PF, ed: *Operative Surgery*, 3rd edition. WB Saunders Co, Philadelphia: 1990, Ch 7.

# THYROIDECTOMY

## SURGICAL CONSIDERATIONS

**Description**: Thyroidectomy, partial or total, is performed for benign and malignant conditions. Through a transverse collar incision, the thyroid gland is exposed by dividing the strap muscles in the neck. The thyroid lobe is freed from the strap muscles by sharp/blunt dissection, which exposes the superior thyroid vessels (Fig 7.10-2). The latter are clamped, cut and ligated, with care being taken not to injure the superior laryngeal nerves. Following division of the middle thyroid vein and inferior thyroid vessels, the thyroid gland is retracted medially and its remaining attachments severed. Again, care is taken not to injure the recurrent laryngeal nerve or the parathyroid glands. Any enlarged or suspicious lymph nodes should be excised for biopsy. If a **total thyroidectomy** is to be performed, the isthmus and opposite lobe are removed as described above. Again, it is important to preserve the parathyroid glands. Careful hemostasis is achieved prior to suturing the strap muscle of the neck and wound closure. Drains are optional. When a **subtotal thyroidectomy** is performed, a rim of the posteriorly located thyroid gland is preserved. Clamps are placed across the gland at a safe distance from the region of the recurrent laryngeal nerve. The superior thyroid vessels are mobilized and ligated, with care being taken not to injure the superior laryngeal nerves. Following division of the middle thyroid vein and inferior thyroid vessels, the thyroid gland is removed subtotally or totally, again with care being taken not to injure the recurrent laryngeal nerves or parathyroid glands. Careful hemostasis is achieved prior to suturing the strap muscles of the neck and wound closure.

**Usual preop diagnosis**: Thyroid tumors; thyroiditis

### SUMMARY OF PROCEDURE

| | |
|---|---|
| **Position** | Supine with head elevated to 30° |
| **Incision** | Transverse collar |
| **Surgical time** | 1 - 2 hrs |
| **Closing considerations** | Adequate hemostasis |
| **EBL** | 50-75 ml |
| **Postop care** | Observe for postop respiratory problems, hypocalcemia, bleeding |
| **Mortality** | < 0.5% |
| **Morbidity** | Hypoparathyroidism: 2-3%<br>Bleeding: 0.3-1%<br>Respiratory obstruction<br>Thyroid storm<br>Wound infection<br>Recurrent laryngeal nerve damage: 0.2%<br>Superior laryngeal nerve damage<br>Hoarseness |
| **Procedure code** | 60220 (total thyroid lobectomy, unilateral); 60225 (total thyroid lobectomy, with contralateral); 60240 (thyroidectomy, total); 60245 (subtotal or partial) |
| **Pain score** | 5-7 |

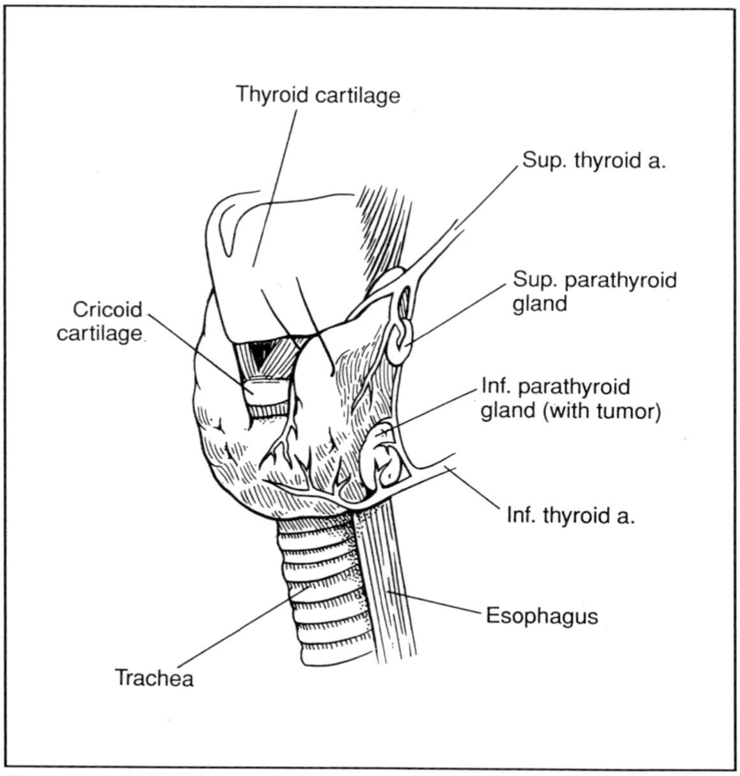

**Figure 7.10-2.** Blood supply to the thyroid gland. (Reproduced with permission from Healey JE Jr: *Surgical Anatomy*, 2nd edition. BC Decker: 1990.)

### PATIENT POPULATION CHARACTERISTICS

**Age range** 20-60 yrs

**Male:Female** 1:6 for hyperthyroidism
5:8 for thyroid cancer

**Incidence** Common

**Etiology** Malignant tumors: 0.1%
Iodine deficiency: >10%

**Associated conditions** Other endocrine disorders (e.g., parathyroid adenoma, gastrinoma, pituitary adenoma, adrenal adenoma)

---

## ANESTHETIC CONSIDERATIONS

### PREOPERATIVE

Hyperthyroidism may be 2° Graves's disease, toxic multinodular goiter, thyroid adenomas, TSH-secreting tumor, thyroiditis or overdosage of thyroid hormone. Common Sx are sweating, intolerance to heat, increased appetite, ↑HR, weight loss or gain, thyroid goiter, exophthalmos. Hypothyroidism may be iatrogenic or 2° autoimmune thyroiditis. Common Sx are intolerance to cold, anorexia, fatigue, weight gain or loss, constipation, ↓HR. Patients presenting for thyroidectomy are usually made euthyroid prior to surgery and may be taking one or more of the following medications: propylthiouracil, methimazole, potassium iodide, glucocorticoids or ß-blockers. The focus of the preop visit is to assure that the patient is in a physiologically euthyroid state.

**Respiratory** Beware of tracheal compression with large goiters.
Hyperthyroid: ↑BMR → ↑$VO_2$ → rapid desaturation on induction.
Hypothyroid: ↓ventilatory response to ↑$CO_2$ and ↓$O_2$ (beware of opioids and sedatives).
**Tests:** CXR; consider preop CT scan of neck to evaluate possible tracheal involvement, especially in patients with large goiters.

**Cardiovascular** Hyperthyroid: Tachycardia, atrial fibrillation, palpitations, CHF. A normal resting HR is helpful in determining whether or not the patient is ready for surgery. If the situation calls for it (e.g., emergency surgery), the patient can be treated with ß-blockers to blunt the sympathomimetic effects of the hyperthyroid state. ß-blocker therapy can be problematic in patients with CHF (titrate while monitoring filling pressures and CO).
Hypothyroid: Bradydysrythmias, diastolic HTN, pericardial effusions, ↓voltage of ECG. Thyroid replacement must be weighed against the risk of precipitating myocardial ischemia. Addison's disease is more common in patients with hypothyroidism; some patients may receive a "stress dose" of steroids (hydrocortisone 300 mg iv) in the perioperative period.
**Tests:** ECG; consider ECHO for evaluation of LV function

**Endocrine**

| | T4 | T3ru | T3 | TSH |
|---|---|---|---|---|
| Hyperthyroid | ↑ | ↑ | ↑ | Normal or ↓ |
| 1° hypothyroid | ↓ | ↓ | ↓ or normal | ↑ |
| 2° hypothyroid | ↓ | ↓ | ↓ | ↓ |

**Tests:** Thyroid function, calcium, Mg, phosphate, alkaline phosphatase, glucose

**Thyroid storm** A life-threatening exacerbation of hyperthyroidism occurring during periods of stress, which is manifested by hyperthermia, cardiac instability, anxiety, altered mental state and tachycardia. Rx: ↑$FiO_2$, sodium iodide (1-2.5 gm iv) + hydrocortisone (100 mg iv) + ß-blockers qs; maintain fluids, electrolytes.

**Myxedema coma** Severe hypothyroidism constituting a medical emergency, with mortality of >50%. Manifestations include stupor or coma, hypothermia, hypoventilation with hypoxemia, bradycardia, hypotension, apathy, hoarseness and hyponatremia. Rx: T4 (400-500 μg loading dose; 50-200 μg maintenance dose qd), hydrocortisone (100-300 mg iv qd).

**Neurological** Hyperthyroid: warm, moist skin, nervousness, anxiety (may require generous sedation).
Hypothyroid: ↓BMR → slow mentation and movement, cold intolerance.

| | |
|---|---|
| **Musculoskeletal** | Hyperthyroid: higher incidence of myasthenia gravis (↑sensitivity to muscle relaxants), skeletal muscle weakness (↑sensitivity to muscle relaxants), clubbing of the fingers, weight loss. Hypothyroid: arthralgias and myalgias. |
| **Renal** | Hypothyroid: impaired renal function 2° amyloidosis, urinary retention, oliguria. **Tests:** BUN; creatinine; electrolytes |
| **Hematologic** | Hyperthyroid: mild anemia, thrombocytopenia. Hypothyroid: coagulation abnormalities, anemia. **Tests:** CBC; PT; PTT |
| **Gastrointestinal** | Hyperthyroid: weight loss and diarrhea. Hypothyroid: GI bleeding, constipation, ileus. **Tests:** CBC; electrolytes; albumin; transaminases |
| **Laboratory** | Other tests as indicated from H&P. |
| **Premedication** | Diazepam 10 mg po or midazolam 0.7-0.8 mg/kg im. Continue antithyroid medications preop. Hyperthyroid patients should be made euthyroid prior to elective surgery and may be on the following drugs: propylthiouracil, methimazole, potassium iodide, ß-blockers and glucocorticoids. Hypothyroid patients can undergo surgery if they have mild-to-moderate disease. If the patient is severely hypothyroid, she/he should be given thyroid replacement prior to elective surgery. |

## INTRAOPERATIVE

**Anesthetic technique:** Normally, GETA; infrequently, under local anesthesia. Hyperthyroid: establish an adequate depth of anesthesia to prevent an exaggerated sympathetic response to surgical stimulation. Avoid agents that stimulate the sympathetic nervous system (e.g., ketamine, pancuronium, meperidine).

| | |
|---|---|
| **Induction** | Standard induction (see Appendix). If the patient has airway compromise 2° a large thyroid goiter, consider an awake fiber optic intubation (see Anesthetic Considerations for "Thoracolumbar Neurosurgical Procedures" in "Neurosurgery" section). |
| **Maintenance** | Standard maintenance (see Appendix). |
| **Emergence** | Airway obstruction 2° recurrent laryngeal nerve damage, tracheomalacia, or hematoma can occur. Consider visualizing vocal cord function prior to extubation. |

| | | |
|---|---|---|
| **Blood and fluid requirements** | Minimal blood loss<br>IV: 18 ga x 1<br>NS/LR @ 5-8 cc/kg/hr<br>Head-up position | Slight head-up position can help make for a bloodless surgical field. |
| **Monitoring** | Standard monitors (see Appendix). | + Others as indicated by patient's status. Maintain temperature, especially in hypothyroid patients. |
| **Positioning** | ✓ and pad pressure points.<br>✓ eyes. | Supine, with head slightly hyperextended, allows for surgical exploration of the neck. |
| **Complications** | Cardiorespiratory depression<br>Sedation | In hypothyroid patients, marked ↓BP, ↓RR and sedation may occur with minimal anesthetic doses. |

## POSTOPERATIVE

| | | |
|---|---|---|
| **Complications** | Recurrent laryngeal nerve damage | Bilateral: patient will be unable to speak and will require re-intubation. Unilateral: characterized by hoarseness. |
| | Tracheomalacia or hematoma with airway compromise | Rx: acute airway obstruction may occur immediately postop, and rapid re-intubation may be life-saving. If airway compromise is 2° hematoma, reopen incision and drain remaining blood; if patient still requires artificial airway, consider awake re-intubation. |
| | Acute hypoparathyroid state (hypocalcemia) | Acute hypocalcemia can present as laryngeal stridor (24-48 hrs postop). Rx: measure $Ca^{++}$; replace if necessary. |
| | Thyroid storm | Can mimic malignant hyperthermia (MH). |
| **Pain management** | PCA morphine (see Appendix). | |
| **Tests** | Vocal cord function | Ability to phonate "e" implies continued vocal cord function. |

**References**

1. Schwartz SI: *Principles of Surgery*, 3rd edition. McGraw-Hill, New York: 1979, Vol 2, Ch 38.
2. Graf G, Rosenbaum SH: Anesthesia and the endocrine system. In *Clinical Anesthesia*. Barash PG, Cullen BF, Stoelting RK, eds. JB Lippincott, Philadelphia: 1992, 1237-65.
3. Sieber FE: Evaluation of the patient with endocrine disease and diabetes mellitus. In *Principles and Practice of Anesthesiology*. Rogers MC, Tinker JH, Covino BG, Longnecker DE, eds. Mosby-Year Book Inc., St. Louis: 1993, 278-84.
4. Brown BR: Anesthetic management of endocrine emergencies. *ASA Annual Refresher Course Lectures* 1992; 224:1-7.
5. Roizen MF: Diseases of the endocrine system. In *Anesthesia and Uncommon Diseases*. Katz J, Benumof JL, Kadis LB, eds. WB Saunders Co, Philadelphia: 1990, 254-62.


# PARATHYROIDECTOMY

## SURGICAL CONSIDERATIONS

**Description:** Through a transverse cervical incision, the thyroid gland is exposed and the strap muscles dissected to increase the exposure of the parathyroid glands. It is necessary to divide the superior thyroid vessels to free the upper lobe for visualization of the superior parathyroid glands. The inferior glands are located near the junction of the inferior thyroid artery and the recurrent laryngeal nerve (Fig 7.10-3). Hemostasis is required in order to visualize the parathyroid glands easily. It is important to identify all four parathyroid glands. When one or more adenomas are present, they are excised, along with one normal gland or part of a normal gland. If the adenoma cannot be found in the neck, tissue from the upper aspect of the superior mediastinum is resected. If one parathyroid cannot be identified on a side, thyroid lobectomy should be performed, since the adenoma may be located within the thyroid substance. If operation is performed for hyperplasia, all glands are removed except for one-half of one gland. Some surgeons preserve parathyroid tissue by freezing it in case subsequent hypoparathyroidism develops. The preserved tissue may be transplanted into various muscles.

**Usual preop diagnosis:** Parathyroid adenoma; parathyroid hyperplasia (primary, secondary or tertiary); parathyroid carcinoma

### SUMMARY OF PROCEDURE

| | |
|---|---|
| **Position** | Supine; roll beneath thoracic spine |
| **Incision** | Transverse cervical |
| **Special instrumentation** | Thyroid retractor |
| **Antibiotics** | Cefotetan 1 gm iv preop |
| **Surgical time** | 1 - 2 hrs |
| **EBL** | 25-50 cc |
| **Postop care** | Monitor serum $Ca^{++}$ (Normal=8.5-10.5 mg% total $Ca^{++}$; 1-1.3 mM ionized $Ca^{++}$) |
| **Mortality** | < 0.5% |
| **Morbidity** | Hypocalcemia: < 15%<br>Hypoparathyroidism: < 5%<br>Recurrent laryngeal paralysis: < 3% |
| **Procedure code** | 60500 |
| **Pain score** | 5-6 |

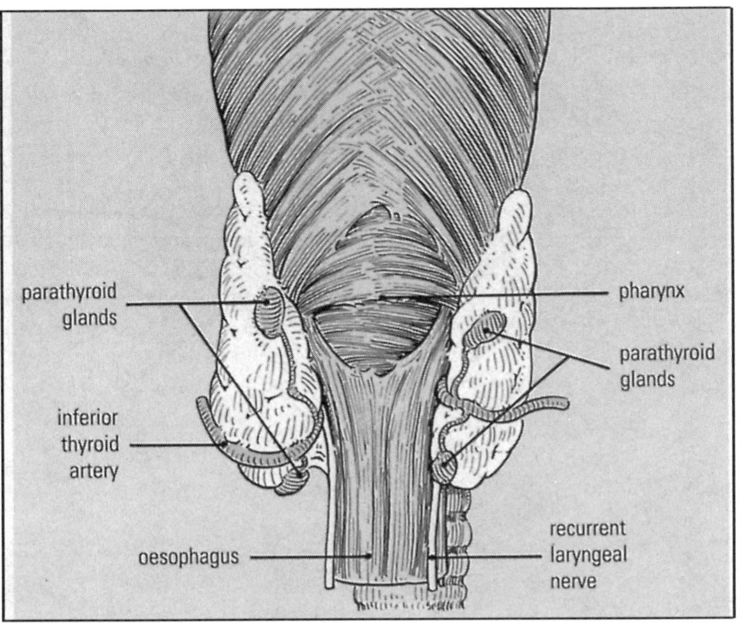


**Figure 7.10-3.** Common position of parathyroid glands (posterior view). (Reproduced with permission from Calne R, Pollard SG: *Operative Surgery*. Gower Medical Pub: 1992)

## PATIENT POPULATION CHARACTERISTICS

| | |
|---|---|
| **Age range** | Increases with age |
| **Male:Female** | 1:2 |
| **Incidence** | 50-100/100,000 |
| **Etiology** | Hyperplasia: 10-15%<br>Cancer: 1% |
| **Associated conditions** | Bone disease: 5-15%<br>Duodenal ulcer: 5-10%<br>Renal calculi |

---

# ANESTHETIC CONSIDERATIONS

## PREOPERATIVE

These patients typically present with hypercalcemia (hyperparathyroidism), which must be controlled prior to surgery. Although 25-50% of cases are asymptomatic, many will present with a variety of Sx, including fatigue, muscle weakness, depression, anorexia, nausea, constipation, abdominal and bone pain, HTN, renal stones and polydipsia. Differential diagnosis for the hypercalcemic patient includes: metastatic disease, multiple myeloma, milk-alkali syndrome, vitamin D intoxication, sarcoidosis, hyperthyroidism, thiazide diuretics, adrenal insufficiency, Paget's disease, immobilization or an exogenous parathyroid hormone-producing tumor.

**Respiratory** — Decreased clearance of secretions from the tracheobronchial tree. Respiratory or metabolic acidosis (will increase the free fraction of calcium, leading to manifestations of hypercalcemia).
**Tests:** As indicated from H&P

**Cardiovascular** — HTN (usually resolves with treatment); ECG may show tachycardia, ↑PR, ↑QRS and ↓QT intervals ± heart block. Patients may have increased sensitivity to digitalis, resistance to catecholamines and hypovolemia (2° anorexia, nausea, vomiting and polyuria). Preop management includes correction of intravascular volume and electrolyte abnormalities. Preop treatment of hypercalcemia may include expansion of intravascular volume and diuresis in order to increase renal calcium excretion, usually accomplished with iv NS and furosemide. Hypophosphatemia can impair myocardial contractility and should be corrected; hemodialysis or peritoneal dialysis can be used to lower dangerously elevated serum calcium levels. Mithramycin is not useful for acute Rx of ↑$Ca^{++}$.
**Tests:** ECG; electrolytes; others as indicated from H&P.

**Neurological** — Patient may present with seizures, hyporeflexia, mental status changes (somnolence, depression, memory loss, psychosis, coma) or peripheral neuropathy. Significant improvement may follow correction of hypercalcemia.

**Musculoskeletal** — These patients may have muscle atrophy and weakness, osteopenia, arthralgia, pathologic fractures (careful laryngoscopy and positioning), osteitis fibrosa cystica. Response to neuromuscular blockers may be enhanced 2° ↑$Ca^{++}$ → muscle weakness.

**Hematologic** — Patients also tend to be hypophosphatemic and may show signs of hemolysis, platelet dysfunction, impaired ventricular contractility and leukocyte dysfunction.
**Tests:** CBC with platelet count; bleeding time

**Endocrine** — Primary hyperparathyroidism is most commonly due to benign parathyroid adenoma (90%), or hyperplasia (9%) and rarely to carcinoma. It may be associated with multiple endocrine adenopathy syndrome. MEA-1 consists of tumors of the parathyroid, pancreatic islets and pituitary. MEA-2 consists of pheochromocytoma, mucosal neuromas, parathyroid tumors and medullary thyroid carcinoma.
**Tests:** As indicated from H&P.

**Renal** — Patients may have renal dysfunction 2° nephrolithiasis, nephrocalcinosis, renal tubular disorders and glomerular disorders. Polyuria 2° ↑$Ca^{++}$ → electrolyte disturbances.
**Tests:** Renal function tests

**Laboratory** — Serum calcium (< 12 mg/dL likely asymptomatic; 12-14 mg/dL, mild symptoms; >16 mg/dL, life-threatening), albumin (increase in albumin by 1 gm/dL will increase total serum calcium by 0.8 mg/dL); electrolytes; glucose; magnesium; phosphate (usually low).

**Premedication** All medications to lower hypercalcemia should be continued unless calcium levels have normalized. If patient has been treated with steroids in the preop period, administer a stress dose (hydrocortisone 100 mg iv q 8 hrs x 24 hrs) prior to induction of anesthesia and continue into the early postop period. Standard premedications (see Appendix) are usually appropriate in this patient group.

## INTRAOPERATIVE

**Anesthetic technique:** GETA, with head slightly hyperextended, allows for surgical exploration of the neck.

**Induction** Standard induction (see Appendix). If patient is clinically hypovolemic, restore intravascular volume prior to induction and titrate induction dose of sedative/hypnotic agents.

**Maintenance** Standard maintenance (see Appendix), with muscle relaxant titrated to effect, using peripheral nerve stimulator. Avoid hyperventilation or hypoventilation (acidosis will increase calcium levels, while alkalosis will lower calcium levels). Maintain adequate hydration and UO throughout the procedure.

**Emergence** No special considerations (see postop complications).

| | | |
|---|---|---|
| **Blood and fluid requirements** | Minimal blood loss<br>IV: 18 ga x 1<br>NS @ 5-8 cc/kg/hr | Avoid calcium-containing iv solution (e.g., LR). |
| **Monitoring** | Standard monitors (see Appendix) | Others as indicated by patient status |
| **Positioning** | ✓ and pad all pressure points.<br>✓ eyes. Carefully protect eyes (ophthalmic ointment and tape). | Patients should be carefully positioned as they tend to be osteopenic and are prone to pathologic bone fractures. Slight head-up position may ↓blood loss and improve surgical visibility. |
| **Complications** | Hypocalcemia | See postop complications (below). |

## POSTOPERATIVE

| | | |
|---|---|---|
| **Complications** | Hypocalcemia<br>Hypophosphatemia<br>Hypocalcemic tetany<br>Seizures | Hypocalcemia may occur in the immediate postop period. Sx include parathesias, muscle spasm, tetany, as well as laryngospasm, bronchospasm and apnea. Rx: includes 10-20 cc calcium gluconate 10% over 10 min. Follow levels and repeat therapy until the clinical signs of hypocalcemia are controlled. |
| | Recurrent laryngeal nerve injury<br>Laryngeal edema 2° surgical manipulation<br>Stridor<br>Laryngospasm<br>Hematoma with airway compromise | Recurrent laryngeal nerve dysfunction can be monitored by having the patient vocalize the letter "e." Unilateral vocal cord dysfunction results in hoarseness, while bilateral vocal cord dysfunction results in aphonia. |
| | Pneumothorax | Dx: pleuritic chest pain, dyspnea, ↑RR, ↓breath sounds, hypoxemia; ✓ CXR. Rx: $O_2$; chest tube and re-intubation as necessary. |
| **Pain management** | PCA (see Appendix). | |
| **Tests** | Serial measurements of:<br>Calcium<br>Phosphate<br>Magnesium<br>Others as clinically indicated<br>CXR to rule out pneumothorax | The lowest calcium level is usually seen after 4-5 d postop. Follow clinical signs of hypocalcemia: Trousseau's sign – carpopedal spasm in response to application of a BP cuff at a level above SBP for 3 min. Chvostek's sign – contracture of the facial muscles produced by tapping on the facial nerve. |

**References**

1. Wang C: The anatomic basis of parathyroid surgery. *Ann Surg* 1976; 183(3):271-75.
2. Graf G, Rosenbaum SH: Anesthesia and the endocrine system. In *Clinical Anesthesia.* Barash PG, Cullen BF, Stoelting RK, eds. JB Lippincott, Philadelphia: 1989. 1191-93.
3. Roizen MF: Diseases of the endocrine system. In *Anesthesia and Uncommon Diseases*, 3rd edition. Katz J, Benumof JL, Kadis LB, eds. W.B. Saunders Co, Philadelphia: 1990, 245-55.


# ADRENALECTOMY

## SURGICAL CONSIDERATIONS

**Description:** **Adrenalectomy** is performed for cortical and medullary tumors or hyperplasia (Fig 7.10-4). The glands are removed by sharp/blunt dissection, with care being taken not to injure the adrenal vein. The latter should be exposed and ligated, avoiding damage to the vena cavae on the right side and the renal vein on the left side. Through a midline or subcostal incision, the left adrenal gland is best exposed by incising the lateral peritoneal attachment of the spleen, allowing it to be mobilized and retracted medially along with the tail of the pancreas. Gerota's fascia is then incised at the upper pole of the left kidney, exposing the adrenal gland. The adrenal is mobilized by sharp/blunt dissection until the prominent adrenal vein is exposed. It is then carefully transected between ligatures and the adrenal gland removed. On the right side, the adrenal is exposed by retracting the right lobe of the liver cephalad and depressing the hepatic flexure inferiorly. After incising the peritoneum lateral to the duodenum, and mobilizing the latter, the IVC is exposed. The right kidney is pulled downward, the adrenal gland is visualized, along with the right adrenal vein entering the vena cava. On occasion, there may be two adrenal veins that require ligating. Once the adrenal vein has been secured, the adrenal gland is easily removed by blunt dissection, ligating any significant vascular attachments.

**Variant procedure or approaches:** The adrenals may be approached **transabdominally** or via a **flank approach**. The flank, or posterior approach is preferred for unilateral adrenalectomy. A portion of the 12th rib is resected, exposing Gerota's fascia. After incising the fascia, the adrenal gland is exposed, mobilized and resected, following ligation of the adrenal vein. The abdominal or posterior approach is indicated for bilateral lesions.

**Usual preop diagnosis:** Cushing's syndrome; aldosteronism; pheochromocytoma; other adrenal tumors

**SUMMARY OF PROCEDURE**

| | Transabdominal | Flank or Posterior |
|---|---|---|
| **Position** | Supine | Nephrectomy or prone jackknife |
| **Incision** | Midline abdominal or bilateral subcostal | Dorsal flank oblique or curved posterior |
| **Special instrumentation** | Denier retractor | None |
| **Unique considerations** | BP monitoring essential for pheochromocytoma patients | ⇐ |
| **Antibiotics** | None | ⇐ |
| **Surgical time** | 1 - 2 hrs | ⇐ |
| **Closing considerations** | Hemostasis | ⇐ |
| **EBL** | 200-300 ml | ⇐ |
| **Postop care** | Continue monitoring BP; PACU → room; ± ICU | ⇐ |
| **Mortality** | 5.6% (Cushing's) | ⇐ |
| **Morbidity** | Respiratory difficulties: 26% | ⇐ |
| | Wound problems: 9% | |
| | Hemorrhage: 3% | ⇐ |
| | Venous thrombosis with embolism (Cushing's): 2% | |
| **Procedure code** | 60540 | ⇐ |
| **Pain score** | 6-8 | 7-9 |

## PATIENT POPULATION CHARACTERISTICS

| | |
|---|---|
| **Age range** | 13-75 yrs |
| **Male:Female** | 1:2.8 |
| **Incidence** | Pheochromocytoma: 0.4-2% of all hypertensive patients<br>Primary hyperaldosteronism: 100/yr<br>Cushing's syndrome: 6/million |
| **Etiology** | Adenoma or adenocarcinoma: 90%<br>Ectopic ACTH: 15% of patients with Cushing's<br>Cushing's syndrome: 10-15% |
| **Associated conditions** | HTN: 75-80%<br>Diabetes: 10-15% |

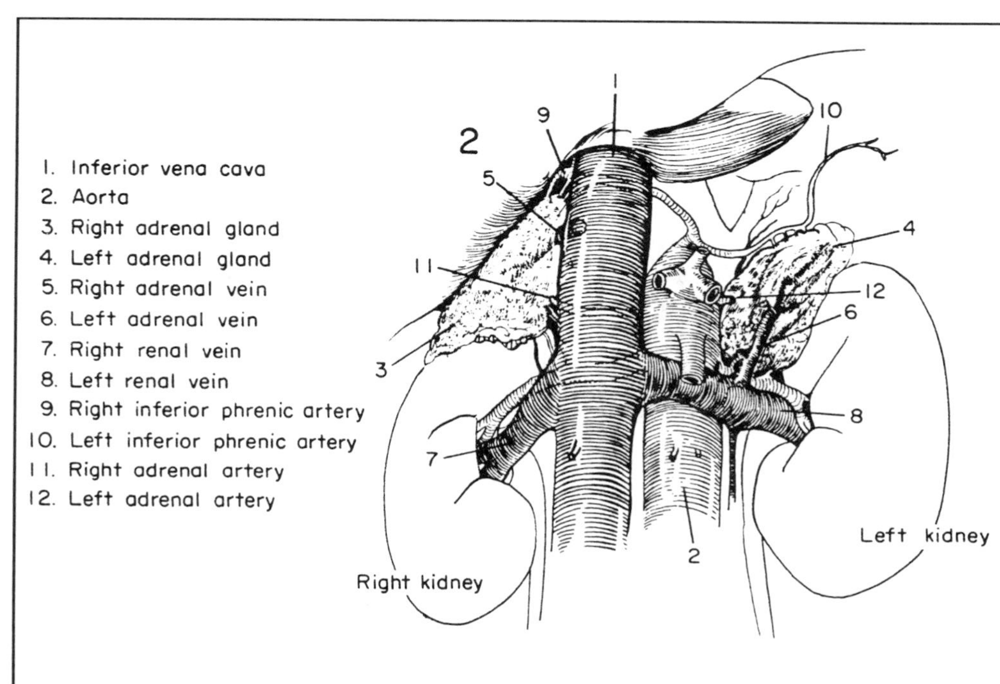


**Figure 7.10-4.** Surgical anatomy for an adrenalectomy. (Reproduced from Zollinger RM Jr, Zollinger RM: *Atlas of Surgical Operations*, 6th edition. Macmillan: 1988.)

---

# ANESTHETIC CONSIDERATIONS

## PREOPERATIVE

**Cushing's syndrome:** Hyperadrenocorticism can be due to adrenal hyperplasia, adrenal carcinoma, pituitary hypersecretion, hypersecretion from exogenous tumor, or exogenous steroid administration. Adrenalectomy is the traditional treatment for hyperadrenocorticism due to adrenal carcinoma.

**Pheochromocytoma:** Tumors of chromaffin tissue origin release massive amounts of catecholamines (norepinephrine > epinephrine) and are responsible for the patient's clinical presentation. The tumor is usually found unilaterally in one of the adrenal glands, but also can be found anywhere in the body that chromaffin tissue arises (e.g., urinary bladder, sympathetic chain). These patients require extensive preop preparation, consisting of α-blockade (phenoxybenzamine 40-100 mg/d) and concomitant volume expansion. Patients with tachydysrhythmias may require ß-blockade only after institution of the α-blockers to prevent serious hypertensive sequelae. Adrenergic blockade and volume expansion may take up to 2 weeks prior to surgical removal of the tumor. Inadequate preop preparation will increase the perioperative morbidity of patients with pheochromocytomas. The adequacy of medical therapy is assessed by the absence of symptoms of catecholamine excess, BP of ≤ 160/90 on 2 measurements in the 36 hours preceding surgery, SBP dropping by ≥ 15% on standing, but not less than an absolute BP of 80/45; no ST-T wave changes for 2 weeks prior to surgery. There is an increased incidence of pheochromocytoma in certain diseases (multiple-endocrine neoplasia II, neurofibromatosis, tuberous sclerosis, Sturge-Weber syndrome, von Hippel-Lindau disease).

**Respiratory** Cushing's syndrome: Patient may be obese with all attendant problems of morbid obesity (see Preoperative Considerations in "Gastroplasty for Morbid Obesity" in "Stomach Surgery").
**Tests:** As indicated from H&P.

**Cardiovascular** Cushing's syndrome: HTN (from hypervolemia), dysrhythmias 2° hypokalemia
Pheochromocytoma: Paroxysmal HTN, tachydysrhythmias, orthostatic hypotension, hypovolemia, myocardial dysfunction, cardiomyopathy, ventricular ectopy, ↓intravascular volume, ↓sensitivity of α-receptors to normal levels of catecholamines, CHF.
**Tests:** ECG; orthostatic vital signs; ECHO or MUGA scan, to evaluate LV function.

**Renal** Cushing's syndrome: Excess steroid production → Na retention and K excretion and glucose intolerance (hyperglycemia).
Pheochromocytoma: HTN from excess catecholamine state may damage kidneys, hyperglycemia.
**Tests:** UA; urine concentrations of catecholamine metabolites; others as appropriate

**Neurological** Cushing's syndrome: Psychiatric changes, headache
Pheochromocytoma: Tremulousness, headache, anxiety, nervousness, paresthesia in arms, hypertensive retinopathy, dilated pupils

**Musculoskeletal** Cushing's syndrome: Striae, muscular wasting, buffalo hump, truncal obesity, thin skin, easy bruisability, osteopenia (compression fractures), weakness
Pheochromocytoma: Weight loss, weakness, fatigue

**Hematologic** Cushing's syndrome: Polycythemia
Pheochromocytoma: Polycythemia (due to hemoconcentration)

**Laboratory** Tests as indicated from H&P.

**Premedication** Cushing's syndrome: Spironolactone often given to inhibit excess aldosterone effects. Midazolam (0.05-0.08 mg/kg), morphine (0.05-0.1 mg/kg im). Hydrocortisone 100 mg q 8 hrs.
Pheochromocytoma: Midazolam (0.05-0.08 mg/kg im); meperidine (0.75-1.5 mg/kg im). Preop steroid replacement if bilateral adrenalectomy is contemplated.

## INTRAOPERATIVE

**Anesthetic technique:** GETA (± epidural for postop analgesia). If postop epidural analgesia is planned, placement of catheter prior to anesthetic induction is helpful in establishing correct placement in the epidural space and assuring a bilateral block (accomplished by placing 5-7 cc of 1% lidocaine via the epidural and eliciting a segmental block).

**Induction** Gentle iv induction (titration to effect with STP or etomidate) and muscle relaxation (vecuronium 0.1 mg/kg). Patient should be adequately anesthetized prior to any stimulation. Unopposed parasympathetic response can occur to laryngoscopy with resultant bradycardia/asystole.

**Maintenance** **Balanced anesthesia:** volatile anesthetic (isoflurane), opiate, muscle relaxant. $N_2O$ can cause bowel distention and is best avoided. Local anesthetic (1.5-2% lidocaine **without** epinephrine (12-15 cc q 60 min) can be injected into the epidural catheter to provide both anesthesia and optimal surgical exposure (contracted bowel and profound muscle relaxation). Some anesthesiologists opt not to use the epidural catheter intraop because chemical "sympathectomy" is more difficult to reverse. The catheter can be effectively utilized for postop administration of opiates with good results. If epidural opiates are used for postop analgesia, a loading dose (e.g., hydromorphone 1.0 mg) should be administered at least 1 hr before the conclusion of surgery. Systemic sedatives (droperidol, opiates, benzodiazepines, etc.) should be minimized during this type of anesthetic as they increase the likelihood of postop respiratory depression. Intraop HTN is best treated with SNP, tachycardia with esmolol, and hypotension with phenylephrine or dopamine. Good communication with surgical team is very important, especially when the adrenal gland is being mobilized.

**Emergence** Depends on ease of the surgical procedure and the hemodynamic stability of the patient intraop. If patient is hemodynamically unstable, hypothermic, or has a large 3rd-space fluid requirement, consider postop ventilation in ICU. (Patients in this group will require postop care in ICU regardless.)

**Blood and fluid requirements**
Anticipate large fluid loss.
IV: 14-16 ga x 2
NS/LR @ 10-15 cc/kg/hr
Warm all fluids.
Humidify inhaled gasses.
Cell saver

Blood loss can be significant, and blood should be immediately available. If procedure does not involve cancer, cell-saving devices can be utilized. Guide fluid management by UO, filling pressures, CO.

| | | |
|---|---|---|
| **Monitoring** | Standard monitors (see Appendix).<br>UO<br>Arterial line<br>± PA catheter | Others as clinically indicated (e.g., PA catheter for patients with pheochromocytoma). |
| **Positioning** | ✓ and pad pressure points.<br>✓ eyes. | Strict attention to patient positioning and padding are important in patients with glucocorticoid excess because of osteopenia and thin, easily bruised skin. |

### POSTOPERATIVE

| | | |
|---|---|---|
| **Complications** | Pneumothorax (incidence approaches 20%)<br>Hypoglycemia<br>Hypoadrenocorticism after tumor resection<br>Cushing's syndrome:<br>Hypoventilation 2° to obesity (hypoxemia, hypercarbia)<br>HTN<br>Pheochromocytoma:<br>BP lability<br>Myocardial dysfunction | Dx: pleuritic chest pain, dyspnea, ↑RR, ↓breath sounds, hypoxemia. ✓ CXR. Rx: $O_2$; chest tube and reintubation as necessary.<br>Consider glucocorticoid and mineralocorticoid replacement – hydrocortisone 100 mg q 8 hrs. |
| **Pain management** | Epidural analgesia (see Appendix).<br>PCA (see Appendix). | Patient should be recovered in an ICU or ward accustomed to treating the side-effects of epidural opiates (e.g., respiratory depression, break-through pain, nausea, pruritus). |
| **Tests** | CXR; ECG; electrolytes; glucose | |

**References**

1. Watson RG, van Heerden JA, Northcutt RC, Grant CS, Ilstrup DM: Results of adrenal surgery for Cushing's syndrome: 10 years' experience. *World J Surg* 1986; 10(4):531-38.
2. Roizen MF, Schreider BD, Hassan SZ: Anesthesia for patients with pheochromocytoma. *Anes Clin North Am* 1987; 5:269.
3. Desmonts JM, le Houelleur J, Remond P, Duvaldedestin D: Anaesthetic management of patients with phaeochromocytoma. A review of 102 cases. *Br J Anaesth* 1977; 49(10):991-98.
4. Roizen MF: Anesthetic implications of concurrent diseases. In *Anesthesia*. Miller RD, ed. Churchill Livingstone, New York: 1990, 804-10.
5. Cousins MJ, Rubin RB: The intraoperative management of pheochromocytoma with total epidural sympathetic blockade. *Br J Anaesth* 1974; 46(1):78-81.
6. Roizen MF, Horrigan RW, Koike M, et al: A perspective randomized trial of four anesthetic techniques for resection of pheochromocytoma. *Anesthesiology* 1982; 57:A43.
7. Sieber FE: Evaluation of the patient with endocrine disease and diabetes mellitus. In *Principles and Practice of Anesthesiology*. Rogers MC, Tinker JH, Covino BG, Longnecker DE, eds. Mosby-Year Book, Inc, St Louis: 1993, 278-98.
8. Christopherson R: Anesthesia for endocrine surgery. In *Principles and Practice of Anesthesiology*. Rogers MC, Tinker JH, Covino BG, Longnecker DE, eds. Mosby-Year Book, Inc, St. Louis: 1993, 2035-48.
9. Roizen MF, Hunt TK, Beaupre PN, et al: The effect of alpha-adrenergic blockade on cardiac performance and tissue oxygen delivery during excision of pheochromocytoma. *Surgery* 1983; 94(6):941-45.

**Surgeons**

**Edward J. Alfrey, MD**
**Donald C. Dafoe, MD**

## 7.11 LIVER/KIDNEY TRANSPLANTATION

**Anesthesiologists**

**Gordon R. Haddow, MB, ChB, FFA(SA)**
**Price Stover, MD**

# KIDNEY TRANSPLANT - CADAVERIC AND LIVING-RELATED DONOR

## SURGICAL CONSIDERATIONS

**Description**: Kidney transplantation offers patients with end-stage renal disease freedom from dialysis. Although kidneys are procured from either cadaveric or living-related donors (LRDs), use of a kidney from a healthy relative provides better histocompatibility, less rejection, fewer infectious complications and better long-term graft survival. During the procedure, a 3-way Foley catheter is placed in the recipient's bladder, and the kidney allograft is placed in the extraperitoneal iliac fossa. A curvilinear incision is made in the right or left lower quadrant. The dissection is maintained in the extraperitoneal space by retracting the peritoneum medial and cephalad; normally a Bookwalter retractor is used. The external iliac artery and vein are identified; surrounding lymphatics are divided after ligation; and the vessels are mobilized for several centimeters. The external iliac vein is clamped first and the renal-vein-to-iliac-vein anastomosis is performed. Then the externaliliac-artery-to-renal-arteryanastomosis is performed, and the clamps are released (Fig 7.11-1). The patient should be euvolemic at this point; mannitol and/or furosemide may be given. The bladder is filled with an antibiotic irrigation solution to allow reimplantation of the ureter, which is performed after the detrusor muscle of the bladder has been dissected away from the mucosa. The wound is closed, normally leaving native kidneys intact.

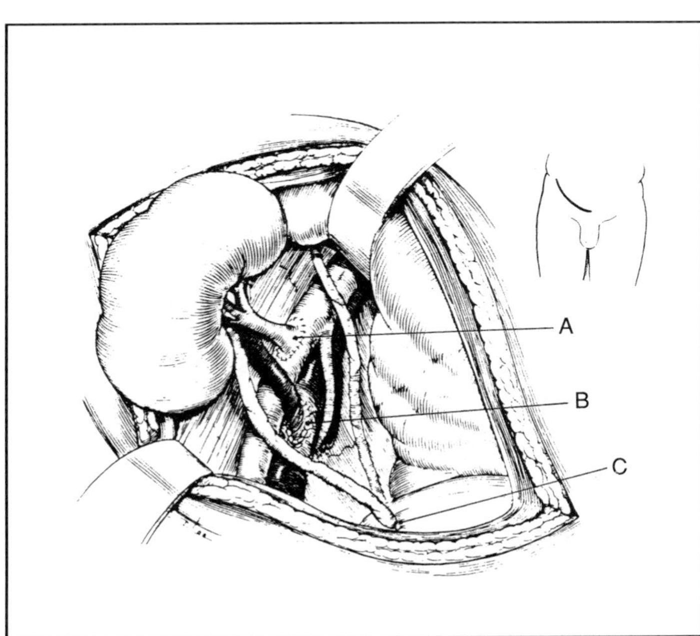


**Figure 7.11-1.** Kidney transplantation, showing anastomoses of: (A) renal artery to external iliac artery; (B) renal vein to iliac vein; and (C) ureter to bladder. To increase exposure of bladder for a ureteroneocystostomy, antibiotic solution is used to fill the bladder. Lower quadrant curvilinear incision is shown in inset. (Reproduced with permission from Hardy JD: *Hardy's Textbook of Surgery*, 2nd edition. JB Lippincott: 1988.)

**Variant procedure or approaches**: Cadaveric or LRD transplant

**Usual preop diagnosis**: End-stage renal disease

### SUMMARY OF PROCEDURE

| | Cadaveric | Living-Related Donor |
|---|---|---|
| **Position** | Supine | ⇐ |
| **Incision** | Lower quadrant curvilinear (Fig 7.11-1 inset) | ⇐ |
| **Special instrumentation** | Bookwalter retractor; vascular instruments; CVP; Foley catheter (3-way) | ⇐ |
| **Unique considerations** | Adequate hydration, CVP 10-12 mmHg; mannitol 12.5-25 gm; intraop immunosuppression prior to reperfusion (steroids, azathioprine 10 mg/kg); potassium-free iv fluid; protection of shunt or fistula important. | ⇐ |
| **Antibiotics** | Gentamicin 1.7 mg/kg; cefazolin 1 gm, 1 hr preop | Cefazolin 1 gm, 1 hr preop |
| **Surgical time** | 2.5 - 3 hrs | 3 hrs |
| **EBL** | 500 cc | ⇐ |

| | Cadaveric | Living-Related Donor |
|---|---|---|
| **Postop care** | Replace UO ml/ml; may have delayed graft function due to preservation and UO or clearance; ICU. | Fluid replacement; delayed graft function unlikely; ICU. |
| **Mortality** | 1% | ⇐ |
| **Morbidity** | Major: 5% | ⇐ |
| | Lymph or serous cell leak: 3-5% | ⇐ |
| | MI: 2-3% | ⇐ |
| | Urinary leak: 2-3% | ⇐ |
| | Wound infection: 2-3% | ⇐ |
| | Arterial thrombosis: 1-2% | ⇐ |
| | Venous thrombosis: 1-2% | ⇐ |
| | Wound hematoma: 1-2% | ⇐ |
| | Postop bleeding: < 1% | ⇐ |
| | Other infectious complications: 15-40% | ⇐ |
| **Procedure code** | 50360 | ⇐ |
| **Pain score** | 5 | 6 |

### PATIENT POPULATION CHARACTERISTICS

| | |
|---|---|
| **Age range** | 3-70 yrs |
| **Male:Female** | 1:1 |
| **Incidence** | 60/1,000,000 |
| **Etiology** | Glomerulonephritis: 25% |
| | HTN: 25% |
| | Diabetes: 25% |
| | Polycystic disease and others: 25% |
| **Associated conditions** | CAD: 40% |
| | HTN: 25% |
| | Uremic and/or diabetic neuropathy: 25% |
| | Hyperparathyroidism: 15-20% |

## ANESTHETIC CONSIDERATIONS

See Anesthetic Considerations following "Cadaveric Kidney/Pancreas Transplant" (below).

**References**

1. Morris PJ, ed: *Kidney Transplantation: principles and practice*, 2nd edition. Grune and Stratton, Orlando, FL: 1984.

# CADAVERIC KIDNEY/PANCREAS TRANSPLANT

## SURGICAL CONSIDERATIONS

**Description:** Patients with or near end-stage renal disease 2° diabetes mellitus (DM) can maintain relative normoglycemia with a successful pancreas transplant. The immunosuppressive requirements are no different than for a kidney transplant alone. The kidney transplant is placed in the iliac fossa on one side and the pancreas transplant is placed in the opposite iliac fossa, with the pancreas normally transplanted first (Fig 7.11-2). The graft is prepared first, on the back table. For the arterial in-flow, either a patch of aorta, including the superior mesenteric and celiac artery trunks, is utilized; or a Y-graft is fashioned, using the donor iliac artery bifurcation anastomosed to the graft splenic and superior mesenteric arteries. The graft portal vein is not reconstructed. The graft duodenal segment, which includes most of the C-loop of the duodenum, is shortened on the back table. The arterial anastomosis is accomplished by anastomosing either the aortic patch or the iliac extension to the donor external iliac artery. The portal vein is anastomosed to the external iliac vein. The bladder should be filled after revascularization of the pancreas to allow good visualization of it while the duodenal segment is sewn to the bladder. Pancreas transplants can have significant blood loss if the graft mesenteric vessels are not occluded properly. Once the pancreas is transplanted, the kidney transplant is placed into the opposite iliac fossa (as described in the preceding segments).

**Variant procedure or approaches**: Isolated islet cells have been transplanted beneath the renal capsule of a renal allograft or into native portal vein, but the success rate has been limited.

**Usual preop diagnosis**: End-stage renal disease 2° DM

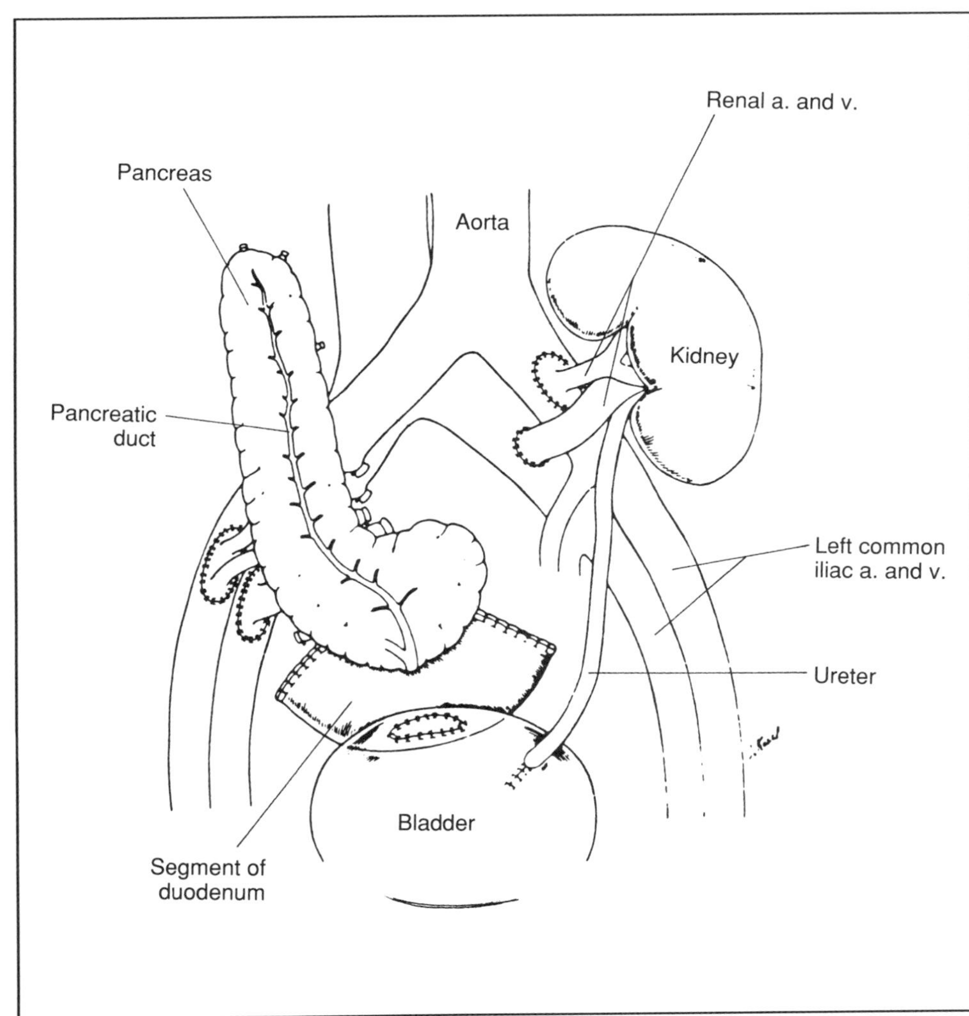


**Figure 7.11-2.** Transplantation of pancreas with bladder drainage through a pancreaticoduodenocystostomy. Renal transplant also shown. (Modified with permission from Moody FG, ed: *Surgical Treatment of Digestive Disease*, 2nd edition. Mosby-Year Book: 1990.)

### SUMMARY OF PROCEDURE

| | |
|---|---|
| **Position** | Supine (cushion heels) |
| **Incision** | Midline or bilateral lower quadrant |
| **Special instrumentation** | Bookwalter retractor; vascular instruments; Foley catheter; NG tube; CVP; arterial line |
| **Unique considerations** | Do not correct hyperglycemia < 300 mg/dL. Maintain adequate hydration, CVP 10-12 mmHg; mannitol 0.25-0.5 gm/kg on unclamping; intraop immunosuppression prior to reperfusion (1 gm methylprednisolone, 10 mg/kg azathioprine after incision); potassium-free iv fluid; protection of shunt or fistula important. |
| **Antibiotics** | Gentamicin (1.7/kg iv slowly), cefazolin (1 gm q 6 hrs for 5 d) |
| **Surgical time** | 5 - 6 hrs |
| **EBL** | 750 cc |
| **Postop care** | ICU x 1-2 d, hourly monitoring of glucose; serum glucose should decline by 50 mg/dL each hr and remain < 200 mg/dL. |
| **Mortality** | 2% |
| **Morbidity** | Infection: 20-60%<br>Major: 15%<br>Thrombosis of graft: 10%<br>Postop bleeding: 2-3% |
| **Procedure code** | 48999, 50360 |
| **Pain score** | 6 |

### PATIENT POPULATION CHARACTERISTICS

| | |
|---|---|
| **Age range** | 15-45 yrs |
| **Male:Female** | 1:1 |
| **Incidence** | 15-20% of all patients with end-stage renal disease |
| **Etiology** | Autoimmune |
| **Associated conditions** | Retinopathy: 100%<br>CAD: 50-70%<br>Uremic and/or diabetic neuropathy: 50%<br>Gastropathy: 25%<br>Hyperparathyroidism: 15-20% |

---

## ANESTHETIC CONSIDERATIONS FOR KIDNEY AND KIDNEY/PANCREAS TRANSPLANTATION

### PREOPERATIVE

Typically, patients presenting for renal transplantation fall into two patient populations: (1) the young and relatively healthy (following dialysis), or (2) an older, more chronically ill group. Rarely, patients will present for transplant surgery without adequate preparation (e.g., $\uparrow K^+$, $\downarrow$pH). Patients presenting for pancreas transplantation are usually severe diabetics with many of the associated problems, such as CAD, autonomic neuropathy, gastroparesis and stiff joint syndrome (difficult intubation).

| | |
|---|---|
| **Respiratory** | Pleuritis and pleural effusions may occur in this patient population. Increased susceptibility to infection is common in the patient with chronic uremia. |
| **Cardiovascular** | Pericarditis (acute or constrictive), HTN, CHF, dysrhythmias, pericardial effusion are common, especially in the un-dialized patient. Diabetes, a common cause of ESRD, is often associated with PVD, CAD and autonomic neuropathy.<br>**Tests:** ECG (rhythm, electrolyte abnormalities, pericarditis, LVH). Other tests (ECHO, stress, etc.) as indicated by H&P. |
| **Gastrointestinal** | Gastroparesis may occur, especially in diabetic patients with autonomic neuropathy. It is safer to assume that these patients will require full-stomach precautions. Ranitidine (50 mg iv) and |

metoclopramide (10 mg iv) should be given 60 min preop to aid gastric emptying and ↓acidity. Na citrate (30 cc, 0.3 M po) should be given immediately before induction.

**Renal** Patients are usually on dialysis. Post-dialysis goals include: $K^+$ = 4-5 mEq/L, BUN < 60 mg%, creatinine < 10 mg%. Metabolic acidosis, hypocalcemia and hypermagnesemia may be present, and require correction preop. Patient may be hypovolemic following dialysis; ✓ pre- and post-dialysis weight (>2 kg loss is significant). Rapid correction of severe hyperkalemia can be achieved by giving iv 50 cc of 50% glucose, together with 12 U regular insulin and 50 mEq $NaHCO_3$.

**Tests:** Creatinine; BUN; creatine clearance; electrolytes

**Hematologic** These patients are typically anemic (Hct = 18-24%). Usually it is not necessary to correct this anemia (unless < 18%). A coagulation disorder may be present with abnormal platelet function (improved by dialysis) and possibly thrombocytopenia, resulting in a prolonged bleeding time. There is a high incidence of post-transfusion hepatitis in this patient population.

**Tests:** Hct; PT; PTT; platelets; bleeding time; hepatic screen

**Neurologic** Peripheral neuropathy may occur and specific deficits should be documented. Autonomic neuropathy can lead to both cardiac (e.g., orthostatic hypotension, ↑HR or ↓HR), silent MI, and gastrointestinal problems.

**Premedication** Patients should continue their routine medications up to the time of surgery. A small dose of midazolam is usually a safe premedication for Rx anxiety. Consider the possibility of a full stomach and use full-stomach precautions (see Appendix).

## INTRAOPERATIVE

**Anesthetic technique:** GETA. Epidural anesthesia may be considered for some cases of renal transplantation.

**Induction** Rapid-sequence induction (see Appendix). ET intubation is aided by succinylcholine (1 mg/kg) if $K^+$ < 5.5 mEq/L; otherwise, use atracurium (0.3 mg/kg) or vecuronium (0.2 mg/kg). Fentanyl (2-5 μg/kg) may be used to suppress the cardiovascular response to intubation.

**Maintenance** Standard maintenance (see Appendix). Maintain muscle relaxation with atracurium or vecuronium, titrated using a nerve stimulator. Avoid meperidine (accumulation of normeperidine may cause CNS toxicity). Anticipate prolonged drug effects, and avoid agents that are primarily excreted by the kidney.

**Emergence** Usually extubated in the OR after protective laryngeal reflexes have returned. Pancreatic transplant patients may be sent to the ICU (e.g., brittle diabetics, hemodynamically unstable).

| | | |
|---|---|---|
| **Blood and fluid requirements** | IV: 14 ga x 1<br>NS qs CVP: 10-15 mmHg<br>Warm fluids.<br>Humidify gasses. | Preop fluid status is highly variable. Fluids should be given to maintain CVP 10-15 mmHg. It is important to maintain adequate vascular volume and BP. Mannitol (0.25-1 g/kg), furosemide (5-20 mg) and low-dose dopamine are often given with reperfusion of the kidney. |
| **Monitoring** | Standard monitors (see Appendix).<br>Arterial line | Arterial pressure is often monitored. Avoid the side of A-V fistulae. Axillary artery is a useful alternate site on occasion. |
| | CVP/PA line | CVP is essential and occasionally a PA line is needed (severe cardiac disease). CVP is kept at 10-15 mmHg, especially after the new kidney is reperfused, to ensure adequate renal blood flow. |
| | Hct, $K^+$ and glucose | In pancreatic transplant patients, glucose should be checked q 30 min and q 10 min for the first hr following reperfusion. Keep glucose < 300 mg % prior to reperfusion. |
| | Neuromuscular | Monitor neuromuscular block to avoid excessive use of neuromuscular relaxants. |
| **Positioning** | ✓ and pad pressure points.<br>✓ eyes. | |
| **Complications** | Hemorrhage<br>Low UO | |

### POSTOPERATIVE

| | | |
|---|---|---|
| **Complications** | Respiratory depression<br>Femoral neuropathy<br>Hemorrhage<br>Electrolyte abnormalities | Monitor UO. Dialysis may be needed until renal function returns. Sudden cardiac arrest can complicate pancreatic transplant (due to autonomic neuropathy). |
| **Pain management** | PCA (see Appendix). | |
| **Tests** | Hct<br>Electrolytes<br>Creatinine, BUN<br>Amylase<br>Glucose | A rise in amylase and blood glucose may indicate failure of the pancreatic transplant. |

**References**

1. Dubernard JM, Sutherland DER, eds: *International Handbook of Pancreas Transplantation.* Kluwer Academic Publishers, Dordrecht, The Netherlands: 1989.
2. Bready LL: Kidney transplantation. *Anesth Clin North Am* 1989; 7(3):487-503.
3. Graybar GB, Deierhoi MH: Anesthesia and pancreatic transplantation. *Anesth Clin North Am* 1989; 7(3)515-49.

# LIVING-RELATED-DONOR NEPHRECTOMY

## SURGICAL CONSIDERATIONS

**Description**: Use of a kidney donated by a healthy relative greatly increases the number and quality of available kidneys for transplantation. The donor/patient is placed in a lateral decubitus position on a flexible OR table with a "kidney rest." (A bean bag or sand bags are also helpful for positioning.) An incision is made from the rectus muscle, angling slightly cephalad to cross into the flank just below the tip of the 12th rib and then past it posteriorly to the paraspinous muscles. The retroperitoneum is exposed using a sternal retractor. The kidney is then mobilized, which takes about 1.5 hours. A clamp is placed across the renal artery at the aorta and the renal vein at the IVC; the renal artery is doubly ligated distally and divided. Just prior to clamping the renal artery, furosemide and/or mannitol may be given to stimulate a diuresis. It is important to keep the vascular volume expanded in these patients prior to removal of the kidney. The ureter is transected and the kidney is removed and taken to the back table where it is flushed with a cold solution (Collin's). It is then transported into the recipient room for re-implantation.

**Usual preop diagnosis**: Donor nephrectomy

### SUMMARY OF PROCEDURE

| | |
|---|---|
| **Position** | Lateral decubitus |
| **Incision** | Flank; may require 12th rib resection |
| **Special instrumentation** | Foley catheter; chest retractor; flexible OR table with "kidney rest"; bean bag or sand bags; SCDs for DVT prophylaxis |
| **Unique considerations** | Possible pneumothorax; avoid ETT dislodgement when turning patient from supine to flank position. |
| **Antibiotics** | Cefazolin 1 gm, 1 hr preop |
| **Surgical time** | 2 - 2.5 hrs |
| **Closing considerations** | Deflex table to facilitate closure |
| **EBL** | 100 cc |
| **Postop care** | CXR to rule out pneumothorax. Epidural is helpful for pain management. PACU → room. |
| **Mortality** | $< 0.1\%$ |

| | |
|---|---|
| **Morbidity** | Ileus: 5-10%<br>Urinary retention: 5-10%<br>Wound infection: 1-3%<br>Pneumothorax: 1%<br>Bleeding: 0.1-0.5% |
| **Procedure code** | 50320 |
| **Pain score** | 7 |

### PATIENT POPULATION CHARACTERISTICS

| | |
|---|---|
| **Age range** | 18-70 yrs |
| **Male:Female** | 1:1 |
| **Incidence** | Up to 20% of all kidney transplants at some centers |
| **Etiology** | Kindness |
| **Associated conditions** | Good health is mandatory for renal donation. |

---

## ANESTHETIC CONSIDERATIONS

### PREOPERATIVE

In order to be a living-related donor (LRD), the donor must be in good health with bilaterally functional kidneys. Diabetes, HIV infection, liver disease and malignancy are all contraindications to kidney donations.

| | |
|---|---|
| **Cardiovascular** | Rule out HTN, CAD. MI in the previous 6 mo is a contraindication. |
| **Renal** | Normal bilateral renal function is required.<br>**Tests:** IVP; creatinine, creatinine clearance |
| **Fluid status** | Adequate hydration is important and UO should be >1.5 ml/kg/hr. Various regimes are used to ensure adequate hydration, usually with iv fluid starting the night before. |
| **Premedication** | Adequate anxiolysis is beneficial. These patients are making a great sacrifice and should be treated with special care. Standard premedication (see Appendix). |

### INTRAOPERATIVE

**Anesthetic technique:** GETA ± epidural for postop pain management.

| | |
|---|---|
| **Induction** | Standard induction (see Appendix). |
| **Maintenance** | Standard maintenance (see Appendix). Avoid long-acting, renally excreted drugs. Ventilate for eucapnia to avoid possible renal artery vasoconstriction caused by hyper- or hypocapnia. Use of an epidural with local anesthetic and/or narcotic may aid both intraop and postop pain relief, but hypotension should be avoided. |
| **Emergence** | Routine extubation in OR. |

| | | |
|---|---|---|
| **Blood and fluid requirements** | IV: 14 ga x 2<br>NS/LR @ 6-8 ml/hr<br>Warm all fluids.<br>Humidify gasses.<br>UO 1.5 ml/kg/hr | Aim for a minimum of 1.5 ml/kg/hr UO. Mannitol (0.25-1 g/kg) given iv once kidney is being manipulated, and if UO decreases. |
| **Monitoring** | Standard monitors (see Appendix). | CVP or invasive arterial monitoring are rarely required. |
| **Positioning** | ✓ and pad pressure points.<br>✓ eyes. | Positioning may impair venous return → ↓BP. Ensure that the head is properly padded and that the cervical spine is in line with thoracic spine. |
| **Complications** | Hemorrhage | Because the vessels are tied close to the aorta and IVC, the possibility of severe hemorrhage exists. |
| | Pneumothorax | Pneumothorax is always possible, especially when the 12th rib is resected. |

## POSTOPERATIVE

| | | |
|---|---|---|
| **Complications** | Pneumothorax<br>Hemorrhage<br>Infection<br>Pulmonary problems<br>Hypokalemia (diuretics)<br>Ileus | |
| **Pain management** | Epidural narcotics (see Appendix).<br>PCA (see Appendix). | Epidural analgesia is quite suitable for these patients and is recommended. |
| **Tests** | CXR<br>Hct | |


**References**

1. Simmons RL, Finch ME, Ascher NL, Najarian JS, eds: *Manual of Vascular Access, Organ Donation and Transplantation.* Springer-Verlag, New York: 1984.
2. Bready LL: Kidney transplantation: in anesthesia for new surgical techniques. *Anesth Clin North Am* 1989; 7(3):503-9.


# ORTHOTOPIC LIVER TRANSPLANT

## SURGICAL CONSIDERATIONS

**Description**: Orthotopic liver transplantation (OLT) is the only curative procedure for end-stage liver disease. The procedure can be divided into three parts: (1) recipient hepatectomy; (2) anhepatic phase; and (3) liver transplant.

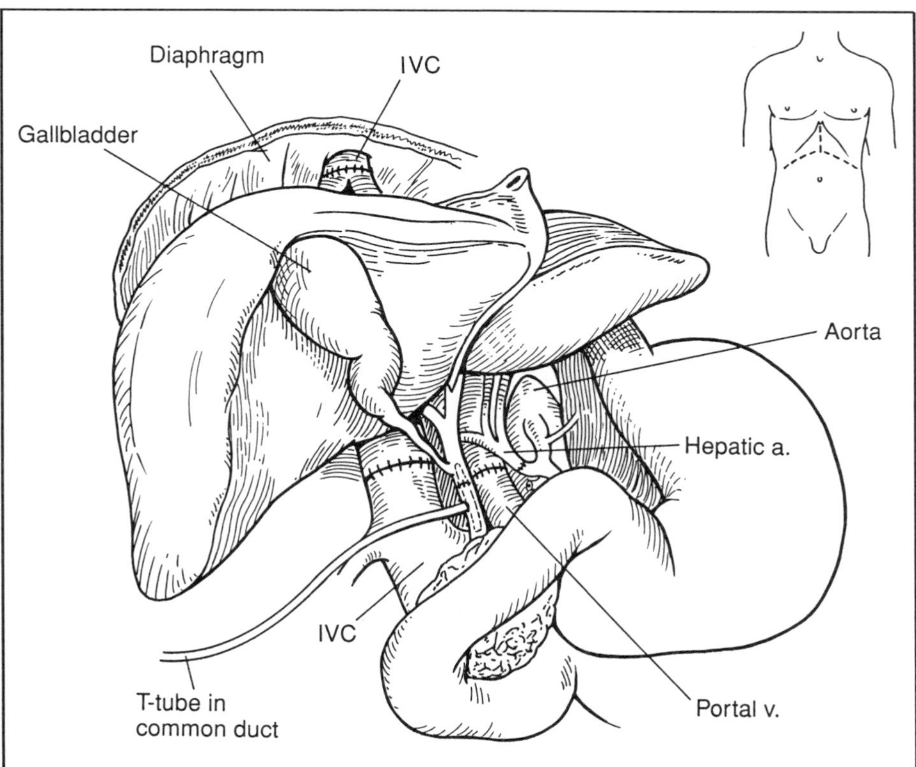


**Figure 7.11-3.** Liver transplantation. Anastomoses – including suprahepatic and infrahepatic IVC, portal vein, hepatic artery and common bile duct – are complete as shown here. Roux-en-Y loop of small intestine is an alternative biliary drainage conduit. Inset shows a chevron incision with midline extension. (Reproduced with permission from Hardy JD: *Hardy's Textbook of Surgery*, 2nd edition. JB Lippincott: 1988.)

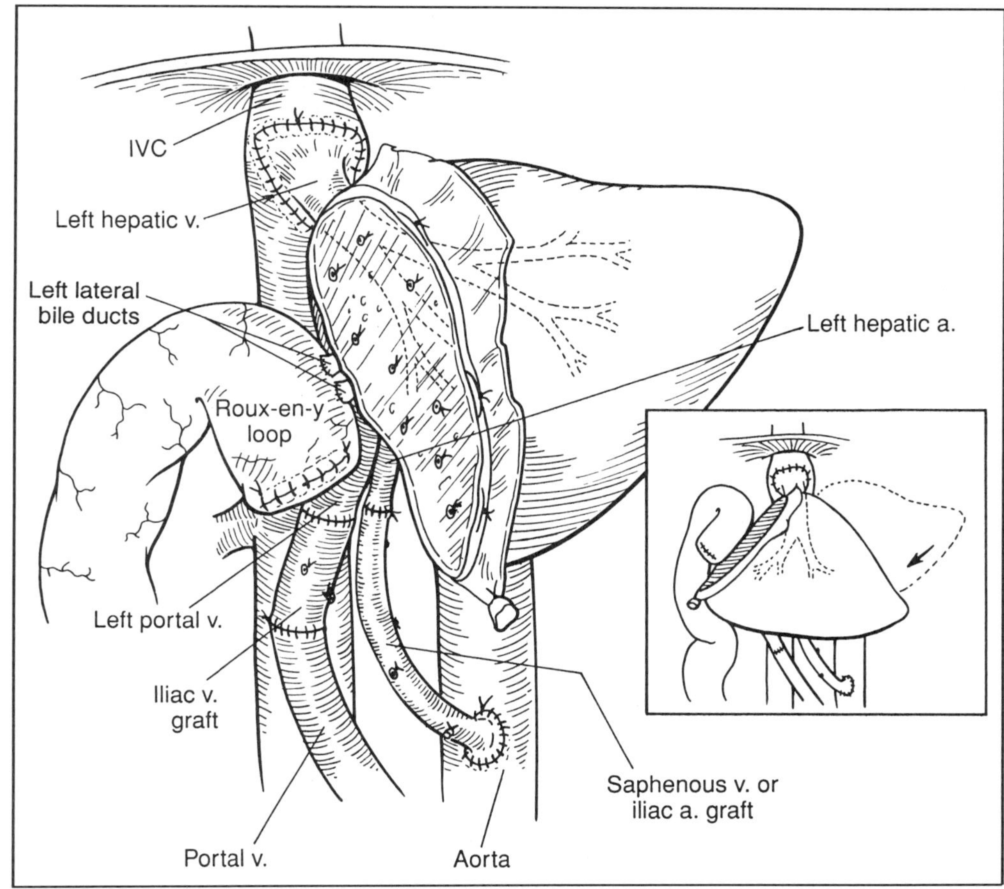


**Figure 7.11-4.** Liver transplantation (child) using left lateral segment from an adult liver. The hepatic artery and portal vein are extended with donor iliac artery and vein, respectively. The final position of the graft is shown (inset). A Roux-en-Y loop of small intestine is used to drain the bile duct(s). The IVC is left intact. The cut surface of the liver can bleed excessively if CVP is too high. (Reproduced with permission from Broelsch CE, et al: "Liver transplantation in children from living related donors: surgical techniques and results. *Ann Surg* 1991; 214(4):432.)

**Recipient hepatectomy** can be relatively straightforward, as in the case of acute hepatic failure, or extremely difficult in a patient with previous multiple procedures and portal HTN. Preparing for the recipient hepatectomy includes mobilization of the suprahepatic vena cava, infrahepatic vena cava and the portal triad. Early in the procedure, veno-venous bypass is established by placing a cannula in the iliac vein through a left groin incision and in the axillary vein via a left axillary incision. The portal vein is cannulated through the inferior mesenteric vein. Veno-venous bypass has greatly reduced the operative blood loss during the recipient hepatectomy phase. It is critical to prevent air from entering the lines during this procedure. Once the liver has been removed, the patient generally is stable, and bleeding can be controlled with suture ligatures.

During the **anhepatic phase**, the new liver graft is brought onto the field and sutured in place. The suprahepatic vena cava anastomosis is sutured first, followed by the infrahepatic vena cava and the portal vein. The hepatic artery is generally re-anastomosed prior to initial revascularization; however, the liver can be revascularized after completion of the portal vein and vena caval anastomoses (Fig 7.11-3). It is critical during the recipient hepatectomy and the anhepatic phase to aggressively replace blood loss because, upon release of the clamps and the reperfusion of the liver, the patient can suffer pulmonary HTN and subsequent cardiac arrest. After the hepatic artery has been anastomosed and the liver is revascularized, the bile duct is connected through either a **choledochojejunostomy** or a **choledocho-choledochostomy**. It is important to remember to clamp and then disconnect the portal venous limb of the veno-venous bypass after reperfusion of the liver to allow adequate portal-vein blood flow into the transplanted graft.

In the pediatric group, segmental grafts are common, particularly left lateral-segment grafts (Fig 7.11-4). The reduction in graft volume is performed on the back table and takes about 3 hours. Occasionally, this results in some blood loss upon revascularization of the graft along the cut segments, but generally this is not a major problem. The CVP should not be excessively high upon revascularization of a segmental graft because the cut segment can bleed excessively.

**Usual preop diagnosis**: End-stage liver disease

### SUMMARY OF PROCEDURE

| | |
|---|---|
| **Position** | Supine; arms out at side for veno-venous bypass. Avoid brachial plexus injury. |
| **Incision** | Chevron with midline extension to xiphoid (Fig 7.11-3 inset) |
| **Special instrumentation** | Upper hand retractor; veno-venous bypass; rapid infuser; cell saver |
| **Unique considerations** | May require massive transfusion; pneumothorax may occur; "reperfusion syndrome" (pulmonary HTN and possible cardiac arrest upon release of clamps and blood flow to liver transplant); protection of OR team from hepatitis A, B, C. If renal failure is present, continuous arteriovenous hemofiltration is advisable. |
| **Antibiotics** | Ampicillin, ceftriaxone 1 gm/each, 1 hr before incision |
| **Surgical time** | 8 - 16 hrs |
| **EBL** | Variable; 8 to >100 U |
| **Postop care** | ICU x 2-5 d; ventilator, may be hypertensive |
| **Mortality** | 15-20% at 1 yr |
| **Morbidity** | Overall: 10-70%<br>Infectious complications, including pneumonia, wound infections and lymphoceles at site of veno-venous bypass: 10-70%<br>Hepatic artery thrombosis: < 7% (greater in pediatric age group)<br>Biliary leak: 3-5% (increased in pediatric age group)<br>Portal venous thrombosis: 3-5% (more common in patients with preop portal venous thrombosis)<br>Perioperative bleeding requiring re-operation: 2-3% |
| **Procedure code** | 47135 |
| **Pain score** | 6 |

### PATIENT POPULATION CHARACTERISTICS

| | |
|---|---|
| **Age range** | Neonate-70 yrs |
| **Male:Female** | 1:1 |
| **Incidence** | 20-30/million/yr (1/3 pediatric) |
| **Etiology** | Adult: Sclerosing cholangitis: 99%<br>Chronic active hepatitis: 20%<br>Alcoholic cirrhosis: 13%<br>Cryptogenic cirrhosis: 11%<br>Primary biliary cirrhosis: 11%<br>Pediatric: Primary biliary atresia: 12%<br>Inborn errors of metabolism: 6% |
| **Associated conditions** | Acquired anemia<br>Coagulopathy<br>Hypoalbuminemia<br>Low systemic vascular resistance<br>High cardiac output<br>Cardiomyopathy in alcoholics<br>Hepatorenal syndrome<br>Massive ascites |

## ANESTHETIC CONSIDERATIONS

### PREOPERATIVE

Patients presenting for liver transplantation present a formidable challenge to the anesthesiologist. Frequently these patients present for surgery with multi-organ system failure. Due to the emergent nature of the surgery, there may be insufficient time available for the customary evaluation and correction of abnormalities in this patient population.

**Respiratory** These patients are often hypoxic because of ascites, pleural effusions, atelectasis, V/Q mismatch and pulmonary AV shunting. As a result, they are usually tachypneic and have a respiratory alkalosis. Evidence of pulmonary infection is usually a contraindication to surgery, but ARDS that may occur with hepatic failure is not.

**Tests:** ABG; PFT, as indicated. CXR: ✓ infection, effusions, atelectasis.

**Cardiovascular** These patients demonstrate a hyperdynamic state with ↑CO and ↓SVR (probably 2° AV fistulae and endogenous vasodilators). This inefficient circulatory state is manifested by a $S_{\bar{v}}O_2$. The SVR usually is not responsive to α-agents. AV fistulae also occur across the pulmonary circulation, so that precautions to prevent air embolism are important. Ejection fraction (EF) is usually high (>60%). Pericardial effusions may be present, and should be drained at surgery. Many of these patients will have dysrhythmias, HTN, pulmonary HTN (very high risk), valvular disease, cardiomyopathy (alcoholic disease, hemochromatosis, Wilson's disease) and CAD. These patients will require appropriate preop consultation and workup.

**Tests:** ECG; ECHO: ✓ EF, contractility, pulmonary HTN, wall motion abnormalities, valve problems. If abnormal, consider a MUGA scan and/or right- and left-heart catheterization with coronary artery angiography.

**Neurological** Patients are often encephalopathic and may be in hepatic coma; however, other organic causes of coma should be ruled out. In fulminant hepatic failure, ↑ICP is common, accounting for 40% of mortality (herniation), and may require prompt treatment (mannitol, hyperventilation, etc.).

**Tests:** Continuous ICP monitoring in fulminant hepatic failure

**Hepatic** Hepatitis serology and the cause of hepatic failure should be determined. Vascular abnormalities, previous RUQ surgery or portal vein decompressive surgery places the patient in a high-risk group. Albumin usually low, with consequent low plasma oncotic pressure → edema, ascites. The magnitude and duration of drug effects may be unpredictable but, generally, these patients have ↑sensitivity to all drugs and their actions are prolonged.

**Tests:** Bilirubin; PT; ammonia level; SGOT; SGPT; albumin

**Gastrointestinal** Portal HTN, esophageal varices and coagulopathies increase the risk of GI hemorrhage. Gastric emptying is often slow and, together with the emergent nature of this surgery, warrants rapid-sequence induction. $H_2$-antagonists are indicated preop.

**Renal** ↓Renal function, especially in fulminant hepatic failure (hepatorenal syndrome). The kidneys often recover after transplantation, but simultaneous kidney transplantation may be justified. These patients are often hypervolemia, hyponatremic and possibly hypokalemic. $Ca^{++}$ is usually normal. Metabolic alkalosis may be present. Consider preop dialysis and intraop continuous AV hemofiltration. Low-dose dopamine (2-4 μg/kg/min) and/or mannitol (0.5-1 gm/kg) is often used intraop to maintain renal function.

**Tests:** BUN; creatinine, creatinine clearance; electrolytes; ABG

**Endocrine** Often glucose intolerant or frankly diabetic, although acute hypoglycemia may be seen in acute hepatic failure. Hyperaldosteronism may be present.

**Tests:** Glucose; electrolytes

**Hematologic** These patients are often anemic due either to blood loss or malabsorption. Coagulation is impaired because of ↓hepatic synthetic function (all factors except VIII and fibrinogen are ↓), abnormal fibrinogen production, ↓/impaired platelets, fibrinolysis, and low-grade DIC.

**Tests:** PT; PTT; platelet count; bleeding time; fibrinogen; fibrin split products (FSP); TEG

**Premedication** Low doses of benzodiazepines may be used judiciously, but often nothing is given prior to surgery. Usually good preop evaluation and discussion suffice. Intramuscular injection should be avoided. Full-stomach precautions are justified. Metoclopramide 10 mg, ranitidine 50 mg iv and Na citrate 0.3 M 30 ml po should be given prior to surgery.

## INTRAOPERATIVE

**Anesthetic technique:** GETA. These patients are extremely complex to manage because of the hemodynamic variability, massive blood loss, coagulopathy and metabolic problems. It is convenient to divide the operation into three stages: pre-anhepatic, anhepatic and neohepatic (discussed below).

**Induction** Often a narcotic (e.g., fentanyl 2-5 μg/kg) is given just prior to induction. Rapid-sequence induction is preferred. STP (3-5 mg/kg) or etomidate (0.3 mg/kg) with succinylcholine (1-2 mg/kg), together with cricoid pressure.

**Maintenance** Standard maintenance (see Appendix) with fentanyl up to 100 μg/kg. A benzodiazepine (e.g., midazolam 0.3 μg/kg) often is given to ensure amnesia during periods of hemodynamic instability when the volatile agent may need to be off. $N_2O$ is avoided because of bowel distention and possible air embolism. Ventilation with $FiO_2 > 0.5$ and $PaCO_2 = \sim 35$ mmHg. Occasionally, PEEP (5 cm $H_2O$) is added. Antibiotics and immunosuppressants should be given per surgeon's direction. Muscle relaxation is usually maintained with pancuronium.

**Pre-anhepatic phase**

The **pre-anhepatic phase** starts at skin incision and ends with removal of the recipient liver. Pleural and pericardial effusions are drained, which may improve oxygenation. Hyperglycemia is common during this period. Decreased filling pressures 2° hemorrhage or vascular compression. Hemorrhage can be severe 2° portal HTN. Coagulation problems usually increase during this period, although fibrinolysis is not usually a problem. Blood loss replacement is accomplished with blood (PRBC) and FFP. Cryoprecipitate and platelets are usually avoided since hypercoagulable states are undesirable once veno-venous bypass is instituted. Hemodynamic instability is not uncommon during the hepatic vascular dissection 2° manipulation of the liver and ↓venous return.

Veno-venous bypass relieves most of the complications of portal and IVC cross-clamping (↓venous return, low CO, tachycardia, acidosis, ↓renal function, intestinal swelling.) Blood is pumped from the femoral vein and the portal system (either portal vein or inferior mesenteric) via a centrifugal pump to the left axillary vein. Generally, no heparin is used, but heparin-bonded cannulae and tubing are used. Bypass flows need to be at least 1 L/min to avoid possible thromboembolism. Bypass flow depends on venous inflow and is drawn into the pump by negative pressure. Low flows may be caused by hypovolemia or obstructed cannulae. Complications include: unexpected decannulation, thromboembolism and air embolism, all of which may need rapid termination of bypass and treatment of hypotension.

Massive blood transfusion is associated with ↓ $Ca^{++}$ and replacement is usually needed (± 500 mg/1000 ml of blood/FFP/plasmalyte mixture). If hyperkalemia occurs, it should be treated aggressively. Metabolic acidosis >5 mEq/L should be treated with bicarbonate. Occasionally, inotropic support is needed, but α-adregenic agents should be avoided because of decreased renal and peripheral perfusion. UO needs to be maintained by ensuring adequate intravascular volume; occasionally, low-dose dopamine and/or mannitol may be needed.

**Anhepatic phase**

The **anhepatic stage** begins with clamping of the hepatic vessels and vena cava and removal of the liver; it ends with the reperfusion of the donor liver. Problems during this period include: hemorrhage, increasing coagulopathy and fibrinolysis, acidosis, hypothermia and ↓renal function. The hemodynamic instability associated with clamping of the hepatic vessels and the congestion of the bowel that occurs can be decreased by veno-venous bypass (see above). Care should be taken to maintain intravascular volume, while avoiding volume overload, since this will worsen fluid overloading on reperfusion. At the completion of vena caval anastomoses, the liver is flushed via the portal vein to remove air, preservation fluid and metabolites. Reperfusion may take place after completion of the portal vein anastomosis or after both portal vein and hepatic artery anastomoses are completed. As in the pre-anhepatic phase, acidosis, ↓$Ca^{++}$, glucose, coagulation and other electrolyte abnormalities should be treated. Fibrinolysis usually starts in this period, but is not usually treated unless severe because of the potential for embolism during veno-venous bypass.

**Neohapatic phase**

The **neohepatic phase** begins with the unclamping of the portal vein, hepatic artery and vena cava and reperfusion of the donor liver. Preparation for this phase is important because this may be a period of great hemodynamic instability. Before removal of the clamps, acidosis should be corrected, ionized $Ca^{++}$ should be normal and $K^+$ should be < 4.5 mEq/L. $CaCl_2$, $NaHCO_3$ and epinephrine should be readily available. Fluid overload prior to declamping should be avoided. Declamping can be attended by ↓BP, ↓HR, dysrhythmias, hypothermia, lactic acidosis, coagulopathy and hyperglycemia.

**Reperfusion syndrome**

**The "reperfusion syndrome"** (which can occur in this phase) is characterized by ↓HR, ↓BP (30% develop MAP < 70% of baseline), conduction defects and ↓SVR in the face of acutely ↑RV fil-ling pressures. Cause unknown. CO is often maintained. A rapid ↑$K^+$ can lead to cardiac arrest. (Rx: ensure normal pH and electrolytes prior to unclamping, rapid therapy when it occurs.) ↓BP and ↓HR are treated with epinephrine (10 $\mu$g increments), while $CaCl_2$ and $NaHCO_3$ are used to correct hyperkalemia and acidosis. Pulmonary edema may occur as a result of fluid overload and may be treated with diuretics, inotropes and phlebotomy. A high venous pressure will cause graft congestion and should be avoided. Reperfusion is associated with severe coagulopathy due to fibrinolysis (usually primary), release of heparin and hypothermia. As liver function returns, there should be an improvement in coagulation, acid-base status (metabolic alkalosis may occur), ↓lactic acidosis, return of glucose to normal and bile production. Hypokalemia may occur 2° uptake by the liver. HTN may be a problem. (Rx: SNP infusion.) Graft failure is associated with coagulopathy, ↑lactic acid, citrate intoxication, hyperglycemia and ↓bile formation.

**Emergence**

Extubation is deferred to ICU, with patient intubated and ventilated. These patients are generally ventilated postop until they are stable and able to be weaned from ventilatory support. Apart from the usual tests, hepatic function needs to be monitored, immunosuppression provided, infection controlled, analgesia ensured (usually morphine) and peptic ulcer prophylaxis given (ranitidine preferred).

<table>
<tr><td>Blood and fluid requirements</td><td>Massive blood loss<br>IV: 10 Fr x 2</td><td>Generally, ivs are placed in the right anti-cubital fossa, left or right IJ or EJ. The left arm is avoided because the axillary vein is used for veno-venous bypass.</td></tr>
<tr><td></td><td>Plasmalyte A® or Normasol®<br>UO >1 ml/kg/hr<br>Warm all fluids.<br>Humidify gasses.<br>Rapid-infusion system<br>Cell savers<br>20 U PRBC<br>20 U FFP<br>20 U PLT</td><td>Plasmalyte A® or Normasol® are preferred (absence of glucose, $Ca^{++}$ and lower $Na^{+}$ content) over NS/LR. Hypernatremia can be a problem due to administration of $NaHCO_3$. The ability to give up to 1.5 L/min of blood should be available. Usually a mixture of Normasol®, PRBC and FFP in the ratio of 250 ml:1 U:1 U is used, yielding Hct = 26-30%. Actual blood loss estimation is extremely difficult, and usually replacement is judged by hemodynamic status, UO and $S_{\bar{v}}O_2$. Cell savers are used to conserve blood. Anticoagulation is with a citrate solution to avoid heparin contamination and cells are washed with Normasol®/Plasmalyte A®. D/C use before biliary reconstruction (infection) or in neoplasms, hepatitis B or spontaneous bacterial peritonitis.</td></tr>
<tr><td>Monitoring</td><td>Standard monitors (see Appendix).<br>ECG (5-lead)<br>Temp-bladder<br>$ETN_2$<br>TEG</td><td>Include 5-lead ECG and bladder temperature. (These patients sustain significant temperature loss.)<br>A full-time anesthesia technologist and lab/blood bank runner are useful. Lab and blood bank should be notified of the expected transplant. An automated data acquisition system also is useful, since there are times during the case when the record may be neglected in favor of working with the patient.</td></tr>
<tr><td></td><td>Arterial lines</td><td>Two arterial lines are placed at the outset– one in the right radial, for ongoing lab and blood gas sampling, with 1 port being designated as heparin-free; another line, in the right femoral artery is utilized for continuous pressure measurement. All flush solutions contain citrate for anticoagulation in order to avoid heparin contamination.</td></tr>
<tr><td></td><td>PA catheter<br>$S_{\bar{v}}O_2$<br>CO</td><td>A PA catheter is essential for management of hemodynamics in these patients because of the rapid changes in vital signs. A catheter capable of measuring mixed-venous $O_2$ sat is very useful, as it gives early clues to impending decompensation. Coagulopathy complicates the placement of central lines and the use of ECHO or ultrasound-guided needles is useful.</td></tr>
<tr><td></td><td>TEE</td><td>TEE is useful to monitor cardiac filling and function and to diagnose problems such as PE or air embolism. Care needs to be taken in placing the TEE, since many of these patients have esophageal varices.</td></tr>
<tr><td></td><td>ICP</td><td>ICP should be measured in patients with fulminant hepatic failure if ↑ICP is a concern.<br>ABG, acid base status, electrolyte, lactate, osmolality, $Ca^{++}$, PT, PTT< platelets, Hct – all should be monitored on a regular basis (hourly or half-hourly and, occasionally, more frequently). The thromboelastograph (TEG) is useful for monitoring coagulation (see discussion of coagulation management, below).</td></tr>
</table>

**Table 7.11-1. Coagulation Therapy Guided by Thrombelastographic Monitoring**

1. Maintenance fluid
   RBC: FFP: Plasmalyte A = 300:200:250 ml
2. Replacement therapy
   a. FFP (2 U) for prolonged reaction time (r > 15 min)
   b. Platelets (10 U) for small MA (MA < 40 mm)
   c. Cryoprecipitate (6-12 U) for persistent slow clot formation rate ($\alpha$ < 40°) with normal MA
3. Pharmacologic therapy
   a. Compare coagulability of whole blood, blood treated with protamine sulfate, and blood treated with epsilon aminocaproic acid.
   b. Epsilon aminocaproic acid (1 gm) for severe fibrinolysis (F < 60 min)
   c. Protamine sulfate (50 mg) for severe heparin effect
   d. Heparin (1000-2000 U) for hypercoagulable state

(Used with permission from Kang YG: Anesthesia for liver transplantation. *Anes Clin North Am* 1989; 7(3): 507.)

**Coagulation management**

TEG
PT
PTT
Platelet counts
Fibrinogen
FSP

Patients are prone to a variety of coagulopathies (↓platelets, ↓coagulation factors, DIC, fibrinolysis, etc.) because of preop factors, massive hemorrhage, anhepatic period and reperfusion of the new liver; therefore, monitoring and treatment are necessary. Also, hypercoagulopathy states need to be avoided because of unheparinized venovenous bypass. While PT, PTT, platelet counts, fibrinogen and FSP may provide relevant information, they may not reflect the true coagulability of patient's blood and tend to take considerable time to perform. Thus, TEG has gained in popularity. It measures whole blood coagulability, not specific factors. TEG works by measuring viscoelastic properties of blood as it forms clot (fibrin connections) between a rotating cuvette and a spindle. Characteristic patterns are formed by the various coagulopathies with the common types shown in Fig 7.11-5. Evaluation of the TEG leads to more rational transfusion therapy, reducing the number of U of blood/blood products used. Comparing specimens of native whole blood vs blood mixed with EACA or protamine can guide pharmacologic therapy of coagulopathies. Table 7.11-1 gives specific recommendations.

**Positioning**

✓ and pad pressure points.
✓ eyes.

Table and arm boards should be well-padded. Head should be placed on a foam rest. Particular care should be taken to pad the retractor supports where they may impinge on the arms and on the radial nerve as it curls around the humerus.

**Temperature control**

Warming blanket
Humidifier

Patient's arms, head and legs should be wrapped in plastic to protect against heat loss. Plastic drapes to protect the ECG electrodes and direct fluid flow off the table are useful to prevent the patient from lying in a pool of fluid.

## POSTOPERATIVE

**Monitoring of hepatic function**

Serial LFTs
PT, PTT
Ammonia level
Lactate
TEG
Bile output

Initial LFTs often show very high liver enzymes, which subside over a period of days. PT generally improves to normal levels, while lactic acidosis usually corrects quickly. Often a metabolic alkalosis follows and may need treatment with HCl.

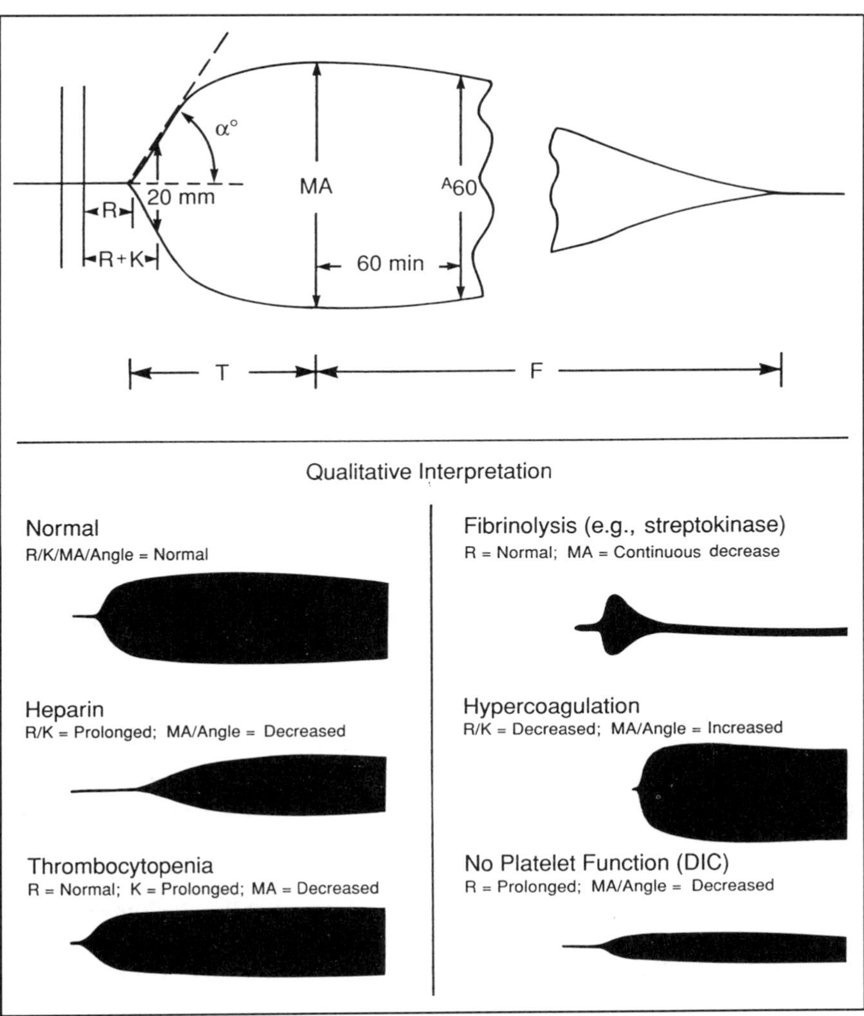


**Figure 7.11-5.** Variables and normal values measured by TEG:
R–reaction time, 6-8 min
R + k–coagulation time, 10-12 min
α–clot formation rate, >50°
MA–maximum amplitude, 50-70 mm
$A_{60}$–amplitude 60 min after MA
$A_{60}$/MA-100–whole blood clot lysis index, >85%
F–whole blood clot lysis time, >300 min
(Reproduced with permission from Kang YG, et al: Intraoperative changes in blood coagulation and thromboelastographic monitoring in liver transplantation. *Anesth Analg* 1985; 64:891.)

**Complications**

- Bleeding
- Partial vein thrombosis
- Hepatic artery thrombosis
- Biliary tract leaks
- Primary non-function
- Rejection
- Infection
- Pulmonary complication
- HTN
- Electrolyte abnormalities (hypokalemia, ↓$Ca^{++}$, ↑Na)
- Alkalosis
- Renal failure
- Peptic ulceration
- Neurologic

This is not a complete list. Feared complications which may result in graft loss include portal vein thrombosis, hepatic artery thrombosis, bile leaks and rejection. These are attended by ↑LFTs, lactic acidosis, coagulopathy, hypoglycemia, ↓renal function and poor bile formation. The reader is referred to Reference 2, below, for a more complete discussion.

**References**


1. Starzl TE, Demetris AJ: Liver transplantation: a 31-year perspective. In *Current Problems in Surgery*. Wells SA Jr, ed. 1990 XXVII: 2-4.
2. Kang YG; Anesthesia for liver transplantation. *Anesthesiology Clin of North Am* 1989; 7(3)551-80.
3. Gelman S, Kang YG, Pearson JD: Anesthetic consideration in liver transplantation. In *Anesthesia for Organ Transplantation*. Fabian JA, ed. JB Lippincott Co, Philadelphia: 1992, Ch 7, 115-39.

4. Paulsen AW, Whitten CW, Ramsay MA, Klintmalm GB: Considerations for anesthetic management during veno-venous bypass in adult hepatic transplantation. *Anesth Analg* 1989; 68(4):489-96.
5. Carmicheal FJ, Lindop MJ, Farman JV: Anesthesia for hepatic transplantation: cardiovascular and metabolic alterations and their management. *Anesth Analg* 1985; 64(2):108-16.
6. Kang YG, Martin DJ, Marguez J, Lewis JH, Bontempo FA, Shaw BW Jr, Starzl TE, Winter PM: Intraoperative changes in blood coagulation and thromboelastic monitoring in liver transplantation. *Anesth analg* 1985; 64(9):888-96.
7. Kang YG, Lewis JH, Navalgund A, Russell MW, Bontempo FA, Niren LS, Starzl TE: Epsilon-aminocaproic acid for treatment of fibrinolysis during liver transplantation. *Anesthesiology* 1987; 66(6):766-73.

# MULTI-ORGAN PROCUREMENT

## SURGICAL CONSIDERATIONS

**Description**: The families of patients who are brain dead (with irreversible cessation of all brain function) may allow donation of the patient's other functioning organs; and this act of altruism can save or enhance the lives of as many as 10 others.

Multi-organ procurement begins with an *in situ* flush used to exsanguinate and cool organs. The donar patient's chest and abdomen are opened from pubis to sternal notch. The chest is opened with a sternal saw, and, generally, an extra large Balfour retractor is used to widely retract the abdomen. The aorta and IVC are dissected first to allow rapid placement of flush line in the event that the patient decompensates. Following this, the liver vasculature is identified in the hepatoduodenal ligament below the liver and dissected out. This part of the procedure generally takes about 1.5 hours.

In cases where the pancreas is procured, an additional 45 minutes to 1 hour is required for mobilization of the pancreas. During pancreas procurement, Betadine® is placed through an NG tube into the stomach and duodenum. A total of about 100-200 cc of Betadine® should be passed. Once the heart, liver, pancreas and kidneys have been mobilized, heparin must be given. For an average-size adult, 30,000 U of heparin is given prior to clamping. The organs are then perfused with Viaspan®. At this point, the ventilator can be turned off and the aorta cross-clamped below the diaphragm.

The heart is the first organ to be removed. If the lungs are removed, an extra 20-30 minutes of perfusion time is required. After removal of the heart and/or lungs, the liver can be removed, followed by the pancreas and kidneys. Total time for multi-organ harvest, including heart, lungs, liver, pancreas and kidneys, is approximately 4 hours, although anesthesia time typically ends with aortic cross-clamping.

**Usual preop diagnosis**: Brain death

### SUMMARY OF PROCEDURE

| | |
|---|---|
| **Position** | Supine |
| **Incision** | Midline only, neck to pubis, ± bilateral transverse extensions |
| **Special instrumentation** | Chest and abdominal retractors |
| **Unique considerations** | Maintain oxygenation and BP as if live patient. May require pressors and/or blood transfusion. Temporarily deflate lungs for sternal sawing. |
| **Antibiotics** | Betadine® via NG tube for pancreas (with duodenal segment) procurement |
| **Surgical time** | ≤ 4 hrs |
| **EBL** | 200 cc |
| **Procedure code** | 47133 (donor hepatectomy); 48155 (pancreatectomy, total); 48160 (with transplantation); 50300 (donor nephrectomy) |

### PATIENT POPULATION CHARACTERISTICS

| | |
|---|---|
| **Age range** | 3-60 yrs |
| **Male:Female** | N/A |
| **Incidence** | Approximately 4530/yr in U.S. |
| **Etiology** | Usually head trauma (e.g., motor vehicle accidents, gunshot wounds to the head) or intracranial bleeding |
| **Associated conditions** | Vasomotor instability<br>Diabetes insipidus<br>Intracranial HTN |

---

## ANESTHETIC CONSIDERATIONS

### PREOPERATIVE

In general, organ donors are previously healthy individuals who have suffered catastrophic, irreversible brain injury of known etiology, most commonly due to blunt head trauma, penetrating head injury, or intracranial hemorrhage. A declaration of brain death by physicians not participating in the organ procurement must be documented. This documentation, together with certification of death and familial consent, should be verified by the anesthesiologist prior to organ procurement. There should be no evidence of disease or trauma involving the organs targeted for donation and, in general, the patient should be hemodynamically stable with minimal inotropic requirements. Once brain death has been declared, it is important to shift the emphasis away from cerebral resuscitation efforts and to focus instead on the maintenance of adequate tissue perfusion and oxygenation. Brain death is frequently followed by a series of pathophysiological events that may complicate the management of these patients.

**Respiratory** Pulmonary dysfunction following brain death has many possible etiologies: aspiration, atelectasis, pneumonia and pulmonary edema. In addition, trauma may cause pulmonary dysfunction related to contusion, pneumothorax or hemothorax. Meticulous pulmonary toilet is essential to prevent atelectasis and pneumonia. Maintenance of adequate oxygenation is requisite to insure preservation of other organs for transplantation. Use mechanical ventilation with TVs of 10-12 cc/kg and a minute ventilation that maintains $PaCO_2$ 35-45 mmHg and pH 7.35-7.45. The $FiO_2$ should insure a $PaO_2$ 75-150 mmHg and arterial saturation >95%. PEEP is usually applied at 3-5 cm $H_2O$ and should not exceed 7.5 cm $H_2O$ because of the deleterious effects on CO, regional blood flow and possible barotrauma. The $FiO_2$ generally should be increased to 100% prior to transport to the OR. An important exception is in the case of heart-lung or lung retrieval where it is important to maintain $FiO_2$ < 40% to minimize possible effects of $O_2$ toxicity. Ideally, PIP should be < 30 cm $H_2O$ to minimize possible barotrauma to the lungs.

**Tests:** Frequent ABGs, including immediate preop period. Proper position of the ETT should be confirmed preop.

**Cardiovascular** Hypotension should be anticipated in all organ donors. This results most commonly from neurogenic shock (derangement of descending vasomotor control → progressive ↓SVR and venous pooling) and hypovolemia. Hypovolemia is usually the result of dehydration therapy for cerebral edema, hemorrhage, diabetes insipidus (DI) or osmotic diuresis due to hyperglycemia. Hypothermia, LV dysfunction and endocrine abnormalities may also contribute to ↓BP. Fluid resuscitation with crystalloid, colloid and PRBCs to maintain Hct >30% should be initiated preop. Hemodynamic goals are: (1) CVP 10-12 cm $H_2O$ (6-8 cm $H_2O$ if lungs are to be procured), MAP between 60-100 mmHg, SBP >100 mmHg, and UO >1 cc/kg/hr. Donors are often placed on inotropic therapy to maintain these parameters; however, following adequate volume resuscitation, preop inotropic therapy often may be gradually decreased or discontinued. If inotropic therapy remains necessary, typically it would consist of dopamine (2-10 μg/kg/min), followed by dobutamine (3-15 μg/kg/min) or epinephrine (0.1-1.0 μg/kg/min), then norepinephrine. The latter 3 agents may be combined with dopamine (2-3 μg/kg/min) in an attempt to augment or preserve renal, mesenteric and coronary arterial blood flow. It should be noted that brain death may be accompanied initially by a transient hypertensive crisis which may require short-term treatment with SNP and/or esmolol.

**Cardiovascular, continued**

ECG abnormalities are common in patients with intracranial injury and are of no pathologic consequence. Atrial and ventricular dysrhythmias and various degrees of conduction block occur frequently in organ donors; the etiology may be electrolyte imbalance, ABG disturbance, ↑ICP, loss of the vagal motor nucleus, inotropic therapy, hypothermia or myocardial contusions or ischemia. Anti-dysrhythmic therapy should follow the usual guidelines except for ↓HR, which is resistant to atropine in this setting. Bradycardia, if accompanied by ↓BP, should be treated with isoproterenol, dopamine, epinephrine or temporary cardiac pacing.

**Tests:** ECG; ECHO (to assess wall motion abnormalities) and possibly coronary angiography (if CAD is suspected).

**Neurological**

DI frequently occurs in brain-dead donors; it is likely the result of destruction of the hypothalamic-pituitary axis. Untreated, it may cause marked hypovolemia and electrolyte disturbances (↑Na, ↑Mg, ↓K, ↓$PO_4$, ↓Ca). Therapy with iv vasopressin (titrated from 2 $\mu$g/kg/min) or desmopressin acetate (DDAVP) (titrated from 0.3 $\mu$g/kg/min) is often initiated to maintain UO $<$ 1.5-3 cc/kg/hr. Many believe the benefits of minimizing electrolyte imbalance, fluid shifts and reduction of core temperature outweigh the risks of vasopressin or desmopressin therapy, including coronary and renal vasoconstriction and possible organ ischemia or uneven distribution of the preservation solutions during flushing. It may be prudent, however, to D/C vasopressin or DDAVP infusions for at least 1 hr prior to aortic cross-clamping and infusion of preservation solutions. Thermoregulation is abnormal in brain-dead donors due to hypothalamic dysfunction; and core temperature should be monitored (bladder, esophageal or rectal). Aggressive warming techniques may have to be employed early to maintain a core temperature $>$ 34-35°C as there are numerous undesirable consequences of significant hypothermia ($<$ 32°C) in the organ donor – e.g., cardiac dysrhythmia, cardiac instability, ↓GFR and cold diuresis, a left shift in the oxyhemoglobin dissociation curve, and pancreatitis. While other endocrine or metabolic disturbances may exist as a result of destruction of the hypothalamic-pituitary axis, currently there is no consistent recommendation for any other hormonal replacement therapy.

**Tests:** Serum electrolytes and osmolality every 4-6 hrs

**Hematologic**

Donors may be anemic from hemodilution and/or hemorrhage. In order to insure adequate tissue $O_2$ delivery, PRBCs are transfused to maintain Hct >30. Some donors may exhibit a coagulopathy; clinically significant bleeding should be treated with clotting factors and platelets. Persistent or severe primary fibrinolysis or DIC may require rapid transfer of the donor to the OR for organ retrieval. Administration of epsilon-aminocaproic acid to treat fibrinolysis is avoided for fear of microvascular thrombosis in the donor organs.

**Tests:** Hb/Hct; PT; PTT; platelet count; DIC screen as clinically indicated.

**Other**

The role of oxygen-free radicals, with regard to reperfusion injury, has prompted the suggested use of mannitol and steroids (and other compounds) as scavengers.

## INTRAOPERATIVE

**Anesthetic technique:** Although anesthesia is unnecessary in brain-dead organ donors, both visceral and somatic reflexes can lead to physiologic responses during the procedure. The goals of intraop management with regard to respiratory, cardiovascular, hematologic and neurologic status are identical to those discussed under preop considerations.

**Induction**

Settings for mechanical ventilation parallel those of the ICU, although it may be advisable to begin with an $FiO_2$ of 100% until the first ABG result is obtained. The exception is when procurement of the lungs or heart-lungs is anticipated; then $FiO_2$ should not exceed 40%. To eliminate reflex neuromuscular activity and to facilitate surgical retraction, a long-acting neuromuscular blocking agent such as pancuronium or pipecuronium (0.15 mg/kg) should be given at the beginning of the procedure and supplemented as necessary.

**Maintenance**

Reflex hypertensive responses to surgical stimulation occur frequently and may lead to excessive intraop blood loss and damage to donor kidneys; management should include the weaning of vasopressors and the initiation of vasodilator therapy with isoflurane, SNP or NTG.

Anesthetic care continues until the proximal aortic cross-clamp is applied. D/C all monitoring and supportive therapy at this point. The notable exception is the case of heart-lung or lung procurement; in this situation, all monitoring except $FiO_2$ should cease with proximal aortic cross-clamping. All supportive care is terminated, with the exception of mechanical ventilation of the lungs at 4 breaths/min or as directed by the transplant team, and suctioning of the ETT after cessation of mechanical ventilation just prior to removal of the tube. Extubation marks the termination of anesthetic care of the heart-lung or lung donor.

| | | |
|---|---|---|
| **Blood and fluid requirements** | IV: 14-16 ga x 1-2<br>NS/LR @ 2-4 ml/kg/hr | Significant 3rd-space losses; may need to administer large volumes of crystalloid, colloid (up to 1 L) and PRBCs (not uncommon to transfuse 2 or more U to maintain Hct >30). Central venous access is necessary for monitoring and for vasoactive drug delivery. |
| **Monitoring** | Standard monitors (see Appendix).<br>Intra-arterial BP<br>CVP line<br>UO | If a PA catheter is in place, it may be used or removed based on concerns of catheter-related, right-side endocardial lesions. Rarely is insertion of a PA catheter warranted in these operations. ABG, Hb/Hct, serum electrolytes and glucose should be monitored hourly; for operations involving procurement of lungs or heart-lungs, ABGs should be obtained at least every 30 min. |
| **Complications** | Hypotension | Most commonly 2° hypovolemia and neurogenic shock (loss of descending vasomotor control). Insure adequate volume repletion as described above, then institute or increase inotropic/vasopressor therapy as previously outlined. |
| | Dysrhythmias | Multiple possible etiologies as described above. Standard treatment and diagnosis should be employed, with the exception of bradycardia, which is atropine-resistant and should be treated with isoproterenol, dopamine, epinephrine or transvenous pacing. |
| | Cardiac arrest | CPR should be instituted in an effort to maintain the viability of the liver, kidneys and other abdominal viscera intended for transplantation. Procurement of the liver and kidneys should proceed rapidly to aortic cross-clamping at the diaphragm and administration of cold preservation fluid into the aorta and portal vein. This series of events will undoubtedly preclude use of the heart and lungs for transplantation. |
| | Oliguria | Insure adequate volume replacement and BP as outlined, then add dopamine (2-3 $\mu$g/kg/min), if not previously instituted to promote renal vasodilation and to increase renal blood flow, glomerular filtration rate and UO. If these measures are ineffective at restoring adequate UO (>1 cc/kg/hr)), then furosemide or mannitol may be used in consultation with the transplant team. |
| | Diabetes insipidus | Fluid and electrolyte therapy as determined by filling pressures and hourly serum electrolyte values. Adjustment of vasopressin or DDAVP infusion to maintain UO < 1.5-3.0 cc/kg/hr; initiation of this infusion should be done in consultation with the transplant team. As previously discussed, it may be advisable to D/C vasopressin or DDAVP at least 1 hr prior to aortic cross-clamping. |
| | Coagulopathy | Transfuse platelets, FFP and cryoprecipitate as necessary for clinical bleeding in the setting of abnormal coagulation studies. Avoid EACA due to risk of microvascular thrombosis in the donor organs. |
| | Hyperglycemia | Avoid dextrose-containing solutions which may aggravate existing hyperglycemia and contribute to osmotic diuresis and electrolyte abnormalities. |
| | Hypothermia | Early aggressive attempts to minimize intraop heat loss are essential and include warming the OR, use of a warming blanket, insulating exposed areas (head, neck, shoulders), warming all fluids, and using heated, humidified inspired gasses. |

| | | |
|---|---|---|
| **Special considerations** | Heart-lung procurement | Division of the mediastinal pleura and tracheal dissection with manipulation of each lung outside the mediastinum may result in profound hypotension and may cause problems with oxygenation and ventilation. Adequate intravascular volume is essential, and inotropic therapy may be required during this period. Problems with ventilation and oxygenation must be communicated immediately to the transplant team. Following aortic cross-clamping and infusion of cardioplegia solution, the lung preservation fluid will be infused via the right and left PAs. During this period, the lungs should be ventilated manually with 4 bpm, or as otherwise directed by the transplant team. It is prudent early on in the procurement procedure to verify the position of the ETT with the transplant surgeon to insure that the tube does not contribute to mucosal injury at the site of the anticipated suture line. |
| | Organ preservation | Therapy aimed at improving organ preservation may require several pharmacologic manipulations as directed by the transplant team. Agents commonly used during organ procurement include dopamine (2-3 $\mu$g/kg/min), furosemide, mannitol, allopurinol (free-radical scavenger), chlorpromazine and phentolamine (vasodilators), heparin (prevents microvascular thrombosis and promotes reperfusion), and $PGE_1$ (vasodilator, membrane stabilizer, anti-platelet effect). Systemic infusion of $PGE_1$ prior to aortic cross-clamping (commonly used in heart-lung or lung procurement) will lead to predictable and profound hypotension; efforts at volume resuscitation toward optimal CVP should continue until the aortic cross-clamp is applied. If heparin is to be administered iv, a catheter should be used after verifying the ability to freely aspirate blood. Methylprednisolone (30 mg/kg) is commonly administered at least 2 hrs before organ retrieval in an effort to protect the heart and kidneys from ischemic injury. |

## POSTOPERATIVE

Not applicable.

**References**

1. Simmons RL, Finch ME, Ascher NL, Najarian JS, eds: *Manual of Vascular Access, Organ Donation and Transplantation.* Springer-Verlag, New York: 1984.
2. Firestone L, Firestone S: Anesthesia for organ transplantation. In *Clinical Anesthesia*, 2nd edition. Barash PG, Cullen BF, Stoelting RK, eds. JB Lippincott Co, Philadelphia: 1992, 1479-82.
3. Gelb AW, Robertson KM: Anaesthetic management for the brain dead for organ donation. *Can J Anaesth* 1990; 37:(7)806-12.
4. Robertson KM, Cook DR: Perioperative management of the multiorgan donor. *Anesth Analg* 1990; 70(5):546-56.
5. Salter DR, Dyke CM: Cardiopulmonary dysfunction after brain death. In *Anesthesia for Organ Transplantation.* Fabian JA, ed. JB Lippincott Co, Philadelphia: 1992, 81-94.

**General References**

1. Terasaki PI, ed: *Clinical Transplants.* UCLA Tissue Typing Laboratory, Los Angeles: 1990.
2. Flye MW, ed: *Principles of Organ Transplantation.* WB Saunders Co, Philadelphia: 1989.
3. Sutherland DER, et al: Results of pancreas transplantation in the United States for 1987-90. *Clin Transplantation* 1991; 5:330-41.

**Surgeon**

**Velerig Selivanov, MD**

## 7.12 TRAUMA SURGERY

**Anesthesiologist**

**Linda Foppiano, MD**

# LAPAROTOMY FOR TRAUMA

## SURGICAL CONSIDERATIONS

**Description**: Indications for laparotomy in the setting of trauma are hemoperitoneum with suspected ongoing significant bleeding, perforated viscus, or shock unexplained by evidence of extremity or chest injury, or pelvic fracture. Clinical manifestations include tenderness and abdominal pain on physical exam, often corroborated by bloody return or positive gram stain on peritoneal lavage. Extravasation of contrast material from hollow viscus on abdominal pelvic CT scan may also be seen. Small amounts of non-contrast fluid from a solid organ (e.g., liver, spleen) laceration may be observed in stable patients.

An **urgent laparotomy** may be indicated in hypotensive patients, who respond poorly to volume resuscitation. Patients may arrive in the OR without benefit of adjunctive diagnostic tests. For stab wounds of the anterior and lateral abdomen, a local exploration of the wound in the emergency department, followed by peritoneal lavage, is usually performed to determine need for formal intraop exploration. For gunshot wounds suspected of penetrating the peritoneum, formal intraop exploration is usually indicated.

The control of hemorrhage under direct vision, with pressure and/or definitive suture repair, requires prompt initiation of the operation, often without preop central or arterial lines in hemodynamically unstable patients. These lines will be essential during the case, but start of the operation should not be delayed by their absence. They should be placed by the anesthesiologist during the case while the surgeons are attempting definitive control of hemorrhage.

The objectives of any laparotomy for trauma are to examine the intraperitoneal space and to control bleeding rapidly. The midline incision is standard in trauma surgery because of its constant anatomic features, rapidity of achieving entry, and its ease of closure. Upon entering the peritoneum through the linea alba, the surgeon and anesthesiologist expect to encounter free blood, and a quick decision must be made as to whether this is an exsanguinating hemorrhage or a mild hemorrhage. If exsanguinating, the source must be identified immediately and tamponaded. Occasionally it may be necessary to clamp the aorta at the level of the diaphragm. This does not decrease any large, venous hemorrhage from the juxtahepatic veins, however, and hepatic and perihepatic packing may be necessary to provide time to catch up with blood loss.

The decision to perform a **Pringle maneuver** and do **veno-veno bypass** or **atrio-caval shunting** must be made early in the case. These modalities of treatment, especially atrio-caval shunting, are reserved for injuries of the liver with massive uncontrollable hemorrhage (e.g., when bleeding is so great that packing cannot staunch it). This circumstance arises from injury and bleeding from intra-hepatic vena cava and juxta-caval hepatic veins. Indecision in the face of such hemorrhage leads to exsanguination. A 500 cc instantaneous blood loss may be expected with each brief attempted look at the area of bleeding. A rapid judgment must be made as to whether packing is still feasible or, if not, to opt for vascular isolation and the increased exposure that atrio-caval shunt provides. This is a wiser course than repeated attempts at placing "the definitive stitch" under poor exposure with torrential hemorrhage. The advent of rapid blood infuser technology has made it easier to keep up with blood loss. Usually the amount of hemorrhage seen upon entering the peritoneum is not life-threatening, and there is time to pack off and systematically examine all quadrants of the abdomen. A cell saver may be utilized to salvage blood from the peritoneum; however, care must be taken not to dislodge any clots.

In penetrating trauma, the retroperitoneum occasionally needs to be explored. In blunt trauma, retroperitoneal hematomas are left alone as they usually will tamponade off in the retroperitoneal tissue planes. Retroperitoneal hematomas may enlarge, requiring blood transfusion. Opening retroperitoneal hematomas from blunt injury risks exsanguination from multiple, simultaneous venous sources. Large tears of the bowel and the colon are clamped or ligated with umbilical tape. Occasionally a small tear is discovered upon running the small bowel and may be repaired at that time. After control of bleeding points, resection of necrotic tissue and/or resection and closure of injured bowel (with appropriate anastomosis or diversions), the abdomen is irrigated with warm NS and closed in a continuous fashion. During the closure, if the bowel has been out of the abdomen for a considerable time, it will be edematous. Often the closure is of such difficulty that it is wiser to leave the fascia open temporarily to minimize increase in abdominal pressure and, consequently, decrease in pulmonary compliance.

The wide variety and severity of injuries dictate the importance of flexibility and cooperation between the anesthesiology and surgical teams involved in the care of trauma patients. The trauma surgeon should keep the anesthesiologist apprised of his estimate of ongoing blood loss and should warn the anesthesiologist of any intraop maneuvers that may cause sudden losses of blood (e.g., manipulating a lacerated liver, dislodging clots near large blood vessels, as in mobilization of a vena cava or aorta). Similarly, the anesthesiologist should keep the surgeon informed of changes in acid/base status, filling pressures, BP, Hct and oxygenation.

**Usual preop diagnosis:** Trauma with ongoing hemoperitoneum or perforated viscus

### SUMMARY OF PROCEDURE

| | |
|---|---|
| **Position** | Supine |
| **Incision** | Midline, usually with chest and proximal thigh prepped |
| **Special instrumentation** | Thompson bar retractor; Level 1 infuser for rapid infusion of warm blood and fluids |
| **Unique considerations** | Potential for fecal contamination may limit use of autotransfusion device (cell saver). Potential for massive blood loss. |
| **Antibiotics** | Cefotetan 1-2 gm (within first hr) |
| **Surgical time** | 1 - 4 hrs |
| **Closing considerations** | Bowel edema and difficulty of abdominal fascial closure often follows massive transfusion. Closure may result in increased intra-abdominal pressure with consequent ↑PIP and ↑atelectasis. DIC and hypothermia may be present. |
| **EBL** | Highly variable. Mortality is high if >20 U of PRBCs are given. |
| **Postop care** | Frequently intubated to ICU. Occasionally, patients will return to CT scan or angiography. |
| **Mortality** | 11% (for an average Injury Severity Score [ISS] = 44). The ISS is statistically superior in predicting mortality, and is the most widely used summary statistic of overall severity of injuries. The maximum ISS is 75. If a fatal lesion is present in only one anatomic area [e.g., brain, skin, abdomen], the ISS is automatically converted to 75. Scores between 20 and 50 on the ISS provide the greatest opportunity for salvaging individual patients through intervention. In one trauma series, no patient with an ISS >60 survived.) |
| **Morbidity** | Wound infection (perforated viscus, skin closed): 50%<br>Wound infection (intact viscus, skin open): 5%<br>Wound infection (other): 5%<br>Abscess: < 10%<br>PE: < 5%<br>Take-back (bleeding, missed injury): < 5%<br>Loss of bowel function common, x 4-8 d |
| **Procedure code** | 49000 |
| **Pain score** | 8 |

### PATIENT POPULATION CHARACTERISTICS

| | |
|---|---|
| **Age range** | 17-93 yrs |
| **Male:Female** | 78:22 |
| **Incidence** | 5% of trauma victims brought to Stanford University Medical Center undergo laparotomy |
| **Etiology** | Penetrating trauma: 53%<br>Blunt trauma: 47% |
| **Associated conditions** | Abdominal injuries only: 72%<br>With orthopedic injuries: 19%<br>With other injuries (neuro, plastics, ENT): 9% |

## ANESTHETIC CONSIDERATIONS

### PREOPERATIVE

**Respiratory**

Associated injuries such as hemo- and/or pneumothorax may be present, requiring thoracostomy tube placement. A widened mediastinum, apical pleural capping or fracture of the 1st or 2nd rib often occur with serious vascular injuries. Multiple rib fractures suggest possible pulmonary contusions, which may not be evident on initial CXR, but can progressively impair oxygenation and ventilation with time and fluid resuscitation.

**Tests:** CXR (PA + lateral views). Upright inspiratory films best delineate chest structures; expiratory films enhance pneumothorax; ABG.

**Cardiovascular** BP and HR should be followed with trends and responses to fluid resuscitation noted. Tachycardia can maintain an adequate BP, with reduced pulse pressure, despite 25-30% loss of blood volume. Attempt to quantitate overt blood loss (e.g., scalp lacerations, open fracture sites). Blunt chest trauma (e.g., steering wheel contact) may result in myocardial contusion with various dysrhythmias, most often premature ventricular or atrial complexes.

**Tests:** Serial Hct; ECG in patients > 50 yrs of age or with blunt chest trauma

**Neurological** Seek physical evidence of open or closed head injuries such as palpable depressions of the skull or scalp lacerations, abrasions or contusions. Pupil size and reactivity should be noted. Intubation in the ER is necessary for patients who are unable to protect their airway, require hyperventilation, or are combative and unable to cooperate with medical staff for exam and treatment. In general, any patient with a Glasgow Coma Scale (GCS) ≤ 7-9 requires intubation. This patient typically has no spontaneous eye opening, inappropriate or incomprehensible speech and only reflexive motor responses. Motor and/or sensory deficits may reflect spinal cord injury and may be associated with neurogenic ("spinal") shock, particularly with upper thoracic or cervical cord injuries.

**Tests:** Cervical spine x-rays – lateral view, including C7, is a good screening exam, looking for altered vertical alignment and unequal disk interspaces. CT scan of head, looking for gross asymmetry, hemorrhage or obliterated ventricles.

**Musculoskeletal** Known or suspected cervical spine injuries require intubation precautions. In urgent cases, intubation without neck extension is achieved with an assistant providing axial traction on the head. If time permits, awake, blind or fiber optically assisted intubation may be attempted. Basilar skull fractures contraindicate passage of nasal ET or OG tubes. Pelvic and femur fractures may represent sources of significant (>1000 cc) occult blood loss.

**Tests:** Radiographs of cervical spine (see above), skull, extremities

**Hematologic** Depending on estimations of prior, ongoing and anticipated surgical blood losses, preop blood T&C may be desired.

**Tests:** Serial Hct; T&C

**Laboratory** Other tests, as indicated from H&P or suspected injuries, including: electrolytes; liver panel; toxicology screen; blood alcohol level.

**Premedication** Premedication is rarely useful due to the urgency of the procedures and the need to have an alert, responsive patient for serial evaluations of mental status or abdominal pain. Sedative premedication should be avoided in patients who are hemodynamically unstable and those with probable head injuries. Virtually all patients are considered to have full stomachs and any compromise of the ability to protect the airway is inappropriate. While Na citrate (30 cc po) may be administered to patients at risk for aspiration, histamine-blockers and metoclopramide may not reach effective levels in the short interval before induction.

## INTRAOPERATIVE

**Anesthetic technique:** GETA with full-stomach precautions.

**Induction** Before induction, a variety of laryngoscope blades (e.g., Miller 1 and 2, Mac 3 and 4) and ETTs with stylets (7.0 and 8.0 mm) should be ready. Equipment for emergent cricothyroidotomy (a 14-ga iv catheter + adapter) and jet ventilation should be in OR.

Most often, preoxygenation is followed by a rapid-sequence iv induction with cricoid pressure (Sellick's maneuver) using STP (3-5 mg/kg) and succinylcholine (1.0-1.5 mg/kg). If hypotension is present or a concern, alternate induction agents (e.g., ketamine 0.5-1.0 mg/kg iv or etomidate 0.1-0.3 mg/kg iv) may be used. Axial head and neck traction is necessary if cervical spine injury is present or suspected.

Patients who are profoundly hypotensive may enter the OR already intubated. Induction consists of verifying ETT placement by auscultation and $ETCO_2$ monitoring. Ventilation with 100% $O_2$ and muscle relaxation with pancuronium or vecuronium (0.1 mg/kg iv) is appropriate. Ongoing fluid resuscitation should be continued during this time.

**Maintenance** $O_2$/air, muscle relaxants, narcotics and volatile agents are titrated as tolerated. Avoid $N_2O$ in the presence of pneumothorax, pneumocephalus, bowel distention, or prolonged procedures. Shorter-acting agents (e.g., volatile agents, fentanyl, vecuronium), carefully titrated, may be preferred in patients with head injuries to facilitate early postop assessment of neurologic status. If hypotension precludes use of volatile agents, low-dose scopolamine (0.1-0.2 mg iv) or ketamine (0.25 mg/kg/15-30 min) can provide amnesia. Heated humidifiers should be used, particularly

| | | |
|---|---|---|
| | in prolonged cases. Heating blankets and elevated room temperatures may also be necessary if hypothermia becomes problematic. | |
| **Emergence** | Prior to extubation, patient should be awake and able to protect his/her airway, and should be hemodynamically stable and spontaneously ventilating with ease through the ETT. Patients who should not be extubated at the end of the case include elderly with rib fractures, hemodynamically unstable patients, those who have received massive fluid and blood product transfusion (e.g., with evidence of intestinal edema), or those with coagulopathy. | |
| **Blood and fluid requirements** | Anticipate large blood loss.<br>IV: 2 (large-bore) 14-16 ga x 2 or 7 Fr x 2<br>NS/LR @ 8-10 ml/kg/hr<br>Fluid warmers<br>Rapid-infusion device<br>Airway humidifier<br>± T&C PRBCs. | Large blood losses may be anticipated, depending on the mechanism of injury (e.g., liver lacerations, major vascular injury, pelvic fractures). Crystalloid, colloid and PRBCs should be given to preserve blood volume as estimated by blood losses, systemic BP, CVP/PCWP and Hct. With massive transfusion, platelets and FFP will also be needed. In general, 2 U FFP and 8-10 U of platelets should be transfused after approximately 10 U of PRBCs (1 blood volume in a 70-kg person) have been given. Postop hypothermia is best minimized by warming all iv and irrigating fluids, maintaining OR temperature @ 78-80°F, warming and humidifying inspired gasses, and using warming blankets. |
| **Monitoring** | Standard monitors (see Appendix).<br>Urinary catheter<br>± Arterial line | Standard monitoring should be applied as soon as the patient enters the OR.<br>Arterial lines may be useful in unstable patients or those in whom frequent blood samples are anticipated. |
| | ± CVP line<br>± PA catheter<br>± TEE | CVP line or PA catheter may be useful if vasoactive drips are needed or if ventricular dysfunction is apparent. In truly emergent cases, the placement of additional monitoring should be accomplished without delay of or interference with the surgical control of hemorrhage and without interrupting aggressive volume resuscitation in progress. |
| **Positioning** | ✓ and pad pressure points.<br>✓ eyes. | If C-spine has not been cleared by radiographs, the neck should remain immobilized intraop and postop. |

## POSTOPERATIVE

| | | |
|---|---|---|
| **Complications** | Hypothermia | Active warming of blood products, warming blankets (Bair-Hugger®) and warm room temperatures should be continued in PACU if hypothermia persists. |
| | Atelectasis, V/Q mismatch | Pulmonary compliance is often increased with large volumes of fluid replacement. Pulmonary contusions may aggravate this problem and severely compromise oxygenation and ventilation, requiring high inspired $O_2$ concentration, high PIP and PEEP. |
| | Coagulopathy | Coagulation products may be necessary, based on platelet counts, PT/PTT, and ongoing RBC transfusion requirements. |
| **Pain management** | PCA or parenteral narcotics (see Appendix). | Patients with rib fractures benefit from epidural narcotic infusions. |
| **Tests** | Hb/Hct<br>CXR, if postop intubation or intraop central line or thoracostomy tubes were placed. | PT/PTT, platelet counts, if unexplained bleeding postop. Fibrinogen, fibrin split products, if DIC is suspected. |

## References


1. Trunkey D, Federle MP: Computed tomography in perspective. *J Trauma* 1986; 26(7):660-61.
2. Trunkey D, et al: Abdominal trauma and indications for celiotomy. In *Trauma*, 2nd edition. Moore EE, Mattox KL, Feliciano DV, eds. Appleton & Lange, Norwalk, CT: 1991.
3. Oreskovich MR, Carrico CJ: Stab wounds of the anterior abdomen. Analysis of a management plan using local wound exploration and quantitative peritoneal lavage. *Ann Surg* 1983; 198(4):411-19.
4. Blaisdell WF: General assessment, resuscitation and exploration of penetrating and blunt abdominal trauma. In *Trauma Management*, Vol 1. Blaisdell WF, Trunkey D, eds. Thieme-Stratton, New York: 1981.
5. Carmona RH, et al: The role of packing and planned reoperation in severe hepatic trauma. *J Trauma* 1984; 24(9):779-84.
6. Cogbill JH, et al: Severe hepatic trauma: a multicenter experience with 1335 liver injuries. *J Trauma* 1988; 28:1433-38.
7. Stanford Trauma Center registry data. June 1990-June 1992.

**Surgeons**

**Babak Edraki, MD** *(Gynecological Oncology, Obstetric Surgery)*
**Nelson Teng, MD, PhD** *(Gynecological Oncology Surgery)*
**Padma Malipedi, MD** *(Gynecological Oncology Surgery)*
**Daniel S. Kapp, MD, PhD** (*Gynecological Oncology Surgery*)
**W. Leroy Heinrichs, MD, PhD** (*Gynecology/Infertility Surgery*)
**Jan T. Rydfors, MD** (*Gynecology/Infertility Surgery*)
**Yasser El-Sayed, MD** (*Obstetric Surgery*)
**Ronald N. Gibson, MD** (*Obstetric Surgery*)
**R. Harold Holbrook, Jr, MD** (*Obstetric Surgery*)

---

# 8. OBSTETRIC & GYNECOLOGIC SURGERY

---

**Anesthesiologists**

**Jon W. Propst, MD, PhD** *(Gynecological Oncology Surgery)*
**Myer H. Rosenthal, MD, FACCP** *(Gynecological Oncology Surgery)*
**Emily Ratner, MD** *(Gynecology/Infertility Surgery)*
**Sheila E. Cohen, MB, ChB, FRCA** *(Obstetric, Gynecology/Infertility Surgery)*
**Carter Cherry, MD** *(Obstetric, Gynecology/Infertility Surgery)*

**Surgeons**

**Babak Edraki, MD**
**Nelson Teng, MD, PhD**
**Padma Malipedi, MD**
**Daniel S. Kapp, MD, PhD**

## 8.1 GYNECOLOGICAL ONCOLOGY

**Anesthesiologists**

**Jon W. Propst, MD, PhD**
**Myer H. Rosenthal, MD, FACCP**

# STAGING LAPAROTOMY FOR OVARIAN CANCER

## SURGICAL CONSIDERATIONS

**Description**: Ovarian carcinoma has the highest mortality rate of all gynecologic malignancies because it is usually discovered in advanced stages, with pelvic mass and ascites being common findings at presentation. Surgery is used for staging as well as therapy. Studies have demonstrated an inverse relationship between postop residual tumor mass and survival; therefore, the goals of surgery are accurate staging and optimal tumor debulking (< 1 cm residual disease). The standard procedure consists of meticulous exploration of the abdominopelvic cavity, abdominopelvic cytology, multiple random and targeted biopsies, **total abdominal hysterectomy (TAH)**, **bilateral salpingo-oophorectomy (BSO)**, **pelvic** and **para-aortic lymph node dissection**, **infracolic omentectomy** and **appendectomy**. After access to the abdomen is obtained through a midline or paramedian abdominal incision, cytologic washings of the pelvis, paracolic gutters, lesser sac and hemidiaphragms are done. The peritoneal cavity is carefully explored. A TAH/BSO is then performed by ligating and transecting the round, infundibulopelvic, broad, cardinal and uterosacral ligaments on both sides. The specimen is cut away from the vagina and the cuff closed. The pelvic and para-aortic lymph nodes are dissected in a manner similar to that described under "Radical Hysterectomy." All residual tumor is removed, using sharp dissection and/or CUSA and/or Argon Beam Coagulator. An appendectomy is usually performed. The omentum is clamped, transected and ligated along its attachment to the transverse colon. A bowel resection with possible colostomy formation may be necessary to achieve optimal cytoreductive surgery (see "Pelvic exenteration"). The peritoneal cavity is copiously irrigated with warm water. Targeted and random biopsies of bladder, cul-de-sac of Douglas, pericolic gutters, hemidiaphragms, small bowel, large bowel and anterior abdominal wall are performed. A permanent peritoneal port may be placed subcutaneously for use in future dose-intensive intraperitoneal chemotherapy. A less extensive surgical procedure may be appropriate if a large volume of unresectable tumor is discovered. Surgery in these cases must be individualized.

In some Stage I lesions a **unilateral salpingo-oophorectomy** is sufficient therapy. The decision to use this approach depends on cell type, age, reproductive status and extent of disease. Generally, a retroperitoneal **lymph node dissection**, **omentectomy** and **appendectomy** are also performed. Approximately 25% of patients undergoing **cytoreductive surgery** for advanced stages of ovarian carcinoma require bowel resection with either primary re-anastomosis or colostomy. Some centers include a routine **splenectomy** in their surgical approach to ovarian cancer; some place a permanent central venous infusion port for convenient venous access. This is usually done at the completion of the abdominal surgery following skin closure.

**Usual preop diagnosis**: Ovarian cancer

### SUMMARY OF PROCEDURE

| | |
|---|---|
| **Position** | Supine |
| **Incision** | Midline or paramedian abdominal |
| **Special instrumentation** | CUSA, Vital View® (suction-irrigation device combined with light source) helpful; laparoscopic Bx forceps (laparoscope, laparoscopic instruments for evaluation of upper abdomen through lower vertical abdominal incision); Argon Beam Coagulator; TA, GIA, EEA stapling devices |
| **Unique considerations** | Removal of large amounts of ascites may result in fluid shifts and intravascular volume depletion intraop and postop. |
| **Antibiotics** | Cefotetan 2 gm iv on call to OR; then q 12 hrs x 2 d |
| **Surgical time** | 1 - 4 hrs; 4 - 5 hrs including splenectomy and bowel surgery for more advanced stages. |
| **Closing considerations** | NG tube placement by anesthesiologist; permanent peritoneal or central venous access for subsequent chemotherapy |
| **EBL** | 500-1000 cc; 250-500 cc for Stage I lesions; 1300 cc for more advanced stages |
| **Postop care** | Extensive peritoneal raw surfaces lead to intraperitoneal fluid 3rd-spacing. Patients require good hydration to maintain intravascular volume. Central hemodynamic monitoring and ICU admission are useful in selected patients. Use SCDs and mini-dose heparin for DVT prophylaxis. |
| **Mortality** | 1-2/1000 |
| **Morbidity** | Postop fever: 14-19%<br>Wound infection: < 5%<br>PE: 1-2%<br>Wound dehiscence: 0.3-3%<br>Ureteral injury: < 1%<br>Vaginal vault prolapse: Rare |

**Procedure code** 58950, 58951
**Pain score** 7-8

### PATIENT POPULATION CHARACTERISTICS

| | |
|---|---|
| **Age range** | All age groups; most common, 50-59 yrs. |
| **Incidence** | 20/100,000 (18,500+ new cases/yr); 1.4% lifetime risk of ovarian cancer |
| **Etiology** | Unknown |
| **Predisposing factors** | Family history<br>↑age at first pregnancy<br>Gonadal dysgenesis<br>Exposure to radiation<br>Environmental factors |
| **Associated conditions** | Familial cancer syndromes (e.g., endometrial, colon, breast)<br>Peutz-Jeghers syndrome – 5% of cases develop gonadal stromal tumor<br>XY gonadal dysgenesis – gonadoblastomas<br>Multiple nevoid basal cell carcinoma (Gorlin's syndrome)<br>Ataxia telangiectasia (hereditary, progressive cerebellar lack of muscular coordination associated with recurrent pulmonary infections and ocular and cutaneous telangiectasias) |

---

## ANESTHETIC CONSIDERATIONS

### PREOPERATIVE

Ovarian carcinoma is usually diagnosed at a relatively late stage and, therefore, the patient may have significant ascites and a fairly large tumor mass. Surgery is indicated for cure of localized tumor and for staging of distant and local metastases. Additional procedures, such as bowel resection or lymph node dissection, are sometimes performed at the same time.[7,8]

| | |
|---|---|
| **Respiratory** | Significant ascites may distend the abdomen and produce respiratory compromise. The presence of orthopnea, tachypnea or other signs of impaired ventilation need to be investigated. Underlying lung diseases such as asthma may also be exacerbated by the abdominal distension. Ask whether patient has received bleomycin (>200 mg/m$^2$), which produces lung injury (Table 8.1-1).<br>**Tests:** CXR; others as indicated from H&P. |
| **Cardiovascular** | If patient has received cardiotoxic drugs such as daunorubicin (>550 mg/m$^2$), a cardiology consultation is indicated. An ECHO, MUGA scan or other studies may be requested to evaluate cardiac function. Exercise tolerance should be evaluated in every patient and any pre-existing cardiac disease explored in the preop visit.<br>**Tests:** As indicated from H&P. |
| **Gastrointestinal** | Patient should have adequate preop iv hydration if given a bowel prep overnight.<br>**Tests:** Serum electrolytes |
| **Neurological** | Not usually significant unless there is neurotoxicity from chemotherapy (see Table 8.1-1). Cyclophosphamide prolongs neuromuscular blockade. |
| **Hematologic** | **Tests:** Hct; WBC: platelets; PT; PTT |
| **Laboratory** | Electrolytes; renal function test; LFT; UA; CT scan of abdomen and pelvis; ECG |
| **Premedication** | Anxiolytic such as lorazepam (1 mg po) on the night before surgery. Midazolam 1-2 mg iv on the morning of surgery. |

### INTRAOPERATIVE

**Anesthetic technique:** GETA. Typically, a balanced anesthetic with inhalational agents and narcotics. An epidural catheter may be placed for postop pain management, and may also be used intraop to decrease anesthetic requirements.

| | |
|---|---|
| **Induction** | Standard induction (see Appendix). |
| **Maintenance** | Standard maintenance (see Appendix). Continue muscle relaxant based on nerve stimulator response. Epidural 2% lidocaine with epinephrine 1:200,000 (~10 ml/hr) if catheter is placed preop. A NG tube should be placed after induction and kept on low suction to help prevent postop N&V. Patients with functioning epidural catheters may require increased fluids due to vasodilation. |

| | | |
|---|---|---|
| **Emergence** | The patient may be extubated at the conclusion of surgery unless hemodynamically unstable or severely edematous from fluid resuscitation. Reverse muscle relaxant with neostigmine (0.07 mg/kg with glycopyrrolate 0.01 mg/kg) and give supplemental $O_2$ after extubation. It is reasonable to schedule a postop ICU bed for unstable patients or those who require invasive monitoring for fluid management. | |
| **Blood and fluid requirements** | ± Significant blood loss<br>IV: 16 ga x 2<br>NS/LR @ 4-6 mg/kg/hr<br>5% albumin<br>6% hetastarch | Blood loss may be 1-2 L. Give PRBCs to keep Hct ~30%. 5% albumin or 6% hetastarch are useful for rapid volume replacement if the Hct is acceptable. If large volumes of ascites are removed, significant hypotension can develop from fluid shifts. Third-space losses, therefore, may be 10-15 ml/kg/hr. |
| **Monitoring** | Standard monitors (see Appendix).<br>± Arterial catheter<br>± CVP/PA catheter<br>Foley catheter<br>NG tube | Arterial and PA catheters are indicated for extensive surgery and/or patients with underlying medical conditions (e.g., CAD, COPD). The measurements of cardiac filling pressures helps to guide fluid replacement when surgery is extensive. |
| **Positioning** | ✓ and pad pressure points.<br>✓ eyes.<br>Anti-embolism stockings and SCD | |
| **Complications** | Hypothermia | These patients tend to become hypothermic, so it is important to warm all iv fluids and inspired gasses. A heating blanket on the bed is helpful, as is wrapping the head with towel or plastic. Keep the OR as warm as practical. Central temperature should be monitored in the bladder or esophagus during surgery. |
| | Renal failure | Renal dose dopamine (1-3 $\mu$g/kg/min) may be indicated to maintain UO >0.5 ml/kg/hr in patients with borderline renal function. |

## POSTOPERATIVE

| | | |
|---|---|---|
| **Complications** | Excess fluid requirement | If patient required large volumes of fluid, extubation may need to be delayed until a diuresis can be started. IPPV with PEEP may be beneficial in maintaining lung volumes and decreasing lung water accumulation. Measurement of cardiac filling pressures is helpful in guiding therapy. |
| **Pain management** | PCA (see Appendix).<br>Epidural narcotics (see Appendix). | Meperidine or morphine work well with PCA. Fentanyl, hydromorphone or morphine are acceptable drugs for epidural analgesia. |

**Table 8.1-1. Toxicities of selected anti-neoplastic chemotherapeutic agents**

| Agent | Site of Toxicity |
|---|---|
| Vincristine, Vinblastine | Neuropathies, SIADH, Myelotoxicity |
| Cytoxan, Mechlorethamine | Prolong neuromuscular block |
| Bleomycin | Pulmonary toxicity |
| Doxorubicin, Daunorubicin | Cardiotoxicity |
| Methotrexate | Bone marrow depression, GI upset, ulcerative stomatitis, pulmonary infiltrates |
| Fluorouracil | Bone marrow depression, hepatic and GI alterations, nervous system dysfunction. |
| Mercaptopurine, thioguanine | Bone marrow depression |
| Actinomycin D | GI upset, bone marrow suppression, oral ulcerations |
| Mitomycin | Myelosuppression, GI upset |
| Cisplatin | GI upset, peripheral neuropathy, electrolyte disturbances |

**References**

1. Heintz APM, Hacker NF, Berek JS, et al: Cytoreductive surgery in ovarian carcinoma: feasibility and morbidity. *Obstet Gynecol* 1986; 67(6):783-88.
2. Halpin TF, McCann TO: Dynamics of body fluids following the rapid removal of large volumes of ascites. *Am J Obstet Gynecol* 1971; 110(1):103-6.
3. Cruikshank DP, Buchsbaum HJ: Effects of rapid paracentesis. Cardiovascular dynamics and body fluid composition. *JAMA* 1973; 225(11):1361-62.
4. Burghardt E, et al: Pelvic lymphadenectomy in operative treatment of ovarian cancer. *Am J Obstet Gynecol* 1986; 155(2):315-19.
5. DiSaia PJ, Creasman WT: Advanced epithelial ovarian cancer. In *Clinical Gynecologic Oncology*. DiSaia PJ, Creasman WT, eds. CV Mosby, St Louis: 1989, 325-416.
6. Wheeless CR Jr: Staging of gynecologic oncology patients with exploratory laparotomy. In *Atlas of Pelvic Surgery*, 2nd edition. Lea & Febiger, Philadelphia: 1988, 378-79.
7. Roizen MF: Anesthetic implications of concurrent diseases. In *Anesthesia*, 3rd edition. Miller RD, ed. Churchill Livingstone, New York: 1990; 793-893.
8. Morrow CP: Malignant and borderline epithelial tumors of the ovary: clinical features, staging, diagnosis, operative assessment and review of management. In *Gynecologic Oncology: Fundamental Principles and Clinical Practice*. Coppleson M, ed. Churchill-Livingstone, New York: 1981, 655-79.

# RADICAL VULVECTOMY

## SURGICAL CONSIDERATIONS

**Description:** ***En bloc* dissection** of the inguinal-femoral region and the vulva is the time-honored treatment for invasive vulvar carcinoma. The surgery involves bilateral excision of lymphatic and areolar tissue in the inguinal and femoral regions, combined with removal of the entire vulva between the labia-crural folds, from the perineal body to the upper margin of mons pubis (Fig 8.1-1). A large surgical wound is created and, if 1° closure without tension is not possible, a skin graft may be necessary. Deep pelvic nodes are almost never involved with metastases when the superficial and deep groin nodes are free of disease; therefore, a **pelvic lymphadenectomy** is no longer routinely performed. If presence of tumor is documented in the groin nodes, particularly in Cloquet's sentinel nodes (the most cephalad, deep inguinal nodes), a **deep pelvic lymphadenectomy** may be performed. **Postop radiation therapy**, however, is widely used instead of a pelvic lymph node dissection to minimize operative morbidity and confer a survival advantage.

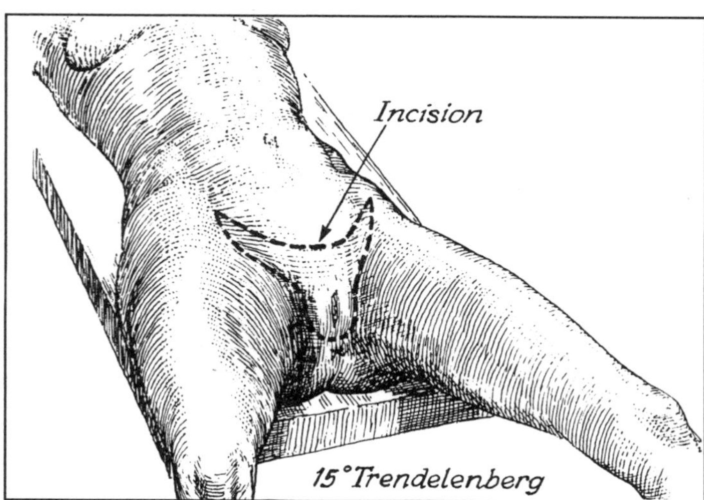

**Figure 8.1-1.** *En bloc* radical vulvectomy and bilateral groin lymph node dissection; with bull's head incision. (Reproduced with permission from Wheeless CR Jr: *Atlas of Pelvic Surgery*. Lea & Febiger: 1988.)

A skin incision in the shape of a bull's head (Fig 8.1-1) allows access to the inguinal-femoral region. (The incision ideally should extend 2+ cm beyond the tumor margin.) The inguinal ligament and rectus fascia should be cleared bilaterally of all nodal tissues. The fossae ovalis on both sides are then identified. The lateral aspect of the femoral sheath is incised along the sartorius muscle, with care being taken not to injure the femoral nerve or vessels. The cribriform fascia is cleaned off the femoral artery. The external pudendal artery, which marks the entrance of the saphenous vein into the fossa ovalis, should be identified and ligated. The proximal and distal segments of the saphenous vein should be ligated and excised as the fibrofatty, lymph-bearing tissue of the femoral sheath is resected. The Cloquet's nodes at the femoral ring beneath the inguinal ligaments on both sides should be resected and submitted for frozen-section pathology evaluation. The deep inguinal lymphatic chain is removed on both sides by opening the inguinal canal from the external inguinal ring. The vulvar incision is carried down through the labia-crural folds. The internal pudendal vessels at the posterior lateral margin of the vulvar incision are identified as they emerge from Alcock's canal, then are ligated and incised. Use of electrocautery in this portion of the procedure usually tends to decrease operative blood loss. The dissection is continued along the periosteum of the symphysis at the level of the fascia of the deep muscles of the urogenital diaphragm. The bulbocavernosus, ischiocavernosus and superficial transverse perinei muscles are removed. A circumferential vaginal incision, excluding the urethral meatus, is then performed and the vulva is removed. The incisions overlying the groin node dissections should be closed with minimal tension after placement of closed-suction Jackson-Pratt drains. The vulvar surgical wound is closed by slightly undermining the skin of the edges of the incision and suturing them to the vaginal mucosa. A **vulvar reconstruction**, using myocutaneous flaps, also can be performed at this time (see "Pelvic exenteration," below).

**Variant procedure or approaches:** In 1962, Byran and associates popularized a **3-incision technique** first described by Kehrer in 1918. Separate incisions are made in each groin and the vulva (Fig 8.1-2). This operative approach has led to a significant decrease in wound infection and breakdown, apparently without increasing tumor recurrence in the inguinal dermal bridge above the symphysis pubis. Another variant is the **hemivulvectomy** (Fig 8.1-3), in which unilateral radical hemivulvectomy and groin node dissection are performed in selected stage I, non-midline, unifocal vulvar cancer patients. This procedure will minimize morbidity, disfigurement and sexual dysfunction. The **deep inguinal node dissection** is performed only if tumor is documented in the superficial nodes by frozen-section evaluation. The observation that almost no contralateral groin metastases occur in the absence of positive ipsilateral groin nodes allows the surgeon to perform only a **unilateral groin node dissection.**

**Usual preop diagnosis:** Invasive vulvar cancer

## SUMMARY OF PROCEDURE

| | *En Bloc* Dissection | 3-Incision | Hemivulvectomy |
|---|---|---|---|
| **Position** | Modified dorsolithotomy in Allen universal stirrups | ⇐ | ⇐ |
| **Incision** | Bull's head, from iliac crest to iliac crest and along labia-crural folds (Fig 8.1-1) | 2 separate groin incisions from iliac crest to pubic tubercle, 1 vulvar incision (Fig 8.1-2) | 1 or 2 separate groin incisions from iliac crest to pubic tubercle; vulvar incision (Fig 8.1-3) |
| **Special instrumentation** | Argon Beam Coagulator | ⇐ | ⇐ |
| **Unique considerations** | Two-team approach to minimize surgical time. Preop bowel prep and constipating medications (e.g. Lomotil®) to decrease postop bowel movements. | ⇐ | ⇐ |
| **Antibiotics** | Cefotetan 2 gm iv on call to OR; then 2 gm iv q 12 hrs x 72 hrs | ⇐ | ⇐ |
| **Surgical time** | 3 - 4 hrs | ⇐ | 2 - 3 hrs |
| **Closing considerations** | Possible skin graft; vulvar and groin suction drains | ⇐ | ⇐ |
| **EBL** | 500-1000 cc | ⇐ | 250-1000 cc |
| **Postop care** | PACU or ICU, if necessary. SCDs and mini-dose heparin for DVT prophylaxis. (**NB:** trauma to femoral vessels at time of groin lymph node dissection increases risk of thrombophlebitis and PE. Aggressive local wound care. | ⇐ | ⇐ |
| **Mortality** | 1-2% | ⇐ | ⇐ |

| | *En Bloc* Dissection | 3-Incision | Hemivulvectomy |
|---|---|---|---|
| **Morbidity** | Wound infection and breakdown: 40-80% | 15% | < 15% |
| | Introital stenosis and dyspareunia: 50% | ⇐ | ⇐ |
| | Lymphedema of lower extremities: 25-30% | ⇐ | < 25% (if deep groin nodes not dissected) |
| | Lymphocysts: 10% | ⇐ | ⇐ |
| | Genital prolapse: 7% | ⇐ | 1-2% |
| | Stress incontinence: 5% | ⇐ | 1-2% |
| | Thrombophlebitis: 3-5% | ⇐ | 1-2% |
| | Hernia: 1-2% | ⇐ | ⇐ |
| | PE: 1-2% | ⇐ | ⇐ |
| **Procedure code** | 56637 | ⇐ | 56631 |
| **Pain score** | 8 | 8 | 7 |

## PATIENT POPULATION CHARACTERISTICS

**Age range** Median 70 yrs

**Incidence** 2.5/100,000; 3-5% of female genital malignancies

**Etiology** Exact etiology unknown; risk factors include:
- Vulvar dystrophies
- Granulomatous disease of vulva
- Bowen's disease
- Condyloma acuminata

**Associated conditions**
- Diabetes
- Obesity
- HTN
- Arteriosclerosis
- Nulliparity
- Positive serology for syphilis
- Cervical malignancy

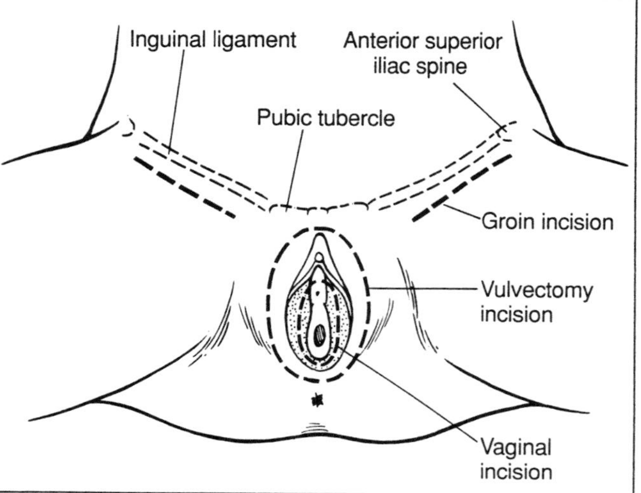


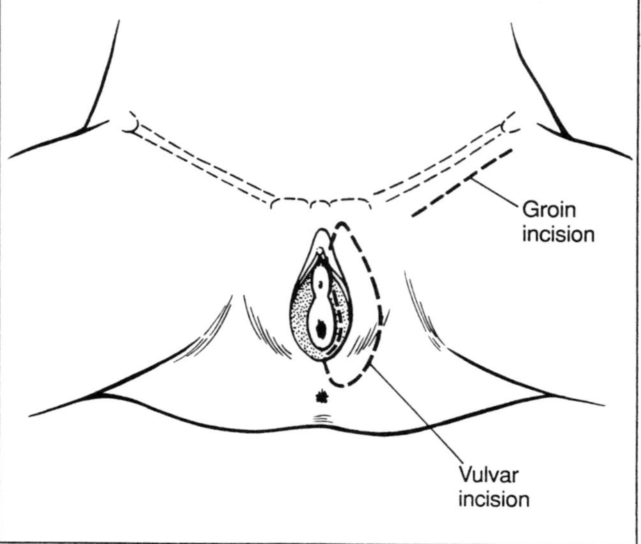


**Figure 8.1-2 (Top).** 3-incision radical vulvectomy and bilateral groin lymph node dissection.
**Figure 8.1-3 (Bottom).** Radical hemivulvectomy with unilateral groin lymph node dissection through a separate incision. (Both figures reproduced with permission from Mattingly RF, Woodruff JD, eds: *TeLinde's Operative Gynecology*. JB Lippincott: 1985.)

# ANESTHETIC CONSIDERATIONS

## PREOPERATIVE

Patients with vulvar carcinoma are typically in the 6th or 7th decade of life and, hence, have a high incidence of concurrent medical problems such as HTN, CAD and diabetes. Radical vulvectomy is performed for invasive tumor which has not metastasized to distant sites. An ICU bed should be reserved for patients with a significant medical history.

**Respiratory** — The presence of lung disease and smoking Hx should be discussed with the patient preop. CXR or PFTs are indicated for patients with significant respiratory disease. The response to bronchodilators should be tested in patients with bronchospastic disease or COPD.
**Tests:** CXR; PFT; ABG

**Cardiovascular** — There is an increased incidence of HTN and atherosclerosis in these patients. A cardiology consultation is indicated for angina, recent MI, CHF or heart murmurs. An ECG should be ordered for all patients >50 yrs old.
**Tests:** ECG; others as indicated from H&P.

**Renal** — In old age, creatinine clearance is decreased due to decreased renal mass, but serum creatinine also decreases because of decreased muscle mass. A preop creatinine clearance, therefore, should be checked in patients >70 yrs old or with known renal dysfunction to assess the degree of impairment.
**Tests:** UA; renal function test

**Gastrointestinal** — Patients should have iv hydration preop if given bowel prep overnight.
**Tests:** Serum electrolytes

**Neurological** — Document a neurological exam if Hx of stroke, seizures or other neurologic disease. Hx of peripheral neuropathy or autonomic dysfunction should be assessed in diabetic patients.
**Tests:** As indicated from H&P.

**Musculoskeletal** — Elderly patients are prone to arthritis and osteoporosis. Inquire about NSAID usage in the last 4 wks preop.

**Endocrine** — Diabetes, obesity and hypothyroidism are common in this population.
**Tests:** Fasting blood sugar; thyroid function; others as indicated from H&P.

**Hematologic** — Chronic anemia may be present. Encourage autologous blood donation if Hct is adequate.
**Tests:** Hb/Hct; PT; PTT; platelets

**Laboratory** — Electrolytes; bleeding time if recent NSAID usage; LFTs if indicated.

**Premedication** — Usually no premedication is needed, but occasionally small doses of midazolam (1-3 mg iv) are useful for anxiety.

## INTRAOPERATIVE

**Anesthetic technique:** GETA ± epidural. Regional anesthesia may be used if there are contraindications to GA.

**General anesthesia:**

**Induction** — Standard induction (see Appendix). Elderly patients usually require reduced dosages of medications. Titration to effect is advised when using any induction agent.

**Maintenance** — Standard maintenance (see Appendix). Continue muscle relaxant based on nerve stimulator response.

**Emergence** — No special considerations

**Regional anesthesia:**

**Epidural** — 2% lidocaine ± epinephrine 1:200,000 (10-15 cc) or 0.5% bupivacaine (10-15 ml) are used; then @ ~10 cc/hr. Narcotics such as morphine (4 mg) or hydromorphone (0.5 mg) may be given in the epidural for postop pain control.

**Blood and fluid requirements**

IV: 16 ga x 2
NS/LR @ 6-8 ml/kg/hr
Warm iv fluids.
UO >0.5 ml/kg hr
PRBCs for Hct < 25% in healthy patients and < 30% in patients with cardiac or pulmonary disease

Occasionally, femoral vessels may be injured, requiring rapid blood replacement. Renal dose dopamine at 3 μg/kg/min may be helpful. Controlled hypotension to MAP = 60-70 mmHg may be helpful in minimizing blood loss (in patients without cardiac or cerebrovascular disease).

| | | |
|---|---|---|
| **Monitoring** | Standard monitors (see Appendix).<br>± Arterial line<br>± CVP line<br>Foley catheter | Invasive monitors indicated for patients in poor condition or with cardiovascular or respiratory disease. An arterial catheter is useful for drawing labs in surgery to check Hct, glucose or ABGs. |
| **Positioning** | √ and pad pressure points.<br>√ eyes.<br>Anti-embolism stockings and SCD | |

**POSTOPERATIVE**

| | | |
|---|---|---|
| **Complications** | Hypothermia<br>Nerve injury<br>Bleeding<br>Atelectasis | <br>Diagnosis of nerve injury may be delayed by epidural anesthesia.<br>Give supplemental $O_2$ postop. |
| **Pain management** | PCA (see Appendix).<br>Epidural narcotics (see Appendix). | Incisions may be left open to granulate in or be covered with skin grafts. Epidural analgesia allows earlier ambulation with less sedation in elderly patients. |
| **Tests** | CXR; ABG; Hct | Tests as indicated from postop clinical findings. |

**References**

1. DiSaia PJ, Creasman WT: Invasive cancer of the vulva. In *Clinical Gynecologic Oncology*. DiSaia PJ, Creasman WT, eds. CV Mosby, St. Louis: 1989, 241-72.
2. Wheeless CR Jr: Radical vulvectomy with bilateral inguinal lymph node dissection. In *Atlas of Pelvic Surgery*. Lea & Febiger, Philadelphia: 1988, 405-11.
3. Mattingly RF, Woodruff JD: Invasive carcinoma of the vulva. In *TeLinde's Operative Gynecology*. Mattingly RF, Thompson JD, eds. JB Lippincott, Philadelphia: 1985, 715-41.
4. DiSaia PJ, Creasman WT, Rich WM: An alternate approach to early cancer of the vulva. *Am J Obstet Gynecol* 1979; 133(7):825-32.
5. Benedet JL, et al: Squamous carcinoma of the vulva; results of treatment, 1938 to 1976. *Am J Obstet Gynecol* 1979; 134(2):201-7.

# CONIZATION OF THE CERVIX

## SURGICAL CONSIDERATIONS

**Description:** Conization of the cervix can be used for both diagnostic and therapeutic purposes. It is performed in cases of biopsy-proven dysplasia with unsatisfactory colposcopy (inadequate visualization of the endocervical canal) or following endocervical curettage showing dysplasia or atypical glandular epithelial cells. Persistent abnormal cytology associated with normal colposcopy, colposcopic suspicion of invasion or cervical biopsy showing micro-invasive cancer are also indications for this procedure. The surgery consists of the annular removal of a cone-shaped wedge of tissue from the cervix with a scalpel.

**Variant procedure or approaches:** In selected patients, a **laser** is used in place of the scalpel. This procedure can be performed under local anesthesia with less blood loss, but operative time is usually longer. The thermal effect of the laser at the cone margins, although usually minimal, may interfere with pathologic interpretation. In pregnant patients, a **shallower cone** is done to minimize complications. Approximately 1% of women with cervical carcinoma are pregnant at the time of diagnosis, and 1/1240 pregnancies is complicated by cervical cancer. Recognition and therapy of pre-invasive cervical lesions during pregnancy, therefore, are of paramount importance. Because of the increased vascularity of the pregnant uterus and cervix, conization is usually associated with increased blood loss and morbidity.

**Usual preop diagnosis:** Cervical dysplasia

### SUMMARY OF PROCEDURE

| | Conization | Laser Conization | Shallow Cone In Pregnancy |
|---|---|---|---|
| **Position** | Lithotomy | ⇐ | Lithotomy; with left lateral tilt in 3rd trimester. |
| **Incision** | Cervical | ⇐ | ⇐ |
| **Special instrumentation** | Colposcope | $CO_2$ laser; protective eyewear; colposcope | Colposcope |
| **Unique considerations** | Infiltration of cervix with dilute vasopressin or phenylephrine solution. A solution of 1:200,000 epinephrine also can be used. Vaginal pack necessary in selected patients. | ⇐ | Phenylephrine, vasopressin or epinephrine should not be used during pregnancy. Liberal use of hemostatic sutures should be made. |
| **Surgical time** | 30 - 60 min | 30 - 90 min | ⇐ |
| **EBL** | 50-200 cc | 50 cc | 100-350 cc |
| **Postop care** | Be aware of postop bleeding. | ⇐ | ⇐ |
| **Mortality** | < 0.01% | ⇐ | ⇐ |
| **Morbidity** | Hemorrhage: 5-10% | ⇐ | 10-15% |
| | Cervical incompetence: 2-3% | ⇐ | ⇐ |
| | Cervical stenosis: 2-3% | ⇐ | ⇐ |
| | Dysmenorrhea: Rare | ⇐ | ⇐ |
| | Infertility: Rare | ⇐ | ⇐ |
| | Injury to rectum and bladder: Rare | ⇐ | ⇐ |
| | Pelvic cellulitis: Rare | ⇐ | Fetal loss: 10-15% (up to 30% in 1st trimester)* |
| | Uterine perforation: Rare | ⇐ | Premature labor: 5-10% (controversial) |
| | | | Rupture of membrane: 2-5% |
| **Procedure code** | 57520 | ⇐ | ⇐ |
| **Pain score** | 3 | 3 | 3 |

*The naturally higher incidence of spontaneous miscarriages in the 1st trimester contributes to this figure.

### PATIENT POPULATION CHARACTERISTICS

| | |
|---|---|
| **Age range** | Reproductive and post-reproductive years |
| **Incidence** | ~5% of Pap smears (+ for dysplasia); 10-17% of patients who undergo colposcopic exams |
| **Etiology** | Smoking<br>Human papilloma virus (HPV)<br>Herpes simplex virus (HSV)<br>Multiple sexual partners<br>Early age of onset of coitus<br>Multiparity<br>Lower socio-economic status<br>Human immunodeficiency virus (HIV)<br>Immuno-compromised hosts |

## ANESTHETIC CONSIDERATIONS

### PREOPERATIVE

Conization is done for diagnosis and treatment of cervical lesions. Occasionally it is necessary to perform the procedure during pregnancy, which increases the risk of bleeding complications. The effect of anesthetic agents on the fetus also needs to be considered.[8]

| | |
|---|---|
| **Respiratory** | Not usually a problem, unless there is Hx of lung disease or smoking. |
| **Cardiovascular** | These patients are generally young and, therefore, less likely to have significant heart disease. |
| **Neurological** | Usually not significant, unless there is Hx of seizure disorder or other neurologic illness. |
| **Hematologic** | **Tests:** Hct; PT; PTT |
| **Laboratory** | Pregnancy test; UA; consider platelet count if regional anesthetic used. |
| **Premedication** | Usually none, although an anxiolytic may be given if not pregnant. Na citrate 0.3 M 30 cc po should be given 30 min prior to induction in all pregnant patients. |

## INTRAOPERATIVE

**Anesthetic technique:** Usually can be a local or MAC anesthetic. The minimalist approach to pharmacologic intervention is appropriate in a pregnant patient. Occasionally, patient may request either GA or regional technique. Pregnancy makes it desirable to perform the procedure under local anesthesia if possible.

**General anesthesia:**

| | |
|---|---|
| **Induction** | Standard induction (see Appendix). In pregnant patients, rapid-sequence induction with cricoid pressure is appropriate. Fentanyl 2-3 $\mu$g/kg iv, morphine 0.05-0.1 mg/kg iv or meperidine 0.5-1 mg/kg iv for analgesia. If patient is to be intubated, use either succinylcholine 1 mg/kg iv or vecuronium 0.1 mg/kg iv for muscle relaxation; otherwise, in non-pregnant patients, mask ventilation may suffice. |
| **Maintenance** | Standard maintenance (see Appendix). It is not necessary to maintain muscle relaxation throughout the case; and either controlled or spontaneous ventilation can be used. |
| **Emergence** | Reverse muscle relaxants with neostigmine or edrophonium and insure that the patient is awake and able to protect her airway prior to extubation. It may be prudent to give an anti-emetic, such as metoclopramide 10 mg iv or droperidol 0.5-1 mg iv, 30 min prior to emergence in non-pregnant patients. |

**Regional anesthesia:** Both spinal and epidural techniques are acceptable, and may be preferred for pregnant patients who cannot tolerate local anesthesia. Prehydration with 1000 cc LR prior to the block is recommended. Treat hypotension with ephedrine 5-10 mg iv, titrated to effect.

| | | |
|---|---|---|
| **Blood and fluid requirements** | Minimal blood loss<br>IV: 18 ga x 1<br>NS/LR @ 2-4 cc/kg/hr | |
| **Monitoring** | Standard monitors (see Appendix).<br>Fetal monitoring may be indicated for pregnancies > 16 wk. | A nurse trained in labor and delivery should accompany patients receiving fetal monitoring. Magnesium or terbutaline may be necessary to suppress the sudden onset of premature labor. Consult with obstetrician on the need for these tocolytic agents. Any evidence of fetal distress should be communicated to the surgeon immediately. |
| **Positioning** | ✓ and pad pressure points.<br>✓ eyes.<br>Left uterine displacement | **NB**: peroneal nerve compression at lateral fibular head → foot drop.<br>Left uterine displacement with a wedge under mattress should be used for pregnant patients (after ~20 wks). |
| **Complications** | Laser eye damage<br>Fire<br>Premature labor | If a laser is used, eye protection is required for the patient and all OR personnel; be alert for fire hazards when using a laser. |

## POSTOPERATIVE

| | | |
|---|---|---|
| **Complications** | Peroneal nerve injury (2° lithotomy position<br>N&V<br>Post-dural puncture headache<br>Premature labor<br>Bleeding | Nerve injury manifested as foot drop and loss of sensation over dorsum of foot.<br>Rx: 10 mg metoclopramide iv<br>May require epidural blood patch later.<br>Tocolytic agents (e.g., terbutaline, magnesium) may be needed, administered in consultation with obstetrician. |
| **Pain management** | Oral analgesic for non-pregnant patients | |

**References**


1. Averette HE, Nasser N, Yankow SL, Little WA: Cervical conization in pregnancy. Analysis of 180 operations. *Am J Obstet Gynecol* 1970; 106(4):543-49.
2. Delmore J, Horbelt DV, Kallail KJ: Cervical conization: cold knife and laser excision in residency training. *Obstet Gynecol* 1992; 79(6):1016-19.
3. Kristensen GB, Jensen LK, Holund B: A randomized trial comparing two methods of cold knife conization with laser conization. *Obstet Gynecol* 1990; 76(6):1009-13.
4. Tabor A, Berget A: Cold knife and laser conization for cervical intra-epithelial neoplasia. *Obstet Gynecol* 1990; 76(4):633-35.
5. DiSaia PJ, Creasman WT: Cancer in pregnancy. In *Clinical Gynecologic Oncology*. DiSaia PJ, Creasman WT, eds. CV Mosby, St. Louis: 1989, 511-22.
6. Samuels F, Landon MB: Medical complications. In *Obstetrics. Normal and Problem Pregnancies*. Gabbe SG, Niebyl JR, Simpson JL, eds. Churchill Livingstone, New York: 1986, 855-57.
7. Jones HW III: Cone biopsy in the management of cervical intra-epithelial neoplasia. In *Clinical Obstetrics and Gynecology*. Pitkin RM, Scott JR, Weingold AB, Stafl A, eds. Harper & Row, Philadelphia: 1983, 26(4):968-79.
8. Levinson G, Shnider SM: Anesthesia for surgery during pregnancy. In *Anesthesia for Obstetrics*. Shnider SM, Levinson G, eds. Williams and Wilkins, Baltimore: 1987, 188-205.


---

# ANESTHETIC CONSIDERATIONS FOR LASER THERAPY TO VULVA, VAGINA, CERVIX

## PREOPERATIVE

Laser therapy is indicated for pre-invasive lesions of the vulva, vagina or cervix. It destroys tissues by the selective application of light energy focused into a beam. Vaporized tissues tend to heal without scarring, and blood loss is minimal due to the cauterizing effect of the laser.[1] Most gynecological laser procedures are done with local anesthesia in the clinic setting and do not require the services of an anesthesiologist.

**Respiratory** Not significant unless there is underlying lung disease.
**Tests:** CXR if >40 yrs old.

**Cardiovascular** In elderly patients, exercise tolerance should be assessed; drug therapy should be given for HTN, CAD or dysrhythmias.
**Tests:** ECG if >50 yrs old.

**Hematologic** **Tests:** Consider platelet count or bleeding time if regional anesthesia to be used; Hct; PT; PTT

**Laboratory** UA; electrolytes; renal function test; pregnancy test in young women

**Premedication** Anxiolytic such as midazolam 1-2 mg iv, if needed.

## INTRAOPERATIVE

**Anesthetic technique:** Either GETA or regional technique may be used. Small lesions may be performed under local anesthesia or MAC.

**General anesthesia:**

**Induction** Standard induction (see Appendix). Muscle relaxation may be accomplished with succinylcholine or a short- or intermediate-acting, non-depolarizing agent.

**Maintenance** Standard maintenance (see Appendix). Continued muscle relaxation is not necessary. A technique with a relatively rapid emergence (e.g. propofol) is useful for outpatient surgery.

**Emergence** No special considerations

**Regional anesthesia:** Spinal or epidural anesthesia may be used with a sensory level to T10. Either lidocaine, tetracaine, or bupivacaine are acceptable, depending on anticipated length of surgery. Provide supplemental $O_2$ if sedation given.

**Spinal** A T10 sensory level is desirable; and lidocaine 75 mg, tetracaine 10 mg or bupivacaine 12 mg can be used. Small-diameter spinal needles (e.g., 25-ga Quincke or 24-ga Sprotte needles) minimize chance of post-dural puncture headache (PDPH).

**Epidural** 2% lidocaine, ± epinephrine 1:200,000 (10-15 cc) or 0.5% bupivacaine (10-15 ml) are used; then @ ~10 cc/hr. Narcotics such as morphine (4 mg) or hydromorphone (0.5 mg) may be given in the epidural for postop pain control.

| | | |
|---|---|---|
| **Blood and fluid requirements** | Minimal blood loss<br>IV: 18 ga x 1<br>NS/LR @ 2-4 cc/kg/hr | Give 1000 cc LR prior to regional block to compensate for vasodilatation. |
| **Monitoring** | Standard monitors (see Appendix). | |
| **Positioning** | √ and pad pressure points.<br>√ eyes. | |
| **Complications** | Eye injury<br>OR fires<br>Aerosolization of viral particles | Goggles should be worn by both patient and all OR personnel during laser use to prevent injury to eyes from light. If the patient is asleep, cover eyes with saline-soaked gauze. Whenever laser is in use, be prepared for fires: know where fire extinguisher is located, and watch for improper handling of lasers. Vaporization of condyloma may produce aerosolization of viral particles; therefore, appropriate ventilation is suggested to disperse smoke. |

### POSTOPERATIVE

| | | |
|---|---|---|
| **Complications** | N&V<br>PDPH | N&V may respond well to 10 mg iv metoclopramide.<br>PDPH may require epidural blood patch for treatment. |
| **Pain management** | Oral analgesics (e.g., Vicodin® or Tylenol® #3 (1-2 tablets po q 4-6 hr) | |

**References**

1. McKenzie AL, Carruth JA: Lasers in surgery and medicine. *Phys Med Biol* 1984; 29(6):619-41.

# SUCTION CURETTAGE FOR GESTATIONAL TROPHOBLASTIC DISEASE

## SURGICAL CONSIDERATIONS

**Description:** Suction curettage is the most efficient method of evacuating a gestational trophoblastic neoplasm (mole). The procedure involves dilation of the cervix by instruments or by laminaria tents, followed by insertion of suction cannula of appropriate diameter into the uterine cavity. Standard negative pressures used are in the range of 30-70 mmHg. Intravenous oxytocin to maintain uterine contraction and minimize blood loss is started after a moderate amount of tissue has been removed. This procedure is followed by gentle, sharp curettage of the uterus. Paracervical injection of dilute vasopressin solution or 1% xylocaine with 1:200,000 epinephrine may decrease operative blood loss (in cases not complicated by thyrotoxicosis or HTN).

**Variant procedure or approaches:** Evacuation of a mole >16 weeks' gestation size is associated with a significant risk of trophoblastic embolization and cardiorespiratory embarrassment (2° pulmonary HTN/edema, cyanosis, ↓CO, ↓BP, right heart failure). Central hemodynamic monitoring using a PA catheter is useful in the management of cardiovascular changes associated with trophoblastic embolization and to prevent inadvertent fluid overload.

**Usual preop diagnosis:** Gestational trophoblastic disease (GTD)

### SUMMARY OF PROCEDURE

| | Small Mole < 16 Weeks Size | Large Mole >16 Weeks Size |
|---|---|---|
| **Position** | Lithotomy | ⇐ |
| **Incision** | None | ⇐ |
| **Special instrumentation** | Suction evacuation kit | ⇐ |
| **Unique considerations** | If mole >12 wks' size, laparotomy setup should be readily available. Oxytocin drip. In some cases, thyrotoxicosis may be present, requiring control with ß-blockers. | ⇐ + Central hemodynamic monitoring with PA catheter; avoid overzealous use of crystalloids and blood transfusions. Preop ABG. |
| **Antibiotics** | Cefotetan 2 gm iv on call to OR | ⇐ |
| **Surgical time** | 30 - 60 min | ⇐ |
| **EBL** | 200-400 cc | ⇐ |
| **Postop care** | Outpatient (usually) | ICU admission in selected cases |
| **Mortality** | Rare | ⇐ |
| **Morbidity** | Trophoblastic embolization: 2.6% | 11-27% |
| | Excessive bleeding: 2% | 10% |
| | Infection: < 2% | ⇐ |
| | Uterine perforation: < 1% | 1-2% |
| | | Acute pulmonary edema: 2-11% |
| **Procedure code** | 59870 | ⇐ |
| **Pain score** | 3 | 3 |

### PATIENT POPULATION CHARACTERISTICS

| | |
|---|---|
| **Age range** | Reproductive age group |
| **Incidence** | 1/1200 deliveries in U.S. |
| **Etiology** | Genetics, androgenous (all chromosomes in true moles are paternal in origin)<br>Nutritional deficiency: protein, folic acid, carotene (vitamin A) |
| **Associated conditions** | Lower socioeconomic status<br>Oriental, Hispanic populations<br>Hyperemesis gravidarum (due to ↑levels of HCG)<br>Pre-eclampsia in first trimester<br>Thyrotoxicosis (Because of its analogy to TSH molecule, ↑levels of HCG can bind TSH receptors and cause thyrotoxicosis.)<br>Prior GTD (incidence ↑ to 0.6-2.0%) |

## ANESTHETIC CONSIDERATIONS

### PREOPERATIVE

Some 80% of cases are diagnosed at the 12th-18th week of development.[9] Most patients have an unusually large uterus for the length of the pregnancy and vaginal bleeding is common. Trophoblastic disease is classified by the degree of invasiveness: retained mole is the most common type and the least invasive. Invasive mole involves the wall of the uterus, and metastatic mole involves more distant sites. Chemotherapy with methotrexate and actinomycin D are usually given postop for invasive or metastatic disease.[10] (See section on TAH/BSO for toxicities of chemotherapeutic agents.)

**Respiratory** — Pulmonary edema may complicate pre-eclampsia, which occurs in 25% of patients with gestational trophoblastic disease. If respiratory distress is present, it also may be due to embolization of tumor to lungs.[7] Avoid over-hydration → pulmonary complications in patients with large moles. **Tests:** ABGs should be obtained preop if there is a question about the pulmonary function of the patient or in patients at high risk of developing trophoblastic embolization. CXR; others as indicated by H&P.

**Cardiovascular** — Blood volume is often depleted due to hyperemesis and vaginal bleeding. Patients may be dehydrated 2° hyperemesis gravidarum preop and adequate hydration should be given preop if patient shows signs of hypovolemia (e.g., tachycardia, orthostatic hypotension, low UO). Pre-

| | |
|---|---|
| | eclampsia may also complicate this disease and can be diagnosed by HTN, proteinuria and edema. If the patient has pre-eclampsia, invasive monitoring of BP may be advisable. Also, if patient is receiving magnesium therapy, a serum level should be checked preop. Magnesium therapy may inhibit myocardial contractility in high doses. Calcium is the preferred antidote for myocardial depression. $MgSO_4 \rightarrow$ uterine atony $\rightarrow$ ↑blood loss. |
| **Neurological** | Seizure prophylaxis with $Mg^{++}$ is indicated for women with severe pre-eclampsia. If seizures occur, a small dose of STP (50-100 mg) or diazepam (10-20 mg) should be given iv and respiration assisted with supplemental $O_2$ by mask. The trachea should be intubated for airway protection in patients with a full stomach and in those who are difficult to ventilate by mask. |
| **Musculoskeletal** | Check reflexes if patient has received $Mg^{++}$. Reduce amount of non-depolarizing muscle relaxant to compensate for the effects of $Mg^{++}$ on muscle strength. |
| **Hematologic** | Anemia may be masked by hypovolemia. Rh – patients with Rh+ partners should receive 300 μg of Rh immune globulin (RhoGAM®) within 72 hrs postop to ↓possibility of Rh iso-immunization in future pregnancies.<br>**Tests:** If patient has received chemotherapy recently, ✓ complete blood count for levels of white cells, and platelets. Bleeding time and platelet count should also be checked in women who have pre-eclampsia or who are having regional anesthesia. |
| **Endocrine** | Hyperthyroidism occurs in 5% of women with hydatidiform moles,[4] and is due to the thyroid-stimulating effects of HCG.<br>**Tests:** Thyroid function tests should be checked preop in women with Sx of hyperthyroidism, and corrected prior to surgery. |
| **Laboratory** | Electrolytes; renal function test; Hct; serum HCG level. Consider thyroid function tests; LFTs; PT; PTT; platelet count; bleeding time; $Mg^{++}$ level; UA, as indicated from H&P. |
| **Premedication** | Usually an anxiolytic such as diazepam 10 mg po or midazolam 5 mg im or 1-2 mg iv. A non-particulate antacid (Na citrate 30 cc 0.3 M) should be given po just before induction. |

## INTRAOPERATIVE

**Anesthetic technique:** Usually GETA, although may be carried out under spinal or epidural anesthesia.

**General anesthesia:**

| | |
|---|---|
| **Induction** | A rapid-sequence induction with cricoid pressure should be used; STP 5 mg/kg iv or propofol 2-3 mg/kg iv is usually recommended. Analgesia is provided by fentanyl 1-3 μg/kg iv or sufentanil 0.1-0.3 μg/kg iv. Succinylcholine 1 mg/kg iv or vecuronium 0.2 mg/kg iv provides muscle relaxation for intubation. |
| **Maintenance** | Standard maintenance (see Appendix). Succinylcholine drip or intermediate-duration, non-depolarizing muscle relaxant may be used depending on anticipated duration of surgery. Prophylaxis for N&V (e.g., metoclopramide 10 mg iv or droperidol 0.5-1.25 mg iv) is recommended. Control BP, if pre-eclamptic, with labetalol, hydralazine or SNP. Try to keep DBP @ 90-100 mmHg. |
| **Emergence** | Extubate when fully awake and protective airway reflexes have returned. Watch for emesis after extubation. Give supplemental $O_2$. |

**Regional anesthesia:**

| | |
|---|---|
| **Spinal** | A T6 sensory level is desirable; and lidocaine (75 mg), tetracaine (10-12 mg) or bupivacaine (10-12 mg) can be used. Small-diameter spinal needles (e.g., 25-ga Quincke or 24-ga Sprotte needles) will minimize the chances of post-dural puncture headache (PDPH). |
| **Epidural** | Use 2% lidocaine ± epinephrine 1:200,000 (10-15 cc) or 0.5% bupivacaine (10-15 cc). Narcotics such as morphine (4 mg) or hydromorphone (0.5 mg) may be given for postop pain control. |

| | | |
|---|---|---|
| **Blood and fluid requirements** | Possible large blood loss<br>IV: 16 ga x 2<br>NS/LR @ 2-4 cc/kg/hr | Two large-volume iv lines should be placed and blood readily available. The usual causes of bleeding are uterine perforation, cervical laceration or uterine atony. |
| **Control of bleeding** | Oxytocin (30 U/L) infusion<br>Isoflurane < 1%<br>Ergonovine maleate 0.2 mg im | Oxytocin is begun about halfway through procedure at 30-60 drops/min (consult obstetrician). Try to keep isoflurane < 1% to prevent uterine relaxation. Ergonovine may be given for severe bleeding. Since this drug can cause HTN, it is contraindicated in cases of pre-eclampsia with elevated BP. |

| | | |
|---|---|---|
| **Monitoring** | Standard monitors (see Appendix).<br>± Arterial catheter<br>± CVP/PA catheter<br>Foley catheter | An arterial catheter and CVP are indicated in cases of thyrotoxicosis, pre-eclampsia or significant hemorrhage. The use of vasodilators such as SNP is also an indication for invasive monitors. |
| **Positioning** | ✓ and pad pressure points.<br>✓ eyes. | **NB**: peroneal nerve compression at lateral fibular head → foot drop.<br>Lifting the legs may cause the level of spinal or epidural anesthesia to move cranially if performed too quickly after the block. |
| **Complications** | Embolization of trophoblastic material | Embolization may occur, especially if >16 wks' gestation. Significant respiratory compromise can occur, requiring postop ventilation and PEEP. |

**POSTOPERATIVE**

| | | |
|---|---|---|
| **Complications** | Bleeding<br>N&V<br>HTN<br>Hypotension | Continue oxytocin infusion. Significant hemorrhage should be evaluated by surgeons for possible perforation, laceration or atony. Anti-emetics such as droperidol (0.6 mg), Compazine® (5-10 mg) or metoclopramide (10 mg) may be useful. BP should be monitored closely in pre-eclamptics. Consider ICU admission if unstable. |
| | Peroneal nerve injury (2° to lithotomy position) | Nerve injury manifested as foot drop and loss of sensation over dorsum of foot. |
| **Pain management** | Epidural, iv, im narcotics (see Appendix). | Other analgesics appropriate for outpatient procedures. |

**References**

1. DiSaia PJ, Creasman WT: Gestational trophoblastic neoplasia. In *Clinical Gynecologic Oncology*. DiSaia PJ, Creasman WT, eds. CV Mosby, St. Louis: 1989, 214-40.
2. Hammond CB, Weed JC Jr, Currie JL: The role of operation in the current therapy of gestational trophoblastic disease. *Am J Obstet Gynecol* 1980; 136(7):844-58.
3. Wheeless CR Jr: Suction curettage for abortion. In *Atlas of Pelvic Surgery*. Lea & Febiger, Philadelphia: 1988, 208-9.
4. Kohorn EI: Clinical management and the neoplastic sequelae of trophoblastic embolization associated with hydatiform mole. In *Obstet Gynecol Surv*, Vol 42(8). Williams & Wilkins, Baltimore: 1987, 484-88.
5. Curry SL, Hammond CB, Tyrey L, Creasman WT, Parker RT: Hydatiform mole: Diagnosis, management and long-term followup of 347 patients. *Obstet Gynecol* 1975; 45(1):1-8.
6. Twiggs LB, Morrow CP, Sehlaerth JB: Acute pulmonary complications of molar pregnancy. *Am J Obstet Gynecol* 1979; 135:(2) 189-94.
7. Lipp RG, Kindrchi JD, Selmitz R: Death from pulmonary embolism associated with hydatiform mole. *Am J Obstet Gynecol* 1962; 83(12):1644-47.
8. Trotter RF, Tieche HL: Maternal death due to pulmonary embolism of trophoblastic cells. Am *J Obstet Gynecol* 1956; 71(5):1114-18.
9. Baird AM, et al: The ultrasound diagnosis of hydatidiform mole. *Clin Radiol* 1977; 28(6):637-645.
10. Jones WB: Gestational trophoblastic neoplasms. The role of chemotherapy and surgery. *Surg Clin North Am* 1978; 58(1):167-79.
11. Bruun T, Kristoffersen K: Thyroid function during pregnancy with special reference to hydatidiform mole and hyperemesis. *Acta Endocrinol* 1978; 88(2)383-89.

# SECOND-LOOK/REASSESSMENT LAPAROTOMY FOR OVARIAN CANCER

## SURGICAL CONSIDERATIONS

**Description**: The clinical evaluation of an ovarian cancer patient's response to chemotherapy may be unreliable because tumor that may defy detection by non-invasive methods can be present in the abdominopelvic cavity. Surgery in the form of "second-look" laparotomy is the most accurate method of evaluation of ovarian cancer patients' response to chemotherapy. It is usually undertaken to determine whether the patient is surgically and pathologically free of disease, after an appropriate number of treatment cycles with platinum-based (CDDP or carboplatin) chemotherapy. In addition, in cases where 1° optimal debulking could not be performed, a "second look"/2° debulking laparotomy is done to achieve optimal cytoreduction. The surgery involves methodical and meticulous exploration of all of the abdomen and pelvis, multiple cytologies and biopsies, lysis of adhesions, resection of the residual tumor, as well as the pelvic and periaortic lymph nodes (if not done at time of first surgery).

**Usual preop diagnosis**: Ovarian carcinoma

### SUMMARY OF PROCEDURE

| | |
|---|---|
| **Position** | Supine |
| **Incision** | Midline or paramedian vertical abdominal |
| **Antibiotics** | Cefotetan 2 gm preop; then q 12 hrs x 2 d |
| **Surgical time** | 2 - 3 hrs |
| **Closing considerations** | Placement of permanent central venous or intraperitoneal access |
| **EBL** | 350-700 cc |
| **Postop care** | PACU → room |
| **Mortality** | 1-2/1000 |
| **Morbidity** | Vaginal vault granulation: 26-44%<br>Postop fever: 14-19%<br>Wound infection: < 5%<br>Wound dehiscence: 0.3-3%<br>PE: 1-2%<br>Incisional hernia: 0.5-1%<br>Ureteral injury: 0.5-1%<br>Necrotizing fasciitis: Rare<br>Post-hysterectomy prolapse of vaginal vault: Rare |
| **Procedure code** | 58960 |
| **Pain score** | 7-8 |

### PATIENT POPULATION CHARACTERISTICS

| | |
|---|---|
| **Age range** | All ages; most common, 50-59 yrs |
| **Incidence** | 10-13/100,000; 18,500+ new cases/yr; 1.4% lifetime risk of ovarian cancer |
| **Etiology** | Risk factors include:<br>Positive family Hx<br>Nulliparity<br>↑age at first pregnancy<br>Gonadal dysgenesis<br>Exposure to radiation<br>Environmental factors |
| **Associated conditions** | Familial cancer syndromes (e.g., endometrial, colon, breast)<br>Peutz-Jeghers syndrome (5% of cases develop gonadal stromal tumor)<br>XY gonadal dysgenesis (gonadoblastomas)<br>Multiple, nevoid basal-cell carcinoma (Gorlin's syndrome)<br>Ataxia telangiectasia |

## ANESTHETIC CONSIDERATIONS

### PREOPERATIVE

Patients having a second-look laparotomy have undergone surgical resection of a tumor with lymph node biopsies, usually followed by chemotherapy and/or radiation therapy. Depending on the type of adjunctive treatment given, the patient may come to surgery in poor physical condition from malnutrition, or toxicity from chemotherapy. Vascular access may be difficult to obtain due to sclerosis or thrombosis of peripheral veins.

**Respiratory** Pulmonary function may be impaired by several chemotherapeutic drugs – most commonly bleomycin. Patients often have a Hickman catheter or other central line already in place which can be used for induction of anesthesia. A preop CXR is mandatory to assess the presence of lung injury. Patients who have dyspnea at rest or with mild exertion, or who have known pulmonary fibrosis, should be evaluated by PFTs, including FVC, $FEV_1$, $MMF_{25-75}$, and ABGs. Patients who have received bleomycin should not receive $O_2$ >39% intraop, but arterial $O_2$ saturation should be kept at least 95%.[5] The pulmonary toxicity of bleomycin is dose-related, with a much higher incidence occurring if over 200 mg/m[6]. Combination chemotherapy with vincristine or cisplatin also increases pulmonary toxicity.[2] Severe lung disease is an indication for the use of spinal or epidural anesthesia whenever possible; otherwise, postop mechanical ventilation may be necessary.

**Tests:** CXR; PFTs; ABGs; others as indicated from H&P.

**Cardiovascular** Cardiotoxicity is seen with several anti-neoplastic agents, especially daunorubicin and doxorubicin. The cardiomyopathy produced by these drugs occurs in two forms: (1) acute – ST- T-wave changes and dysrhythmias, which are transient and usually not a serious problem; and (2) chronic – a dose-related toxicity manifested by CHF. Total doses of doxorubicin as low as 250 $mg/m^2$ can cause myocardial damage, but is more common at doses >550 $mg/m^2$. Cardiac irradiation, or combination chemotherapy with cyclophosphamide, increases the risk of cardiac toxicity.[2] Patients who have received cardiotoxic drugs are usually followed by serial ECHOs or MUGA scans, and the results of these tests should be reviewed preop. Patients with CHF or ECG changes should have a cardiology consultation to optimize their medical condition preop.

**Tests:** ECG; others as indicated from H&P.

**Neurological** Peripheral neuropathies are produced by vincristine, cyclophosphamide, taxol, 5-fluorouracil and several other drugs. Vincristine can also produce SIADH. Other CNS effects include N&V, seizures and cerebellar dysfunction. A preop neurologic exam is required for those patients with evidence of neurotoxicity. It is important to document the presence of neurologic deficits preop for subsequent comparisons.

**Endocrine** Steroids such as prednisone are commonly used as chemotherapeutic agents, and as treatment for pulmonary fibrosis and other complications of chemotherapy. The use of steroids for several wks suppresses the endogenous secretion of the adrenal cortex, which may take up to 6 mo to recover fully. Hydrocortisone 100 mg iv, therefore, is given perioperatively every 8 hrs to cover the stress associated with surgery. The dose is tapered rapidly over 2 or 3 d postop. If patient is receiving hormone replacement for hypothyroidism, it may be continued as scheduled perioperatively. Diabetics should be managed to keep blood sugar @ 150-250 mg/dl. A glucose and insulin infusion (100 U regular insulin/L D5W) is useful for maintaining proper blood glucose levels intraop. Infuse at 10-20 ml/hr, based on the results of hourly blood glucose determinations during surgery; 20 mEq KCl/L may be added in patients with normal renal function to prevent hypokalemia. Oral hypoglycemic agents should be withheld on the day of surgery.

**Tests:** Fasting blood sugar

**Renal** Many chemotherapeutic drugs have renal toxicity; therefore, a preop set of renal function tests is mandatory. Patients with impaired renal function should be given appropriate dosages of medications (e.g., antibiotics) which depend on renal excretion.

**Tests:** Renal function tests; UA

**Musculoskeletal** Vincristine produces a neurotoxicity manifested by numbness and tingling in the extremities, weakness, foot drop, loss of reflexes, ataxia and muscle pains. Muscle weakness in the arms and legs indicates that the drug should be discontinued. Muscle weakness can also sometimes involve the larynx and extraocular muscles of the eye. Reduced amounts of neuromuscular blocking drugs should be used intraop and a nerve stimulator used to follow twitches.

**Gastrointestinal** Consider hydration overnight if given a bowel prep or if there is significant N&V.

**Tests:** Serum electrolytes

**Hematologic** Bone marrow suppression is a very common side effect of anti-neoplastic drugs. The toxicity usually produces a reversible drop in leukocytes, erythrocytes and platelets with a nadir 10-14-d post treatment. Patients with a total neutrophil count of < 1,000 should be kept in isolation until counts improve. A low platelet count (< 50-100,000) is an indication for platelet transfusion preop. Regional anesthesia in patients with thrombocytopenia needs to be carefully considered due to the increased risk of bleeding complications. It is useful to check a bleeding time preop when in doubt about the coagulation status of a patient. A preop transfusion of platelets and/or RBCs is recommended if lab values are below acceptable limits (platelets < 100,000, Hct< 26). **Tests:** Hb/Hct; WBC; PLT; PT; PTT; bleeding time

**Laboratory** LFTs

**Premedication** Anxiolytic such as midazolam 1-5 mg im or iv. Stress-dose hydrocortisone (100 mg) if indicated.

## INTRAOPERATIVE

**Anesthetic technique:** GETA usually indicated. Surgery may be done under regional anesthesia in selected cases of pulmonary toxicity. Combined GETA/epidural is also an excellent choice.

**General anesthesia:**

**Induction** Standard induction (see Appendix). Consider renal function and surgery duration when deciding on agent.

**Maintenance** Standard maintenance (see Appendix). An epidural may be used to reduce GA requirements. Analgesia with fentanyl, morphine, meperidine or epidural local anesthetic, combined with narcotic.

**Emergence** Extubate when patient is responsive and neuromuscular block is fully reversed. In patients with borderline pulmonary function, extubation may be delayed until patient is in the PACU or ICU, and after ABG is checked while the patient breathes spontaneously.

**Regional anesthesia:**

**Epidural** 2% lidocaine ± epinephrine 1:200,000 (10-15 cc) or 0.5% bupivacaine (10-15 ml) are used; then @ ~10 cc/hr. Narcotics such as morphine (4 mg) or hydromorphone (0.5 mg) may be given in the epidural for postop pain control.

**Blood and fluid requirements**

IV: 14-16 ga x 2
NS/LR @ 7-10 ml/kg/hr
Keep UO >0.5 ml/kg/hr.
PRBC for Hct < 30%
5% albumin
6% hetastarch
FFP/PLT

Excessive use of NS can lead to hyperchloremic metabolic acidosis; therefore, alternating NS and LR solutions makes sense when giving large volumes of iv fluids. 5% albumin or 6% hetastarch may be used as volume replacement when Hct >30%, although they have no proven advantages over crystalloid solutions. FFP and platelets are used if there is evidence of coagulopathy (↑PT/PTT, ↓PLT).

**Monitoring**

Standard monitors (see Appendix).
± CVP/PA catheter
Foley catheter
NG tube
± Arterial line

Arterial and CVP catheters are indicated for patients with compromised cardiac or pulmonary function or patients having extensive surgical procedures.

**Positioning**

√ and pad pressure points.
√ eyes.
Anti-embolism stockings and SCD

It is useful to maintain access to at least one arm for blood drawing and additional iv access.

**Complications**

Hypothermia — Warm all fluids and humidify inspired gasses. Heating pad on the bed. Wrap head in plastic or towels.

Bleeding — √ PT; PTT, PLTs periodically for large blood loss.

## POSTOPERATIVE

**Complications**

Bleeding
Nausea — Anti-emetics (i.e., metoclopramide 10 mg iv) should be given for nausea.
Infection
Respiratory insufficiency — Supplemental $O_2$ should be given in PACU.

| | | |
|---|---|---|
| **Pain management** | PCA (see Appendix).<br>Epidural narcotics (see Appendix). | Surgeons may infiltrate wound edges with 0.25% bupivacaine in those patients without epidurals. |
| **Tests** | CXR; ABG | As indicated by postop clinical findings. |


**References**

1. DiSaia PJ, Creasman WT: Advanced epithelial ovarian cancer. In *Clinical Gynecologic Oncology*. DiSaia PJ, Creasman WT, eds. CV Mosby, St. Louis: 1989, 325-416.
2. Barnhill DR, Hoskins WJ, Heller PB, Park RC: The second-look surgical reassessment for epithelial ovarian carcinoma. *Gynecol Oncol* 1984; 19(2):148-54.
3. Copeland LJ, Gershenson DM, Wharton JT, Atkinson EN, Sneige N, Edwards CL, Rutledge FN: Microscopic disease at second-look laparotomy in advanced ovarian cancer. *Cancer* 1985; 55(2):472-78.
4. Dauplat J, Ferriere JP, Gorbinet M, Legros M, Chollet P, Giraud B, Plagne R: Second-look laparotomy in managing epithelial ovarian carcinoma. *Cancer* 1986; 57(8):1627-31.
5. Roizen MF: Anesthetic implications of concurrent diseases. In *Anesthesia*, 3rd edition. Miller RD, ed. Churchill Livingstone, New York: 1990, 793-893.
6. Calabresi P, Chabner BA: Antineoplastic agents. In *Goodman and Gilman's: The Pharmacologic Basis of Therapeutics*, 8th edition. Gilman AG, Rall TW, Nies AS, Taylor P, eds. Pergammon Press, New York: 1990, 1209-63.


# PELVIC EXENTERATION

## SURGICAL CONSIDERATIONS

**Description:** Pelvic exenteration was introduced by Brunschwig as an ultra-radical surgical approach for advanced and radio-resistant cervical cancer. Although advanced vaginal and vulvar carcinoma have occasionally been treated with this procedure, its most important role is in the management of centrally recurrent, surgically resectable, radio-resistant cervical carcinoma. Pelvic exenteration involves ***en bloc* resection** of all pelvic tissues, including uterus, cervix, vagina, bladder and rectum. Involvement of distal vagina may require resection of vulva and groin nodes. The goal of this procedure is curative, with removal of all cancer tissue and reconstruction of appropriate diversions for the urine and stool if the colon cannot be re-anastomosed to the rectum. It is rare for cervical and vaginal cancer to involve the lower 5 cm of the rectum and anus. It is, therefore, possible to mobilize the descending colon and anastomose it primarily to the distal rectum. An **ileal loop urinary conduit, omental pelvic carpet** or **sling** and **gracilis myocutaneous flaps** for vaginal and perineal reconstruction are then performed. A rectus abdominis muscle flap also can be used for vaginal reconstruction. This type of flap yields excellent aesthetic and functional results. In cases where an omental sling (shown in Fig 8.1-4) cannot be developed, an absorbable synthetic mesh is sutured to the pelvic

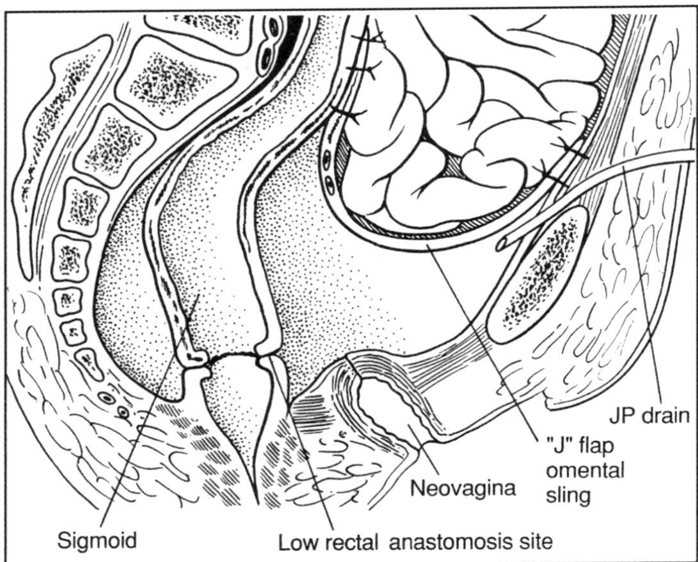


**Figure 8.1-4.** Sagittal section of the pelvis after a total pelvic exenteration. Note that all the reproductive organs, along with their supporting structures, the rectum and the bladder, have been resected. Drains can be placed through separate stab incisions in the abdomen. The small bowel is kept away from the operative site by a pelvic lid. The urinary and fecal diversions are not diagrammed. (Reproduced with permission from Wheeless CR: *Atlas of Pelvic Surgery*. Lea & Febiger: 1988.)

peritoneum to create a pelvic lid (like a hammock) to keep the small bowel off the denuded pelvic peritoneum, and thus decreasing the possibility of small bowel obstruction. In general, an additional 2-3 hours of surgical time and an additional 300 cc of estimated blood loss are expected when a vaginal reconstruction is undertaken. An exploratory laparotomy is needed prior to initiation of the exenterative procedure to rule out spread of disease outside the pelvis and/or extension to pelvic sidewalls and pelvic lymph nodes, all of which are absolute contraindications to this procedure.

Resectability is evaluated by palpation of pelvic and para-aortic lymph nodes, liver, hemidiaphragms and peritoneal surfaces of the upper abdomen and pelvis. Washings should be obtained for cytology. A thorough lymph node dissection should then be performed and all suspicious nodes should be submitted for frozen-section pathologic examination. The pararectal, paravesical and presacral spaces should then be developed. If the patient is found to be inoperable, CUSA can be used to decrease the tumor burden. Consideration also should be given to IORT. If the patient is deemed operable, the space of Retzius is developed. The round ligaments are then transected close to the pelvic sidewall bilaterally; and the infundibulopelvic ligaments are also ligated and transected. The ureters are divided as close to the bladder as possible. The superior hemorrhoidal vessel is ligated and transected; and the colon is transected at the appropriate level. The anterior divisions of the internal iliac artery on both sides are ligated and divided; and the web of tissue is clamped close to the pelvic sidewall, transected and suture-ligated. Following this, sharp dissection can be done to free up the specimen from the low attachments to the levator muscles. In larger tumors, the levator muscle is partially removed with the specimen to provide adequate margins. From a combined perineal and abdominal approach, the distal vagina, urethra and perineum (± rectum) can be resected. The specimen is handed off the field, hemostasis is achieved, an ileal loop or other urinary conduit is performed, low rectal anastomosis is done, vaginal reconstruction is undertaken, and the pelvic floor is covered. (Figs 8.1-4 and 1-5 show the completed exenteration.)

**Variant procedure or approaches: Anterior pelvic exenteration** involves preservation of rectosigmoid, while **posterior pelvic exenteration** involves preservation of bladder. Posterior exenteration has proved more useful in cancer of vulva or vagina than in cervical cancer. Anterior and posterior exenterations are used in selective cases because of the increased risk of an incomplete tumor resection and multiple complications and malfunctioning of the preserved organ.

**Usual preop diagnosis:** Recurrent cervical carcinoma following radiotherapy

## SUMMARY OF PROCEDURE

| | |
|---|---|
| **Position** | Modified dorsolithotomy with Allen stirrups |
| **Incision** | Midline longitudinal, perineal |
| **Special instrumentation** | Vital View® & Argon Beam Coagulator (may be helpful); EEA, GIA, TA staplers; Robo-retractor® or similar devices |
| **Unique considerations** | Full and thorough mechanical and antibiotic intestinal prep. NG tube placement intraop. SCD and mini-dose heparin intraop for DVT prophylaxis. Preop PFTs. Consider preop Greenfield IVC filter placement to avoid PE for high-risk patients. Consider intraop radiation of tumor bed and/or of resection margins. Abort case if extrapelvic metastases and/or tumor extension to pelvic sidewalls noted. |
| **Antibiotics** | Cefotetan 2 gm iv q 12 hrs to begin, 12 hrs preop, and continue 72 hrs postop. |
| **Surgical time** | 8 - 12 hrs (2-team approach); 5 - 10 hrs (for anterior and posterior exenteration) |
| **Closing considerations** | Abdominal drains; colostomy; ureteral stents; urostomy; intraop radiation therapy. Triple-lumen central line placement. Copious irrigation of the operative sites. |
| **EBL** | 1200-4000 cc |
| **Postop care** | ICU: 2-3 d. Correction of electrolyte imbalance. Extensive peritoneal raw surfaces lead to intraperitoneal fluid 3rd-spacing. Patients require good hydration to maintain intravascular volume. SCDs and mini-dose heparin for DVT prophylaxis. Consider concentrated albumin infusion to maintain intravascular volume. Early and aggressive use of TPN is important. Maintain Hct in the low 30s as concentrated blood may lead to sludging and contribute to flap necrosis and wound breakdown. Remove ureteral stents 1-2 wks postop, when the edema at the ureterointestinal site has subsided. |
| **Mortality** | 5-11% |

| | | |
|---|---|---|
| **Morbidity** | Intraop hemorrhage requiring a median of 5 U PRBC transfusion | |
| | Infectious: | Non-specific: 25% |
| | | Flap necrosis: 20% |
| | | Pelvic cellulitis: 19% |
| | | Pyelonephritis: 17% |
| | | Wound infection: 6% |
| | | Sepsis: 3% |
| | Psychiatric: | Confusion: 24% |
| | Intestinal: | Ileus: 18% |
| | | GI fistula: 13% |
| | | Stoma breakdown: 3% |
| | | Small bowel obstruction: 5% |
| | Renal: | Ureteral fistulae: 14% |
| | | Failure: 5% |
| | Cardiovascular: | CHF: 8% |
| | | Venous thrombosis: 3-7% |
| | | DIC: 3% |
| | | Dysrhythmia: 3% |
| | | MI: 3% |
| | Pulmonary: | Pneumonia: 3% |
| | | PE: 2% |
| | Neurologic: | CVA: 2% |
| | | Spinal cord infarction: < 2% |
| **Procedure code** | 58240 | |
| **Pain score** | 7-8 | |

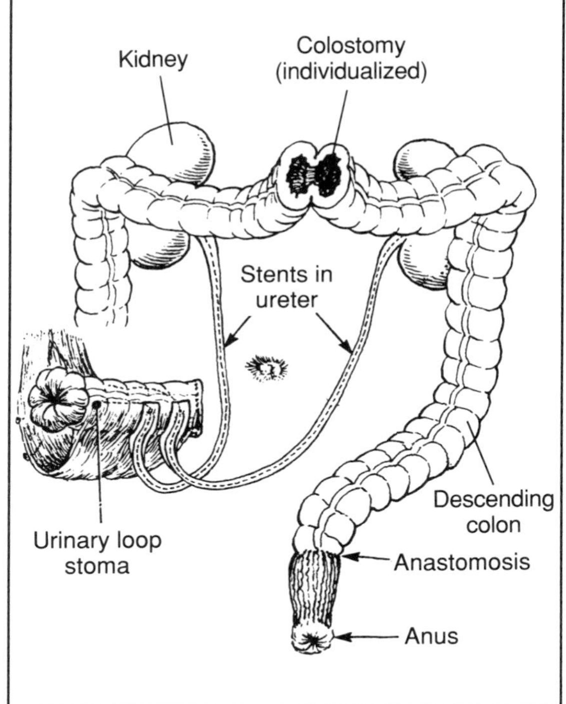


**Figure 8.1-5.** Conceptual drawing shows the urinary and fecal diversions after a total pelvic exenteration. (Reproduced with permission from Wheeless CR: *Atlas of Pelvic Surgery*. Lea & Febiger: 1988.)

### PATIENT POPULATION CHARACTERISTICS

**Age range** All age groups

**Incidence** 1.5-17% of cervical cancers treated with radiation therapy (depending on stage and cell type)

**Associated conditions** Advanced or recurrent gynecologic malignancies
Radiation injury

---

## ANESTHETIC CONSIDERATIONS

### PREOPERATIVE

This procedure is performed for recurrent central cervical or other gynecologic carcinomas, and involves removal of all pelvic tissues. Occasionally, the bladder or rectum is preserved, if not involved with tumor. Most patients have undergone preop radiation therapy.

**Respiratory** Usually not significant unless there is Hx of smoking or lung disease. Ask about prior chemotherapy. (See Anesthetic Considerations for "Second-Look Laparotomy for Ovarian Cancer.")
**Tests:** CXR; ABG; PFTs, if indicated from H&P.

**Cardiovascular** Exercise tolerance should be assessed. Underlying CAD or CHF should be medically optimized preop in consultation with a cardiologist. Any exposure to cardiotoxic chemotherapy should be investigated and may require further tests, such as an ECHO. (See "Second-Look Laparotomy for Ovarian Cancer.")
**Tests:** ECG; ECHO or exercise stress test as indicated from H&P. Cardiac catheterization for patients with Hx of pulmonary HTN manifesting increased dyspnea or right-side CHF (pedal edema, LFTs, etc.), unstable angina or recent MI.

| | |
|---|---|
| **Neurological** | Any Hx of stroke, seizure, carotid artery disease or other neurologic disease should be evaluated and documented. |
| **Endocrine** | Any endocrine disease, such as diabetes, should be optimized in consultation with the patient's primary care physician or endocrinologist. Ask about recent corticosteroid use.<br>**Tests:** Fasting blood sugar; thyroid function tests, as indicated from H&P. |
| **Gastrointestinal** | Patients should have iv hydration if given a bowel prep. A long intestinal tube (Miller-Abbot or Cantor tube) should be placed preop for bowel decompression.<br>**Tests:** Serum electrolytes |
| **Hematologic** | Many patients will be anemic from chronic disease and malnutrition. Preop transfusion of packed cells to increase Hct >30% is indicated. Ask about recent NSAID usage.<br>**Tests:** CBC; PT; PTT; bleeding time, if indicated. |
| **Laboratory** | Renal function tests; LFTs; calcium; magnesium; UA; CT scan of pelvis |
| **Premedication** | Anxiolytic (e.g., valium 10 mg po) given the night before and the morning of surgery. Careful explanation about the procedure and the potential for postop intubation and mechanical ventilation. |

## INTRAOPERATIVE

**Anesthetic technique:** GETA ± supplemental epidural anesthesia. Inhalation anesthetics may be used in relatively healthy patients. A high-dose narcotic technique should be used for patients with significant CAD or in poor overall physical condition.

**General anesthesia:**

| | |
|---|---|
| **Induction** | Standard induction (see Appendix), unless otherwise indicated by patient condition. Long-acting muscle relaxants (e.g., pancuronium or pipecuronium) should be used unless patient has significant renal dysfunction, in which case an atracurium (~10 μg/kg/min) infusion should be used. |
| **Maintenance** | $O_2$/isoflurane or high-dose fentanyl (50-75 μg/kg) combined with midazolam (0.1 - 0.5 mg/kg). Epidural local anesthetic and/or narcotic (morphine or hydromorphone) can be given to reduce anesthetic requirements when using inhalation agents. |
| **Emergence** | If patient is hemodynamically stable, warm and responsive at the end of surgery, extubation may be appropriate. Any patient who is unstable, hypothermic, has had a high-dose narcotic, or who has significant edema of the face or airway should be ventilated overnight in the ICU prior to an attempt at extubation. All patients need to be monitored in an ICU postop 2-3 d due to the large fluid shifts that can occur. |

**Regional anesthesia:**

| | |
|---|---|
| **Epidural** | 2% lidocaine, with or without epinephrine 1:200,000 (10-15 cc) or 0.5% bupivacaine (10-15 ml) are used; then at ~10 cc/hr. Narcotics such as morphine (4 mg) or hydromorphone (0.5 mg) may be given in the epidural for postop pain control. |

| | | |
|---|---|---|
| **Ventilation** | 5 cm $H_2O$ PEEP may help prevent atelectasis. | √ ABGs during surgery; adjust ventilation accordingly to keep normocarbic. $HCO_3$ is given for metabolic acidosis when base deficit >5 and pH < 7.20. |
| **Blood and fluid requirements** | Possible large blood loss<br>IV: 14-16 ga x 2<br>NS/LR @ 10-15 ml/kg/hr | Renal ultrafiltration is improved by NS/LR, but bowel edema is also increased.[15] LR is useful when acidosis is present and NS is better when giving blood products or when metabolic alkalosis is present. |
| | Colloid solutions<br>PRBCs when Hct < 30%<br>FFP/PLT<br>Keep PAWP < 20 mmHg.[17]<br>Ionized Ca<br>Maintain UO of 0.5-1 ml/kg/hr. | Colloid solutions are superior in restoring hemodynamic stability when large fluid volumes are required. UO should guide fluid therapy, in addition to PA pressures and cardiac output. Dopamine 3-5 μg/kg/hr also may be used to maintain UO. Use of furosemide or mannitol is controversial and probably a last resort to prevent anuric renal failure. Controlled hypotension to a MAP of 60-70 mmHg is useful in healthy patients to reduce blood loss. Measure ionized calcium after rapid administration of blood products; replace calcium as necessary. Platelets or FFP may be given for coagulation abnormalities studies as necessary to treat significant bleeding. |

| | | |
|---|---|---|
| **Monitoring** | Standard monitors (see Appendix).<br>± Arterial line<br>± TEE<br>Foley catheter ± PA catheters | Invasive hemodynamic monitoring with arterial and PA catheters usually is required.<br>TEE allows intraop assessment of myocardial function and may be appropriate in selected patients. |
| **Positioning** | √ and pad pressure points.<br>√ eyes.<br>Anti-embolism stockings and SCD | **NB:** peroneal nerve compression at lateral fibular head → foot drop. |
| **Complications** | Hypothermia<br>Bleeding<br>Coagulopathy<br>Trauma to kidney | Warm OR. Humidify gasses. Wrap head in towels. Warm saline lavage of abdomen. Warm-water bladder irrigation through Foley catheter.<br>Watch for hematuria or ↓UO. |

**POSTOPERATIVE**

| | | |
|---|---|---|
| **Complications** | Bleeding<br>Fluid therapy | √ Hct and coags periodically. Be prepared for continued increased fluid requirements for 24 hrs postop. It is essential to maintain optimal cardiac filling pressures. After 24 hrs, fluid mobilization will begin, usually requiring some diuretic therapy. |
| | Peroneal nerve injury 2° lithotomy position | Nerve injury manifested as foot drop and loss of sensation over dorsum of foot. |
| **Pain management** | Epidural or iv opiates (see Appendix). | |
| **Tests** | Hct | Others as indicated from H&P. |


**References**

1. Wheeless CR Jr: Total pelvic exenteration. In *Atlas of Pelvic Surgery*. Lea & Febiger, Philadelphia: 1988, 445-55.
2. DiSaia PJ, Creasman WT: Invasive cervical cancer. In *Clinical Gynecologic Oncology*. DiSaia PJ, Creasman WT, eds. CV Mosby, St. Louis: 1989, 67-132.
3. Matthews CM, Morris M, Burke TW, Gershenson DM, Wharton TJ, Rutledge FN: Pelvic exenteration in the elderly patient. *Obstet Gynecol* 1992; 79(5):773-77.
4. Anthopoulos AP, Manetta A, Larson JE, Podczaski ES, Bartholomew MJ, Mortel R: Pelvic exenteration: a morbidity and mortality analysis of a seven year experience. *Gynecol Oncol* 1989; 35(2):219-23.
5. Jackowatz JG, Porudominsky D, Riihimaki DU, Kemeny M, Kokal WA, Braly PS, Terz JJ, Beatty DJ: Complications of pelvic exenteration. *Arch Surg* 1985; 120:(11)1261-65.
6. Rutledge FN, Smith JP, Wharton JT, O'Quinn AG: Pelvic exenteration: Analysis of 296 patients. *Am J Obstet Gynecol* 1977; 129(8):881-92.
7. Morley GW, Lindenauer SM: Pelvic exenterative therapy for gynecologic malignancy: an analysis of 70 cases. *Cancer* 1976; 38(1 Suppl):581-86.
8. Eisenkop SM, Nalick RH, Teng NH: Modified posterior exenteration for ovarian cancer. *ObstetGynecol* 1991; 78(5P+1):879-85.
9. Fiorica JV, Roberts WS, Hoffman MS, Barton DP, Finan MA, Lyman G, Cavanagh D: Concentrated albumin infusion as an aid to postoperative recovery after pelvic exenteration. *Gynecol Oncol* 1991; 43(3):265-69.
10. Symmonds RE, Pratt JH, Webb MJ: Exenterative operations: experience with 198 patients. *Am J Obstet Gynecol* 1975; 121(7):907-18.
11. Hatch KD, Gelder MS, Soong SJ, Baker VV, Shingleton HM: Pelvic exenteration with low rectal anastomosis: survival, complications, and prognostic factors. *Gynecol Oncol* 1990; 38(3):462-67.
12. Stanhope CR, Webb MJ, Podratz KC: Pelvic exenteration for recurrent cervical cancer. *Clin Obstet Gynecol* 1990; 33(4):897-909.
13. Counts RB, Haisch C, Simon TL, Maxwell NG, Heimbach DM, Carrico CJ: Hemostasis in massively transfused trauma patients. *Ann Surg* 1979; 190(1):91-9.
14. Tweedie IE, Baxter JN, Taylor GT, Keens SJ, Campbell IT: Intraoperative fluids - How much and of what? (Abstract) *Br J Anaesth* 1986; 58:1329P.
15. Bevan DR, Dudley HA, Horsey PJ: Renal function during and after anaesthesia and surgery: significance for water and electrolyte management. *Br J Anaesth* 1973; 45(9):968-75.
16. Skillman JJ, Restall S, Salzman EW: Randomized trial of albumin vs. electrolyte solutions during abdominal aortic operations. *Surgery* 1975; 78(3):291-303.
17. Shires GT III, Peitzman AB, Albert SA, Illner H, Silane MF, Perry MO, Shires GT: Response of extravascular lung water to intraoperative fluids. *Ann Surg* 1983; 197(5):515-19.

# EXPLORATORY LAPAROTOMY, TAH/BSO FOR UTERINE CANCER

## SURGICAL CONSIDERATIONS

**Description**: Currently, endometrial cancer is the most common gynecologic malignancy in the U.S. The first step in the management of this cancer is an **exploratory laparotomy**, concurrent with a **hysterectomy**. The objective, aside from 1° therapy, is to obtain as much surgical and pathological staging data as feasible for determination of adjuvant postop therapy. Careful exploration is carried out for evidence of omental, liver, peritoneal and adnexal metastases. Aortic and pelvic areas are palpated for metastases and suspicious nodes are removed. If no suspicious nodes are present, some pelvic and periaortic lymph nodes are sampled. Note that this is less extensive than the more complete lymph node dissection of a radical hysterectomy. The lymph node sampling may be omitted in the treatment of some uterine sarcomas. A **total hysterectomy** with **BSO** is then performed in the usual manner (see discussion of TAH/BSO in "Staging Laparotomy for Ovarian Cancer").

**Usual preop diagnosis**: Endometrial carcinoma

### SUMMARY OF PROCEDURE

| | |
|---|---|
| **Position** | Supine |
| **Incision** | Midline longitudinal abdominal |
| **Unique considerations** | Minimal possible manipulation of the uterus |
| **Antibiotics** | Cefotetan 2 gm iv on call to OR; then 2 gm iv q 12 hrs x 2 d |
| **Surgical time** | 2 - 3 hrs |
| **Closing considerations** | NG tube placement |
| **EBL** | 400-750 cc |
| **Postop care** | Consider using SCDs and mini-dose heparin for DVT prophylaxis. |
| **Mortality** | 0.1% |
| **Morbidity** | Hemorrhage requiring transfusion: 15%<br>Thrombophlebitis: 7%<br>UTI: 7%<br>Paralytic ileus: 2-5%<br>Wound infection: 3%<br>PE: 1-2%<br>Pelvic infection: 1.5%<br>Wound dehiscence: 1%<br>Bowel injuries: < 1%<br>Urinary tract injuries: < 1%<br>Note: complication rates may vary, depending on disease, age, prior history of XRT and pre-existing medical conditions.) |
| **Procedure code** | 58200 |
| **Pain score** | 7 |

### PATIENT POPULATION CHARACTERISTICS

| | |
|---|---|
| **Age range** | Reproductive and post-reproductive ages (average = 61 yrs) |
| **Incidence** | 70-80/100,000 |
| **Etiology** | Exposure to unopposed endogenous or exogenous estrogen<br>Increased extraglandular conversion of androstenedione to estrone<br>Sequential oral contraceptive pills<br>Exposure to radiation (sarcomas) |
| **Associated conditions** | Obesity<br>Diabetes<br>HTN<br>Nulliparity<br>Late menopause<br>Early menarche |

| | |
|---|---|
| **Associated conditions (cont...)** | Family Hx<br>Stein Leventhal syndrome<br>Chronic anovulation<br>Ovarian and colon cancer<br>Granulosa cell ovarian tumors<br>Arthritis<br>Hypothyroidism |

## ANESTHETIC CONSIDERATIONS

### PREOPERATIVE

Endometrial cancer is usually diagnosed in post-menopausal women who present with vaginal bleeding. Exploratory laparotomy and TAH/BSO are commonly performed for removal of the primary tumor as well as staging of metastatic disease. Occasionally, preop radiation therapy may be in progress, with consequent systemic effects.

| | |
|---|---|
| **Respiratory** | Check for Hx of lung disease or smoking.<br>**Tests:** CXR if >40 yrs; others as indicated from H&P. |
| **Cardiovascular** | If there is Hx of CAD, HTN or CHF, Sx (e.g., angina, dyspnea or peripheral edema) should be investigated. Assess patient's exercise tolerance and current medications. Tests such as an exercise treadmill or ECHO may be indicated if patient has significant angina or CHF.<br>**Tests:** All patients >50 years old should have a preop ECG. Any further testing should be ordered in consultation with a cardiologist or patient's primary care physician. |
| **Neurological** | Seldom a significant problem unless there is Hx of cerebrovascular disease, seizures or other neurologic disease. |
| **Endocrine** | Ask about use of estrogen supplements or birth control pills as these are risk factors for endometrial cancer.[4] Also inquire about the presence of endocrine diseases, such as diabetes and hypothyroidism, which have been associated with this tumor. If the patient has received corticosteroids within the previous 6 mo, a supplemental dose of hydrocortisone (100 mg iv q 12 hrs x 2 d) should be given for surgery.<br>**Tests:** Glucose and thyroid function tests, if indicated from H&P. |
| **Neuromuscular** | Osteoarthritis and osteoporosis common in this patient population. Ask about NSAID usage.<br>**Tests:** Bleeding time is indicated if considering regional anesthesia. |
| **Hematologic** | If vaginal bleeding has been profuse or of long duration, significant anemia may occur. Consider preop iron supplements if there are several days until surgery.<br>**Tests:** CBC; PT; PTT; reticulocyte count |
| **Laboratory** | Electrolytes; renal function tests; LFTs; UA; CT scan of abdomen and pelvis |
| **Premedication** | Anxiolytic, such as diazepam 10 mg po or midazolam 1-5 mg im or iv, if necessary. Discuss anesthetic plan and options for postop pain management with patient. |

### INTRAOPERATIVE

**Anesthetic technique:** GETA ± epidural for postop pain control.[5,6,7] In unusual circumstances (e.g., severe lung disease) surgery may be done under spinal or epidural anesthesia.

**General anesthesia:**

| | |
|---|---|
| **Induction** | Standard induction (see Appendix). |
| **Maintenance** | Standard maintenance (see Appendix). Continued muscle relaxation is usually required to facilitate surgery. Epidural 2% lidocaine with epinephrine 1:200,000 at 10 ml/hr may be given to reduce anesthetic requirements. |
| **Emergence** | Reverse muscle relaxant with neostigmine (0.07 mg/kg with glycopyrrolate 0.01 mg/kg). Patient should awaken at the end of surgery and be extubated in the OR; provide supplemental $O_2$ until patient is fully recovered from anesthesia. |

**Regional anesthesia:**

| | |
|---|---|
| **Epidural** | 2% lidocaine, ± epinephrine 1:200,000 (10-15 cc) or 0.5% bupivacaine (10-15 ml) are used; then @ ~10 cc/hr. Narcotics such as morphine (4 mg) or hydromorphone (0.5 mg) may be given in the epidural for postop pain control. |

| | | |
|---|---|---|
| **Blood and fluid requirements** | IV: 16 ga x 1<br>NS/LR @ 4-6 cc/kg/hr<br>PRBC for Hct < 25% | Crystalloid is used for volume replacement. If anemia is present preop it may be necessary to give PRBCs to keep Hct >25%. |
| **Monitoring** | Standard monitors (see Appendix).<br>Foley catheter<br>± Arterial line<br>± CVP/PA catheters<br>NG tube | Direct monitoring of arterial pressure is indicated in patients with CAD, severe HTN or lung disease.<br>CVP or PA catheters may be appropriate in selected patients. |
| **Positioning** | ✓ and pad pressure points.<br>✓ eyes.<br>Anti-embolism stockings and SCD | |
| **Complications** | Hypothermia (mild)<br><br>Trauma or obstruction of ureter | Warm iv fluids and inspired gasses. Heating pad on OR table. Wrap head in towels or plastic.<br>Watch for hematuria or decreased urine flow. |

**POSTOPERATIVE**

| | |
|---|---|
| **Pain management** | PCA (see Appendix).<br>Epidural narcotics (see Appendix). |


**References**

1. Berman ML, Ballon SC, Lagasse LD, Watring WG: Prognosis and treatment of endometrial cancer. *Am J Obstet Gynecol* 1980; 136(5):679-88.
2. DiSaia PJ, Creasman WT: Adenocarcinoma of the uterus. In *Clinical Gynecologic Oncology*. DiSaia PJ, Creasman WT, eds. CV Mosby, St. Louis: 1989, 161-97.
3. Dicker RC, Greenspan JR, Straus LT, et al: Complication of abdominal and vaginal hysterectomy among women of reproductive age in the United States. The Collaborative Review of Sterilization. *Am J Obstet Gynecol* 1982; 144(7):841-48.
4. Gray LA Sr, Christopherson WM, Hoover RN: Estrogens and endometrial carcinoma. *Obstet Gynecol* 1977; 49:(4)385-9.
5. Cousins MJ, Mather LE: Intrathecal and epidural administration of opioids. *Anesthesiology* 1984; 61(3):276-310.
6. Bromage PR, Camporesi E, Chestnut D: Epidural narcotics for postoperative analgesia. *Anesth Analg* 1980; 59(7):473-80.
7. Rawal N, Sjostrand U, Dahlstrom B: Postoperative pain relief by epidural morphine. *Anesth Analg* 1981; 60(10):726-31.


# RADICAL HYSTERECTOMY

## SURGICAL CONSIDERATIONS

**Description**: Radical hysterectomy is the preferred mode of therapy for young women with Stage IA, IB or IIA cervical carcinoma who want to preserve ovarian function. It is also appropriate with Stage II endometrial and Stage I vaginal carcinoma. The operation involves the removal of the uterus, along with the upper vagina and all the parametrial tissues to the pelvic sidewall. A pelvic and para-aortic **lymph node dissection** is usually performed at the beginning of the procedure. Suspicious nodes are submitted for pathological frozen-section evaluation. The paravesical and pararectal spaces are then developed. The "web" of tissue between these two spaces should be palpated carefully (Fig 8.1-6). If parametrial tumor extension is noted and/or the lymph nodes are positive on frozen section, the hysterectomy may be aborted. The **radical hysterectomy** is performed after the pararectal and paravesical spaces have been developed. The uterine arteries are divided at their origin from the anterior division of the internal iliac artery. The ureters are dissected free of the parametrial tissues. The parametrial tissues are then transected close to the pelvic sidewall. The rectovaginal space is then developed (Fig 8.1-7). The uterosacral ligaments are transected between their uterine and sacral attachments. The upper third of the vagina is then cross-clamped and divided in such a manner as to provide a 3 cm margin. The specimen is delivered *en bloc*. Note that during this procedure, the ureters and bladder are dissected free and left intact. In selected women younger than 45 years who may require postop radiotherapy, ovarian function is preserved by performing an **oopheropexy**. This is accomplished by severing the utero-ovarian ligament and mobilizing the ovarian vessels as they course through the infundibulopelvic ligament. The ovaries are then sutured outside the radiation therapy field and marked with metal clips for future identification.

**Variant procedure or approaches**: **Stallworthy, Dolstad, Novak, Rutledge, Wertheim** and other surgeons have proposed several modifications in an effort to reduce the incidence of ureteral and bladder fistulae. These approaches include preservation of blood supply to the terminal 2 cm of the pelvic ureter by widely displacing ureters (not dissecting them from their fascial beds) and limiting parametrial dissection to the proximal 1/3 or 1/2.

**Usual preop diagnosis**: Stage IA, IB or IIA cervical carcinoma; Stage II endometrial or Stage I vaginal carcinoma (less common)

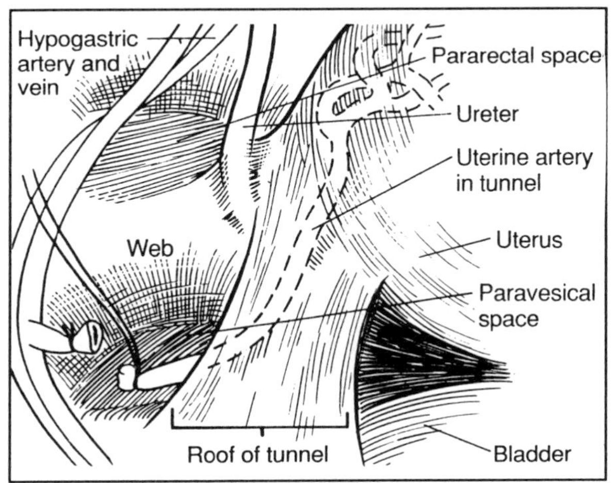


**Figure 8.1-6.** View of parametrial area, showing positions of ureter and uterine artery to web, hypergastric vessels, paravesical and pararectal spaces. (Reproduced with permission from Wheeless CR: *Atlas of Pelvic Surgery*. Lea & Febiger: 1988.)

## SUMMARY OF PROCEDURE

| | |
|---|---|
| **Position** | Supine |
| **Incision** | Midline longitudinal or low transverse abdominal (Maylard) |
| **Special instrumentation** | Argon Beam Coagulator, Vital View® (suction, irrigation and light source combined in 1 instrument) helpful |
| **Unique considerations** | Abort case if positive para-aortic lymph nodes found on frozen section, or if obvious parametrial involvement noted. Consider intraop radiation therapy (investigational), if patient is inoperable. |
| **Antibiotics** | Cefotetan 2 gm iv on call to OR; then q 12 hrs x 3 doses |
| **Surgical time** | 3 - 6 hrs |
| **Closing considerations** | Vaginal and abdominal drains; NG tube placement; suprapubic bladder catheter placement; oophoropexy; copious irrigation |
| **EBL** | 750-1500 cc |
| **Postop care** | Transient ileus very common. Advance diet very slowly. Transient bladder dysfunction very common; therefore, continued bladder drainage for 1+ wks may be necessary. Consider using SCDs and mini-dose heparin for DVT prophylaxis. |
| **Mortality** | 0.3-2.0% |
| **Morbidity** | Paralytic ileus: 3-11%<br>Pelvic lymphocyst: 6.4%<br>Intraop hemorrhage: 5.6%<br>Thrombophlebitis: 5%<br>Pneumonia: 1.5-4%<br>Wound infection: 3.5%<br>Pelvic infection: 2.2%<br>PE: 2.2%<br>Vesical injury: 2-3.5%<br>Vesical fistulae: 1.8%<br>Small bowel obstruction: 1.5%<br>Ureteral fistulae: 1.1%<br>Ureteral injury: 1.1%<br>Wound dehiscence: 1%<br>Postop lymphedema: < 1%<br>Rectal injury: < 1%<br>Pelvic urinoma: Rare |
| **Procedure code** | 58210 |
| **Pain score** | 8 |

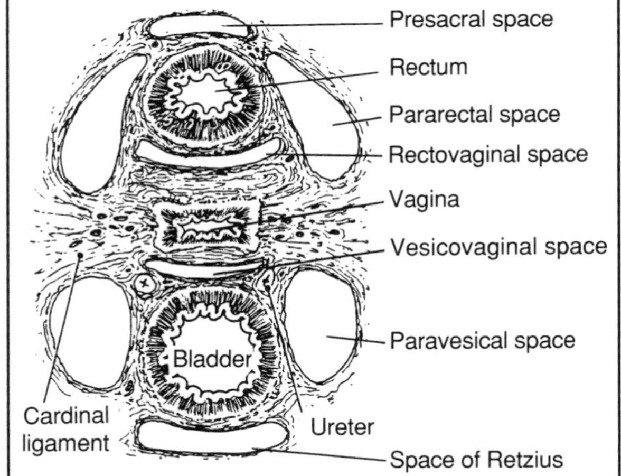


**Figure 8.1-7.** Schematic diagram of a cut in the antero-posterior plane with positions of all spaces in relation to pelvic organs. (Reproduced with permission from Wheeless CR: *Atlas of Pelvic Surgery*. Lea & Febiger: 1988.)

## PATIENT POPULATION CHARACTERISTICS

| | |
|---|---|
| **Age range** | Reproductive and post-reproductive yrs |
| **Incidence** | 10/100,000 |
| **Etiology** | Human Papilloma Virus (HPV), subtypes 16, 18 (most common) and others |
| **Associated conditions** | Smoking<br>Venereal warts<br>Genital herpes<br>Multiple sexual partners<br>Early-age onset of coitus<br>Multiparity<br>Lower socio-economic status<br>HIV infection |

---

# ANESTHETIC CONSIDERATIONS

## PREOPERATIVE

This surgery is usually performed for cervical or endometrial carcinoma in young women who wish to preserve ovarian function, and whose tumor has not spread beyond local invasion. Lymph nodes are removed to confer a therapeutic advantage and to plan postop adjuvant therapy, if any.

| | |
|---|---|
| **Respiratory** | These tumors have been associated with cigarette smoking. ✓ for pre-existing lung disease.<br>**Tests:** As indicated from H&P. |
| **Cardiovascular** | Patients >50 yrs need a preop ECG. ✓ for Hx of heart disease such as rheumatic fever, mitral valve prolapse or CAD.<br>**Tests:** As indicated from H&P. |
| **Neurological** | Not usually significant unless Hx of neurologic disease. |
| **Musculoskeletal** | Question patient about any joint or muscle disease and their exercise tolerance. |
| **Gastrointestinal** | Consider supplemental iv hydration in patients given a bowel prep. |
| **Endocrine** | Not usually important unless pre-existing disease. Check for corticosteroid use in the previous 6 mo. |
| **Hematologic** | Ask about NSAID usage in the previous month. Encourage autologous blood donation.<br>**Tests:** Consider checking a bleeding time if regional anesthetic planned. Hb/Hct; PT; PTT; platelet count. |
| **Laboratory** | Electrolytes; renal panel; UA; CT scan of pelvis and abdomen (helpful but not necessary) |
| **Premedication** | Anxiolytic such as diazepam 10 mg po |

## INTRAOPERATIVE

**Anesthetic technique:** GETA + epidural for postop pain control. (Surgery may be performed in patient with respiratory compromise, under regional block.)

| | |
|---|---|
| **Induction** | Standard induction (see Appendix). |
| **Maintenance** | Standard maintenance (see Appendix). Muscle relaxation usually required to assist with surgical exposure. |
| **Emergence** | No special considerations |

| | | |
|---|---|---|
| **Blood and fluid requirements** | Occasional blood loss >1500 ml<br>IV 14-16 ga x 2<br>NS/LR @ 6-8 cc/kg/hr<br>Maintain UO >0.5 ml/kg/hr.<br>Warm iv fluids.<br>Humidify inspired gasses. | Good iv access is necessary to deal with potential for bleeding. Controlled hypotension to a MAP of 60-70 mmHg may help reduce blood loss. A lymph node dissection will increase 3rd-space losses and should be accounted for in fluid management. Fluid requirements generally are increased by a functioning epidural catheter due to vasodilation. Controversy exists with regard to recurrence of cancer in patients who have received non-autologous blood transfusions. |

| | | |
|---|---|---|
| **Monitoring** | Standard monitors (see Appendix).<br>Foley catheter<br>CVP catheter<br>± Arterial catheter | Invasive monitoring is indicated for patients with underlying cardiopulmonary disease, advanced age, or where controlled hypotension is planned. |
| **Positioning** | √ and pad pressure points.<br>√ eyes.<br>Anti-embolism stockings and SCD | |
| **Complications** | Injury to ureters | Watch for hematuria or decreased urine flow. |

## POSTOPERATIVE

| | | |
|---|---|---|
| **Complications** | Atelectasis<br>Hypothermia<br>Bleeding | Give supplemental $O_2$ postop. Encourage use of incentive spirometer. |
| **Pain management** | PCA (see Appendix).<br>Epidural narcotics (see Appendix). | Add ketorolac 30-60 mg im q 6 hr for breakthrough pain, or add dilute local anesthetic to epidural infusion. |


**References**

1. Wertheim E: The extended abdominal operation for carcinoma uteri (based on 500 operative cases). *Am J Obstet* 1912; 66:169-232.
2. Lee YN, Wang KL, Lin MH, Liu CH, Wang KG, Lan CC, Chuang JT, Chen AC, Wu CC: Radical hysterectomy with pelvic lymph node dissection for treatment of cervical cancer: a clinical review of 954 cases. *Gynecol Oncol* 1989; 32:135-42.
3. Meigs JV: Radical hysterectomy with bilateral pelvic lymph node dissections. A report of 100 patients operated on five or more years ago. *Am J Obstet Gynecol* 1951; 62:854-70.
4. Hoskins WJ, Ford JH Jr, Lutz MH, Averette HE: Radical hysterectomy and pelvic lymphadenectomy for the management of early invasive cancer of the cervix. *Gynecol Oncol* 1976; 4(3):278-90.
5. Symmonds RE, Pratt JH: Prevention of fistulas and lymphocysts in radical hysterectomy. *Obstet Gynecol* 1961; 17:57-64.
6. Lerner HM, Jones HW III, Hill EC: Radical surgery for the treatment of early invasive cervical carcinoma (Stage IB): Review of 15 years experience. *Obstet Gynecol* 1980; 56(4):413-18.
7. Kindermann G, Debus-Thiede G: Postoperative urological complication after radical surgery for cervical cancer. In *Baillière's Clinical Obstetrics and Gynaecology, Operative Treatment of Cervical Cancer.* Baird DT, et al, eds. Baillière Tindall/WB Saunders Co, London: 1988; 2(4):933-41.
8. Ayhan A, Tuncer ZS: Radical hysterectomy with lymphadenectomy for treatment of early stage cervical cancer: clinical experience of 278 cases. *J Surg Oncol* 1991; 47(3):175-77.
9. Ayhan A, Tuncer ZS, Yarali H: Complications of radical hysterectomy in women with early stage cervical cancer: clinical analysis of 270 cases. *Eur J Surg Oncol* 1991; 17(5):492-94.
10. DiSaia PJ, Creasman WT: Invasive cervical cancer. In *Clinical Gynecologic Oncology.* DiSaia PJ, Creasman WT, eds. CV Mosby, St. Louis: 1989, 67-132.

# INTERSTITIAL PERINEAL IMPLANTS

## SURGICAL CONSIDERATIONS

**Description: Radiotherapy** is the treatment modality of choice for International Federation of Gynecology and Obstetrics (FIGO) Stage IIB-IVA carcinoma of the cervix, Stage I, II, III and IVA vaginal cancers, selected vulvar cancers and pelvic recurrences of gynecologic cancers. Often, **external-beam therapy** is combined with **brachytherapy**, either in the form of **intracavitary insertion** or as an **interstitial perineal template implant**. Intracavitary radiotherapy utilizes devices such as Fletcher suits or cylinders that are fitted into the vagina and provide a therapeutic boost to the vaginal apex region after external beam irradiation. In general, these devices do not require a laparotomy or laparoscopy for guidance. For selected patients with distorted anatomy and/or bulky tumors, interstitial implants provide superior dose distribution and better local tumor control. The two most widely used systems are the **Martinez Universal Perineal Interstitial Template (MUPIT)** and the **Syed-Neblett applicator**. These systems have similar efficacy and both are performed in the OR with the patient under local or GA. A **laparotomy** is frequently performed at the time of interstitial implant placement to accurately guide the needles into their target tissues and to avoid radiation injury to bowel and/or other pelvic organs not involved with tumor. To minimize postop patient discomfort, some centers use **laparoscopy** instead of laparotomy for needle guidance. A two-team approach is used: gynecologic/oncology team performs the laparotomy or laparoscopy and guides the needles from above; radiation/oncology team inserts the implants from below. The implants are afterloaded with the appropriate radiation source when the patient has returned to her shielded room. If a hysterectomy has been done before, an omental pelvic carpet, or a pelvic lid made of delayed, absorbable mesh, is performed to provide additional space between the radiation source and bowel.

### SUMMARY OF PROCEDURE

| | Laparotomy-Guided | Laparoscopy-Guided |
|---|---|---|
| **Position** | Modified dorsolithotomy; Allen stirrups | ⇐ |
| **Incision** | Midline longitudinal abdominal | Vertical infraumbilical and multiple small transverse incisions at the pubic hairline |
| **Special instrumentation** | Syed-Neblett template or MUPIT systems, or modifications thereof | ⇐ + Video-laparoscopy equipment, preferably with a 3-chip camera |
| **Unique considerations** | MRI and/or CT scans + information from physical exam are used to pre-plan implant with a computer dosimetry program. Patients require thorough preop mechanical and antibiotic bowel prep. Preop epidural placement or postop PCA (see Appendix) may prove helpful for pain control. Foley catheter needs to be inserted through an opening at the top of the clear plastic template prior to implant positioning. | ⇐ + Adhesions of variable severity may be present from prior surgery or radiation. Care should be taken to avoid possible bowel injury at time of trocar insertion. Patient needs to be in steep Trendelenburg position for duration of procedure. |
| **Antibiotics** | Cefotetan 2 gm iv on call to OR; then q 12 hrs x 3 doses | ⇐ |
| **Surgical time** | 1.5 - 3 hrs | ⇐ |
| **EBL** | 150-350 cc | Minimal |
| **Closing considerations** | Suture template to perineum. Perform rectal exam and adjust any needles that are too close to, or have protruded through, at the rectal mucosa. Pack any space between template and perineum with Vaseline® gauze. Obtain A-P and lateral orthogonal localization films with the patient in the supine bed rest position. Insert Hypaque® dye into bladder (via Foley catheter) prior to localization films. Consider insertion of a large Foley into the rectum and attach to a drainage bag. Consider NG tube placement. | ⇐ + Release the pneumoperitoneum completely. Consider insertion of 1 L heparinized LR to cause the bowel to float and remain mobile, thus minimizing the risk of radiation injury. |

| | | |
|---|---|---|
| **Postop care** | Patient is confined to bed while interstitial implants are in place. SCDs and mini-dose heparin for DVT prophylaxis. Vigorous use of incentive spirometry. Consider constipating medications (e.g., Lomotil®). Patient must be placed in a shielded room. Visitors and medical personnel should interact with patient from behind a lead shield until radiation sources have been removed. | ⇐ |
| **Mortality** | 0.1-0.3% | ⇐ |
| **Morbidity** | Rectovaginal fistula: 10-20% | ⇐ |
| | Vesicovaginal fistula: 6-20% | ⇐ |
| | Hemorrhagic proctitis with diarrhea and tenesmus: 7-18% | ⇐ |
| | Radiation cystitis: 7-10% | ⇐ |
| | Cervical necrosis: 5-6% | ⇐ |
| | Vaginal vault necrosis: 3-5% | ⇐ |
| | Rectal fibrosis: 2-5% | ⇐ |
| | Pelvic infection: 2-3% | ⇐ |
| **Procedure code** | 77778, 49000 | 77778, 56300 |
| **Pain score** | 8-9 | 8-9 |

### PATIENT POPULATION CHARACTERISTICS

| | |
|---|---|
| **Age range** | Reproductive and post-reproductive yrs; childhood rare |
| **Etiology** | Cervical, vaginal or vulvar carcinomas<br>Pelvic recurrence of gynecologic malignancies |

---

## ANESTHETIC CONSIDERATIONS

**(Procedures covered: intracavity devices, interstitial devices)**

### PREOPERATIVE

Radiation implants are used for palliation or cure in cervical, endometrial and ovarian carcinoma. The implants concentrate the radiation close to the site of the tumor, and may be supplemented by external beam radiation as well. The unusual tolerance of the uterus and vagina to radiation permit large doses to be given, and accounts for the success in treating cervical lesions.[11] The sigmoid, rectum and large bowel are much more sensitive to radiation injury and limit the dose of radiation that may be given to the pelvis.

| | |
|---|---|
| **Respiratory** | Usually not significant unless underlying lung disease is present. |
| **Cardiovascular** | Many patients with pelvic tumors are elderly and prone to cardiovascular disease. There are no specific recommendations except to check a preop ECG in all patients >50 yrs who are otherwise asymptomatic.<br>**Tests:** ECG; others as indicated from H&P. |
| **Neurological** | Usually not significant unless there is Hx of neurologic disease. |
| **Musculoskeletal** | Inquire about any Hx of arthritis. Osteoporosis is also common among elderly patients. |
| **Hematologic** | **Tests:** Hb/Hct; PT; PTT; platelets |
| **Laboratory** | UA; electrolytes; renal panel |
| **Premedication** | An anxiolytic such as midazolam (1-5 mg iv) may be used if necessary. |

### INTRAOPERATIVE

**Anesthetic technique:** Typically GETA. A postop epidural is useful for pain management.

| | |
|---|---|
| **Induction** | Standard induction (see Appendix) |
| **Maintenance** | Standard maintenance (see Appendix). It is not necessary to maintain neuromuscular blockade after intubation. |

| | |
|---|---|
| **Emergence** | Metoclopramide (10 mg iv) or droperidol (0.5-1 mg iv) can be given for prophylaxis against nausea 30 min before emergence. |
| **Blood and fluid requirements** | Small blood loss<br>IV: 18 ga x 1<br>NS/LR @ 2-4 cc/kg/hr |
| **Monitoring** | Standard monitors (see Appendix). |
| **Positioning** | √ and pad pressure points.<br>√ eyes.<br>Anti-embolism stockings and SCD |

## POSTOPERATIVE

| | | |
|---|---|---|
| **Pain management** | Epidural narcotics (see Appendix).<br>PCA (see Appendix). | Ketorolac 30-60 mg im q 6 hrs is useful for breakthrough pain, unless the patient has peptic ulcer disease or renal insufficiency. |

## References


1. Fu KK, Snead PK, Leibel SA, Nori D, Peschel RE: Carcinoma of the cervix. In *Interstitial Brachytherapy: Physical, Biological, and Clinical Considerations*. Anderson LL, Nath R, Weaver KA, Nori D, Phillips TL, Son YU, Chin-Tsao ST, Meigooni AS, Meli JA, Smith V, eds. Interstitial Collaborative Working Group. Raven Press, New York: 1990, 179-88.
2. Phillips TL, Nori D, Peschel RE: Carcinoma of the vagina and vulva. In *Interstitial Brachytherapy: Physical, Biological, and Clinical Considerations*. Anderson LL, Nath R, Weaver KA, Nori D, Phillips TL, Son YU, Chin-Tsao ST, Meigooni AS, Meli JA, Smith V, eds. Interstitial Collaborative Working Group. Raven Press, New York: 1990, 189-97.
3. Sharma SK, Forgione H, Isaacs JH: Iodine - 125 interstitial implants as salvage therapy for recurrent gynecologic malignancies. *Cancer* 1991; 67(10):2467-71.
4. Hockel M, Knapstein PG: The combined operative and radiotherapeutic treatment (CORT) of recurrent tumors infiltrating the pelvic wall: first experience with 18 patients. *Gynecol Oncol* 1992; 46(1):20-8.
5. Ampuero F, Doss LL, Khan M, Skipper B, Hilgers RD: The Syed-Neblett interstitial template in locally advanced gynecological malignancies. *Int J Radiat Oncol Biol Phys* 1983; 9(12):1897-1903.
6. Martinez A, Edmundson GK, Cox RS, Gunderson LL, Howes AE: Combination of external beam irradiation and multiple-site perineal application (MUPIT) for treatment of locally advanced or recurrent prostatic, anorectal, and gynecologic malignancies. *Int J Radiat Oncol Biol Phys* 1985; 11(2):391-98.
7. Montana GS, Fowler WC, Varia MA, Walton LA, Mack Y, Shemanski L: Carcinoma of the cervix, Stage III. Results of radiation therapy. *Cancer* 1986; 57(1):148-54.
8. Feder BH, Syed AM, Neblett D: Treatment of extensive carcinoma of the cervix with the "transperineal parametrial butterfly," a preliminary report on the revival of Waterman's approach. *Int J Radiat Oncol Biol Phys* 1978; 4(7-8):735-42.
9. Rotman M, Aziz H: Techniques in the radiation treatment of carcinoma of the uterine cervix. *Int J Radiat Oncol Biol Phys* 1991; 20(1):173-75.
10. Aristizabal SA, Surwit EA, Hevezi JM, Heusinkveld RS: Treatment of advanced cancer of the cervix with transperineal interstitial irradiation. *Int J Radiat Oncol Biol Phys* 1983; 9(7):1013-17.
11. DiSaia PJ, Nolan JF, Arneson AN: Radiation therapy in gynecology. In *Obstetrics and Gynecology*, 4th edition. Danforth DN, ed. Harper and Row, Philadelphia: 1982, 1214-30.

**Surgeons**

**W. Leroy Heinrichs, MD PhD**
**Jan T. Rydfors, MD**

---

# 8.2 GYNECOLOGY/INFERTILITY SURGERY

---

**Anesthesiologists**

**Emily Ratner, MD**
**Sheila E. Cohen, MB, ChB, FRCA**
**Carter Cherry, MD**

# DILATATION AND CURETTAGE

## SURGICAL CONSIDERATIONS

**Description:** During dilatation and curettage (D&C), the endometrial lining of the uterus and coexisting lesions (myoma, polyp) are removed. This procedure is performed to diagnose and treat bleeding from uterine and cervical lesions, to complete an incomplete or missed spontaneous abortion (SAB), or to treat cervical stenosis. It is used infrequently as a primary method for pregnancy termination. A D&C is performed less frequently with the advent of the office endometrial biopsy and medical management of bleeding problems.

With the patient in the dorsal lithotomy position, the surgeon initially performs a bimanual examination under anesthesia to obtain information about both the presence of adnexal pathology and anatomic detail of the uterus. A speculum is inserted into the vagina, and the cervix is grasped with a clamp. The cervix is pulled gently toward the operator, who then uses a uterine probe to delineate the length of the uterus and the angulation between the cervical canal and uterus. The uterine cavity is reached by dilating the cervical canal with progressively larger dilators (Hegar's or Pratt) to 8-9 mm diameter. A ureteral stone forceps is often used at this stage to remove existing polyps. A curette is used to systematically remove the endometrial lining (Fig 8.2-1).

**Usual preop diagnosis**: Uncontrolled uterine bleeding refractory to hormonal treatment in young women; abnormal uterine bleeding in perimenopausal/postmenopausal women; incomplete, missed or induced abortion; cervical stenosis causing dysmenorrhea or infertility

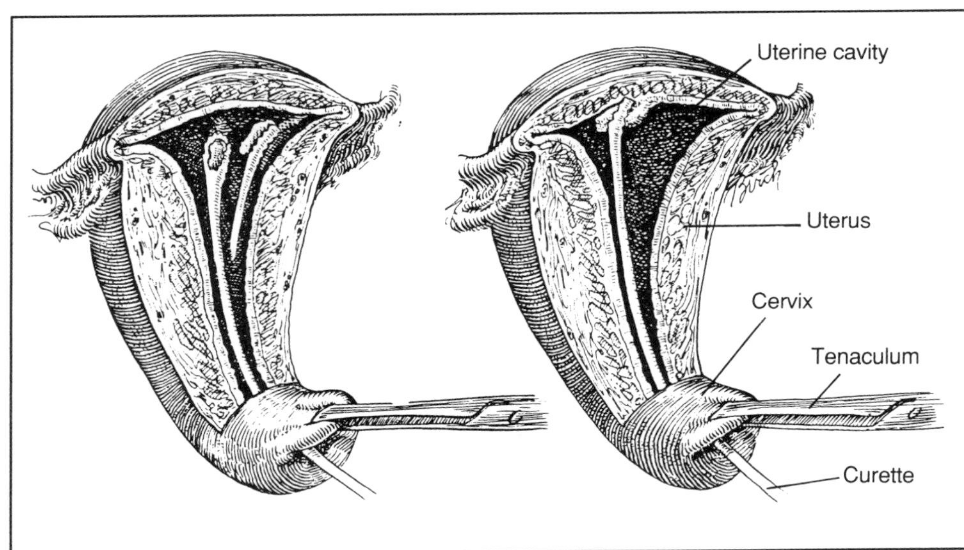


←**Figure 8.2-1.** Curettage of endometrial lining. (Reproduced with permission from Thompson JD, Rock JA, eds: *TeLinde's Operative Gynecology*, 7th edition. JB Lippincott: 1992.)

### SUMMARY OF PROCEDURE

| | |
|---|---|
| **Position** | Dorsal lithotomy with stirrups |
| **Incision** | None |
| **Special instrumentation** | To prevent peroneal nerve injury, the area of the leg leaning against the stirrup should be well-cushioned. Following induction, perineum is positioned at the very end of the table to ensure optimum exposure. During the cervical dilatation, a vasovagal response can occur, with subsequent bradycardia and hypotension. Uterine perforations will often cause severe postop pain. |
| **Surgical time** | 5 - 15 min |
| **EBL** | 50-100 cc |
| **Mortality** | Minimal |
| **Morbidity** | Postop fever: 1.7%<br>Uterine perforation: 0.63%<br>Severe immediate postop bleeding (usually caused by cervical injury): < 1% |
| **Procedure code** | 58120 |
| **Pain score** | 3-5 |

## PATIENT POPULATION CHARACTERISTICS

| | |
|---|---|
| **Age range** | 20-80 yrs |
| **Incidence** | >1/50 females |
| **Etiology** | Dysfunctional uterine bleeding |
| **Associated conditions** | Obesity<br>HTN |

## ANESTHETIC CONSIDERATIONS

See Anesthetic Considerations following "Therapeutic Abortion, Dilatation and Evacuation" (below).

**References**

1. Mackenzie IZ, Bibby JG: Critical assessment of dilatation and curettage in 1029 women. *Lancet* 1978; 2(8089):566-68.
2. Thompson JD, Rock JA, eds: *TeLinde's Operative Gynecology*, 7th edition. JB Lippincott, Philadelphia: 1992, 303-16.

# THERAPEUTIC ABORTION, DILATATION AND EVACUATION

## SURGICAL CONSIDERATIONS

**Description**: **Therapeutic abortion (TAB)** is the elective termination of a pregnancy prior to viability (usually considered to be 24 weeks). In 1982, 1,574,000 legal abortions were performed in the U.S., a ratio of 426 abortions per 1000 live births. **Suction curettage** is the most efficient method to terminate pregnancies during the first trimester (< 12 weeks), and the great majority of abortions are performed this way. Few (< 5%) of first trimester abortions in the U.S. are performed with a sharp curette. Increased operative time and blood loss is seen with this method, resulting in its being practiced mainly in locations where a suction apparatus is not available. Suction curettage for a spontaneous abortion is performed in a manner identical to a regular TAB, except that a cervical dilatation might not be needed and the blood loss is usually 2-3 times greater. Very early termination (< 4 weeks following LMP) can be performed without anesthesia, using a method called "menstrual regulation."

The **TAB procedure** consists of a standard cervical dilatation (required for gestations >6 weeks), followed by vacuum aspiration of the uterine contents, using a plastic suction curette (Fig 8.2-2). Alternatively, the cervical canal can be dilated >6 hours prior to the operation with laminaria or synthetic osmotic dilators which, after insertion, swell to provide dilatation. A sharp curette is often used at the very end to gently verify the emptiness of the cavity, followed by re-aspiration. Due to the risk of missing the pregnancy, most physicians wait until 7-8 weeks following the LMP before performing the operation. Ergonovine maleate and oxytocin (Pitocin®) are often used (20-30 U oxytocin/1000 cc iv or 0.2 mg ergonovine maleate im) during the procedure to reduce bleeding, although their efficacy has been questioned. The procedure is performed under either local or GA; it is general-

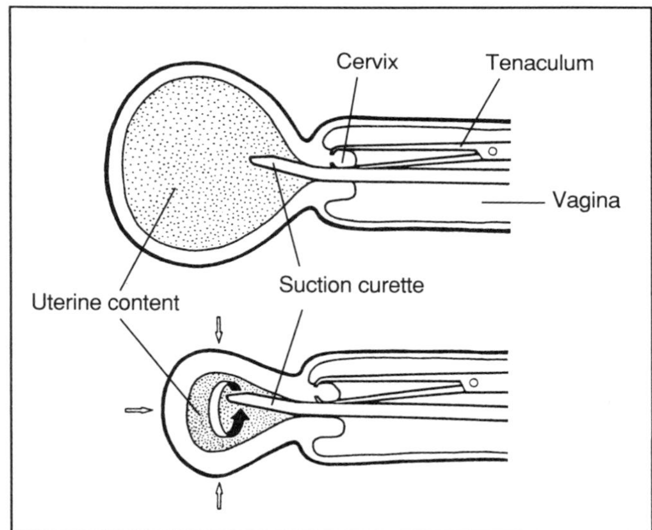

**Figure 8.2-2.** Uterine aspiration. Top – uterus at beginning of procedure; bottom – at conclusion of procedure. (Reproduced with permission from Thompson JD, Rock JA, eds: *TeLinde's Operative Gynecology*, 7th edition. JB Lippincott: 1992.)

ly felt that local is safer. Regardless of the method used, the obtained product of conception (POC) is sent for histological examination to exclude the presence of trophoblastic tissue or ectopic pregnancy.

**Variant procedure: Dilatation and evacuation (D&E)** remains the safest method for mid-trimester pregnancy termination.[1] It is performed similarly to first-trimester suction curettage, with the addition of using large-ring forceps to grasp and remove fetal parts intermittently. This procedure is often performed under paracervical block.

**Usual preop diagnosis**: Pregnancy (viable or non-viable): 52% within 8 weeks estimated gestational age; 90% within 12 weeks estimated gestational age

## SUMMARY OF PROCEDURE

| | 1st-Trimester Suction Curettage | | 2nd-Trimester D&E | |
|---|---|---|---|---|
| **Position** | Dorsal lithotomy with patient in Allen stirrups. Following induction, perineum positioned at the end of the table to ensure optimum exposure. | | ⇐ | |
| **Incision** | None | | ⇐ | |
| **Special instrumentation** | Suction | | ⇐ + Large-ring forceps | |
| **Unique considerations** | To prevent peroneal nerve injury, the area of the leg leaning against the stirrup should be well-cushioned. During cervical dilatation, a vasovagal reaction can occur → bradycardia and hypotension. During injection of lidocaine for the paracervical block, seizures may occur if >12 cc of 1% solution are injected. Uterine perforations will often cause excessive postop pain. | | ⇐ | |
| **Surgical time** | 5 - 15 min | | 15 - 45 min | |
| **EBL**[2] | No. weeks gestation: | | 300-500 cc | |
| | 1-4 | 10 cc | | |
| | 5-8 | 10-30 cc | | |
| | 9-10 | 30-80 cc | | |
| | 11-12 | 80-200 cc | | |
| | 13-14 | 200-400 cc | | |
| **Postop care** | PACU – severe immediate postop bleeding usually caused by cervical injury. Excessive postop pain can be caused by a uterine perforation. | | ⇐ | |
| **Mortality** | 0-3.1/100,000[3,4] | | 13/100,000[1] | |
| **Morbidity** | Mild infection | 1/216 | T >38° for > 1 d | 13.4/1,000 |
| | Resuctioned day of surgery | 1/553 | Cervical injury | 11.6/1,000 |
| | Resuctioned subsequently | 1/596 | Cervical tear | 10/1,000 |
| | Cervical stenosis causing amenorrhea | 1/6,071 | Retained POC | 9/1,000 |
| | Cervical tear | 1/9,444 | Hemorrhage | 7.1/1,000 |
| | Underestimation of gestational age | 1/15,454 | UTI | 1.8/1,000 |
| | Convulsive seizure (after local anesthesia) | 1/25,086 | | |
| | Total | 1/118 | | |
| **Complications requiring hospitalization** | Incomplete abortion | 1/3,617 | Endometritis | 8,5/1,000 |
| | Sepsis | 1/4,722 | Uterine perforation | 3.2/1,000 |
| | Uterine perforation | 1/10,625 | Need for laparotomy | 2.1/1,000 |
| | Vaginal bleeding | 1/14,166 | Need for blood transfusion | 1.9/1,000 |
| | Inability to complete | 1/28,333 | | |
| | Coexisting tubal pregnancy | 1,42,500 | | |
| | Total | 1/1,405 | | |

| | | |
|---|---|---|
| **Procedure code** | 59812 (spontaneous abortion, any trimester)<br>59820 (missed abortion, 1st trimester)<br>59821 (missed abortion, 2nd trimester)<br>59830 (septic abortion)<br>59840 (1st trimester elective termination, suction curettage/D&C) | 59841 (D&E) |
| **Pain score** | 5 | 5 |

**PATIENT POPULATION CHARACTERISTICS**

| | |
|---|---|
| **Age range** | 15-45 yrs |
| **Incidence** | >1/5 females |
| **Etiology** | Wishing pregnancy termination |

---

## ANESTHETIC CONSIDERATIONS

**(Procedures covered: dilatation and curettage [D&C], therapeutic abortion [TAB], dilatation and evacuation [D&E])**

### PREOPERATIVE

These are among the most common procedures performed in gynecology. Patients presenting for these procedures are generally healthy; however, bleeding and sepsis may alter ASA status.

| | |
|---|---|
| **Cardiovascular** | Hemodynamic status may be impaired 2° preop uterine bleeding, and patient may be septic from retained uterine products. ✓ BP, HR, orthostatic vital signs.<br>**Tests:** As indicated from H&P. |
| **Laboratory** | Hb/Hct; other tests as indicated from H&P. |
| **Premedication** | Anxiolytic (e.g., midazolam 1-2 mg iv) as needed. |

### INTRAOPERATIVE

**Anesthetic technique:** Local, regional or GA all may be appropriate. In the younger patient population, spinal anesthesia may be less desirable because of increased incidence of post-dural puncture headache (PDPH).

**Local anesthesia:** Some obstetricians/gynecologists perform these procedures under local anesthesia. Paracervical block has the potential for inadvertent iv administration with consequent toxic reaction.

**Regional anesthesia:** A T10 sensory level is sufficient to provide anesthesia for procedures on the uterus.

| | |
|---|---|
| **Spinal** | 5% lidocaine 75-100 mg; 0.75% bupivacaine 10-15 mg in 7.5% dextrose. (See Anesthetic Considerations for "Cesarean Section.") |
| **Epidural** | 1.5-2.0% lidocaine with epinephrine 5 $\mu$g/cc, 15-25 cc; supplement with 5-10 cc as needed. Supplemental iv sedation. (See Anesthetic Considerations for "Cesarean Section.") |

**General anesthesia:**

| | |
|---|---|
| **Induction** | Standard induction (see Appendix). |
| **Maintenance** | Standard maintenance (see Appendix) used commonly, although frequently done by mask with $O_2/N_2O$ + volatile anesthetic and spontaneous respiration. May also use propofol infusion (100-250 $\mu$g/kg/min), with $N_2O$, without volatile anesthetic. A small amount of opiate may be used. High incidence of postop N&V warrant prophylactic treatment with metoclopramide (5-10 mg iv). Ondansetron (4 mg iv) may prove useful in these patients. |
| **Emergence** | Be ready with suction in the event of vomiting on emergence. |

| | | |
|---|---|---|
| **Blood and fluid requirements** | Minimal blood loss<br>IV: 18 ga x 1 (unless hypovolemic)<br>NS/LR @ 2 cc/kg/hr | Usual replacement of maintenance fluids and overnight deficit with crystalloid. Blood replacement rarely indicated. |
| **Control of blood loss** | Oxytocin (Pitocin®) 20-30 U<br>Ergonovine maleate (0.2 mg) | Oxytocin causes uterine contraction, with a consequent decrease in blood loss. Rapid iv bolus may lead to |

| | | |
|---|---|---|
| **Monitoring** | Standard monitors (see Appendix). | hypotension. Oxytocin is usually diluted in 1 L of crystalloid and then infused. Ergonovine maleate also causes uterine contraction and is usually given im. Side effects include HTN, myocardial ischemia and dysrhythmias, especially if given iv.[6] |
| **Monitoring** | Standard monitors (see Appendix). | |
| **Positioning** | √ hip, leg, hand position.<br>√ and pad pressure points.<br>√ eyes.<br>Shoulder abducted < 90° | Lithotomy position can be deleterious to pulmonary function, as it may impair respiratory mechanics. Rarely, hemodynamic changes can occur on elevation of the legs into the stirrups, as this increases venous return to the heart. Problems with hypotension on lowering legs post-op are more common.[7] |
| **Vagal stimulation** | When cervix is grasped and dilated, patient may have excessive vagal stimulation, which can be treated by prompt cessation of stimulation and with atropine (0.4 mg), if indicated. | |
| **Complications** | Nerve injury | Be sure that no peripheral nerve injury (e.g., foot drop) occurs. Common peroneal nerve palsy is possible if pressure on the nerve over the fibula is not prevented by adequate padding or positioning. Hyperflexion of the hip joint can cause femoral and lateral femoral cutaneous nerve palsy. Obturator and saphenous nerve injury are also complications of the lithotomy position[3]. |
| | Finger trauma | Take care to insure safety of patient's fingers when manipulating foot of the bed. Avoid finger injury by placing patient's arms on arm boards or by wrapping her hands.[6] |

## POSTOPERATIVE

| | | |
|---|---|---|
| **Complications** | High incidence of N&V<br>Uterine rupture with severe abdominal pain (rare)<br>Severe hemorrhage, necessitating blood transfusion (rare) | Anti-emetics, including metoclopramide 10 mg iv, droperidol 1 mg iv and ondansetron 4 mg iv, can be useful in this setting.<br>Severe bleeding may be 2° cervical injury. |
| **Pain management** | Small amount of iv opiate<br>Ketorolac 60 mg im also works well, although it is best not used in an actively bleeding patient. | Extreme pain may be caused by uterine perforation. Patients usually tolerate oral pain medications. |
| **Tests** | Hb/Hct, if hemorrhage | |


**References**

1. Grimes DA et al: Mid-trimester abortion by dilatation and evacuation. *N Engl J Med* 1977; 296(20):1141-45.
2. Pernoll ML, ed: *Current Obstetrics and Gynecologic Diagnosis and Treatment.* Appleton & Lange, Norwalk, CT: 1991, 686-91.
3. Grimes DA, Cates W Jr: Complications from legally-induced abortion: a review. *Obstet Gynecol Surv* 1979; 34(3):177-91.
4. Hakim-Elahi E: Complications of first-trimester abortion: a report of 170,000 cases. *Obstet Gynecol* 1990; 76(1):129-35.
5. Thompson JD, Rock JA, eds: *TeLinde's Operative Gynecology*, 7th edition. JB Lippincott, Philadelphia: 1992, 317-42.
6. *Physician's Desk Reference*, 46th edition. Medical Economics Data, Inc, Montvale NJ: 1992.
7. Welborn, SG: The lithotomy position, anesthesiologic considerations. In *Positioning in Anesthesia and Surgery.* WB Saunders Co, Philadelphia: 1978, 156-61.
8. Courtney, MA: Neurologic sequelae of childbirth and regional anesthesia. In *Manual of Obstetric Anesthesia.* Churchill Livingstone, New York: 1992.
9. Hodgkinson CP, Drukker BH: Operative Gynecology. In *Obstetrics and Gynecology.* Danforth DN, ed. Harper and Row, Philadelphia: 1982, 1247.

# HYSTEROSCOPY

## SURGICAL CONSIDERATIONS

**Description:** **Hysteroscopy** is a procedure in which the endometrial cavity can be examined, allowing for direct visualization of lesions. The procedure is used primarily to investigate abnormal uterine bleeding, often caused by intrauterine submucous myoma and polyps. After the diagnosis, these lesions can be removed using a variety of techniques. For example, ablation of the endometrial lining may be carried out with a rollerball, resectoscope or Nd:YAG laser.

**Variant procedure or approaches:** **Diagnostic hysteroscopies** can be performed under both GA and local anesthesia, while **operative hysteroscopies** are usually performed under GA. An examination under anesthesia is performed, followed by the insertion of open speculum and the attachment of a tenaculum to the cervix. The cervical canal is dilated until the hysteroscope with its sheath can be introduced (Fig 8.2-3). A distention medium is then used to provide adequate visualization. Several different distention media are used (e.g., $CO_2$ is frequently used for diagnostic cases). The flow is limited to 1200 cc/min and the intrauterine pressure is kept < 200 mmHg in order to prevent cardiac dysrhythmias.[1]

For optimum operative hysteroscopy in the presence of bleeding, dextran 70 is the most frequently used medium. It is highly viscous and not miscible with blood; thus, it provides superb visibility. Although fatal anaphylaxis has been noted only rarely, an attempt should be made to keep the amount used to < 50 cc. Dextrose, 4-6% dextran and 3% sorbitol in water have also been used; but due to their miscibility with blood, fewer operative cases are performed with this media. A view camera can be attached to the hysteroscope to allow for easier visualization. During operative cases, an accompanying laparoscope (see "Laparoscopy") is often introduced from above to evaluate the progress of the hysteroscopy and to safeguard against uterine perforation and potential bowel injury.

Choice of distention media[2] (++ = preferred; + = satisfactory; – = not used):

| | $CO_2$ | Hyskon® | Low-viscosity fluid |
|---|---|---|---|
| Office use | ++ | – | + |
| OR use | ++ | ++ | ++ |
| Diagnostic | ++ | ++ | + |
| Operative | – | ++ | – |

**Usual preop diagnosis:** Abnormal uterine bleeding; infertility; recurrent pregnancy loss

### SUMMARY OF PROCEDURE

| | |
|---|---|
| **Position** | Dorsal lithotomy (Allen stirrups) |
| **Incision** | None |
| **Special instrumentation** | $CO_2$ insufflator; Hyskon® or fluid pump; laser; electrocautery equipment |
| **Unique considerations** | Accelerated fluid absorption with prolonged procedures or with resections may lead to pulmonary edema. Laparoscopy often accompanies this procedure (see "Laparoscopy"). |
| **Surgical time** | 15 min - 2 hrs |
| **EBL** | 0-100 cc |
| **Postop care** | Excessive postop bleeding can be controlled by using a 5 cc Foley balloon catheter in the uterus for several hrs.[3] |
| **Mortality** | 1/10,000 anaphylaxis to Hyskon®[4] |
| **Morbidity** | Shoulder pain can occur from $CO_2$ used as a distention medium. Pleural effusion can be seen with use of low-viscosity medium.[5] |
| **Procedure code** | 58990 (diagnostic hysteroscopy); 58992 (hysteroscopy with adhesiolysis or septum resection); 58994 (hysteroscopy with submucous myomata resection); 58996 (hysteroscopy with endometrial ablation) |
| **Pain score** | 3-5 |

**PATIENT POPULATION CHARACTERISTICS**

| | |
|---|---|
| **Age range** | 20-80 yrs |
| **Incidence** | >1/50 |
| **Etiology** | Unexplained uterine bleeding<br>Infertility |
| **Associated conditions** | Obesity |

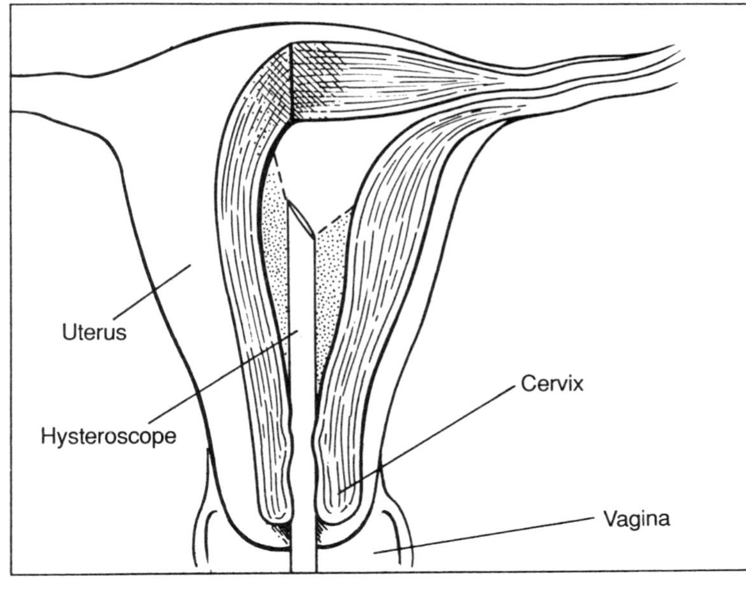


**Figure 8.2-3.** Hysteroscopy.

## ANESTHETIC CONSIDERATIONS

### PREOPERATIVE

Hysteroscopy may be performed for diagnostics or treatment of intrauterine pathology. Patients presenting for this procedure are generally healthy.

| | |
|---|---|
| **Cardiovascular** | Patient may be undergoing hysteroscopy for uterine bleeding; so BP, HR and orthostatic vital signs should be noted.<br>**Tests:** As indicated from H&P. |
| **Laboratory** | Hb/Hct if bleeding Hx. Other tests as indicated from H&P. |
| **Premedication** | Anxiolytic (e.g., midazolam 1-2 mg iv) as needed. |

### INTRAOPERATIVE

**Anesthetic technique:** Local, regional or GA may be used. In the younger patient population, spinal anesthesia may be less desirable because of increased incidence of post-dural puncture headache (PDPH).

**Local anesthesia:** Some procedures may be done under local, especially if they are diagnostic. Paracervical block has the potential for an inadvertent intravenous administration with consequent toxic reaction.

**Regional anesthesia:** A T10 sensory level is sufficient to provide anesthesia for procedures on the uterus.

| | |
|---|---|
| **Spinal** | 5% lidocaine 75-100 mg; 0.75% bupivacaine 10-15 mg in 7.5% dextrose. (See Anesthetic Considerations for "Cesarean Section.") |
| **Epidural** | 1.5-2.0% lidocaine with epinephrine 5 μg/cc, 15-25 cc; supplement with 5-10 cc as needed. Supplemental iv sedation. (See Anesthetic Considerations for "Cesarean Section.") |

**General anesthesia:**

| | |
|---|---|
| **Induction** | Standard induction (see Appendix). |
| **Maintenance** | Standard maintenance (see Appendix). Patients have a high incidence of vomiting, so prophylaxis (e.g., metoclopramide 10 mg iv), as in patients for D&C, is warranted. |
| **Emergence** | Be ready with suction in the event of vomiting on emergence. |

| | | |
|---|---|---|
| **Blood and fluid requirements** | Minimal blood loss<br>IV: 18 ga x 1 (unless hypovolemic)<br>NS\LR @ 2cc/kg/hr | Usual replacement of maintenance fluids and overnight deficit in the form of crystalloid. Blood replacement is almost never indicated. |

| | | |
|---|---|---|
| **Positioning** | √ hip, leg and hand positions.<br>√ and pad pressure points.<br>√ eyes.<br>Shoulder abduction < 90° | Lithotomy position can be deleterious to pulmonary function, as it may impair respiratory mechanics. Rarely, hemodynamic changes occur on elevation of legs into the stirrups, as this increases venous return to the heart. Problems with hypotension on lowering legs postop are common.[8] Take care to insure that no peripheral nerve injury occurs. Common peroneal nerve palsy is possible if pressure on the nerve over the fibula is not prevented by adequate padding or positioning. Hyperflexion of hip joint can cause femoral and lateral femoral cutaneous nerve palsy. Obturator and saphenous nerve injury are also complications of the lithotomy position.[2] Take care to insure safety of patient's fingers when manipulating the foot of the bed. Avoid finger injury by placing patient's arms on arm boards or by wrapping her hands.[1] |
| **Monitoring** | Standard monitors (see Appendix). | |
| **Surgical stimulation** | When cervix is grasped and dilated, patient may have excessive vagal nerve stimulation. | RX: prompt cessation of stimulation by surgeons and treatment with atropine if indicated. |
| **Complications** | Pulmonary edema<br>Coagulopathy<br>Anaphylactoid reactions<br>Finger injury | Dextran 70 (Hyskon®) and dextran 40 are frequently infused into the uterus during hysteroscopy to facilitate visualization of intrauterine structures. Case reports of ARDS, pulmonary edema, DIC, as well as platelet dysfunction, have been reported when large volumes have been used.[10,11,12] It has been recommended that no more than 300 ml of this solution be infused to avoid these potentially serious complications. Anaphylactoid reactions have also occurred after exposure to Hyskon®. |

## POSTOPERATIVE

| | | |
|---|---|---|
| **Complications** | High incidence of N&V<br>Respiratory compromise from excessive dextran absorption. | Anti-emetics, including metoclopramide 10 mg iv, droperidol 1 mg iv and ondansetron 4 mg iv, can be useful in this setting. |
| **Pain management** | Small dose of titrated opiate | Patients usually tolerate oral pain medications. |
| **Tests** | Consider CXR and ABG. | If respiratory compromise. |


**References**

1. Semm K: *Atlas of Gynecologic Laparoscopy and Hysteroscopy.* WB Saunders Co, Philadelphia: 1977.
2. Pellicer A, Diamond MP: Distending media for hysteroscopy. In *Obstet Gynecol Clin North Am.* 1988; 15:23-8.
3. DeCherney A, Polan ML: Hysteroscopic management of intrauterine lesions and intractable uterine bleeding. *Obstet Gynecol* 1983; 61(3):392-97.
4. Borten M, Seibert CP, Taymor ML: Recurrent anaphylactic reaction to intraperitoneal dextran 75 used for prevention of postsurgical adhesions. *Obstet Gynecol* 1983; 61(6):755-57.
5. Adoni A, et al: Postoperative pleural effusion caused by dextran. *Int J Gynaecol Obstet* 1980; 18(4):243-44.
6. Thompson JD, Rock JA, eds: *TeLinde's Operative Gynecology*, 7th edition. JB Lippincott, Philadelphia: 1992, 385-410.
7. Bagget M, ed: Clinical obstetrics and gynecology. In *Gynecologic Endoscopy and Instrumentation.* Harper & Row, Philadelphia: 1983, 318.
8. Welborn, SG: The lithotomy position, anesthesiologic considerations. In *Positioning in Anesthesia and Surgery.* WB Saunders Co, Philadelphia: 1978, 156-61.
9. Courtney MA: Neurologic sequelae of childbirth and regional anesthesia. In *Manual of Obstetric Anesthesia.* Churchill Livingstone, New York: 1992.
10. Leake JF, Murphy AA, Zacur HA: Noncardiogenic pulmonary edema: a complication of operative hysteroscopy. *Fertil Steril* 1987; 48(3):497-99.
11. Vercellini P, Rossi R, Pagnoni B, Fedele L: Hypervolemic pulmonary edema and severe coagulopathy after intrauterine dextran instillation. *Obstet Gynecol* 1992; 79(5[P + 2]):838-39.
12. Jedeikin R, Olsfanger D, Kessler I: Disseminated intravascular coagulopathy and adult respiratory distress syndrome: life-threatening complications of hysteroscopy. *Am J Obstet Gynecol* 1990; 162(1):44-5.

# LAPAROSCOPY

## SURGICAL CONSIDERATIONS

**Description: Laparoscopy** is an endoscopic technique frequently used in gynecological surgery to visualize the pelvic structures. It is rapidly becoming the most common surgical procedure in gynecology, with its ability to substitute for laparotomy, thus cutting down postop recovery and hospital bed time. Laparoscopy is used most frequently to perform sterilization and diagnose the etiology of pelvic pain. Pelvic adhesions and endometriosis are frequently found and can be treated endoscopically at the time of diagnosis. Finally, laparoscopy is becoming a major surgical tool in the infertility workup and for treatment of ectopic pregnancies. A steady improvement in equipment over the last decade has allowed more challenging cases to be done with the laparoscope. **Laparoscopic linear salpingostomies** and **salpingectomies** are frequently performed for ectopic pregnancies. It is now common to remove ovarian cysts, ovaries and fibroid tumors through the laparoscope.

A uterine manipulator (Hulka, Acorn or a Harris-Kronner Uterine Manipulator Injector [HUMI]) is inserted into the cervical canal. A small infraumbilical incision is made for the insertion of the Verres needle, through which approximately 3 L of $CO_2$ is insufflated. The needle is promptly replaced by a larger trocar which hosts the laparoscope and attached fiber optic light source. One or more suprapubic incisions are made to allow the use of a variety of instruments (grasping forceps, biopsy, suction, irrigation, cutting and coagulation) needed to perform the operation. A laser source can be attached to the laparoscope.

**Usual preop diagnosis:** Elective sterilization; pelvic pain; infertility; pelvic mass (adnexal or uterine); ectopic pregnancy; vaginal hysterectomy (laparoscopically assisted)

### SUMMARY OF PROCEDURE

| | |
|---|---|
| **Position** | Dorsal lithotomy (Allen stirrups). Shoulder braces help prevent movement upwards during Trendelenburg positioning for pelvic exposure. |
| **Incision** | Infraumbilical + 1 - 4 suprapubic incisions (Fig 8.2-4) |
| **Special instrumentation** | Often, laser or Argon Beam Coagulator |
| **Unique considerations** | The operating table is brought down during Verres needle and trocar insertion. Pneumoperitoneum usually dictates need for tracheal intubation. Dysrhythmias such as sinus tachycardia and bradydysrhythmia frequently occur during or shortly after $CO_2$ insufflation and also with traction of pelvic structures.[1] Hypercapnia from excessive $CO_2$ absorption (intra-abdominal pressure >20 mmHg) may cause cardiac dysrhythmias or cardiac arrest (2/1000[2]). Often during ectopic pregnancy operations, vasopressin (Pitressin®) solution (1-5 U vasopressin in 10 cc physiologic solution), 1-5 cc, is injected into the mesosalpinx to reduce bleeding. Changes in cardiac output can be seen then. Monitoring of fluid status may be hampered by no urine drainage, and by the fact that aspirated fluid contains blood plus irrigation. |
| **Surgical time** | Sterilization: 10 - 20 min<br>Pelvic pain: 20 min - 3 hrs<br>Ectopic pregnancy: 1 - 3 hrs<br>Laparoscopy-assisted vaginal hysterectomy: 2 - 3 hrs |
| **Closing considerations** | Often 1-2 L of fluid (usually 5000 U heparin in 1000 cc LR) is left in the pelvis at the end of the case to prevent adhesion formation. Fluid overload with pulmonary edema can occur. An effort is made to remove as much $CO_2$ as possible at the end of the operation to prevent postop abdominal and shoulder pain. |
| **EBL** | Sterilization: < 10 cc; pelvic pain: < 300 cc; ectopic pregnancy: < 500 cc |
| **Postop care** | Outpatient |
| **Mortality** | Tubal sterilization 1.7-10.8/100,000 cases[3,4,5]<br>Postop shoulder and chest pain from unabsorbed gas/peritoneal irritation: 30% |
| **Morbidity** | Bleeding or tissue damage:<br>With sterilization[7]: 1.6/1,000<br>With diagnostic laparoscopy[7]: 3.1/1,000<br>Intra-abdominal complications: 85/10,000[2]<br>Vessel damage: 30/10,000[6] |

**Procedure code** 58980 (diagnostic laparoscopy); 58982 (laparoscopy with fulguration of oviducts); 58983 (laparoscopy with oviduct occlusion); 58984 (laparoscopy with fulguration/excision of superficial pelvic lesions); 58985 (laparoscopy with lysis of adhesion); 58986 (laparoscopy with biopsy); 58987 (laparoscopy with aspiration); 58988 (laparoscopy with removal of adnexal structures)

**Pain score** 5-8

## PATIENT POPULATION CHARACTERISTICS

**Age range** 20-60 yrs

**Incidence** >1/20 females

**Etiology** Multiparous women wanting permanent sterilization
Pelvic pain
Pelvic mass
Infertility
Ectopic pregnancy

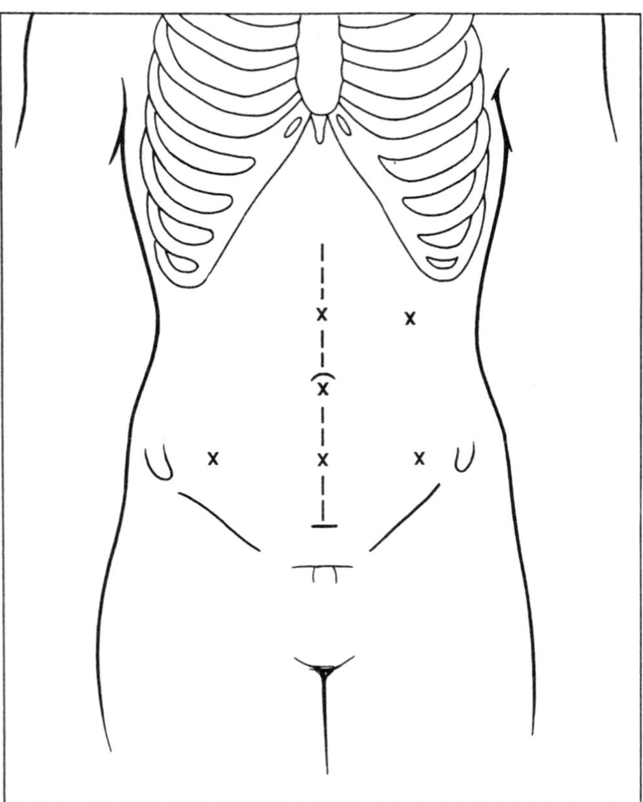

**Figure 8.2-4.** Possible sites for laparoscopic incisions. (Reproduced with permission from Gomel V, Taylor PJ, Yuzpe AA, Rioux JE: *Laparoscopy and Hysteroscopy in Gynecologic Practice*. Year Book Medical Pub: 1986.)

## ANESTHETIC CONSIDERATIONS

See Anesthetic Considerations following "Infertility Operations" (below).

**References**


1. Myles PS: Bradyarrhythmia and laparoscopy: a prospective study of HR changes with laparoscopy. *Aust N Z J Obstet Gynaecol* 1991; 31(2):171-73.
2. Destefano F, et al: Complications of interval laparoscopic tubal sterilization. *Obstet Gynecol* 1983; 61(2):153-58.
3. Aubert JM, Lubell I, Schima M: Mortality risk associated with female sterilization. *Int J Gynaecol Obstet* 1980; 18(6):406-10.
4. Peterson HB, DeStefano F, Rubin GL et al: Deaths attributable to tubal sterilization in the United States, 1977 to 1981. *Am J Obstet Gynecol* 1983; 146(2):131-36.
5. Chi IC, Potts M, Wilkens L: Rare events associated with tubal sterilizations: an international experience. *Obstet Gynecol Surv* 1986; 41(1):7-19.
6. Bhiwandiwala PP, Mumford SD, Kennedy KI: Comparison of the safety of open and conventional laparoscopic sterilization. *Obstet Gynecol* 1985; 66(3):391-94.
7. Hulka JF, et al: American Association of Gynecologic Laparoscopists' 1985 Member Survey. *J Reprod Med* 1987; 32(10):732-35.

# PELVIC LAPAROTOMY

### (FOR MYOMECTOMY, OVARIAN CYSTECTOMY, OOPHORECTOMY, ECTOPIC PREGNANCY, ABDOMINAL COLPOPEXY, MOSCHOWITZ ENTEROCELE REPAIR, PRESACRAL NEURECTOMY)

## SURGICAL CONSIDERATIONS

**Description:** These are all common gynecological procedures. **Laparotomy** is most frequently performed via a Pfannenstiel incision, which permits good pelvic exposure. A vertical incision is used in oncological surgery or in the presence of a large uterus. A knife or Bovie® is used to cut through the skin and underlying tissue until the rectus fascia is reached. The fascia is nicked, and then sharply incised bilaterally 2-4" with scissors or electrocautery (Bovie®). The rectus muscle is sharply separated in the midline down to the pubis and the peritoneum is entered. The peritoneal incision is then extended vertically or transversely. The pelvis and entire abdominal cavity is first explored by palpation. The bowels are then usually packed in a cephalad direction with surgical laparotomy sponges (laps) to prevent them from falling back into the pelvis. Good muscle relaxation is important during this stage to ensure optimum packing. A self-retaining retractor is frequently used to keep the laps in place and to enhance exposure. After the desired operation has been performed, the retractor and packs are removed. During the peritoneal closure, abdominal muscle relaxation is once again critical in order to minimize tension on this layer and risk of bowel injury with the needle. The rectus fascia, the subcutaneous tissue and finally the skin, are closed in succession.

**Variant procedures: Myomectomies** are performed to remove myomata that are causing pain, abnormal bleeding or infertility. Myomata are heavily vascularized at the base, and the surgeon has several ways to minimize this bleeding. A clamp can be placed across the uterine vasculature, thus minimizing the blood flow to the uterus. A common alternative is the use of a vasoconstrictor such as diluted epinephrine (1:200,000) or vasopressin solution (1-5 U/10 cc NS). The solution (2-10 cc) is injected around the myoma prior to incising the uterus, which invariably → ↑HR and ↑BP. Gonadotropin releasing hormone (GNRH) agonists may be used for a few months prior to the operation in order to render the patient hypoestrogenic, and thus decrease the vascularity of the myomata. After the myomata have been removed, the uterine defects are closed with several layers of suture, and the uterine serosa is closed.

**Ovarian cystectomies** are performed to alleviate related pain and to diagnose the identity of asymptomatic cysts. Small, single-functional ovarian cysts are found at different stages in a woman's menstrual cycle. At times, due to hormonal imbalance, these cysts can increase in size and quantity, which may cause severe pain. The ovary can also contain various non-functional cysts (i.e., tumors) which have to be removed if found, even if asymptomatic, in order to rule out malignancy. After the pelvic structures are well-visualized, the cystic ovary is stabilized with instruments or surgical laps. Sharp or blunt dissection is used to shell out the cyst intact. If there is any suspicion about the nature of the cyst, an intraop frozen section is obtained. The ovary is then reapproximated and the abdomen closed. If the cyst is large and little healthy ovarian stroma remains, an **oophorectomy** is performed.

**Ectopic pregnancies** are usually medical emergencies. Increasingly, laparoscopy is being used to treat this condition (see "Laparoscopy"), although laparotomies for ectopic pregnancies are still widely performed. The abdomen is entered, and the pregnancy located quickly. An attempt is made to control the bleeding with the surgeon's hand, clamp or suture. Frequently, large amounts of blood in the pelvis are suctioned and the ectopic pregnancy is removed via a partial tubal resection, salpingostomy or salpingectomy; then the abdomen is closed. A D&C is often performed at the end to prevent late bleeding from the pregnancy-induced endometrial proliferation (see "D&C").

In **abdominal colpopexy** (fixation of vagina), the patient is initially placed in the lithotomy position in order to perform an examination under anesthesia, as well as to insert a vaginal pack needed to identify the vaginal apex. A urethral catheter is inserted prior to staging the laparotomy. A rectus fascia graft is obtained during the opening of the abdomen (a Marlex® mesh can be used instead). The bowel is packed and the defect is examined from the abdominal perspective. Frequently there is an accompanying enterocele which is closed initially (see Moschowitz procedure, below). The peritoneum over the vaginal apex is then entered and the neighboring rectum and bladder are dissected a distance away from the vaginal apex. The peritoneum over the sacrum is incised and the cephalad end of the graft is sutured to the anterior sacral ligament of the 3rd vertebrae. The caudal end of the graft is attached to the vaginal apex, with the surgeon frequently using a vaginal hand to place these last sutures. The peritoneum and abdomen are closed, and the patient is placed back in the dorsal lithotomy position for a high posterior colporrhaphy (repair of vagina).

The **Moschowitz procedure** is used to reduce enteroceles via an abdominal approach. The abdomen is entered in the usual fashion, the uterus held up with a traction suture, the bowel packed, and the patient placed in the Trendelenburg position. Multiple, concentric, purse-string sutures close the defect in the pouch of Douglas; and the abdomen is closed.

The **presacral neurectomy** is an operation performed for women with severe chronic midline pelvic pain. Usually the patient has a history of prior surgeries to diagnose and treat the problem. A laparotomy is initially performed with packing of the bowels. The rectosigmoid is brought over to the left in order to make a vertical, posterior, parietal, peritoneal incision over the sacral area. The anatomy is examined closely and the presacral nerves are ligated; then the peritoneum and abdomen are closed. Severe bleeding can be seen intraop from the hemorrhoidal and sacral veins, but usually can be controlled with pressure.

**Usual preop diagnosis:** Myomata (pelvic pain, hypermenorrhea, infertility); ovarian cysts and oophorectomy (pelvic pain, undiagnosed ovarian mass); ectopic pregnancy; vaginal vault prolapse; enterocele; presacral neurectomy (chronic pelvic pain)

## SUMMARY OF PROCEDURE

| | |
|---|---|
| **Position** | Supine or lithotomy |
| **Incision** | Pfannenstiel or low midline abdominal |
| **Unique considerations** | Muscle relaxation is important during bowel packing and abdominal closure. Vasoconstrictor substances for controlling myomata bleeding (1:200,000 epinephrine and 1-5 U vasopressin/10 cc NS) are often used and can alter BP and HR. |
| **Antibiotics** | 1-2 gm iv cefoxitin or cefotetan |
| **Surgical time** | 45 min - 2 hrs<br>Abdominal colpopexy: 4 - 5 hrs |
| **EBL** | 150-1000 cc (maximum related to procedure) |
| **Postop care** | PACU |
| **Mortality** | Minimal |
| **Morbidity**[2] | Gastric dilatation: 3%<br>Thrombophlebitis: 3%<br>PE: 2%<br>Ureteral stenosis: 1% |
| **Procedure code** | 58410 (laparotomy with presacral sympathectomy); 58925 (ovarian cystectomy, unilateral or bilateral); 58940 (oophorectomy, partial or total, unilateral or bilateral); 58140 (myomectomy, excision of fibroid tumor of uterus, single or multiple); 57270 (repair of enterocele, abdominal approach); 57280 (colpopexy, abdominal approach) |
| **Pain score** | 8 |

## PATIENT POPULATION CHARACTERISTICS

| | Myomectomy | Ovarian Cystectomy, Oophorectomy | Ectopic Pregnancy | Abdominal Colpopexy, Moschowitz | Presacral Neurectomy |
|---|---|---|---|---|---|
| **Age range** | 20-45 yrs | 20-85 yrs | 15-45 yrs | 40-80 yrs | 20-50 yrs |
| **Incidence** | >1/5 females | ⇐ | 1/100 females | 1/500 females | ⇐ |
| **Etiology** | Congenital | Endometriosis<br>Anovulation<br>Adenoma | Pre-existing salpingitis | Multiparous obesity<br>Chronic cough | Endometriosis |
| **Associated conditions** | Menorrhagia | Endometriosis | Pelvic adhesions | Pelvic relaxation | Endometriosis |

# ANESTHETIC CONSIDERATIONS

See Anesthetic Considerations following "Infertility Operations" (below).

**References**

1. Thompson JD, Rock JA, eds: *TeLinde's Operative Gynecology*, 7th edition. JB Lippincott, Philadelphia: 1992.
2. Uyttenbroeck F: *Gynecologic Surgery - Treatment of Complications and Prevention of Injuries*. Masson Publishing, New York: 1980.
3. Tovell HM, Dank LD: *Gynecologic Operations: As Performed by Members of the Staff of the Woman's Hospital, St. Luke's Hospital Center, New York*. Harper and Row, Hagerstown, Md; 1978.

# INFERTILITY OPERATIONS

## (FIMBRIOPLASTY, TUBAL REANASTOMOSIS, METROPLASTY, TUBAL CANNULATION, ADVANCED REPRODUCTIVE TECHNOLOGY)

## SURGICAL CONSIDERATIONS

**Description:** These operations all deal with reproductive problems. The general trend is to avoid laparotomies and to perform operations using outpatient laparoscopy and hysteroscopy techniques whenever possible.

**Fimbrioplasty** is used to repair distal fallopian tubal occlusion, a common cause for infertility, which is usually a consequence of pelvic inflammatory disease. The operation is performed most often via a **pelvic laparotomy** (see "Pelvic Laparotomy"). A urethral catheter is inserted to empty the bladder, followed by the insertion of a transcervical uterine catheter for chromopertubation (dye injection). The abdomen is opened and the pelvic structures are exposed. Emphasis is made during the operation to follow microsurgical techniques in order to minimize trauma. Meticulous hemostasis is important. A wound protector is often used instead of self-retaining retractors. The peritoneum and pelvic structures are kept moist with intermittent irrigation. An overhead salpingolysis and ovariolysis are performed microsurgically. Once the adnexae have been freed, they are elevated by loosely packing the pouch of Douglas with insulated pads (plastic sheathed covered laps). Chromopertubation is then performed and, if occlusion is present, a new stoma is created using microsurgical instruments and sutures. The abdomen is then closed.

**Tubal reanastomosis**, performed to restore fertility, is very similar to fimbrioplasty with microsurgical techniques followed diligently. After the tubal segments have been freed slightly from their underlying mesosalpinx, the occluded ends are cut and chromopertubation is performed to ensure patency. After patency has been established, anastomosis is performed in two layers. The mesosalpinx is reapproximated to the tubal serosa and the abdomen closed.

The uterus is embryologically formed by the fusion of two paramesonephric tubes. At times, the fusion is incomplete and a septated uterus or bicornuate uterus is formed. The malformed uterus is associated with an increased risk for miscarriages and pre-term labor. **Metroplasty** is used to correct this condition. The **Strassmann procedure** for bicornuate uteri uses a standard pelvic laparotomy. Following uterine exposure, an incision is made on the medial side of each hemicorpus and carried down until the uterine cavity is entered. The edges are reapproximated to form a single uterus. The **Tompkins procedure** for septated uteri also uses the standard pelvic laparotomy approach. A uterine wedge containing the septum is removed, followed by closure of the uterus. More recently, septated uteri have been repaired via a hysteroscopic approach (see "Hysteroscopy") with scissors or laser.

**Proximal tubal cannulation** is a relatively new technique with great promise, in which proximal tubal occlusion can be repaired through either a fluoroscopic or a hysteroscopic approach. The hysteroscopic approach, usually performed under GA, allows the surgeon to insert a small cannula to restore tube patency. This procedure is often done with laparoscopy in order to follow the progress of the cannulization and to visualize the chromopertubation (see "Hysteroscopy and Laparoscopy").[2]

**Gamete intra-fallopian transfer**[3] (GIFT) and **tubal embryo transfer** (TET) are methods of advanced reproductive technology. Couples who have undergone extensive infertility workups and treatment without success eventually become candidates for GIFT and TET procedures. Ovarian follicles are stimulated to grow with the help of gonadotropins. These follicles are then punctured with a needle transvaginally to "harvest" the eggs. These eggs can be mixed with semen and placed directly into the distal end of the fallopian tube using laparoscopic techniques and a small tubal catheter (see "Laparoscopy"). In the TET procedure, the semen and eggs are allowed to incubate a few days *in vitro*; embryos form and are transferred to the fallopian tubes in a manner similar to the GIFT procedure.

**Usual preop diagnosis:** Infertility; history of multiple spontaneous abortion and pre–term labor (see "Laparotomy," "Laparoscopy" and "Hysteroscopy")

### SUMMARY OF PROCEDURE

(For summaries of specific procedures, see "Laparoscopy," "Hysteroscopy," and "Pelvic Laparotomy" sections, above.)

### PATIENT POPULATION CHARACTERISTICS

| | |
|---|---|
| **Age range** | 20–40 yrs |
| **Incidence** | 1/20 females |

| | |
|---|---|
| **Etiology** | PID<br>Endometriosis<br>Idiopathic |
| **Associated conditions** | Obesity |

---

## ANESTHETIC CONSIDERATIONS

**(Procedures covered: pelvic laparotomy/laparoscopy for myomectomy; ovarian cystectomy; oophorectomy; ectopic pregnancy; abdominal colpopexy; Moschowitz enterocele repair; presacral neurectomy; infertility operations)**

### PREOPERATIVE

This is generally a healthy patient population; however, this procedure can be performed for a wide variety of pathologic conditions.

| | |
|---|---|
| **Cardiovascular** | Patients undergoing myomectomy and, especially, ectopic pregnancy removal, may have had a significant amount of preop bleeding; therefore, BP, HR and orthostatic vital signs should be noted.<br>**Tests:** As indicated from H&P. |
| **Laboratory** | Hb/Hct. Patients with ectopic pregnancy may have urine/serum pregnancy tests, as well as pelvic ultrasound. |
| **Premedication** | Patients with ruptured ectopic pregnancies may come to the OR urgently, and should be treated as for full stomach. This includes premedication with a non-particulate antacid, Na citrate (bicarb) 30 ml po, metoclopramide 10 mg iv, and ranitidine 50 mg iv. |

### INTRAOPERATIVE

**Anesthetic technique:** GETA is preferred in patients undergoing laparoscopic surgery and in patients presenting for emergency surgery. Regional anesthesia is best avoided in hemodynamically unstable patients (i.e., ectopic pregnancies), and for laparoscopy where breathing difficulty may develop 2° to pneumoperitoneum and Trendelenburg position. GA may be suitable for simple laparotomies. In the younger patient population, spinal anesthesia is less desirable because of increased incidence of post-dural puncture headache (PDPH).

**General anesthesia:**

| | |
|---|---|
| **Induction** | Standard induction (see Appendix). A patient with an intact ectopic pregnancy undergoing laparoscopy should have an ETT placed and be mechanically ventilated to assure adequate oxygenation, ventilation and acid-base balance.[4] In a patient with a ruptured ectopic pregnancy, ketamine 1-2 mg/kg or etomidate 0.1-0.4 mg/kg may be preferable if a large blood loss has occurred. These patients may also have full stomachs; and, in this case, they require a rapid-sequence induction with cricoid pressure and immediate ET intubation (succinylcholine 1.5 mg/kg). |
| **Maintenance** | Standard maintenance (see Appendix). A high incidence of N&V warrants prophylaxis with metoclopramide 10 mg iv or droperidol 1 mg iv. |
| **Emergence** | Be ready with suction in the event of vomiting on emergence. |

**Regional anesthesia:** A T6-8 sensory level is recommended for pelvic/lower abdominal surgery.

| | |
|---|---|
| **Spinal** | 5% lidocaine 75-100 mg; 0.75% bupivacaine 10-15 mg in 7.5% dextrose. (See Anesthetic Considerations for "Cesarean Section.") |
| **Epidural** | 1.5-2.0% lidocaine with epinephrine 5 μg/cc, 15-25 cc; supplement with 5-10 cc as needed. Supplemental iv sedation. (See Anesthetic Considerations for "Cesarean Section.") |

| | | |
|---|---|---|
| **Blood and fluid requirements** | Possible heavy blood loss<br>IV: 16-18 ga x 1-2<br>NS/LR @ 5-7 cc/kg/hr | Patients with ectopic pregnancies may have large blood loss both preop and intraop. Adequate iv access is imperative in these patients, as is the availability of blood. |

| | | |
|---|---|---|
| **Control of blood loss** | Epinephrine<br>Vasopressin | During myomectomies, surgeons may inject vasopressors into the area surrounding myomata prior to excision. This can cause HTN and cardiac dysrhythmias. |
| **Monitoring** | Standard monitors (see Appendix).<br>± Foley catheter<br>Ectopic pregnancy:<br>± Arterial catheter | Patients with ectopic pregnancies may need intra-arterial monitoring if major hemorrhage is anticipated. |
| **Positioning** | ✓ and pad pressure points.<br>✓ eyes. | During abdominal colpopexy, patient is placed intermittently in both the lithotomy and supine positions. (See "D&C" for concerns regarding the lithotomy position.) |
| **Complications** | Respiratory:<br>Pneumoperitoneum<br>↑$PaCO_2$, ↓$PaO_2$<br>ETT Migration | Pneumoperitoneum with $CO_2$ and steep Trendelenburg position cause cephalad displacement of diaphragm with ↓FRC, ↓pulmonary compliance, and ↑airway closure/atelectasis. Hypercarbia and hypoxia, due to respiratory compromise, can result unless ventilation is controlled during GA. Check for endobronchial migration of ETT upon assumption of Trendelenburg position. |
| | Pneumothorax | Pneumothorax due to retroperitoneal dissection of insufflated gas into the mediastinum can cause hypoxemia, ↑airway pressure, subcutaneous emphysema and hypotension. |
| | Cardiovascular:<br>↓BP<br>Hemorrhage<br>Dysrhythmias | ↓BP can result from ↓venous return caused by pneumoperitoneum. Hemorrhage can result from blood vessel injury or rapid reversal of head-down position. Unintended intravascular injection of $CO_2$ gas can lead to hypotension and dysrhythmias. |
| | Neurological:<br>Nerve injury<br>Brachial plexus injury<br>Nerve root compression | Use of Trendelenburg position incurs risk of nerve injury. Hyperextension of arm may result in brachial plexus injury and careful padding of vulnerable points is necessary. Shoulder brace can compress nerve roots in retroclavicular region. |

### POSTOPERATIVE

| | | |
|---|---|---|
| **Complications** | N&V<br>Anemia | Rx: metoclopramide 10 mg 1-2 hr |
| | Shoulder pain | Postop pain may be referred to the shoulder, due to irritation of diaphragm by residual pneumoperitoneum or bleeding. |
| **Pain Management** | PCA (see Appendix). | |
| **Tests** | Hb/Hct, if hemorrhage occurs. | |

---

## ANESTHETIC CONSIDERATIONS FOR *IN VITRO* FERTILIZATION

### PREOPERATIVE

This is generally a fit, healthy patient population. Little is required beyond routine tests, unless otherwise indicated.

| | |
|---|---|
| **Laboratory** | Hct; other tests as indicated from H&P. |
| **Premedication** | Standard premedication (see Appendix). |

### INTRAOPERATIVE

**Anesthetic technique:** Local, regional (e.g., spinal and epidural), and GA all have been employed for laparoscopic *in vitro* fertilization. Rapid recovery is desirable as the procedure is frequently done on an outpatient basis. Local anesthesia may result in inadequate pain relief and require heavy iv sedation. Regional anesthesia provides better pain relief, but breathing difficulty can develop due to pneumoperitoneum and Trendelenburg position. GETA with controlled ventilation is, therefore, most commonly used.

| | | |
|---|---|---|
| **Induction** | Standard induction (see Appendix). Avoidance of succinylcholine may decrease postop myalgia. | |
| **Maintenance** | Standard maintenance (see Appendix). $N_2O$ does not appear to adversely affect success of fertilization.[5] | |
| **Emergence** | No special considerations | |
| **Blood and fluid requirements** | Minimal blood loss<br>IV: 18 ga x 1<br>NS/LR @ 2 cc/kg/hr | Blood loss minimal, unless trauma to vasculature. Rarely, trauma to blood vessels or organs following laparoscopy may necessitate laparotomy. |
| **Monitoring** | Standard monitors (see Appendix). | |
| **Positioning** | √ and pad pressure points.<br>√ eyes. | |
| **Complications** | Respiratory:<br>Pneumoperitoneum:<br>↑$PaCO_2$, ↓$PaO_2$<br>ETT migration<br>Pneumothorax | Pneumoperitoneum with $CO_2$ and steep Trendelenburg position cause cephalad displacement of diaphragm with ↓FRC, ↓pulmonary compliance, and ↑airway closure/atelectasis. Hypercarbia and hypoxia, due to respiratory compromise, can result unless ventilation is controlled during GA. Check for endobronchial migration of ETT upon assumption of Trendelenburg position. Pneumothorax due to retroperitoneal dissection of insufflated gas into the mediastinum can cause hypoxemia, ↑airway pressure, subcutaneous emphysema and hypotension. |
| | Cardiovascular:<br>↓BP<br>Hemorrhage<br>Dysrhythmias | ↓BP can result from ↓venous return caused by pneumoperitoneum. Hemorrhage can result from blood vessel injury or rapid reversal of head-down position. Unintended intravascular injection of $CO_2$ gas can lead to hypotension and dysrhythmias. |
| | Neurological:<br>Nerve injury<br>Brachial plexus injury<br>Nerve root compression | Use of Trendelenburg position incurs risk of nerve injury. Hyperextension of arm may result in brachial plexus injury and careful padding of vulnerable points is necessary. Shoulder brace can compress nerve roots in retroclavicular region. |

**POSTOPERATIVE**

| | | |
|---|---|---|
| **Complications** | Shoulder pain | Postop pain may be referred to the shoulder, due to irritation of diaphragm by residual pneumoperitoneum or bleeding. |
| **Pain management** | Oral analgesics are usually sufficient. | |

**References**

1. Thompson JD, Rock JA, eds: *TeLinde's Operative Gynecology*, 7th edition. JB Lippincott, Philadelphia: 1992, 437-62, 603-46.
2. Confino ET: Transcervical balloon tuboplasty: a multicenter study. *JAMA* 1990; 264:2079-82.
3. Tanbo T: Assisted fertilization in infertile women with patient tubes: a comparison of *in vitro* fertilization, gamete intra-fallopian transfer and tubal embryo stage transfer. *Hum Reproduction* 1990; 5:266-70.
4. Resiner, LS. The pregnant patient and the disorders of pregnancy. In *Anesthesia and Uncommon Diseases*. WB Saunders Co, Philadelphia: 1990, 165-66.
5. Rosen MA, Roizen MF, Eger EI II, Glass RH, Martin M, Dandekar PV, Dailey PA, Litt L: The effect of nitrous oxide on *in vitro* fertilization success rate. *Anesthesiology* 1987; 67(1):42-4.

# HYSTERECTOMY – VAGINAL OR TOTAL ABDOMINAL

## SURGICAL CONSIDERATIONS

**Description:** After cesarean section (C-section), **hysterectomy** is the most commonly performed operation in the U.S. (650,000/year). Two approaches are possible: vaginal and abdominal. The **vaginal approach**, performed with the patient in a dorsal lithotomy position, is preferred since it offers significantly less morbidity and mortality. Its use is limited by situations in which uterine size, pelvic adhesions, or the presence of gynecological cancers require an **abdominal approach**. Often the approach is decided upon in the OR, where a pelvic examination under anesthesia will determine the true uterine size, degree of prolapse and the presence of pelvic pathology. A laparoscopy may very well be performed at the outset of surgery in order to evaluate the pelvis and free up adhesions which would have made a vaginal approach initially unsafe. In patients ≥ 45 years, **bilateral salpingo-oophorectomy** (BSO) is often performed in addition to the hysterectomy to provide ovarian cancer prophylaxis. Pelvic relaxation syndrome is the most frequent preop diagnosis in patients having a vaginal hysterectomy. Pelvic relaxation includes one or more of the following: prolapse of the uterus; intestine into the pouch of Douglas (enterocele); bladder into the anterior vaginal wall (cystocele); urethra into the anterior vaginal wall (urethrocele); and rectum into the posterior vaginal wall (rectocele). In these cases, the hysterectomy is often accompanied by an anterior/posterior colporrhaphy, anterior bladder neck suspension, and perineoplasty.

**Variant approaches: Abdominal hysterectomy** is performed through a Pfannenstiel or midline incision, depending on the uterine size and the need to perform a lymph node dissection for cancer. A Pfannenstiel incision often can be improved with two types of muscle-splitting steps: the **Maylard**, in which the rectus muscles are cut just above the pubis, or a **Cherney rectus muscle detachment** performed at the pubic insertion. After entering the abdomen, a self-retaining retractor is placed and the round, ovarian and broad ligaments clamped, cut and tied, in that order. The uterine vessels are identified and ligated, followed by the creation of a bladder flap and, finally, the cutting and ligation of the uterosacral and cardinal ligaments. The vagina is entered and the cervix removed. Then the vaginal cuff is closed in a way to incorporate the uterosacral ligaments for support. The visceral peritoneum is reapproximated, the retractor removed, and the abdominal layers closed.

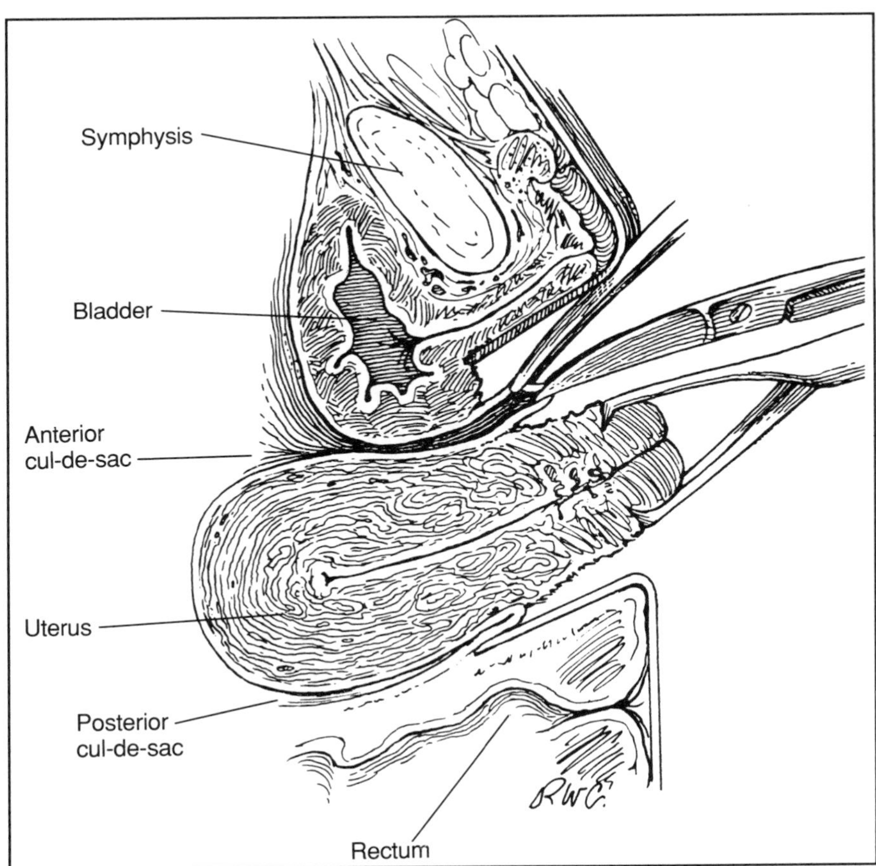

**Figure 8.2-5.** Surgical anatomy for vaginal hysterectomy. (Reproduced with permission from Thompson JD, Rock JA, eds: *TeLinde's Operative Gynecology*, 7th edition. JB Lippincott: 1992.)

In a **vaginal hysterectomy**, the cervix is retracted, a paracervical incision is made, and the anterior and posterior cul de sacs are entered (Fig 8.2-5). The uterosacral and cardinal ligaments and the uterine vessels are cut and ligated. With steady downward traction, the broad ligament is ligated in a step-wise manner until either the ovarian or infundibulopelvic ligament is reached, and one of the two is ligated, depending on whether the ovaries are to be removed or not. After the uterus has been removed, the peritoneum is reapproximated, followed by the closing of the vaginal cuff, which often includes the uterosacral and cardinal ligaments for support. A vaginal pack is often left in place. An increasingly frequent combination of laparoscopically assisted vaginal hysterectomy is being practiced to evaluate the pelvis for unrecognized disease and to ensure prophylactic adnexectomy in women ages ≥ 40-45 yrs.

**Usual preop diagnosis:** Uterine myoma; pelvic relaxation syndrome; pelvic pain 2° endometriosis or adhesions; uncontrolled uterine bleeding/dysmenorrhea; endometrial hyperplasia; gynecological cancers

## SUMMARY OF PROCEDURE

| | Abdominal Approach | | Vaginal Approach |
|---|---|---|---|
| **Position** | Supine | | Lithotomy. Following induction, position patient so that the perineum is at end of operating table to ensure optimum surgical exposure. |
| **Incision** | Pfannenstiel or low midline. The Pfannenstiel incision can be extended with a Maylard muscle-splitting procedure or a Cherney rectus muscle detachment at pubic insertion. | | Pericervical vaginal |
| **Special instrumentation** | None | | Stirrups |
| **Unique considerations** | None | | To prevent peroneal nerve injury, the area of leg leaning against stirrup should be well-cushioned. Often, vasoconstriction agents (1:200,000 epinephrine and vasopressin) are used to cut down perioperative vaginal cuff bleeding.[1] |
| **Antibiotics** | 1-2 gm cefoxitin or cefotetan | | ⇐ |
| **Surgical time** | 1 - 2 hrs | | 0.75 - 1.5 hrs |
| **EBL** | 1500 cc | | 750-1000 cc |
| **Postop care** | PACU | | ⇐ |
| **Mortality**[2] | Overall 14.6/10,000[3] | | 0.2%[4] |
| | < 25 yrs | 8.9/10,000 | 0/10,000 |
| | 25-34 | 4.7 | 0.9 |
| | 35-44 | 3.8 | 0.5 |
| | 45-54 | 6.5 | 2.7 |
| | 55-64 | 41.3 | 1.9 |
| | 65-74 | 93.0 | 18.3 |
| | >75 | 255.8 | 56.8 |
| **Morbidity**[4-7] | Febrile morbidity | 32.3/100 | 15.3/100 |
| | Hemorrhage requiring transfusion | 15.4/100 | 8.3/100 |
| | Femoral nerve injury | 11.6/100 | – |
| | Wound infection | 7/100 | – |
| | Unintended major surgical procedure | 1.7/100 | 5.1/100 |
| | Vaginal cuff infection | 3.1/100 | 2.1/100 |
| | Re-hospitalization | 2.8/100 | 1.8/100 |
| | Bladder injury | 0.5/100 | |
| | Ureter injury | 0.4/100 | |
| | Life-threatening event | 0.4/100 | |
| **Procedure code** | 58150 (TAH ± adnexectomy)<br>58152 (TAH with colpourethropexy)<br>58180 (supracervical abdominal hysterectomy ± adnexectomy) | | 58260 (total vaginal hysterectomy ± adnexectomy) |
| **Pain score** | 5-8 | | 4-6 |

## PATIENT POPULATION CHARACTERISTICS

| | |
|---|---|
| **Age range** | 30-80 yrs |
| **Incidence** | >1/5 females; 650,000/yr in U.S. |

| | |
|---|---|
| **Etiology** | Uterine myomata<br>Endometriosis<br>Uterine prolapse<br>Uterine cancer |
| **Associated conditions** | Stress urinary incontinence<br>Obesity |

---

# ANESTHETIC CONSIDERATIONS

## PREOPERATIVE

Although many patients presenting for this procedure are otherwise healthy, others may have metastatic cancer.

**Respiratory** — CXR may be indicated to rule out pleural effusion or other lung pathology in cancer patients. Additionally, ABGs, ± PFTs, may be indicated preop in patients with significant pulmonary involvement.
**Tests**: As indicated from H&P.

**Cardiovascular** — Patient may have blood loss from the primary problem. Additionally, she may have undergone bowel prep, which can cause dehydration and electrolyte abnormalities. Assessment of volume status, using BP and orthostatic vital signs, is important.
**Tests**: As indicated from H&P.

**Hematologic** — Hb/Hct. Patients with Hx of easy bruising or bleeding should have coagulation parameters evaluated (PT, PTT, platelet count, bleeding time).

**Laboratory** — Electrolytes; BUN; creatinine

**Premedication** — Anxiolytic (e.g., midazolam 1-2 mg iv) as needed.

## INTRAOPERATIVE

**Anesthetic technique:** GA is commonly used; however, either spinal or epidural anesthesia is appropriate for adequately hydrated patients who are undergoing simple hysterectomy through a Pfannenstiel incision, or vaginal hysterectomy. In the younger patient population, spinal anesthesia may be less desirable because of the increased incidence of post-dural puncture headache (PDPH) in using this technique. Patients with extensive cancer who undergo exploratory laparotomy with lymph node dissections may benefit from combined epidural/GA with decreased postop pulmonary complications and early ambulation. Some studies advocate the use of epidural anesthesia in order to decrease intraop blood loss.[1]

**General anesthesia:**

**Induction** — Standard induction (see Appendix).

**Maintenance** — Standard maintenance (see Appendix). Muscle relaxation is necessary if the procedure is performed abdominally. These patients have a high incidence of N&V, and prophylaxis with metoclopramide 10 mg iv or droperidol 1 mg iv is indicated.

**Emergence** — Be ready with suction in the event the patient vomits on emergence.

**Regional anesthesia:** A T6-8 sensory level is sufficient to provide anesthesia for procedures on the uterus.

**Spinal** — 5% lidocaine 75-100 mg; 0.75% bupivacaine 10-15 mg in 7.5% dextrose. (See Anesthetic Considerations for "Cesarean Section.")

**Epidural** — 1.5-2.0% lidocaine with epinephrine 5 μg/cc, 15-25 cc; supplement with 5-10 cc as needed. Supplemental iv sedation. (See Anesthetic Considerations for "Cesarean Section.")

| | | |
|---|---|---|
| **Blood and fluid requirements** | Possible heavy blood loss<br>IV: 16-18 ga x 2<br>Warm all fluids.<br>Heat, humidify gasses.<br>Autologous blood donation | Preop autologous blood transfusion may not be possible in patients who are already anemic. Blood and evaporative losses are usually greater in patients undergoing abdominal, rather than vaginal, hysterectomy. Patients having a Pfannenstiel incision should also have smaller fluid requirements than those having a larger midline incision. |

| | | |
|---|---|---|
| **Control of blood loss** | Vaginal hysterectomy:<br>Moderate blood loss - NS/LR @ 4-5 cc/kg/hr.<br><br>Abdominal hysterectomy:<br>Moderate-to-heavy blood loss<br>NS/LR @ 6-10 cc/kg/hr | In order to avoid blood transfusion, consider colloid infusion in patients who have a good cardiac function and can tolerate a low Hct. May need blood transfusion. |
| **Monitoring** | Vaginal hysterectomy:<br>Standard monitors (see Appendix).<br>± Foley catheter<br><br>Abdominal hysterectomy:<br>Standard monitors (see Appendix).<br>Foley catheter<br>± Arterial line<br>± CVP line | A Foley catheter may be helpful (to monitor fluid status) during vaginal hysterectomy if the procedure is expected to be longer than usual. During abdominal hysterectomy, a Foley catheter is useful, since this procedure is longer, involves more fluid shifts and may involve a significant blood loss. Intra-arterial and CVP monitoring are useful in patients undergoing large tumor resections and in whom large blood losses are anticipated. |
| **Positioning** | √and pad pressure points.<br>Shoulder abduction < 90° | The lithotomy position has several considerations for safety. (See previous section on D&C for details.) |
| **Complications** | Vaginal hysterectomy:<br>Cervical stimulation<br>Epinephrine/vasopressin injection<br>→ HTN on cardiac dysrhythmias<br><br>Abdominal hysterectomy:<br>Cervical stimulation<br>Epinephrine/vasopressin injection<br><br>Abdominal hysterectomy:<br>Blood loss | Vagal stimulation may occur when the surgeons grasp the cervix; subsequent bradycardia may ensue. This can be treated by cessation of the surgical stimulus and treatment with atropine if indicated. The surgeons may use epinephrine or vasopressin to decrease local bleeding. Either of these agents may cause HTN or cardiac dysrhythmias.[10] Hemorrhage is possible with large tumor resections, and must be treated with adequate fluid and blood replacement. Attention must be given to associated problems such as hypothermia, hypocalcemia and dilutional coagulopathy. |

**POSTOPERATIVE**

| | | |
|---|---|---|
| **Complications** | N&V<br>Anemia | Rx with metoclopramide 5-10 mg q 1-2 hrs |
| **Pain management** | Epidural opiates (see Appendix).<br>PCA (see Appendix). | If catheter to be used postop |
| **Tests** | Hct; CXR (if CVP catheter placed intraop) | To evaluate line placement and rule out pneumothorax. |

**References**


1. England GT, Randall HW, Graves WL: Impairment of tissue defenses by vasoconstrictors in vaginal hysterectomies. *Obstet Gynecol* 1983; 61(3):271-74.
2. Wingo PA, et al: The mortality risk associated with hysterectomy. *Am J Obstet Gynecol* 1984; 152(7):803-8.
3. *Hospital Mortality, PAS Hospitals, United States, 1972-1973.* Commission of Professional and Hospital Activities, Ann Arbor: 1975.
4. Dicker RC, Greenspan Jr, Strauss LT et al: Complications of abdominal and vaginal hysterectomy among women of reproductive age in the United States. The Collaborative Review of Sterilization. *Am J Obstet Gynecol* 1982; 144(7):841-48.
5. Kvist-Poulsen H, Borel J: Iatrogenic femoral neuropathy subsequent to abdominal hysterectomy: incidence and prevention. *Obstet Gynecol* 1982; 60(4):516-20.
6. Daly JW, Higgins KA: Injury to the ureter during gynecological surgical procedures. *Surg Gynecol Obstet* 1988; 167(1):19-22.
7. Georgy FM: Femoral neuropathy following abdominal hysterectomy. *Am J Obstet Gynecol* 1975; 123(8):819-22.
8. Thompson JD, Rock JA, eds: *TeLinde's Operative Gynecology*, 7th edition. JB Lippincott, Philadelphia: 1992, 663-738.
9. Modig, J: Regional anaesthesia and blood loss. *Acta Anaesthesiol Scand Suppl:1988, 89*; 44-8.
10. *Physician's Desk Reference*, 46th edition. Medical Economics Data, Inc, Montvale, NJ:1992.

# ANTERIOR AND POSTERIOR COLPORRHAPHY, ENTEROCELE REPAIR, VAGINAL SACROSPINOUS SUSPENSION

## SURGICAL CONSIDERATIONS

**Description:** Cystocele (Fig 8.2-6A) and rectocele (Fig 8.2-6B) are prolapses (relaxation) of the anterior and posterior vaginal wall, respectively. They occur 2° multiparity and congenital weakening of pelvic tissue. The term "pelvic relaxation syndrome" includes the often coexisting anatomical "relaxations" (e.g., enterocele [Fig 8.2-6C] and uterine prolapse). Cystoceles are often symptomatic due to bladder protrusion past the introitus during straining. Often this relaxation will allow the bladder neck to lose its important anatomical relationship to the urethra and the rest of the bladder. The result can be bothersome stress urinary incontinence for the patient (see "Operations for Stress Urinary Incontinence"). The rectocele is often experienced as a vaginal bulge during straining, and tends to cause severe constipation. Enteroceles herniation of the small bowel into the rectovaginal septum, is often experienced as pelvic pain. The goal of the colporrhaphy is to restore the original anatomy. Due to the frequent coexisting relaxations, a posterior colporrhaphy (vaginal repair), enterocele repair and vaginal hysterectomy are frequently performed at the same time.

In an **anterior colporrhaphy**, the patient is placed in a high dorsal lithotomy position with the perineum at the end of the operating table for surgical access. The bladder is emptied and a weighted speculum is inserted into the vagina. A **vaginal hysterectomy** is performed at this point, if indicated (see "Vaginal Hysterectomy"). The extent of the urethrocystocele is determined manually and the vaginal mucosa is grasped at its cephalic border with two clamps. From this point to the external urethral meatus, the mucosa is undermined with a vasoconstrictive solution (epinephrine 5-10 cc, 1:200,000), phenylephrine (1:200,000) or vasopressin (1-5 U/10 cc NS). This decreases blood loss significantly and helps to determine the depth of the vaginal mucosa. The mucosa is cut over this undermined area and, with the help of sharp and blunt dissection, the mucosa is dissected laterally from its underlying fascia. A series of fascial plication sutures are placed to reduce the cystourethrocele. The redundant mucosa is excised and the edges are reapproximated. A suprapubic catheter is most often inserted at the end to prevent bladder over-distention. If necessary, a **posterior colporrhaphy** may be performed. A small portion of perineum posterior to the introitus is removed initially. The vaginal mucosa over the rectocele is undermined with vasoconstrictor fluid prior to incision, followed by dissection of the overlying mucosa in a manner nearly identical to anterior colporrhaphy. One or several layers of stitches are placed to plicate the pararectal fascia, allowing for reduction of the rectocele. Sometimes, part of the levator ani muscle is included to provide better

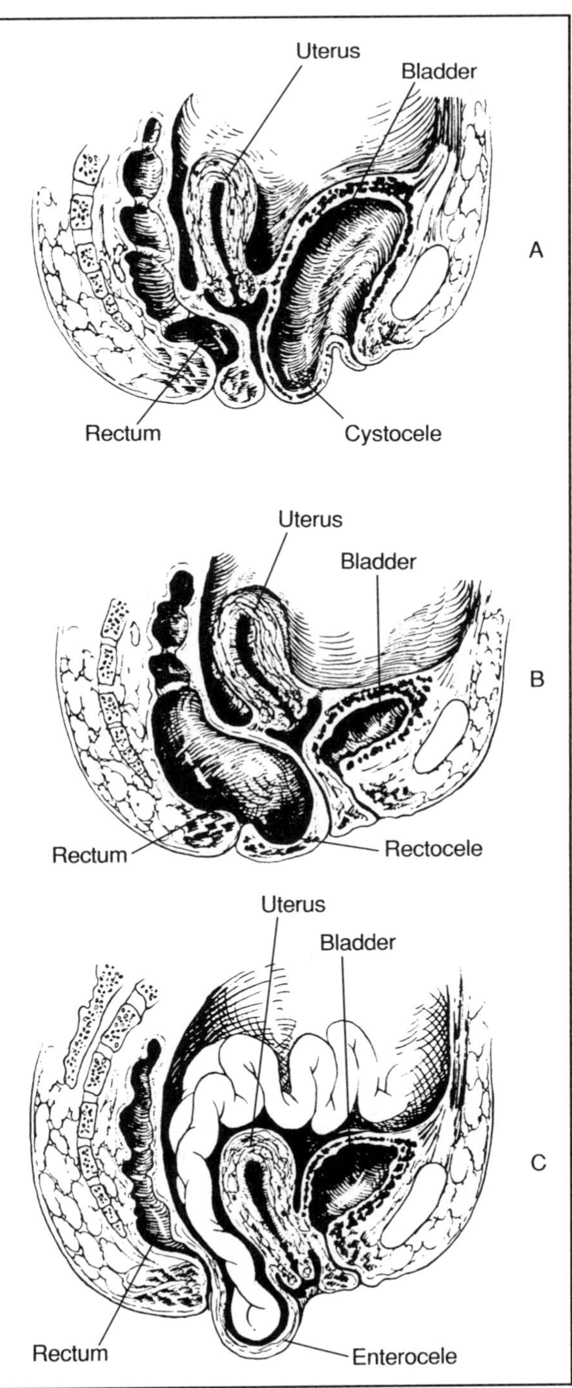


**Figure 8.2-6.** (A) Anatomy of cystocele. (B) Anatomy of rectocele. (C) Anatomy of enterocele. (Reproduced with permission from Pernoll ML, ed: *Current Obstetrics and Gynecological Diagnosis and Treatment.* Appleton & Lange: 1991.)

support. Redundant mucosa is excised and the edges reapproximated. A vaginal pack is usually placed in order to minimize bleeding.

An **enterocele** often is first noticed during a posterior colporrhaphy procedure, and is repaired prior to finishing the posterior repair. The enterocele is well-identified and dissected away from the surrounding tissue. Two or more parallel purse-string stitches are used to close the enterocele. The enterocele tissue distal to the purse-string closure is excised. In order to reduce the enterocele in an optimum fashion, intra-abdominal pressure has to be at a minimum.

**Variant procedure or approaches: Vaginal sacrospinous suspension** with the Miya hook is an elegant alternative to the abdominal colpopexy procedure for women with severe uterine and/or vaginal vault prolapse. The patient is placed in a dorsal lithotomy position and an examination under anesthesia is performed. A vasoconstrictive solution is injected (usually 1:200,000 epinephrine 3-5 cc) in the posterior vaginal wall. A vertical incision is made and the mucosa is bluntly dissected off the rectum in an anterolateral direction. An enterocele, if found, is repaired at this time. The pararectal tissue is then bluntly pierced to enter the pararectal space. The anatomy surrounding the sacrospinous ligament is well palpated and, with the help of the special Miya hook, a large suture is placed into the sacrospinous ligament. The other end of the suture is placed at the apex of the vagina which, after tying, is pulled in a lateral cephalad direction. The mucosa is finally closed.

The **Le Fort procedure** is now a rare operation and is performed in very old women with complete prolapse of the uterus and/or vagina who do not desire to remain sexually active. With the patient in a dorsal lithotomy position, a rectangular strip from the anterior and posterior vaginal wall is removed initially, followed by closure of the margins each to the other. The result is a near-complete closure of the vagina.

**Usual preop diagnosis:** Symptomatic cystocele or stress urinary incontinence; symptomatic uterine prolapse; enterocele; rectocele causing severe constipation; dyspareunia

## SUMMARY OF PROCEDURE

| | | |
|---|---|---|
| **Position** | Dorsal lithotomy | |
| **Incision** | Vaginal mucosal; peritoneum for enterocele repair | |
| **Unique considerations** | To prevent peroneal nerve injury, the area of the leg leaning against the stirrup should be well-cushioned. Putting the legs in a high position increases venous return to the heart. Infiltration with epinephrine and vasopressin are often used to reduce intraop bleeding. This causes changes in cardiac output, HR and BP. Low intra-abdominal pressure (good muscle relaxation) is needed during the enterocele reduction. A urethral catheter is not used intraop. | |
| **Antibiotics** | 1-2 gm iv cefoxitin/cefotetan | |
| **Surgical time** | 45 min (anterior colporrhaphy)<br>30 min (posterior colporrhaphy/enterocele repair) | |
| **Closing considerations** | Suprapubic catheter (anterior colporrhaphy); vaginal pack (enterocele repair) | |
| **EBL** | 20-500 cc | |
| **Postop care** | PACU | |
| **Mortality** | 1% | |
| **Morbidity** | Anterior colporrhaphy[1] | Vaginal sacrospinous suspension (Miya hook) |
| | Delayed voiding 1-7 d: 30%<br>Foul vaginal discharge: 14%<br>Bacteriuria: 13%<br>Pyrexia (>100.4F): 11%<br>Atelectasis: 3%<br>Delayed voiding > 7 d: 0.6%<br>Need for blood transfusion: 0.6%<br>Urethrovaginal fistula: 0.4%<br>Acute gastric dilatation: 0.2% | Bleeding in gluteal and pudendal vessels<br>Pararectal burning pain ≥ 2 mo<br>Sciatic pain (indicating misplaced sutures which must be removed)<br>Peritoneal tear (during Miya hook insertion) |
| **Procedure code** | 57282 (sacrospinous ligament fixation); 57260 (combined anteroposterior colporrhaphy); 57265 (combined anteroposterior colporrhaphy, with enterocele repair); 57268 (repair of enterocele, vaginal approach); 57240 (anterior colporrhaphy, repair of cystocele); 57250 (posterior colporrhaphy, repair of rectocele) | |
| **Pain score** | 5-8 | |

### PATIENT POPULATION CHARACTERISTICS

| | |
|---|---|
| **Age range** | 40-80 yrs |
| **Incidence** | >1/5 |
| **Etiology** | Multiparous state<br>Obesity<br>Chronic cough |
| **Associated conditions** | Pelvic relaxation syndrome |

## ANESTHETIC CONSIDERATIONS

See Anesthetic Considerations following "Operations for Stress Urinary Incontinence" (below).

**References**

1. Beck RP, et al: A 25-year experience with 519 anterior colporrhaphy procedures. *Obstet Gynecol* 1991; 78(6):1011-18.
2. Thompson JD, Rock JA, eds: *TeLinde's Operative Gynecology*, 7th edition. JB Lippincott, Philadelphia: 1992.
3. Miyazaki F: Miya hook ligature carrier for sacrospinous ligament suspension. *Obstet Gynecol* 1987; 70(2):286-88.
4. Pernoll ML, ed: *Current Obstetrics and Gynecological Diagnosis and Treatment.* Appleton & Lange, Norwalk, Ct: 1991, 830-50.
5. Corson S, Sedlacek T, Hoffman J: *Greenhill's Surgical Gynecology*, 5th edition. Year Book Medical Pub, Chicago: 1986.

# OPERATIONS FOR STRESS URINARY INCONTINENCE

## SURGICAL CONSIDERATIONS

**Description:** Stress urinary incontinence is a common condition affecting mostly older and multiparous women. It is a disorder of the musculofascial support to the bladder neck and pelvic floor. These patients usually have extensive preop workup to exclude urge incontinence and almost all have been treated with pelvic floor exercises (Kegel) and estrogen prior to surgery. Two surgical approaches exist: **abdominal suspension** procedures and **suspension by the vaginal route**. Ongoing controversy exists concerning which approach is best. Patient position is crucial for all vaginal surgery.

**Vaginal approaches:** The **Kelly urethral plication** is often the primary surgical treatment, especially when other vaginal surgery needs to be performed. The patient initially is placed in a high dorsal lithotomy position with the perineum at the end of the operating table for surgical exposure. The bladder is emptied and a weighted speculum is inserted into the vagina. The extent of the cystourethrocele is determined and the vaginal mucosa is grasped at its cephalic border with two clamps. From this point to the external urethral meatus, the mucosa is usually undermined with 5-10 cc of a vasoconstrictive solution (epinephrine 1:200,000), phenylephrine (1:200,000) or vasopressin (1-5 U/10 cc NS). This decreases blood loss significantly and helps to determine the depth of the mucosa. With the help of sharp and blunt dissection, the mucosa is freed laterally from its underlying adherent fascia. A series of vertical mattress sutures are placed in the mobilized paraurethral and paravesicle fascia in order to reduce the cystourethrocele and elevate the posterior urethra to a high retropubic position. The redundant mucosa is excised and the edges are reapproximated. A suprapubic catheter is often inserted at the end of the surgery to prevent bladder over-distention.

**Anterior vesicle neck suspension** (**Stamey** and **Pereyra**) are two very similar procedures wherein the vaginal mucosa is incised and dissected off the underlying paravesicle and paraurethral fascia much the same way as in the Kelly plication. Instead of using a layer of mattress sutures, both suspension methods use two lateral sutures that suspend the vesicle neck on each side (Fig 8.2-7A). The ends of the sutures are tied over the rectus fascia to provide support. The Stamey method uses a small Dacron® cuff to prevent the suture from tearing through the paravesicle fascia, while in the Pereyra method, the posterior loop is firmly attached to the pubourethral ligament. One or two small suprapubic abdominal incisions must be made to allow for the tying of the sutures. Specialized long needles are used to help the placement of these sutures, and a cystoscope is often used to verify their placement. Finally, a suprapubic catheter is placed at the end of the operation. (See Urology section.)

**Abdominal approaches:** The **Marshall-Marchetti-Krantz (M-M-K)** and **Burch** are probably the most common abdominal suspension procedures. The patient is placed in the frog-leg position with a urethral catheter in place. A Pfannenstiel incision is used to enter the space of Retzius, which lies between the parietal peritoneum and the rectus fascia under the pubic bone. Blunt dissection is used to open and extend this space. The surgeon then inserts two fingers into the vagina to raise the anterior vagina and bladder neck. This enables the surgeon to place two or more sutures in the tissue just lateral to the urethra and attach them to the pubic fibrocartilage or Cooper's ligament (Burch).

The **urethral sling procedure** is reserved for women with low urethral pressure and/or for whom other incontinence operations have failed. The goal of the sling procedure is to produce extrinsic compression of the urethrovesical junction with the help of a strip anchored to the rectus fascia (Fig 8.2-7B). With the patient in the dorsal lithotomy position, a urethral catheter is placed and the vaginal mucosa incised and dissected off the underlying paravesicle and paraurethral fascia similar to the Kelly plication. The retropubic space is entered through a Pfannenstiel incision and a strip of rectus fascia is obtained. The strip is then brought through the vagina, around the urethra and back to the abdomen, where it is fastened to the rectus fascia, creating a sling under the urethra at the junction of the bladder neck. The vaginal and abdominal incisions are closed, and a suprapubic catheter is place.

**Usual preop diagnosis:** Stress urinary incontinence

### SUMMARY OF PROCEDURE

| | Kelly Plication | M-M-K/Burch |
|---|---|---|
| **Position** | Dorsal lithotomy | Frog leg |
| **Incision** | Vaginal mucosa | Pfannenstiel |
| **Unique considerations** | Cushion area of leg against stirrup to prevent peroneal injury. Epinephrine (1:200,000) or vasopressin are often infiltrated to reduce intraop bleeding for vaginal approaches. This causes changes in cardiac output, bleeding, HR and rhythm. The urethral catheter is frequently removed and reinserted during surgery. | ⇐ |
| **Antibiotics** | Cefoxitin/cefotetan 1-2 gm iv | ⇐ |
| **Surgical time** | 1 hr | ⇐ |
| **Closing considerations** | Suprapubic catheter | ⇐ |
| **EBL** | 50 cc | 100-200 cc |
| **Postop care** | Inpatient | ⇐ |
| **Mortality** | Minimal | ⇐ |
| **Morbidity** | Prolonged catheter time: 54% | Rare |
| | Bladder perforation: 24% | Rare |
| | Outlet obstruction: 2% | Rare |
| | Urethral perforation: 2% | Rare |
| | Detrusor instability: Rare (due to vaginal approach) | 14% |
| | Enterocele: Rare | 4% |
| | Incisional hernia: Rare | 0.09% |
| | Osteitis pubis: Rare | 3.2% |
| | Uterine prolapse: Rare | 4% |
| | UTI: Rare | 10.4% |
| | Voiding difficulties: Rare | 2% |
| | Wound infection: Rare | 8.7% |
| **Procedure code** | 51845 (abdominovaginal vesical neck suspension, e.g. Stamey/Pereyra) | 51840 (urethropexy, e.g. M-M-K or Burch) |
| **Pain score** | 6-8 | 6-8 |

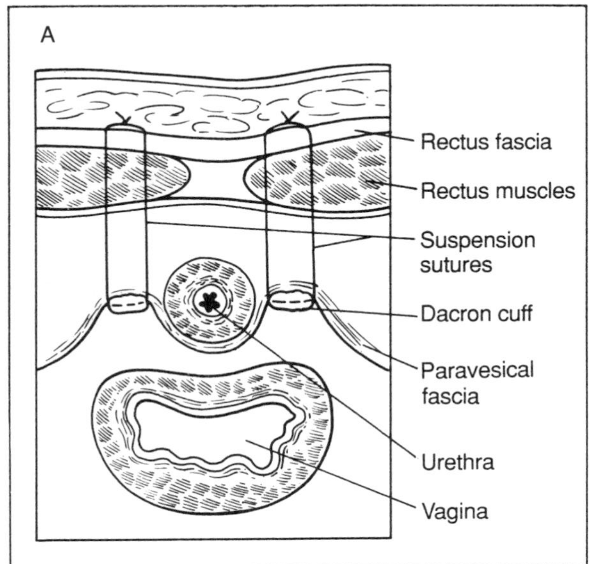


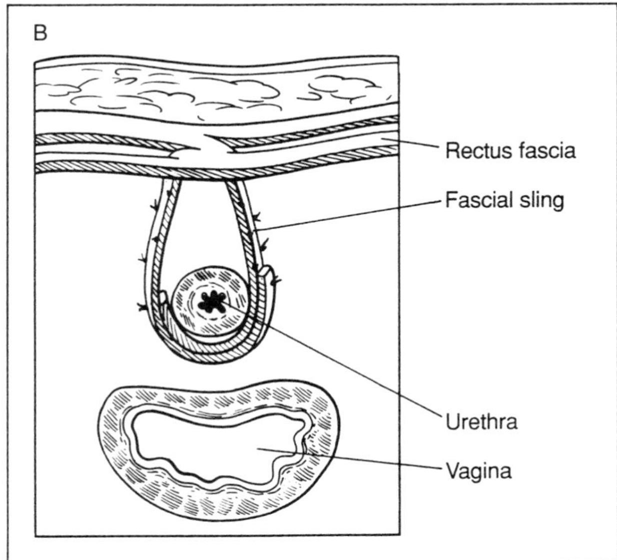


**Figure 8.2-7.** (A) Stamey procedure. (B) Urethral sling procedure. (Reproduced with permission from Varner RE, Sparks JM: Surgery for Stress Urinary Incontinence. *Surg Clin North Am* 1991; 71(5):1124, 1128.)

### PATIENT POPULATION CHARACTERISTICS

| | |
|---|---|
| **Age range** | 40-80 yrs |
| **Incidence** | >1/5 females |
| **Etiology** | Multiparous state<br>Obesity<br>Chronic cough |
| **Associated conditions** | Other components of pelvic relaxation syndrome (rectocele, uterine prolapse, enterocele) |

---

## ANESTHETIC CONSIDERATIONS

**(Procedures covered: anterior and posterior colporrhaphy; enterocele repair; vaginal sacrospinous suspension; operations for stress incontinence)**

### PREOPERATIVE

This is usually an older patient population, past child-bearing age. Patient may be relatively healthy otherwise. √ for concurrent disease.

| | |
|---|---|
| **Laboratory** | Hb/Hct, as indicated from H&P. |
| **Premedication** | Anxiolytic (e.g., midazolam 1-2 mg iv) as needed. |

### INTRAOPERATIVE

**Anesthetic technique:** Regional or GA may be used. In the younger patient population, spinal anesthesia may be less desirable because of increased incidence of post-dural puncture headache (PDPH).

**Regional anesthesia:** A T10 sensory level is sufficient to provide anesthesia for procedures on the uterus and bladder, but a T6 level is recommended if the peritoneum is opened.

| | |
|---|---|
| **Spinal** | 5% lidocaine 75-100 mg; 0.75% bupivacaine 10-15 mg in 7.5% dextrose. (See Anesthetic Considerations for "Cesarean Section.") |
| **Epidural** | 1.5-2.0% lidocaine with epinephrine 5 μg/cc, 15-25 cc; supplement with 5-10 cc as needed. Supplemental iv sedation. (See Anesthetic Considerations for "Cesarean Section.") |

**General anesthesia:**

| | | |
|---|---|---|
| **Induction** | Standard induction (see Appendix). | |
| **Maintenance** | Standard maintenance (see Appendix). | |
| **Emergence** | No special considerations | |
| **Blood and fluid requirements** | Normally minimal blood loss<br>IV: 16-18 ga x 1<br>NS/LR @ 2-4 cc/kg/hr | Only 1 iv is normally necessary for adequate intraop hydration. |
| **Control of blood loss** | Epinephrine, vasopressin, phenylephrine used by surgeons. | Surgeons may inject vasopressors into the submucosa to minimize blood loss. This may cause intraop and cardiac dysrhythmias.[1] |
| **Monitoring** | Standard monitors (see Appendix). | Although bladder catheterization prior to incision is normal, the catheter is not left in place throughout surgery in those patients undergoing anterior and posterior colporrhaphy, enterocele repair and Kelly urethral plication. Suprapubic bladder catheters are placed toward the end of surgery in these procedures, as well as in the Stamey, Pereyra and urethral sling procedures. |
| **Positioning** | √ and pad pressure points.<br>√ eyes. | See "D&C" for concerns regarding the lithotomy position. |

**POSTOPERATIVE**

| | | |
|---|---|---|
| **Complications** | N&V | Rx: metoclopramide 5-10 mg iv |
| **Pain management** | IV opiates<br>Usually rapid conversion to po pain medications. | |
| **Tests** | None indicated. | |

**References**

1. Stamey TA: Endoscopic suspension of the vesical neck for urinary incontinence in females. *Ann Surg* 1980; 192(4):465-71.
2. Pereyra AJ, et al: Pubourethral supports in perspective: modified Pereyra procedure for urinary incontinence. *Obstet Gynecol* 1982; 59(5):643-48.
3. Lee RA, et al: Surgical complications and results of modified Marshall-Marchetti-Krantz procedure for urinary incontinence. *Obstet Gynecol* 1979; 53(4):447-450.
4. Galloway NT, et al: The complications of colposuspension. *Br J Urol* 1987; 60(2):122-24.
5. Blaivas JG, et al: Pubovaginal fascial sling for the treatment of complicated stress urinary incontinence. *J Urol* 1991; 145(6):1214-18.
6. Thompson JD, Rock JA, eds: *TeLinde's Operative Gynecology*, 7th edition. JB Lippincott, Philadelphia: 1992, 887-941.
7. Varner RE, Sparks JM: Surgery for stress urinary incontinence. *Surg Clin North Am* 1991; 71(5):1111-34.
8. *Physician's Desk Reference*, 46th edition. Medical Economics Data, Inc, Montvale, NJ: 1992.

**Surgeons**

**Yasser El-Sayed, MD**
**Ronald N. Gibson, MD**
**Babak Edraki, MD**
**R. Harold Holbrook Jr, MD**

## 8.3 OBSTETRIC SURGERY

**Anesthesiologists**

**Sheila E. Cohen, MB, ChB, FRCA**
**Carter Cherry, MD**

# CESAREAN SECTION – LOWER SEGMENT AND CLASSICAL

## SURGICAL CONSIDERATIONS

**Description**: Cesarean section (C-section) is the delivery of the fetus through a horizontal or vertical incision into the **lower uterine segment**. The skin incision is made either as a Pfannenstiel (transverse in the crease above the pubis) or vertical midline from umbilicus to pubis. The peritoneal cavity is entered as in any laparotomy. A retractor is placed inferiorly and the reflection of visceral peritoneum from the bladder dome to the anterior lower segment of the uterus (bladder flap) is incised and displaced inferiorly, along with the bladder. The uterus is entered sharply and the incision extended with digital pressure and/or bandage scissors. The fetal head is elevated out of the pelvis and delivered through the uterine incision. In cases of non-vertex lie, the infant's breech is grasped and brought out of the incision. After the delivery of the fetus, the cord is double-clamped and cut, and cord blood is obtained for analysis. The placenta is removed manually and the uterine cavity cleared of all debris and clots. The uterine incision is closed with a running, interlocking stitch, followed by a 2nd imbricating layer. The bladder flap and parietal peritoneum do not require closure. Finally, the fascia is closed and the skin re-approximated with staples. **Classical C-section** usually involves a vertical skin incision and fundal vertical uterine incision (Fig 8.3-1). Patients with a history of prior classical C-section should be delivered abdominally via a repeat C-section, since the risk of uterine rupture with labor of vaginal delivery is 2%.

**Usual preop diagnosis**: Failure to progress in labor; elective repeat C-section; fetal distress

**SUMMARY OF PROCEDURE**

| | Lower-Segment C-Section | Classical C-Section |
|---|---|---|
| **Position** | Supine with left lateral tilt. (In obese patients, the pannus may be lifted superiorly by tape or towel clips.) | ⇐ |
| **Incision** | Skin: transverse low abdominal (Pfannenstiel) or repeat vertical. Uterus: transverse (Kerr) or low vertical (for premature infants or non-vertex lie) | Skin: Pfannenstiel or, more commonly, vertical midline. Uterus: vertical fundal |
| **Special instrumentation** | Bladder blade retractor; small ring forceps; bandage scissors; suction bulb; DeLee suction trap (if meconium) | ⇐ |
| **Unique considerations** | ✓ fetal heart tones before procedure. If for CPD: cervical exam within last 15 min before procedure. If for fetal distress: continuous monitoring until skin incision. | ⇐ |
| **Antibiotics** | If in labor or membranes ruptured: cefotetan 2 gm iv, immediately after cord clamping. | ⇐ |
| **Surgical time** | 20 - 90 min | 40 - 90 min |
| **Closing considerations** | Low transverse: closed in 2 layers. Low vertical: 2 layers; may require additional operative time for repair of incision if extension into cervix or fundus. | 3-layer closure requires additional time. |
| **EBL** | 750-1000 cc | 1000-2000 cc |
| **Postop care** | Observation for bleeding and hypotension | Special attention to vital signs needed due to additional blood loss. |
| **Mortality** | < 0.1% | ⇐ |
| **Morbidity** | Infection: | |
| | Not in labor: < 5% | ⇐ |
| | In labor/ruptured membranes: ≤ 50% (antibiotics reduce to 15%) | ⇐ |
| | Small bowel obstruction: Rare | ⇐ |
| **Procedure code** | 59515 | ⇐ |
| **Pain Score** | 4 | 7 |

### PATIENT POPULATION CHARACTERISTICS

**Age range** 14-40+ yrs

**Incidence**[1] 10-25%

**Etiology**[2] Failure to progress: 30%
Repeat C-section: 30%
Fetal anomaly/other: 20%
Abnormal presentation: 10%
Fetal distress: 10%

**Associated conditions** Pre-eclampsia/eclampsia
DIC
Hemolysis, elevated liver enzyme, low platelet count (HELLP) syndrome
Obstetrical hemorrhage/shock
Chorioamnionitis

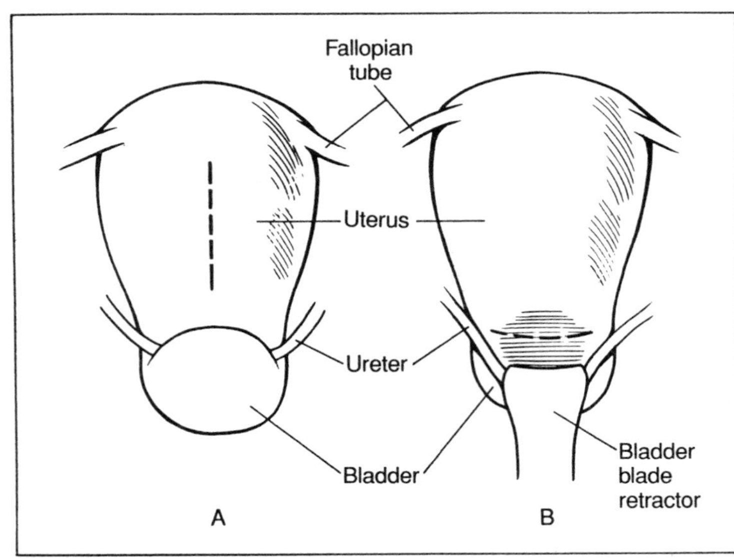


**Figure 8.3-1.** Typical cesarean section incisions. (A) Classic incision, in upper uterine segment. (B) Low transverse incision.

---

## ANESTHETIC CONSIDERATIONS

**(Procedures covered: cesarean section; emergent obstetrical hysterectomy; repair of uterine rupture)**

### PREOPERATIVE

In general, these patients are young and healthy, although the pregnant patient has undergone profound physiologic changes which affect the conduct of anesthesia. Patients present for emergency cesarean section (C-section) for fetal distress and hemorrhage (placenta previa, abruptio placenta and, rarely, uterine rupture).

**Respiratory** The pregnant patient frequently will have a compensated respiratory alkalosis ($PCO_2$=32-34). ↑minute ventilation (MV) (↑50%), and ↓FRC (↓20%). ↑$O_2$ consumption (↑20%) with ↓FRC results in rapid onset of hypoxemia if ventilation is compromised. Small airway closure due to elevation of diaphragm (exaggerated by obesity and supine position) can result in shunting and ↓$PaO_2$. ↑MV and ↓FRC enhance uptake of inhalational anesthetics. Mucosal capillary engorgement in upper airways may necessitate a smaller ETT and mandates careful airway suctioning to avoid bleeding.
**Tests:** As indicated from H&P.

**Cardiovascular** Typically, there is a ↓SVR (↓15%), ↓diastolic pressure and MAP (↓15%) with ↑HR (↑30%) and cardiac output (↑30%). To avoid aortocaval compression and hypotension, the supine position should be managed by the use of left lateral tilt. Immediately postpartum, 600-800 ml blood enters the central circulation, due to placental transfusion, with further increase in cardiac output.
**Tests:** As indicated from H&P.

**Hematologic** These patients have ↑blood volume (↑35%), ↑plasma volume (↑45%), ↑red cell mass (↑20%). WBC count increases to 15,000/$mm^3$. Iron deficiency anemia often is superimposed on the dilutional anemia of pregnancy (Hct 33%). The typical blood loss of 500-800 ml is usually well-tolerated. Excessive blood loss is possible with multiple gestation, previous C-section, PIH, placenta previa, abruptio placenta and uterine atony.
**Tests:** Hb/Hct

**Gastrointestinal** Abnormalities, including decreased gastric motility (after onset of labor), gastroesophageal reflux, raised intragastric pressure and gastric hyperacidity, predispose to aspiration pneumonitis. All parturients should be considered to have full stomachs and should receive clear antacid (e.g., 0.3 M Na citrate 30 cc) immediately prior to GA or regional anesthesia. Administer iv metoclopramide 10 mg and ranitidine 50 mg before emergent C-section. Before elective C-section, parturients at high risk for aspiration (e.g., planned or potential GA, difficult airway, or any patient with reflux esophagitis, or obesity) should receive an $H_2$-blocker (e.g., ranitidine 150 mg po) the night before and the morning of surgery.

**Hepatic** Liver enzymes can be mildly elevated and plasma protein concentration is diminished (increased unbound drug levels); however, liver function is usually normal.
**Tests:** As indicated from H&P.

**Renal** These patients have ↑renal blood flow (↑50%), glomerular filtration rate and creatinine clearance, and ↓serum creatinine and blood urea $N_2$. Dependent edema results from increased water and sodium retention 2° resetting of the osmotic threshold for thirst and vasopressin secretions.
**Tests:** As indicated from H&P.

**Laboratory** Type and screen maternal blood (cross-match unnecessary unless significant blood loss is anticipated). Routine autologous blood donation is not recommended. Coagulation studies, bleeding time and/or platelet count recommended with PIH, abruptio placenta, heavy maternal bleeding. BUN; creatinine; UA; fasting blood glucose; others as indicated from H&P.

**Premedication** Agents to decrease risk of aspiration pneumonitis have been discussed. Sedatives are not routinely administered. In extremely anxious patients, however, 0.5-1.0 mg midazolam iv is an excellent anxiolytic without apparent affect on maternal memory or alertness or neonatal condition.

## SPECIAL CONSIDERATIONS

**Pregnancy-induced hypertension (PIH)** PIH is characterized by generalized vasoconstriction with relative intravascular volume depletion and, occasionally, diffuse capillary leak. There is an increased risk of hypotension with regional anesthesia. Cautious hydration prior to regional anesthesia is necessary to prevent hypotension or pulmonary edema. Hepatic dysfunction may be present (HELLP syndrome: hemolysis, elevated liver enzymes, and low platelet count). Epidural anesthesia is preferred over spinal because of lower risk of hypotension. Cardiovascular stability is better with regional than GA, provided intravascular volume is adequate. Abnormal bleeding time (↓platelet count or dysfunctional platelets) contraindicates regional anesthesia. If GA is necessary, control BP with small doses of labetalol (10-20 mg iv over 3-5 min) or esmolol (0.5 mg/kg over 1 min) prior to induction to blunt hypertensive response to laryngoscopy. There is a potential for difficult intubation in PIH due to airway edema; therefore, a small ETT (6.0 mm) should be available. $MgSO_4$ potentiates neuromuscular blocking agents; avoid defasiculating dose of muscle relaxant prior to induction and use smaller than normal doses of non-depolarizing agents.
**Tests:** PT; PTT; platelets; bleeding time; LFTs

**Eclampsia** Treat eclamptic seizures with adequate oxygenation and a small dose of STP (50-100 mg) or diazepam (5 mg). Intubate if necessary to protect airway.

**Massive maternal hemorrhage: Placenta previa, Abruptio placenta, Ruptured uterus** Insert 2 large-bore iv catheters (14-16 ga). Assure immediate availability of cross-matched blood. Rapidly restore intravascular volume with crystalloid, colloid or both. Induction of GA with ketamine (1-1.5 mg/kg) is preferred in hypovolemic patients. DIC can follow abruptio placenta or amniotic fluid embolism. Dilutional thrombocytopenia following massive blood loss might require platelet transfusion. Uterine atony is treated with oxytocin 20-40 U/L (risk of hypotension with boluses); methylergonovine, 0.2 mg im (risk of HTN); or prostaglandin $F_2$-alpha, 0.25 mg im or intramyometrially (risk of pulmonary HTN, bronchospasm). Emergency hysterectomy following cesarean delivery may be the only solution to continued bleeding. Induction of GA may be necessary if massive bleeding occurs during regional anesthesia.

**Diabetes** Diabetic patients have an increased propensity to hypotension following regional anesthesia, with the fetus becoming more acidotic than normal as a result. Determine blood glucose hourly and maintain at 80-100 mg/dL. Insulin requirements decrease drastically after delivery, and insulin dosage must be reduced to prevent maternal hypoglycemia.
**Tests:** Fasting blood glucose; UA

**Response to anesthetic drugs** In pregnant patients, MAC is ↓ $\leq$ 40% for inhaled agents; combined with more rapid uptake, this predisposes to anesthetic overdose. Sensitivity to local anesthetics also increased. Epidural space capacity decreased, due to engorgement of epidural veins; this decreases requirements for local anesthetics and increases possibility of intravascular injection of drugs. Increased sensitivity to non-depolarizing muscle relaxants (especially in patients receiving $MgSO_4$) mandates careful monitoring and use of reduced doses. Decreased protein binding may increase toxicity of highly protein-bound drugs such as bupivacaine.

## INTRAOPERATIVE

**Anesthetic technique:** General considerations involve primarily the choice of anesthetic. Compared with regional anesthesia, the risks of aspiration and difficult intubation with GA significantly increase maternal morbidity and mortality.[3] Anesthetic choice in specific circumstances depends on maternal and fetal conditions and degree of urgency. Properly conducted GA or regional anesthesia probably are equally safe for the fetus.[4]

**Epidural or spinal anesthesia** are preferred for elective or semi-elective C-section when no contraindications to regional anesthesia exist (e.g., patient refusal, coagulopathy, active neurological disease, hypovolemia, sepsis). Spinal anesthesia is increasingly popular in obstetrics coincident with the use of pencil-point needles (e.g., Sprotte, Whitacre). Risk of headache with these needles is low (1-2%). Advantages of spinal over epidural anesthesia include: technical ease, more rapid onset of block, more solid anesthesia, and less shivering. Hypotension, however, is more common with spinal anesthesia. Vigorous fluid loading (e.g., 1000-2000 cc LR) is essential to minimize the risk of hypotension.

**General anesthesia** normally is used when regional anesthesia is contraindicated or when there is inadequate time to institute regional blockade. Obstetric emergencies for which rapid induction of GA may be indicated include: severe maternal hemorrhage, prolapsed umbilical cord, severe fetal bradycardia, severe persistent fetal decelerations, or the need for intrauterine manipulations. Less dire situations often permit the performance of a "quick spinal" or extension of a functioning epidural block with an agent having a rapid onset (e.g., 10-20 cc 3% 2-chloroprocaine). Continuous monitoring of the fetal heart rate (FHR) in the OR may allow use of regional anesthesia if the FHR tracing is reassuring. Constant communication with the obstetrician regarding maternal and fetal condition is essential. Although situations exist in which a GA is preferable to regional, the risks must be weighed against the benefits for patients with greater potential for complications. If difficult intubation is anticipated, rapid-sequence induction of GA should not be undertaken. Alternative approaches include awake intubation, spinal anesthesia or local infiltrations by the obstetrician. Sometimes, a non-reassuring FHR pattern is diagnosed as "fetal distress" and the patient is delivered immediately. Fetal distress is an imprecise and nonspecific term with little positive predictive value. The severity of any FHR abnormality should be considered when the urgency of delivery and type of anesthesia are determined. C-section performed for a non-reassuring FHR pattern does not necessarily preclude the use of regional anesthesia.[4]

**Regional anesthesia:**

**Epidural**

Apply monitors, fluid load and place the patient in the sitting or lateral decubitus position. A 3 ml test dose of 1.5% lidocaine (45 mg) with 1:200,000 epinephrine (15 $\mu$g) is given through the epidural needle or catheter to exclude intravascular injection (symptoms: dizziness, tinnitus, new taste in mouth) or subarachnoid placement (motor/sensory block in lower extremities). After 3-5 min, inject 15-20 cc 2% (300-400 mg) lidocaine with 1:200,000 epinephrine (75-100 $\mu$g) incrementally over 5 min. Sodium bicarbonate, 1 mEq/10 cc lidocaine, hastens onset of block, but increases risk of hypotension. Bupivacaine 0.5%, 15-20 ml (75-100 mg), with or without epinephrine 1:200,000 and bicarbonate 0.05 mEq/20 ml, or 3% 2-chloroprocaine, 15-20 ml (450-600 mg) also can be used. To ensure a T4 level of anesthesia throughout surgery, additional local anesthetic is often needed. If a functioning epidural catheter is in place and an urgent C-section becomes necessary, 15-20 ml 3% 2-chloroprocaine (450-600 mg) should produce adequate surgical anesthesia within 5-10 min.

Administer $O_2$ by mask or nasal cannula and check FHR prior to abdominal prep. Monitor BP every min until stable, then every 3-5 min. Treat ↓20% in BP or SBP < 95-100 mmHg with further uterine displacement, additional fluids, and ephedrine 5-10 mg iv. For inadequate anesthesia, give additional epidural local anesthetic, 50 $\mu$g fentanyl iv or epidurally, 50% $N_2O/O_2$, ketamine 5-10 mg iv, or infiltrate with local anesthetic. The patient must remain conscious to avoid risk of aspiration. If anesthesia is still inadequate, induce GA (see below).

After delivery of infant and placenta, rapidly infuse oxytocin 20-30 U/L. Antibiotics given at surgeon's request. Observe for excessive blood loss. Chest pain, mild oxyhemoglobin desaturation and SOB after delivery may be due to irritation of diaphragm by blood or packs, too high or inadequate level of anesthesia, or venous air or amniotic fluid embolization. S-T segment changes on ECG occur, but do not usually signify myocardial ischemia.[5]

**Spinal**

Apply monitors, administer fluid, and position as for epidural anesthesia. Metoclopramide 10 mg iv, 5-10 min prior to block decreases intraop N&V. Insert 24-25 ga pencil-point needle (or small diamond-tip needle) and verify free flow of CSF. In urgent situations, a larger pencil-point needle (e.g., 22 ga Sprotte) is easier and faster to place with minimal increase in headache.[6] Inject hyperbaric 0.75% spinal bupivacaine, 11.25-12.0 mg (1.5-1.6 ml), and position the patient with left uterine displacement. Prophylactic ephedrine, 5-10 mg iv, at time of spinal injection decreases the incidence of hypotension. Monitor and treat BP as for epidural. Adjust operating table position to insure a T4 level of anesthesia. If anesthesia is inadequate and time permits, consider repeating spinal block or placement of an epidural catheter. Treat persistent inadequate anesthesia as for epidural. Induce GA if other measures fail.

**General anesthesia:**

**Induction** Tilt table or use left hip displacement and administer 500-1000 ml dextrose-free crystalloid prior to induction. Preoxygenation for 3 min is optimal; however, 4 maximal inspiratory breaths in 30 sec is a satisfactory substitute in an emergency. Place patient in maximal "sniff" position with elevation of shoulders, if necessary, to optimize position for intubation. After patient is prepped and draped, and obstetric team is ready to begin, perform rapid-sequence induction with cricoid pressure. Administer thiopental, 3-5 mg/kg (or ketamine, 1-1.5 mg/kg, in hypovolemic patients) and succinylcholine 1 mg/kg to induce GA and facilitate intubation. Inflate cuff of ETT and verify tracheal placement by $ETCO_2$ waveform and auscultation of bilateral breath sounds.

**Failed intubation**[7] If tracheal intubation is unsuccessful, monitor $O_2$ saturation and mask ventilate, maintaining cricoid pressure. Summon experienced help and quickly decide whether surgery must proceed. The risks of continuing with mask GA and cricoid pressure must be weighed against the risk of allowing the mother to awaken. If ventilation is impossible, attempt emergency transtracheal ventilation using a 12-14-ga iv catheter and appropriate tubing to connect to a high-pressure $O_2$ source (e.g., $O_2$ flush valve on anesthesia machine); or an emergency cricothyrotomy or tracheostomy should be performed by experienced personnel. **Planning for a failed intubation must occur before it actually happens.** A difficult intubation tray, including equipment for emergency jet ventilation, must be immediately accessible in the delivery room.

**Maintenance** 50% $N_2O/O_2$ with 0.7-1.0% isoflurane or enflurane, or 0.5% halothane. Control ventilation, avoiding extreme hypocapnia ($PCO_2$ 30 mmHg) which decreases umbilical blood flow. After delivery, substitute an opioid (e.g., fentanyl 50-100 $\mu$g) for volatile agent and increase concentration of $N_2O$ to 70%. Administer small doses of muscle relaxants (e.g., vecuronium 1-2 mg) as needed. Reverse with neostigmine 0.05 mg/kg and glycopyrrolate 0.01 mg/kg or atropine 0.02 mg/kg. Maternal awareness occasionally occurs with this anesthetic technique.

**Emergence** Delay extubation until patient is fully awake and muscle strength has returned to normal.

| | | |
|---|---|---|
| **Blood and fluid requirements** | Moderate blood loss<br>IV: 16-18 ga x 1<br>NS/LR 1-3 L typical replacement | Infuse 1-2 L dextrose-free crystalloid immediately prior to regional anesthesia. Typical blood loss = 500-800 cc. |
| **Monitoring** | Standard monitors (see Appendix).<br>FHR monitor<br>± CVP or PA catheter | Arterial BP monitoring via automated BP device or arterial line for severe or labile HTN. CVP or PA catheter useful in oliguric patients unresponsive to fluid challenges. PA catheter indicated for pulmonary edema. |
| **Positioning** | Left uterine displacement (blanket under right hip and/or table tilt) | Minimizes aortocaval compression. |
| **Complications** | Amniotic fluid embolism | Rare cause of hemodynamic instability, hypoxemia and DIC. Usually fatal. Rx: supportive – 100% $O_2$, PEEP and vasopressors. |

## POSTOPERATIVE

| | | |
|---|---|---|
| **Complications** | PE | DX: pleuritic chest pain, hypoxemia, ↑RR, ↑HR, ↑A-a gradient. Rx: supportive – 100% $O_2$, volume expansion and vasopressors. |
| | Postpartum hemorrhage | See Anesthetic Considerations for "Removal of Retained Placenta." |
| **Pain management** | **Epidural:** 3-5 mg preservative-free morphine in 10 cc after delivery.<br>**Intrathecal:** morphine 0.1-0.25 mg given with spinal local anesthetic. Chloroprocaine interferes with analgesia from epidural opioids. | Common side effects include: pruritus 70%, nausea 30-40% and respiratory depression. Nalbuphine (2.5-5.0 mg) and naloxone (0.2-0.4 mg) are used for reversal of these side effects. |

| | | |
|---|---|---|
| | **Parenteral opioids:** iv or im opioids or PCA instituted in recovery room. | Risk of delayed respiratory depression in healthy patients is small; however, adequately trained nursing staff and a protocol for treatment of complications are mandatory if intraspinal opioids are used. These patients should not routinely receive sedatives or other systemic opioids for 12 hrs, and close monitoring of RR and level of consciousness is necessary. Pulse oximetry is recommended in high-risk patients. |
| **Tests** | None indicated routinely. | |


**References**

1. Placek PJ, Taffel SM: Trends in cesarean section rates for the United States, 1970–78. *Public Health Rep* 1980; 95(6):540-48.
2. O'Driscoll K, Foley M: Correlation of decrease in perinatal mortality and increase in cesarian section rates. *Obstet Gynecol* 1983; 61(1):1-5.
3. Chadwick HS, Posner K, Caplan RA, Ward RJ, Cheney FW: A comparison of obstetric and nonobstetric anesthesia malpractice claims. *Anesthesiology* 1991; 74(2):242-49.
4. Marx GF, Luykx WM, Cohen S: Fetal-neonatal status following caesarean section for fetal distress. *Br J Anaesth* 1984; 56(9):1009-13.
5. McLintic AJ, Pringle SD, Lilley S, Houston AB, Thorburn J: Electrocardiographic changes during cesarean section under regional anesthesia. *Anesth Analg* 1992; 74(1):51-6.
6. Leeman MI, Sears DH, O'Donnell LA, Reisner LS, Jassy LJ, Harmon TW, O'Donnell RH, Kelleher JF, Santos GC: The incidence of postdural puncture headache in obstetrical patients comparing the 24-gauge and 22-gauge Sprotte needles. *Anesthesiology* 1991; 75:A853.
7. Benumof JL: Management of the difficult adult airway: With special emphasis on awake tracheal intubation. *Anesthesiology* 1991; 75(6):1087-1110.


# EMERGENT OBSTETRICAL HYSTERECTOMY

## SURGICAL CONSIDERATIONS

**Description**: The most common indications for emergency obstetrical hysterectomy are rupture of the gravid uterus and intractable postpartum bleeding. Causes of uterine rupture include breakdown of a previous uterine scar, obstructed labor or trauma. Causes of intractable postpartum bleeding include uterine rupture after a vaginal delivery, placenta accreta or previa, and postpartum uterine atony non-responsive to other interventions, either medical (oxytocin, methylergonovine, prostaglandins) or surgical (ligation of uterine or internal iliac arteries). The emergent nature of these conditions requires rapid intervention by the anesthesiologist, including iv fluid resuscitation, as well as blood and blood product administration, if necessary. The patient's oxygenation and coagulation parameters must be monitored closely, given the risk of hypoxia and DIC 2° massive blood loss; and prompt transfer to a well-equipped OR should be undertaken.

The technique for an emergent obstetrical hysterectomy is largely similar to a hysterectomy for other indications. Of note is the engorged and prominent nature of the vessels supplying the gravid uterus. The edematous tissues surrounding the uterus are very friable and may bleed profusely if improperly manipulated. A **supracervical** or **total hysterectomy** may be performed. Through a midline or Pfannenstiel incision, the uterus is elevated out of the abdominal cavity. The round ligaments are clamped, transected and ligated; and the anterior leaf of the broad ligament is incised bilaterally from the transected round ligaments to the vesicouterine reflection. The posterior leaf of the broad ligament adjacent to the uterus is entered at a level just below that of the fallopian tubes and utero-ovarian ligaments. These are then clamped, transected and ligated. Next, incision of the posterior leaf of the broad ligament toward the cardinal ligaments is performed. With gentle blunt dissection, the bladder and attached vesicouterine peritoneal flap are dissected off the lower uterine segment. The ascending uterine arteries and veins are identified bilaterally, then clamped, transected and ligated. If a subtotal hysterectomy is planned, the body of the uterus is amputated at this level, and the cervical stump is closed with interrupted sutures. If a total hysterectomy is planned, dissection of the bladder off the cervix is continued until the cervicovaginal margin is identified. The cardinal and uterosacral ligaments are clamped, transected and ligated, with clamps placed as close to the cervix as possible without including cervical tissue. Once the level of the lateral vaginal fornix is reached, a clamp is swung below the cervix, across the lateral vaginal fornix. The cervix is then amputated off the vaginal cuff. Throughout the procedure, it is vital to clamp and ligate any bleeding vessels, and to take extra care to avoid damage to the ureter or bladder. Following removal of the uterus and cervix, the vaginal cuff angles are sutured to the ipsilateral cardinal ligament stumps, and the vaginal cuff is closed with a running locked stitch. The abdominal wall is closed in layers.

**Usual preop diagnosis**: Rupture of gravid uterus; intractable postpartum bleeding

### SUMMARY OF PROCEDURE

| | |
|---|---|
| **Position** | Supine, with left lateral tilt |
| **Incision** | Pfannenstiel or midline longitudinal |
| **Unique considerations** | Monitoring of coagulation parameters and correction of DIC. Consider central venous hemodynamic monitoring. Pediatrics team present, if indicated. |
| **Antibiotics** | Cefotetan 2 gm iv q 12 hrs; total 3 doses |
| **Surgical time** | 2 - 3 hrs |
| **Closing considerations** | Subcutaneous intraperitoneal drains, if indicated. |
| **EBL** | 3000-4000 cc |
| **Postop care** | ICU if blood loss severe; patient may require continued intubation and mechanical ventilatory support. Monitor for infectious morbidity and acute renal failure. |
| **Mortality** | < 1% |
| **Morbidity** | Hemorrhage<br>Postop febrile morbidity<br>DIC<br>Wound infection<br>Sheehan's syndrome<br>Bladder injury<br>Intraperitoneal bleeding requiring re-operation<br>Vesicovaginal fistula<br>Ureterovaginal fistula<br>Post-transfusion infectious morbidity |
| **Procedure code** | 59525 |
| **Pain score** | 7 |

### PATIENT POPULATION CHARACTERISTICS

| | |
|---|---|
| **Age range** | Reproductive age |
| **Incidence** | 0.11% of obstetric patients |
| **Etiology** | Unknown |
| **Associated conditions** | Placenta accreta<br>Uterine atony non-responsive to medical or other surgical intervention<br>Extension of cervical tear to lower uterine segment<br>Placenta previa<br>Uterine rupture<br>Uterine inversion |

## ANESTHETIC CONSIDERATIONS

See Anesthetic Considerations following "Cesarean Section" (above).

**References**


1. Cunningham FG, MacDonald PC, Gant NF, eds: *Williams Obstetrics*, 18th edition. Appleton & Lange, Norwalk CT: 1989, 453-55.
2. Creasy RK, Resnik R, eds: *Maternal-Fetal Medicine: Principles and Practice*, 2nd edition. WB Saunders, Philadelphia: 1989, 864-66.
3. Plauche WC: Peripartum hysterectomy. *Obstet Gynecol Clin North Am* 1988; 15(4):783-95.
4. Chestnut DH, Dewan DM, Redick LF, Caton D, Spielman FJ: Anesthetic management for obstetric hysterectomy: a multi-institutional study. *Anesthesiology* 1989; 70(4):607-10.
5. Suchartwatnachai C, Linasmita V, Chaturachinda K: Obstetric hysterectomy: Ramathibodi's experience 1969-87. *Int J Gynaecol Obstet* 1991; 36(3):183-86.
6. Al-Sibai MH, Rahman J, Rahman MS, Butalack F: Emergency hysterectomy in obstetrics – a review of 117 cases. *Aust NZ J Obstet Gynaecol* 1987; 27(3):180-84.
7. Chestnut DH, Eden RD, Gall SA, Parker RT: Peripartum hysterectomy: a review of cesarean and postpartum hysterectomy. *Obstet Gynecol* 1985; 65(3):365-70.
8. Clark SL, Yeh SY, Phelan JP, Bruce S, Paul RH: Emergency hysterectomy for obstetric hemorrhage. *Obstet Gynecol* 1984; 64(3):376-80.
9. Plauche WC, Wychek JS, Iannessa M, Rousset KM, Mickal A: Cesarean hysterectomy at Louisiana State University (Service of Charity Hospital), 1975 through 1981. *South Med J* 1983; 76(10):1261-63.
10. Schneider GT, Tyrone CH: Cesarean total hysterectomy: experience with 160 cases. *South Med J* 1966; 59(8):927-29.


# REPAIR OF UTERINE RUPTURE

## SURGICAL CONSIDERATIONS

**Description:** Rupture of the gravid uterus is considered a true obstetric emergency and can be catastrophic, with significant maternal and fetal mortality. The classic symptoms are "shearing" pain, cessation of uterine contractions, loss of fetal heart tones and the onset of vaginal bleeding. Unfortunately, these warning symptoms occur only in a minority of uterine rupture cases. Extrusion of the placenta through the uterine rupture may result in late decelerations due to uteroplacental insufficiency. Extrusion of the umbilical cord may be manifested by recurrent variable decelerations. Suprapubic pain as the only symptom has not been associated with uterine rupture. In cases where the uterine rupture occurs at the site of a prior uterine scar, the clinical course is usually less severe and the blood loss less than in cases of primary rupture of an intact uterus. The incidence of uterine rupture at the site of the old scar is 0.5% for lower-uterine transverse cesarean sections, and 2% for classic cesarean sections. Uterine rupture mimics abruptio placenta in its presentations; however, once the diagnosis is made, prompt surgical intervention is mandated. **Total abdominal hysterectomy** (see previous section), or **supracervical hysterectomy**, is the definitive therapy; however, depending on the clinical situation and patient's wishes for future fertility, a **uterine repair** may be undertaken. This consists of a 2-3-layered closure of the defect, using synthetic absorbable sutures. A transverse abdominal incision is made approximately 3 cm above the symphysis pubis and carried to the anterior rectus fascia. The fascia is incised and the muscles of the anterior abdominal wall separated from the midline sharply and bluntly. The peritoneum is elevated and entered sharply. Because of the emergent nature of this condition and the possible massive blood loss associated with rupture of a gravid uterus, the anesthesiologist must act quickly. Prompt, aggressive $O_2$ administration, together with iv fluid resuscitation, is indicated. Serious consideration should be given to the use of unmatched O-negative blood until cross-matched blood becomes available. Intraop hypogastric-artery ligation may help minimize blood loss. Patient's coagulation parameters must be monitored, since hypoxia and massive blood loss are associated with DIC.

**Usual preop diagnosis:** Uterine rupture

### SUMMARY OF PROCEDURE

| | |
|---|---|
| **Position** | Supine with left-lateral tilt |
| **Incision** | Pfannenstiel (low, transverse abdominal) or midline longitudinal |
| **Unique considerations** | Pediatrics team present for infant resuscitation, if necessary. Thorough surgical exploration of the urinary tract (bladder and ureters) since ~10% of cases are associated with bladder lacerations. Cell saver may be helpful. |

| | |
|---|---|
| **Antibiotics** | Cefotetan 2 gm iv q 12 hrs x 3 doses |
| **Surgical time** | 1 - 2 hrs |
| **EBL** | 500-3000 cc |
| **Postop care** | ICU if blood loss severe; continued intubation and mechanical ventilatory support if aggressive fluid resuscitation results in pulmonary edema. Acute renal failure may occur 2° hypoxic and hypovolemic renal injury at time of acute uterine rupture with massive bleeding; monitor UO and serial renal function tests. |
| **Mortality** | Fetal: 35-45%<br>Maternal: 5% |
| **Morbidity** | Blood transfusion >5 U: 58.3%<br>Postop wound infection: 33%<br>Pelvic abscess: 8.3%<br>Repeat uterine rupture with subsequent pregnancies: 5% |
| **Procedure code** | 59350 |
| **Pain score** | 6 |

### PATIENT POPULATION CHARACTERISTICS

| | |
|---|---|
| **Age range** | Reproductive age |
| **Incidence** | 1/1400 deliveries |
| **Etiology** | Prior uterine surgery<br>Grand multiparity<br>Obesity<br>Manual removal of placenta<br>Injury from tools of abortion<br>Direct or indirect violence<br>Oxytocin use<br>Intra-amniotic or vaginal prostaglandins<br>Breech extractions<br>Internal or external version<br>Forceps rotation<br>Shoulder dystocia<br>Fundal pressure<br>Neglect (cephalopelvic disproportion, etc.)<br>Congenital uterine anomaly<br>Cornual pregnancy<br>Gestational trophoblastic neoplasia<br>Placenta percreta<br>Abruptio placenta |

## ANESTHETIC CONSIDERATIONS

See Anesthetic Considerations following "Cesarean Section" (above).

**References**


1. Chazotte C, Cohen WR: Catastrophic complications of previous cesarean section. *Am J Obstet Gynecol* 1990; 163(3):738-42.
2. Plauche WC, VonAlmen W, Muller R: Catastrophic uterine rupture. *Obstet Gynecol* 1984; 64(6):792-97.
3. Eden RD, Parker RT, Gall SA: Rupture of the pregnant uterus: a 53-year review. *Obstet Gynecol* 1986; 68(5):671-74.
4. Akasheh F: Rupture of the uterus. Analysis of 104 cases of rupture. *Am J Obstet Gynecol* 1968; 101(3):406-8.
5. Yussman MA, Haynes DM: Rupture of the gravid uterus. A 12-year study. *Obstet Gynecol* 1970; 36(1):115-20.
6. Golan A, Sandbank O, Rubin A: Rupture of the pregnant uterus. *Obstet Gynecol* 1980; 56(5):549-54.
7. Reyes-Ceja L, Cabrera R, Insfran E, Herrera-Lasso F: Pregnancy following previous uterine rupture. Study of 19 patients. *Obstet Gynecol* 1969; 34(3):387-89.
8. Claman P, Carpenter RJ, Reiter A: Uterine rupture with the use of vaginal prostaglandin $E_2$ for induction of labor. *Am J Obstet Gynecol* 1984; 150(7):889-90.
9. Sawyer MM, Lipshitz J, Anderson GD, Dilts PV Jr: Third-trimester uterine rupture associated with vaginal prostaglandin $E_2$. *Am J Obstet Gynecol* 1981; 140(6):710-11.-9

# POSTPARTUM TUBAL LIGATION

## SURGICAL CONSIDERATIONS

**Description**: Postpartum tubal ligation (PPTL) is female surgical sterilization performed at the time of cesarean section (C-section) after delivery of the infant and repair of the uterine incision or within the first several days after a vaginal delivery. Although PPTL can be performed immediately postpartum, problems in the neonate may not be immediately evident and a delay in surgery may be appropriate. If performed after a vaginal delivery, a small infraumbilical incision is made in the skin and carried down through the parietal peritoneum. The fallopian tubes are identified, grasped with a Babcock clamp and brought out of the incision. It is important to identify the fimbriated end to insure the structure being ligated is the fallopian tube and not the round ligament. A midsegment portion of the tube over an avascular portion of mesosalpinx is selected and tubal patency is disrupted by a variety of methods (**Pomeroy, Parkland, Irving, Uchida,** etc.). The Pomeroy, or a modification of it, is the most common technique used. The segment of tube grasped is ligated with absorbable suture and the knuckle of tube formed is excised. The cut ends of the tubes should be hemostatic before replacing the tubes into the abdomen. The wound is closed in layers in the usual fashion.

**Usual preop diagnosis:** Patient desires permanent sterilization.

### SUMMARY OF PROCEDURE

| | |
|---|---|
| **Position** | Supine; steep Trendelenburg often required to allow bowel to fall away for exposure. |
| **Incision** | Infraumbilical |
| **Special instrumentation** | Small Richardson and Army/Navy retractors; Babcock clamp; vein retractor |
| **Unique considerations** | A sterilization consent form must be in the chart and signed by the patient by the required date. The procedure must be considered permanent even though reversal may be possible. The newborn should be healthy and stable before proceeding. The bladder should be drained prior to the procedure. |
| **Antibiotics** | None recommended. |
| **Surgical time** | 15 - 25 min |
| **EBL** | 10 cc |
| **Postop care** | Routine postpartum care after recovery from anesthesia |
| **Mortality** | 3/100,000 |
| **Morbidity** | Hemorrhage<br>Infection<br>Incidental damage to bowel or bladder |
| **Procedure code** | 58605 (after vaginal delivery); 59611 (with C-section) |
| **Pain score** | 3 |

### PATIENT POPULATION CHARACTERISTICS

| | |
|---|---|
| **Age range** | Reproductive age |
| **Incidence** | The most common contraceptive procedure in the U.S. |

## ANESTHETIC CONSIDERATIONS

### PREOPERATIVE

Optimal timing of tubal ligation is controversial. The patient with a functioning epidural catheter may benefit from having surgery immediately after delivery. Many surgeons, however, favor waiting 8-24 hrs, when adequate assessment of the neonate should be complete and risk of maternal hemorrhage lessened. Alternatively, the epidural catheter can be left in place and re-injected later. Because aspiration remains a risk, initiation of GA or spinal anesthesia often is delayed 8-24 hrs until the acute GI changes of pregnancy have regressed. There is no benefit to delaying surgery beyond this time.

| | |
|---|---|
| **Respiratory** | FRC returns to normal almost immediately after delivery.<br>**Tests:** As indicated from H&P. |

**Cardiovascular** The physiologic changes of pregnancy return to normal at varying intervals after delivery. For example, risk of aortocaval compression disappears immediately. Blood volume returns to pre-pregnant values over several days. Postpartum hemorrhage can occur without warning.
**Tests:** As indicated from H&P.

**Gastrointestinal** Postpartum patients continue to be at risk for acid aspiration, although it is not known exactly when normal GI function returns. Precautions for prevention of acid aspiration should be followed as discussed in "Cesarean Section."

**Neurological** Local anesthetic requirements for spinal anesthesia remain decreased after delivery.[4]

**Laboratory** Hct; other tests as indicated from H&P.

**Premedication** Precautions should be taken to decrease risk of aspiration pneumonitis, as discussed under "Cesarean Section."

## INTRAOPERATIVE

**Anesthetic technique:** Spinal anesthesia is preferred if a functioning epidural catheter is not in place. Epidural catheters frequently become dislodged after patient becomes ambulatory. GA is acceptable if patient has a strong preference or if contraindications to regional anesthesia exist. These patients may be at risk for aspiration of gastric contents at least 8-24 hrs post-delivery.

**Regional anesthesia:**

**Spinal** For technique and monitoring for spinal anesthesia, see "Cesarean Section," above. Hyperbaric 5% lidocaine, 70-80 mg, with 10 μg fentanyl if more prolonged analgesia desired.[5] With the patient supine, adjust position of the operating table to obtain a T6 level of anesthesia. Most procedures for PPTL last 30-40 min, but some (e.g., Uchida, Irving) may last about 1 hr. If more prolonged surgery is likely (e.g., obese patient, or patient with adhesions) bupivacaine (10-12 mg) may be preferable. Sedate patient as necessary with small doses of iv midazolam 0.5-1.0 mg, or opioid.

**Epidural** A 3 ml epidural test dose, followed after 3-5 min by 15-20 cc 3% 2-chloroprocaine or 1.5-2% lidocaine with 1:200,000 epinephrine injected incrementally. Additional local anesthetic as needed to ensure adequate level of anesthesia.

**General anesthesia:**

**Induction** Rapid-sequence induction with thiopental (3-5 mg/kg) and succinylcholine (1 mg/kg) for ET intubation.

**Maintenance** Standard maintenance (see Appendix).

**Emergence** Extubation should be delayed until patient is fully awake and protective airway reflexes have returned.

**Blood and fluid requirements** Minimal blood loss
IV: 16-18 ga x 1
NS/LR @ 2-4 cc/kg/hr

1-1.5 L dextrose-free crystalloid immediately prior to regional anesthesia

**Monitoring** Standard monitors (see Appendix).

**Positioning** √ and pad pressure points.
√ eyes.

**Complications** None specific

## POSTOPERATIVE

**Complications** Minimal bleeding

**Pain management** **Intraspinal opioids**: 10 μg fentanyl
**Parenteral opioids**: IV or im opioids (e.g., meperidine 10-20 mg iv q 10-15 min titrated to RR and patient's level of pain) instituted in recovery room.

Intrathecal fentanyl 10 μg, given with spinal local anesthetic, enhances intraop anesthesia and provides several hrs postop analgesia.[5]

**Tests** None routinely indicated.

**References**

1. Cunningham FG, MacDonald PC, Grant NF, eds: *Williams Obstetrics*, 8th edition. Appleton & Lange, Norwalk, CT: 1989, 921-43.
2. Wheeless CR Jr: *Atlas of Pelvic Surgery*, 2nd edition. Lea & Febiger, Philadelphia: 1988, 282-88.
3. Hatcher RA, Stewart F, Trussell J, et al: *Contraceptive Technology*, 15th revised edition. Irvinton Publishers, New York: 1990, 387-421.
4. Abouleish EI: Postpartum tubal ligation requires more bupivacaine for spinal anesthesia than does cesarean section. *AnesthAnalg* 1986; 65(8):897-900.
5. Malinow AM, Mokriski BL, Nomura MK, Kaufman MA, Snell JA, Sharp GD, Howard RA: Effect of epinephrine on intrathecal fentanyl analgesia in patients undergoing postpartum tubal ligation. *Anesthesiology* 1990; 73:(3):381-85.

# REPAIR OF VAGINAL/CERVICAL LACERATIONS

## SURGICAL CONSIDERATIONS

**Description**: Vaginal and cervical lacerations occur 2° trauma of spontaneous or operative vaginal delivery. Adequate repair requires optimal surgical assistance, exposure and patient comfort. Repair may be performed in a birthing bed, or may require patient positioning, lighting, anesthesia or monitoring capabilities available only in an OR. Vaginal and cervical lacerations can extend into the perineum, rectum, urethra, bladder, lower uterine segment, broad ligament or peritoneal cavity.

**Lacerations of the lower vagina** are generally easy to identify and repair. Small superficial lacerations that do not bleed often do not need repair, while larger ones should be approximated. Deep lacerations may cause profuse bleeding, especially when the area of the clitoris is involved. If bleeding persists despite placement of multiple stitches, brief tamponade may be adequate to achieve hemostasis or vaginal packing may be required. Lacerations involving the perineum are classified as follows. First degree: involves break in mucosa and skin. Second degree: involves deeper tissue (bulbocavernosus and levator ani fascia and muscle). Third degree: involves anal sphincter. Fourth degree: extends into rectal mucosa. First- and second-degree lacerations are repaired in layers with continuous or interrupted stitches. The skin is usually closed with a subcuticular stitch. When the anal sphincter is lacerated it often retracts. The ends are grasped with Allis clamps and approximated with multiple figure-of-eight stitches. When the laceration extends into the rectum, the rectal mucosa is closed in two layers, with the second layer imbricating the first. With periurethral lacerations, a catheter may need to be placed in the urethra to prevent passing a stitch through it. A laceration involving the urethra or bladder should be closed in multiple layers, followed by bladder drainage for several days.

**Lacerations of the upper vagina** are often difficult to visualize. Uterine bleeding and the umbilical cord of an undelivered placenta can obscure the field. It can be difficult to determine if bleeding is vaginal or uterine. It is helpful to deliver the placenta and control uterine bleeding before proceeding. Once visualization is adequate, it is important to place the first stitch above the apex of the laceration to control bleeding from vessels that may have retracted. Again, vaginal packing may be required if oozing of blood persists.

Superficial **lacerations of the cervix** occur with most deliveries but usually require no treatment. Deep lacerations can cause significant blood loss, especially when they involve branches from the uterine artery or extend into the lower uterine segment. Again, the first stitch must be placed above the apex of the laceration to control bleeding from vessels that may have retracted. A **laparotomy** may be necessary if a laceration extends into the lower uterine segment or broad ligament and is causing significant bleeding that cannot be controlled otherwise.

**Usual preop diagnosis**: Vaginal or cervical laceration

### SUMMARY OF PROCEDURE

| | |
|---|---|
| **Position** | Dorsal lithotomy |
| **Incision** | None (unless exploratory laparotomy is performed). |

| | |
|---|---|
| **Special instrumentation** | Right-angle retractors; ring forceps; weighted speculum; Gelpi retractor; vaginal packing |
| **Antibiotics** | May be used for lacerations involving entry into the peritoneal cavity or the rectal mucosa: cefotetan 1 gm iv q 12 hrs; total of 2 doses may be considered. |
| **Surgical time** | 10 - 45 min (possibly longer if exploratory laparotomy is performed). |
| **EBL** | Variable. Possible need for transfusion. Areas that persistently ooze after repeated placement of suture may be managed with vaginal packing. |
| **Postop care** | PACU → ward |
| **Mortality** | Rare |
| **Morbidity** | Hemorrhage<br>Infection<br>Rectovaginal fistula<br>Vesicovaginal fistula |
| **Procedure code** | 12001-12047 |
| **Pain score** | 3 |

### PATIENT POPULATION CHARACTERISTICS

| | |
|---|---|
| **Age range** | Reproductive age |
| **Incidence** | Not uncommon |
| **Etiology** | Trauma 2° spontaneous or operative vaginal delivery: 98%<br>Other vaginal/pelvic trauma: 2% |
| **Associated conditions** | Major blood loss possible<br>With nonobstetric etiology, the possibility of sexual assault needs to be explored. |

---

## ANESTHETIC CONSIDERATIONS

### PREOPERATIVE

Vaginal and cervical lacerations may go undetected until a considerable loss of blood has occurred. Patients should be examined carefully for Sx of hypovolemia with appropriate volume resuscitation prior to anesthesia.

| | |
|---|---|
| **Respiratory** | FRC returns to normal almost immediately after delivery.<br>**Tests:** As indicated from H&P. |
| **Cardiovascular** | The physiologic changes of pregnancy return to normal at varying intervals after delivery. For example, risk of aortocaval compression disappears immediately. Blood volume returns to pre-pregnant values over several days. Postpartum hemorrhage can occur without warning. Ensure adequate fluid resuscitation prior to induction of GA or regional anesthesia.<br>**Tests:** As indicated from H&P. |
| **Gastrointestinal** | Postpartum patients continue to be at risk for acid aspiration, although it is not known exactly when normal GI function returns. Precautions for prevention of acid aspiration should be followed as discussed in "Cesarean Section." |
| **Neurological** | Local anesthetic requirements for spinal anesthesia remain decreased after delivery. |
| **Laboratory** | Hct; other tests as indicated from H&P. |
| **Premedication** | Precautions should be taken to decrease risk of aspiration pneumonitis, as discussed under "Cesarean Section." |

### INTRAOPERATIVE

**Anesthetic technique:** In many patients, a functioning epidural catheter will be in place, and supplemental doses of anesthetic may be given to provide adequate analgesia for the surgery. If no epidural is placed and the patient is hemodynamically stable, a spinal anesthetic may be satisfactory. Occasionally GA may be required.

**Regional anesthesia:**

| | |
|---|---|
| **Epidural** | Supplemental doses of local anesthetic (2-chloroprocaine or 2% lidocaine 10-15 cc) injected incrementally with patient in sitting position (if tolerated) to promote perineal anesthesia. |

| | | |
|---|---|---|
| **Spinal** | Hyperbaric lidocaine 5% 50-70 mg with patient in sitting position, if tolerated. 24-ga pencil-point needle (Sprotte or Whitacre) to decrease incidence of spinal headache. Anesthesia to T10 is usually adequate. Repair of larger lacerations may require a higher level and, consequently, a higher dose; therefore, a longer-acting agent such as hyperbaric bupivacaine 0.75% 1.5 ml is used. | |
| **General anesthesia:** | | |
| **Induction** | Rapid-sequence induction with thiopental (3-5 mg/kg) and succinylcholine (1 mg/kg) for ET intubation. | |
| **Maintenance** | Standard maintenance (see Appendix). | |
| **Emergence** | Extubation should be delayed until patient is fully awake and protective airway reflexes have returned. | |
| **Blood and fluid requirements** | IV: 16-18 ga x 1<br>NS/LR @ 2-4 cc/kg/hr | 1-1.5 L dextrose-free crystalloid immediately prior to regional anesthesia. Blood loss may be extensive until laceration is repaired. |
| **Monitoring** | Standard monitors (see Appendix). | |
| **Complications** | Bleeding | |
| **Positioning** | √ and pad pressure points.<br>√ eyes. | **NB:** peroneal nerve compression at lateral fibular head→ foot drop. |

### POSTOPERATIVE

| | | |
|---|---|---|
| **Complications** | Bleeding<br>Peroneal nerve injury (2° lithotomy position) | Nerve injury manifested as foot drop and loss of sensation over dorsum of foot. |
| **Pain management** | **Intraspinal opioids**: 10 μg fentanyl<br>**Parenteral opioids**: IV or im opioids (e.g., meperidine 10-20 mg iv q 10-15 min up to 50 mg instituted in recovery room. | Intrathecal fentanyl 10 μg given with spinal local anesthetic – enhances intraop anesthesia and provides several hrs postop analgesia.[2] |
| **Tests** | Hct | |

References

1. Zuspan P, Quilligan EJ, eds: *Douglas-Stromme: Operative Obstetrics*, 5th edition. Appleton & Lange, New York: 1988.
2. Golan A, David MP: Repair of birth injuries. In *Operative Perinatology: Invasive Obstetric Techniques*. Iffy L, Charles D, eds. Macmillan, New York: 1984, 730-50.
3. Cunningham FG, MacDonald PC, Grant NF, eds: *Williams Obstetrics*, 8th edition. Appleton & Lange, Norwalk, CT: 1989, 307-26, 405-14.

# CERVICAL CERCLAGE - ELECTIVE AND EMERGENT

## SURGICAL CONSIDERATIONS

**Description**: Cervical cerclage is the reinforcement of the cervix to prevent premature cervical dilation in patients with an incompetent cervix. With cervical incompetence there is painless dilation of the cervix in the midtrimester of pregnancy. The membranes bulge through the cervix and rupture, followed by delivery of a severely premature infant.

An **elective cerclage** is performed prophylactically before pregnancy or after the first trimester of pregnancy on patients with a past history of cervical incompetence. If cerclage is performed before pregnancy it may need to be removed because of spontaneous abortion or fetal anomalies. It is generally performed between 14-16 weeks gestation, but may be performed as early as 10 weeks gestation. An **emergent cerclage** is performed in patients who present in the second trimester with painless cervical dilation and/or effacement. Ultrasound is performed before the procedure to confirm viability and to rule out major congenital anomalies. An emergent cerclage should not be performed if there is advanced cervical dilation, or any evidence of infection, contractions or uterine bleeding.

There are two types of cerclage procedures generally performed: the McDonald and the Shirodkar. The **McDonald cerclage** is technically easier, and the one most commonly performed. A purse-string stitch with non-absorbable monofilament suture is placed high around the cervix near the level of the internal os and tied at the twelve o'clock position. The end of the suture is cut long to facilitate removal. The cerclage is removed electively at term or earlier if there is rupture of membranes, persistent contractions, bleeding or evidence of infection. The **Shirodkar cerclage** involves incising the cervix transversely, anteriorly and posteriorly, and advancing the bladder off the cervix. A nonabsorbable monofilament suture is placed submucosally between the incisions and the mucosa is closed, thus burying the stitch. A Shirodkar cerclage may be left for future pregnancies if abdominal delivery is performed.

**Usual preop diagnosis:** Cervical incompetence

### SUMMARY OF PROCEDURE

| | |
|---|---|
| **Position** | Dorsal lithotomy, with use of cane stirrups. Left lateral pelvic tilt (if performed during pregnancy); Trendelenburg. |
| **Incision** | None with McDonald cerclage; transverse cervical with Shirodkar cerclage. |
| **Special instrumentation** | Right-angle retractors; monofilament, non-absorbable stitch |
| **Unique considerations** | For emergent cerclage, when prolapsing membranes are present, they may be reduced by filling the bladder and/or possibly removing amniotic fluid transabdominally. |
| **Antibiotics** | None recommended. |
| **Surgical time** | 30 min - 1 hr (longer for Shirodkar cerclage) |
| **EBL** | 25-50 cc (may be higher with the Shirodkar cerclage) |
| **Postop care** | PACU → ward; tocolysis with indomethacin or other agent can be considered. |
| **Mortality** | Rare |
| **Morbidity** | Morbidity is increased for emergent cerclage, especially when performed later in 2nd trimester. The McDonald cerclage is associated with less trauma and bleeding than the Shirodkar cerclage.<br>Cervical trauma<br>Rupture of membranes<br>Chorioamnionitis<br>Preterm labor<br>Spontaneous abortion |
| **Procedure code** | 59320 |
| **Pain score** | McDonald – 2; Shirodkar – 3 |

### PATIENT POPULATION CHARACTERISTICS

| | |
|---|---|
| **Age range** | Reproductive age |
| **Incidence** | Not uncommon |
| **Etiology** | Cervical trauma from previous vaginal delivery<br>Cervical trauma at time of previous D&C<br>Previous treatment for cervical dysplasia: laser therapy, cryotherapy, LEEP/large loop excision of transitional zone (LLETZ), cone Bx<br>Congenital anomalies<br>Idiopathic |

## ANESTHETIC CONSIDERATIONS

### PREOPERATIVE

This is a generally fit and healthy patient population. Little will need to be done other than routine tests, unless otherwise indicated. Cerclage is usually performed between 14-24 weeks of pregnancy. When performed after 20 wks, relevant physiologic changes are as discussed under "Cesarean Section." Patient may receive drugs such as ß-sympathomimetics (e.g., terbutaline), nifedipine, or indomethacin to decrease uterine irritability.

| | |
|---|---|
| **Laboratory** | Hct; other tests as indicated from H&P. |
| **Premedication** | None usually. If >18 wks gestation, precautions should be taken to decrease risk of aspiration pneumonitis, as discussed under "Cesarean Section." |

## INTRAOPERATIVE

**Anesthetic technique:** Drug exposure during the critical period of organogenesis (15-56 d) should be minimized, although no particular anesthetic techniques or agents have proven teratogenic in humans. Through an action on vitamin $B_{12}$, $N_2O$ inhibits methionine synthetase, which is involved in thymidine synthesis. This may explain why $N_2O$ is teratogenic in rodents. There is no evidence, however, that $N_2O$ is teratogenic when used for cervical cerclage or other operations in humans.[6-8] Avoid diazepam during the period of organogenesis because of reports of cleft lip.[9] Ensure adequate uteroplacental perfusion and fetal oxygenation by maintaining normal maternal BP and oxyhemoglobin saturation. Use left uterine displacement after 20 wks gestation. Maternal hyperventilation and IPPV may diminish uteroplacental and umbilical blood flow. Monitoring FHR may permit optimization of fetal well-being by adjustment of anesthetic technique or patient position. Spinal anesthesia is ideal as it minimizes fetal drug exposure and provides good operating conditions. Risk of headache is low with the use of pencil-point needles (e.g., Sprotte, Whitacre). Epidural anesthesia is an appropriate alternative for this procedure. GA may be used if regional anesthesia is contraindicated.

**Regional anesthesia:**

| | |
|---|---|
| **Spinal** | Hyperbaric 5% spinal lidocaine 70-80 mg (or bupivacaine 7-9 mg if prolonged procedure anticipated). Position patient to obtain T8 block. Monitor BP every min until stable, then every 3-5 min. Treat >20% decrease in BP or SBP < 95-100 mmHg with additional fluids and ephedrine 5-10 mg iv. |

**General anesthesia:**

| | |
|---|---|
| **Induction** | Standard induction (see Appendix). If >18 wks gestation, then rapid-sequence induction is indicated. |
| **Maintenance** | Standard maintenance (see Appendix). If < 15-18 wks gestation, the use of mask anesthesia with $O_2/N_2O$/volatile agent/opioid is appropriate. If >18 wks gestation, ET intubation will be necessary. |
| **Emergence** | If >18 wks gestation, extubate patient when fully awake and protective airway reflexes have returned. |

| | | |
|---|---|---|
| **Blood and fluid requirements** | Minimal blood loss<br>IV: 16-18 ga x 1<br>NS/LR @ 4 mg/kg/hr | 1-1.5 L dextrose-free crystalloid immediately prior to regional anesthesia |
| **Monitoring** | Standard monitors (see Appendix). | |
| **Positioning** | Left uterine displacement, if >20 wks gestation.<br>✓ and pad pressure points.<br>✓ eyes. | Left uterine displacement with a wedge under mattress should be used for pregnant patients (after ~20 wks).<br>**NB:** peroneal nerve compression at lateral fibular head→ foot drop. |

## POSTOPERATIVE

| | | |
|---|---|---|
| **Complications** | Preterm labor<br>Maternal dysrhythmias<br>Hypotension | Observe for preterm labor in recovery area. Tocolytic agents (ß-adrenergic agents) given to inhibit uterine contractions can cause maternal dysrhythmias or hypotension. |
| | Peroneal nerve injury | Nerve injury manifested as foot drop and loss of sensation over dorsum of foot. |
| **Pain management** | **Intraspinal opioids:** 5-10 μg fentanyl<br>**Parenteral opioids:** iv or im opioids (e.g., meperidine 10-20 mg q 15 min up to 50 mg) instituted in recovery room. | Intrathecal fentanyl given with spinal improves intraop analgesia and provides short-period postop analgesia. Risk of delayed respiration depression minimal in healthy patients. |

**References**

1. Parisi VM: Cervical incompetence. In *Maternal - Fetal Medicine: Principles and Practice*, 2nd edition. Creasy RK, Resnik R, eds. WB Saunders Co, Philadelphia: 1989, 447-62.
2. Barth WH Jr, Yeomans ER, Hankins GD: Emergent cerclage. *Surg, Gynecol Obstet* 1990; 170(4):323-26.
3. Jewelewicz R: Incompetent cervix: pathogenesis, diagnosis and treatment. *Semin Perinatol* 1991; 15(2):156-61.
4. Wesseley AC: Early cerclage for cervical incompetence. *The Female Patient* 1991; 16:21.
5. Harger JH: Cervical cerclage: patient selection, morbidity, and success rates. *Clin Perinatol* 1983; 10(2):321-41.
6. Crawford JS, Lewis M: Nitrous oxide in early human pregnancy. *Anaesthesia* 1986; 41(9):900-5.
7. Aldridge LM, Tunstall ME: Nitrous oxide and the fetus. A review and the results of a retrospective study of 175 cases of anaesthesia for insertion of a Shirodkar suture. *Br J Anaesth* 1986; 58(12):1348-56.
8. Mazze RI, Kallen B: Reproductive outcome after anesthesia and operation during pregnancy: a registry study of 5405 cases. *Am J Obstet Gynecol* 1989; 161(5):1178-85.
9. Safra MJ, Oakley GP Jr: Association between cleft lip with or without cleft palate and prenatal exposure to diazepam. *Lancet* 1975; 2(7933):478-84.

# REMOVAL OF RETAINED PLACENTA

## SURGICAL CONSIDERATIONS

**Description**: In most deliveries, the placenta is easily removed with gentle cord traction and uterine massage. If, after 30 min, the placenta remains undelivered, **manual removal**, following either parenteral analgesia or GA, must be initiated. A possible alternative to manual removal involves injection of 10 cc of oxytocin (10 U/cc) into the umbilical vein; however, the success of this procedure is unpredictable. A retained placental fragment may cause immediate or late postpartum hemorrhage. An ultrasound evaluation of the uterus may help in the detection of a retained fragment. If retained products are found, **curettage** is recommended. Frequently, the retained product will already have been flushed out of the uterus by brisk bleeding. In such cases, iv oxytocin, intramuscular prostaglandins or methylergonovine may be administered to contract the uterus prior to curettage.

Bleeding from a retained placenta or fragment is frequently brisk, so the anesthesiologist must be ready to administer iv fluids and $O_2$, and to correct any coagulopathy. Cross-matched blood must be available. Placenta accreta, if extensive, can cause profuse bleeding at delivery, and a hysterectomy is often necessary.

Oxytocin 20 U in 1000 cc of LR should be administered after manual removal of the placenta or after sharp/suction curettage of a retained placental fragment.

**Usual preop diagnosis**: Retained placenta

### SUMMARY OF PROCEDURE

| | |
|---|---|
| **Position** | Dorsal lithotomy |
| **Incision** | None |
| **Special instrumentation** | Banjo curette/suction cannula |
| **Unique considerations** | IV fluids; use of blood and blood products, as needed; monitoring of vital signs |
| **Antibiotics** | Cefotetan 2 gm iv q 12 hrs; 3 total doses |
| **Surgical time** | 30 min |
| **EBL** | Variable – 300-900 cc |
| **Postop care** | PACU → ward. Monitor for infection and further bleeding. |
| **Mortality** | Rare |
| **Morbidity** | Hemorrhage<br>Endometritis<br>Uterine perforation 2° curettage<br>Asherman's syndrome<br>Transfusion-related morbidity (hepatitis, HIV, transfusion reactions) |

| | |
|---|---|
| **Procedure code** | 59414 |
| **Pain score** | 5 |

### PATIENT POPULATION CHARACTERISTICS

| | |
|---|---|
| **Age range** | Reproductive age |
| **Incidence** | 0.25-0.8% of vaginal deliveries |
| **Etiology** | Unknown |
| **Associated conditions** | Placenta accreta<br>Mismanagement of third stage of labor<br>Avulsed cotyledon<br>Succenturiate lobe |

---

## ANESTHETIC CONSIDERATIONS

### PREOPERATIVE

The degree of urgency associated with these patients may vary dramatically. Some patients may be hemodynamically unstable as a result of continued bleeding in the postpartum period; others may have a retained placenta with minimal bleeding. Patient's volume status should be carefully assessed.

| | |
|---|---|
| **Respiratory** | FRC returns to normal almost immediately after delivery.<br>**Tests:** As indicated from H&P. |
| **Cardiovascular** | Restore intravascular volume prior to institution of analgesia or anesthesia. Extension of existing lumbar epidural blockade may aggravate hypovolemia and should proceed with caution. Consider possibility of placenta accreta (placental villi are attached to myometrium). |
| **Gastrointestinal** | Postpartum patients continue to be at risk for acid aspiration, although it is not known exactly when normal GI function returns. Precautions for prevention of acid aspiration should be followed as discussed in "Cesarean Section." |
| **Neurological** | Local anesthetic requirements for spinal anesthesia remain decreased after delivery. |
| **Hematologic** | Coagulopathy can develop with retained placenta if bleeding is severe and persistent.<br>**Tests:** PT; PTT; platelets; FSP, as indicated. |
| **Laboratory** | Other tests as indicated from H&P. T&C for 2 U+ if time permits. Emergency transfusion with O– blood may be necessary. |
| **Premedication** | Precaution should be taken to decrease risk of aspiration, as discussed under "Cesarean Section." |

### INTRAOPERATIVE

**Anesthetic technique:** Anesthesia for the removal of a retained placenta may vary from MAC to GA performed as an emergency. In the multiparous patient, MAC may be sufficient to enable the obstetrician to empty the uterus. If additional uterine relaxation is needed, however, then GA may be required. The incidence of retained placenta is about 1%. If intravascular volume has been restored and an existing epidural catheter is in place, the block can be extended to provide adequate anesthesia. Initiating spinal anesthesia is also an option if: intravascular volume status is adequate; there is no active bleeding; and uterine relaxation is not required. Small doses of opioids and midazolam sometimes provide sufficient analgesia and sedation to allow removal of a retained placenta without compromising maternal safety. If this proves inadequate or hemorrhage is severe, however, GA with ET intubation is required. Preliminary experience suggests that NTG 50-100 μg iv provides uterine relaxation and delivery of retained placenta in normovolemic patients receiving iv analgesia.[9]

**Regional anesthesia:**

| | |
|---|---|
| **Spinal** | For technique and monitoring of spinal anesthesia, see "Cesarean Section," above. Hyperbaric 5% spinal lidocaine, 50-75 mg; adjust the position of operating table to obtain T8 level of anesthesia. |
| **Epidural** | For technique and monitoring, see "Cesarean Section." Administer increments of 3% 2-chloroprocaine or 2% lidocaine with 1:200,000 epinephrine until block level adequate. Additional local anesthetic as needed to ensure adequate level of anesthesia. |

| | | |
|---|---|---|
| **MAC** | Titrate small doses opioid (e.g., fentanyl 25-50 μg) and midazolam 0.5-1.0 mg. Ensure patient is awake and responsive throughout. Consider NTG 50-100 μg iv for uterine relaxation. Hypotension may follow vasodilation due to NTG, and should be treated with volume and pressors if necessary. | |
| **General anesthesia:** | | |
| **Induction** | Preoxygenation, rapid-sequence induction with cricoid pressure, and hydration, as discussed in "Cesarean Section." Ketamine (1 mg/kg) preferred for induction of hypotensive patient, but in larger doses (>1.5 mg/kg) theoretically may increase uterine tone and make removal of placenta more difficult. Anesthesia with $N_2O/O_2$ + opioid (but no volatile agent) often permits delivery of the placenta. | |
| **Maintenance** | If uterine relaxation is necessary, administer volatile agent (>1 MAC) until uterine tone decreases. | |
| **Emergence** | Extubation should be delayed until patient is fully awake and protective airway reflexes have returned. | |
| **Blood and fluid requirements** | Anticipate large blood loss<br>IV: 16-18 ga x 1-2<br>NS/LR @ 6-8 cc/kg/hr | Infuse crystalloid solution to maintain BP (1-1.5 L iv) prior to regional anesthesia. Treat hypotension with fluids and ephedrine, and by decreasing concentration of volatile agent. Surgery is usually brief in duration; additional muscle relaxation not usually necessary. |
| **Monitoring** | Standard monitors (see Appendix). | |
| **Complications** | Bleeding | |
| **Positioning** | ✓ and pad pressure points.<br>✓ eyes. | **NB:** peroneal nerve compression at lateral fibular head→ foot drop. |

## POSTOPERATIVE

| | | |
|---|---|---|
| **Complications** | Peroneal nerve injury (2° lithotomy position)<br>Bleeding | Nerve injury manifested as foot drop and loss of sensation over dorsum of foot. |
| **Pain management** | IV or im opioids, titrated to effect as usual, instituted in recovery room. | |
| **Tests** | Hct | |


**References**

1. Huber MG, Wildschut HI, Boer K, Kleiverda G, Hoek FJ: Umbilical vein administration of oxytocin for the management of retained placenta: is it effective? *Am J Obstet Gynecol* 1991; 164(5 P+1):1216-19.
2. Cunningham FG, MacDonald PC, Gant NF, eds: *Williams Obstetrics*, 18th edition. Appleton & Lange, Norwalk CT: 1989, 482-83.
3. Pernoll LM, ed: *Current Obstetric and Gynecologic Diagnosis and Treatment*, 7th edition. Appleton & Lange, Norwalk CT: 1991, 568-73.
4. Creasy RK, Resnik R, eds: *Maternal-Fetal Medicine: Principles and Practice*, 2nd edition. Saunders, Philadelphia: 1989, 862-63.
5. Wilken-Jensen C, Strom V, Nielsen MD, Rosenkilde-Gram B: Removing a retained placenta by oxytocin -- a controlled study. *Am J Obstet and Gynecol* 1989; 161(1):155-56.
6. Lee CY, Madrazo B, Drukker BH: Ultrasonic evaluation of the postpartum uterus in the management of postpartum bleeding. *Obstet Gynecol* 1981; 58(2):227-32.
7. Schenker JG, Margalroth EJ: Intrauterine adhesions: an updated appraisal. *Fertil Steril* 1982; 37(5):593-610.
8. Robinson HP: Sonar in the puerperium. A means of diagnosing retained products of conception. *Scott Med J* 1972; 17(11):364-66.
9. Desimone CA, Norris MC, Leighton BL: Intravenous nitroglycerin aids manual extraction of a retained placenta. [Letter] *Anesthesiology* 1990; 73(4):787.

# MANAGEMENT OF UTERINE INVERSION

## SURGICAL CONSIDERATIONS

**Description**: Uterine inversion is associated with fundal implantation of the placenta whereby a thinning of the uterine wall, together with placental separation, causes an invagination of the myometrium, resulting in inversion. Vigorous fundal pressure or cord traction also can contribute to uterine inversion, which can be complete or incomplete. Complete inversion results in the inverted fundus extending beyond the cervix and appearing at the vaginal introitus, whereas in an incompletely inverted uterus, the fundus does not extend beyond the external cervical os. Uterine inversion can cause hemorrhage and shock, and must be managed as an obstetrical emergency. An anesthesiologist must be called to the delivery room as soon as a diagnosis of uterine inversion is made. The ready availability of GA is paramount. Intravenous access with two infusion systems and appropriate fluid resuscitation must be initiated emergently. Whole blood should be available to support cardiac output, if necessary.

Frequently, reinversion can be accomplished with iv tocolytics such as terbutaline and magnesium sulfate; however, GA (preferably halothane) may be necessary. Three primary methods for uterine reinversion are the Johnson, Huntington, and Haultain procedures. Normally, the **Johnson method** is attempted first. Persistent pressure applied to the fundus is used to elevate the uterus into the vagina. The placenta, if attached, is not removed until iv resuscitation has been initiated, and iv tocolytics (or anesthesia) have been administered. Oxytocin is given when the uterus has been reinverted. **Laparotomy** must be performed if reinversion with the Johnson method is unsuccessful. The **Huntington procedure** involves grasping the round ligaments and applying upward traction on them, while an assistant exerts upward pressure on the uterus via a hand in the vagina. If the inverted uterus is trapped below the cervical ring, the **Haultain procedure** is used. This procedure involves making a longitudinal fundal incision posteriorly to allow easier reinversion of the fundus.

**Usual preop diagnosis**: Uterine inversion

### SUMMARY OF PROCEDURE

| | Manual Reinversion | Huntington/Haultain |
|---|---|---|
| **Position** | Dorsal lithotomy | Supine |
| **Incision** | None | Pfannenstiel or midline longitudinal |
| **Unique considerations** | Prompt $O_2$ and iv fluid resuscitation; use of blood and blood products as necessary. | ⇐ |
| **Antibiotics** | Cefotetan 2 gm iv q 12 hrs; total 3 doses | ⇐ |
| **Surgical time** | 30 min | 1 - 2 hrs |
| **EBL** | 150-4000 cc | ⇐ |
| **Postop care** | ± ICU. ARDS may necessitate mechanical ventilation. Monitor for acute renal failure 2° hypoxia and hypovolemia. | ⇐ |
| **Mortality** | Rare | ⇐ |
| **Morbidity** | Febrile morbidity | ⇐ |
| | Clinical shock | ⇐ |
| | Infectious morbidity from blood transfusion | ⇐ |
| **Procedure code** | 58999 | ⇐ |
| **Pain score** | 5 | 7 |

### PATIENT POPULATION CHARACTERISTICS

| | |
|---|---|
| **Age range** | Reproductive age |
| **Incidence** | 1/2000-6000 deliveries |
| **Etiology** | Unknown |
| **Associated conditions** | Fundal implantation of the placenta<br>Primiparity<br>Intrapartum oxytocin<br>Placenta accreta<br>Therapy of pre-eclampsia with magnesium sulfate<br>Macrosomic fetus |

# ANESTHETIC CONSIDERATIONS

## PREOPERATIVE

These patients often present in shock out of proportion to blood loss. Immediate resuscitation may be necessary.

| | |
|---|---|
| **Respiratory** | FRC returns to normal almost immediately after delivery.<br>**Tests:** As indicated from H&P. |
| **Cardiovascular** | Massive hemorrhage and pain usual with complete inversion. Prior to induction insert large-bore iv and rapidly infuse fluids, including colloid to treat hypotension. Blood transfusion may be necessary, although is seldom available until after surgery. |
| **Gastrointestinal** | Postpartum patients continue to be at risk for acid aspiration, although it is not known exactly when normal GI function returns. Precautions for prevention of acid aspiration should be followed as discussed in "Cesarean Section." |
| **Neurological** | Local anesthetic requirements for spinal anesthesia remain decreased after delivery.[1] |
| **Laboratory** | Other tests as indicated from H&P. T&C for 2 U; keep 2 U ahead. |
| **Premedication** | Na citrate 30 cc po within 30 min of induction. If time permits, other agents to decrease risk of acid aspiration, as discussed under "Cesarean Section." |

## INTRAOPERATIVE

**Anesthetic technique:** Induction of anesthesia should not await intravascular volume replacement. Bleeding usually stops when uterus is replaced. Usually, GETA is required, often with increasing concentrations of volatile agents to facilitate uterine replacement. If regional anesthesia (e.g., epidural or spinal) was used for delivery, replacement of uterus may be accomplished with little further anesthetic intervention. If regional anesthesia was not used for delivery, iv analgesia with small doses of fentanyl (25-50 μg iv) occasionally allows reduction.

| | |
|---|---|
| **Induction** | Rapid-sequence induction with ketamine (1.0 mg/kg) preferred. Higher dose may adversely increase uterine tone. |
| **Maintenance** | Halothane, enflurane and isoflurane, all effective uterine relaxants, but isoflurane is most rapidly eliminated. Hypotension should be treated with fluids + vasopressors. |
| **Emergence** | Extubation should be delayed until patient is fully awake and protective airway reflexes have returned. |

| | | |
|---|---|---|
| **Blood and fluid requirements** | Significant blood loss<br>IV: 16-18 ga x 1 or 2 | Possible continued blood loss after reduction of uterus, due to uterine atony. |
| **Monitoring** | Standard monitors (see Appendix). | Arterial line may be useful if time allows. |
| **Positioning** | √ and pad pressure points.<br>√ eyes. | |
| **Complications** | Uterine atony<br>Massive blood loss | Rx: ↓volatile anesthetic concentrations. Oxytocin infusion, uterine massage, ± methylergonovine (0.2 mg iv/im → ↑BP. |

## POSTOPERATIVE

| | |
|---|---|
| **Complications** | Bleeding |
| **Pain management** | Parenteral opiates |
| **Tests** | Hct |


**References**

1. Cunningham FG, MacDonald PC, Gant NF, eds: *Williams Obstetrics*, 18th edition. Appleton & Lange, Norwalk: 1989, 422-23.
2. Creasy RK, Resnik R, eds: *Maternal-Fetal Medicine: Principles and Practice*, 2nd edition. Saunders, Philadelphia: 1989, 519-20.
3. Brar HS, Greenspoon JS, Platt LD, Paul RH: Acute puerperal uterine inversion. New approaches to management. *J Repro Med* 1989; 34:(2)173-77.
4. Shah-Hosseini R, Evrard JR: Puerperal uterine inversion. *Obstet and Gynecol* 1989; 73(4):567-70.
5. Kitchin J, Thiagarajah S, May HV Jr, Thornton WN Jr: Puerperal inversion of the uterus. *Am J Obstet Gynecol* 1975; 123:51-8.
6. Platt LD, Druzin ML: Acute puerperal inversion of the uterus. *Am J Obstet Gynecol* 1981; 141(2):187-90.
7. Lee WK, Baggish MS, Lashgari M: Acute inversion of the uterus. *Obstet Gynecol* 1978; 51(2):144-47.

**Surgeon**

**Fuad S. Freiha, MD, FACS**

# 9. UROLOGY

**Anesthesiologists**

**Steven Deem, MD**
**Ronald G. Pearl, MD, PhD**

# DIAGNOSTIC TRANSURETHRAL (ENDOSCOPIC) PROCEDURES

## SURGICAL CONSIDERATIONS

**Description:** Many urologic diseases are diagnosed and evaluated endoscopically through the urethra with the use of specialized instruments such as cystoscopes and resectoscopes. With the patient in a lithotomy position, the cystoscope is introduced into the urethra and advanced under direct vision all the way into the bladder (Figs 9-1A,B), allowing inspection of the urethra (**urethroscopy**) and bladder (**cystoscopy**). If pathology is noted, a biopsy can be obtained easily through the cystoscope. It is also possible to introduce small catheters into the ureteral orifices and advance them up to the kidneys for radiologic evaluation (**retrograde pyelography**), to collect urine specimens, or to bypass areas of obstruction. If the upper urinary tract needs to be visualized, a ureteroscope is introduced through the urethra into the bladder and through the ureteral orifice into the ureter and advanced up to the kidney, allowing inspection of the ureter (**ureteroscopy**) and intra-renal collecting system (**nephroscopy**). Often, these procedures precede a major surgical operation.

**Usual preop diagnosis:** Hematuria; hydronephrosis; benign prostatic hypertrophy; cancer of the urethra, prostate, ureter and renal pelvis; urinary tract stones; strictures; ureteropelvic junction obstruction; hemorrhagic or interstitial cystitis

### SUMMARY OF PROCEDURE

| | Urethroscopy/ Cystoscopy | Ureteroscopy/ Nephroscopy |
|---|---|---|
| **Position** | Lithotomy | ⇐ |
| **Incision** | None | ⇐ |
| **Special instrumentation** | Cystoscope | Ureteroscope |
| **Unique considerations** | Use of x-ray and fluoroscopy | ⇐ |
| **Antibiotics** | Gentamicin 80 mg iv, slowly | ⇐ |
| **Surgical time** | 15 min | 45 min |
| **EBL** | None | ⇐ |
| **Postop care** | PACU → home | ⇐ |
| **Mortality** | Minimal | ⇐ |
| **Morbidity** | Infection: 5% | ⇐<br>Ureteral perforation: < 5% |
| **Procedure code** | 52000 | 52320, 50551 |
| **Pain score** | 1 | 1 |

### PATIENT POPULATION CHARACTERISTICS

| | | |
|---|---|---|
| **Age range** | All ages | ⇐ |
| **Male:Female** | 1:1 | ⇐ |
| **Incidence** | 30% of all urologic procedures | ⇐ |
| **Etiology** | Hematuria | ⇐ |
| | Urethral and bladder tumors | ⇐ |
| | Stones | ⇐ |
| | Urethral strictures | ⇐ |
| | | Ureteropelvic junction obstruction |
| **Associated conditions** | Prostatic hypertrophy | Hydronephrosis |
| | Cystitis | ⇐ |

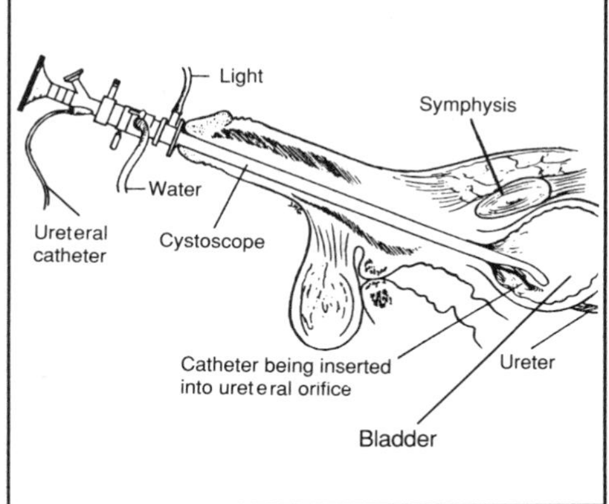


**Figure 9-1A.** Cystoscope introduced into bladder via urethra, male anatomy. (Reproduced with permission from Hardy JD: *Textbook of Surgery*. JB Lippincott: 1988.)

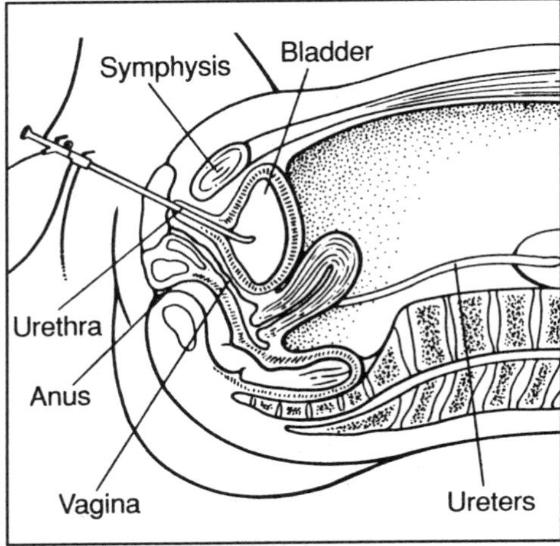


**Figure 9-1B.** Cystoscope introduced into bladder, female anatomy. (Reproduced with permission from Govan DE: *Roche Manual of Urologic Procedures*. Hoffmann-LaRoche: 1976.)

## ANESTHETIC CONSIDERATIONS

See Anesthetic Considerations following "Therapeutic Transurethral Procedures (Except TURP)" (below).

**References**

1. Ballentine Carter H: The Urologic Examination and Diagnostic Techniques. In *Campbell's Urology*, 6th edition. Walsh PC, et al, eds. WB Saunders Co, Philadelphia: 1992, Vol 1, Ch 8, 331-41.
2. Huffman JL: Ureteroscopy. In *Campbell's Urology*, 6th edition. WB Saunders Co, Philadelphia: 1992, Vol 3, Ch 61, 2195-2230.

# THERAPEUTIC TRANSURETHRAL PROCEDURES (EXCEPT TURP)

## SURGICAL CONSIDERATIONS

**Description**: Therapeutic transurethral procedures, the most common urologic operations, require the use of specialized instruments such as cystoscopes and resectoscopes. Because of continuously improving instrumentation and fiber optics, the range and complexity of these operations are widening, and more operations are being done transurethrally now than ever before. These operations are: **transurethral resection (TUR)** of any urethral, prostatic or bladder pathology; **fulguration** of bleeding vessels; **instillation of chemicals** such as oxychlorosene (chloropactin) and formalin into the bladder; **extraction** of stones; and **incision and dilation** of strictures.

With the patient in the lithotomy position, the cystoscope or resectoscope is introduced into the urethra and advanced under direct vision into the bladder, allowing inspection of the urethra and bladder (Figs 9-1A,B). The pathology is identified. If a tumor, it is resected piecemeal with the electrode of the resectoscope, using the cutting current and cauterizing the base of the tumor with the coagulating current. If the pathology is a stone, it is extracted with special forceps or stone basket. Occasionally, a stone needs to be crushed either with a lithotrite or with electrohydraulic probes before it can be extracted. Chemicals can be instilled through the cystoscope to control interstitial and hemorrhagic cystitis. Bleeding vessels can be coagulated with the electrode. Strictures can be dilated, or incised and dilated.

**Variant procedure or approaches**: Occasionally, access to the intrarenal collecting system (renal pelvis and calyces) and upper ureter is easier and more appropriately done through a **percutaneous nephrostomy** than a transurethral procedure. The patient is placed in a prone or flank position, a percutaneous stab wound is made at the costovertebral angle and a tube is introduced into the kidney under fluoroscopic control.

**Usual preop diagnosis**: Tumors of the urinary tract; stones; interstitial or hemorrhagic cystitis; strictures

**SUMMARY OF PROCEDURE**

| | Transurethral | Percutaneous |
|---|---|---|
| **Position** | Lithotomy | Flank or prone |
| **Incision** | None | Stab wound |
| **Special instrumentation** | Cystoscope; resectoscope; catheters; stents | Percutaneous nephrostomy kit; nephroscope; urethroscope; catheters; stents |
| **Unique considerations** | Use of x-rays, fluoroscopy and electrocautery | ⇐ |
| **Antibiotics** | Gentamicin 80 mg iv, slowly | ⇐ |
| **Surgical time** | 1 hr | 2 - 3 hrs |
| **EBL** | 100 cc | 500 cc |
| **Postop care** | Irrigation of tubes and catheters to clear clots and prevent obstruction | ⇐ |
| **Mortality** | < 1% | ⇐ |

| | Transurethral | Percutaneous |
|---|---|---|
| **Morbidity** | Bleeding: 10% | ⇐ |
| | Infection: 5% | ⇐ |
| | Perforation: 2% | ⇐ |
| | Retained stones: 2% | ⇐ |
| **Procedure code** | 52234, 52235, 52240 (TUR bladder tumors) | ⇐ |
| | 50650 (ureteral tumor) | |
| | 50200 (renal tumor) | |
| | 52330 (stone extraction) | |
| | 52250 (instillation of chloropactin) | |
| | 51700 (instillation of formalin) | |
| | 52281 (dilation and incision strictures) | |
| | 50551 (nephroscopy) | |
| | 50060 (percutaneous nephrolithotomy) | |
| **Pain score** | 1 | 3 |

### PATIENT POPULATION CHARACTERISTICS

| | | |
|---|---|---|
| **Age range** | All ages | ⇐ |
| **Male:Female** | 1:1 | ⇐ |
| **Incidence** | 10% of urologic diseases involve these procedures | ⇐ |
| **Etiology** | Urethral and bladder tumors | Kidney stones |
| | Bladder and ureteral stones | Upper ureteral stones |
| | Interstitial cystitis | Ureteropelvic junction obstruction |
| | Hemorrhagic cystitis | |
| | Urethral stricture | |

---

## ANESTHETIC CONSIDERATIONS

**(Procedures covered: diagnostic transurethral procedures; therapeutic transurethral procedures [except TURP])**

### PREOPERATIVE

Patients of all ages may present for ureteral stone extraction. Paraplegics and quadriplegics have a predilection for nephrolithiasis, and may present for repeated cystoscopies. Bladder tumors usually seen in the older population, who may present for cystoscopy or transurethral resection. These patients are likely to have pre-existing medical problems, including: CAD, CHF, PVD, cerebrovascular diseases, COPD and renal impairment. Preop evaluation should be directed toward the detection and treatment of these conditions prior to anesthesia.

**Neurological** Paraplegics and quadriplegics may present for repeated cystoscopies and stone extractions. Note Hx of autonomic hyperreflexia (AH); Sx may include flushing, headache and nasal stuffiness, associated with voiding or noxious stimuli below the level of spinal cord injury (see below).

**Musculoskeletal** Contractures, pressure sores may make positioning difficult in paraplegics or quadriplegics.

**Laboratory** Tests as indicated from H&P.

**Premedication** Sedation prn anxiety (e.g. lorazepam 1-2 mg po 1-2 hrs before surgery; midazolam 1-2 mg iv in preop area).

### INTRAOPERATIVE

**Anesthetic technique:** Spinal, continuous lumbar epidural and GA are acceptable, with the choice dependent on type and length of procedure, age and co-existing disease, and patient preference. Simpler transurethral procedures (e.g., cystoscopy) are amenable to topical anesthesia, while longer and more complex procedures (e.g., ureteral stone extraction) will require regional or GA (see discussion below regarding AH). Note that many of these procedures are done on an outpatient basis; and the anesthetic should be planned appropriately. For regional anesthesia, a sacral block is required for urethral procedures, T9-T10 level for procedures involving the bladder, and as high as T8 for procedures involving the ureters.

**Regional anesthesia:**

| | |
|---|---|
| **Topical** | 2% lidocaine jelly |
| **Spinal** | 5% lidocaine 50-75 mg, 0.75% bupivacaine 10-12 mg |
| **Lumbar epidural** | 1.5-2.0% lidocaine with epinephrine 5 μg/cc, 15-25 cc; supplement with 5-10 cc boluses as needed. Supplemental iv sedation. |

**General anesthesia:**

| | |
|---|---|
| **Induction** | Standard induction (see Appendix). ET intubation may not be necessary for shorter procedures. Succinylcholine should be avoided in paralysed patients 2° hyperkalemia → VF or asystole. |
| **Maintenance** | Pure inhalation anesthetic (e.g., $N_2O$, isoflurane) for short cases. IV technique (e.g., propofol 100-200 μg/kg/min; supplement with $N_2O$, ± isoflurane ± narcotic). Muscle relaxation not essential. Narcotics not essential since postop pain is usually minimal. |
| **Emergence** | No specific considerations |

| | | |
|---|---|---|
| **Blood and fluid requirements** | Usually minimal blood loss<br>IV: 18 ga x 1<br>NS/LR @ 2-4 cc/kg/hr | |
| **Monitoring** | Standard monitors (see Appendix). | |
| **Positioning** | ✓ and pad pressure points.<br>✓ eyes. | **NB**: peroneal nerve compression at lateral fibular head → foot drop. |
| **Complications** | Anticipate hypotension upon returning from lithotomy position at end of procedure.<br>Autonomic hyperreflexia (AH):<br>-Severe HTN<br>-Bradycardia<br>-Dysrhythmias<br>-Cardiac arrest | Rx: volume (200-500 cc NS/LR) or ephedrine (5 mg iv) may be necessary. Patients with spinal cord injury level above T10 are at risk for AH associated with stimulation below the level of transection. T6-T10 transection levels may be associated with less severe manifestations. AH can be prevented by GA, spinal or epidural anesthesia. If AH occurs intraop it should be treated by deepening the level of anesthesia, and iv anti-hypertensive agents (e.g., SNP 0.5-5.0 μg/kg/min, labetalol 5-10 mg iv, phentolamine, 2-5 mg iv), if necessary. |

## POSTOPERATIVE

| | | |
|---|---|---|
| **Complications** | Peroneal nerve injury 2° lithotomy position<br>Fever/bacteremia<br>Bladder perforation | Peroneal nerve injury manifested as foot drop with loss of sensation over dorsum of foot. Seek neurology consultation.<br>Bladder perforation may present as shoulder pain in the awake patient, but may go unnoticed in a patient under GA. Sx include unexplained HTN, tachycardia, hypotension (rare). |
| **Pain management** | Pain usually mild; Rx: morphine 2-4 mg iv q 10-15 min prn. | |

**References**

1. Mebust WK: Transurethral Surgery. In *Campbell's Urology*, Vol 3, 6th edition. Walsh PC, Retite AB, Stamey TA, Vaughn ED Jr, eds. WB Saunders Co, Philadelphia: 1992, Ch 80, 2900-22.
2. Lambert DH, Deane RS, Mazuzan JE Jr: Anesthesia and the control of blood pressure in patients with spinal cord injury. *Anesth Analg* 1982; 61(4):344-48.

# TRANSURETHRAL RESECTION OF THE PROSTATE (TURP)

## SURGICAL CONSIDERATIONS

**Description:** **TURP** is one of the most common urologic operations, performed to relieve bladder outlet obstruction by an enlarging prostate gland. It is often preceded by **cystoscopy** to evaluate the size of the prostate gland and to rule out any other pathology, such as bladder tumor or stone. The operation is performed with the resectoscope, a specialized instrument with an electrode capable of transmitting both cutting and coagulating currents. The resectoscope is introduced into the bladder (Fig 9-2) and the tissue protruding into the prostatic urethra is resected in small pieces called "chips." Bleeding vessels are coagulated with the coagulating current. The resection is performed with continuous irrigation using an isotonic solution such as sorbitol 2.7% with mannitol 0.54%. Once the obstructing prostatic tissues are completely resected and bleeding vessels coagulated, the chips are irrigated out of the bladder and the resectoscope removed. An indwelling Foley catheter is introduced into the bladder. The time of transurethral resection should not exceed 2 hrs because excessive absorption of the irrigating fluid may lead to dilutional hyponatremia, seizures and heart failure. The size of the enlarged prostate or adenoma, therefore, needs to be carefully assessed preop to determine if it is possible to complete the resection within a time limit of 2 hrs. If not, an open prostatectomy is performed. This variant approach is discussed under "Open Prostate Operations."

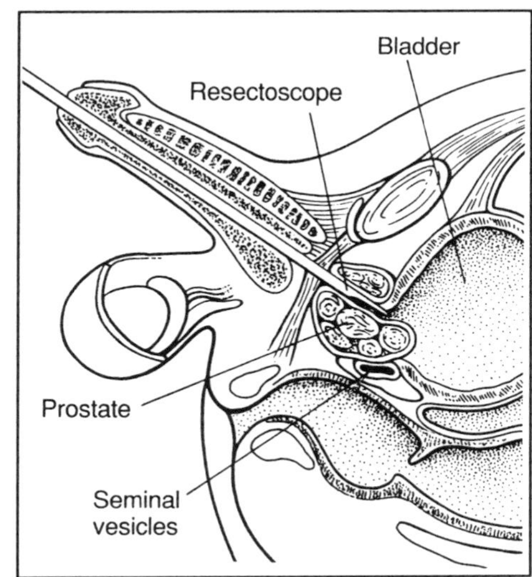


**Figure 9-2.** Transurethral resection of prostate using a resectoscope. (Reproduced with permission from Govan DE: *Roche Manual of Urologic Procedures*. Hoffmann-LaRoche: 1976.)

**Variant procedure or approaches:** Although **laser resection/ prostatectomy** is still an investigational operation, it has several demonstrated advantages over a regular resection. These include: decreased time of surgery, significantly less blood loss, and the fact that it can be done as an outpatient procedure.

**Usual preop diagnosis**: Benign prostatic hypertrophy; prostate cancer

### SUMMARY OF PROCEDURE

| | TURP | Laser TURP |
|---|---|---|
| **Position** | Lithotomy | ⇐ |
| **Incision** | None | ⇐ |
| **Special instrumentation** | Cystoscope; resectoscope; catheters; electrocautery | Cystoscope; resectoscope; catheters; electrocautery (stand-by); laser equipment |
| **Unique considerations** | During resection, the patient should be absolutely still because any movement may lead to perforation or injury to the external sphincter, leading to postop incontinence. | During resection, the patient and all personnel should wear protective eyeglasses. |
| **Antibiotics** | Gentamicin 80 mg iv, slowly | ⇐ |
| **Surgical time** | 1 - 2 hrs (not to exceed 2 hrs) | 1 hr |
| **EBL** | 500 cc | None |
| **Postop care** | Irrigation of the Foley catheter to clear it of clots and keep it from being blocked. Determination of serum Na. | ⇐ |
| **Mortality** | < 1% | Unknown (investigational procedure) |
| **Morbidity** | Significant intraop bleeding: 10%<br>Intraop perforation which may require a laparotomy: 5%<br>Postop bleeding which may necessitate a return to OR for fulguration of bleeding vessels: 5% | Unknown |

| | TURP | Laser TURP |
|---|---|---|
| **Morbidity, continued** | Absorption of irrigating fluid which may lead to dilutional hyponatremia, mental confusion and heart failure: 2% | |
| **Procedure code** | 52601 | Investigational |
| **Pain score** | 1 | 1 |

### PATIENT POPULATION CHARACTERISTICS

| | |
|---|---|
| **Age range** | 49-90 yrs; typically 70s and 80s |
| **Incidence** | Very common; 90% of men will develop benign hypertrophy; 20% may need surgical intervention |
| **Etiology** | Aging<br>Benign prostatic hypertrophy<br>Prostate cancer |
| **Associated conditions** | Chronic obstructive pulmonary disease: 10%<br>Heart disease: 10%<br>HTN: 10%<br>Diabetes: 5%<br>DIC – patients with prostate cancer may also have a low-grade, subclinical DIC, which becomes clinically manifest postop: 1-2% |

---

## ANESTHETIC CONSIDERATIONS

### PREOPERATIVE

Patients presenting for prostate surgery are generally elderly and are likely to have pre-existing medical problems, including: CAD, CHF, PVD, cerebrovascular disease, COPD and renal impairment. Preop evaluation should be directed toward the detection and treatment of these conditions prior to anesthesia.

| | |
|---|---|
| **Respiratory** | COPD common in this age group. Patients with >10 pack-year smoking Hx or with any respiratory Sx may need PFTs. For dyspnea with moderate exercise, ✓ VC, $FEV_1$, MMEF. If VC < 80%, $FEV_1$ < 60%, or MMEF < 40% predicted, ✓ ABG. If ABG and PFT markedly abnormal, consider postponing surgery until patient's respiratory condition has been optimized.<br>**Tests**: PFT; CXR; ABG, as indicated from H&P. |
| **Cardiovascular** | HTN, CAD common in this age group. Assess exercise tolerance by H&P (e.g., should be able to climb a flight of stairs without difficulty or SOB).<br>**Tests**: ECG; others as indicated from H&P. |
| **Neurological** | Cerebrovascular disease, Alzheimer's, and other neurologic problems may be present in this age group. Assess mental status to guide evaluation of any intraop or postop changes. |
| **Renal** | Anticipate renal impairment 2° chronic obstruction.<br>**Tests**: BUN; creatinine; electrolytes. If ↑BUN and ↑creatinine, ✓ creatinine clearance (normal= 95-140 ml/min). |
| **Musculoskeletal** | Various arthritides in this age group may cause problems with positioning for regional anesthesia and surgery. |
| **Endocrine** | Increased incidence of diabetes mellitus.<br>**Tests**: blood glucose; UA |
| **Hematologic** | Moderate blood loss expected with larger glands. If gland < 30 gm, no cross-match necessary; gland 30-80 gm, cross-match 2 U of blood; gland >80 gm, cross-match 4 U blood.<br>**Tests:** Hct |
| **Laboratory** | Other tests as indicated from H&P. |
| **Premedication** | Continue commonly used drugs (e.g., digitalis, β-blockers, NTG) to prevent cardiovascular problems. Sedation prn anxiety (e.g., lorazepam 1-2 mg po on call to OR). |

### INTRAOPERATIVE

**Anesthetic technique:** Regional or GA. Choice of technique depends on co-existing disease and patient preference. Regional anesthesia may hold some advantage over GA for TURP in that it allows evaluation of mental status, and, thus, earlier detection of TURP syndrome. The incidence of post-dural headache is very low in this age group (< 1%).

A T9 level is optimal. Continuous lumbar epidural anesthesia has no advantage over spinal anesthesia for TURP, since sacral block may be less reliable, the procedure is relatively short, and supplemental doses are usually not necessary.

**Regional anesthesia:**

| | |
|---|---|
| **Spinal** | 0.75% bupivacaine, 12 mg in 7.5% dextrose solution (1.6 cc) |

**General anesthesia:**

| | |
|---|---|
| **Induction** | Standard induction (see Appendix). |
| **Maintenance** | Standard maintenance (see Appendix). Muscle relaxation is not mandatory, although patient movement during the procedure must be avoided. |
| **Emergence** | Postop pain is usually not significant. Anticipate hypotension when legs are repositioned from lithotomy. Avoid stress on lumbar spine by slowly and simultaneously bringing legs together and returning to supine position. |

| | | |
|---|---|---|
| **Blood and fluid requirements** | Moderate blood loss<br>IV: 16-18 ga x 1<br>NS/LR @ 2-4 cc/kg/hr | Blood loss can be large if venous sinuses are entered; it can also be difficult to quantify because of irrigant. To flush away blood and tissue and to promote visibility during TURP, continuous irrigation is used. Irrigating fluid must be non-electrolytic to prevent dispersion of current, but near-iso-osmotic to prevent hemolysis of blood. For these reasons, sorbitol (2.7%) with mannitol (0.54%) or glycine (1.5%) are added to distilled water to produce solutions which are slightly hypo-osmolar to blood. |
| **Monitoring** | Standard monitors (see Appendix).<br>Regional anesthesia allows monitoring of mental status. Invasive monitoring if indicated from H&P. | |
| **TURP syndrome** | Intravascular volume overload<br>Hyponatremia<br>Hypotonicity 2° absorption of irrigant<br>Symptoms include:<br>-N&V<br>-Visual disturbances<br>-Mental status changes<br>-Coma<br>-Seizures<br>-HTN<br>-Angina<br>-Cardiovascular collapse | Factors which influence the absorption of irrigant include: hydrostatic pressure of irrigant (height of bag), number of venous sinuses opened, peripheral venous pressure, duration of surgery, and experience of the surgeon. Resections should optimally be limited to 1 hr or less. Some CNS manifestations are 2° glycine and its metabolites. Rx may include observation, diuresis (e.g., furosemide 5-20 mg iv), and administration of hypertonic saline (e.g., 100 cc 3% saline over 1-2 hrs). Serum sodium < 120 is associated with more severe symptoms, and the goal of therapy is to restore sodium to >120. In milder cases, observation and water restriction may be sufficient. |
| **Positioning** | ✓ and pad pressure points.<br>✓ eyes. | **NB**: peroneal nerve compression at lateral fibular head $\rightarrow$ foot drop. |
| **Complications** | Bladder perforation<br>TURP syndrome | Bladder perforation may produce shoulder pain in the awake patient. Bladder perforation (and TURP syndrome) may go unnoticed under GA; Sx: $\uparrow$BP, $\uparrow$HR (occasionally $\downarrow$BP). |

## POSTOPERATIVE

| | | |
|---|---|---|
| **Complications** | TURP syndrome<br>Bladder perforation<br>Fever/bacteremia/sepsis<br>Hypothermia | (See discussion of TURP syndrome, above.) |
| **Pain management** | Minimal postop pain | Rx: Morphine 1-4 mg iv prn until comfortable. |
| **Tests** | Hct; electrolytes<br>Blood cultures if febrile | Consider serum osmolarity, CXR, ECG in TURP syndrome. |

**References**

1. Mebust WK: Transurethral Surgery. In *Campbell's Urology*, 6th edition. Walsh PC, Retite AB, Stamey TA, Vaughn ED Jr, eds. WB Saunders Co, Philadelphia: 1992, Vol 3, Ch 80, 2900-22.
2. Jensen V: The TURP syndrome. *Can J Anaesth* 1991; 38(1):90-96.
3. Abrams PH, Shah PJ, Bryning K, et al: Blood loss during transurethral resection of the prostate. *Anaesthesia* 1982; 37(1):71-73.

# OPEN PROSTATE OPERATIONS

## SURGICAL CONSIDERATIONS

**Description**: Open (in contrast to transurethral or endoscopic) operations on the prostate gland are common. They include: **simple prostatectomy**; **radical prostatectomy**; and **retropubic exposure** of the prostate for brachytherapy through either a midline extraperitoneal incision which extends from the umbilicus to the symphysis pubis or through a Pfannenstiel incision (Fig 9-3, inset).

**Simple prostatectomy**: When the benign prostatic hypertrophy or adenoma is too large to be resected transurethrally, it is removed by a simple prostatectomy. The prostate gland is exposed through a retropubic approach (Fig 9-3A) and the anterior capsule is incised, exposing the adenoma — the central part of the prostate — which is excised, "shelled" out by finger dissection (Fig 9-3B), leaving behind the peripheral prostate and all the associated structures. A Foley catheter is left indwelling in the urethra, and the incision in the prostate capsule is closed. In a **suprapubic prostatectomy**, the incision is made in the bladder and the adenoma shelled from within the bladder.

**Radical prostatectomy**: The term "radical prostatectomy" may be misleading. It is used to differentiate this cancer operation from a simple prostatectomy (used for benign prostatic hypertrophy). Radical prostatectomy can be achieved through either a **retropubic** or **perineal approach**, the choice being a matter of training, expertise and surgeon's preference. In radical prostatectomy, all of the prostate gland is removed, together with the bladder neck, the seminal vesicles and the ampullae of the vas deferens. A **limited pelvic lymphadenectomy** is also performed. After the prostate gland and its associated structures are removed, the bladder neck is reduced to 1 cm diameter and anastomosed to the membranous urethra over an indwelling Foley catheter. The majority of the blood loss occurs during control of the dorsal vein complex. In the past 10 yrs, attempts have been made to preserve potency by preserving the nerves to the corpora cavernosa.

**Retropubic exposure of the prostate** is performed in preparation for brachytherapy (interstitial irradiation). The anterior aspect of the prostate glad is exposed through an extraperitoneal suprapubic incision

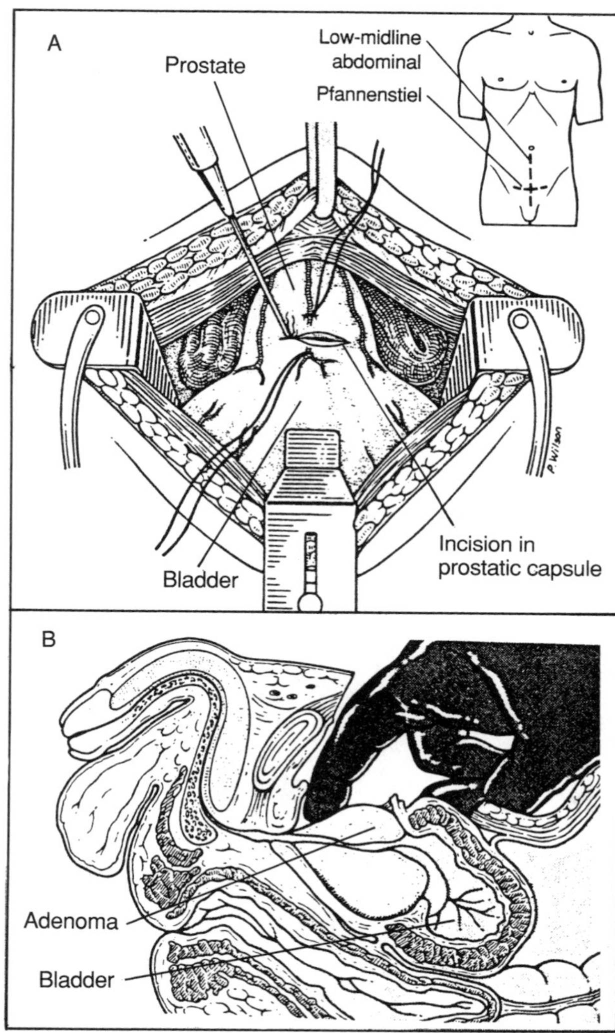


**Figure 9-3.** Simple retropubic prostatectomy: (A) incision made in the anterior prostatic capsule; (B) adenoma is "shelled out" by finger dissection. (Reproduced with permission from: *Atlas of General Surgery*. Butterworths: 1986.) Inset shows midline abdominal and Pfannenstiel incisions.

(Pfannenstiel) and the gland is implanted with radioactive material, either directly through the incision, or perineally through a template.

**Usual preop diagnosis:** Benign prostatic hypertrophy; prostate cancer

**SUMMARY OF PROCEDURE**

| | Simple Prostatectomy | Radical–Retropubic | Radical–Perineal | Retropubic Exposure |
|---|---|---|---|---|
| **Position** | Supine | ⇐ | Lithotomy | Supine |
| **Incision** | Extraperitoneal, low midline or Pfannenstiel (Fig 9-3, inset) | ⇐ | Perineal (Fig 9-4) | Extraperitoneal, low midline or Pfannenstiel (Fig 9-3, inset) |
| **Unique considerations** | None | ⇐ | Extreme hip flexion | Use of radioactive material |
| **Antibiotics** | Gentamicin 80 mg iv, slowly | ⇐ | ⇐ | ⇐ |
| **Surgical time** | 1 hr | 3 hrs | ⇐ | 2 hrs |
| **EBL** | 500 cc | 1500 cc | 500 cc | Minimal |
| **Postop care** | Irrigate catheter to clear blood clots and prevent obstruction, frequently if urine is bloody. | ⇐ | ⇐ | ⇐ |
| **Mortality** | < 1% | ⇐ | ⇐ | ⇐ |
| **Morbidity** | Bleeding: 2% | ⇐ | ⇐ | ⇐ |
| | DVT: 2% | ⇐ | ⇐ | ⇐ |
| | Infection: 2% | ⇐ | ⇐ | ⇐ |
| | PE: 1% | ⇐ | ⇐ | ⇐ |
| | | Impotence:<br>-Non nerve-sparing: 100%<br>-Nerve-sparing: 50%<br>Lymphocele: 4% | | |
| **Procedure code** | 55831 | 55840 | 55810 | 55860 |
| **Pain score** | 8 | 8 | 6 | 8 |

**PATIENT POPULATION CHARACTERISTICS**

| | |
|---|---|
| **Age range** | 40-80 yrs |
| **Incidence** | 20% of men will develop symptomatic benign prostatic hypertrophy; 9% will develop clinically evident prostate cancer. |
| **Etiology** | Aging |
| **Associated conditions** | COPD: 10%<br>CAD: 10%<br>HTN: 10%<br>Diabetes mellitus: 5%<br>Renal failure: 1% |

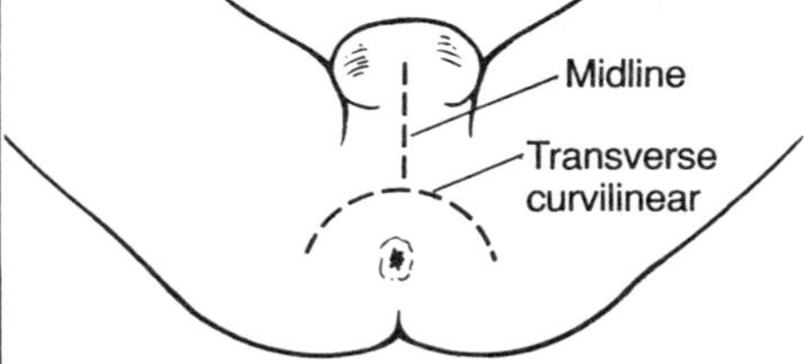


**Figure 9-4.** Perineal incisions.

# ANESTHETIC CONSIDERATIONS

## PREOPERATIVE

Patients presenting for prostate surgery are generally elderly and are likely to have pre-existing medical problems, including: CAD, CHF, PVD, cerebrovascular disease, COPD and renal impairment. Preop evaluation should be directed toward the detection and treatment of these conditions prior to anesthesia.

| | |
|---|---|
| **Respiratory** | COPD common in this age group. Patients with Hx of >10 pack-year smoking or with respiratory Sx may require PFTs. For dyspnea with moderate exercise, check VC, $FEV_1$, MMEF. If VC < 80%, $FEV_1$ < 60%, or MMEF < 40% predicted, check ABG. If ABG and PFT are markedly abnormal, consider postponing surgery until patient's respiratory condition has been optimized.<br>**Tests**: PFT; CXR; ABG, as indicated from H&P. |
| **Cardiovascular** | HTN, CAD common in this age group. Assess exercise tolerance by H&P (e.g., should be able to climb a flight of stairs without difficulty or SOB).<br>**Tests**: ECG; others as indicated from H&P. |
| **Neurological** | Cerebrovascular disease, Alzheimer's and other neurologic problems may be present in this age group. Assess mental status to guide evaluation of any intraop or postop changes. |
| **Renal** | Anticipate renal impairment 2° chronic obstruction.<br>**Tests**: BUN; creatinine; electrolytes. If ↑BUN and ↑creatinine: check creatinine clearance (normal=95-140 ml/min). |
| **Musculoskeletal** | Various arthritides may cause problems with positioning for regional anesthesia and surgery. |
| **Endocrine** | Increased incidence of diabetes mellitus.<br>**Tests**: blood glucose; UA |
| **Hematologic** | Moderate blood loss expected with larger glands. For glands < 30 gm, no cross-match necessary; for glands 30-80 gm, cross-match 2 U of blood; for glands >80 gm, cross-match 4 U blood.<br>**Tests:** Hct |
| **Laboratory** | Other tests as indicated from H&P. |
| **Premedication** | Continue commonly used drugs (e.g., digitalis, β-blockers, diuretics, NTG) to prevent cardiovascular complications. Sedation prn anxiety (e.g., lorazepam 1-2 mg po on call to OR). |

## INTRAOPERATIVE

**Anesthetic technique:** Regional (spinal, continuous spinal, continuous lumbar epidural) or GA are acceptable techniques. If regional anesthesia used, optimal block level is T8-T10 (depending on incision site). Advantages of regional anesthesia include potential for lower intraop blood loss, and possible lower incidence of DVT postop. Disadvantages include positioning considerations (see below).

**Regional anesthesia:**

| | |
|---|---|
| **Spinal** | Hyperbaric tetracaine 10-15 mg with epinephrine 200 $\mu g$ (0.2 cc of 1:1000 solution). |
| **Epidural** | 1.5-2% lidocaine with epinephrine 5 $\mu g$/cc, 15-25 cc, supplemental iv sedation as necessary. Additional epidural lidocaine (5-10 cc boluses) may be needed, depending on length of procedure. |

**General anesthesia:**

| | |
|---|---|
| **Induction** | Standard induction (see Appendix). |
| **Maintenance** | Standard maintenance (see Appendix). |
| **Emergence** | No special considerations |

| | | |
|---|---|---|
| **Blood and fluid requirements** | Moderate-to-large blood loss<br>IV: 14-16 ga x 1-2<br>NS/LR @ 4-6 cc/kg/hr | Additional requirements dependent on type of anesthesia. Regional techniques are associated with higher fluid requirement because of sympathectomy and systemic vasodilation; it also may be associated with lower blood loss than GA.[4] |
| **Monitoring** | Standard monitors (see Appendix).<br>Depending on underlying disease:<br>± CVP<br>± Arterial line | Some patients require CVP to aid in assessment of volume status. Arterial line is often useful for continuous BP monitoring and frequent blood draws. Patients at particularly high risk (e.g., history of pre-existing cardiopulmonary disease) should probably have both. |
| **Positioning** | Anticipate hypotension on return from lithotomy position.<br>✓ and pad pressure points.<br>✓ eyes. | Rx: volume (200-500 cc NS/LR) or ephedrine (5 mg iv) may be necessary. Elderly patients with arthritis or respiratory impairment may not tolerate the extreme positioning associated with perineal prostatectomy for extended periods of time, thus precluding the use of regional anesthesia (a combined technique with GA may be considered). **NB**: peroneal nerve compression at lateral fibular head → foot drop. |

## POSTOPERATIVE

| | | |
|---|---|---|
| **Complications** | Peroneal nerve injury 2° lithotomy position | Manifested by foot drop with loss of sensation on dorsum of foot. Seek neurology consultation. |
| | DVT | Incidence of DVT less with regional than GA. Sx: variable, with pain and tenderness over involved area. |
| **Pain management** | Significant postop pain. Rx: morphine 0.1-0.3 mg/kg iv in incremental doses (e.g., 2-4 mg q 10-15 min prn). | Consider epidural narcotic or PCA (see Appendix). |
| **Tests** | Hct | |


**References**

1. Stutzman RE, Walsh PC: Suprapubic and Retropubic Prostatectomy. In *Campbell's Urology*, 6th edition. Walsh PC, et al, eds. WB Saunders Co, Philadelphia: 1992, Vol 3, Ch 77, 2851-64.
2. Walsh PC: Radical Retropubic Prostatectomy. In *Campbell's Urology*, 6th edition. WB Saunders Co, Philadelphia: 1992, Vol 3, Ch 78, 2865-86.
3. Paulson DF: Perineal Prostatectomy. In *Campbell's Urology*, 6th edition. WB Saunders Co, Philadelphia: 1992, Vol 3, Ch 79, 2887-99.
4. Hendolin H, Mattila MA, Poikolainen E: The effect of lumbar epidural analgesia on the development of deep vein thrombosis of the legs after open prostatectomy. *Acta Chir Scand* 1981; 147(6):425-29.
5. Donald JR: The effect of anaesthesia, hypotension, and epidural analgesia on blood loss in surgery for pelvic floor repair. *Br J Anaesth* 1969; 41(2):155-66.


# NEPHRECTOMY

## SURGICAL CONSIDERATIONS

**Description**: Nephrectomies fall into three basic groups: simple, partial and radical. (Surgical anatomy is illustrated in Fig 9-5.)

**Simple nephrectomy**, performed for benign conditions, is the surgical excision of the kidney and only a small segment of proximal ureter. The dorsal approach is well-suited for this operation, and begins with an incision extending from the 12th rib to the iliac crest along the lateral edge of the sacrospinalis muscle and quadratus lumborum muscle. The dorsolumbar fascia is opened, exposing Gerota's fascia and the perinephric fat. The kidney is mobilized until the hilum is exposed. The artery and vein are tied, suture-ligated and transected. The ureter is followed distally as far as possible, tied and transected; and the kidney is delivered out of the incision, which is then closed by approximating the dorsolumbar fascia and the fascia of the sacrospinalis muscle.
**Usual preop diagnosis:** Chronic hydronephrosis; hypoplastic kidney; renovascular HTN; double collecting system

**Partial nephrectomy** is the surgical excision of the segment of the kidney harboring the pathology. It is performed for small renal-cell carcinomas and benign tumors of the kidney, such as angiomyolipomas, and for duplicated collecting systems with a diseased moiety. If the partial nephrectomy is being done for renal-cell carcinoma, it may be accompanied with a **regional lymphadenectomy**. The flank approach is well-suited for this operation, and begins with an incision over the 12th or 11th rib, or in between, and extends anteriorly over the external and internal oblique muscles, which are transected. The transversalis muscle and fascia are opened, exposing Gerota's fascia. The renal capsule is exposed at the planned site of resection. Control of the renal vessels is advised for control of bleeding, if excessive. Incision in the renal parenchyma is made by sharp and blunt dissection, suture-ligating all bleeders. If the collecting system is opened, it should be closed with absorbable sutures. After complete hemostasis, Gelfoam® or perinephric fat is used to cover the raw surface of the kidney.
**Usual preop diagnosis:** Renal-cell carcinoma; double collecting system

**Radical nephrectomy** is the surgical excision of the kidney, with its surrounding perinephric fat and Gerota's fascia,

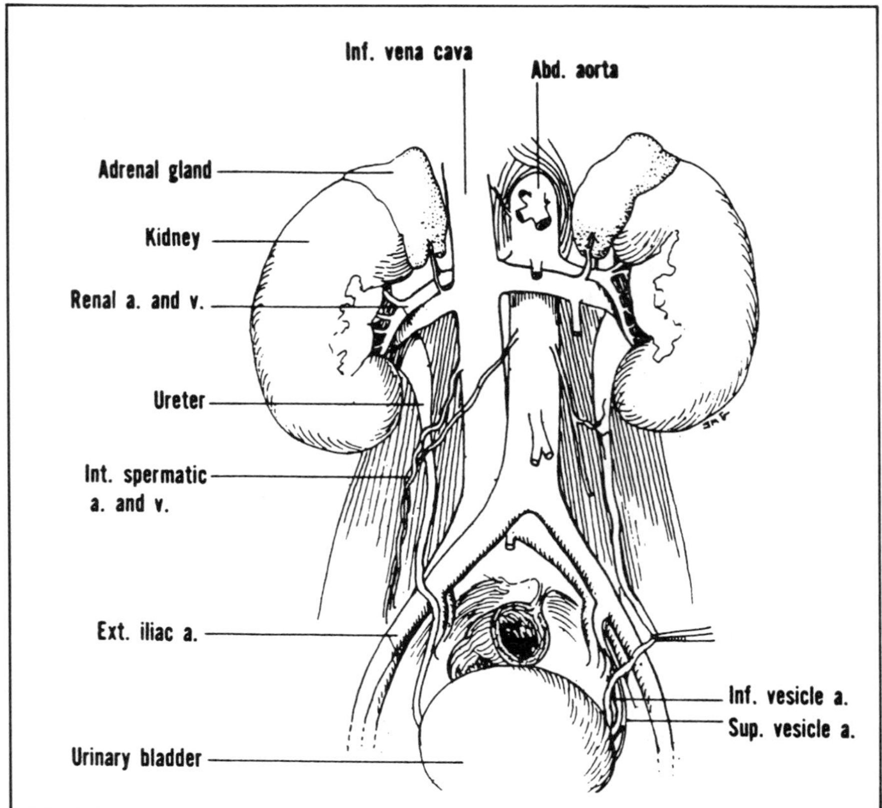


**Figure 9-5.** Surgical anatomy of the urinary tract. (Reproduced with permission from Hardy JD: *Textbook of Surgery*. Lippincott: 1988.)

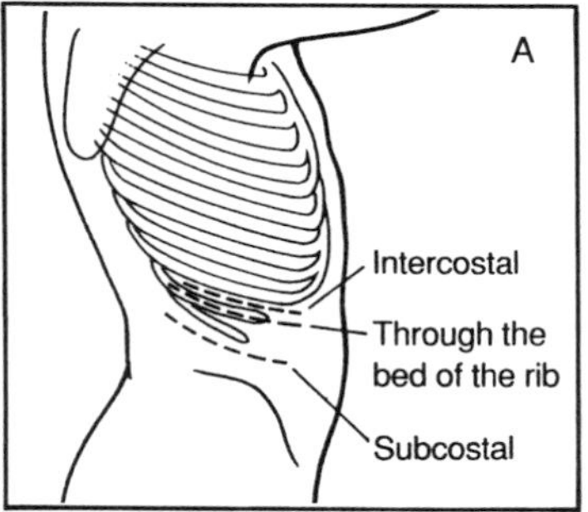


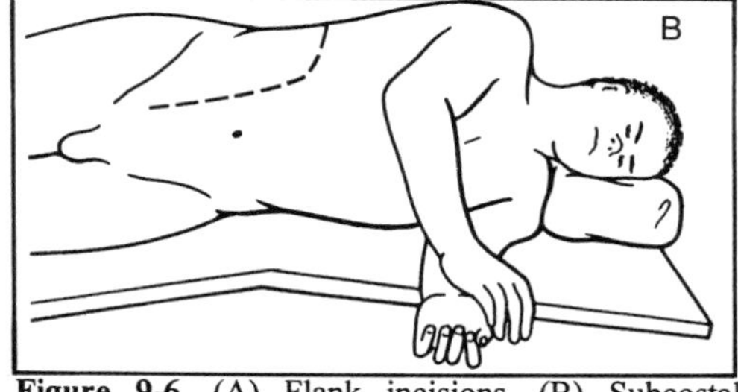


**Figure 9-6.** (A) Flank incisions. (B) Subcostal transabdominal incision.

and the proximal 2/3rds of the ureter, accompanied by paracaval or para-aortic **lymphadenectomy**. It is performed for renal-cell carcinoma. Early control of renal vessels is advised before excessive manipulation of the tumor, to minimize blood loss and hematogenous spread. Transabdominal or flank approaches are best suited for this operation. **Nephroureterectomy** is a radical nephrectomy with ureter resection, including the ureteral orifice and a cuff of bladder wall around it. It is accompanied by a regional lymphadenectomy since it is performed for a cancerous condition. The approach is either transabdominal or extra-peritoneal through an extended flank incision, starting at the tip of the 11th rib and curving caudally along the lateral edge of the rectus abdominis muscle down to the pubic bone. Some surgeons prefer two separate incisions: a flank incision for the radical nephrectomy part and a lower abdominal incision for the ureterectomy.

**Usual preop diagnosis**: Renal-cell carcinoma; Wilms' tumor; transitional-cell carcinoma of the renal collecting system or ureter

## SUMMARY OF PROCEDURE

| | Simple Nephrectomy | Partial Nephrectomy | Radical Nephrectomy |
|---|---|---|---|
| **Position** | Flank or prone | Flank | Supine or flank |
| **Incision** | Flank (Fig 9-6A) or dorsal along paraspinous muscles | Flank (Fig 9-6A) | Midline or subcostal transabdominal (Fig 9-6B) or flank; subcostal or intercostal or through bed of 11th or 12th rib (Fig 9-6A). |
| **Unique considerations** | None | ⇐ | If tumor involves renal vein and/or IVC, clamp IVC. |
| **Antibiotics** | None | ⇐ | ⇐ |
| **Surgical time** | 2 - 3 hrs | 3 - 4 hrs | ⇐ |
| **Closing considerations** | Chest tube may be required if pleura opened with flank incision. | ⇐ | ⇐ |

| | Simple Nephrectomy | Partial Nephrectomy | Radical Nephrectomy |
|---|---|---|---|
| **EBL** | 500 cc | 1200 cc | 500 cc |
| **Mortality** | < 1% | ⇐ | 1% |
| **Morbidity** | Prolonged ileus: 5%<br>Pneumothorax 2° unrecognized pleural perforation: 2% | ⇐ | ⇐ |
| **Procedure code** | 50220 | 50240 | 50234 |
| **Pain score** | 10 | 10 | 10 |

### PATIENT POPULATION CHARACTERISTICS

| | | | |
|---|---|---|---|
| **Age range** | All ages | ⇐ | ⇐ |
| **Male:Female** | 1:1 | ⇐ | ⇐ |
| **Incidence** | < 1% | ⇐ | ⇐ |
| **Etiology** | Double collecting system<br>Chronic hydronephrosis<br>Hypoplastic kidney<br>Renovascular HTN | ⇐<br>Localized renal-cell carcinoma | Wilms' tumor: 8% of all childhood malignancies<br>Transitional-cell carcinoma: 7% of all kidney tumors<br>Renal-cell carcinoma: 3% of adult malignancies |
| **Associated conditions** | HTN if nephrectomy is used for renovascular HTN. | | |

## ANESTHETIC CONSIDERATIONS

See Anesthetic Considerations following "Operations on the Renal Pelvis and Upper Ureter" (below).


**References**

1. Novic AC, Streem SB: Surgery of the Kidney. In *Campbell's Urology*, 6th edition. WB Saunders Co, Philadelphia: 1992, Vol 3, Ch 65, 2413-2500.
2. Coleman DL: Control of postoperative pain: non-narcotic and narcotic alternatives and their effect on pulmonary function. *Chest* 1987; 92(3):520-28.


# OPERATIONS ON THE RENAL PELVIS AND UPPER URETER

## SURGICAL CONSIDERATIONS

**Description:** Operations on the renal pelvis and upper ureter are becoming less common because of the increasing use of endoscopic and percutaneous procedures. The basic surgical approach is the same as that for nephrectomy (see previous procedure). Specific procedures include:

**Pyeloplasty** is the surgical correction of congenital ureteropelvic junction stenosis to relieve obstruction. The most commonly used is the **dismembered pyeloplasty**, or **Anderson-Heinz pyeloplasty**, wherein the diseased ureteropelvic junction is excised, the redundant renal pelvis is reduced, and an anastomosis is established between the renal pelvis and ureter (Fig 9-7).

**Usual preop diagnosis:** Ureteropelvic junction obstruction

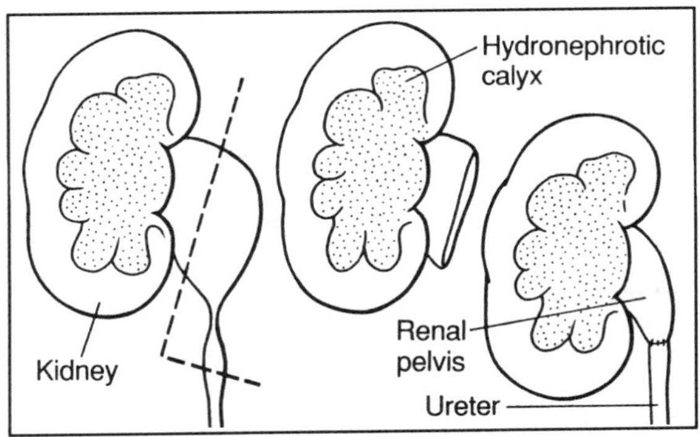


**Figure 9-7.** Dismembered pyeloplasty.

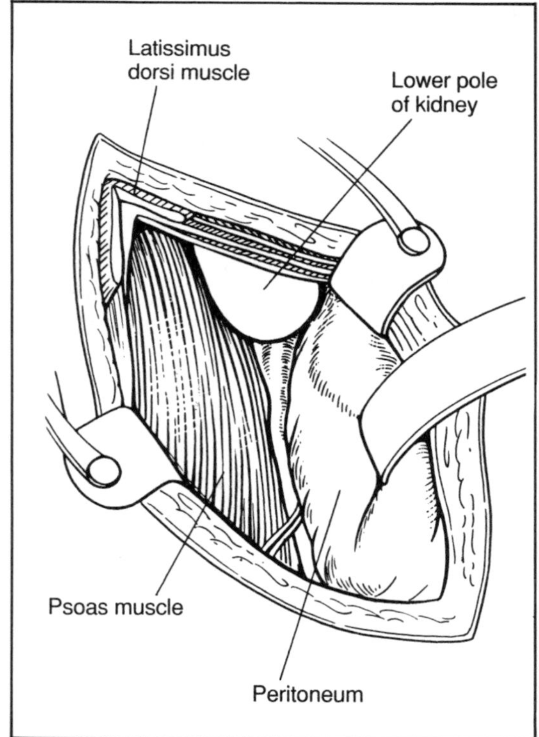


**Figure 9-8.** Surgical exposure of the lower pole of kidney, renal pelvis and proximal ureter. (Reproduced with permission from *Atlas of General Surgery*. Butterworths: 1986.)

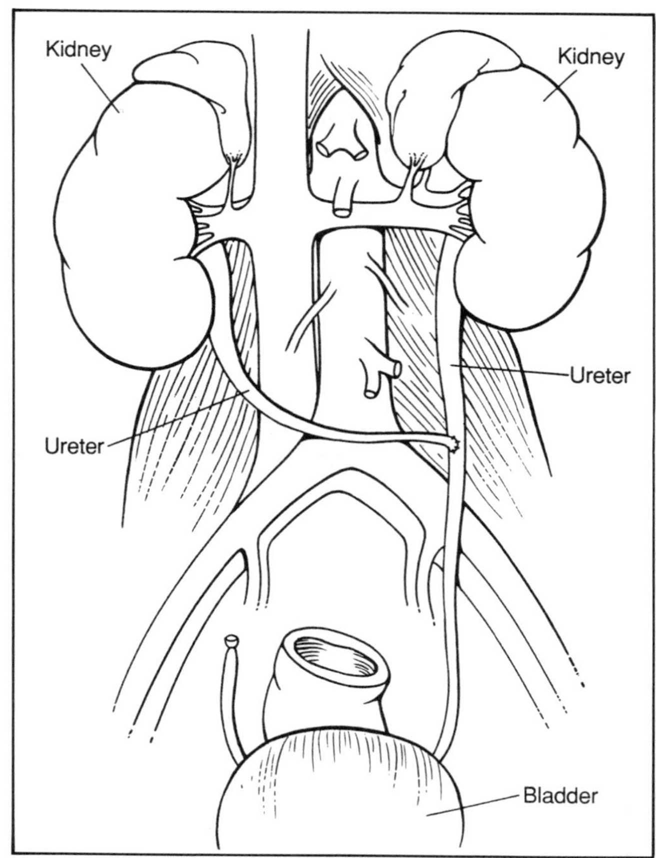


**Figure 9-9.** Transureteroureterostomy.

**Pyelolithotomy and ureterolithotomy** are used to remove calculi from the renal pelvis or ureter. The upper ureter and renal pelvis are exposed (Fig 9-8), usually through a flank approach, the calculus is palpated and an incision is made in the ureter or renal pelvis over the calculus, which is then delivered. The incision is closed with fine, absorbable sutures.

**Usual preop diagnosis:** Renal pelvic or ureteral stone

**Transureteroureterostomy** is the transposition of one ureter across the midline and anastomosing it to the other ureter (Fig 9-9). This operation is performed whenever the distal ureter is traumatized or diseased, and the proximal ureter is not long enough to re-implant into the bladder. The recipient ureter should be normal.

**Usual preop diagnosis**: Traumatic loss of distal ureter; distal ureteral tumor requiring distal ureterectomy

## SUMMARY OF PROCEDURE

| | Pyeloplasty | Pyelolithotomy/ Ureterolithotomy | Transuretero-ureterostomy |
|---|---|---|---|
| **Position** | Flank or prone | ⇐ | Supine |
| **Incision** | Flank (Fig 9-6) or dorsal | ⇐ | Midline abdominal (Fig 9-3, inset) |
| **Antibiotics** | None | ⇐ | ⇐ |
| **Surgical time** | 3 hrs | 1 - 2 hrs | 3 hrs |
| **EBL** | Minimal | ⇐ | ⇐ |
| **Mortality** | < 1% | ⇐ | ⇐ |
| **Morbidity** | Urinary leakage: 5%<br>Infection: 2% | ⇐ | ⇐ |
| **Procedure code** | 50405 | 50130, 50610 | 50770 |
| **Pain score** | 10 | 10 | 10 |

### PATIENT POPULATION CHARACTERISTICS

| | Pyeloplasty | Pyelolithotomy/ Ureterolithotomy | Transuretero-ureterostomy |
|---|---|---|---|
| **Age range** | All ages | ⇐ | ⇐ |
| **Male:Female** | 1:1 | ⇐ | ⇐ |
| **Incidence** | Rare | Extremely rare | ⇐ |
| **Etiology** | Ureteropelvic junction obstruction: 80% (of causes of dilated collecting system in the newborn) | Renal pelvic and upper ureteral stone | Traumatic loss of lower ureter<br>Lower ureteral tumor |
| **Associated conditions** | Renal failure: 1% | ⇐ | ⇐ |

## ANESTHETIC CONSIDERATIONS

### PREOPERATIVE

**Respiratory** Increased postop pulmonary complications because of location of incision. If Hx of pulmonary disease (e.g., asthma, COPD), consider postop respiratory therapy.
**Tests:** PFTs, ABG – as indicated from H&P.

**Cardiovascular** Consider possibility of renal HTN.

**Hematologic** Polycythemia may be seen in association with polycystic kidney disease, renal-cell carcinoma. Consider preop blood donation for autologous transfusion.
**Tests**: Hct

**Laboratory** Electrolytes; BUN; creatinine; other tests as indicated from H&P.

**Premedication** Standard premedication (see Appendix).

### INTRAOPERATIVE

**Anesthetic technique:** GA is recommended for these procedures; technique depends on underlying disease. Regional techniques (spinal or epidural) are alternatives, but are less than optimal because of awkward positioning which may lead to patient discomfort and pain resulting from diaphragmatic stimulation.

**Induction** Standard induction (see Appendix).

**Maintenance** Standard maintenance (see Appendix). If intraperitoneal approach is used, consider limiting $N_2O$ to avoid distention of bowel and interference with operative field. If IVC must be cross-clamped, the resulting hypotension should be treated with fluids and vasopressors.

**Emergence** No specific considerations

**Blood and fluid requirements**
Mild-to-moderate blood loss
IV: 14-16 ga x 1
NS/LR @ 6-8 cc/kg/hr
Warm all fluids.

Intraperitoneal approach associated with higher fluid requirements (8-10 cc/kg/hr). When renal vessels are to be cross-clamped, mannitol (0.5 gm/kg) is often given prior to occlusion (20 min maximum).

**Monitoring**
Standard monitors (see Appendix).
Urinary catheter

Invasive monitoring if indicated from H&P.

**Positioning**
Use axillary roll if lateral.
Avoid stretching brachial plexus – limit abduction to 90°.
If prone, repeatedly ✓ eyes and pressure points.
Assure free excursion of abdomen.

The lateral position with kidney rest and table flexion may lead to hypotension, possibly 2° vena cava obstruction. Moderate iv volume administration, as well as gradual assumption of the position, are recommended to avoid this complication.

**Complications**
Pneumothorax
Hypotension with positioning (see above).
Indigo carmine → ↑BP, ↑SVR
Methylene blue → ↓BP

Sx of pneumothorax include: ↑RR, ↑PIP, hypoxemia, hypercarbia. If in doubt, ✓ CXR.

### POSTOPERATIVE

| | | |
|---|---|---|
| **Complications** | Post-nephrectomy syndrome<br>Eye injury (if prone)<br>Brachial plexus injury (if lateral)<br>Pneumothorax<br>Atelectasis<br>Pneumonia | Post-nephrectomy syndrome 2° retractor injury. L1 nerve root damage with resulting pain, dysesthesia and sensory loss in L1 dermatome distribution. |
| **Pain management** | Morphine 0.1-0.3 mg/kg iv in incremental doses<br>Consider epidural narcotic, PCA (see Appendix). | Postop analgesia critical to minimize pulmonary complications. |
| **Tests** | Hct; CXR | Others dependent on operative course, co-existing disease. |

References

1. Greenstein A, Vernon Smith MJ, Koontz WW Jr: Surgery of the Ureter. In *Campbell's Urology*, 6th edition. Walsh PC, et al, eds. WB Saunders Co, Philadelphia: 1992, Vol 3, Ch 68, 2552-70.

# CYSTECTOMY

## SURGICAL CONSIDERATIONS

**Description**: Open (in contrast to transurethral or endoscopic) bladder operations (cystectomies) account for 15-20% of all urological procedures. They are grouped as simple, partial and radical procedures.

**Simple cystectomy** is performed for benign conditions of the bladder, such as severe hemorrhagic cystitis, radiation cystitis, and contracted bladder. It involves the removal of the bladder only. The operation is performed through a lower abdominal incision. The peritoneal reflections are incised down to the pouch of Douglas; the vasa deferentia are identified, cross-clamped, transected and tied. The superior vesical arteries are identified, cross-clamped near their origin, transected and tied. The ureters are identified, separated from the surrounding tissues, cross-clamped near the bladder, transected and tied. The bladder is bluntly separated from the anterior rectal wall all the way to the apex of the prostate. The lateral pedicles of the bladder are cross-clamped, cut and tied. The endopelvic fascia is incised, separating the prostate from the lateral pelvic wall. The puboprostatic ligaments are transected and the dorsal vein of the penis is suture-ligated. The tied dorsal vein and urethra are incised just distal to the apex of the prostate. The specimen is delivered out of the incision and hemostasis secured with electrocautery. An ileal conduit is then performed (see below).

**Partial cystectomy** is the excision of only the part of the bladder containing the pathology. This is not a commonly performed operation and is reserved for tumors located in the dome of the bladder of older patients who are poor surgical risks for major operations such as radical cystectomy. The operation is preceded by a cystoscopy to identify the site of pathology. Beginning with a lower abdominal incision, the dome and lateral walls of the bladder are separated from the surrounding tissues, which are covered by wet packs in order to minimize contamination. An incision is made in the dome of the bladder at least 2 cm away from the pathology. The inside of the bladder is inspected and the pathology identified. The incision in the bladder is continued around, and at least 2 cm away from, the pathology, until the latter is completely excised. Bleeders in the wall of the bladder are electrocoagulated. The bladder wall is then closed in 2 layers — a through-and-through layer and an inverting layer — using absorbable material. Wet packs are removed, a drain is left in the region and the abdominal incision is closed.

**Radical cystectomy** (or **radical cystoprostatectomy**) is performed for treatment of invasive bladder cancer. It encompasses the removal of the bladder and the lower ureters, the prostate gland and seminal vesicles in men, and the uterus, ovaries and anterior vaginal wall in women (Fig 9-10, A&B). Accompanied by a **pelvic lymphadenectomy**, it is performed in the supine position, except when a concomitant **urethrectomy** is required, wherein a lithotomy position is used.

Following cystectomy, whether radical or simple, some form of **urinary diversion** is required. This can be accomplished with either a standard ileal conduit or a bladder substitution. The **ileal conduit** is constructed from 6-8 inches of terminal ileum isolated from the small intestine with its blood supply. The continuity of the small intestine is accomplished by a simple anastomosis. The ureters are implanted into the proximal end of the conduit and the distal end is brought through the abdominal wall as a stoma (Fig 9-11). **Bladder substitution** is a more complex operation wherein a longer segment of bowel is isolated, with its blood supply, and fashioned into a pouch. The ureters are implanted in the pouch and the most dependent part of the pouch is connected to the membranous urethra, avoiding a stoma (Fig 9-12). Not all patients undergoing cystectomies are candidates for bladder substitution. For example, patients who require a urethrectomy are not candidates because of the need to remove the urethra.

**Usual preop diagnosis**: Bladder cancer; contracted bladder; hemorrhagic cystitis; radiation cystitis; bladder diverticulum

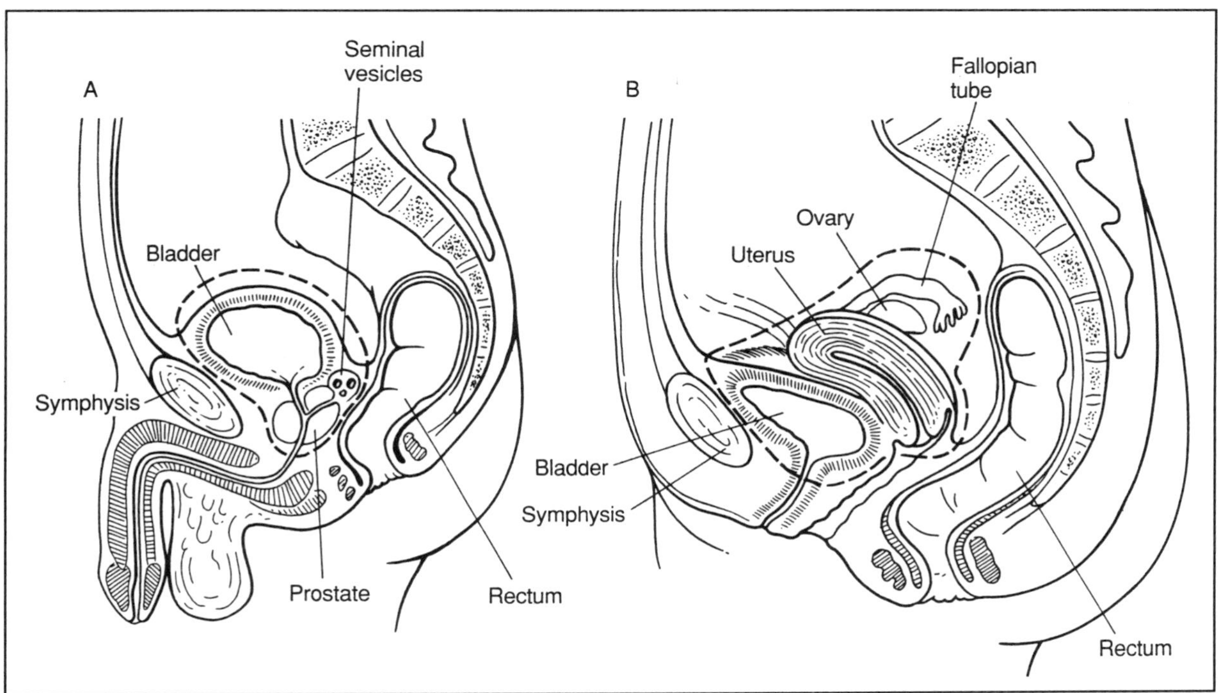


**Figure 9-10.** Anatomy of the pelvis with tissue to be excised outlined by dashed line: (A) male; (b) female. (Reproduced with permission from *Atlas of General Surgery*. Butterworths: 1986.)

## SUMMARY OF PROCEDURE

| | Simple Cystectomy | Partial Cystectomy | Radical Cystectomy |
|---|---|---|---|
| **Position** | Supine | ⇐ | Supine or lithotomy |
| **Incision** | Transperitoneal, midline | ⇐ | ⇐ |
| **Antibiotics** | Parenteral broad spectrum (e.g., gentamicin 80 mg im) | ⇐ | ⇐ |
| **Surgical time** | 4 hrs | 2 hrs | 6 hrs |
| **EBL** | 1000 cc | Minimal | 1500 cc |
| **Postop care** | Care of the stoma | Catheter care | Care of the stoma |
| **Mortality** | 1% | < 1% | 2% |
| **Morbidity** | Prolonged ileus: 5% | – | 5% |
| | Infection: 2% | – | 2% |
| | | Hematuria: 5% | |
| **Procedure code** | 51570 | 51550 | 51596 |
| **Pain score** | 10 | 10 | 10 |

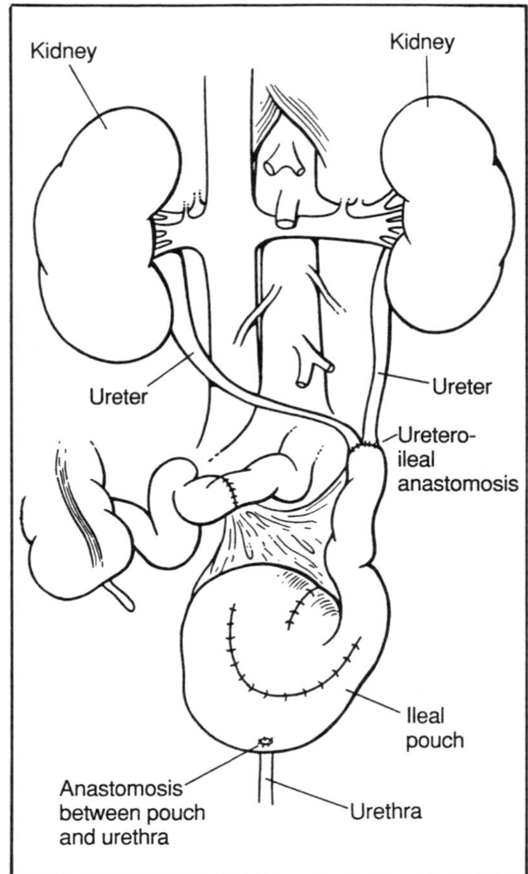


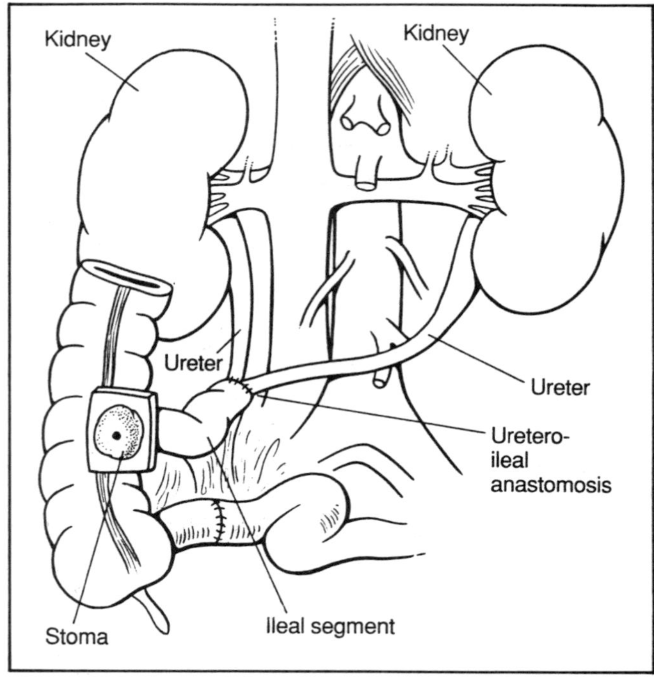


↑**Figure 9-11.** Ileal conduit. A segment of ileum is isolated from terminal ileum and continuity of the bowel is re-established with an end-to-end anastomosis. Ureters are joined to the proximal end of the ileal segment and the distal end is brought out to the skin as a stoma.

←**Figure 9-12.** Bladder substitution. A segment of ileum is fashioned into a pouch and anastomosed to the urethra. The ureters are joined to the proximal, non-detubularized segment.

### PATIENT POPULATION CHARACTERISTICS

| | Simple Cystectomy | Partial Cystectomy | Radical Cystectomy |
|---|---|---|---|
| **Age range** | 40-80 yrs | ⇐ | ⇐ |
| **Male:Female** | 3:1 | ⇐ | ⇐ |
| **Incidence** | 40,000 new cases of bladder cancer diagnosed/yr; 20% treated with cystectomy. | ⇐ | ⇐ |
| **Etiology** | Contracted bladder<br>Hemorrhagic and radiation cystitis | Bladder cancer<br>Bladder diverticulum | ⇐ |
| **Associated conditions** | Heart disease: 10%<br>HTN: 10%<br>COPD: 5%<br>Diabetes mellitus: 5% | ⇐ | ⇐ |

---

## ANESTHETIC CONSIDERATIONS

### PREOPERATIVE

**Respiratory** Note Hx of pulmonary disease in older patients.
**Tests:** As indicated from H&P.

**Cardiovascular** Note Hx of cardiac disease, HTN in older patients.
**Tests:** ECG; others as indicated from H&P.

| | | |
|---|---|---|
| **Gastrointestinal** | Bowel prep likely and may cause dehydration and electrolyte disturbances.<br>**Tests:** Electrolytes | |
| **Hematologic** | T&C for 2-4 U PRBC.<br>**Tests:** Hct; PT; PTT | |
| **Laboratory** | Other tests as indicated from H&P. | |
| **Premedication** | Sedation prn anxiety in adults; lorazepam 1-2 mg po 1-2 hrs preop; midazolam 1-2 mg iv in preop area. | |

## INTRAOPERATIVE

**Anesthetic technique:** Spinal, continuous lumbar epidural or GA are acceptable, with choice dependent on length of procedure, co-existing disease and patient preference. A combined technique using GA and regional anesthesia may be preferable. A T4 sensory level is recommended since peritoneal stimulation is likely during this procedure.

**Regional anesthesia:**

| | | |
|---|---|---|
| **Spinal** | 0.75% bupivacaine 12-15 mg in 7.5% dextrose; hyperbaric tetracaine 10-15 mg with 200 μg epinephrine for procedures longer than 3 hrs. | |
| **Epidural** | 1.5-2% lidocaine with epinephrine 5 μg/15-25 cc; supplement with 5-10 cc as needed. Supplemental iv sedation (e.g., midazolam 1.0 mg iv prn, fentanyl 50 μg iv prn) | |

**General anesthesia:**

| | | |
|---|---|---|
| **Induction** | Standard induction (see Appendix). These patients may be significantly dehydrated and require volume replacement before induction. | |
| **Maintenance** | Standard maintenance (see Appendix). | |
| **Emergence** | No specific considerations | |
| **Blood and fluid requirements** | Significant blood loss possible<br>IV: 16 ga x 1<br>NS/LR @ 6-10 cc/kg/hr<br>Warm fluids.<br>Humidify gasses. | Blood loss may be less with regional than GA. |
| **Monitoring** | Standard monitors (see Appendix).<br>Arterial line<br>CVP line | Consider PA catheter in patients with cardiopulmonary disease. UO as measure of volume status may be lost during procedure. |
| **Complications** | Major blood loss<br>3rd-space losses<br>Hypothermia | |

## POSTOPERATIVE

| | | |
|---|---|---|
| **Complications** | Hypothermia | |
| **Pain management** | Morphine 0.1-0.3 mg/kg iv in incremental doses<br>Consider epidural narcotics or PCA (see Appendix). | |
| **Tests** | Hct | Others as indicated by intraop course. |

**References**

1. Freiha FS: Open Bladder Surgery. In *Campbell's Urology*, 6th edition. Walsh PC, et al, eds. WB Saunders Co, Philadelphia: 1992, Vol 3, Ch 74, 2750-73.

# OPEN BLADDER OPERATIONS (OTHER THAN CYSTECTOMY)

## SURGICAL CONSIDERATIONS

**Description**: Open bladder operations include:

**Augmentation cystoplasty** (or **enterocystoplasty**): Small, contracted bladders can be enlarged and their size and capacity augmented with a segment of intestine. The bladder is opened widely, anteroposteriorly, or from side-to-side, or with a cruciate incision. A segment of intestine — either small bowel, cecum or colon — is isolated from the intestinal tract, detubularized and added on to the bladder.
**Variant procedure:** The antrum of the stomach can also be used (**gastrocystoplasty**).
**Usual preop diagnosis:** Contracted bladder from chronic cystitis

**Repair of vesicovaginal or enterovesical fistulas**: The communication between the vagina and bladder or bladder and bowel is identified and excised, and the edges freshened until normal, non-inflamed tissues are exposed. The openings in the bladder and in the vagina or bowel are closed and omentum is interposed in between to promote healing and prevent recurrences. With enterovesical fistulas, often the diseased segment of the intestine is excised and an end-to-end anastomosis of the intestine performed.
**Variant procedure:** Transvaginal repair of vesicovaginal fistula (see "Vaginal Operations").
**Usual preop diagnosis:** Vesicovaginal or enterovesical fistula

**Ureteral re-implantation,** performed to correct vesicoureteral reflux, is more commonly used in the pediatric group than in adults. In adults, it is performed mainly for lower ureteral injuries, iatrogenic or traumatic. The lower ureter is identified and dissected proximally until adequate length is obtained. The bladder is opened and a 2-3 cm submucosal tunnel is created in or near the trigone, and the ureter is brought into the tunnel and fixed with sutures. In children, if the ureter is dilated, its diameter is reduced by imbrication before re-implantation. In adults, a non-refluxing implantation is usually not necessary if the operation is being performed for ureteral injury.
**Usual preop diagnosis**: Vesicoureteral reflux; lower ureteral injuries

### SUMMARY OF PROCEDURE

| | Augmentation Cystoplasty | Repair of Fistulas | Ureteral Re-implantation |
|---|---|---|---|
| **Position** | Supine | Supine or lithotomy | Supine |
| **Incision** | Low abdominal | ⇐ | ⇐ |
| **Antibiotics** | Gentamicin 80 mg iv, slowly | ⇐ | ⇐ |
| **Surgical time** | 4 hrs | 3 hrs | ⇐ |
| **EBL** | Minimal | ⇐ | ⇐ |
| **Postop care** | Care of catheters and stents | ⇐ | ⇐ |
| **Mortality** | < 1% | ⇐ | ⇐ |
| **Morbidity** | Infections: 5%<br>Urinary leakage: 1% | ⇐ | ⇐ |
| **Procedure code** | 51800 | 57301, 51900 | 50781 |
| **Pain score** | 10 | 10 | 10 |

### PATIENT POPULATION CHARACTERISTICS

| | | | |
|---|---|---|---|
| **Age range** | All ages | ⇐ | ⇐ |
| **Male:Female** | 1:4 | ⇐ | ⇐ |
| **Incidence** | Rare | ⇐ | ⇐ |
| **Etiology** | Contracted bladders from chronic cystitis | Traumatic vesicovaginal fistulas<br>Regional enteritis<br>Diverticulitis<br>Colon cancer | Vesicoureteral reflux<br>Injury to lower ureters |

# ANESTHETIC CONSIDERATIONS

## PREOPERATIVE

| | |
|---|---|
| **Respiratory** | Note Hx of pulmonary disease in elderly patients.<br>**Tests:** CXR, PFT, ABG, if indicated from H&P. |
| **Cardiovascular** | Note Hx of cardiac disease in elderly patients.<br>**Tests:** ECG; others, if indicated from H&P. |
| **Neurological** | Paraplegics and quadriplegics may present for operations on the bladder and urinary tract. Obtain Hx of autonomic hyperreflexia (AH). Sx are: flushing, headache, nasal stuffiness, HTN associated with voiding and noxious stimuli below level of transection. |
| **Laboratory** | Other tests as indicated from H&P. |
| **Premedication** | Sedation prn anxiety (e.g., lorazepam 1-2 mg po 1-2 hrs prior to surgery; midazolam 1-2 mg iv in preop area). |

## INTRAOPERATIVE

**Anesthetic technique:** Spinal, continuous lumbar epidural or GA are acceptable, with choice dependent on length of procedure, co-existing disease and patient preference. A combined technique using light GA with a regional anesthesia is also acceptable. A T10 sensory level is sufficient to provide anesthesia for procedures on the bladder, but a T4 level is recommended if the peritoneum is opened. (See "Diagnostic Transurethral [Endoscopic] Procedures" for considerations in patients with AH.)

**Regional anesthesia:**

| | |
|---|---|
| **Spinal** | 5% lidocaine 75-100 mg; 0.75% bupivacaine 10-15 mg in 7.5% dextrose |
| **Epidural** | 1.5-2.0% lidocaine with epinephrine 5 $\mu$g/cc, 15-25 cc; supplement with 5-10 cc as needed. Supplemental iv sedation. |

**General anesthesia:**

| | |
|---|---|
| **Induction** | Standard induction (see Appendix). |
| **Maintenance** | Standard maintenance (see Appendix). Consider limiting $N_2O$ for prolonged intraperitoneal procedures. |
| **Emergence** | No specific considerations |

| | | |
|---|---|---|
| **Blood and fluid requirements** | Minimal-to-moderate blood loss<br>IV: 16-18 ga x 1<br>NS/LR @ 2-4 cc/kg/hr<br>Warm fluids.<br>Humidify gasses for lengthy procedures. | Intraperitoneal procedures have considerably higher requirements (e.g., NS/LR @ 6-10 cc/kg/ hr). |
| **Monitoring** | Standard monitors (see Appendix) for simpler procedures.<br>± Arterial/CVP lines | UO as a measure of volume status may be lost during the procedure. Consider arterial line, CVP for longer, more complex procedures. |
| **Positioning** | ✓ and pad pressure points.<br>✓ eyes. | **NB**: peroneal nerve compression at lateral fibular head → foot drop. |
| **Complications** | Autonomic hyperreflexia (AH) | See discussion in "Diagnostic Transurethral (Endoscopic) Procedures." |

## POSTOPERATIVE

| | | |
|---|---|---|
| **Complications** | Hypothermia<br>Fever, bacteremia | |
| **Pain management** | Morphine 0.1-0.3 mg/kg in incremental doses.<br>Consider epidural narcotics or PCA (see Appendix). | |
| **Tests** | Hct<br>Blood cultures if febrile | Others as indicated by intraop course. |

**References**

1. Freiha FS: Open Bladder Surgery. In *Campbell's Urology*, 6th edition. Walsh PC, et al, eds. WB Saunders Co, Philadelphia: 1992, Vol 3, Ch 74, 2750-73.

# INGUINAL OPERATIONS

## SURGICAL CONSIDERATIONS

**Description**: Inguinal operations are very common, and are usually performed on an outpatient basis. Groin dissection, however, may necessitate inpatient care.

**Inguinal herniorrhaphy**: A 3" inguinal incision is made, starting 1" medial to the anterior superior iliac spine, and ending at the pubic tubercle. The external oblique aponeurosis is excised, opening the external inguinal ring. The spermatic cord and the hernial sac are freed off the inguinal canal (Fig 9-13); then the hernial sac is dissected off the spermatic cord and followed proximally into the internal inguinal ring where it is suture-ligated and excised. The floor of the inguinal canal is strengthened by approximating the conjoined tendon to the reflected part of the inguinal ligament.
**Usual preop diagnosis:** Inguinal hernia

**Orchiopexy** is performed through the same incision as used in herniorrhaphy. Once the inguinal canal is exposed, a search for the undescended testis begins. The testis and cord are dissected free from all surrounding tissue until adequate length is obtained to bring the testis down to the scrotum. Next, a pouch is created in the wall of the scrotum by incising the scrotal skin and dissecting it off dartos fascia. The testis is brought down into the pouch and fixed to the dartos fascia with sutures, and the incisions are closed. Often a **herniorrhaphy** is performed at the same time.
**Usual preop diagnosis:** Undescended testis

**Radical orchiectomy** is performed through a herniorrhaphy incision (described above). The spermatic cord is freed and cross-clamped at the internal inguinal ring, transected and suture-ligated. The testis, with its tunica vaginalis, is then delivered through the incision by blunt and sharp dissection and the inguinal incision is closed. Sometimes, a testicular prosthesis is inserted and fixed in the scrotum before the inguinal incision is closed.
**Usual preop diagnosis:** Testicular cancer

**Ligation of spermatic vein** is performed through a small, transverse incision 1-2" above the internal inguinal ring. Muscles are split and peritoneum reflected medially to expose the spermatic vessels; the vein is identified and ligated.
**Usual preop diagnosis:** Varicocele causing infertility

**Groin dissection**, or **inguino-femoral lymphadenectomy** (lymph node dissection), is the most critical of the inguinal operations. It is performed

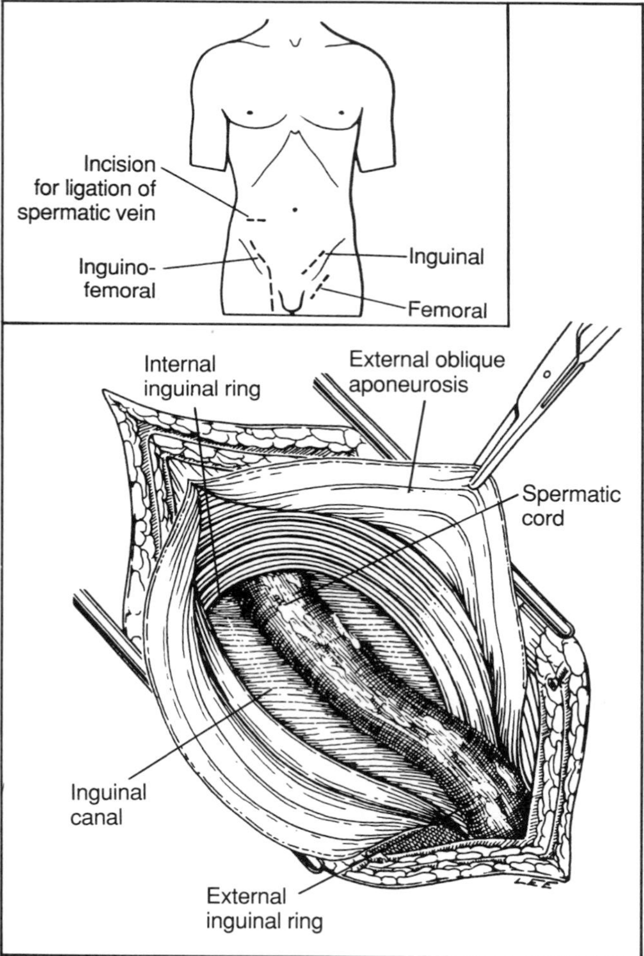


**Figure 9-13.** Surgical anatomy of the inguinal canal. (Reproduced with permission from *Atlas of General Surgery*. Butterworths: 1986.) Inset shows groin incisions.

through either an inguinal incision (Fig 9-13) curved distally over the femoral vessels or through 2 incisions, inguinal and upper-thigh (Fig 9-13), over the femoral triangle. A complete inguinal and femoral lymphadenectomy is performed.
**Usual preop diagnosis**: Penile cancer

### SUMMARY OF PROCEDURE

| | Herniorrhaphy, Orchiopexy, Orchiectomy | Ligation of Spermatic Vein | Groin Dissection |
|---|---|---|---|
| **Position** | Supine | ⇐ | ⇐ |
| **Incision** | Inguinal (Fig 9-13, inset) | Transverse groin (Fig 9-13, inset) | Inguinal and upper thigh (Fig 9-13, inset) |
| **Antibiotics** | None | ⇐ | ⇐ |
| **Surgical time** | 1 hr | ⇐ | 3 hrs |
| **EBL** | Minimal | ⇐ | 200 cc |
| **Postop care** | PACU → home | ⇐ | PACU → ward; leg elevation |
| **Mortality** | < 1% | ⇐ | ⇐ |
| **Morbidity** | Wound infection: 2% | ⇐ | ⇐<br>Necrosis of skin: 20% |
| **Procedure code** | 49505 (herniorrhaphy)<br>54640 (orchiopexy)<br>54530 (orchiectomy) | 55530 | 38760 |
| **Pain score** | 7 | 5 | 7 |

### PATIENT POPULATION CHARACTERISTICS

| | | | |
|---|---|---|---|
| **Age range** | All ages | Young adults | Middle age |
| **Incidence** | Hernia: 5% of population<br>Undescended testis: 0.8% of male children<br>Testis cancer: 6/100,000 | 1% of young men | Extremely rare, < 1% of all males |
| **Etiology** | Unknown | Varicocele | Penile cancer: Very rare |

## ANESTHETIC CONSIDERATIONS

### PREOPERATIVE

Consider causes of increased intra-abdominal pressure during H&P. (Pediatric inguinal operations are discussed in "Pediatric General Surgery.")

**Respiratory** Chronic cough is a common precipitating factor.
**Gastrointestinal** Constipation may be a precipitating factor.
**Laboratory** Tests as indicated from H&P.
**Premedication** Sedation for adults prn anxiety (e.g., lorazepam 1-2 mg po 1-2 hrs before surgery; midazolam 1-2 mg iv in preop area).

### INTRAOPERATIVE

**Anesthetic technique:** Local anesthesia (with sedation), spinal, epidural or GA are acceptable techniques, with choice dependent on patient age and co-existing disease, type and length of procedure and patient preference. Local anesthesia is acceptable for simple herniorrhaphy, although discomfort may be elicited if the peritoneum is manipulated. If a spinal or epidural anesthesia is chosen, a T6 level should be sought. Most inguinal procedures are done on an outpatient basis, and the anesthetic should be planned appropriately.

**Regional anesthesia:**

**Spinal** 5% lidocaine, 75 mg; 0.75% bupivacaine, 12-15 mg
**Epidural** 1.5-2.0% lidocaine with epinephrine 5 μg/cc, 15-25 cc; supplement with 5-10 cc as needed. Supplemental iv sedation with local or regional technique in adults; e.g., midazolam (1-2 mg iv), fentanyl (25-50 μg iv prn anxiety or discomfort); or propofol infusion (25-50 μg/kg/min).

**General anesthesia:**

| | | |
|---|---|---|
| **Induction** | Standard induction (see Appendix). ET intubation and/or controlled ventilation may not be needed for shorter cases. | |
| **Maintenance** | Standard maintenance (see Appendix); consider iv technique. Muscle relaxation usually not imperative. | |
| **Emergence** | No specific considerations | |
| **Blood and fluid requirements** | Usually minimal blood loss<br>IV: 18 ga x 1<br>NS/LR @ 1-2 cc/kg/hr | Minimize NS/LR to avoid postop urinary retention after herniorrhaphy. |
| **Monitoring** | Standard monitors (see Appendix). | |

**POSTOPERATIVE**

| | | |
|---|---|---|
| **Complications** | N&V<br>Failure to void | May delay discharge from PACU → home. |
| **Pain management** | Local anesthesia<br>Ketorolac 60 mg im in adults<br>± Morphine 2-4 mg iv or fentanyl 50-100 μg iv. | Instillation or infiltration of wound with 0.25% bupivacaine or ilioinguinal nerve block provides prolonged postop analgesia and decreases need for narcotics in outpatients. This can be used in both adult and pediatric patients. |


**References**

1. Howards SS: Surgery of the Scrotum and Testis in Childhood. In *Campbell's Urology*, 6th edition. WB Saunders Co, Philadelphia: 1992, Vol 3, Ch 52, 1939-50.
2. Goldstein M: Surgery of Male Infertility and Other Scrotal Disorders. In *Campbell's Urology*, 6th edition. WB Saunders Co, Philadelphia: 1992, Vol 3, Ch 87, 3114-49.
3. Herr HW: Surgery of Penile and Urethral Carcinoma. In *Campbell's Urology*, 6th edition. WB Saunders Co, Philadelphia: 1992, Vol 3, Ch 85, 3073-89.
4. Casey WF, Rice LJ, Hannallah RS, et al: A comparison between bupivacaine instillation versus ilioinguinal/iliohypogastric nerve block for postoperative analgesia following inguinal herniorrhaphy in children. *Anesthesiology* 1990; 72(4):637-39.


# PENILE OPERATIONS

## SURGICAL CONSIDERATIONS

**Penectomy** is the total or partial resection of the penis for squamous-cell carcinoma of the penile skin. If the tumor can be resected with a safe margin of at least 2 cm, partial penectomy is usually enough. A tourniquet is placed at the base of the penis, which is amputated at least 2 cm proximal to the tumor. The corpora cavernosa are sutured and the tourniquet released, followed by inspection for bleeding. The edges of the urethra are sutured to the ventral skin and the lateral and dorsal skin edges are approximated over the ends of the corpora cavernosa. Often, an inguinal lymph node biopsy follows the penectomy.
**Usual preop diagnosis:** Squamous-cell carcinoma of the penile skin

**Insertion of penile prosthesis** is performed for impotence. The prosthesis is inserted into the corpora cavernosa (Fig 9-14) through a small lateral or dorsolateral incision made at the base of the penis and carried down through the tunica albuginea into the corpus tissue. Inflatable prostheses require an inguinal incision for placement of reservoir and pump.

**Usual preop diagnosis:** Impotence

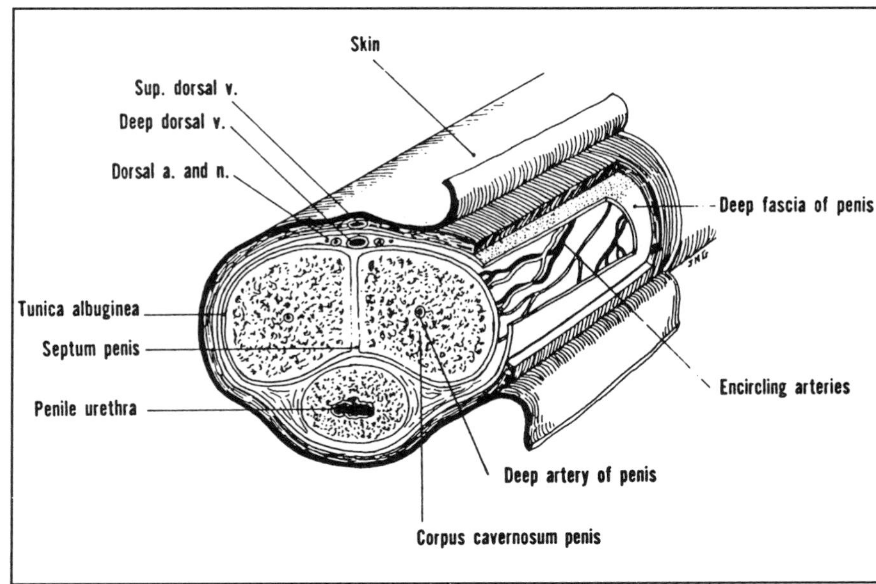


**Figure 9-14.** Anatomy of the penis. (Reproduced with permission from Hardy JD: *Textbook of Surgery*. JB Lippincott, 1988.)

**Hypospadias repair** is performed primarily on children before the age of 5 years. There are many different procedures described, and each has its own application. The aim of any repair is to advance the urethral meatus from its aberrant position to the tip of the glans penis and, at the same time, correct any curvature. These operations require meticulous and careful dissection; magnifying loupes are commonly used.

**Usual preop diagnosis:** Hypospadias

## SUMMARY OF PROCEDURE

| | Penectomy | Insertion of Penile Prosthesis | Hypospadias Repair |
|---|---|---|---|
| **Position** | Supine | ⇐ | ⇐ |
| **Incision** | Circumferential penile | Bilateral incisions at base of penis | Ventral aspect of penis |
| **Special instrumentation** | None | ⇐ | Magnifying loupes |
| **Unique considerations** | None | ⇐ | Children < 5 yrs |
| **Antibiotics** | None | Gentamicin 80 mg iv, slowly; ampicillin 2 gm iv | None |
| **Surgical time** | 2 hrs | ⇐ | 4 hrs + |
| **Closing considerations** | None | ⇐ | Elaborate pressure dressings |
| **EBL** | 200 cc | ⇐ | 50 cc |
| **Postop care** | PACU → home | ⇐ | PACU → ward; good sedation |
| **Mortality** | < 1% | ⇐ | ⇐ |
| **Morbidity** | Penile hematoma: 5% | Malfunction: 10%<br>Edema: 5%<br>Infection: 2%<br>Extrusion of the prosthesis: 1% | Urethrocutaneous fistula: 5%<br>2%<br>⇐<br>Hematoma: 2% |
| **Procedure code** | 54120 | 54460 | 54360 |
| **Pain score** | 5 | 5 | 5 |

## PATIENT POPULATION CHARACTERISTICS

| | | | |
|---|---|---|---|
| **Age range** | Adults | ⇐ | Children |
| **Incidence** | < 1% of all males | 1-2% of all males | 1:200 |
| **Etiology** | Poor hygiene | Organic or psychogenic impotence | Congenital |

## ANESTHETIC CONSIDERATIONS

### PREOPERATIVE

**Neurological** Patients presenting for insertion of a penile prosthesis often have Hx of diabetes or spinal cord injury. Note presence of neuropathy or Hx of autonomic hyperreflexia (AH) (see "Diagnostic Transurethral [Endoscopic] Procedures"). Sx suggestive of AH include headache, flushing, nasal stuffiness, HTN associated with voiding or noxious stimuli below the level of transection. It is important to document neurological deficits prior to regional anesthesia.

**Hematologic** Coagulation defects may be present in patients with priapism. There is a high incidence of priapism in patients with sickle-cell anemia.
**Tests**: Hct, PT, PTT, if indicated from H&P.

**Laboratory** Other tests as indicated from H&P.

**Premedication** Sedation prn anxiety in adults (e.g., lorazepam 1-2 mg po 1-2 hrs prior to surgery; midazolam 1-2 mg iv in preop area).

### INTRAOPERATIVE

**Anesthetic technique:** Spinal, caudal, continuous lumbar epidural and GA are acceptable, with choice dependent on length of procedure, patient age, co-existing disease and patient preference. Sacral anesthesia (saddle block) is sufficient; lumbar epidural anesthesia may be less reliable than spinal or caudal at blocking sacral fibers.

**Regional anesthesia:**

**Spinal** 5% lidocaine 50 mg; 0.75% bupivacaine 10 mg in 7.5% dextrose; hyperbaric tetracaine 10 mg with epinephrine for longer procedures.

**Caudal** 0.5% bupivacaine with epinephrine 5 μg/cc 15-20 cc

**Epidural** 1.5% lidocaine with epinephrine 5 μg/cc 15-25 cc; supplement with 5-10 cc as needed. Supplemental iv sedation.

**General anesthesia:**

**Induction** Standard induction (see Appendix). ET intubation may not be necessary for shorter procedures.

**Maintenance** Standard maintenance (see Appendix). Deeper levels of anesthesia are usually required to obtund autonomic reflexes (e.g., HTN, laryngospasm) resulting from intense surgical stimulation that may occur during these procedures.

**Emergence** No specific considerations

**Blood and fluid requirements** Minimal blood loss
IV: 18 ga x 1
NS/LR at 2 cc/kg/hr

**Monitoring** Standard monitors (see Appendix).

**Complications** Autonomic hyperreflexia (AH) — See "Diagnostic Transurethral (Endoscopic) Procedures."

### POSTOPERATIVE

**Complications** Urinary retention

**Pain management** Morphine 0.05-0.1 mg/kg iv or fentanyl 1.0 μg/kg iv prn

**References**

1. Herr HW: Surgery of Penile and Urethral Carcinoma. In *Campbell's Urology*, 6th edition. WB Saunders Co, Philadelphia: 1992, Vol 3, Ch 85, 3073-89.
2. Goldstein I, Krane RJ: Diagnosis and Therapy of Erectile Dysfunction. In *Campbell's Urology*, 6th edition. WB Saunders Co, Philadelphia: 1992, Vol 3, Ch 84, 3033-72.
3. Duckett JW: Hypospadias. In *Campbell's Urology*, 6th edition. WB Saunders Co, Philadelphia: 1992, Vol 3, Ch 50, 1893-1919.

## SCROTAL OPERATIONS

### SURGICAL CONSIDERATIONS

**Description**: Scrotal operations are minor, common urologic procedures, performed on an outpatient basis.

**Simple orchiectomy** is performed as an alternative to medical castration using either estrogens or LH-RH agonists on men with metastatic prostate cancer for androgen ablation. It is always bilateral. A small scrotal incision is made and the testis delivered. The spermatic cord is cross-clamped, transected and suture-ligated.
**Usual preop diagnosis:** Metastatic prostate cancer

**Vasovasostomy** is the re-establishment of the continuity of the vas deferens and fertility following a previously performed vasectomy. Through a small scrotal incision, the testis and spermatic cord are delivered. The site of previous vasectomy is identified and excised and the two ends of the vas deferens anastomosed. It is bilateral and requires the use of either the operating microscope or magnifying loupes.
**Usual preop diagnosis:** Infertility 2° vasectomy

**Hydrocelectomy**: The testis, with the surrounding hydrocele (Fig 9-15), is delivered through a scrotal incision. The wall of the hydrocele is excised and the edges sutured around the epididymis to prevent recurrence.
**Variant procedure or approach:** Aspiration used as a temporizing approach since recurrence is almost 100%.
**Usual preop diagnosis:** Hydrocele

**Spermatocelectomy**: A spermatocele is a cyst of the epididymis which is usually excised with that part of the epididymis from which it arises.
**Variant procedure:** Aspiration as a temporizing maneuver until the operation can be performed.
**Usual preop diagnosis:** Spermatocele or epididymal cyst

**Insertion of testicular prosthesis**: A small incision is made in the scrotal skin and a pouch is created by blunt dissection in dartos fascia. The prosthesis is placed in the pouch and fixed to dartos fascia to prevent prosthesis migration.
**Usual preop diagnosis:** Absent testis, either congenitally or following orchiectomy

**Reduction of testicular torsion** is an emergency operation which must be performed within 6 hrs of occurrence in order to prevent irreversible ischemic damage to the testis. Through a small scrotal incision, the testis is reduced and fixed to the dartos fascia to prevent re-torsion.
**Usual preop diagnosis:** Acute testicular torsion

#### SUMMARY OF PROCEDURE

| | |
|---|---|
| **Position** | Supine |
| **Incision** | Scrotal (Fig 9-15, inset) |
| **Special instrumentation** | Operating microscope; magnifying loupe for vasovasostomy |
| **Antibiotics** | None |
| **Surgical time** | 1 hr |
| **EBL** | Negligible |
| **Postop care** | PACU → home |
| **Mortality** | < 1% |
| **Morbidity** | Scrotal hematoma: 2%<br>Wound infection: 2% |
| **Procedure code** | 54520 (simple orchiectomy)<br>55400 (vasovasostomy)<br>49515 (hydrocelectomy)<br>54840 (spermatocelectomy)<br>54660, 54661 (insertion of testicular prosthesis)<br>54600 (reduction of testicular torsion) |
| **Pain score** | 4 |

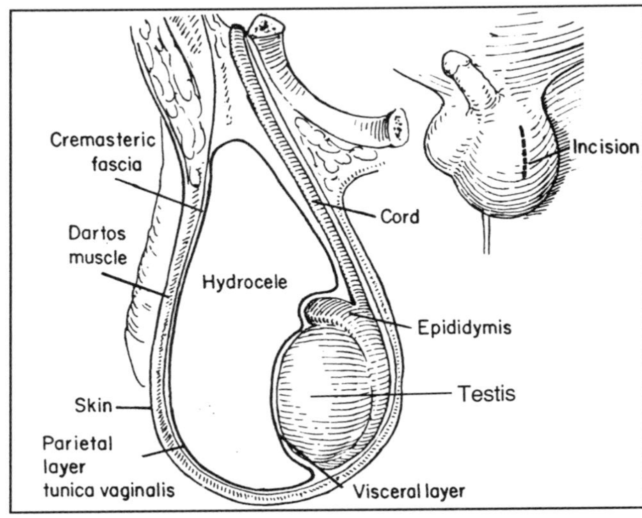


**Figure 9-15.** Scrotal hydrocele; scrotal incision. (Reproduced with permission from Zollinger RM, Zollinger RM Jr: *Atlas of Surgical Operations*. MacMillan Pub Co: 1983.)

### PATIENT POPULATION CHARACTERISTICS

| | |
|---|---|
| **Age range** | All ages |
| **Incidence** | Common |
| **Etiology** | (See preop diagnosis for each procedure, above.) |

---

## ANESTHETIC CONSIDERATIONS

### PREOPERATIVE

| | |
|---|---|
| **Respiratory** | Note Hx of pulmonary disease in elderly patients presenting for orchiectomy. **Tests:** Consider CXR, PFT, ABG, if indicated from H&P. |
| **Cardiovascular** | Note Hx of cardiac disease in elderly patients presenting for orchiectomy. **Tests:** ECG; others, if indicated from H&P. |
| **Neurological** | Document neurological exam prior to regional anesthetic in patients with metastatic prostate carcinoma (spinal-cord or nerve-root compression may be present preop). |
| **Musculoskeletal** | Note presence of spinal metastases if orchiectomy is done for palliation of prostate carcinoma. Extensive lumbar metastases may preclude the use of spinal or epidural anesthesia (relative contraindication). **Tests**: L-spine films if Hx suggestive of spinal metastases. |
| **Laboratory** | Other tests as indicated from H&P. |
| **Premedication** | Sedation prn anxiety (e.g., lorazepam 1-2 mg po 1-2 hrs prior to surgery; midazolam 1-2 mg iv in preop area). |

### INTRAOPERATIVE

**Anesthetic technique:** Local anesthesia (with sedation) is acceptable for simpler operations (vasectomy, orchiectomy). Procedures which are longer or more complex may require spinal, epidural or GA. A sensory level of T10 is required to block pain 2° testicular manipulation. For children undergoing orchiopexy, GA, with or without supplemental caudal blockade, is preferred. Many of these procedures are done on an outpatient basis, and the anesthetic should be appropriately planned.

**Regional anesthesia:**

| | |
|---|---|
| **Spinal** | 0.75% bupivacaine 10-12 mg in 7.5% dextrose (1.6 cc); lidocaine 75-100 mg (5% in dextrose) for shorter procedures. |
| **Epidural** | 1.5-2.0% lidocaine with epinephrine 5 μg/cc, 15-20 cc; supplement with 5-10 cc as needed. Supplemental iv sedation with local or regional techniques (e.g., midazolam 1-2 mg, fentanyl 25-50 μg iv prn anxiety or discomfort). |

**General anesthesia:**

| | |
|---|---|
| **Induction** | Standard induction (see Appendix). |
| **Maintenance** | Standard maintenance (see Appendix). Muscle relaxation usually not imperative. Deeper levels of anesthesia are usually required to obtund autonomic reflexes (e.g., HTN, laryngospasm) resulting from intense surgical stimulation that may occur during these procedures. |
| **Emergence** | No specific considerations |

| | | |
|---|---|---|
| **Blood and fluid requirements** | Minimal blood loss<br>IV: 18 ga x 1<br>NS/LR @ 2 cc/kg/hr | |
| **Monitoring** | Standard monitors (see Appendix). | |
| **Positioning** | ✓ and pad pressure points.<br>✓ eyes. | **NB**: peroneal nerve compression at lateral fibular head → foot drop. |

### POSTOPERATIVE

| | | |
|---|---|---|
| **Complications** | Peroneal nerve injury 2° lithotomy position | Peroneal nerve injury manifested by foot drop and loss of sensation on dorsum of foot. Seek neurology consultation. |

| | | |
|---|---|---|
| **Pain management** | Ketorolac 60 mg im in adults ± Morphine 2-4 mg iv or fentanyl 50-100 μg iv prn. | Following orchiopexy, high incidence of postop pain, N&V, which may be reduced by ilioinguinal/ilio-hypogastric nerve blocks. |

**References**

1. Howards SS: Surgery of the Scrotum and Testis in Childhood. In *Campbell's Urology*, 6th edition. WB Saunders Co, Philadelphia: 1992, Vol 3, Ch 52, 1939-50.
2. Hannallah RS, Broadman LM, Belman AB, et al: Comparison of caudal and ilioinguinal/iliohypogastric nerve blocks for control of post-orchiopexy pain in pediatric ambulatory surgery. *Anesthesiology* 1987; 66(6):832-34.

# PERINEAL OPERATIONS

## SURGICAL CONSIDERATIONS

**Urethroplasty**: Urethral strictures which do not respond to transurethral dilation and incision are corrected with urethroplasty. A transverse, or longitudinal perineal incision is made and carried down to the urethra, which is dissected free from surrounding tissues. The strictured area is excised and end-to-end anastomosis performed over a catheter.
**Variant procedure:** Transurethral incision and dilation, which is associated with a 30-50% recurrence rate.
**Usual preop diagnosis:** Urethral stricture, usually post-traumatic

**Urethrectomy**: Partial or total urethrectomy is done through a longitudinal perineal incision. The urethra is dissected free of surrounding tissues and followed proximally and distally from the membranous urethra to the external urethral meatus. In total urethrectomy, a tubularized skin graft is interposed between membranous urethra and perineal skin.
**Usual preop diagnosis:** Urethral carcinoma

**Insertion of artificial urinary sphincter** is performed for incontinence. The operation consists of a perineal incision through which a cuff is inserted around the bulbar urethra. A scrotal incision is made to implant the pump that inflates and deflates this cuff.
**Usual preop diagnosis**: Urinary incontinence

### SUMMARY OF PROCEDURE

| | Urethroplasty | Urethrectomy | Insertion of Sphincter |
|---|---|---|---|
| **Position** | Lithotomy | ⇐ | ⇐ |
| **Incision** | Perineal (Fig 9-4) | ⇐ | Perineal (Fig 9-4) and scrotal (Fig 9-15, inset) |
| **Antibiotics** | Parenteral broad spectrum (e.g., gentamicin 80 mg im) | ⇐ | ⇐ |
| **Surgical time** | 3 hrs | 2 hrs | 3 hrs |
| **EBL** | 100 cc | 300 cc | Minimal |
| **Postop care** | PACU → room | ⇐ | ⇐ |
| **Mortality** | < 1% | ⇐ | ⇐ |
| **Morbidity** | Wound infection: 2% | ⇐ | ⇐<br>Erosion of the urethra: 10%<br>Extrusion of sphincter: 2% |
| **Procedure code** | 53410 | 53210 | 53440 |
| **Pain score** | 3 | 3 | 4 |

### PATIENT POPULATION CHARACTERISTICS

| | | | |
|---|---|---|---|
| **Age range** | All ages | Adults | Older adults |
| **Incidence** | < 1% of urologic procedures | ⇐ | 2% of radical prostatectomy |
| **Etiology** | Traumatic strictures | Unknown | Radical prostatectomy: 2% Incontinence |

# ANESTHETIC CONSIDERATIONS

## PREOPERATIVE

This is a generally healthy patient population; preop considerations should be based on H&P.

| | |
|---|---|
| **Laboratory** | Tests as indicated from H&P. |
| **Premedication** | Sedation prn anxiety in adults (e.g., lorazepam 1-2 mg po 1-2 hrs prior to surgery; midazolam 1-2 mg iv in preop area). |

## INTRAOPERATIVE

**Anesthetic technique:** Spinal or GA are acceptable, with choice dependent on length of procedure, position, patient age, co-existing disease and patient preference. A sacral sensory level (saddle block) is usually sufficient. Lumbar epidural anesthesia may be less reliable at providing sacral anesthesia, and offers no advantages over the above techniques for shorter procedures, although caudal anesthesia may be an acceptable alternative.

**Regional anesthesia:**

| | |
|---|---|
| **Spinal** | 0.75% bupivacaine 10 mg in 7.5% dextrose; hyperbaric tetracaine 10 mg (with epinephrine (200 μg) for longer procedures) |
| **Caudal** | 0.5% bupivacaine with epinephrine 5 μg/cc 15-20 cc. Supplemental iv sedation. |

**General anesthesia:**

| | | |
|---|---|---|
| **Induction** | Standard induction (see Appendix). | |
| **Maintenance** | Standard maintenance (see Appendix); muscle relaxation usually not imperative. Deeper levels of anesthesia are usually required to obtund autonomic reflexes (e.g., HTN, laryngospasm) resulting from intense surgical stimulation that may occur during these procedures. | |
| **Emergence** | No specific considerations | |
| **Blood and fluid requirements** | Minimal blood loss<br>IV: 18 ga x 1<br>NS/LR at 2 cc/kg/hr | |
| **Monitoring** | Standard monitors (see Appendix). | |
| **Positioning** | ✓ and pad pressure points.<br>✓ eyes. | **NB**: peroneal nerve compression at lateral fibular head → foot drop.<br>Patients with arthritis or other musculoskeletal disorders may not tolerate the exaggerated lithotomy position, thus precluding the use of a regional technique. |
| **Complications** | Anticipate hypotension on return from lithotomy position. | Rx: volume (200-500 cc NS/LR) or ephedrine (5 mg iv) may be necessary. |

## POSTOPERATIVE

| | | |
|---|---|---|
| **Complications** | Peroneal nerve injury 2° lithotomy position) | Peroneal nerve injury manifested as foot drop with loss of sensation over dorsum of foot. Seek neurology consultation. |
| **Pain management** | Mild-to-moderate pain<br>Morphine 0.05-0.1 mg/kg iv prn | |

**References**

1. Devine CJ Jr, Jordan GH, Schlossberg SM: Surgery of the Penis and Urethra. In *Campbell's Urology*, 6th edition. WB Saunders Co, Philadelphia: 1992, Vol 3, Ch 83, 2957-3032.

# VAGINAL OPERATIONS

## SURGICAL CONSIDERATIONS

**Description**: Vaginal operations are performed by both urologists and gynecologists. They include the following:

**Repair of vesicovaginal fistulas**: The vaginal approach is usually recommended for small and distally located vesicovaginal fistulas; otherwise, a transabdominal repair is performed (see "Open Bladder Operations"). An incision is made in the anterior vaginal wall around the fistula, which is excised. Bladder and vaginal walls are separated and closed with interposition of tissues or flaps to separate the incisions and prevent recurrence. A Foley catheter is left indwelling.
**Variant approach:** Transabdominal repair of vesicovaginal fistula (see "Open Bladder Operations").
**Usual preop diagnosis:** Vesicovaginal fistula

**Operations to correct urinary stress incontinence**: Many procedures have been described to correct female urinary stress incontinence. They all achieve the purpose of restoring the posterior ureterovesical angle and lifting the bladder neck behind the symphysis pubis. The operation most commonly used by urologists is the **Stamey Procedure** (Fig 9-16), or **endoscopic vesical neck suspension**, which has the advantage of placing the sutures under cystoscopic guidance to insure their proper placement and position and to prevent them from transversing the bladder. The operation is performed through two small suprapubic incisions, one on either side of the midline and an anterior vaginal incision. A nylon suture is placed in a loop form on either side of the bladder neck and not around it. When these sutures are pulled up and tied over the anterior rectus sheath, they pull the bladder neck up to its original position behind the symphysis pubis and restore the acute nature of the posterior ureterovesical angle.
**Variant approach:** The **Marshall-Marchetti-Krantz operation**, which is performed retropubically, sutures the anterior portion of the urethra, bladder neck and bladder to the pubic bone.
**Usual preop diagnosis:** Urinary stress incontinence

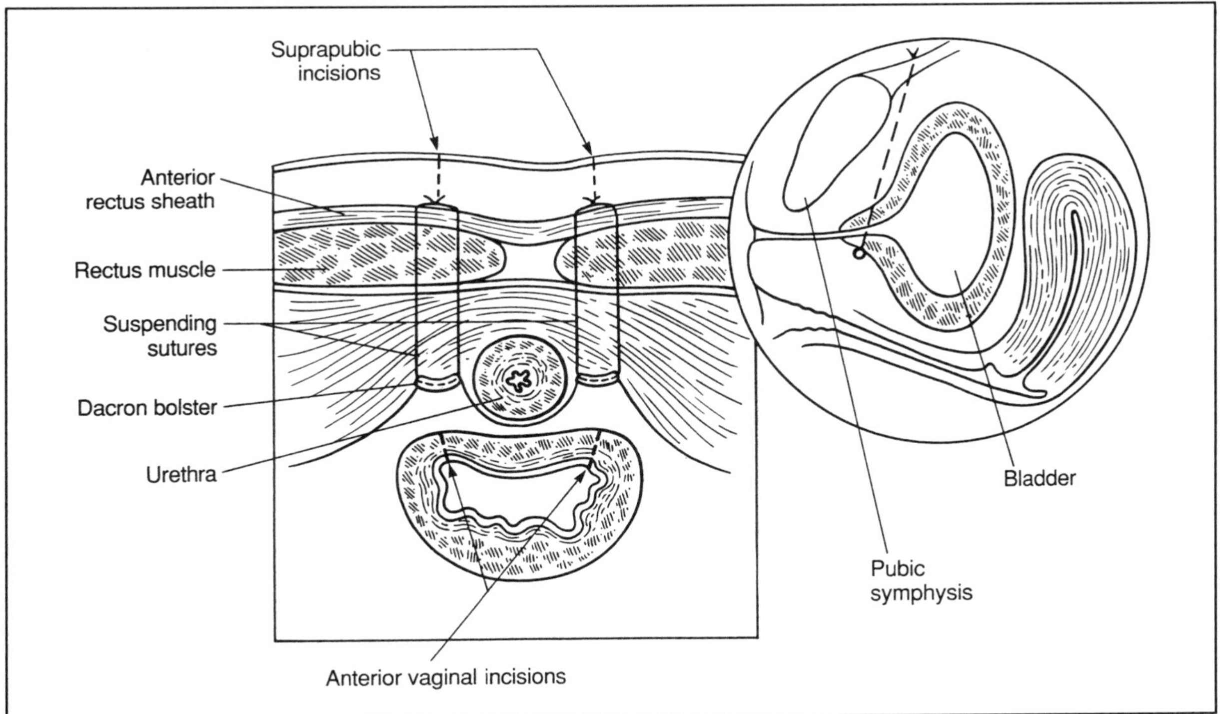


**Figure 9-16.** Stamey procedure, sectional view; inset shows lateral view.

**Excision of urethral diverticulum**: Urethral diverticula are extremely rare and need excision only if they are the cause of recurrent urinary tract infections. An incision is made in the anterior vaginal wall over the urethral diverticulum, which is dissected all around until it is attached only by its neck. It is excised and the neck closed. A Foley catheter is left indwelling, and the vaginal incision is closed.
**Usual preop diagnosis:** Recurrent urinary tract infections 2° infected urethral diverticulum

### SUMMARY OF PROCEDURE

| | Repair of Vesicovaginal Fistula | Correction of Stress Incontinence | Excision of Urethral Diverticulum |
|---|---|---|---|
| **Position** | Lithotomy | ⇐ | ⇐ |
| **Incision** | Anterior vaginal | Anterior vaginal; suprapubic | Anterior vaginal |
| **Special instrumentation** | None | Cystoscope | None |
| **Antibiotics** | Gentamicin 80 mg iv, slowly | ⇐ | ⇐ |
| **Surgical time** | 2 hrs | 1 hr | ⇐ |
| **EBL** | 200 cc | 500 cc | 200 cc |
| **Postop care** | PACU → room | ⇐ | ⇐ |
| **Mortality** | < 1% | ⇐ | ⇐ |
| **Morbidity** | Infection: 2% | ⇐ | ⇐ |
| | Recurrence: 2% | 10% | |
| **Procedure code** | 57300 | 51845 | 53230 |
| **Pain score** | 3 | 5 | 3 |

### PATIENT POPULATION CHARACTERISTICS

| | | | |
|---|---|---|---|
| **Age range** | 20-80 yrs | ⇐ | ⇐ |
| **Incidence** | < 1% of urologic procedures | 5% of urologic procedures | < 1% of urologic procedures |
| **Etiology** | Traumatic delivery<br>Iatrogenic following hysterectomy: < 1% | Childbirth | Congenital: Extremely rare |

---

## ANESTHETIC CONSIDERATIONS

### PREOPERATIVE

This is a generally healthy patient population. Preop considerations should be based on H&P.

**Laboratory** Tests as indicated from H&P.

**Premedication** Standard premedication (see Appendix).

### INTRAOPERATIVE

**Anesthetic technique:** Spinal, continuous lumbar epidural, or GA are acceptable, with choice dependent on age, coexisting disease and patient preference. A block level of T9-T10 is recommended for operations involving the bladder, whereas somewhat higher levels of anesthesia may be necessary if a suprapubic incision is made. Epidural anesthesia may be less reliable than spinal at providing sacral anesthesia.

**Regional anesthesia:**

**Spinal** 0.75% bupivacaine 12 mg (1.6 cc)

**Epidural** 2% lidocaine with epinephrine 5 $\mu$g/cc, 15-20 cc. Supplemental iv sedation.

**General anesthesia:**

**Induction** Standard induction (see Appendix).

**Maintenance** Standard maintenance (see Appendix). Muscle relaxation not imperative.

**Emergence** No specific considerations

**Blood and fluid requirements** Minimal blood loss
IV: 18 ga x 1
NS/LR @ 2-4 cc/kg/hr

**Monitoring** Standard monitors (see Appendix).

**Positioning** √ and pad pressure points.
√ eyes.

**NB**: peroneal nerve compression at lateral fibular head → foot drop.

| | | |
|---|---|---|
| **Complications** | Anticipate hypotension when returning from lithotomy.<br>Bladder perforation | Rx: volume (200-500 cc NS/LR) or ephedrine (5 mg iv) may be necessary.<br>Bladder perforation may present as shoulder pain in the awake patient, but may go unnoticed in the patient under GA. Sx include unexplained HTN, tachycardia, hypotension (rare). |

**POSTOPERATIVE**

| | | |
|---|---|---|
| **Complications** | Peroneal nerve injury 2° lithotomy position<br>Bladder perforation (see above) | Peroneal nerve injury is manifested as foot drop with loss of sensation on dorsum of foot. Seek neurology consultation. |
| **Pain management** | Consider ketorolac 60 mg iv/im in adults; supplement with morphine 0.05-0.1 mg/kg iv prn. | |

References

1. Raz S, Little NA, Juma S: Female Urology. In *Campbell's Urology*, 6th edition. WB Saunders Co, Philadelphia: 1992, Vol 3 Ch 75, 2782-2828.

## 10. ORTHOPEDIC SURGERY

**Surgeons**

**Gordon A. Brody, MD** *(Hand Surgery)*
**Lawrence A. Rinsky, MD** *(Hand Surgery)*
**Amy L. Ladd, MD** *(Shoulder Surgery)*
**John J. Csongradi, MD** *(Surgery of the Lower Extremities)*
**Stuart B. Goodman, MD, MSc, FRCS(C), FACS** *(Surgery of the Lower Extremities)*
**Eugene J. Carragee, MD** *(Spine Surgery)*

**Anesthesiologists**

**Talmage D. Egan, MD** *(Hand, Shoulder Surgery)*
**Peter S. Kosek, MD** *(Surgery of the Lower Extremities)*
**Frederick G. Mihm, MD** *(Surgery of the Lower Extremities)*

**Surgeons**

**Gordon A. Brody, MD**
**Lawrence A. Rinsky, MD**

## 10.1 HAND SURGERY

**Anesthesiologist**

**Talmage D. Egan, MD**

# DARRACH PROCEDURE

## SURGICAL CONSIDERATIONS

**Description:** The Darrach procedure is a resection of the distal ulna. The distal 2 cm of the ulna is resected subperiosteally, and local soft tissues are used to stabilize and cover the remaining ulna. It is commonly performed in patients who have had a disruption of the distal radioulnar joint with subluxation of the ulna. It is also indicated for patients who have had a malunion of a distal radius fracture such that the radius has shortened relative to the ulna or is abnormally angulated, resulting in dorsal subluxation of the ulna and impingement of the ulnar head upon the carpus. This causes painful motion of the wrist and forearm and post-traumatic degenerative arthritis of the ulnar head, carpus and sigmoid notch of the distal radius. Disorders of the distal radioulnar joint and degeneration of the ulnar head, which may lead to attrition rupture of the overlying extensor tendons, are common in rheumatoid arthritis. This dorsal prominence of the ulnar head is treated by **Darrach resection**, combined with a soft-tissue procedure to stabilize the remaining ulna. Osteoarthritic degeneration of the distal radioulnar joint, either 2° trauma (see above) or due to idiopathic osteoarthritis, responds well to this procedure.

**Variant procedure or approaches**: Modifications of the Darrach procedure, such as the **hemi-resection interposition technique of Bowers**, are performed for the same indications as above.

**Usual preop diagnosis**: Arthritis or derangement of the distal radioulnar joint; rheumatoid arthritis; ulnar impingement syndrome; malunion of Colles' fracture or other fracture of the distal radius

### SUMMARY OF PROCEDURE

| | |
|---|---|
| **Position** | Supine, with arm extended on hand-surgery table |
| **Incision** | Dorsal-ulnar, over distal ulna |
| **Special instrumentation** | Pneumatic tourniquet |
| **Antibiotics** | Cefazolin 1 gm iv |
| **Surgical time** | 1 - 2.5 hrs, depending on associated procedures |
| **Tourniquet** | 150 mm above systolic; max time = 120 min |
| **Closing considerations** | Routine skin closure; postop splint placed at conclusion of procedure. |
| **EBL** | Minimal; performed under tourniquet control. |
| **Postop care** | Elevation to minimize swelling. PACU → home, or overnight stay in observation bed. |
| **Mortality** | Minimal |
| **Morbidity** | Ulnar nerve injury<br>Postop swelling |
| **Procedure code** | 25999 |
| **Pain score** | 5-7 |

### PATIENT POPULATION CHARACTERISTICS

| | |
|---|---|
| **Age range** | Late teens-elderly |
| **Male:Female** | Slight predominance of females, due to incidence of malunion of Colles' fractures in women with senile osteoporosis. |
| **Incidence** | Not uncommon |
| **Etiology** | See Usual Preop Diagnosis, above. |
| **Associated conditions** | Rheumatoid arthritis |

## ANESTHETIC CONSIDERATIONS

See Anesthetic Considerations following "Thumb Carpometacarpal Joint Fusion/Arthroplasty/Stabilization" (below).

**References**

1. Dingman PVC: Resection of the distal end of the ulna. *J Bone Joint Surg [Am]* 1952; 34:893-900.

# DORSAL STABILIZATION AND EXTENSOR SYNOVECTOMY OF THE RHEUMATOID WRIST

## SURGICAL CONSIDERATIONS

**Description:** This procedure is indicated for patients with rheumatoid arthritis and extensor tenosynovitis refractory to medical treatment, as well as extensor tendon ruptures, and/or intercarpal synovitis. The procedure is performed under tourniquet control through a straight dorsal incision over the wrist. A **radical tenosynovectomy** of the extensor tendons in all six extensor compartments is carried out. Tendon ruptures or impending ruptures are repaired with tendon grafts or side-to-side anastomoses. Bone spurs are removed and a synovectomy of the distal radioulnar joint is carried out. A **modified Darrach procedure**, with resection or osteoplasty of the distal ulna, is usually performed. If there is evidence of synovitis within the wrist joint, a synovectomy is performed through a dorsal arthrotomy. A flap of the extensor retinaculum is transposed beneath the extensor tendons to reinforce the dorsal wrist ligaments and, thus, stabilize the wrist to prevent volar subluxation of the carpus. A posterior interosseous neurectomy is carried out at the same time. The remaining extensor retinaculum is divided into two transverse strips and one is used to stabilize the distal ulna. The second strip is placed dorsal to the extensor tendons so they will not bowstring during wrist extension.

**Usual preop diagnosis**: Rheumatoid arthritis with extensor tendon tenosynovitis; extensor tendon rupture; distal radioulnar joint synovitis and/or subluxation

### SUMMARY OF PROCEDURE

| | |
|---|---|
| **Position** | Supine, with arm extended on hand-surgery table |
| **Incision** | Dorsal wrist (Fig 10.1-1) |
| **Special instrumentation** | Pneumatic tourniquet |
| **Antibiotics** | Cefazolin 1 gm iv |
| **Surgical time** | 2 hrs |
| **Tourniquet** | 150 mm above systolic; max time = 120 min |
| **Closing considerations** | Postop splint |
| **EBL** | Minimal; tourniquet used until dressing in place. |
| **Postop care** | Admitted overnight for pain control and limb elevation. |
| **Mortality** | Minimal |
| **Morbidity** | Extremity swelling<br>Delayed healing 2° immunosuppression and steroid use<br>Wound infection |
| **Procedure code** | 25116 |
| **Pain score** | 3-5 |

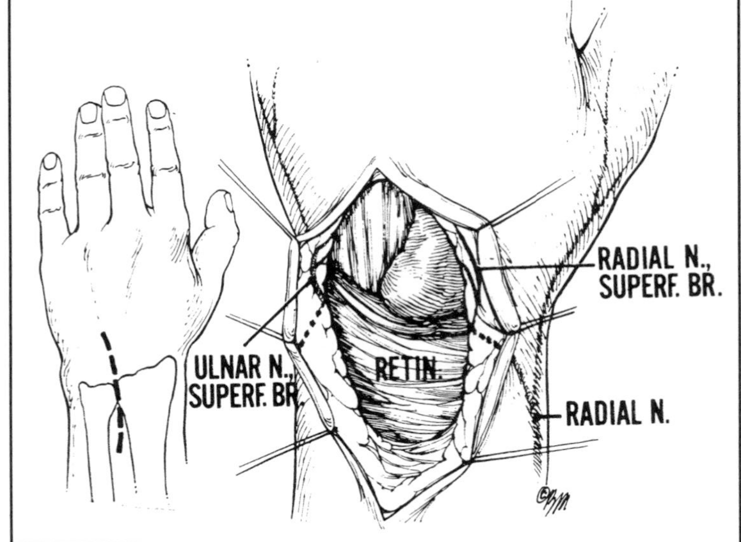


**Figure 10.1-1.** Incision and exposure for dorsal tenosynovectomy. Note superficial branches of radial and ulnar nerves protected in skin flaps. (Illustration by Elizabeth Roselius, © 1988. Reproduced with permission from Green DP: *Operative Hand Surgery*, 2nd edition. Churchill Livingstone: 1988.)

### PATIENT POPULATION CHARACTERISTICS

| | |
|---|---|
| **Age range** | Procedure uncommon before 4th decade |
| **Male:Female** | As in all patients with rheumatoid arthritis, females more common. |
| **Incidence** | Not uncommon |
| **Etiology** | Connective tissue disorder; rheumatoid arthritis or variant |
| **Associated conditions** | All conditions associated with connective tissue disorders, including: active rheumatoid arthritis, steroid dependency, immunosuppressive remittive therapy, and/or skin fragility. |

## ANESTHETIC CONSIDERATIONS

See Anesthetic Considerations following "Thumb Carpometacarpal Joint Fusion/Arthroplasty/Stabilization" (below).

**References**

1. Millender LH, Nalebuff FA: Preventive surgery – tenosynovectomy and synovectomy. *Orthop Clin North Am* 1975; 6(3):765-92.

# METACARPOPHALANGEAL AND INTERPHALANGEAL JOINT ARTHROPLASTY

## SURGICAL CONSIDERATIONS

**Description: Joint replacement** in the hand is most commonly indicated in patients with rheumatoid arthritis with severe joint destruction leading to pain and dysfunction. It is rarely indicated in patients with osteoarthritis. The most common prostheses, made of silicone rubber and popularized by Swanson, differ from total joint replacement in the hip or knee in that they do not function as true joints, but rather as spacers in a **resection arthroplasty**. Most of the stability and motion of these joints depend on meticulous soft-tissue reconstructions involving tendon and ligament transfers, as well as intensive postop physical therapy. To obtain good results, patients must be well-motivated and understand their disease process and what will be asked of them during the recovery period. The results for **metacarpophalangeal (MP) arthroplasty** are far better than those obtained in the proximal interphalangeal joints. **Proximal interphalangeal joint arthroplasty** is now indicated only for the central middle and ring digits in patients with good ligamentous and tendinous structures. **Distal interphalangeal (DIP) arthroplasty** is rarely performed, since these patients do well with fusions. The procedure for the MP joints is performed through a dorsal transverse incision under tourniquet control. The metacarpal heads are removed with an oscillating saw and the intramedullary canals reamed to accept the stems of the prostheses. Once they have been placed with a no-touch technique, the capsule is closed and the supporting ligaments are reconstructed with centralization of extensor tendons. A splint with support for each finger is placed at the conclusion of surgery. Reconstructive procedures of the wrist and fingers can be combined with arthroplasty.

**Variant procedure or approaches**: Some surgeons favor longitudinal incisions rather than a transverse incision for the approach to the MP joints.

**Usual preop diagnosis**: Rheumatoid arthritis or other connective-tissue disorder

### SUMMARY OF PROCEDURE

| | |
|---|---|
| **Position** | Supine, with arm extended on hand-surgery table |
| **Incision** | Dorsal hand, transverse or longitudinal |
| **Special instrumentation** | MP or PIP joint prostheses and associated instruments for preparing the medullary canal; pneumatic tourniquet |
| **Antibiotics** | Cefazolin 1 gm iv |
| **Surgical time** | 2.5 hrs |
| **Tourniquet** | 150 mm above systolic; max time = 120 min |
| **Closing considerations** | Critical postop splinting |
| **EBL** | Minimal; tourniquet used throughout procedure. |
| **Postop care** | Admitted to hospital for pain control and limb elevation. |
| **Mortality** | Minimal |
| **Morbidity** | Swelling<br>Wound infection<br>Prosthesis infection (rare) |
| **Procedure code** | 26531 |
| **Pain score** | 7 |

### PATIENT POPULATION CHARACTERISTICS

| | |
|---|---|
| **Age range** | > 50 yrs |
| **Male:Female** | As in rheumatoid arthritis, females predominate. |
| **Incidence** | Uncommon |
| **Etiology** | Rheumatoid arthritis or other connective-tissue disorder |
| **Associated conditions** | As in rheumatoid arthritis (e.g., skin fragility, steroid dependency, immunosuppression) |

## ANESTHETIC CONSIDERATIONS

See Anesthetic Considerations following "Thumb Carpometacarpal Joint Fusion/Arthroplasty/Stabilization" (below).

# ARTHRODESIS OF THE WRIST

## SURGICAL CONSIDERATIONS

**Description:** A variety of arthrodeses can be performed about the wrist. These include **radiopancarpal arthrodesis** (total wrist fusion), radiolunate, radioscapholunate, and intercarpal arthrodeses (partial wrist fusions). Radiopancarpal is generally performed as a salvage procedure for wrist pathology that cannot be treated with a procedure that preserves wrist motion. These indications include post-traumatic degenerative arthritis following fractures and dislocations, idiopathic osteoarthritis, and/or rheumatoid arthritis. In the non-rheumatoid patient, an effective procedure is an arthrodesis using an iliac crest bone graft fixed with plate and screws. Alternative techniques with other forms of fixation are also used. It has been shown that a position of fusion in 10°-15° of dorsiflexion provides the greatest grip strength. In the rheumatoid patient, a technique using intramedullary fixation with a large-diameter Steinmann pin is preferred. Rheumatoid bone is osteoporotic, 2° disuse and chronic steroid administration. Screw fixation is not ideal in this soft bone. Bone graft is obtained locally in these patients, usually from the resected ulnar head. **Radiolunate fusion** is also indicated in rheumatoid patients who have progressive ulnar translation of the carpus. The lunate acts to block this translation of the carpus. **Radioscapholunate fusion** is indicated in patients with radiocarpal arthritis. This procedure preserves about 50% of wrist motion which occurs at the midcarpal joint. Bone graft is necessary and is easily obtained from the distal radius through the same incision. There are a variety of **intercarpal arthrodeses**, including **triscaphe** (scaphotrapezialtrapezoid), **scaphocapitate**, **lunotriquetrel**, and **four-corner** (capitate-hamate-triquetral-lunate). These procedures are indicated for the treatment of intercarpal arthritis, carpal instabilities due to intercarpal ligament tears and Kienbock's disease. Each procedure requires bone graft, which may be obtained from the distal radius or the iliac crest. The **Cloward cervical spine fusion instrumentation** is useful for obtaining a bicortical plug of bone from the iliac crest with minimal dissection.

**Usual preop diagnosis:** Post-traumatic arthritis; osteoarthritis or rheumatoid arthritis; Kienbock's disease; carpal instability

### SUMMARY OF PROCEDURE

| | |
|---|---|
| **Position** | Supine, with arm extended on hand-surgery table. The iliac crest may be prepped and elevated with a sandbag beneath the ipsilateral buttock. |
| **Incision** | Dorsal wrist, transverse (for intercarpal fusion) or longitudinal |
| **Special instrumentation** | Pneumatic tourniquet |
| **Unique considerations** | Bone-graft donor site |

| | |
|---|---|
| **Antibiotics** | Cefazolin 1 gm iv |
| **Surgical time** | 2 hrs |
| **Tourniquet** | 150 mm above systolic; max time = 120 min |
| **Closing considerations** | Immobilization with splints |
| **EBL** | Minimal; procedure is performed under tourniquet control. If iliac crest bone graft is used, there may be up to 500 cc of blood loss. |
| **Postop care** | PACU → room for pain and edema control |
| **Mortality** | Minimal |
| **Morbidity** | Nonunion of fusion ≤ 20% |
| **Procedure code** | 25800-25810 |
| **Pain score** | 7-9 |

### PATIENT POPULATION CHARACTERISTICS

| | |
|---|---|
| **Age range** | >40 yrs |
| **Male:Female** | Females predominate in rheumatoid arthritis; males in post-traumatic arthritis. |
| **Incidence** | Common |
| **Etiology** | Trauma: Common<br>Rheumatoid arthritis: Common |
| **Associated conditions** | Typical for rheumatoid arthritis (e.g., skin fragility, steroid dependency, immunosuppression) |

## ANESTHETIC CONSIDERATIONS

See Anesthetic Considerations following "Thumb Carpometacarpal Joint Fusion/Arthroplasty/Stabilization" (below).

**References**

1. Green DP: *Operative Hand Surgery*, 2nd edition. Churchill Livingstone, New York: 1988.

# TOTAL WRIST REPLACEMENT

## SURGICAL CONSIDERATIONS

**Description:** The major indication for this procedure is rheumatoid arthritis of the wrist. **Total wrist replacement (TWR)** is often recommended in patients with bilateral wrist disease. An arthrodesis will be carried out on the non-dominant helping hand and a TWR on the dominant hand to preserve dexterity. Many surgeons prefer to avoid **bilateral wrist arthrodesis**, although some patients with bilateral fusions have been able to function relatively well. Currently available protheses are suitable only for low-demand patients, and are not indicated for high-demand patients with post-traumatic arthritis. These patients will do better with wrist arthrodesis. Silastic® wrist prostheses are associated with a high failure rate and silicone synovitis, and their use has been abandoned by many surgeons. The most commonly used prostheses today are metal on ultra-high-molecular-weight polyethylene articulations that are fixed with methy-methacrylate cement or bone ingrowth into porous stems. All of these prostheses depend on intact, normally functioning wrist extensor tendons, especially the extensor carpi radialis brevis, for balance and function. Absence of this tendon is felt by many to be an absolute contraindication to this procedure. Because these tendons are so commonly affected by rheumatoid arthritis, the patient population for this procedure is limited. In addition to functioning tendons, meticulously accurate placement of the components in relation to the centers of rotation of the wrist is critical for success. If the centers of rotation of the prosthesis do not duplicate those of the normal wrist, early component loosening and failure is likely. Intraop radiographs are useful in verifying component position. These patients frequently have other upper extremity deformities which will require reconstruction. Because of the complexity of TWR, other reconstructive procedures are not carried out at the same time.

**Usual preop diagnosis**: Rheumatoid arthritis

### SUMMARY OF PROCEDURE

| | |
|---|---|
| **Position** | Supine, with arm extended on hand-surgery table |
| **Incision** | Dorsal wrist |
| **Special instrumentation** | TWR instrumentation; pneumatic tourniquet |
| **Antibiotics** | Cefazolin 1 gm iv |
| **Surgical time** | 2 hrs |
| **Tourniquet** | 150 mm above systolic; max time = 120 min |
| **Closing considerations** | Postop splint |
| **EBL** | Minimal; procedure performed under tourniquet control. |
| **Postop care** | PACU → room |
| **Mortality** | Minimal |
| **Morbidity** | Infection<br>Poor wound healing |
| **Procedure code** | 25446 |
| **Pain score** | 4-8 |

### PATIENT POPULATION CHARACTERISTICS

| | |
|---|---|
| **Age range** | Rare before 4th decade; most in 6th and 7th decades |
| **Male:Female** | Females outnumber males, as in rheumatoid arthritis. |
| **Incidence** | Rare |
| **Etiology** | Rheumatoid arthritis |
| **Associated conditions** | Rheumatoid arthritis |

## ANESTHETIC CONSIDERATIONS

See Anesthetic Considerations following "Thumb Carpometacarpal Joint Fusion/Arthroplasty/Stabilization" (below).

**References**

1. Green DP: *Operative Hand Surgery*, 2nd edition. Churchill Livingstone, New York: 1988.

# THUMB CARPOMETACARPAL JOINT FUSION/ ARTHROPLASTY/STABILIZATION

## SURGICAL CONSIDERATIONS

**Description:** Patients with degenerative arthritis of the carpometacarpal (CMC) joint of the thumb present with subluxation, pain and synovitis of the joint. A **synovectomy and ligament reconstruction** to restore stability will treat pain and prevent further degeneration. This procedure is performed through a curvilinear incision over the joint. A distally attached graft of the radial 1/2 of the flexor carpi radialis tendon is passed through a drill hole in the base of the metacarpal and woven into the joint capsule. In the later stages of degeneration, patients must be treated either with an arthroplasty or an arthrodesis. A variety of **arthroplasty techniques** are available to the surgeon. The most successful methods involve resection of all or part of the trapezium and replacement with a biological spacer – usually a rolled up tendon graft commonly referred to as an "anchovy." These procedures also stabilize the first metacarpal with a tendon transfer through a drill hole in the bone. **Arthrodesis** (fusion) is another alternative. Fixation may be obtained with Kirschner wires and intraosseous compression wires. The time to fusion with this technique is six weeks. These patients have very few limitations and perform almost all normal activities of daily living. This procedure requires very little postop hand therapy, compared with arthroplasty techniques. It is also well-suited to active patients. In some patients with extensive bone loss and cyst formation, bone graft is necessary and can be obtained form the distal radius.

**Usual preop diagnosis**: Osteoarthritis of CMC joint; basal joint arthritis; synovitis of CMC joint; CMC joint dislocation; trauma

### SUMMARY OF PROCEDURE

| | |
|---|---|
| **Position** | Supine, with arm extended on hand-surgery table |
| **Incision** | Curvilinear over joint at base of thumb. Tendon graft for interposition can be obtained through multiple small transverse incisions. |
| **Special instrumentation** | Pneumatic tourniquet |
| **Antibiotics** | Cefazolin 1 gm iv |
| **Surgical time** | 1.5 - 2 hrs |
| **Tourniquet** | 150 mm above systolic; max time = 120 min |
| **EBL** | Minimal; procedures performed under tourniquet control. |
| **Postop care** | Postop splintage; overnight hospital stay for pain control |
| **Mortality** | Minimal |
| **Morbidity** | Nonunion of arthrodesis occurs as frequently as 20% in some series. Newer techniques, such as the tension-band intraosseous wire and sliding cortical graft, have much lower failure rates. Silicone rubber prostheses are associated with particulate synovitis. |
| **Procedure code** | 26841 |
| **Pain score** | 8-9 |

### PATIENT POPULATION CHARACTERISTICS

| | |
|---|---|
| **Age range** | Joint stabilization in 3rd - 5th decades; arthroplasty and arthrodesis in 5th - 8th decades |
| **Male:Female** | Basal joint instability and arthritis much more prevalent in women. |
| **Incidence** | Common |
| **Etiology** | Trauma may play a role in producing instability. Patients who have had an intra-articular fracture of the base of the first metacarpal with a nonanatomic reduction will have incongruence of the joint and develop post-traumatic arthritis. Rheumatoid arthritis leads to instability and degeneration of the joint. Many patients with congenital ligamentous laxity will have unstable basal joints and will develop arthritis. |
| **Associated conditions** | Rheumatoid arthritis<br>Osteoarthritis<br>Carpal tunnel syndrome (CTS) |

## ANESTHETIC CONSIDERATIONS FOR WRIST PROCEDURES

**(Procedures covered: Darrach procedure; dorsal stabilization and extensor synovectomy of the rheumatoid wrist; metacarpophalangeal and interphalangeal joint arthroplasty; arthrodesis of the wrist; total wrist replacement; thumb carpometacarpal joint fusion [arthroscopy and stabilization])**

### PREOPERATIVE

**Airway** Rheumatoid involvement of the cervical spine, TMJ and cricoarytenoid joint (CAJ) are common in this patient population. Erosion of cervical vertebrae → unstable cervical spine (e.g., atlantoaxial subluxation) necessitates extreme care in head and neck manipulation. Cervical spine fusion (↓neck ROM), TMJ arthritis (↓mouth opening) and CAJ arthritis (laryngeal narrowing, hoarseness, DOE, stridor) portend difficult intubation and may necessitate awake fiber optic intubation. In the case of CAJ arthritis, use of a smaller ETT may be required.

**Respiratory** Rheumatoid patients may exhibit Sx of pleural effusion (✓ CXR) or pulmonary fibrosis (dyspnea, diffuse rales, ↓diffusing capacity, honeycomb appearance in CXR.

**Tests:** Consider CXR, PFTs, ABGs in affected patients.

**Cardiovascular** Rheumatoid patients may suffer from pericarditis, myocarditis, valvular disease and cardiac conduction defects. Because of the physical limitations imposed by the disease process, it may prove difficult to evaluate these patients' cardiovascular status; hence, cardiology consultation, ECG and ECHO may be useful in preparing for surgery.

**Tests:** Consider ECG and ECHO, especially in patients with severe rheumatoid arthritis.

**Neurological** Rheumatoid patients may have cervical or lumbar radiculopathies that should be documented carefully preop. In addition, peripheral neuropathy with consequent sensory/motor defects may be present.

**Tests:** Consider C-spine radiographs to rule out occult subluxations in rheumatoid patients with neck pain or upper extremity radiculopathy.

**Musculoskeletal** Bony deformities or muscle contractures may necessitate special attention to positioning.

**Hematologic** Anemia, eosinophilia and thrombocytosis may be present. Venous access may be difficult 2° vasculitis and ↑skin fragility (steroid-induced). Virtually all of these patients will be on some type of anti-inflammatory medication that may result in anemia or platelet inhibition. Ideally, patients should discontinue NSAIDs at least 5 d preop.

**Endocrine** Rheumatoid patients are likely to be on oral corticosteroids and require supplemental perioperative steroids (e.g., 100 mg hydrocortisone q 8 hr iv) to treat adrenal suppression.

**Laboratory** Hb/Hct serves as a minimum in otherwise healthy rheumatoid patients. Severe rheumatoid patients require more extensive testing to screen for drug effects, etc. (e.g., serum electrolytes; glucose; kidney function tests; LFTs).

**Premedication** Standard premedication (see Appendix).

### INTRAOPERATIVE

**Anesthetic technique:** Regional anesthesia, GA, or a combination of the two are commonly used. A brachial plexus block via the axillary approach is excellent for this procedure; it is a means of avoiding tracheal intubation for GA if airway difficulty is anticipated. Intravenous regional anesthesia (Bier block) is most useful for short procedures (< 1 hr). If regional anesthesia is contraindicated, rheumatoid patients may require awake fiber optic intubation.

**Regional anesthesia:**

**Axillary block** 1.5% mepivacaine 40-50 ml for routine cases; 1% etidocaine 40 ml for procedures estimated to last > 2.5 hrs. The medial aspect of the upper arm is innervated by the intercostobrachial nerve (T2) and requires a separate subcutaneous field block in the axilla, especially when a tourniquet is used. The lateral cutaneous nerve of the forearm, a sensory branch of the musculocutaneous nerve supplying sensation to the lateral forearm, is frequently missed by the axillary approach to the brachial plexus. Thus, a block of this nerve at the elbow is sometimes necessary. If sedation is necessary, propofol (50-150 μg/kg/min) by continuous infusion or intermittent bolus injection of opioid/benzodiazepine are good choices.

**General anesthesia:**

**Induction** Standard induction (see Appendix) in patients with normal airways.

**Maintenance** Standard maintenance (see Appendix).

| | | |
|---|---|---|
| **Emergence** | Skin closure is frequently followed by application of a splint, and the patient should remain anesthetized during the splinting procedure. Cases with difficult airways require awake extubation. | |
| **Blood and fluid requirements** | Minimal blood loss<br>IV: 18 ga x 1<br>NS/LR @ 1.5-3 cc/kg/hr | Catheter placed in the non-operated upper extremity. |
| **Monitoring** | Standard monitors (see Appendix). | |
| **Positioning** | Special handling required.<br>✓ and pad pressure points.<br>✓ eyes.<br>✓ C-spine instability. | As with nearly all orthopedic cases, positioning is a subtle, yet crucial aspect of anesthetic management. Rheumatoid patients may have contractures that require special attention. Steroid-dependent patients require special handling because of fragile skin. |
| **Axillary block complications** | Inadequate block<br>Intravascular injection<br>Peripheral nerve damage<br>Axillary hematoma<br>Axillary artery thrombosis<br>Pneumothorax | Very minimal doses of local anesthetic can cause CNS toxicity if reverse flow occurs during an intra-arterial injection. Axillary thrombosis and pneumothorax are extremely rare. |

## POSTOPERATIVE

| | | |
|---|---|---|
| **Pain management** | PCA (see Appendix), in combination with regional block. | Combined regional-general anesthetic techniques are excellent for wrist procedures, especially with respect to postop pain management. |
| **Tests** | None routinely indicated. | |


**References**

1. Green DP: *Operative Hand Surgery*, 2nd edition. Churchill Livingstone, New York: 1988.
2. Vandam LD: Anesthesia for Hand Surgery. In *Flynn's Hand Surgery*, 4th edition. Jupiter JB, ed. Williams and Wilkins, Baltimore: 1991, 46-54.
3. Ramamurthy S: Anesthesia. In *Operative Hand Surgery*, 2nd edition. Green DP, ed. Churchill Livingstone, New York: 1988, 27-60.
4. White RH: Preoperative evaluation of patients with rheumatoid arthritis. *Semin Arthritis Rheum* 1985; 14(4):287-99.
5. Keenan MA, Stiles CM, Kaufman RL: Acquired laryngeal deviation associated with cervical spine disease in erosive polyarticular arthritis. *Anesthesiology* 1983; 58(5):441-49.
6. Goldberg ME, et al: A comparison of three methods of axillary approach to brachial plexus blockade for upper extremity surgery. *Anesthesiology* 1987; 66(6):814-16.
7. Brockway MS, Wildsmith JA: Axillary brachial plexus block: method of choice? *Br J Anaesth* 1990; 64(2):224-31.
8. Tuominen MK, Pitkanen MT, Numminen MK, Rosenberg PH: Quality of axillary brachial plexus block. Comparison of success rate using perivascular and nerve stimulator techniques. *Anesthesia* 1987; 42(1):20-2.
9. Cockings E, Moore PL, Lewis RC: Transarterial brachial plexus blockade using high doses of 1.5% mepivacaine. *Reg Anesth* 1987; 12(4):159-64.

# EXCISION OF GANGLION OF THE WRIST

## SURGICAL CONSIDERATIONS

**Description:** Ganglion cysts about the wrist most commonly occur dorsally, originating from the scapholunate joint. The second most common site is volar to the scaphotrapezial joint. To prevent recurrence, these synovial fluid-filled outpouchings of the joint capsule must be excised completely. This requires isolating the stalk of the cyst to its origin, and excising a small cuff of normal joint capsule with the cyst. The joint, therefore, must be entered for a complete excision. Older studies found that the recurrence rate was decreased by the use of general anesthesia, as opposed to local or regional anesthetics. This was due to the fact that a more complete excision was performed when the patient was under a general anesthetic. Hand specialists today feel that regional anesthetics are quite acceptable for this procedure, as long as the surgeon performs a meticulous excision. Volar wrist ganglions commonly involve the radial artery, which is at risk during excision. A preop Allen test should be performed to ensure that, if the radial artery is interrupted, there will not be ischemia in the hand.

**Usual preop diagnosis**: Ganglion cyst, primary or recurrent

### SUMMARY OF PROCEDURE

| | |
|---|---|
| **Position** | Supine, with arm extended on hand-surgery table |
| **Incision** | Longitudinal or transverse directly over cyst |
| **Special instrumentation** | Pneumatic tourniquet |
| **Antibiotics** | Cefazolin 1 gm iv |
| **Surgical time** | 0.5 - 1.5 hrs |
| **Tourniquet** | 150 mm above systolic; max time = 120 min |
| **Closing considerations** | Routine skin closure. Large recurrent cysts may require a repair of the wrist capsule. Splint applied in OR. |
| **EBL** | Minimal; performed under tourniquet control. |
| **Postop care** | Elevation to prevent swelling |
| **Mortality** | Minimal |
| **Morbidity** | Injury to radial artery: Rare |
| **Procedure code** | 25111, 25112 |
| **Pain score** | 2-4 |

### PATIENT POPULATION CHARACTERISTICS

| | |
|---|---|
| **Age range** | Infants-elderly |
| **Male:Female** | 1:1 |
| **Incidence** | Very common |
| **Etiology** | Unknown. Trauma has been associated with about 50% of ganglion cysts. Underlying carpal instabilities, such as scapholunate instability, have been implicated. |
| **Associated conditions** | Carpal instability<br>Trauma (wrist sprains and strains) |

---

## ANESTHETIC CONSIDERATIONS

See Anesthetic Considerations following "Repair of Flexor Tendon Laceration" (below).

# PALMAR AND DIGITAL FASCIECTOMY

## SURGICAL CONSIDERATIONS

**Description:** This procedure is indicated for the treatment of Dupuytren's contractures of the digits, which produces a neoplastic thickening of the palmar and digital fascia. These pathologic cords (whose active cell is the myofibroblast) contract and, through their connections with the skin, tendon sheath and phalangeal bone, cause flexion contractures of the metacarpophalangeal, proximal interphalangeal and distal interphalangeal joints. The disease is progressive; and the only treatment is surgical excision of the fascia. In addition to the pathologic changes in the fascia of the hands, many patients also have thickening of the plantar fascia of the foot (Ledderhose's disease) and the dorsal fascia of the penis (Peyronie's disease). Patients with severe contractures that have been neglected may require amputation. Because the pathologic fascia is so intimately connected to the skin, it is sometimes necessary to excise the skin and replace it with full-thickness skin grafts. The groin is an excellent donor site for these grafts.

There are many different surgical approaches, most requiring the creation of Z-plasties for a tension-free closure. The **McCash technique** has been quite successful for the excision of palmar disease. This method consists of excising the palmar fascia through transverse incisions that are not sutured closed, but rather are left open to granulate and contract over a three-week postop period. These patients have a very low complication rate.

**Usual preop diagnosis**: Dupuytren's contracture

### SUMMARY OF PROCEDURE

| | |
|---|---|
| **Position** | Supine, with arm extended on hand-surgery table |
| **Incision** | Transverse or longitudinal palmar. Groin may be used as a full-thickness skin graft donor site. |
| **Antibiotics** | None |
| **Surgical time** | 1 - 3 hrs |
| **Tourniquet** | 150 mm above systolic; max time = 120 min. Because of the need to deflate tourniquet so that hemostasis can be obtained, Bier block is not suitable. |
| **Closing considerations** | Must obtain meticulous hemostasis. Z-plasties and skin grafts used frequently. |
| **EBL** | Minimal; dissection done under tourniquet control. A small amount of blood loss occurs when tourniquet is released and hemostasis is obtained. |
| **Postop care** | Pain control is essential. Patient may be admitted for initial postop period. Limb elevation to minimize swelling. Regional techniques that provide postop pain relief are very useful. |
| **Mortality** | Minimal |
| **Morbidity** | Hematoma<br>Skin necrosis<br>Infection<br>Digital nerve and artery injury<br>Reflex-sympathetic dystrophy |
| **Procedure code** | 26121, 26123 |
| **Pain score** | 7-8 |

### PATIENT POPULATION CHARACTERISTICS

| | |
|---|---|
| **Age range** | Typically, 40-60 yrs; can occur in teens. |
| **Male:Female** | More common in males |
| **Incidence** | Common |
| **Etiology** | Definite heritance – associated with strong family Hx. Ethnic diathesis for northern Europeans with fair hair and skin, blue eyes. Almost never seen in Blacks. Experimental studies suggest that microhematomas 2° repetitive trauma may be important in the disease process. |
| **Associated conditions** | Cigarette smoking<br>Alcoholism<br>Anti-seizure medications |

## ANESTHETIC CONSIDERATIONS

See Anesthetic Considerations following "Repair of Flexor Tendon Laceration" (below).

# REPAIR OF FLEXOR TENDON LACERATION

## SURGICAL CONSIDERATIONS

**Description:** The prognosis and difficulty of a flexor tendon repair depends on the anatomic site of the laceration. There are five zones of injury in the upper extremity (Fig 10.1-2). Zone I is distal to the flexor digitorum superficialis (FDS) tendon insertion and involves only the flexor digitorum profundus (FDP) tendon. Zone II extends from the entrance to the fibro-osseous sheath at the metacarpal head to the FDS insertion. Lacerations usually involve both the FDS and FDP. These are the most difficult to repair and have the worst prognosis as the tendons are apt to become scarred to each other and limit gliding. Zone III is the palm; Zone IV is within the carpal canal; and Zone 5 is in the forearm. Lacerations in these areas are easier to repair and have good prognoses for restoration of tendon gliding and, thus, digit motion. Associated injuries to the neural structures are common. Digital nerve lacerations are seen in Zone II; median nerve injuries, in Zone IV. Occasionally, nerve injuries occur in Zone V.

In general, nerve injuries are repaired at the time of the tendon repair. Tendons lacerated in the finger are often pulled back into the palm by muscular contraction. A palmar incision is required to retrieve the tendon, which must then be threaded carefully through the pulleys in the digit. Suture techniques for tendon repair create a juncture that is far weaker than an intact tendon. For this reason, the juncture must be protected from mechanical stress for a period of eight weeks or more. This is done by splinting the hand with the wrist and digits flexed so that the pull on the tendon by its muscle is limited by the tenodesis effect. It is important that the patient emerges gently from anesthesia to limit the stress upon the tendon. The best results are obtained when repair is carried out within seven days of the injury, although primary repair can be performed up to three weeks. After seven days, the muscle begins to undergo irreversible contracture. If the flexor tendon is advanced after this has occurred, a flexion contracture results. If a flexor tendon laceration is neglected, a palm-to-fingertip tendon graft, using a different flexor tendon, should be performed. If the tendon bed is suitable for gliding, the graft can be accomplished in one stage. If not, a Silastic® tendon spacer (rubber rod) must be placed at the first stage. Six-to-eight weeks later, a palm-to-fingertip graft is placed in the bed prepared with the Silastic® rod. Tendon graft donor sites include the palmaris longus tendon and toe extensors.

A variant of the sharp flexor tendon laceration is the FDP avulsion from its insertion in Zone 1. This is the so-called "jersey finger." This injury occurs during forceful grasp, and most commonly affects the ring finger. A common mechanism is the football or rugby player who is grasping the jersey of a ball carrier. The FDP tendon retracts and should be repaired within seven days. If neglected, these patients should be treated with a **distal interphalangeal (DIP) arthrodesis**. A flexor tendon graft through an intact FDS tendon usually is not indicated, as tendon adhesions will commonly interfere with the function of the FDS, leading to decreased overall active motion of the digit. The most common complication is the development of tendon adhesions, which limit tendon gliding and digit motion. If these patients fail to improve within a three-to-six-month course of physical therapy, they require an operative tenolysis to lyse the adhesions.

**Usual preop diagnosis**: Flexor tendon laceration; FDP avulsion ("jersey finger"); digital nerve laceration; median nerve laceration

### SUMMARY OF PROCEDURE

| | |
|---|---|
| **Position** | Supine, with arm extended on hand-surgery table. The foot may be prepped for a tendon graft. |
| **Incision** | Zig-zag hand or wrist |
| **Special instrumentation** | Pneumatic tourniquet |
| **Antibiotics** | Cefazolin 1 gm iv |

| | |
|---|---|
| **Surgical time** | 1-2 hrs; may be extended for nerve repair and treatment of associated injuries. |
| **Closing considerations** | Tendon and nerve repairs must be protected with splints prior to emergence from GA. Smooth extubation (see "Emergence"). |
| **EBL** | Minimal; procedure performed under tourniquet control. |
| **Postop care** | PACU → home |
| **Mortality** | Minimal |
| **Morbidity** | Tendon adhesions: 25%<br>Rupture of tendon repair: < 5%<br>Infection: Rare |
| **Procedure code** | 26350-26373 |
| **Pain score** | 2-4 |

### PATIENT POPULATION CHARACTERISTICS

| | |
|---|---|
| **Age range** | Infant-elderly |
| **Male:Female** | Slight male predominance, due to occupational injuries |
| **Incidence** | Not uncommon |
| **Etiology** | Trauma |

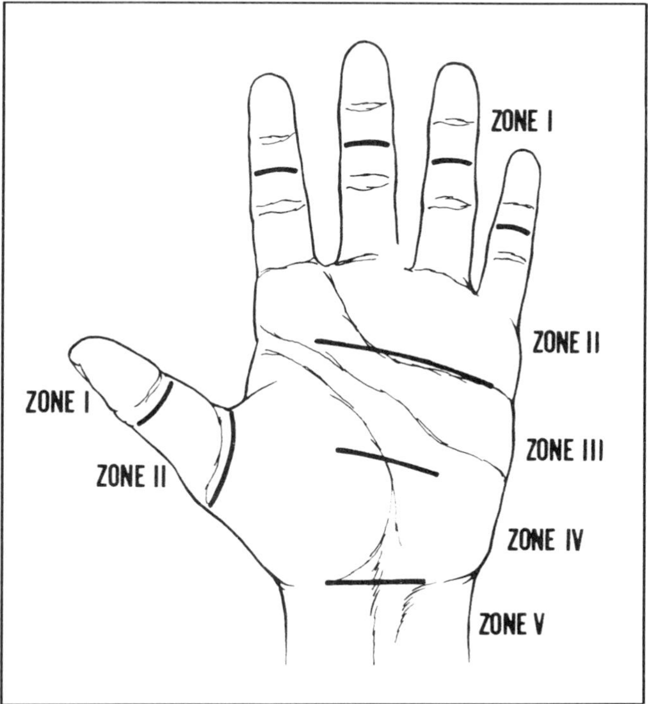


**Figure 10.1-2.** Zone classification of flexor tendon injuries. (Reproduced with permission from Green DP: *Operative Hand Surgery*, 2nd edition. Churchill Livingstone: 1988.)

---

## ANESTHETIC CONSIDERATIONS

**(Procedures covered: excision of ganglion of the wrist; palmar and digital fasciectomy; flexor tendon laceration)**

### PREOPERATIVE

The majority of patients presenting for these procedures are usually otherwise healthy. Many of them present for elective surgery as a result of progressive functional impairment and pain, and preop workup is routine.

| | |
|---|---|
| **Neurological** | If regional anesthesia is contemplated, pre-existing sensory or motor defects should be carefully documented. |
| **Laboratory** | Hb/Hct (healthy patients); otherwise, as indicated from H&P. |
| **Premedication** | Moderate-to-heavy premedication (e.g., midazolam 0.5-1.0 mg iv q 5 min titrated to effect) is often desirable if regional block is done. |

### INTRAOPERATIVE

**Anesthetic technique:** Regional anesthesia (most common), GA or a combination of the two may be used. Intravenous regional anesthesia (Bier block) is most useful for short procedures such as these which last for < 1 hr (see "Wrist Arthroscopy"). A brachial plexus block via the axillary approach is excellent for this procedure. Because most of these procedures are done on an outpatient basis, brachial plexus block without GA is usually preferred in order to promote early "street-readiness."

**Regional anesthesia:**

**Axillary block** 1.5% mepivacaine 40-50 ml for routine cases; 1% etidocaine 40 ml for procedures that may last >2.5 hrs. The medial aspect of the upper arm is innervated by the intercostobrachial nerve (T2) and requires a separate subcutaneous field block in the axilla, especially when a tourniquet is

**Axillary block, continued** used. The lateral cutaneous nerve of the forearm, a sensory branch of the musculocutaneous nerve supplying sensation to the lateral forearm, is frequently missed by the axillary approach to the brachial plexus. Thus, a block of this nerve at the elbow is sometimes necessary. If sedation is necessary, propofol (50-150 μg/kg/min) by continuous infusion or intermittent bolus injection of opioid/benzodiazepine are good choices.

**General anesthesia:**

**Induction** Standard induction (see Appendix).

**Maintenance** Standard maintenance (see Appendix).

**Emergence** Standard emergence (see Appendix). Skin closure is frequently followed by application of a splint; patient should remain anesthetized during splinting procedure.

**Blood and fluid requirements**

Minimal blood loss
IV: 18 ga x 1
NS/LR @ 1.5-3 cc/kg/hr

An 18-ga iv catheter placed in the non-operated upper extremity should be adequate.

**Monitoring** Standard monitors (see Appendix).

**Positioning**

√ and pad pressure points.
√ eyes.

**Axillary block complications**

Intravascular injection
Inadequate block
Peripheral nerve damage
Axillary hematoma

Minimal doses of local anesthetic can cause CNS toxicity during an accidental intravascular injection. Seizures should be treated with STP or midazolam titrated to effect, accompanied by airway control. If there is any question of a full stomach, intubation should be accomplished rapidly.

Axillary artery thrombosis
Pneumothorax

Axillary thrombosis and pneumothorax very rare.

## POSTOPERATIVE

**Pain management** Oral analgesics are usually sufficient.

The lingering analgesia of the brachial plexus block is often sufficient for pain relief in the recovery room; oral analgesic therapy can be instituted prior to discharging patient to home.

**Tests** None routinely indicated.

**References**

1. Green DP: *Operative Hand Surgery*, 2nd edition. Churchill Livingstone, New York: 1988.
2. Vandam LD: Anesthesia for Hand Surgery. In *Flynn's Hand Surgery*, 4th edition. Jupiter JB, ed. Williams and Wilkins, Baltimore: 1991, 46-54.
3. Ramamurthy S: Anesthesia. In *Operative Hand Surgery*, 2nd edition. Green DP, ed. Churchill Livingstone, New York: 1988, 27-60.
4. Goldberg ME, et al: A comparison of three methods of axillary approach to brachial plexus blockade for upper extremity surgery. *Anesthesiology* 1987; 66(6):814-16.
5. Brockway MS, Wildsmith JA: Axillary brachial plexus block: method of choice? *Br J Anaesth* 1990; 64(2):224-31.
6. Tuominen MK, Pitkanen MT, Numminen MK, Rosenberg PH: Quality of axillary brachial plexus block. Comparison of success rate using perivascular and nerve stimulator techniques. *Anesthesia* 1987; 42(1):20-2.
7. Cockings E, Moore PL, Lewis RC: Transarterial brachial plexus blockade using high doses of 1.5% mepivacaine. *Reg Anesth* 1987; 12(4):159-64.
8. Davis WJ, Lennon RL, Wedel DJ: Brachial plexus anesthesia for outpatient surgical procedures on an upper extremity. *Mayo Clin Proc* 1991; 66(5):470-73.

# WRIST ARTHROSCOPY

## SURGICAL CONSIDERATIONS

**Description:** Wrist arthroscopy may be performed for either diagnostic or therapeutic indications. A smaller diameter version of the standard arthroscope is used for visualizing the wrist joint. All of the entry portals are on the dorsum of the wrist and course between the extensor compartments. Irrigation is used during the procedure and a cannula is routinely placed ulnar to the extensor carpi ulnaris tendon. Unlike the knee joint, where visualization is obtained by distention of the joint, in-the-wrist visualization is obtained by distraction. The digits are placed in finger traps and up to 10 pounds of traction can be placed on the wrist. Specialized instrumentation is available to resect and debride intra-articular structures and to place sutures to repair torn ligaments. Arthroscopic techniques can also be used to irrigate and debride the infected wrist joint. At Stanford University Medical Center, we have performed over 50 wrist arthroscopies, both diagnostic and therapeutic, under Bier block. All patients tolerated the surgery well and were able to view the procedure on the monitor, and to discuss the findings with the surgeon intraop. Anesthesia time of up to 80 minutes was well-tolerated. If an open procedure, such as repair of an intercarpal ligament, is contemplated following diagnostic arthroscopy, either a general anesthetic or regional block is preferred.

**Variant procedure or approaches**: The standard approach is to suspend the forearm vertically in traction. The forearm can also be placed horizontally on the hand table in traction.

**Usual preop diagnosis**: Internal derangement of the wrist of unknown etiology; tears of the triangular fibrocartilage complex; intercarpal instability due to intercarpal ligament tears; rotatory subluxation of the scaphoid; scapholunate dissociation; luno-triquetral dissociation; fracture of distal radius ulnar impingement syndrome; rheumatoid synovitis; intra-articular infection

### SUMMARY OF PROCEDURE

| | |
|---|---|
| **Position** | Supine, with arm extended on hand-surgery table |
| **Incision** | Small incisions are made on the dorsum of the wrist for instrument insertion. |
| **Special instrumentation** | 2.7 mm diameter arthroscope, 0 or 30-degree field of view; light source and video camera; television monitor; surgical power shaver; joint irrigation system; traction device for forearm; pneumatic tourniquet |
| **Unique considerations** | Patient is often awake and observes surgery on monitor. |
| **Antibiotics** | Cefazolin 1 gm iv |
| **Surgical time** | 30 min - 2 hrs |
| **Tourniquet** | 150 mm above systolic; max time = 120 min |
| **Closing considerations** | Arthroscopic portals are each closed with a single skin suture. |
| **EBL** | Minimal; procedure performed with tourniquet control. |
| **Postop care** | PACU → home |
| **Mortality** | Minimal |
| **Morbidity** | Infection: < 1%<br>Swelling (2° to irrigation fluid): Common<br>Nerve and artery damage: Uncommon |
| **Procedure code** | 29843, 29848 |
| **Pain score** | 1-3 |

### PATIENT POPULATION CHARACTERISTICS

| | |
|---|---|
| **Age range** | Adolescent-elderly. This procedure is not indicated in children. |
| **Male:Female** | 1:1 |
| **Incidence** | Least common form of arthroscopy |
| **Etiology** | See Usual Preop Diagnosis, above. |
| **Associated conditions** | Degenerative arthritis (post-traumatic and osteo); rheumatoid arthritis |

## ANESTHETIC CONSIDERATIONS

See Anesthetic Considerations following "Carpal Tunnel Release" (below).

**References**

1. Green DP: *Operative Hand Surgery*, 2nd edition. Churchill Livingstone, New York: 1988.

# CARPAL TUNNEL RELEASE

## SURGICAL CONSIDERATIONS

**Description:** This is the most commonly performed procedure in hand surgery. It consists of the transection of the transverse carpal ligament through either an open-palmar or an endoscopic approach. The procedure may include synovectomy of the flexor tendons, tendon transfers to restore thumb opposition and the excision of masses from within the carpal canal. In patients with severe synovitis, as in rheumatoid arthritis, a synovectomy should be performed at the same time. If there is advanced thenar atrophy and weakness of thumb opposition, a tendon transfer also should be done at that time. The most common transfer is the **Camitz Opponensplasty**, in which the palmaris longis tendon is prolonged with palmar fascia and transferred to the thumb. Transfers of the extensor indicis proprius and superficial flexor tendons also can be performed. Because of the great danger of lacerating a nerve during endoscopic carpal tunnel release, it is recommended that the procedure be performed under a local anesthetic with infiltration only into the skin. Thus, the nerves remain sensate and can be probed and identified by the awake patient. Short-acting sedation can be used during the insertion of the trocar and sheath into the carpal canal.

**Usual preop diagnosis**: Carpal tunnel syndrome (CTS); median nerve compression at the wrist

**SUMMARY OF PROCEDURE**

| | Open Carpal Tunnel Release | Endoscopic Carpal Tunnel Release |
|---|---|---|
| **Position** | Supine | ⇐ |
| **Incision** | Longitudinal incision in palm; may extend to forearm | 2 cm transverse at proximal flexion crease of wrist; 1 cm, mid-palm |
| **Special instrumentation** | Pneumatic tourniquet | Endoscopic carpal tunnel release system: endoscope, sheath and trocar, special cutting tools |
| **Unique considerations** | None | Danger of intraop injury to digital nerves, median nerve, tendons, superficial vascular arch |
| **Antibiotics** | Cefazolin 1 gm iv | ⇐ |
| **Surgical time** | 0.5 - 1.5 hrs | 30 min |
| **Closing considerations** | Simple skin closure | ⇐ |
| **EBL** | Minimal; performed under tourniquet control. | Minimal |
| **Postop care** | Splint, elevation | No splint, early motion, elevation |
| **Mortality** | Minimal | ⇐ |
| **Morbidity** | Overall complication rate: 4% | ⇐ |
| | Reflex sympathetic dystrophy (RSD): < 5% | Rare |
| | Hematoma: Rare | Complications of ulnar nerve palsy |
| | Infection: Uncommon | Tendon and nerve laceration: Rare (< 1%) |
| | | Vascular injury: Less common than nerve injury |
| **Procedure code** | 64721 | ⇐ |
| **Pain score** | 1-2 | 1-2 |

### PATIENT POPULATION CHARACTERISTICS

**Age range** 20-80 yrs; 50% are 40-60 yrs

**Male:Female** 1:2

**Incidence** Common

**Etiology** Compression of the median nerve within the carpal tunnel by synovitis
Mass effect 2° tumor or fracture fragments, peripheral neuropathy, gout, anomalous structures, thrombosis of a persistent median artery and idiopathic.
Repetitive trauma (e.g., computer use.)

**Associated conditions**
Rheumatoid arthritis
Thyroid imbalance
Diabetes
Amyloidosis
Multiple myeloma
Alcoholism
Hemophilia
Pregnancy
Menopause
Gout
Fractures of the distal radius
Kienbock's disease

---

## ANESTHETIC CONSIDERATIONS

**(Procedures covered: wrist arthroscopy; carpal tunnel release)**

### PREOPERATIVE

In general, there are two patient populations involved: (1) healthy patients with a history of wrist trauma, and (2) rheumatoid patients. (See Anesthetic Considerations for "Dorsal Stabilization and Extensor Synovectomy of the Rheumatoid Wrist" for discussion of preop concerns in the rheumatoid patient.)

**Laboratory** Hb/Hct (healthy patients); otherwise, as indicated from H&P.

**Premedication** Moderate-to-heavy premedication (e.g., midazolam 0.5-1.0 mg iv q 5 min titrated to effect) is often desirable if regional block is done.

### INTRAOPERATIVE

**Anesthetic technique:** Intravenous regional anesthesia is an excellent technique for procedures that are < 1 hr. For longer procedures, an axillary brachial plexus block is a good alternative. Both of these techniques are especially appropriate for outpatients.

**Intravenous regional block** 40-50 cc of 0.5% lidocaine is injected intravenously into the exsanguinated limb. This will usually provide up to 1 hr of anesthesia before tourniquet pain becomes severe. The use of a double-cuffed tourniquet may help minimize tourniquet pain. For procedures < 40 min, the tourniquet should be deflated briefly (~10 sec), then reinflated while observing the patient for signs of toxicity (60-90 sec) before final deflation. If sedation is needed, propofol (50-150 $\mu$g/kg/min) by continuous infusion, or intermittent bolus injection of opioid/benzodiazepine, are good choices.

**Blood and fluid requirements**
Minimal blood loss
IV: 18 ga x 1
NS/LR @ 1.5-2 cc/kg/hr

An 18-ga iv catheter placed in the non-operated upper extremity should be adequate.

**Monitoring** Standard monitors (see Appendix).

**Positioning**
✓ and pad pressure points.
✓ eyes.

| | | |
|---|---|---|
| **Intravenous regional block complications** | Systemic toxicity:<br>- Tinnitus<br>- Dizziness<br>- Blurred vision<br>- Seizure<br>- ↓HR, ↓BP<br>Inadequate block<br>Thrombophlebitis | Systemic toxic reaction to the local anesthetic may occur as a result of tourniquet leak or inadvertent premature (< 20 min) tourniquet release. Treatment is supportive. Seizures are controlled with STP or midazolam with appropriate airway protection. Even with a functioning tourniquet, it is possible to overcome tourniquet pressure by injecting too vigorously. Care must be taken when switching from proximal to distal tourniquet; never deflate proximal tourniquet until verifying that distal tourniquet is working. Finally, never deflate tourniquet(s) until at least 20 min have elapsed. |

## POSTOPERATIVE

| | | |
|---|---|---|
| **Pain management** | Oral analgesics usually sufficient. | Residual analgesia with intravenous regional anesthesia is minimal; some iv opioid is usually necessary until the patient is tolerating fluids in the recovery room. |
| **Tests** | None routinely indicated. | |

## References


1. Vandam LD: Anesthesia for Hand Surgery. In *Flynn's Hand Surgery*, 4th edition. Jupiter JB, ed. Williams and Wilkins, Baltimore: 1991, 46-54.
2. Ramamurthy S: Anesthesia. In *Operative Hand Surgery*, 2nd edition. Green DP, ed. Churchill Livingstone, New York: 1988, 27-60.
3. Brown EM, McGriff JT, Malinowski RW: Intravenous regional anaesthesia (Bier block): a review of 20 years' experience. *Can J Anaesth* 1989; 36(3 Pt 1):307-10.
4. Grice SC, Morell RC, Balestrieri FJ, et al: Intravenous regional anesthesia: evaluation and prevention of leakage under the tourniquet. *Anesthesiology* 1986; 65(3):316-20.
5. Davies JA, Wilkey AD, Hall ID: Bupivacaine leak past inflated tourniquets during intravenous regional analgesia. *Anaesthesia* 1984; 39(10):996-99.
6. Rosenberg PH, Kalso EA, Tuominen MK, Linden HB: Acute bupivacaine toxicity as a result of venous leakage under the tourniquet cuff during a Bier block. *Anesthesiology* 1983; 58(1):95-8.
7. Duggan J, Mckeown DW, Scott DB: Venous pressures generated during IV regional anaesthesia. *Br J Anaesth* 1983; 55:1158P-59P.
8. Sukhani R, Garcia CJ, Munhall RJ, et al: Lidocaine disposition following intravenous regional anesthesia with different tourniquet deflation technics. *Anesth Analg* 1989; 68(5):633-37.

# REPAIR OF FRACTURES AND DISLOCATIONS OF THE DISTAL RADIUS, CARPUS AND METACARPALS

## SURGICAL CONSIDERATIONS

**Description:** Patients with fractures of the distal radius, carpus and/or metacarpals, which cannot be treated adequately with closed methods, require **open reduction and fixation** (ORIF). The criteria for adequate treatment include anatomic reduction of the fracture fragments and stable maintenance of this reduction. Closed, unstable, distal radius fractures often are treated by traction and application of an external fixator in the OR to maintain the reduction by ligamentotaxis. Patients with wrist dislocation and distal radius fractures frequently have signs of neurologic compromise, such as carpal tunnel syndrome (CTS). Vascular compromise of the hand associated with these injuries is rare, usually occurring in patients with severe crush or high-energy injuries. The devascularized hand is a surgical emergency, and revascularization must be carried out as soon as possible. Fractures of these structures are associated with blast and crush injuries, as well as low-velocity gunshot wounds. These injuries have significant soft-tissue components which must be treated. The possibility of a coexisting compartment syndrome should be considered; and a fasciotomy may be needed at the time of surgery. Treatment of these fractures often involves a bone graft from the iliac crest to augment the reduction. A variety of fixation devices, including screws and plates, as well as Kirschner wires, are used. Open fractures are, by definition, contaminated and should be irrigated and debrided within eight hours of the injury. Surgical approaches are direct through longitudinal or transverse incisions. Some fractures of the articular surface of the distal radius are amenable to arthroscopically guided percutaneous pin fixation. Screw fixation of the scaphoid can be accomplished also by arthroscopy. Fluoroscopy is often utilized, as are standard portable radiographs to monitor and assess the quality of the reduction of the fracture. Soft-tissue coverage of these injuries may be problematic and **local flaps** or **free microvascular tissue transfers** may be indicated. Free transfers can come from the same limb (radial forearm flap, based on the radial artery; lateral upper arm flap, based on the posterior radial collateral artery) or a remote site (latissimus dorsi muscle, based on the thoracodorsal artery; or scapular skin flap, based on the circumflex scapular artery). Remote flaps require special patient positioning and draping. Microsurgical tissue transfers may also need special pharmacological considerations, such as the administration of heparin or dextran to prevent thrombosis of the anastomosis.

**Usual preop diagnosis**: Fractures of the distal radius (Colles', Barton's, Smith's are common eponyms); wrist dislocations (perilunate, lunate); fractures of the metacarpals; gunshot wounds; crush injuries; blast injuries

### SUMMARY OF PROCEDURE

| | |
|---|---|
| **Position** | Supine, with arm extended on hand-surgery table. Iliac crest bone graft may be indicated and should be prepped with a sandbag beneath the ipsilateral buttock. |
| **Incision** | Longitudinal or transverse |
| **Special instrumentation** | Fluoroscopy; wrist arthroscopy instrumentation; internal and external fixation devices and power tools; operating microscope; pneumatic tourniquet |
| **Unique considerations** | Associated injuries and soft-tissue problems in high-energy fractures |
| **Antibiotics** | Indicated during the treatment of infected fractures. Treatment of both open and closed fractures requires broad spectrum cephalosporin prophylaxis. Special cases of contamination, such as soil and human bite injuries, require specific extended coverage. |
| **Surgical time** | 30 min - 3 hrs. Microsurgical tissue transfers can have surgical times of 8 hrs or more. |
| **Tourniquet** | 150 mm above systolic; max time = 120 min |
| **Closing considerations** | Some injuries require local flaps or free microsurgical tissue transfers for closure. Fasciotomy wounds are usually left open. Splint applied at surgery. |
| **EBL** | Minimal for fracture treatment, as tourniquet control is used. Iliac crest or free-tissue donor sites can result in blood loss of 500-2000 cc. |
| **Postop care** | Monitor free-tissue transfers with temperature monitoring and visual inspection. |
| **Mortality** | Usually due to associated injuries |
| **Morbidity** | Loss of reduction, requiring repair<br>Nonunion<br>Infection |
| **Procedure code** | 25500-25695 |
| **Pain score** | 3-9 |

### PATIENT POPULATION CHARACTERISTICS

| | |
|---|---|
| **Age range** | All ages. More conservative approaches are used with elderly patients. |
| **Male:Female** | 1:1 |
| **Incidence** | Very common |
| **Etiology** | Trauma |
| **Associated conditions** | Traumatic injuries |

---

## ANESTHETIC CONSIDERATIONS

### PREOPERATIVE

The majority of patients presenting for these procedures are relatively young and healthy. Most of these patients present for elective repair of a traumatic injury, and preop workup is routine. Replantation and some wrist procedures, such as repair of a compound fracture, require immediate attention and necessitate emergency surgery and full-stomach considerations.

**Neurologic** — If regional anesthesia is contemplated, pre-existing sensory or motor defects should be documented carefully preop.

**Laboratory** — Hb/Hct (healthy patients); otherwise, as indicated from H&P.

**Premedication** — Moderate-to-heavy premedication (e.g., midazolam 0.5-1.0 mg iv q 5 min titrated to effect) is often desirable if regional block is done.

### INTRAOPERATIVE

**Anesthetic technique:** GETA or regional anesthesia are commonly used. A brachial plexus block via the axillary approach is excellent for short (1-2 hr) procedures on the wrist and hand. Regional anesthesia alone is a means of avoiding the risk of aspiration pneumonitis associated with GA in the patient with a full stomach whose operation must be done emergently (see "Rapid-Sequence Induction of Anesthesia," in Appendix). Unfortunately, because these cases often require the use of bone grafts harvested from the iliac crest, regional anesthesia alone usually is not feasible. For similar reasons, regional anesthesia also is not appropriate for cases that require a free-tissue transfer.

**General anesthesia:**

**Induction** — Standard induction (see Appendix).

**Maintenance** — Standard maintenance (see Appendix).

**Emergence** — Skin closure is frequently followed by application of a splint; patient should remain anesthetized during splinting procedure.

**Regional anesthesia:**

**Axillary block** — 1.5% mepivacaine or 1.5% lidocaine 40 ml for routine cases; 1% etidocaine 40 ml for procedures that may last >2.5 hrs. The medial aspect of the upper arm is innervated by the intercostobrachial nerve (T2) and requires a separate subcutaneous field block in the axilla, especially when a tourniquet is used. The lateral cutaneous nerve of the forearm, a sensory branch of the musculocutaneous nerve supplying sensation to the lateral forearm, is frequently missed by the axillary approach to the brachial plexus. Thus, a block of this nerve at the elbow is sometimes necessary. If sedation is needed, propofol (50-150 μg/kg/min) by continuous infusion or intermittent bolus injection of opioid/benzodiazepine (e.g., midazolam 0.5-1.0 mg iv q 5 min and alfentanil 5-10 μg/kg iv q min titrated to effect) can be used.

| | | |
|---|---|---|
| **Blood and fluid requirements** | Minimal-to-moderate blood loss<br>IV: 18 ga x 1<br>NS/LR @ 1.5-3 cc/kg/hr | Minimal-to-moderate blood loss unless an iliac crest bone graft becomes necessary; these graft donor sites can lose 250-500 ml of blood. An 18-ga iv catheter placed in the non-operated upper extremity should be adequate. |
| **Monitoring** | Standard monitors (see Appendix). | |
| **Positioning** | ✓ and pad pressure points.<br>✓ eyes. | |

| | | |
|---|---|---|
| **Axillary block complications** | Inadequate block<br>Intravascular injection<br>Peripheral nerve damage<br>Axillary hematoma<br>Axillary artery thrombosis<br>Pneumothorax | Minimal doses of local anesthetic can cause CNS toxicity during an accidental intravascular injection. Seizures should be treated with STP or midazolam titrated to effect, accompanied by airway control. If there is any question of a full stomach, then intubation should be accomplished rapidly. Axillary thrombosis and pneumothorax are extremely rare. |

### POSTOPERATIVE

| | | |
|---|---|---|
| **Pain management** | PCA (see Appendix), in combination with regional block. | Combined regional-general anesthetic techniques are excellent for wrist procedures, especially with respect to postop pain management. |
| **Tests** | None routinely indicated. | |

**References**


1. Green DP: *Operative Hand Surgery*, 2nd edition. Churchill Livingstone, New York: 1988.
2. Vandam LD: Anesthesia for Hand Surgery. In *Flynn's Hand Surgery*, 4th edition. Jupiter JB, ed. Williams and Wilkins, Baltimore: 1991, 46-54.
3. Ramamurthy S: Anesthesia. In *Operative Hand Surgery*, 2nd edition. Green DP, ed. Churchill Livingstone, New York: 1988, 27-60.
4. Goldberg ME, et al: A comparison of three methods of axillary approach to brachial plexus blockade for upper extremity surgery. *Anesthesiology* 1987; 66(6):814-16.
5. Brockway MS, Wildsmith JA: Axillary brachial plexus block: method of choice? *Br J Anaesth* 1990; 64(2):224-31.
6. Tuominen MK, Pitkanen MT, Numminen MK, Rosenberg PH: Quality of axillary brachial plexus block. Comparison of success rate using perivascular and nerve stimulator techniques. *Anesthesia* 1987; 42(1):20-2.
7. Cockings E, Moore PL, Lewis RC: Transarterial brachial plexus blockade using high doses of 1.5% mepivacaine. *Reg Anesth* 1987; 12(4):159-64.
8. Davis WJ, Lennon RL, Wedel DJ: Brachial plexus anesthesia for outpatient surgical procedures on an upper extremity. *Mayo Clin Proc* 1991; 66(5):470-73.


# DIGIT AND HAND REPLANTATION

## SURGICAL CONSIDERATIONS

**Description:** Patients with traumatic amputations of digits and the hand are candidates for emergency microsurgical replantation of these parts. In children, replantation is attempted for essentially all amputations. In the adult, replantation is carried out for amputations of the thumb, multiple digits, and amputations through the palm. In general, amputations of a single digit are not candidates for replantation because of the minimal loss of function in relation to the long rehabilitation period and expected outcome. Certainly, a single digit amputated proximal to the insertion of the flexor digitorum superficialis (FDS) tendon (Zone II) (Fig 10.1-2) should not be replanted. The condition of the amputated part plays an important role in the decision to proceed with replantation. A severely crushed, contaminated, or burned part cannot be expected to survive and function. The patients may also have associated traumatic injuries which will take preference over replantation (i.e., intra-abdominal bleeding with a positive peritoneal lavage, chest injuries). The patient's overall health status must be assessed. A patient with unstable angina should probably not be subjected to a lengthy microsurgical procedure.

There are a variety of reasons that people suffer amputations. Many of these patients are substance abusers or intoxicated at the time of injury. Studies of these patients also have shown a high incidence of psychopathology, along with substance abuse. Because these procedures are emergent, patients often arrive at the hospital with full stomachs. While regional anesthesia techniques provide peripheral vasodilation through their sympatholytic effect, many surgeons prefer general anesthesia because of the unpredictable length of the procedures. While the patient is being readied for induction, the surgeon prepares the amputated part in the OR. At this time, the structures to be repaired are tagged, which saves a great deal of anesthetic time. When the patient is prepped and draped, the hand is irrigated and debrided, and the corresponding structures are tagged in similar manner. The amputated part is brought to the field and the actual replantation is performed. Once arterial blood flow is reestablished, the patient must be kept warm to prevent vasospasm. As with other microsurgical procedures, pharmacologic intervention is indicated to prevent thrombosis; intravenous heparin and dextran are normally administered. Skin grafts for soft-tissue coverage and vein grafts to replace segmental vascular defects are commonly used. Vein grafts can be obtained from the ipsilateral upper extremity or from the lower extremity, especially the dorsum of the foot. The lateral thigh or abdomen are excellent donor sites for split-thickness skin grafts. Rarely is an immediate microsurgical free-tissue transfer indicated for soft-tissue coverage.

**Usual preop diagnosis**: Traumatic amputation of the digits or hand

### SUMMARY OF PROCEDURE

| | |
|---|---|
| **Position** | Supine, with arm extended on hand-surgery table |
| **Incision** | Extensile exposures of neurovascular structures. Lower extremity prepped and draped as donor site for vein grafts from dorsum of foot, split-thickness skin graft from the thigh. |
| **Special instrumentation** | Operating microscope; microsurgical instrumentation |
| **Unique considerations** | Emergency procedure |
| **Antibiotics** | Cefazolin 1 gm iv |
| **Surgical time** | 3 - 12 hrs |
| **Tourniquet** | 150 mm above systolic; max time = 120 min |
| **Closing considerations** | Routine volar hand splint |
| **EBL** | < 500 cc |
| **Postop care** | ICU → requires monitoring in intensive nursing environment. Should be kept pain-free for extended period postop to minimize vessel spasm. Patients will benefit from postop sedation. |
| **Mortality** | Minimal |
| **Morbidity** | Loss of replanted part (vessel thrombosis): 10%<br>Infection: Rare |
| **Procedure code** | 20816-20823 |
| **Pain score** | 3-5 |

### PATIENT POPULATION CHARACTERISTICS

| | |
|---|---|
| **Age range** | All ages, infant-8th decade |
| **Male:Female** | 1:1 |
| **Incidence** | Uncommon |
| **Etiology** | Trauma |
| **Associated conditions** | Substance abuse<br>Alcoholism |

---

## ANESTHETIC CONSIDERATIONS

### PREOPERATIVE

In general, there are two patient populations for hand replantation: (1) isolated hand injury patients (common), and (2) multiple trauma victims (rare).

**Respiratory** As suggested by coexisting disease or acute trauma injuries. Evidence of occult chest injury, including pneumothorax and pulmonary contusion, should be sought.
**Tests:** Consider CXR, ABGs in victims of significant trauma.

**Cardiovascular** As suggested by coexisting disease or acute trauma injuries. Look for evidence of occult cardiac or mediastinal injuries, such as myocardial contusion or great vessel rupture.
**Tests:** Consider CXR (with NG tube in place to assess mediastinal widening), and ECG in victims of significant trauma.

**Neurological** As suggested by co-existing disease or acute trauma injuries. The possibility of closed head injury should be addressed in multiple-trauma victims. Verify integrity of C-spine.
**Tests:** Consider head CT prior to beginning a long procedure under GA in a patient with evidence of head trauma; C-spine x-ray.

**Gastrointestinal** All patients should be considered to have full stomachs and, therefore, at increased risk for aspiration pneumonitis. In general, they should receive preop medication to reduce stomach volume and acidity (e.g., metoclopramide 10 mg iv and ranitidine 50 mg iv).

**Hematologic** Multiple-trauma victims are likely to suffer from acute blood loss. Although blood loss from these procedures is generally modest, a preop T&C for several U PRBCs is wise for trauma patients.
**Tests:** CBC

**Metabolic** Approximately 1/2 of trauma victims are intoxicated. Anesthesia-related implications of ethanol intoxication include: decreased anesthetic requirements, diuresis, vasodilation and hypothermia.

**Laboratory** As suggested by co-existing disease or acute trauma injuries. In general, most victims of significant trauma are best-served by obtaining a wide variety of baseline lab studies to screen for unrecognized injury. These studies normally include: ABGs; UA; renal function tests; LFTs; serum amylase; tox screen.

**Premedication** Full-stomach precautions: Na citrate 0.3 M 30 cc, metoclopramide 10 mg iv; $H_2$-blocker

## INTRAOPERATIVE

**Anesthetic technique:** GETA, after rapid-sequence induction. Because of the unpredictable length of these procedures and the possible need for bone and/or vessel grafts, regional anesthesia is not feasible as the primary technique. A concurrent, continuing brachial plexus block, however, will provide sympathetic blockade, as well as postop analgesia, and catheter placement should be considered prior to inducing GA. The hand injury repair may be done concurrently with other procedures in multiple-trauma victims.

**Induction** Rapid-sequence induction is mandatory in emergency cases, unless awake intubation is performed. C-spine fracture patients or those with facial injuries may require awake fiber optic intubation. Hemodynamically unstable, acute-trauma patients may be more safely induced with etomidate or ketamine.

**Maintenance** Standard maintenance (see Appendix) for stable patients. Hemodynamically unstable, acute-trauma victims undergoing emergency surgery may be better-served by using a combination of medications designed to have minimal hemodynamic consequences (e.g., fentanyl for analgesia, vecuronium for muscle relaxation and scopolamine or midazolam for amnesia). $N_2O$ is best avoided in the unstable patient because of its myocardial depressant effects.

**Emergence** Difficult airway or full-stomach cases require awake extubation. Trauma victims who have undergone a prolonged procedure or who have significant associated cardiopulmonary injuries are usually left intubated for postop mechanical ventilation.

| | | |
|---|---|---|
| **Blood and fluid requirements** | Significant blood loss<br>IV: 16 ga x 1<br>NS/LR @ 1.5-3 cc/kg/hr + replacement of blood loss<br>Fluid/blood warmers, heating blanket, warmed circuit humidifier | A 16-ga iv catheter in non-operated upper extremity should be adequate in hemodynamically stable patients. Acute-trauma victims who are unstable require a minimum of 2 large-bore iv catheters. |
| **Monitoring** | Standard monitors (see Appendix). | Invasive hemodynamic monitoring should be considered in acute, multiple-trauma victims. |
| **Positioning** | ✓ and pad pressure points.<br>✓ eyes. | |
| **Complications** | Hemodynamic instability | Previously unrecognized injuries (e.g., pneumothorax, cardiac tamponade, intracranial bleeding) should be considered as a cause of unexplained intraop hemodynamic instability in all acute-trauma victims. |

### POSTOPERATIVE

| | | |
|---|---|---|
| **Complications** | Sepsis<br>ARDS | Many trauma victims survive the initial insult only to die later of sepsis or ARDS. |
| **Pain management** | PCA (see Appendix). | |
| **Tests** | None routinely indicated. | |

**References**

1. Green DP: *Operative Hand Surgery*, 2nd edition. Churchill Livingstone, New York: 1988.
2. Vandam LD: Anesthesia for Hand Surgery. In *Flynn's Hand Surgery*, 4th edition. Jupiter JB, ed. Williams and Wilkins, Baltimore: 1991, 46-54.
3. Ramamurthy S: Anesthesia. In *Operative Hand Surgery*, 2nd edition. Green DP, ed. Churchill Livingstone, New York: 1988, 27-60.
4. Nicholls BJ, Cullen BF: Anesthesia for trauma. *J Clin Anesth* 1988; 1(2):115-29.
5. Soderstrom CA, Cowley RA: A national alcohol and trauma center survey. Missed opportunities, failures of responsibility. *Arch Surg* 1987; 122(9):1067-71.
6. Cullings HM, Hendee WR: Radiation risks in the orthopaedic operating room. *Contemp Orthop* 1984; 8:48-52.

# POLLICIZATION OF A FINGER

## SURGICAL CONSIDERATIONS

**Description:** This procedure is indicated in the infant with congenital absence or hypoplasia of the thumb. A normal finger with its tendon, nerve and vascular supply is shortened and rotated into the position of the thumb (Fig 10.1-3). Tendon transfers are performed to substitute for the absent or hypoplastic thenar muscles. These patients may have many other associated congenital anomalies, which should be ruled out prior to surgery.

**Variant procedure or approaches**: There are several different surgical techniques. They all share the basic transposition and rotation of the finger to the thumb position.

**Usual preop diagnosis**: Aplastic thumb; hypoplastic thumb; radial club hand

### SUMMARY OF PROCEDURE

| | |
|---|---|
| **Position** | Supine, with arm extended on hand-surgery table |
| **Incision** | Multiple incisions on the hand |
| **Special instrumentation** | Pneumatic tourniquet |
| **Antibiotics** | Cefazolin 1 gm iv |
| **Surgical time** | 2 - 3 hrs |
| **Tourniquet** | 150 mm above systolic; max time = 120 min |
| **Closing considerations** | Complex skin flaps are necessary. A plaster shell dressing (cast) is placed while the patient is still anesthetized. |
| **EBL** | Minimal; performed under tourniquet control. |
| **Postop care** | PACU → overnight admission for observation |
| **Mortality** | Minimal |
| **Morbidity** | Ischemia (loss of digit): Rare<br>Skin flap necrosis: Moderately common |
| **Procedure code** | 26550 |
| **Pain score** | 1-2 |

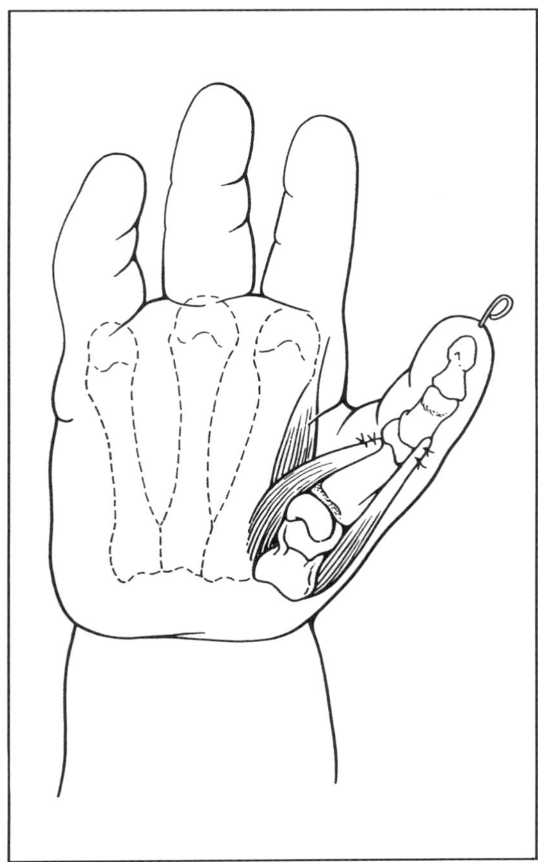

## PATIENT POPULATION CHARACTERISTICS

| | |
|---|---|
| **Age range** | 1-4 yrs is ideal time for surgery. Procedure should be done before patient begins school. |
| **Male:Female** | 1:1 |
| **Incidence** | Overall, about 1/20,000 live births require a variant of this procedure. |
| **Etiology** | Unknown; also associated with thalidomide ingestion. |
| **Associated conditions** | Associated congenital anomalies of the upper extremity, spine and lower extremities<br>Absence of radius (radial club hand), common<br>Various forms of syndactylies, common<br>Abnormalities of the hematopoietic system (Fanconi's syndrome), cardiovascular system (ASDs in Holt-Oram syndrome), spine, and GI system, along with hypothyroidism, are frequently associated. |

←**Figure 10.1-3.** Pollicization of a finger. (Reproduced with permission from Green DP: *Operative Hand Surgery*, 2nd edition. Churchill Livingstone: 1988.)

## ANESTHETIC CONSIDERATIONS

See Anesthetic Considerations following "Pediatric Orthopedic Surgery for Extremities."

# SYNDACTYLY REPAIR

## SURGICAL CONSIDERATIONS

**Description:** Syndactyly refers to congenital failure of separation of two or more fingers. It is complete if it extends to the ends of the fingers; incomplete syndactyly extends short of the finger ends. A **simple syndactyly repair** joins fingers by only skin and fibrous tissues. A **complex syndactyly repair** signifies fusion of adjacent phalanges or interposition of accessory phalanges, with frequent abnormalities of the neurovascular structures.[2,4] Surgical separation is performed in the first few years of life for functional, as well as aesthetic, reasons. The technique involves creation of a dorsal, proximally based skin flap to recreate the web.[1] A zigzag dorsal and palmar incision is then created, separating from the distal end in a proximal direction. The digital nerve and arteries are dissected proximally as far as possible. Primary closure is almost never possible, and supplemental full-thickness skin graft harvested from the groin is used to complete the closure. Usually only one site is done at a time per hand; and, never should both sides of a digit be released because of risk to the vascular supply. It is not always possible to save all the bony elements.[2]

**Usual preop diagnosis**: Syndactyly of fingers; bifid finger, thumb/finger

## SUMMARY OF PROCEDURE

| | |
|---|---|
| **Position** | Supine |
| **Incision** | Zigzag between digits; skin graft donor site from groin |
| **Special instrumentation** | Magnification loupes always necessary. Tourniquet is mandatory. |
| **Unique considerations** | Groin skin also must be taken for graft closure. |
| **Antibiotics** | Usually none |
| **Surgical time** | 2 - 4 hrs |
| **Closing considerations** | Above-the-elbow cast to keep incision away from mouth and other hand of the infant or child |
| **EBL** | < 20 cc |
| **Postop care** | PACU → home, if simple syndactyly |
| **Mortality** | Rare |
| **Morbidity** | Partial slough of flaps or skin graft<br>Scarring and some stiffness of fingers<br>Angulatory deformities late, occasionally depending on bony elements |
| **Procedure code** | 22561 (simple); 22562 (complex) |
| **Pain score** | 1-3 |

## PATIENT POPULATION CHARACTERISTICS

| | |
|---|---|
| **Age range** | 6 mo-5 yrs |
| **Male:Female** | 2:1 |
| **Incidence** | 1/2000 births (the most common significant congenital hand anomaly) |
| **Etiology** | Family Hx: 10-40%<br>Failure of differentiation in the 6th-8th wk of intrauterine life |
| **Associated conditions** | Polydactyly, accessory phalanges<br>Apert's syndrome<br>Poland's syndrome |

#### References


1. Bauer TB, Tondra JM, Trusler HM: Technical modification in repair of syndactylism. *Plast Reconstr Surg* 1956; 17:385-92.
2. Chapman MW: *Operative Orthopaedics*, 2nd edition. JB Lippincott, Philadelphia: 1993, 1555-58.
3. Flatt AE: *The Care of Congenital Hand Anomalies*. CV Mosby, St. Louis: 1977, 170-212.
4. Morrissy RT: *Atlas of Pediatric Orthopaedic Surgery*. JB Lippincott, Philadelphia: 1992, 703-6.

**Surgeon**

**Amy L. Ladd, MD**

## 10.2 SHOULDER SURGERY

**Anesthesiologist**

**Talmage D. Egan, MD**

# SHOULDER ARTHROSCOPY

## SURGICAL CONSIDERATIONS

**Description**: The use of shoulder arthroscopy has grown significantly in the past decade, due largely to technical advances in knee arthroscopy. Many procedures are now performed primarily or adjunctively through the arthroscope, replacing open techniques. The advantages include minimal incisions, decreased postop morbidity, and potentially faster rehabilitation. Arthroscopy is frequently employed for diagnostic purposes prior to an open procedure. Diagnostically, the most common uses include verifying a tear of the rotator cuff, capsule or labrum. Examination of the glenohumeral joint and the subacromial bursa can also be performed. Therapeutically, arthroscopy may be employed for irrigation in sepsis, synovectomy for rheumatoid arthritis, or synovial chondromatosis. It may assist an open procedure, such as limited rotator cuff repair, after identifying the deep and superficial aspects of the tear. Definitive procedures may include anterior stabilization procedures and subacromial decompression in conjunction with a distal clavicle resection. Most surgeons use the lateral decubitus position with the arm abducted approximately 45°, elevated approximately 20° with 5-15 lbs. of traction applied. The semi-sitting position, also known as the "beach chair" or "barber chair" position,[1] has gained popularity in the past few years, due to problems of positioning and traction on the brachial plexus. This entails the patient being seated upright, approximately 70° to the horizontal, somewhat more upright than for open shoulder procedures.[1]

Initially, an 18-gauge spinal needle is inserted into the glenohumeral joint, passing through the posterior deltoid and infraspinatus muscle and the posterior capsule of the joint (see shoulder anatomy, figure 10.2-1). Placement is verified by injecting saline to inflate the joint capsule. A stab incision is made using a No. 11 blade in the direction previously defined by the finder needle. Sharp, then blunt trocars are used to gain access to the joint and permit insertion of the arthroscopic device. Improper insertion of the instruments can injure the axillary or suprascapular nerves and the cartilage of the glenohumeral joint. An additional anterior portal is used for instrumentation; an anterolateral portal is employed for access to the subacromial space. The joint is continuously irrigated with a LR solution, usually containing epinephrine (1 mg/3 L). At the end of the procedure the portals are infiltrated with local anesthetic and a drain may be placed within the depth of the wound. The arm is typically placed in a sling-and-swathe-type immobilization and neurovascular integrity is assessed.

**Usual preop diagnosis**: Rotator cuff tear; subacromial impingement; glenohumeral instability

### SUMMARY OF PROCEDURE

| | |
|---|---|
| **Position** | Lateral decubitus or semi-sitting (barber chair)[1] |
| **Incision** | Posterior arthroscopic portal, anterior instrumentation portal, lateral instrumentation portal for visualizing subacromial bursa; superior portal for semi-sitting position |
| **Special instrumentation** | Arthroscope; power burrs; cutting devices; holmium laser |
| **Unique considerations** | Rigid eye patch over ipsilateral eye to prevent corneal abrasion suggested. Positioning of the head with appropriate support, removing upper section of operating table, if possible, for better access with semi-sitting position. ETT taped to opposite side of face. |
| **Antibiotics** | Cefazolin 1 gm iv preop, particularly if bone work performed. |
| **Surgical time** | Positioning the patient is time-intensive; can add as much as 45 min.<br>Diagnostic: < 1 hr<br>Reconstructive: 2 - 4 hrs |
| **EBL** | Minimal-200 cc (less with use of epinephrine, electrocautery and laser) |
| **Postop care** | Frequently outpatient; overnight if interscalene or supraclavicular block is given or reconstructive procedure performed. |
| **Mortality** | Minimal |
| **Morbidity** | Extravasation of fluid (NS or LR): >50%<br>Brachial plexus neuritis (lateral decubitus position): 10-30%<br>Breakage of instruments: < 1%<br>Infection: 0.04-3.49% |
| **Procedure code** | 23700 (examination and manipulation under anesthesia); 29815 (diagnostic); 29821 (synovectomy); 29822, 29823 (debridement); 29826 (decompression of subacromial space) |
| **Pain score** | 5 (diagnostic); 7-8 (reconstruction) |

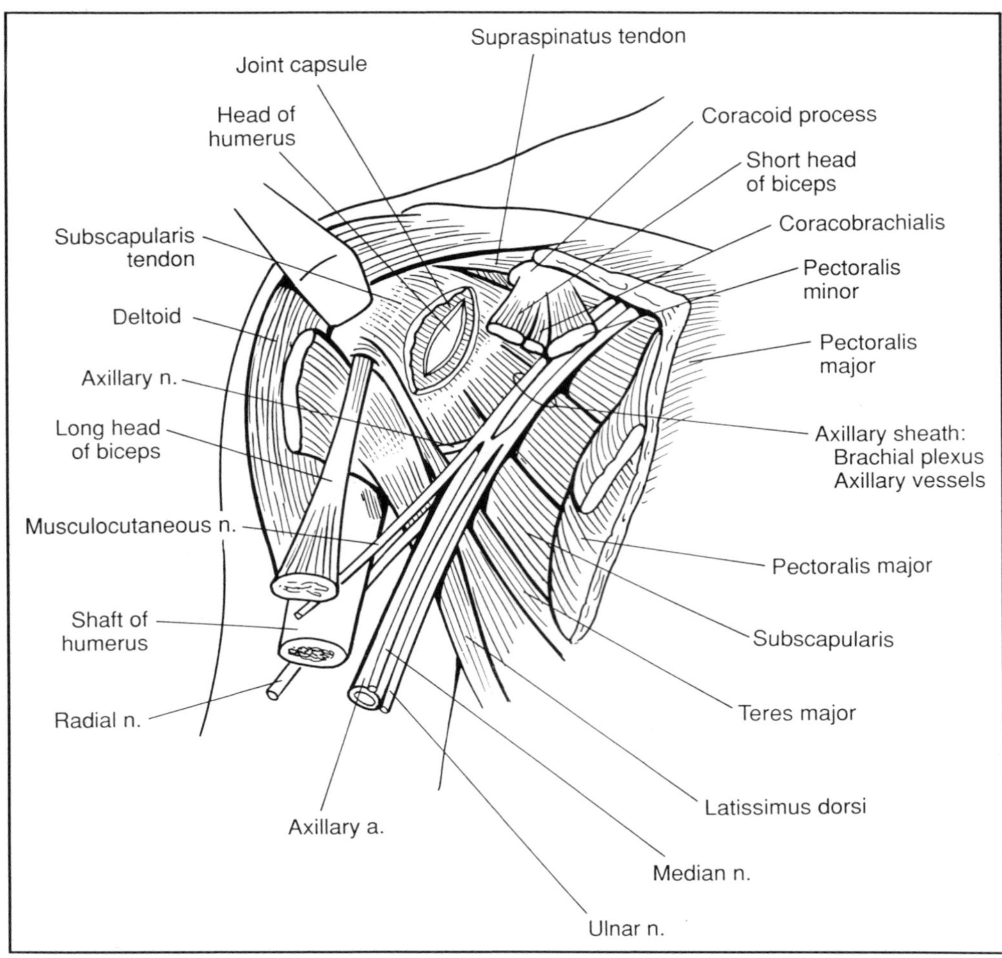


**Figure 10.2-1.** Anatomy of the shoulder joint, anterior. (Reproduced with permission from Hoppenfeld S, deBoer P, eds: *Surgical Exposures in Orthopaedics: The Anatomic Approach.* JB Lippincott: 1984.)

### PATIENT POPULATION CHARACTERISTICS

| | |
|---|---|
| **Age range** | 15-35 yrs (instability)<br>40-75 yrs (rotator cuff and acromial pathology) |
| **Male:Female** | 2:1-4:1 |
| **Incidence** | Very common |
| **Etiology** | Young patients: usually sports-related<br>Older patients: cuff and acromial pathology; age-wear phenomenon<br>Rotator cuff pathology and acromial impingement (frequently coexist) |
| **Associated conditions** | Cervical arthritis and radiculopathy with rotator cuff pathology |

---

## ANESTHETIC CONSIDERATIONS

See Anesthetic Considerations following "Surgery for Shoulder Dislocations or Instability" (below).

**References**

1. Altchek DW, Warren RF, Skyhar MJ: Shoulder arthroscopy. In *The Shoulder*. Rockwood CA Jr, Matsen FA III, eds. WB Saunders Co, Philadelphia: 1990, 258-77.
2. Bigliani LU, Flatow EL, Deliz ED: Complications of shoulder arthroscopy. *Orthop Rev* 1991; 20(9):743-51.
3. Matthews LS, Fadale PD: *Technique and Instrumentation for Shoulder Arthroscopy: Instructional Course Lectures.* American Academy of Orthopedic Surgeons, Park Ridge, IL: 1989, Vol 38.

# SURGERY FOR ACROMIAL IMPINGEMENT, ROTATOR CUFF TEARS AND ACROMIOCLAVICULAR DISEASE

## SURGICAL CONSIDERATIONS

**Description**: The terms "acromial impingement," "rotator cuff disease" and "acromioclavicular disease" are frequently used interchangeably, representing a continuum of disease and co-existing conditions, manifest in the fifth decade or later. "Bursitis," "rotator cuff tendinitis" or "bicipital tendinitis" are frequently the first presenting symptoms before a frank rotator cuff tear occurs.

**Acromial impingement:** Subacromial spurs are associated with subacromial or subdeltoid bursitis and possibly related to outer-thickness rotator cuff tears.

**Rotator cuff tears:** The rotator cuff is a confluence of four tendons supporting the glenohumeral joint – the subscapularis anteriorly, and the supraspinatus, including infraspinatus and teres minor posteriorly. The most common site for rotator cuff tear is the supraspinatus tendon. Rotator cuff repair requires a deltoid-splitting incision. Care is taken not to extend the split more than 5 cm distal to the acromion because of possible injury to the axillary nerve, which innervates the deltoid 5 cm or more from the lateral aspect of the acromion.

**Acromioclavicular disease:** Acromioclavicular arthritis is frequently associated with this disease, particularly in the older population. "Acromioclavicular arthritis" may also occur in athletes as a result of trauma. An oblique, lateral or saber-type incision is used (see Fig 10.2-1 for shoulder anatomy). Traction of the arm is typically required to identify the extent of acromial impingement or acromioclavicular disease. Similarly, rotation of the arm is required to visualize the extent of the rotator cuff tear. The shoulder girdle is well-vascularized; blood loss from these procedures is greater than that from arthroscopy, but usually less than 500 cc. On completion of the procedure, a drain is placed, and a sling-and-swathe-type immobilization splint is applied. Care must be taken in moving the patient. Adequate neuromuscular relaxation permits safe application of dressing and splints (particularly important for rotator cuff repairs).

**Usual preop diagnosis**: Rotator cuff tears (partial or complete); acromioclavicular disease; impingement; bursitis; bicipital tendinitis

### SUMMARY OF PROCEDURE

| | |
|---|---|
| **Position** | Semi-sitting, somewhat less flexed than for arthroscopy, approximately 40-70°; or lateral decubitus |
| **Incision** | Oblique, saber-type incision anteriorly over distal acromion; lateral or deltopectoral incision for wider exposure. Deltoid-splitting incision for rotator cuff tears. |
| **Special instrumentation** | Power equipment for bone work; self-retaining retractors for cuff repairs |
| **Unique considerations** | Rigid eye protection for ipsilateral eye and careful head positioning |
| **Antibiotics** | Cefazolin 1 gm iv preop |
| **Surgical time** | 1 - 3 hrs |
| **Closing considerations** | Muscle relaxation when mobilizing cuff and during closure. Arm in sling and swathe, or abduction pillow. Immobilizer should be positioned prior to awakening patient to minimize potential for rupture of repair. |
| **EBL** | 200-400 cc |
| **Postop care** | Maintenance of position in sling and swathe; no active motion of shoulder girdle for 2 d - 6 wks, depending on procedure. |
| **Mortality** | Minimal |
| **Morbidity** | Infection: 1-5%<br>Breakage of instruments: < 1% |
| **Neurologic morbidity** | Axillary nerve damage: < 2%<br>Musculocutaneous nerve damage: < 2%<br>Brachial plexus damage (position-dependent) |
| **Procedure code** | 23700 (examination and manipulation under anesthesia); 23130 (acromioplasty); 23120 (partial excision of distal clavicle); 23420 (rotator cuff repair) |
| **Pain score** | 5-8 |

### PATIENT POPULATION CHARACTERISTICS

| | |
|---|---|
| **Age range** | Rotator cuff tears >40 yrs (younger for athletes) |
| **Male:Female** | 3:1 |
| **Incidence**[1,2] | 5-30% of general population affected by rotator cuff and acromial conditions, depending on age, thickness of tear, associated conditions |
| **Etiology** | Age-related<br>Trauma (70% involved in light work) |
| **Associated conditions** | Bursitis<br>Tendinitis<br>Impingement<br>Rotator cuff disease (especially in first-time glenohumeral dislocations >40 yrs)<br>Diabetes and renal failure<br>Hypermobility |

## ANESTHETIC CONSIDERATIONS

See Anesthetic Considerations following "Surgery for Shoulder Dislocations or Instability" (below).

**References**

1. Neer CS II: Impingement lesions. *Clin Orthop* 1983; 173:70-7.
2. Ionnotti JP, ed. : *Rotator cuff disorders: evaluation and treatment.* American Academy of Orthopaedic Surgeons, Park Ridge, 1991.
3. Ellman H, Hanker G, Bayer M: Repair of the rotator cuff. End-result study of factors influencing reconstruction. *J Bone Joint Surg* 1986; 68(8): 1136-44.
4. Tubiana R, McCullough CJ, Masquelet AC: *An Atlas of Surgical Exposures of the Upper Extremity.* JB Lippincott, Philadelphia: 1990.

# SURGERY FOR SHOULDER DISLOCATIONS OR INSTABILITY

## SURGICAL CONSIDERATIONS

**Description**: Younger patients, particularly athletes and patients with hypermobility problems, are the most prone to this condition. Recurrent anterior dislocations are the most common, followed by anterior-inferior (A-I) and posterior dislocations, frequently a manifestation of multi-directional instability. First-time dislocators >40 yrs have a high incidence of associated rotator cuff tears, while second-time dislocators have a significantly increased chance of recurrent dislocations. Posterior dislocation is most commonly associated with grand mal seizures, significant trauma and multi-directional instability. Frequently, examination under anesthesia will precede the open procedure to better assess the plane of instability.

Typically, the patient is in the semi-sitting position to allow access to the anterior, lateral and posterior aspects of the glenohumeral joint. Most commonly, the joint is accessed through a deltopectoral (anterior) incision, between the level of the coracoid proximally and the deltopectoral interval distally. Access to the posterior aspect of the glenohumeral joint is through a longitudinal posterolateral incision. In the case of the anterior approach (Fig 10.2-1), the coracobrachialis tendon is retracted medially, and the deltoid is retracted laterally. The joint is entered through a capsular incision and stabilization is performed. Stabilization may require repair of the torn capsule and labrum (**Bankart repair**). Or, less frequently, a bone block of the tip of the coracoid with its tendon may be moved to the front of the joint, serving as a sling to prevent dislocations (**Bristow repair**). A drain is placed, and the arm is immobilized. The surgeon will identify special considerations before awakening the patient, including the placement of a special brace or splint, and careful positioning to prevent a dislocation.

**Usual preop diagnosis:** Fractures; Hill-Sachs lesion; glenohumeral instability; A-I dislocation; posterior dislocation

### SUMMARY OF PROCEDURE

| | Glenohumeral Instability | Anterior-Inferior, Posterior Dislocations |
|---|---|---|
| **Position** | "Beach chair" or semi-sitting | Lateral decubitus for posterior stabilization |
| **Incision**[1,2] | Deltopectoral | A-I, posterior – splitting of the infraspinatus and teres minor; transverse or longitudinal; posterior – inferior axillary incision |
| **Special instrumentation** | Power equipment; special bone-anchoring sutures; glenoid and humeral instrumentation | – |
| **Antibiotics** | Cefazolin 1 gm iv preop if bone work performed. | ⇐ |
| **Surgical time** | 2 - 4 hrs | ⇐ |
| **Closing considerations** | Repair of cuff, sling and swathe or abduction pillow, as dictated by surgical findings. | ⇐ |
| **EBL** | 200-400 cc | ⇐ |
| **Postop care** | No active motion for 6 wks | ⇐ |
| **Mortality** | Minimal | ⇐ |
| **Morbidity** | Axillary nerve palsy: 15% | Suprascapular nerve injury |
| **Procedure code** | 23700 (examination and maniupulation under anesthesia) | ⇐ |
| | | ⇐ |
| | 23455 (Bankart operation) | ⇐ |
| | 23460 (capsulorrhaphy with bone block) | ⇐ |
| | 23462 (capsulorrhaphy using coracoid, Bristow) | 23465 (posterior capsulorrhaphy) |
| **Pain score** | 8 | 8 |

### PATIENT POPULATION CHARACTERISTICS

| | |
|---|---|
| **Age range** | 15-35 yrs |
| **Male:Female** | 1:1 |
| **Incidence** | Common |
| **Etiology** | Trauma<br>Hypermobility<br>Seizures |
| **Associated conditions** | Rotator cuff tears<br>Hypermobility syndrome<br>Seizure disorder |

## ANESTHETIC CONSIDERATIONS

**(Procedures covered: shoulder arthroscopy; surgery for acromial impingement, rotator cuff tears and acromioclavicular disease; surgery for shoulder dislocations or instability)**

### PREOPERATIVE

Typically, three patient populations present for repair of rotator cuff tears or arthroscopy: (1) healthy post-trauma, (2) non-rheumatoid arthritic, and (3) rheumatoid arthritic. Individuals presenting for repair of shoulder dislocations may also include those with a joint hypermobility syndrome (e.g., Marfan or Ehlers-Danlos) or seizure disorder patients.

**Respiratory** Arthritic patients may exhibit Sx of pleural effusion or pulmonary fibrosis. Hoarseness may indicate cricoarytenoid joint (CAJ) involvement → difficult intubation. (See Anesthetic Considerations for "Dorsal Stabilization and Extensor Synovectomy of the Rheumatoid Wrist" in "Hand Surgery" section.) Seizure disorder patients who suffer from recurrent shoulder dislocation as a result of frequent grand mal seizures may also suffer from occult aspiration pneumonia or pneumonitis.

**Tests:** CXR; PFTs; ABGs in debilitated rheumatoid patients

**Cardiovascular** Arthritic patients may suffer from chronic pericardial tamponade, valvular disease and cardiac conduction defects. Patients presenting for shoulder stabilization because of joint hypermobility syndromes are likely to have valvular dysfunction and are vulnerable to aortic dissection 2° HTN. These patients should receive antibiotic prophylaxis for bacterial endocarditis.
**Tests:** ECG, ECHO in patients with severe rheumatoid arthritis. Recent ECHO to assess valve function and aortic root size indicated in most patients with Marfan syndrome.

**Neurological** Arthritic patients may have cervical or lumbar radiculopathies that should be documented carefully preop. For example, head flexion may cause cervical cord compression. Patients with severe seizure disorders can suffer from recurrent shoulder dislocations 2° frequent violent grand mal seizures. Such patients should be maximally treated for seizure disorder prior to elective surgery. Be aware that as many as 15% of shoulder dislocations can be accompanied by axillary nerve palsy, which should be documented carefully preop.
**Tests:** C-spine radiographs to rule out occult subluxations in arthritic patients with neck complaints or upper extremity radiculopathy. Verify therapeutic levels of anti-epileptic medication in seizure disorder patients.

**Musculoskeletal** Arthritic patients may have limited neck and jaw ROM and may require fiber optic intubation techniques. Bony deformities or muscle contractures may necessitate special attention to positioning. Patients with joint hypermobility syndromes presenting for shoulder surgery may also suffer other joint dislocations 2° positioning problems.

**Hematologic** Virtually all patients will be on some type of anti-inflammatory medication that may result in anemia or platelet inhibition. Ideally, patients should discontinue NSAIDs at least 5 d preop. In addition, selected patients with Ehlers-Danlos are known to have severe coagulation defects that may preempt the use of regional anesthesia.
**Tests:** A coagulation profile is mandatory in Ehlers-Danlos patients.

**Endocrine** Rheumatoid patients are likely to be on oral corticosteroids and, thus, require supplemental perioperative steroids (e.g., 100 mg hydrocortisone q 8 hr iv) to treat adrenal suppression.

**Laboratory** Hb/Hct (in healthy patients); other tests as indicated from H&P. Patients with Ehlers-Danlos syndrome should always have banked blood available for surgery, except for the most trivial of procedures.

**Premedication** Moderate-to-heavy premedication (e.g., in adults, midazolam 1 mg iv q 5 min titrated to effect) is often desirable prior to placement of regional block.

## INTRAOPERATIVE

**Anesthetic technique**: GETA or regional anesthesia, or a combination of the two techniques can be used. The interscalene approach to the brachial plexus is excellent for surgical procedures on the shoulder, either alone or in combination with GA. When logistically feasible, the combined technique is ideal.

**General anesthesia:**

**Induction** Standard induction (see Appendix). Arthritic patients may require awake fiber optic intubation.

**Maintenance** Standard maintenance (see Appendix).

**Emergence** Management of emergence and extubation should be routine, except in difficult airway cases which require awake extubation.

**Regional anesthesia:**

**Interscalene block** Anesthetics and doses:
- 3% 2-chloroprocaine 30-40 ml for procedures lasting < 1 hr.
- 1.5% lidocaine 30-40 ml for procedures lasting up to 2.5 hrs.
- 1% etidocaine 30-40 ml for procedures lasting >2.5 hrs.

The skin on the top of the shoulder (C3-C4) and the medial aspect of the upper arm (T2) often require separate subcutaneous field blocks. Phrenic nerve block → hemidiaphragmatic paralysis is an inevitable consequence of the interscalene block, which may not be tolerated by patients with significant pre-existing respiratory compromise. Major complications, such as total spinal or pneumothorax resulting from interscalene block, are extremely rare; therefore, this technique is suitable for use in outpatients. Interscalene block is contraindicated in patients with contralateral recurrent laryngeal nerve or phrenic nerve palsy. If sedation is needed, midazolam (0.5-1.0 mg boluses), alfentanil (0.125-0.25 μg/kg/min by infusion) or propofol (50-100 μg/kg/min by infusion), given initially in subanesthetic doses and thereafter titrated to effect, are good choices.

| | | |
|---|---|---|
| **Blood and fluid requirements** | Minimal-to-moderate blood loss<br>IV: 18 ga x 1<br>NS/LR @ 1.5-3 cc/kg/hr | IV catheter placed in contralateral upper extremity. |
| **Monitoring** | Standard monitors (see Appendix).<br>± Precordial Doppler<br>± Arterial line | To help avoid VAE, consider precordial Doppler monitoring when semi-sitting position used. Consider intra-arterial BP monitoring for patients with hypermobility disorders because of risk for aortic dissection 2° HTN. |
| **Positioning** | ✓ and pad pressure points.<br>✓ eyes.<br>↑VAE risk in semi-sitting position | Postural hypotension is the most common complication of the semi-sitting position. Changing to this position gradually can help prevent hypotension, as can the use of anti-embolism stockings, plus fluid-loading the patient. Marfan and Ehlers-Danlos patients require very gentle positioning to prevent joint dislocations. |
| **Interscalene block complications** | Total spinal<br>Accidental epidural injection<br>IV injection (seizures/dysrhythmias)<br>Stellate ganglion block (Horner's syndrome)<br>Laryngeal nerve block<br>Phrenic nerve block<br>Pneumothorax | Resuscitative equipment, including airway management tools, should be immediately available. |
| **Other complications** | Hypotension during surgical prep and positioning | Hypotension during long surgical preps normally can be avoided by using light inhalation anesthesia (e.g., isoflurane 0.3-0.5%) to ensure amnesia, with moderate muscle relaxation to prevent bucking on the ETT, and maintaining adequate hydration. Anti-embolism stockings will help prevent venous pooling in lower limbs. |
| | Cardiac dysrhythmia<br>VAE | Dysrhythmias may be 2° to irrigation fluids containing epinephrine. |

## POSTOPERATIVE

| | | |
|---|---|---|
| **Pain management** | PCA (see Appendix) or regional block techniques. | Combined regional-general anesthetic techniques are excellent for shoulder procedures, especially with respect to postop pain management. |
| **Tests** | None indicated routinely. | |

**References**


1. Hoppenfeld S: *Surgical Exposures in Orthopaedics: The Anatomic Approach.* Hoppenfeld S, deBoer P, eds. JB Lippincott, Philadelphia: 1984.
2. Tubiana R, McCullough CJ, Masquelet AC: *An Atlas of Surgical Exposures of the Upper Extremity.* JB Lippincott, Philadelphia: 1990.
3. Balas GI: Regional anesthesia for surgery on the shoulder. *Anesth Analg* 1971; 50(6):1036-41.
4. Urmey WF, Talts KH, Sharrock NE: One hundred percent incidence of hemidiaphragmatic paresis associated with interscalene brachial plexus anesthesia as diagnosed by ultrasonography. *Anesth Analg* 1991; 72(4):498-503.
5. White RH: Preoperative evaluation of patients with rheumatoid arthritis. *Semin Arthritis Rheum* 1985; 14(4):287-99.
6. Reginster JY, Damas P, Franchimont P: Anaesthetic risks in osteoarticular disorders. *Clin Rheum* 1985; 4:30-8.
7. Keenan MA, Stiles CM, Kaufman RL: Acquired laryngeal deviation associated with cervical spine disease in erosive polyarticular arthritis. *Anesthesiology* 1983; 58(5):441-49.
8. Salathe M, Johr M: Unsuspected cervical fractures: a common problem in ankylosing spondylitis. *Anesthesiology* 1989; 70(5):869-70.
9. Winnie AP: Interscalene brachial plexus block. *Anesth Analg* 1970; 49(3):455-66.
10. Verghese C: Anaesthesia in Marfan's syndrome. *Anaesthesia* 1984; 39(9):917-22.
11. Wells DG, Podolakin W: Anaesthesia and Marfan's syndrome: case report. *Can J Anaesth* 1987; 34(3+Pt 1):311-14.
12. Dolan P, Sisko F, Riley E: Anesthetic considerations for Ehlers-Danlos syndrome. *Anesthesiology* 1980; 52(3):266-69.
13. Carron H: Regional anesthesia for upper extremity surgery symposium. *Reg Anaesth* 1980; 5:2-9.

# SHOULDER (GLENOHUMERAL) ARTHROPLASTY

## SURGICAL CONSIDERATIONS

**Description.** Shoulder joint replacement is most commonly performed for end-stage arthritis or following trauma. Osteoarthritis is far less common in the glenohumeral joint than in the hip and knee joints. Inflammatory conditions, such as rheumatoid arthritis and psoriatic arthritis, may require shoulder replacement for correction and pain relief, and are frequently associated with massive rotator cuff tears.

**Hemi-arthroplasty**, or replacement of the humeral side only, is commonly done for osteoarthritis. Comminuted fractures about the shoulder joint may require **arthroplasty**, particularly in the older patient. As with total hip and total knee replacements, bone cement (polymethylmethacrylate), as well as special implants for improved bone fixation, may be used.

The most common type of arthroplasty is the **unconstrained** (separate glenoid and humeral components), while **constrained** or **hinged devices** rarely are used. During arthroplasty, the humeral component is placed within the shaft of the humerus, after the humeral head is removed. The glenoid component requires re-surfacing of the glenoid, the most difficult aspect of this procedure. Similar to other total joint replacements, revision surgery may be required, adding to the operative time and blood loss.

Through a deltopectoral incision (Fig 10.2-1), the interval between the coracoid and the deltoid insertion are developed. This is followed by making an oblique incision of approximately 10 cm between the deltoid muscle and the pectoralis muscle. The coracobrachialis tendon is retracted, the capsule of the glenohumeral joint is divided and the joint is identified. Removal of the humeral head is performed, and the humeral component is replaced. If the glenoid is replaced, the surface is fashioned to accept a glenoid component. Similar to total hip surgery, this requires sizing of the canal of the humerus, as well as determining the size and position of the humeral head and the size of the glenoid cavity. A provisional reduction is performed, with the humeral component or the humeral and glenoid components in place, at which time the fit is preliminarily assessed. Cement (polymethylmethacrylate) may be used for fixing the components in place. Following final positioning, the joint is reduced and the wound is closed over suction drainage. The shoulder girdle is well-vascularized and blood loss may exceed a unit. A sling-and-swathe-type immobilization is applied; revision surgery may require a special splint. A specific program of protected rehabilitation typically lasts 6-12 weeks.

**Usual preop diagnosis:** Osteoarthritis; inflammatory arthritis; trauma

### SUMMARY OF PROCEDURE

| | |
|---|---|
| **Position** | Semi-sitting |
| **Incision** | Deltopectoral incision or extended incision |
| **Special instrumentation** | Glenoid and humeral instrumentation, in addition to usual shoulder instruments; mixing and introduction of cement |
| **Unique considerations** | Systemic illnesses of the patient; systemic complications of use of cement in the patient; precautions in pregnant staff working with methylmethacrylate; usage of laminar flow or UV lighting for total joint precautions, depending on the surgeon's preference and capabilities of the OR. |
| **Antibiotics** | Cefazolin 1 gm iv preop, if bone work performed. |
| **Surgical time** | 2 - 5 hrs |
| **Closing considerations** | Drain; sling and swathe |
| **EBL** | 200-1000 cc |
| **Postop care** | No postop active motion for approximately 4-6 wks |
| **Mortality** | < 1% |
| **Morbidity** | Blood loss<br>Nerve injury<br>Hypotension<br>Infection |
| **Procedure code** | 23700 (examination and manipulation under anesthesia); 23472 (total shoulder replacement); 23470 (hemi-arthro-plasty) |
| **Pain score** | 8 |

### PATIENT POPULATION CHARACTERISTICS

| | |
|---|---|
| **Age range**[1] | 45-80 yrs |
| **Male:Female** | 1:1 |
| **Incidence** | Uncommon |
| **Etiology** | Osteoarthritis<br>Inflammatory arthritis<br>Trauma<br>Avascular necrosis<br>Systemic disease |
| **Associated conditions** | Inflammatory disease<br>Systemic disease<br>Alcoholism<br>Rotator cuff pathology<br>Arthritis and radiculopathy<br>Cervical arthritis |

---

## ANESTHETIC CONSIDERATIONS

### PREOPERATIVE

Typically, three patient populations present for shoulder arthroplasty: (1) healthy post-trauma, (2) non-rheumatoid arthritic, and (3) rheumatoid arthritic.

| | |
|---|---|
| **Respiratory** | Rheumatoid arthritic patients may exhibit Sx of pleural effusion or pulmonary fibrosis. Hoarseness may indicate cricoarytenoid joint (CAJ) involvement → difficult intubation. (See Anesthetic Considerations for "Dorsal Stabilization and Extensor Synovectomy of the Rheumatoid Wrist" in "Hand Surgery" section.)<br>**Tests:** CXR; PFTs; ABGs in debilitated rheumatoid patients |
| **Cardiovascular** | Rheumatoid arthritic patients may suffer from chronic pericardial tamponade, valvular disease and cardiac conduction defects.<br>**Tests:** ECG and ECHO in patients with severe rheumatoid arthritis |
| **Neurological** | Arthritic patients may have cervical or lumbar radiculopathies that should be documented carefully preop. For example, head flexion may cause cervical cord compression.<br>**Tests:** C-spine radiographs to rule out occult subluxations in rheumatoid patients with neck complaints or upper extremity radiculopathy |
| **Musculoskeletal** | Arthritic patients may have limited neck and jaw ROM that may require special intubation techniques. Bony deformities or muscle contracture may necessitate special attention to positioning. |
| **Hematologic** | Virtually all non-trauma patients will be on some type of anti-inflammatory medication that may result in anemia or platelet inhibition. Ideally, patients should discontinue NSAIDs at least 5 d preop. |
| **Endocrine** | Rheumatoid patients are likely to be on oral corticosteroids and, thus, require supplemental perioperative steroids (e.g., 100 mg hydrocortisone q 8 hr iv) to treat adrenal suppression. |
| **Laboratory** | Hb/Hct (healthy patients); other tests as indicated from H&P. |
| **Premedication** | Moderate-to-heavy premedication (e.g., midazolam 0.5-1 mg iv q 5 min titrated to effect) is desirable if regional block is done. |

### INTRAOPERATIVE

**Anesthetic technique**: GETA or regional anesthesia, or a combination of the two, can be used. The interscalene approach to the brachial plexus is excellent for surgical procedures on the shoulder, either alone or in combination with GA.

**General anesthesia:**

| | |
|---|---|
| **Induction** | Standard induction (see Appendix). Rheumatoid patients may require awake fiber optic intubation. |

| | |
|---|---|
| **Maintenance** | Standard maintenance (see Appendix). Because of the typically long duration of these cases, the opioid selected as part of the balanced anesthetic technique is best given, perhaps, by continuous infusion (e.g., iv sufentanil [0.25-1.0 μg/kg/hr]). Some surgeons prefer muscle relaxation beyond that provided by volatile anesthetic. |
| **Emergence** | Management of emergence and extubation should be routine except in difficult airway cases which require awake extubation. Emergence from anesthesia should be delayed until patient's shoulder is securely immobilized in the sling and swathe to prevent undesired movement of the newly placed prosthesis. |

**Regional anesthesia:**

| | |
|---|---|
| **Interscalene block** | Anesthetics and doses:<br>- 1.5% lidocaine 30-40 ml for procedures lasting up to 2.5 hrs.<br>- 1% etidocaine 30-40 ml for procedures lasting >2.5 hrs.<br>The skin on the top of the shoulder (C3-C4) and the medial aspect of the upper arm (T2) often require separate subcutaneous field blocks. Phrenic nerve block → hemidiaphragmatic paralysis is an inevitable consequence of the interscalene block, which may not be tolerated by patients with significant pre-existing respiratory compromise. Major complications, such as total spinal or pneumothorax resulting from interscalene block, are extremely rare. Interscalene block is contraindicated in patients with contralateral recurrent laryngeal nerve or phrenic nerve palsy. If sedation is needed, midazolam (0.5-1.0 mg boluses), alfentanil (0.125-0.25 μg/kg/min by infusion) or propofol (50-100 μg/kg/min by infusion), given initially in subanesthetic doses and thereafter titrated to effect, are good choices. |

| | | |
|---|---|---|
| **Blood and fluid requirements** | Moderate-to-significant blood loss<br>IV: 16 ga x 1<br>NS/LR @ 1.5-3.0 cc/kg/hr | RBC recovery and reinfusion techniques (e.g., cell saver) are advisable because blood loss can be considerable. Catheter in non-operated upper extremity. |
| **Monitoring** | Standard monitors (see Appendix). | Consider invasive, hemodynamic monitoring in the debilitated or elderly patient. |
| | Precordial Doppler | Since VAE is a possible complication of the semi-sitting position, consider using precordial Doppler for cases done in this position. |
| **Positioning** | ✓ and pad pressure points.<br>✓ eyes.<br>↑VAE risk | Postural hypotension is the most common complication of the semi-sitting position. Changing patient to this position gradually can help prevent hypotension, as can the use of anti-embolism stockings and fluid-loading the patient. |
| **Interscalene block complications** | Total spinal<br>Epidural anesthesia<br>IV injection (seizures/dysrhythmias)<br>Stellate ganglion block (Horner's syndrome)<br>Laryngeal nerve block<br>Phrenic nerve block<br>Pneumothorax | Resuscitative equipment, including airway management tools, should be immediately available. |
| **Other complications** | Potential for embolic event<br>Hypotension during prep and positioning<br>VAE | Because of the increased risk of VAE during shoulder arthroplasty, $N_2O$ may be discontinued during placement of the humeral component. The use of methylmethacrylate cement has been associated with the sudden onset of hypotension and even cardiac arrest, presumably due to profound vasodilation ± associated VAE. ↓BP during long surgical prep can usually be avoided by using light inhalation anesthesia (isoflurane 0.3-0.5%) to ensure amnesia, with moderate muscle relaxation to prevent bucking on the ETT, and maintaining adequate hydration. |

### POSTOPERATIVE

| | | |
|---|---|---|
| **Pain management** | PCA (see Appendix) or regional block techniques. | Combined regional-general anesthetic techniques are excellent for shoulder procedures, especially with respect to postop pain management. |
| **Tests** | None indicated routinely. | |

**References**

1. Cofield RH: Degenerative and arthritic problems of the glenohumeral joint. In *The Shoulder*. Rockwood CA Jr, Matsen FA III, eds. WB Saunders Co, Philadelphia: 1990, 678-749.
2. Neer CS II, Watson KC, Stanton FJ: Recent experience in total shoulder replacement. *J Bone Joint Surg* [Am] 1992; 64:319-37.
3. Balas GI: Regional anesthesia for surgery on the shoulder. *Anesth Analg* 1971; 50(6):1036-41.
4. White RH: Preoperative evaluation of patients with rheumatoid arthritis. *Semin Arthritis Rheum* 1985; 14(4):287-99.
5. Salathe M, Johr M: Unsuspected cervical fractures: a common problem in ankylosing spondylitis. *Anesthesiology* 1989; 70(5):869-70.
6. Reginster JY, Damas P, Franchimont P: Anaesthetic risks in osteoarticular disorders. *Clin Rheum* 1985; 4:30-8.
7. Keenan MA, Stiles CM, Kaufman RL: Acquired laryngeal deviation associated with cervical spine disease in erosive polyarticular arthritis. *Anesthesiology* 1983; 58(5):441-49.
8. Andersen KH: Air aspirated from the venous system during total hip replacement. *Anaesthesia* 1983; 38(12):1175-78.
9. Newens AF, Volz RG: Severe hypotension during prosthetic hip surgery with acrylic bone cement. *Anesthesiology* 1972; 36(3):298-300.

# SHOULDER GIRDLE PROCEDURES

## SURGICAL CONSIDERATIONS

**Description.** Trauma about the shoulder girdle in young patients ranges from athletic injuries to life-threatening trauma. Some of these injuries include: common athletic injuries such as **acromioclavicular joint separations** which rarely require surgery unless there is associated **acromial** or **clavicular fractures. Posterior sternoclavicular dislocations** may warrant surgical stabilization if the trachea is compressed. **Clavicle fractures**, frequently associated with **scapular fractures**, occasionally require open reduction.

**Scapular fractures** involving the glenoid also may require surgical stabilization. Extreme fractures involving the shoulder girdle (**scapulothoracic dissociations**) include scapular fracture, clavicle fracture, subclavian or axillary artery disruption and brachial plexus injury. These may coexist with **proximal humerus fractures**, rib fractures and pneumothorax. In the older, debilitated patient, the most common injury is proximal humeral fracture, which may be amenable to surgical stabilization, or may be so comminuted as to warrant hemi- or total arthroplasty.

For each of these fractures, the incision is made over the appropriate site, the fracture or dislocation is identified and reduced under manual or manipulative traction, and appropriate fixation proceeds. For instance, a displaced proximal humerus fracture in a young person may require fixation with a plate and screws through a deltopectoral approach (see "Surgery for Shoulder Dislocation or Instability" and "Shoulder Arthroplasty" sections). A scapular fracture in a scapulothoracic dissociation would be stabilized with a plate and screws via a posterior approach (see "Instability") after vascular repair of the subclavian artery and fixation of the clavicle, if necessary. Typically, a sling or sling-and-swathe-type immobilization is required. As with other shoulder procedures, relaxation is necessary upon awakening the patient.

**Usual preop diagnosis:** Trauma about the shoulder girdle

SUMMARY OF PROCEDURE

| | Anterior | Posterior |
|---|---|---|
| **Position** | Semi-sitting or prone | Lateral decubitus (scapula) |
| **Incision** | Anterior, superior or oblique for acromioclavicular; supraclavicular for clavicle; deltopectoral for proximal humerus and glenoid | Posterior lateral border or medial border of scapula, spinous scapula, depending on location. |
| **Special instrumentation** | Plates and screws; tension band wiring for comminuted fractures | ⇐ |
| **Unique considerations** | Multiple trauma warrants early stabilization; may require vascular repair and brachial plexus exploration. | ⇐ |
| **Surgical time** | 2 - 10 hrs | ⇐ |
| **Closing considerations** | Fracture-dependent; most commonly requires application of sling-and-swathe | ⇐ |
| **EBL** | 200-1200 cc or greater, depending on trauma. | ⇐ |
| **Postop care** | May require ICU for multiple-trauma patients. | ⇐ |
| **Mortality** | Mortality dependent on associated conditions:<br>Infection<br>Neurologic injury<br>Respiratory failure<br>Massive blood loss<br>Unrecognized pneumothorax<br>Cardiac tamponade | ⇐ |
| **Morbidity** | Nerve injury (axillary, brachial plexus) | Axillary and suprascapular |
| | Stiffness | ⇐ |
| | Poor healing | ⇐ |
| **Procedure code** | 23700 (examination and manipulation under anesthesia) | ⇐ |
| | 23515 (ORIF of clavicle fracture) | |
| | 23525 (reduction of sternoclavicular dislocation) | |
| | 23550 (ORIF of acromioclavicular dislocation) | |
| | 23615 (ORIF of proximal humeral fracture) | 23585 (ORIF of scapular fracture) |
| | 23800 (shoulder arthrodesis) | |
| | 23802 (with bone graft) | |
| **Pain score** | 6-10 | 6 (clavicle and AC joint); 8 (scapula and proximal humerus) |

PATIENT POPULATION CHARACTERISTICS

| | |
|---|---|
| **Age range** | 15-80 yrs, depending on nature of trauma |
| **Male:Female** | 5:1 |
| **Incidence** | Common |
| **Etiology** | Trauma |
| **Associated conditions** | Axillary nerve palsy<br>Musculocutaneous nerve palsy<br>Brachial plexus injury<br>Arterial disruption in high-energy trauma<br>Brachial and great vessel injuries and posterior sternoclavicular dislocation pneumothorax |

## ANESTHETIC CONSIDERATIONS

See Anesthetic Considerations following "Brachial Plexus Surgery" (below).

**References**

1. Imatani RJ: Fractures of the scapula: a review of 53 fractures. *J Trauma* 1975; 15(6):473-78.
2. Neer CS II: Fractures about the shoulder. In *Fractures in Adults*. Rockwood CA Jr, Green DP, eds. JB Lippincott, Philadelphia: 1984, 713-21.
3. Neviaser RJ: Injuries to the clavicle and acromioclavicular joint. *Orthop Clin North Am* 1987; 18(3):433-38.
4. Rockwood CA Jr: Injuries to the sternoclavicular joint. In *Fractures in Adults*. Rockwood CA Jr, Green DP, eds. JB Lippincott, Philadelphia: 1992, 910-48.
5. Neer CS II and Rockwood CA Jr: Fractures and dislocations of the shoulder. In *Fractures in Adults*. Rockwood CA Jr, Green DP, eds. JB Lippincott, Philadelphia: 1984, 675-985.
6. Rockwood CA Jr, Matsen FA III, eds: *The Shoulder*. WB Saunders Co, Philadelphia, 1990.
7. Richards RR, Sherman RM, Hudson AR, Waddell JP: Shoulder arthrodesis using a pelvic-reconstruction plate. A report of eleven cases. *J Bone Joint Surg* [Am] 1988; 70(3):416-21.


# BRACHIAL PLEXUS SURGERY

## SURGICAL CONSIDERATIONS

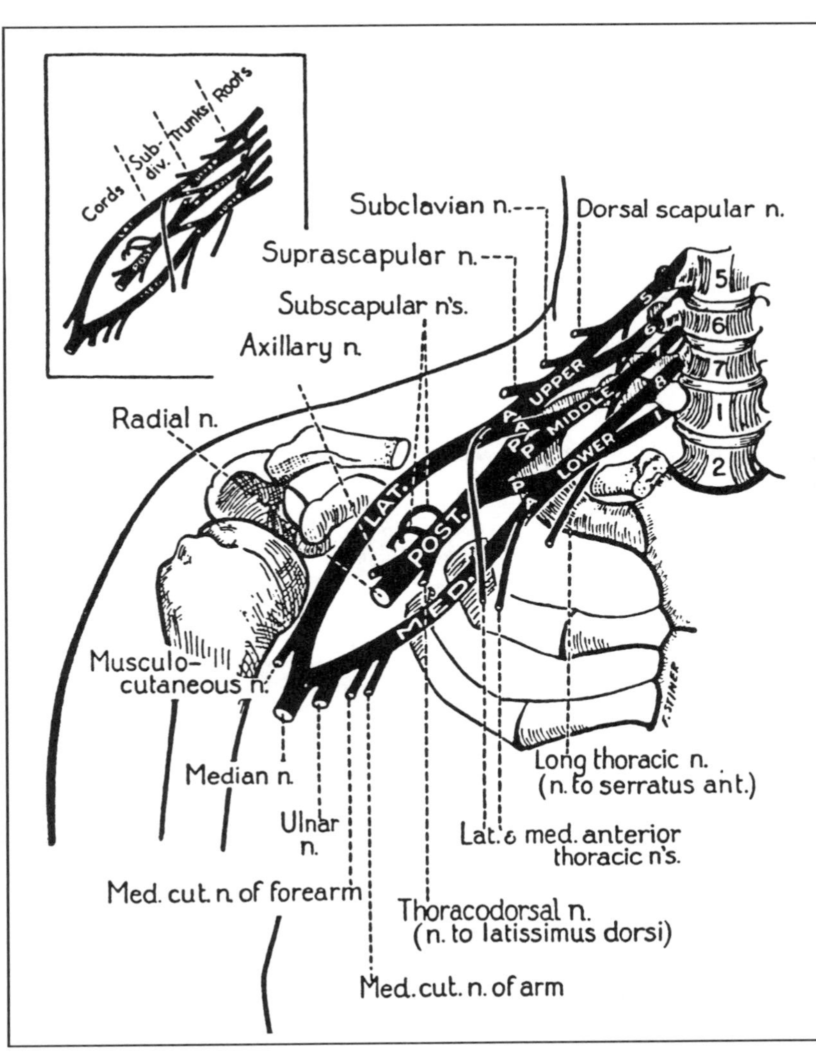


←**Figure 10.2-2.** Diagram of the branchial plexus. (Reproduced with permission from Haymaker W, Woodhall B: *Peripheral Nerve Injuries*. WB Saunders: 1956.)

**Description:** Brachial plexus injuries occur most commonly in two groups: traumatic birth injuries and high-energy trauma. Surgery ranges from exploration with neurolysis to repairs to cable nerve grafting. Typically, the latter requires grafting with the sural nerve, and nerve pedicle transfer, such as transfer of the spinal accessory nerve to denervated paralyzed muscle, combined with muscle transfers. C5-C-6 is most commonly injured in obstetrical (Erb's) palsy. Injuries in adults are more commonly closed-traction injuries. Similar to obstetrical palsy, they occur with an outstretched, abducted arm with the neck rotated in the opposite direction. The most severe form includes complete avulsion at the preganglionic level, presenting with a Horner's syndrome, winging of the scapula and a flail arm. These are typically "supraclavicular" injuries, and have a poorer prognosis. Surgical exposure may proceed above the clavicle similar to an anteriorneck dissection, or may require an extension below the clavicle. Occasionally, an osteotomy of the clavicle for extensive dissection is required. For axillary nerve dissection, a posterior approach is also used. Open injuries, such as gunshot or knife wounds are typically "infraclavicular" and have a better prognosis. (See diagram of brachial plexus, Fig 10.2-2.)

**Usual preop diagnosis:** Obstetrical palsy; adult trauma – most commonly motorcycle accident

### SUMMARY OF PROCEDURE

| | |
|---|---|
| **Position** | Lateral decubitus or semi-sitting |
| **Incision** | Supra- or infraclavicular, extensile to include deltopectoral incision. Clavicle osteotomy incision will provide for improved exposure. Supraclavicular incision used for supraclavicular brachial plexus. |
| **Special instrumentation** | Nerve stimulator |
| **Unique considerations** | Associated trauma |
| **Surgical time** | 4 - 10 hrs |
| **Closing considerations** | Other incisions if nerve grafts obtained. |
| **EBL** | 400-2000 cc |
| **Mortality** | Minimal |
| **Morbidity** | Bleeding<br>Hematoma<br>Pneumothorax<br>Clavicular nonunion |
| **Procedure code** | 23700 (examination and manipulation under anesthesia); 64713 (exploration of brachial plexus); 64861 (repair); 64872 (delayed repair); 64874, 64876 (extensive mobilization); 64897 (nerve grafting); 64905 (nerve pedicle transfer) |
| **Pain score** | 8 |

### PATIENT POPULATION CHARACTERISTICS

| | |
|---|---|
| **Age range** | Infants and children: 3 mo-8 yrs<br>Adults: 20-40 yrs |
| **Male:Female** | Adult: 5:1 |
| **Incidence** | Infant: 0.3-8/1000 births<br>Adult: Commonly associated with motercycle accidents |
| **Etiology** | Obstetrical palsy<br>Trauma |
| **Associated conditions** | None known |

## ANESTHETIC CONSIDERATIONS

**(Procedures covered: shoulder girdle procedures; brachial plexus surgery)**

### PREOPERATIVE

With the exception of traumatic birth injuries, most of these patients are healthy males who have suffered major blunt or penetrating trauma. For the acute and subacute trauma victim, the major anesthesia-related concerns center around associated traumatic injuries. Many adult trauma victims with brachial plexus injuries will be operated on in the first few days after their injury. For infants (usually operated on at 6-12 mo), the major anesthesia-related concerns are those routinely associated with pediatric anesthesia. Approximately half of all trauma victims are intoxicated. The anesthesia-related implications of ethanol intoxication include: decreased anesthetic requirements, diuresis, vasodilation and hypothermia.

**Respiratory** As suggested by coexisting disease or acute trauma injuries. Look for evidence of occult chest injury, including pneumothorax (tachypnea, wheezing, ↓BP, ↓$PaO_2$, CXR changes) and pulmonary contusion (multiple rib fracture, ↓$PaO_2$).

**Tests:** Consider CXR and ABGs in victims of significant trauma; other tests as indicated from H&P.

**Cardiovascular** As suggested by coexisting disease or acute trauma injuries. Look for evidence of occult cardiac or mediastinal injuries, such as myocardial contusion (e.g., ECG abnormalities typically consistent with ischemia) or great vessel rupture (e.g., widened mediastinum).

**Tests:** Consider CXR (with NG tube in place to access mediastinal widening) and ECG in victims of significant trauma; others as indicated from H&P.

**Neurological** Victims of shoulder trauma are vulnerable to brachial plexus damage. Look for evidence of upper extremity nerve dysfunction and document any injuries preop. The possibility of closed-head injury also should be considered.

**Tests:** Head CT prior to beginning a procedure under GA in a patient with evidence of head trauma.

**Musculoskeletal** As suggested by coexisting disease or acute trauma injuries. The amount of force necessary to produce a brachial plexus injury mandates a C-spine series to rule out C-spine fracture in all victims of brachial plexus trauma.

**Laboratory** In general, most victims of significant trauma are best served by obtaining a wide variety of baseline lab studies to screen for unrecognized injury. These studies should generally include: Hct; CBC; ABGs; UA; renal function tests; LFTs; serum amylase.

**Premedication** None

## INTRAOPERATIVE

**Anesthetic technique:** Because of the unpredictable and prolonged length of these procedures, GETA is preferred over regional techniques.

**Induction** Rapid-sequence induction is mandatory in unscheduled cases, unless awake FOL intubation is performed (see "Anesthetic Considerations for Thoracolumbar Neurosurgical Procedures" in "Neurosurgery" section). C-spine fracture patients or those with facial injuries may require awake fiber optic intubation or other special airway techniques as indicated from H&P. Hemodynamically unstable, acute-trauma patients may be more safely induced with etomidate (0.3-0.4 mg/kg iv) or ketamine (1-3 mg/kg iv).

**Maintenance** Balanced anesthesia with low-dose isoflurane (0.4-0.6%), iv sufentanil (0.25-1.0 $\mu$g/kg/hr) and $N_2O$ in $O_2$ is suitable for stable patients. Hemodynamically unstable, acute-trauma victims undergoing emergency surgery are not likely to tolerate this regimen and are better served by using a combination of medications designed to have minimal hemodynamic consequences (e.g., fentanyl for analgesia, vecuronium for muscle relaxation and scopolamine or midazolam for amnesia). $N_2O$, with its myocardial depressant effects, is best avoided in the unstable patient. For brachial plexus surgery, some surgeons prefer minimal muscle relaxation after tracheal intubation so that a nerve stimulator can be used to help identify surgical anatomy.

**Emergence** Management of emergence and extubation should be routine except in difficult airway or full-stomach cases which require that extubation be delayed until patient's airway reflexes have returned and patient is fully awake.

**Blood and fluid requirements**

Significant blood loss
IV: 14-16 ga x 1-2
NS/LR @ 1.5-3 cc/kg/hr + replacement of blood loss @ 3 x volume
Fluid warmer
Airway humidifier

IV catheter placed in the non-operated upper extremity is usually adequate in hemodynamically stable patients. Unstable, acute-trauma victims require a minimum of 2 large-bore iv catheters.

**Monitoring**

Standard monitors (see Appendix).
± SSEP

Invasive hemodynamic monitoring should be considered in acute, multiple-trauma victims. Some surgeons request SSEP to make continuous assessment of preop intact brachial plexus possible. When using SSEP monitoring, high doses of volatile anesthetic agents should generally be avoided because they adversely affect SSEP readings.

| | | |
|---|---|---|
| **Positioning** | ✓ and pad pressure points.<br>✓ eyes.<br>VAE risk | Postural hypotension is the most common complication of the semi-sitting position, particularly during the surgical prep period. SCD or anti-embolism stockings may be beneficial. VAE is a potential complication of this position. |
| **Complications** | Hemodynamic instability | Previously unrecognized injuries (e.g., pneumothorax, cardiac tamponade, intracranial bleeding) should be considered as a cause of unexplained intraop hemodynamic instability in all acute-trauma victims. |
| | Possible VAE | VAE risk is increased with patient in semi-sitting position. |

**POSTOPERATIVE**

| | | |
|---|---|---|
| **Complications** | Sepsis<br>ARDS | Many trauma victims survive the initial insult only to die later of sepsis or ARDS. |
| **Pain management** | PCA (see Appendix). | |
| **Tests** | None routinely indicated. | |

**References**


1. Nanakas AO: Injuries to the brachial plexus. In *The Pediatric Upper Extremity: Diagnosis and Treatment.* Bora FW Jr, ed. WB Saunders Co, Philadelphia: 1986, 247-58.
2. Leifert RD: Neurological problems. In *The Shoulder*. Rockwood CA Jr, Matsen FA III, eds. WB Saunders Co, Philadelphia: 1990, 750-58.
3. Nicholls BJ, Cullen BF: Anesthesia for trauma. *J Clin Anesth* 1988; 1(2):115-29.
4. Soderstrom CA, Cowley RA: A national alcohol and trauma center survey. Missed opportunities, failures of responsibility. *Arch Surg* 1987; 122(9):1067-71.
5. Mahla ME, Long DM, McKennett J, Green C, McPherson RW: Detection of brachial plexus dysfunction by somatosensory evoked potential monitoring--a report of two cases. *Anesthesiology* 1984; 60(3):248-52.
6. Grundy BL: Intraoperative monitoring of sensory-evoked potentials. *Anesthesiology* 1983; 58(1):72-87.
7. Balas GI. Regional anesthesia for surgery on the shoulder. *Anesth Analg* 1971; 50(6):1036-41.


# ARM SURGERY

## SURGICAL CONSIDERATIONS

**Description.** Surgical procedures on the arm are primarily for trauma or tumor surgery. Other procedures include extended approaches from the shoulder for significant trauma or tendon transfer. Exploration of peripheral nerves, most commonly of the radial nerve, are also included in this category, as are distal extensile approaches from the elbow for trauma or for lateral epicondylitis (tennis elbow). Depending on the lesion or fracture, the incision is developed through an internervous or intramuscular compartment. Procedures include **excisional biopsy** for soft tissue or bone tumors of the arm; **tumor excision**, which may be marginal, wide or radical, depending on the tumor encountered; **tendon transfers**, such as pectoralis transfer to replace biceps function, used primarily for brachial plexus injuries; **fractures and non-union fractures of the humerus** and other bony procedures. Depending on the location of pathology, appropriate incisions as outlined are used.

**Usual preop diagnosis:** Trauma; tumor

### SUMMARY OF PROCEDURE

| | |
|---|---|
| **Position** | Supine; semi-sitting position for extended deltopectoral; lateral decubitus |
| **Incision** | Anterolateral approach; posterior approach in the lateral decubitus position |
| **Special instrumentation** | Plate and screws; external fixators; IM rods; occasionally, PMMA (methylmethacrylate cement) for tumor surgery |
| **Unique considerations** | CT-guided sclero-therapy preop for vascular tumors. Longitudinal incisions for Bx and tumor excisions (not violating fascial planes). |
| **Surgical time** | 45 min - 4 hrs |
| **Closing considerations** | Drain frequently required. |
| **EBL** | Minimal-500+ cc, depending on pathology |
| **Mortality** | Varies with pathology |
| **Morbidity** | Bleeding<br>Shoulder stiffness<br>Nerve injury |
| **Procedure code** | 23700 (examination and manipulation under anesthesia); 24076 (excisional Bx deep tissue upper arm); 24077 (radical resection of tumor); 24301 (tendon transfer); 24430 (repair of non-union humerus); 24515 (ORIF of humeral shaft); 24400 (osteotomy of humerus) |
| **Pain score** | 4-7 |

### PATIENT POPULATION CHARACTERISTICS

| | |
|---|---|
| **Age range** | Varies with procedure |
| **Male:Female** | Varies with procedure |
| **Incidence** | Procedure-dependent |
| **Etiology** | Fractures<br>Nerve entrapment (radial) following trauma<br>Tumors |
| **Associated conditions** | Radial nerve injury with humeral fractures |

## ANESTHETIC CONSIDERATIONS

### PREOPERATIVE

The majority of patients presenting for arm procedures are relatively young and healthy. Most of these patients present for elective repair of a traumatic injury; thus, the preop workup is routine. Some arm procedures, such as repair of a compound fracture, require immediate attention and necessitate emergency surgery and full-stomach considerations.

| | |
|---|---|
| **Laboratory** | Hb/Hct (healthy patients); other tests as indicated from H&P. |
| **Premedication** | Moderate-to-heavy premedication (e.g., midazolam 0.5-1.0 mg iv q 5 min titrated to effect) is often desirable if regional block is used. |

### INTRAOPERATIVE

**Anesthetic technique:** GETA or regional anesthesia, or a combination of the two, can be used for surgical procedures on the arm. A brachial plexus block via the supraclavicular approach is excellent for procedures on the distal arm. The interscalene approach to the brachial plexus is perhaps best for more proximal procedures near the shoulder. Regional anesthesia alone is a means of avoiding the risk of aspiration pneumonitis associated with GA in the patient with a full stomach.

**General anesthesia:**

| | |
|---|---|
| **Induction** | Standard induction (see Appendix) except in acute-trauma patients, where rapid-sequence induction is appropriate. |
| **Maintenance** | Standard maintenance (see Appendix). |
| **Emergence** | Management of emergence and extubation should be routine, except in difficult airway cases, which require awake extubation. Skin closure is frequently followed by application of a splint; patient should remain anesthetized during splinting procedure. |

**Regional anesthesia:**

| | |
|---|---|
| **Interscalene block** | Anesthetics and doses:<br>3% 2-chloroprocaine 30-40 ml for procedures lasting < 1 hr.<br>1.5% lidocaine 30-40 ml for procedures lasting up to 2.5 hrs.<br>1% etidocaine 30-40 ml for procedures lasting >2.5 hrs.<br>Skin on the top of the shoulder (C3-C4) and the medial aspect of the upper arm (T2) often require separate subcutaneous field blocks. Phrenic nerve block → hemidiaphragmatic paralysis is an inevitable consequence of the interscalene block, which may not be tolerated by patients with significant pre-existing respiratory compromise. Major complications (e.g., total spinal or pneumothorax) resulting from interscalene block, are very rare; therefore, this technique is suitable for outpatients. Interscalene block is contraindicated in patients with contralateral recurrent laryngeal nerve or phrenic nerve palsy. If sedation is needed, midazolam (0.5-1.0 mg boluses), alfentanil (0.125-0.25 μg/kg/min by infusion) or propofol (50-100 μg/kg/min by infusion) given initially in subanesthetic doses, and thereafter titrated to effect, are good choices. |
| **Supraclavicular block** | 1.5% mepivacaine or lidocaine 40 ml for routine cases. 1% etidocaine 40 ml for procedures estimated to last >2.5 hrs. The upper arm medial aspect is innervated by the intercostobrachial nerve (T2) and requires a separate subcutaneous field block in the axilla, especially with tourniquet use. |
| **Supplemental sedation** | Supplemental sedation may be accomplished with use of propofol by continuous infusion (50-150 μg/kg/min) or intermittent bolus injection of opioid/benzodiazepine (e.g., midazolam 0.5-1.0 mg iv q 5 min and alfentanil 5-10 μg iv q 5 min) titrated to effect. |

| | | |
|---|---|---|
| **Blood and fluid requirements** | Minimal blood loss<br>IV: 18 ga x 1<br>NS/LR @ 1.5-3 cc/kg/hr | IV catheter should be placed in the contralateral upper extremity. |
| **Monitoring** | Standard monitors (see Appendix). | |
| **Positioning** | ✓ and pad pressure points.<br>✓ eyes. | |
| **Interscalene block complications** | Total spinal<br>Epidural anesthesia<br>IV injection (seizures/dysrhythmias)<br>Stellate ganglion block (Horner's syndrome)<br>Laryngeal nerve block<br>Phrenic nerve block<br>Pneumothorax | Resuscitative equipment, including airway management tools, should be immediately available. |
| **Supraclavicular block complications** | Inadequate block<br>Intravascular injection<br>Peripheral nerve damage<br>Hematoma<br>Horner's syndrome<br>Phrenic nerve paralysis<br>Recurrent laryngeal nerve paralysis<br>Pneumothorax | If accidental intra-arterial injection occurs, minimal doses of local anesthetic can cause CNS toxicity. Pneumothorax is an important concern when the supraclavicular approach is used. A large pneumothorax may become symptomatic quickly; most take many hours to develop and may be without Sx. The possibility of pneumothorax associated with the supraclavicular block makes this approach less suitable for use with outpatient procedures. |

## POSTOPERATIVE

| | | |
|---|---|---|
| **Pain management** | PCA (see Appendix).<br>± Regional block | Combined regional-GA is excellent for arm procedures, especially with respect to postop pain management. |
| **Tests** | None routinely indicated. | |

**References**


1. Henry AK: *Extensile Exposure*, 2nd edition, Churchill Livingstone, Edinburgh: 1973.
2. Hoppenfeld S, deBoer, eds: *Surgical Exposures in Orthopaedics: The Anatomic Approach.* JB Lippincott, Philadelphia: 1984.
3. Moorthy SS, Schmidt SI, Dierdorf SF, Rosenfeld SH, Anagnostou JM: A supraclavicular lateral paravascular approach for brachial plexus regional anesthesia [see comments]. *Anesth Analg* 1991; 72(2):241-44.

**Surgeons**

**John J. Csongradi, MD**
**Stuart B. Goodman, MD, MSC, FRCS(C), FACS**

# 10.3 SURGERY OF THE LOWER EXTREMITIES

**Anesthesiologists**

**Peter S. Kosek, MD**
**Frederick G. Mihm, MD**

# OPEN REDUCTION AND INTERNAL FIXATION (ORIF) OF PELVIS OR ACETABULUM

## SURGICAL CONSIDERATIONS

**Description**: ORIF procedures of the acetabulum and pelvis are some of the most challenging operations in orthopedic surgery. They are long and tedious procedures, requiring special training, several surgical assistants, and a whole armamentarium of plates, screws, reduction clamps and different devices. The patient usually arrives in OR in balanced traction, with either a tibial or femoral traction pin. Stabilization of anterior pelvic ring (pubic symphysis) may be performed acutely by the orthopedic surgeon using plates and screws applied to the pubic rami during **exploratory laparotomy** by a general/trauma surgeon. The procedures involve obtaining a reduction by open means through one or more long incisions. **Anterior approaches** to the pelvis include the suprapubic Pfannenstiel incision for plating the symphysis, and the ilioinguinal and iliofemoral incisions for reaching the anterior and medial portion of the acetabulum. Lateral approaches to the acetabulum may be combined with a **trochanteric osteotomy**, for wider exposure. Posterior incisions over the buttock expose the posterior column and also can be combined with a trochanteric osteotomy for wider exposure of the acetabular dome. **Extensile exposures** utilize larger dissections in order to visualize both anterior and posterior columns of the acetabulum and pelvis. The aim is to secure a congruous, anatomically sound reduction that is maintained by the application of plates and screws. Bone grafting is used to bridge defects. The patient is usually on protected weight-bearing crutches for several months in the postop period. (Also see "Closed Reduction and External Fixation of Pelvis.")

**Usual preop diagnosis**: Fractures of pelvis/acetabulum; nonunion/malunion of the pelvis/acetabulum

### SUMMARY OF PROCEDURE

| | |
|---|---|
| **Position** | Supine (anterior approach); lateral decubitus (with transtrochanteric); lateral decubitus or prone (posterior approach) |
| **Incision** | Ilioinguinal, iliofemoral over hip joint (anterior); straight lateral, posterior with anterior extension (with transtrochanteric); posterolateral (posterior) |
| **Special instrumentation** | Plates, screws, reduction clamps, etc. Cell saver recommended. |
| **Unique considerations** | Fracture table |
| **Antibiotics** | Broad-spectrum cephalosporin (e.g., cefamandole 1 gm iv q 6 hrs x 48 hrs) |
| **Surgical time** | ≥3 - 6 hrs (anterior); ≥4 - 6 hrs (with transtrochanteric); ≥3 - 6 hrs (posterior) |
| **Closing considerations** | May require re-application of balanced traction. |
| **EBL** | 1000 cc or more |
| **Postop care** | Multiple-trauma victim → ICU; others → PACU |
| **Mortality** | 10%+, dependent on extent of multiple trauma |
| **Morbidity** | Ileus: Virtually 100%<br>Sacroiliac pain (pelvic fractures): 25-50%<br>Lumbosacral plexus or sciatic nerve injury (usually peroneal branch): 15-25%<br>Heterotrophic ossification: 10-25% (↓ with NSAIDs)<br>Avascular necrosis: 5-20%<br>Genitourinary problems, including bladder and urethral rupture: 5-15%<br>Gynecological and colorectal injuries: 3-7%<br>Leg-length discrepancy: 3-5%<br>Nonunion: 3-5%<br>Vascular complications: 1%<br>Respiratory distress: Common<br>Delayed union: Not uncommon<br>Osteomyelitis<br>↓BP 2° to retroperitoneal hematoma: Not uncommon<br>Malunion: Not uncommon<br>Residual instability: Not uncommon<br>Rupture of diaphragm: Rare |

**Procedure code** 27217 (ORIF anterior pelvis); 27218 (ORIF posterior pelvis); 27226 (acetabular fixation)
**Pain score** 9

### PATIENT POPULATION CHARACTERISTICS

**Age range** Any age, but predominance of males < 30 yrs
**Male:Female** 5:1
**Incidence** 1-2%
**Etiology** Motorcycle and motor vehicle accidents: 60-80%
Falls: 10-15%
Crush injury: 5%
Others: 5%

**Associated conditions** Frequently associated with trauma to other organ systems, including head and neck, chest, abdomen and extremities. These often will be addressed concurrently with the pelvic or acetabular fracture.

## ANESTHETIC CONSIDERATIONS

See Anesthetic Considerations following "Amputations About the Hip and Pelvis: Disarticulation of the Hip and Hind-quarter Amputation" (below).

**References**


1. Bucholz RW, Brumback RJ: Fractures of the shaft of the femur. In *Rockwood and Green's Fractures in Adults*, 3rd edition. Rockwood CA Jr, Green DP, Bucholz RW, eds. JB Lippincott, Philadelphia: 1991, 1653-1723.
2. Burgess AR, Tile M: Fractures of the pelvis. In *Rockwood and Green's Fractures in Adults*, 3rd edition. Rockwood CA Jr, Green DP, Bucholz RW, eds. JB Lippincott, Philadelphia 1991, 1399-1479.
3. Crenshaw AH: Delayed union and nonunion of fractures. In *Campbell's Operative Orthopaedics*. Crenshaw AH, ed. CV Mosby, St. Louis: 1987, Vol 3, 2053-2118.
4. Kane WJ: Complications of pelvic fractures and their treatment. In *Complications in Orthopaedic Surgery*. Epps CH Jr, ed. JB Lippincott, Philadelphia: 1986, 795-814.
5. Sisk TD: Fractures of the hip and pelvis. In *Campbell's Operative Orthopaedics*. Crenshaw AH, ed. CV Mosby, St. Louis: 1987, Vol 3, 1719-81.
6. Mears DC, Rubash HE: *Pelvic and Acetabular Injuries*. Slack Inc., Thorofare NJ: 1986.
7. Tile M: *Fractures of the Pelvis and Acetabulum*. Williams and Wilkins, Baltimore: 1984.


# OSTEOTOMY AND BONE GRAFT AUGMENTATION OF THE PELVIS

## SURGICAL CONSIDERATIONS

**Description**: Patients undergoing this procedure have acetabular insufficiency (acetabular dysplasia), i.e., poor coverage of the femoral head by the acetabulum without advanced arthrosis of the hip. The aim of the operation is to expand the bony roof of the acetabulum to enable a broader contact surface for the hip joint. In children, bone grafting alone may be sufficient; in adults, however, cutting of the pelvis (osteotomy) to reorient or broaden the weight-bearing surface is necessary. A supplemental bone graft to expand the weight-bearing surface may be added. The osteotomy is usually internally fixed with screws or pins to allow early mobilization without displacement. Weight-bearing is permitted after healing of the osteotomy – about 8 weeks postop.

**Usual preop diagnosis**: Acetabular dysplasia or deficiency; subluxation of the hip

## SUMMARY OF PROCEDURE

| | |
|---|---|
| **Position** | Supine |
| **Incision** | Anterior: ilioinguinal or iliofemoral |
| **Special instrumentation** | Pelvic retractors; power or Gigli saw; screws and other instrumentation |
| **Unique considerations** | Intraop radiographs |
| **Antibiotics** | Broad-spectrum cephalosporin (e.g., cefamandole 1 gm iv q 6 hrs x 48 hrs) |
| **Surgical time** | 3 hrs |
| **EBL** | 500+ cc |
| **Postop care** | PACU → room; usually on protected weight-bearing x 8 wks |
| **Mortality** | Minimal |
| **Morbidity** | Ileus: 100%<br>Leg-length discrepancy: Uniformly present after pelvic osteotomy<br>Neurological deficit:<br>Injury to lateral cutaneous nerve: Common (50%)<br>Sciatic nerve: Uncommon (1%)<br>Thromboembolism: 5-10%<br>Wound infection: septic arthritis, osteomyelitis: 1-7%<br>Delayed union, nonunion, malunion: 1-2%<br>Genitourinary problems: urinary retention requiring catheterization: Common<br>Hematoma: Common<br>Hypotension 2° to retroperitoneal hematoma: Rare<br>Vascular complications: Rare |
| **Procedure code** | 27120, 27146 |
| **Pain score** | 8 |

### PATIENT POPULATION CHARACTERISTICS

| | |
|---|---|
| **Age range** | 20-50 yrs |
| **Male:Female** | 3-4 x higher incidence in females for congenital hip dysplasia; equal incidence for other causes |
| **Etiology** | Congenital hip dysplasia<br>Neuromuscular disorders – cerebral palsy, meningomyelocele<br>Pediatric trauma to acetabular growth plate |
| **Associated conditions** | Depends on diagnosis |

## ANESTHETIC CONSIDERATIONS

See Anesthetic Considerations following "Amputations About the Hip and Pelvis: Disarticulation of the Hip and Hind-quarter Amputation" (below).

**References**

1. Chiari K: Iliac osteotomy in young adults. In *The Hip: Proceedings of the 7th Open Meeting of the Hip Society*. CV Mosby, St. Louis: 1979, 260-77.
2. Salter RB, Thompson GH: The role of innominate osteotomy in young adults. *In The Hip: Proceedings of the 7th Open Meeting of the Hip Society*. CV Mosby, St. Louis: 1979, 278-312.
3. Sutherland DH, Greenfield R: Double innominate osteotomy. *J Bone Joint Surg* [Am] 1977; 59(8):1082-91.

# ARTHRODESIS OF THE SACROILIAC JOINT

## SURGICAL CONSIDERATIONS

**Description**: In this procedure, a painful and/or unstable sacroiliac (SI) joint is fused, usually by excising the joint through a **posterior approach**, and employing an iliac crest bone graft. Supplemental screw fixation of the joint is often used. The SI joint may be exposed through a dorsal vertical incision directly over the posterior pelvis. The posterior muscles are reflected from the medial aspect of the pelvis, and the SI joint is easily identified. The joint is debrided of cartilage and packed with strips of cancellous bone. Alternatively, the procedure may be performed through an **anterior approach**, sweeping the abdominal contents medially and approaching the SI joint anteriorly. The incision follows just inferior to the iliac crest; the abdominal muscle insertions are detached from the iliac crest. The pelvis is exposed subperiosteally, posterior to the SI joint. Then the joint cartilage is excised and packed with cancellous bone strips.

**Variant procedure or approaches**: Anterior or posterior approach

**Usual preop diagnosis**: Arthritis or arthrosis of the SI joint; pelvic instability

### SUMMARY OF PROCEDURE

| | |
|---|---|
| **Position** | Usually prone; rarely supine (when concomitantly fixing an acetabular fracture through an anterior approach) |
| **Incision** | Posterior, usually; anterior, rarely |
| **Special instrumentation** | Special pelvic retractors, screws and plates; intraop x-ray |
| **Unique considerations** | Intraop radiographs or use of image intensifier |
| **Antibiotics** | Broad-spectrum cephalosporin (e.g., cefamandole 1 gm iv q 6 hrs x 48 hrs) |
| **Surgical time** | 2 - 3 hrs |
| **EBL** | 250-500 cc |
| **Postop care** | Usually on protected weight-bearing walker or crutches for 6-8 wks |
| **Mortality** | Extremely low |
| **Morbidity** | Ileus: Virtually always<br>Osteomyelitis: < 1%<br>Wound infection: < 1%<br>Genitourinary problems; urinary retention requiring catheterization: Common<br>Delayed union, nonunion, malunion, leg-length discrepancy: Not uncommon<br>Neurological deficit; injury to lumbosacral plexus: Rare, unless present preop; L5 nerve root susceptible in anterior approaches<br>Hypotension 2° to retroperitoneal hematoma: Rare<br>Injury to bowel: Rare<br>Vascular complications; injury to iliac arteries: Rare<br>Thromboembolism |
| **Procedure code** | 27280 |
| **Pain score** | 7 |

### PATIENT POPULATION CHARACTERISTICS

| | |
|---|---|
| **Age range** | 20-50 yrs |
| **Male:Female** | Increased incidence in males (trauma) |
| **Incidence** | Rare |
| **Etiology** | Trauma: Post-pelvic fracture dislocation<br>Painful septic arthritis |

## ANESTHETIC CONSIDERATIONS

See Anesthetic Considerations following "Amputations About the Hip and Pelvis: Disarticulation of the Hip and Hind-quarter Amputation" (below).

**References**

1. Kane WJ: Complications of pelvic fractures and their treatment. In *Complications in Orthopaedic Surgery*. Epps CH Jr, ed. JB Lippincott, Philadelphia: 1986, 795-814.
2. Russell TA: Arthrodesis of the lower extremity and hip. In *Campbell's Operative Orthopaedics*. Crenshaw AH, ed. CV Mosby, St. Louis: 1987, Vol 2, 1091-1130.
3. Sisk TD: Fractures of hip and pelvis. In *Campbell's Operative Orthopaedics*. Crenshaw AH, ed. CV Mosby, St. Louis: 1987, Vol 3, 1719-81.

# CLOSED REDUCTION AND EXTERNAL FIXATION OF THE PELVIS

## SURGICAL CONSIDERATIONS

**Description**: This procedure entails manipulating the pelvis to obtain an acceptable reduction by closed means under GA, and then applying an anterior external fixation device to maintain the reduction. The pins for the external fixator are inserted into the iliac crest either percutaneously or through small incisions. During this procedure, either radiographs or the image intensifier is used to confirm that an acceptable reduction has been obtained. In some centers, this procedure is done in the emergency department as a life-saving procedure.

**Usual preop diagnosis**: Displaced fracture of the pelvis; unstable fracture of the pelvis

### SUMMARY OF PROCEDURE

| | |
|---|---|
| **Position** | Supine |
| **Incision** | Done percutaneously or through small incisions along the iliac crest |
| **Special instrumentation** | External fixation device of surgeon's choice; often performed on a radiolucent table using the image intensifier. |
| **Antibiotics** | Broad-spectrum cephalosporin (e.g., cefamandole 1 gm iv q 6 hrs x 48 hrs). Combination antibiotics, if multiple severe open fractures or other significant injuries are present. |
| **Surgical time** | 1 - 1.5 hrs |
| **EBL** | Negligible from surgical procedure; however, anticipate large blood losses (4+ U) from the pelvic fracture alone. |
| **Postop care** | Multiple-trauma victim → ICU; others → PACU |
| **Mortality** | 10% or more, depending on extent of multiple trauma; 50% in open fractures. |
| **Morbidity** | Ileus: virtually 100% |
| | Sacroiliac pain: 15-30%+ |
| | Genitourinary problems, including bladder or urethral rupture: 13% |
| | Neurological deficit to lumbosacral plexus: 1-10% |
| | Malunion/severe deformity: 5% |
| | Leg-length discrepancy: 3-5% |
| | Impotence: 1-5% |
| | Residual instability: 1-3% |
| | Vascular complications: 1% |
| | Hypotension 2° to retroperitoneal hematoma: Common |
| | Respiratory distress: Common |
| | Gynecological and colorectal injuries: More common with open fractures/dislocations |
| | Delayed union, nonunion: Not uncommon |
| | Osteomyelitis: Rare |
| | Rupture of diaphragm: Rare |
| **Procedure code** | 27193 (closed reduction); 20690, 20602 (external fixation) |
| **Pain score** | 7-10 |

### PATIENT POPULATION CHARACTERISTICS

**Age range** Any age, but predominance of males < 30 yrs
**Male:Female** 5:1
**Incidence** Common
**Etiology** Motorcycle and motor vehicle accidents: 60-80%
Falls: 10-15%
Crush injury: 5%
Other: 5%

**Associated conditions** Frequently associated with trauma to other organ systems, including head and neck, chest, abdomen and extremities. A patient sustaining a pelvic fracture also has a probability of having other injuries, including:
Musculoskeletal: 85%
Respiratory: 60%
CNS: 40%
GI: 30%
Urologic: 12%
CVS: 6%
These will often be addressed concurrently with the pelvic fracture.

---

## ANESTHETIC CONSIDERATIONS

See Anesthetic Considerations following "Amputations About the Hip and Pelvis: Disarticulation of the Hip and Hindquarter Amputation" (below).

---

**References**

1. Bucholz RW, Brumback RJ: Fractures of the shaft of the femur. In *Rockwood and Green's Fractures in Adults*, 3rd edition. Rockwood CA Jr, Green DP, Bucholz RW, eds. JB Lippincott, Philadelphia: 1991, 1653-1723.
2. Kane WJ: Complications of pelvic fractures and their treatment. In *Complications in Orthopaedic Surgery.* Epps CH Jr, ed. JB Lippincott, Philadelphia: 1986, 795-814.
3. Sisk TD: Fractures of hip and pelvis. In *Campbell's Operative Orthopaedics.* Crenshaw AH, ed. CV Mosby, St. Louis: 1987, Vol 3, 1719-81.
4. Mears DC, Rubash HE: *Pelvic and Acetabular Injuries.* Slack Inc., Thorofare NJ: 1986.
5. Tile M: *Fractures of the Pelvis and Acetabulum.* Williams and Wilkins, Baltimore: 1984.

# AMPUTATIONS ABOUT THE HIP AND PELVIS: DISARTICULATION OF THE HIP AND HINDQUARTER AMPUTATION

## SURGICAL CONSIDERATIONS

**Description**: These surgical procedures accomplish an excision of the entire lower extremity. In a hip disarticulation, the amputation is performed through the hip joint, while in a hindquarter amputation, excision of the lower extremity, hip joint and a portion of the pelvis is performed. In a **hip disarticulation**, an anterior, racquet-shaped incision is made and all muscles crossing the hip joint are incised or detached. The femoral artery, vein and nerve, obturator vessels, sciatic nerve and deep vessels are isolated and ligated. The gluteal flap is brought anteriorly and sewn to the anterior portion of the incision. In a **hindquarter amputation**, anterior and posterior incisions are used. The iliac wing is divided posteriorly and the symphysis pubis is disarticulated anteriorly. Either the common iliac or external iliac vessels are ligated, as are all nerves to the lower extremity. Usually the gluteal flap is drawn anteriorly for closure. These procedures are performed very rarely – for severe trauma, tumor or infection – and are often life-saving surgeries. They are often performed in conjunction with a general surgeon, and standard bowel prep is done. The operations are long and tedious, with extensive blood loss, in patients who are usually systemically ill.

**Usual preop diagnosis**: Malignant tumor of femur, hip or pelvis; traumatic amputation to femur, hip or pelvis; uncontrollable infection to leg, hip or pelvis (e.g., clostridia)

### SUMMARY OF PROCEDURE

| | Hip Disarticulation | Hindquarter Amputation |
|---|---|---|
| **Position** | Supine | Lateral decubitus; stabilized by bean bag and/or kidney rests. |
| **Incision** | Anterior racquet type (rare) | Anterior and posterior |
| **Unique considerations** | Urinary catheter should be placed. | Urinary catheter, NG tube; scrotum strapped to opposite thigh; anus stitched closed/sealed. |
| **Antibiotics** | Broad-spectrum cephalosporin (e.g., cefamandole 1 gm iv q 6 hrs) | ⇐ |
| **Surgical time** | 3 - 4 hrs | 4 - 5 hrs |
| **EBL** | 1000-2000 cc (intraop blood salvage system recommended) | 2000-3000 cc |
| **Postop care** | ICU | ⇐ |
| **Mortality** | Rare in patients undergoing elective amputation for trauma or localized tumor; higher for patients with debilitated trauma, chronic infection or extensive invasive malignant tumor; highest in clostridial infections: ~50%+. | ⇐ |
| **Morbidity** | Anemia: Common | ⇐ |
| | Electrolyte abnormalities: Common | ⇐ |
| | Hematoma: Common | ⇐ |
| | Neurological injury to lumbosacral plexus or peripheral nerves: Common | ⇐ |
| | Paralytic ileus: Common | ⇐ |
| | Psychosocial problems: Common | ⇐ |
| | UTI: Common | ⇐ |
| | Flap necrosis: Not uncommon | ⇐ |
| | Incomplete excision with recurrence of tumor or infection: Not uncommon | ⇐ |
| | Injury to peritoneal or retroperitoneal contents, including bowel and bladder: Not uncommon | ⇐ |
| | Vascular injury – iliac, other vessels: Not uncommon | ⇐ |
| **Procedure code** | 27295 | 27290 |
| **Pain Score** | 10 | 10 |

### PATIENT POPULATION CHARACTERISTICS

| | |
|---|---|
| **Age range** | Any age |
| **Male:Female** | Similar, except higher incidence in males for traumatic etiologies |
| **Incidence** | Uncommon |
| **Etiology** | Malignant tumor<br>Trauma<br>Infection: clostridial myonecrosis, chronic osteomyelitis, etc. |

---

## ANESTHETIC CONSIDERATIONS FOR PROCEDURES ABOUT THE PELVIS AND HIP

**(Procedures covered: ORIF of pelvis or acetabulum; osteotomy and bone graft augmentation of pelvis; arthrodesis of SI joint; closed reduction and external fixation of pelvis; amputations about hip and pelvis: disarticulation of hip and hindquarter amputation)**

### PREOPERATIVE

Patients presenting for pelvic surgery generally fall into two categories: 1) Major trauma – pelvic fracture requires substantial force and seldom occurs alone. These patients require aggressive fluid therapy with large-bore ivs and invasive monitors (arterial line and CVP). If the patient can be made hemodynamically stable with volume resuscitation, a thorough evaluation for coexisting neurological, thoracic or abdominal trauma should be undertaken prior to anesthesia. 2) Tumor resection and amputation of thigh, hip and pelvis. Because of large intraop blood loss and 3rd-spacing of fluids, invasive hemodynamic monitoring is necessary. Although epidural anesthesia is seldom adequate for surgery, postop epidural analgesia is an effective means to control the tremendous pain caused by this type of surgery. Other patient populations covered in this section include otherwise healthy patients with congenital or acquired hip dysplasia presenting for augmentation procedures.

| | |
|---|---|
| **Respiratory** | Trauma patients are at risk for hemothorax, pneumothorax, pulmonary contusion, fat embolism and aspiration. A chest tube will be needed prior to surgery if either a hemothorax or pneumothorax is present. Pulmonary fat embolus occurs in 10-15% of patients with long bone fractures, and can occur after isolated pelvic fractures. Sx include hypoxemia, tachycardia, tachypnea, respiratory alkalosis, mental status changes, conjunctival petechiae, fat bodies in the urine and diffuse pulmonary infiltrates. The Sx of pulmonary aspiration are similar to those of fat embolism. Preop therapy for either should include supplemental $O_2$ to correct hypoxemia (this may necessitate mechanical ventilation) and meticulous fluid management to prevent worsening of pulmonary capillary leak.<br>**Tests:** CXR, or others as indicated from H&P. |
| **Cardiovascular** | Blunt chest trauma can produce both cardiac contusion and aortic tear. Preop ECG and CPK isoenzymes will help evaluate the presence of myocardial injury. A wide mediastinal silhouette suggests aortic tear, which requires evaluation with TEE or angiography.<br>**Tests:** ECG; CPK isoenzymes; others as indicated from H&P. |
| **Neurological** | The possibility of coexistent neurologic trauma necessitates a thorough preop mental status and peripheral sensory exam. A CT scan of the head is indicated for any patient with loss of consciousness prior to anesthesia. |
| **Musculoskeletal** | For trauma patients, cervical spine films will evaluate the stability of the cervical spine prior to neck manipulation during ET intubation. Thoracic and lumbar x-rays should also be evaluated for the presence of traumatic spinal deformity or instability that would require special stabilization in the anesthetized patient.<br>**Tests:** C-spine x-rays or others as indicated from H&P. |
| **Hematologic** | Restore Hct to 25% prior to inducing anesthesia. Have available 1 blood volume (70 cc/kg) or 1 total erythrocyte mass (20 cc/kg) for intraop transfusion. Transfusions of more than 1 blood volume will require monitoring and possible replacement of platelets and coagulation factors. The incidence of DVT is very high in these patients, and prophylaxis with SCDs or low-dose subcutaneous heparin is indicated whenever feasible. |

**Renal** Renal injury commonly results from trauma to the collecting system, myoglobinuria from rhabdomyolysis and ischemic acute tubular necrosis from hypovolemia or aortic dissection. Foley catheters should be placed only after urologic consultation for possible urethral tear. Suprapubic catheters are often necessary. Monitoring of UO is mandatory to detect intraop compromise of the collecting system, and to monitor adequacy of renal perfusion.
**Tests:** UA; BUN; creatinine; others as indicated from H&P.

**Laboratory** Hct; electrolytes; other tests as indicated from H&P.

**Premedication** Pain can be treated with morphine (1-2 mg iv q 10 min titrated to pain relief) prior to anesthesia.

## INTRAOPERATIVE

**Anesthetic technique:** GETA is indicated due to the duration and extent of the surgery, as well as the varied positions that are necessary to accomplish pelvic fixation. Regional anesthesia is generally inadequate for major pelvic surgery; however, in elective surgeries, serious consideration should be given to postop epidural analgesia.

**Induction** A rapid-sequence induction (see Appendix) is necessary for trauma patients to minimize aspiration risk. Elective cases can undergo a standard induction (see Appendix).

**Maintenance** Standard maintenance (see Appendix).

**Emergence** Extubate trauma patients when fully awake and protective airway reflexes have returned. Do not extubate patients with evolving pulmonary injuries (fat embolism, aspiration or contusion). Monitoring in an ICU is usually indicated for trauma and cancer patients. Prolonged stays can be anticipated for patients with severe coexistent trauma.

| | | |
|---|---|---|
| **Blood and fluid requirements** | Large blood loss<br>IV: 14-16 ga x 2<br>NS/LR @ 8-12 cc/kg/hr<br>2-4 U PRBC in OR<br>Warm fluids.<br>Humidify gasses. | Expect large blood losses (from 0.5-2 or more blood volumes) with all but augmentation procedures. Cell scavenging techniques are useful to reduce the requirement for blood. Care should be taken to insure that cells have been adequately washed to minimize ↓BP on reinfusion. |
| **Control of blood loss** | Deliberate hypotension<br>Hemodilution | Patients with severe cardiovascular disease or carotid artery stenosis are not candidates for hypotension. Full replacement of any volume deficit is mandatory prior to inducing hypotension. Commonly used agents are isoflurane (1-3%) or esmolol (50-200 $\mu$g/kg/min) ± SNP (0.25-3 $\mu$g/kg/min). These agents are titrated to produce a 30% ↓ in preop MAP (but not < 60 mmHg). |
| **Monitoring** | Standard monitors (see Appendix).<br>Arterial line<br>CVP line<br>± PA catheter<br>UO | Patients with myocardial dysfunction should have fluid and inotropic/pressor therapy, guided by a PA catheter. Patients for shelf procedures may require only standard monitoring. |
| **Positioning** | ✓ and pad pressure points.<br>✓ eyes. | Meticulous padding of the chest, pelvis and extremities is imperative to prevent nerve injury and ischemia of the extremities. ↓BP → risk of neurovascular injury. |
| **Complications** | Hypothermia<br>Damage to urinary collecting system<br>Major blood loss<br>Coagulopathy | Warming of hypothermic patient may unmask severe volume depletion that will increase fluid requirement to well above apparent losses. |

## POSTOPERATIVE

| | | |
|---|---|---|
| **Complications** | Nerve root damage<br>Peripheral nerve damage | Preop or intraop damage to L4-S5 nerve roots and cauda equina, resulting in hemiplegia and bladder and bowel dysfunction. Neuropathy of the femoral, genitofemoral and lateral femoral cutaneous nerves can result from pressure on the ilioinguinal ligament during surgery. |

| | | |
|---|---|---|
| **Pain management** | IV morphine<br>Spinal opiates | Morphine 1-2 mg iv q 10 min prn<br>Epidural hydromorphone 50 μg/cc infused at 100-250 μg/hr, ± bupivacaine 0.125-0.25 % at 4-8 cc/hr, provides excellent analgesia. |
| **Tests** | Hct, CXR, coagulation profile, as indicated. | |

**References**


1. McCollough NC III: Complications of amputation surgery. In *Complications in Orthopaedic Surgery*. Epps CH Jr, ed. JB Lippincott, Philadelphia: 1986, 1335-67.
2. Tooms RE: Amputations of lower extremity. In *Campbell's Operative Orthopaedics*. Crenshaw AH, ed. CV Mosby, St. Louis: 1987, Vol 1, 607-27.


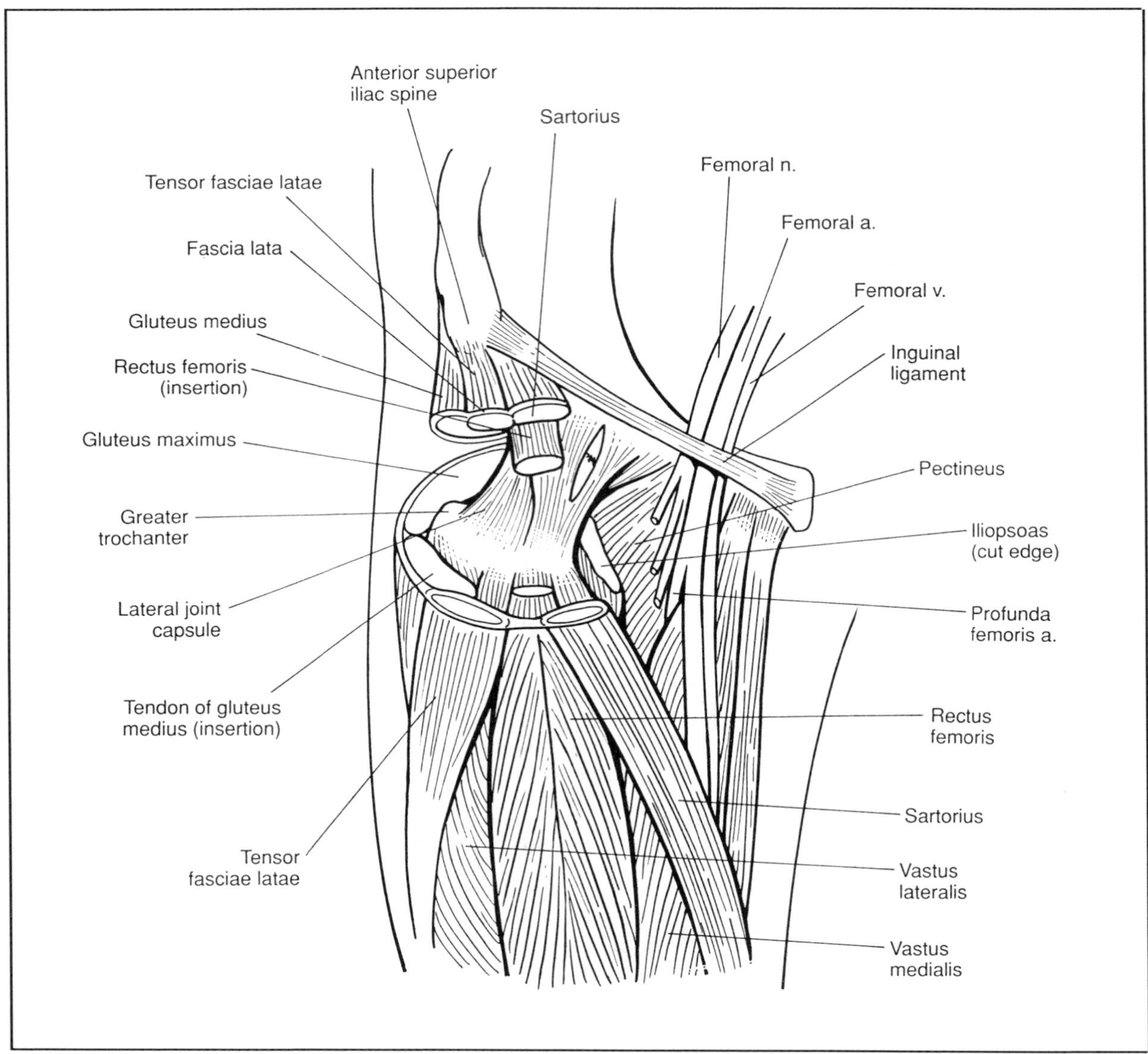


**Figure 10.3-1.** Surgical exposure of the hip joint: The hip joint may be exposed through a number of approaches. The relevant anatomical landmarks are shown here. (Reproduced with permission from Hoppenfeld S, deBoer P: *Surgical Exposures in Orthopaedics*. JB Lippincott: 1984.)

# ARTHROPLASTY OF THE HIP

## SURGICAL CONSIDERATIONS

**Description**: **Total hip arthroplasty** is one of the most successful procedures in orthopedic surgery. In this procedure, the hip joint (Fig 10.3-1) is approached through one of several standard incisions. The femoral head is dislocated from the acetabulum, and the arthritic femoral head and a portion of the neck are excised. The acetabulum is reamed to accept a cemented or cementless cup made of metal and plastic. The femoral stem and head are usually modular, allowing for numerous shapes, sizes, lengths, etc. The metallic femoral component may be cemented or cementless. A hybrid total hip combines a cemented femoral stem and a cementless acetabular cup. After relocation of the new prosthetic hip joint and closure of the tissues, the patient is usually placed in traction or positioning devices to prevent dislocation. Mobilization takes place over the ensuing days.

**Variant procedure or approaches**: **Unipolar** (only the femoral side is replaced); **bipolar** (both the femoral side and the acetabular side are replaced; the acetabular cup is not fixed to the pelvis). **Revision procedures** are more arduous and time-consuming, as the "failed" or loose component(s) must be removed and the bone prepared to accept new cemented or cementless components. These procedures require more specialized equipment for extracting prostheses and cement, and rebuilding the femoral or acetabular bone stock (allografts, autografts, etc.). Often, special components are needed for implantation of a new prosthesis. In the **Girdlestone procedure (resection arthroplasty)**, the components are removed, but not replaced. This procedure is usually performed for infection.

**Usual preop diagnosis**: Fracture of femoral neck; arthritis of hip; arthrosis of hip; loose (or malpositioned) hip prosthesis; chronic dislocation of hip arthroplasty; infected hip arthroplasty

**SUMMARY OF PROCEDURE**

| | Unipolar, Bipolar, Total Hip Replacement | Revision, Total Hip Replacement | Girdlestone Resection Arthroplasty |
|---|---|---|---|
| **Position** | Supine (for anterior or anterolateral approaches); lateral decubitus position (for lateral or posterior approaches) | ⇐ | ⇐ |
| **Incision** | Anterolateral, lateral or posterolateral over hip joint | ⇐ | ⇐ |
| **Special instrumentation** | Appropriate prostheses and instrumentation | Special instruments for excising cement | ⇐ |
| **Unique considerations** | In lateral decubitus position, patient is usually stabilized by bean bag and/or kidney rests. SCDs used. | A trochanteric osteotomy is frequently performed. | ⇐ |
| **Antibiotics** | Broad-spectrum cephalosporin (e.g., cefamandole 1 gm iv q 6 hrs x 48 hrs) | ⇐ | Intraop cultures; then same |
| **Surgical time** | 2 - 3 hrs | 3 - 6 hrs or more | 3 hrs or more |
| **EBL** | 500-750 cc (intraop blood retrieval system recommended) | 1000 cc or more | ⇐ |
| **Postop care** | Patient's legs immobilized between abduction wedge; or operated leg suspended in a splint or placed in traction. | ⇐ | ⇐ |
| **Mortality** | Rare | ⇐ | ⇐ |
| **Morbidity** | DVT: >50% | ⇐ | ⇐ |
| | Without prophylaxis: ≥ 50% | ⇐ | ⇐ |
| | With adjusted-dose heparin, Coumadin®, or SCD, antiembolism stockings: 10-20% | ⇐ | ⇐ |

| | Total Hip Replacement | Revision Hip Replacement | Girdlestone Resection |
|---|---|---|---|
| **Morbidity, continued** | Heterotopic ossification: 3-50% (average, 13%; significant, 4-5%) | >3-50% | ⇐ |
| | Intraop cementless fracture: 5-20% | ⇐ | ⇐ |
| | UTI: 7-14% | ⇐ | ⇐ |
| | Late aseptic loosening requiring revision: 5-10% (after 10 yrs) | >5-10% | – |
| | Wound infection: 1% | 3-10% | – |
| | Primary psoriatic and diabetic patients: 5-10% | | |
| | Primary OA: 1% | | |
| | Hematoma (major): < 5% | ⇐ | 5-10% |
| | Femoral/sciatic nerve injury: 0.7-3.5% | – | – |
| | PE: 1.8-3.4% (if no prophylaxis) | ⇐ | ⇐ |
| | Intraop cemented fracture: 1-3% | 2-3% | 1-3% |
| | Postop subluxation/dislocation: 0.5-3% | ⇐ | – |
| | Vascular injury to iliac vessels: < 0.5% | >0.5% | ⇐ |
| | Urinary retention requiring catheterization: Common | ⇐ | ⇐ |
| | GI bleed, MI, cholecystitis: Rare | ⇐ | – |
| | | | Neurological injury: 3-10% |
| **Procedure code** | 27130 | 27134; 27132; 27137; 27138 | 27122; 27090; 27091 |
| **Pain score** | 7 | 8 | 8 |

### PATIENT POPULATION CHARACTERISTICS

**Age range** Hip fracture and cases of arthrosis of the hip joint, generally >60 yrs; arthritis of the hip (e.g., rheumatoid arthritis or juvenile rheumatoid arthritis, traumatic arthritis), all ages

**Male:Female** Dependent on disease etiology

**Incidence** Common: approximately 150,000/yr in U.S.
Osteoarthritis
Sero-positive or sero-negative arthritis
Avascular necrosis
Traumatic arthritis
Congenital dislocation of the hip

**Associated conditions** Dependent on primary conditions (e.g., rheumatoid arthritis patients may have numerous deformities, cardiorespiratory disease, etc.)

---

## ANESTHETIC CONSIDERATIONS

See Anesthetic Considerations following "Synovectomy of the Hip" (below).

**References**

1. Bierbaum BE, Pomeroy DL, Berklacich FM: Late complications of total hip replacement. In *The Hip and its Disorders*. Steinberg ME, ed. WB Saunders Co, Philadelphia: 1991, 1061-96.
2. Calandruccio RA: Arthroplasty of the hip. In *Campbell's Operative Orthopaedics*. Crenshaw AH, ed. CV Mosby, St. Louis: 1987, Vol 2, 1213-1501.
3. Ranawat CS, Figgie MP: Early complications of total hip replacement. In *The Hip and its Disorders*. Steinberg ME, ed. WB Saunders Co, Philadelphia: 1991, 1042-60.
4. Scheller AD, Turner RH, Lowell JD: Complications of arthroplasty and total joint replacement in the hip. In *Complications in Orthopaedic Surgery*. Epps CH Jr, ed. JB Lippincott, Philadelphia: 1986, 1059-1108.

# ARTHRODESIS OF THE HIP

## SURGICAL CONSIDERATIONS

**Description**: In adults, this procedure is accomplished by fusing the femur to the acetabulum. Some form of internal fixation is usually employed; a spica cast is sometimes placed immediately postop or a few days later. The patient is usually not a good candidate for total hip arthroplasty (e.g., a young, healthy male with unilateral traumatic arthritis). The hip is usually fused in 30° of flexion, 10-30° of external rotation, and neutral-to-slight adduction. The surgical procedure may be performed through anterior, lateral or posterior incisions, with the lateral being most common. A **trochanteric osteotomy** facilitates exposure. After excising the cartilage surfaces, internal fixation, using screws ± a plate, is performed (Fig 10.3-2).

**Usual preop diagnosis**: Arthritis or arthrosis of the hip; previous septic arthritis of the hip; recurrent subluxation or dislocation of the hip

### SUMMARY OF PROCEDURE

| | |
|---|---|
| **Position** | Usually supine; occasionally lateral decubitus |
| **Incision** | Anterior or lateral thigh |
| **Special instrumentation** | Plates and screws or other internal fixation; reamers from surface replacement arthroplasty set may also be useful; intraop x-ray; fracture table |
| **Unique considerations** | Intraop radiographs or image intensifier used with patient on fracture table |
| **Antibiotics** | Broad-spectrum cephalosporin (e.g., cefamandole 1 gm iv q 6 hrs x 48 hrs) |
| **Surgical time** | 3 - 4 hrs |
| **EBL** | 500-1000 cc; cell saver recommended |
| **Postop care** | Spica cast |
| **Mortality** | Extremely low |
| **Morbidity** | Limb shortening: Some shortening is always present<br>Delayed union, nonunion, malunion: 10-15%<br>Femoral shaft fracture: 5-10%<br>Wound infection: < 1%<br>Genitourinary problems: urinary retention requiring catheterization: Common<br>Ileus: Common<br>Late degenerative arthritis of other lower extremity joints or back: Common, many yrs later<br>Injury to iliac or femoral vessels: Rare<br>Neurological deficit; injury to lateral cutaneous nerve, sciatic or femoral nerves: Not uncommon<br>Osteomyelitis: Rare<br>Vascular complications: Rare<br>Superior mesenteric artery syndrome causing duodenal obstruction: Extremely rare<br>Thromboembolism: See discussion in "Arthroplasty of the Hip," above. |
| **Procedure code** | 27284 |
| **Pain score** | 9 |

### PATIENT POPULATION CHARACTERISTICS

| | |
|---|---|
| **Age range** | 18-50 yrs |
| **Male:Female** | Usually males > females |
| **Incidence** | Rare |
| **Etiology** | Trauma, general<br>Neuromuscular disorders: cerebral palsy, meningomyelocele<br>Trauma to acetabular growth plate<br>Congenital hip dysplasia |
| **Associated conditions** | Depends on etiology |

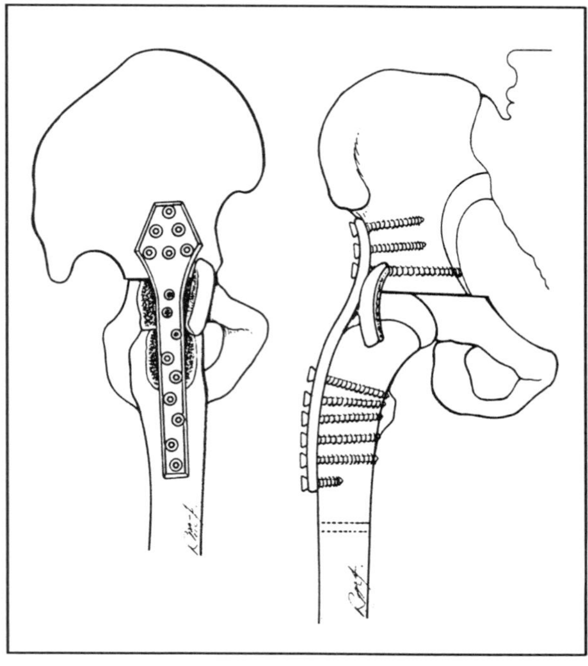

**Figure 10.3-2.** Arthrodesis of the hip using an AO Cobra® plate. (Reproduced with permission from Crenshaw AH: *Campbell's Operative Orthopaedics*, Vol I. Mosby-Year Book: 1992. Redrawn from Muller ME, et al: *Manual of internal fixation.* Techniques recommended by AO group, 2nd edition. Springer-Verlag: 1979. )

## ANESTHETIC CONSIDERATIONS

See Anesthetic Considerations following "Synovectomy of the Hip" (below).

**References**

1. Carnesale PG, Stewart MJ: Complications of arthrodesis surgery. In *Complications in Orthopaedic Surgery*. Epps CH Jr, ed. JB Lippincott, Philadelphia: 1986, 1289-1306.
2. Russell TA: Arthrodesis of the lower extremity and hip. In *Campbell's Operative Orthopaedics*. Crenshaw AH, ed. CV Mosby, St. Louis: 1987, Vol 2, 1091-1130.

# SYNOVECTOMY OF THE HIP

## SURGICAL CONSIDERATIONS

**Description**: An arthrotomy of the hip joint is performed through one of several standard approaches (anterior, anterolateral, lateral, posterior). A **capsulotomy** is performed, and is closed with reabsorbable sutures later in the case. Generally, the hip is not dislocated, but the cartilage surfaces are inspected and documented. The synovium, as well as any loose bodies, cartilage flaps and osteophytes, are excised. Although weight-bearing is usually protected, ROM and strengthening exercises are begun early.

**Usual preop diagnosis**: Chronic synovitis of hip; loose bodies in hip; juvenile and adult rheumatoid arthritis; pigmented villonodular synovitis

### SUMMARY OF PROCEDURE

| | |
|---|---|
| **Position** | Supine for anterior or anterolateral surgical approaches; lateral decubitus for posterior approaches |
| **Incision** | Overlying hip joint, depending on specific surgical approach |
| **Unique considerations** | Patient may have systemic disease (e.g., rheumatoid arthritis); careful positioning of limbs is necessary to avoid fracture or skin slough. |
| **Antibiotics** | Broad-spectrum cephalosporin (e.g., cefamandole 1 gm iv q 6 hrs) |
| **Surgical time** | 2 hrs |
| **EBL** | < 500 cc |
| **Mortality** | Rare |
| **Morbidity** | Thromboembolism: See figures for "Arthroplasty of the Hip."<br>Neurovascular injury – femoral or sciatic nerve, or iliac vessels: < 3%<br>Wound infection or dehiscence: < 3%<br>Septic arthritis and osteomyelitis: < 1% (unless synovectomy is performed for infection)<br>Avascular necrosis of femoral head: Rare (if hip is not dislocated)<br>Hematoma: Rare (if drainage tubes employed)<br>Inability to void, requiring urinary catheterization: Common |
| **Procedure code** | 27054 |
| **Pain score** | 7-8 |

### PATIENT POPULATION CHARACTERISTICS

| | |
|---|---|
| **Age range** | < 60 yrs |
| **Male:Female** | Dependent on disease etiology (e.g., preponderance of females in rheumatoid arthritis) |
| **Incidence** | Rare |
| **Etiology** | Septic arthritis: Very common<br>Rheumatoid arthritis (juvenile/adult): Rare<br>Pigmented villonodular synovitis: Rare<br>Trauma: Rare |
| **Associated conditions** | See Etiology, above. |

## ANESTHETIC CONSIDERATIONS FOR HIP PROCEDURES

**(Procedures covered: arthroplasty; arthrodesis; synovectomy)**

### PREOPERATIVE

Osteoarthritis is the most common indication for hip arthroplasty. These patients are usually elderly and their anesthetic management is tailored to any concurrent disease. Rheumatoid and other inflammatory arthritides form another group of candidates for these procedures, and the special anesthetic considerations for these patients are outlined below. Avascular necrosis of the hip is seen in patients with sickle-cell disease and in heart transplant patients.

| | |
|---|---|
| **Respiratory** | Patients with rheumatoid arthritis frequently have associated pulmonary complications. SOB on performing activities of daily living or exercise such as climbing a flight of stairs warrants further evaluation with PFTs. Pulmonary effusions are common. Pulmonary fibrosis (rare) often manifests as cough and dyspnea. Rheumatoid arthritis involvement of the cricoarytenoid joints may produce glottic narrowing and manifest as hoarseness. Arthritic involvement of the TMJ limits mouth opening and may necessitate special techniques (e.g., fiber optic or light wand) for ET intubation.<br>**Tests:** As indicated from H&P. |
| **Cardiovascular** | The severity of the arthritis often limits exercise, and ECHO and/or dipyridamole/thallium imaging may be necessary for adequate cardiac evaluation in patients with poor exercise tolerance. HTN and cardiovascular disease are common in elderly patients. Rheumatoid arthritis is associated with pericardial effusion, cardiac valve fibrosis, cardiac conduction abnormalities and aortic regurgitation. An ECG is indicated in all rheumatoid arthritis patients, and ECHO is indicated for patients with physical Sx suggestive of tamponade or cardiovascular disease.<br>**Tests:** As indicated from H&P. |

| | |
|---|---|
| **Neurological** | In patients with rheumatoid arthritis, a thorough neurological exam preop often yields evidence of cervical nerve root compression. Patients with arthritis involving the cervical spine should have lateral neck films preop to determine the stability of the atlanto-occipital joint. After the stability of the spine has been established, full ROM of the neck should be evaluated for evidence of further nerve-root compression or cerebral ischemia (suggesting vertebral artery compression). Evidence of cerebral ischemia mandates a full neurovascular evaluation.<br>**Tests:** As indicated from H&P. |
| **Musculoskeletal** | Pain and decreased joint mobility make positioning and regional anesthesia difficult in patients with arthritis. |
| **Hematologic** | Rheumatoid arthritis patients often have anemia. Patients with Hb >12 gm/dl are candidates for preop autologous blood donation. DVT is common after hip surgery, and prophylaxis for its occurrence reduces mortality. Effective preventive measures include SCDs and subcutaneous heparin. NSAID-induced coagulopathy may preclude the use of regional anesthesia.<br>**Tests:** PT; PTT; bleeding time; others as indicated from H&P. |
| **Renal** | In order to predict the clearance of anesthetics and adjuvants in this elderly population, a preop estimation of renal function is useful.<br>**Tests:** Creatinine; BUN |
| **Laboratory** | Other tests as indicated from H&P. |
| **Premedication** | In the absence of limited pulmonary reserve or severe cardiac disease, a standard premedication (see Appendix) is appropriate. |

## INTRAOPERATIVE

**Anesthetic technique**: GETA or regional anesthesia.

**General anesthesia:**

| | |
|---|---|
| **Induction** | The lateral position may mandate ET intubation for patients undergoing GA. A careful preop airway evaluation will determine the need for special airway techniques (e.g., fiber optic intubation or light wand). Aggravation of cricoarytenoid arthritis that is common in rheumatoid arthritis patients can be minimized if a small ETT (6-7 mm cuffed) is used. For otherwise healthy patients, standard induction (see Appendix) is appropriate. |
| **Maintenance** | Standard maintenance (see Appendix). Neuromuscular blockade facilitates the placement and testing of the prosthesis. |
| **Emergence** | No special considerations |

**Regional anesthesia:** Induction of regional anesthesia, with its attendant positioning requirements, can be uncomfortable in patients with limited joint mobility. Rheumatoid arthritis patients, however, rarely have involvement of the lumbar spine, and regional anesthesia offers the advantages of decreased perioperative DVT, decreased intraop blood loss and no need for airway manipulation. Anesthesia to T10 is adequate. Full motor blockade is essential for placement of the prosthesis and assessment of the passive ROM. Lumbar epidural block (15-20 cc 2% lidocaine with epinephrine 1:200,000, administered over 15 min) has the advantage of slow onset, allowing time to treat the induced cardiovascular changes. Postop epidural opiates can provide excellent analgesia. Spinal anesthesia, with 15 mg of bupivacaine 0.5% and morphine 0.2 mg placed at L3-L4, has a more rapid onset than epidural anesthesia and yields analgesia for up to 24 hrs postop.

| | | |
|---|---|---|
| **Blood and fluid requirements** | Major blood loss<br>IV: 14-16 ga x 2<br>NS/LR @ 4-8 cc/kg/hr | Cell scavenging helps reduce total transfusion requirement. Care should be taken to ensure that cells have been adequately washed to minimize ↓BP on re-infusion. |
| **Control of blood loss** | Regional anesthesia<br>Controlled hypotension | These techniques may be appropriate in selected patient populations. |
| **Monitoring** | Standard monitors (see Appendix).<br>± CVP line<br>± Arterial line | Invasive monitoring is indicated in the presence of exercise-limiting cardiac or pulmonary disease. |
| **Positioning** | Axillary roll, bean bag<br>✓ and pad pressure points.<br>✓ eyes. | Meticulous padding of extremities and maintaining a neutral neck position are mandatory. A bean bag and axillary roll are also necessary to stabilize patient in the lateral position and to protect dependent arm from neurovascular compression injuries. |

| | | |
|---|---|---|
| **Complications** | Methylmethacrylate:<br>↓BP 2° vasodilation<br>↓$PaO_2$ 2° embolization<br>Cardiovascular collapse<br>VAE<br>Major blood loss<br>DVT<br>Nerve damage<br>Femur fracture | Embolization of air, fat, bone fragments and cement may occur during insertion of the femoral prosthesis. Systemic hypotension and pulmonary HTN may occur. Care should be taken to insure that the patient is adequately hydrated prior to procedure, and pressors may be necessary to maintain BP (ephedrine 5-20 mg iv or epinephrine 10-100 μg iv and increasing the dose as necessary). |

**POSTOPERATIVE**

| | | |
|---|---|---|
| **Complications** | Nerve damage<br>DVT | Sciatic nerve injury is evidenced by foot drop and an inability to flex the knee. |
| **Pain management** | Spinal opiates<br>Epidural analgesia | Epidural hydromorphone 50 μg/cc infused at 100-250 μg/hr provides excellent analgesia. |
| **Tests** | Hct<br>CXR, if CVP was placed. | |

**References**


1. Richardson EG: Miscellaneous nontraumatic disorders. In *Campbell's Operative Orthopaedics*. Crenshaw AH, ed. CV Mosby, St. Louis: 1987, Vol 2, 1014-15.

# OPEN REDUCTION AND INTERNAL FIXATION (ORIF) OF PROXIMAL FEMORAL FRACTURES

## (FEMORAL NECK, INTERTROCHANTERIC, SUBTROCHANTERIC FRACTURES)

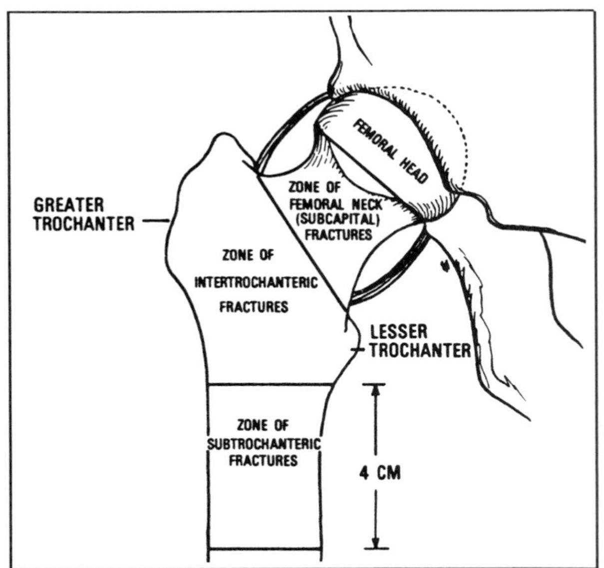


**Figure 10.3-3.** Anatomical classification of fractures of the proximal femur. (Reproduced with permission from Hardy JD: *Hardy's Textbook of Surgery* 2nd edition. JB Lippincott: 1988.)

### SURGICAL CONSIDERATIONS

**Description**: Fractures of the proximal femur are seen in two distinct populations: most commonly, in elderly patients as the result of falls; and younger patients following trauma. In elderly patients, the fracture occurs through osteoporotic bone in the femoral neck, intertrochanteric or subtrochanteric area (Fig 10.3-3). Displaced femoral neck fractures are usually treated by **prosthetic replacement**. Nondisplaced or minimally displaced femoral neck fractures are usually treated by **closed reduction and percutaneous pinning** of the fracture. Intertrochanteric and subtrochanteric fractures, whether displaced or nondisplaced, are usually treated by ORIF with a nail-plate or nail-rod device. Prosthetic replacement is performed only rarely. Elderly patients frequently have numerous medical problems, which means that the fractures require prompt internal fixation/prosthetic replacement to facilitate early mobilization. In younger patients (16-40 yrs), proximal femoral fractures are almost always treated by ORIF with screws, plates and screws, or intramedullary devices. These are normally much higher energy fractures, often associated with multiple trauma.

**Variant procedure or approaches**: **Percutaneous pinning** of nondisplaced femoral neck fracture; **ORIF of displaced femoral neck fracture** (also see "Arthroplasty for the Hip"); **ORIF of intertrochanteric or subtrochanteric fracture** are variants.

**Usual preop diagnosis**: Nondisplaced femoral neck fracture; displaced femoral neck fracture (those not requiring prosthetic replacement); intertrochanteric ± subtrochanteric fracture

**SUMMARY OF PROCEDURE**

| | Nondisplaced Femoral Neck Fracture | Displaced Femoral Neck Fracture | Intertrochanteric ± Subtrochanteric Fracture |
|---|---|---|---|
| **Position** | Supine, on fracture table | ⇐ | ⇐ |
| **Incision** | Proximal lateral thigh | ⇐ | ⇐ |
| **Special instrumentation** | Usually multiple percutaneous pins | Screw and side plate | Screw plate device or intramedullary device |
| **Unique considerations** | Fracture table and image intensifier used. | ⇐ | ⇐ |
| **Antibiotics** | Broad-spectrum cephalosporin (e.g., cefamandole 1 gm iv q 6 hrs x 48 hrs) | ⇐ | ⇐ |
| **Surgical time** | 1 hr | 1.5 - 2 hrs, including placing patient on fracture table and obtaining adequate reduction of fracture | 1.5 - 3 hrs |
| **EBL** | < 100 cc | 250-500 cc | 500+ cc |
| **Postop care** | Generally PACU → room; if medically unstable → ICU | ⇐ | ⇐ |

| | Nondisplaced Femoral Neck Fracture | Displaced Femoral Neck Fracture | Intertrochanteric ± Subtrochanteric Fracture |
|---|---|---|---|
| **Mortality** | 10-30% in first 12 mo postop in elderly; in younger patients, depends on multiple trauma. | ⇐ | ⇐ |
| **Morbidity** | Dysrhythmias: ~50% | ⇐ | ⇐ |
| | MI: ~50% | ⇐ | ⇐ |
| | Respiratory failure: ~50% | ⇐ | ⇐ |
| | Urinary retention requiring catheterization: ~50% | ⇐ | ⇐ |
| | UTI: ~50% | ⇐ | ⇐ |
| | Thromboembolism: 40%+ | ⇐ | ⇐ |
| | Avascular necrosis and late segmental collapse: 10-20% | ≥15-35% | 1% |
| | Infection, deep: 2-17% | ⇐ | ⇐ |
| | Infection, superficial: 2-17% | ⇐ | ⇐ |
| | Septic arthritis: 2-17% | ⇐ | ⇐ |
| | Nonunion: 5-15% | 20-30% | 2% |
| | Malunion: < 10% | ≤ 10% | 10-20% |
| | Loss of reduction: < 5% | ~10% | 10% |
| | Hematoma | – | – |
| | Intraop comminution of the fracture | – | – |
| | Neurological injury: Rare | ⇐ | ⇐ |
| | Vascular injury: Rare | ⇐ | ⇐ |
| **Procedure code** | 27235 | 27236 | 27244 |
| **Pain score** | 5-6 | 7 | 8 |

## PATIENT POPULATION CHARACTERISTICS

| | |
|---|---|
| **Age range** | Usually >60 yrs (patients with an intertrochanteric fracture average 65-70 yrs); occasionally, younger patients, 16-35 yrs (as part of multiple-trauma situation) |
| **Male:Female** | Elderly 1:4-5 |
| **Incidence** | Extremely common – about 5-100 per 100,000; femoral neck fractures are about twice as common as intertrochanteric fractures. |
| **Etiology** | Accidents and falls<br>Pathological fracture<br>Multiple trauma (younger patients)<br>Stress fracture |
| **Associated conditions** | Numerous serious medical conditions often present in elderly<br>Senile dementia<br>Multiple trauma often accompanies this fracture in younger patients. |

# ANESTHETIC CONSIDERATIONS

See "Anesthetic Considerations for Lower-Extremity Procedures" at the end of "Orthopedic Surgery for Lower Extremities" section.

**References**


1. Crenshaw AH: Delayed union and nonunion of fractures. In *Campbell's Operative Orthopaedics*. Crenshaw AH, ed. CV Mosby, St. Louis: 1987, Vol 3, 2053-2118.
2. Sisk TD: Fractures of the hip and pelvis. In *Campbell's Operative Orthopaedics*. Crenshaw AH, ed. CV Mosby, St. Louis: 1987, Vol 3, 1719-81.
3. Wilkins RM, Winter WG: Complications of treatment of fractures and dislocations of the hip. In *Complications in Orthopaedic Surgery*. Epps CH Jr, ed. JB Lippincott, Philadelphia: 1986, 469-511.

# OPEN REDUCTION AND INTERNAL FIXATION (ORIF) OF DISTAL FEMUR FRACTURES

## SURGICAL CONSIDERATIONS

**Description**: ORIF of the distal femur fracture involves a longitudinal incision along the femoral shaft, obtaining reduction by direct visualization of the fracture fragments, and applying plates and screws along the femur for rigid internal fixation. An iliac crest bone graft may be necessary. Some intramedullary devices are also available for fixation of these fractures.

**Usual preop diagnosis**: Fracture of the distal femur; nonunion/malunion of the distal femur; degenerative arthritis of knee, with deformity

### SUMMARY OF PROCEDURE

| | |
|---|---|
| **Position** | Supine. Patient usually arrives at OR in balanced traction if fracture is acute. |
| **Incision** | Lateral or medial thigh along the femoral shaft |
| **Special instrumentation** | Special plates, screws, reduction clamps; radiolucent table; intraop blood salvage. |
| **Unique considerations** | Usually requires intraop radiographs; tourniquet |
| **Antibiotics** | Broad-spectrum cephalosporin (e.g., cefamandole 1 gm iv q 6 hrs x 48 hrs) |
| **Surgical time** | 3 hrs (or more, depending on difficulty) |
| **EBL** | 750 cc or more |
| **Postop care** | Multiple-trauma victim → ICU; others → PACU |
| **Mortality** | ~3-4%, depending on the extent of multiple trauma |
| **Morbidity** | Nonunion: 4-33%<br>Malunion: 4-31%<br>Infection, osteomyelitis, septic arthritis; closed/open:<br>Grade I: 1-5%<br>Grade II: 5-20%<br>Grade III: >20%<br>Delayed union: 0-17%<br>Vascular complications: 2-3%<br>Neurological deficit to peripheral nerves, peroneal nerve: ~3%<br>Compartment syndrome: Rare<br>Hypotension: Rare<br>Leg-length discrepancy: Rare<br>Respiratory distress and fat embolism: Rare |
| **Procedure code** | 27514, 27506, 27470, 27472, 27450 |
| **Pain score** | 8 |

### PATIENT POPULATION CHARACTERISTICS

| | |
|---|---|
| **Age range** | Any age; predominance of males < 40 yrs (trauma); degenerative arthritis of knee < 60 yrs<br>Special rare case is elderly patient with a supracondylar fracture above a total knee replacement |
| **Male:Female** | 5:1 |
| **Incidence** | Common in trauma center patients; rare in cases of degenerative arthritis of knee (osteotomy) or elderly patient with a supracondylar fracture above a total knee replacement |
| **Etiology** | Motorcycle and motor vehicle accidents<br>Falls<br>Industrial injury<br>Degenerative arthritis of knee |
| **Associated conditions** | Frequently associated with trauma to other organ systems |

## ANESTHETIC CONSIDERATIONS

See "Anesthetic Considerations for Lower-Extremity Procedures" at the end of "Orthopedic Surgery for Lower Extremities" section.

**References**

1. Crenshaw AH: Delayed union and nonunion of fractures. In *Campbell's Operative Orthopaedics*. Crenshaw AH, ed. CV Mosby, St. Louis: 1987, Vol 3, 2053-2118.
2. Hohl M, Larson RL: Complications of treatment of fractures and dislocations of the knee. In *Complications in Orthopaedic Surgery*. Epps CH Jr, ed. JB Lippincott, Philadelphia: 1986, 537-84.
3. Hohl M, Johnson EE, Wiss DA: Fractures of the knee. In *Rockwood and Green's Fractures in Adults*, 3rd edition. Rockwood CA Jr, Green DP, Bucholz RW, eds. JB Lippincott, Philadelphia: 1991, 1725-97.
4. Russell TA: Malunited fractures. In *Campbell's Operative Orthopaedics*. Crenshaw AH, ed. Mosby, St. Louis: 1987, 2015-52.
5. Sisk TD: Fractures of lower extremity. In *Campbell's Operative Orthopaedics*. Crenshaw AH, ed. CV Mosby, St. Louis: 1987, Vol 3, 1607-1718.

# OPEN REDUCTION AND INTERNAL FIXATION (ORIF) OF THE FEMORAL SHAFT WITH PLATE

## SURGICAL CONSIDERATIONS

**Description**: ORIF of the femoral shaft involves obtaining a reduction by open means, usually through a longitudinal lateral incision along the length of the femur, and applying plates and screws along the femur to maintain the reduction. An iliac crest bone graft may be necessary.

**Usual preop diagnosis**: Fracture of femur

### SUMMARY OF PROCEDURE

| | |
|---|---|
| **Position** | Supine or lateral decubitus |
| **Incision** | Lateral thigh along length of femur, ± iliac crest incision |
| **Special instrumentation** | Special plates, screws; reduction clamps; blood salvage device |
| **Unique considerations** | Fracture or radiolucent table; image intensifier. Patient usually arrives at OR in balanced traction. |
| **Antibiotics** | Broad-spectrum cephalosporin (e.g., cefamandole 1 gm iv q 6 hrs) |
| **Surgical time** | 3 hrs or more, depending on difficulty |
| **EBL** | 750 cc; cell saver recommended |
| **Postop care** | Multiple-trauma victims: ICU; others: PACU |
| **Mortality** | Dependent on extent of multiple trauma |
| **Morbidity** | Knee stiffness: 20-30%<br>Delayed union, nonunion, malunion: 5-21%<br>Leg-length discrepancy: 0-11%<br>Failure of fixation: 5-10%<br>Infection, osteomyelitis: < 5%<br>Hypotension: Not uncommon<br>Respiratory distress and fat embolism: Not uncommon, often subclinical<br>Compartment syndrome: Rare<br>Neurological deficit to peripheral nerves: Rare<br>Vascular complications: Rare |
| **Procedure code** | 27506 |
| **Pain score** | 9 |

### PATIENT POPULATION CHARACTERISTICS

| | |
|---|---|
| **Age range** | Any age, but predominance of males < 30 |
| **Male:Female** | 5:1 |
| **Incidence** | Unknown |
| **Etiology** | Motorcycle and motor vehicle accidents<br>Falls<br>Industrial injuries |
| **Associated conditions** | Frequently associated with trauma to other organ systems |

## ANESTHETIC CONSIDERATIONS

See "Anesthetic Considerations for Lower-Extremity Procedures" at the end of "Orthopedic Surgery for Lower Extremities" section.

**References**

1. Bucholz RW, Brumback RJ: Fractures of the shaft of the femur. In *Rockwood and Green's Fractures in Adults*, 3rd edition. Rockwood CA Jr, Green DP, Bucholz RW, eds. JB Lippincott, Philadelphia: 1991, 1653-1723.
2. Crenshaw AH: Delayed union and nonunion of fractures. In *Campbell's Operative Orthopaedics*. Crenshaw AH, ed. CV Mosby, St. Louis: 1987, Vol 3, 2053-2118.
3. Rankin EA, Baker GI: Complications of treatment of fractures of the femoral shaft. In *Complications in Orthopaedic Surgery*. Epps CH Jr, ed. JB Lippincott, Philadelphia: 1986, 513-36.
4. Russell TA: Malunited fractures. In *Campbell's Operative Orthopaedics*. Crenshaw AH. ed. Mosby, St. Louis: 1987, 2015-52.

# INTRAMEDULLARY NAILING OF FEMORAL SHAFT

## SURGICAL CONSIDERATIONS

**Description**: This procedure, performed acutely for fracture or later for a nonunion or malunion of the femoral shaft, involves obtaining a reduction by closed or open means, and inserting an intramedullary nail from proximal to distal in the femur, typically through a small incision in the lateral thigh (closed technique). An iliac crest bone graft may be necessary for nonunions. The procedure is usually performed using a fracture table and image intensifier. Through a small incision just proximal to the greater trochanter, the pyriformis fossa (just lateral to the femoral neck) is exposed. Reaming of the medullary canal is performed, and a long nail (rod) is inserted proximal to distal (Fig 10.3-4). Screws may be inserted through the rod if the fracture is comminuted and unstable.

**Usual preop diagnosis**: Femoral shaft fracture; nonunion/malunion of the femur; leg-length discrepancy

### SUMMARY OF PROCEDURE

| | |
|---|---|
| **Position** | Supine (or lateral decubitus) |
| **Incision** | Lateral thigh |
| **Special instrumentation** | Intramedullary nails and interlocking screws; intramedullary saw for closed femoral shortening of femur |
| **Unique considerations** | If fracture is acute, patient may be a multiple-trauma case with other injuries. Most surgeons use fracture table with image intensifier. Patient may arrive at OR in balanced traction. |
| **Antibiotics** | Broad-spectrum cephalosporin (e.g., cefamandole 1 gm iv q 6 hrs x 48 hrs) |
| **Surgical time** | 2 - 3 hrs; 3+ hrs for nonunion/malunion of femur or closed femoral shortening of femur |

| | |
|---|---|
| **EBL** | 250-500 cc; 750 cc or more for nonunion/malunion of femur or closed femoral shortening of femur (cell saver recommended) |
| **Postop care** | If surgery performed acutely, patient is usually a multiple-trauma victim with numerous injuries and extensive blood loss; usually goes to ICU. |
| **Mortality** | Dependent on extent of trauma |
| **Morbidity** | Respiratory distress and fat embolism: 10%<br>Malunion: 5-10%<br>Infection, osteomyelitis:<br>Closed technique: 0-1%<br>Open technique: 1-10%<br>Vascular complication ~2% (up to 15% have occult vascular-flow abnormalities)<br>Neurological deficit to peripheral nerves: 2%<br>Delayed union: 1%<br>Nonunion: 1%<br>Hypotension: Common in multiple-trauma situations<br>Knee stiffness: Common<br>Leg-length discrepancies: Not uncommon<br>Compartment syndrome: Rare<br>Failure of fixation: Rare |
| **Procedure code** | 27506 |
| **Pain score** | 6 |

### PATIENT POPULATION CHARACTERISTICS

| | |
|---|---|
| **Age range** | Any age, but predominance of males < 30 |
| **Male:Female** | 5:1 |
| **Incidence** | Very common |
| **Etiology** | Motorcycle and motor vehicle accidents: 60-80%<br>Falls: 5-10%<br>Industrial injuries: 5-10%<br>Previous trauma: Rare |
| **Associated conditions** | Frequently associated with trauma to other organ systems |

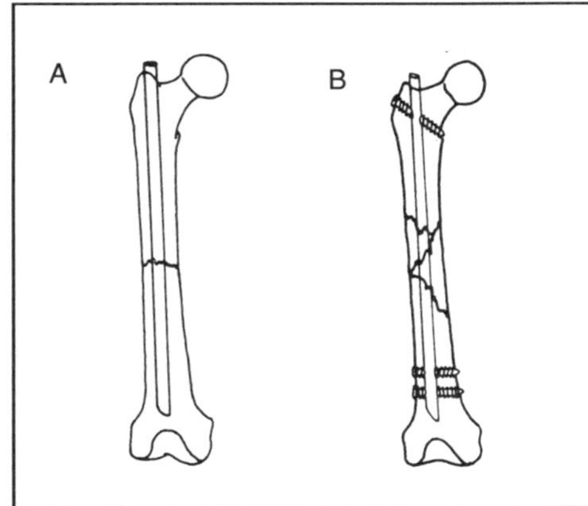


**Figure 10.3-4.** (A) Simple and (B) locked intramedullary fixation of femoral shaft. (Reproduced with permission from Hardy JD: *Hardy's Textbook of Surgery*, 2nd edition. JB Lippincott: 1988.)

## ANESTHETIC CONSIDERATIONS

See "Anesthetic Considerations for Lower-Extremity Procedures" at the end of "Orthopedic Surgery for Lower Extremities" section.

**References**

1. Bucholz RW, Brumback RJ: Fractures of the shaft of the femur. In *Rockwood and Green's Fractures in Adults*, 3rd edition. Rockwood CA Jr, Green DP, Bucholz RW, eds. JB Lippincott, Philadelphia: 1991, 1653-1723.
2. Crenshaw AH: Delayed union and nonunion of fractures. In *Campbell's Operative Orthopaedics*. Crenshaw AH, ed. CV Mosby, St. Louis: 1987, Vol 3, 2053-2118.
3. Rankin EA, Baker GI: Complications of treatment of fractures of the femoral shaft. In *Complications in Orthopaedic Surgery*. Epps CH Jr, ed. JB Lippincott, Philadelphia: 1986, 513-36.
4. Russell TA: Malunited fractures. In *Campbell's Operative Orthopaedics*. Crenshaw AH, ed. CV Mosby, St. Louis: 1987, Vol 3, 2015-52.

# REPAIR OF NONUNION/MALUNION OF PROXIMAL THIRD OF FEMUR, PROXIMAL FEMORAL OSTEOTOMY FOR OSTEOARTHRITIS

## SURGICAL CONSIDERATIONS

**Description**: Operations for nonunion/malunion of the proximal femur entail realigning the bones with a femoral osteotomy (as necessary); stabilizing the reduction with internal fixation (using a nail-plate/nail-rod device); and supplementing this with a bone graft. In young patients (< 50 years) in whom early OA of the hip spares some of the cartilage, the hip may be realigned with **proximal femoral osteotomy**. This entails cutting the bone at the level of the lesser trochanter, realigning the hip, and stabilizing the osteotomy with internal fixation.

**Variant procedure or approaches**: Osteotomy of proximal 1/3 of femur for degenerative arthritis of hip

**Usual preop diagnosis**: Nonunion/malunion of proximal 1/3 of femur; early degenerative arthritis of hip

### SUMMARY OF PROCEDURE

| | Repair Nonunion/Malunion | Proximal Femoral Osteotomy |
|---|---|---|
| **Position** | Supine or lateral decubitus | ⇐ |
| **Incision** | Proximal lateral thigh | ⇐ |
| **Special instrumentation** | Plates, screws; reduction clamps; occasionally an intramedullary device. Cell saver recommended. Some surgeons use fracture or radiolucent table with image intensifier. | ⇐ |
| **Antibiotics** | Broad-spectrum cephalosporin (e.g., cefamandole 1 gm iv q 6 hrs) | ⇐ |
| **Surgical time** | 2 hrs for bone grafting alone; 3 hrs or more if difficult malunion | 3 hrs |
| **EBL** | 500-750 cc or more | 500 cc + |
| **Mortality** | Rare: < 1% | ⇐ |
| **Morbidity** | Leg-length discrepancy: Common | – |
| | Technical complications/fixation failure: 1-5% | ⇐ |
| | Superficial, deep infection/osteomyelitis: 1% | ⇐ |
| | Malunion: Not uncommon | – |
| | Compartment syndrome: Rare | ⇐ |
| | Neurological deficit to peripheral nerves: Rare | ⇐ |
| | Vascular complications: Rare | ⇐ |
| | | Progressive pain/arthritis (by 5-10 yrs): 40-50% |
| | | Delayed union: 5-10% |
| | | Nonunion: 1-5% |
| **Procedure code** | 27170, 27472 (bone graft repair)<br>27470 (without graft) | 27161; 27165 |
| **Pain score** | 8 | 8 |

### PATIENT POPULATION CHARACTERISTICS

| | | |
|---|---|---|
| **Age range** | Any age | ⇐ |
| **Male:Female** | 1:1 | ⇐ |
| **Incidence** | Rare | ⇐ |
| **Etiology** | Previous surgery: Rare<br>Previous trauma: Rare | Early degenerative arthritis of the hip: Not uncommon |
| **Associated conditions** | May accompany multiple traumas | |

## ANESTHETIC CONSIDERATIONS

See "Anesthetic Considerations for Lower-Extremity Procedures" at the end of "Orthopedic Surgery for Lower Extremities" section.

**References**

1. Crenshaw AH: Delayed union and nonunion of fractures. In *Campbell's Operative Orthopaedics*. Crenshaw AH, ed. CV Mosby, St. Louis: 1987, Vol 3, 2053-2118.
2. Russell TA: Malunited fractures. In *Campbell's Operative Orthopaedics*. Crenshaw AH, ed. CV Mosby, St. Louis: 1987, Vol 3, 2015-52.
3. Wilkins RM, Winter WG: Complications of treatment of fractures and dislocations of the hip. In *Complications in Orthopaedic Surgery*. Epps CH Jr, ed. JB Lippincott, Philadelphia: 1986, 469-511.

# CLOSED REDUCTION AND EXTERNAL FIXATION OF FEMUR

## SURGICAL CONSIDERATIONS

**Description**: This procedure entails manipulating the femur to obtain an acceptable reduction by closed or limited-open means, then applying an external fixation device to maintain the reduction. The pins for the external fixator are inserted percutaneously or through small incisions. This method of treatment normally is used for severe open fractures (e.g., Grade II or III) with extensive bone and soft-tissue injury.

**Usual preop diagnosis**: Displaced, open fracture of the femur

### SUMMARY OF PROCEDURE

| | |
|---|---|
| **Position** | Supine or lateral |
| **Incision** | Done percutaneously or through small incisions |
| **Special instrumentation** | External fixation device of surgeon's choice; radiolucent table with image intensifier |
| **Unique considerations** | Fracture is usually an open, extremely comminuted fracture in a multiple-trauma patient. |
| **Antibiotics** | Broad-spectrum cephalosporin (e.g., cefamandole 1 gm iv q 6 hrs until wound closed) + gentamicin (80 mg iv q 8 hrs until wound closed; adjust for renal status) for Grade III open fractures. |
| **Surgical time** | 1 hr |
| **EBL** | Operative blood loss usually 100-200 cc; however, blood loss may be extensive prior to surgery. |
| **Postop care** | Multiple-trauma victims → ICU; others → PACU |
| **Mortality** | Dependent on extent of trauma |
| **Morbidity** | Re-fracture: 2-12% |
| | Hypotension 2° blood loss and other injuries: Common |
| | Stiffness of knee: Common |
| | Delayed union, nonunion, malunion: More common in comminuted, open fractures |
| | Leg-length discrepancy: More common in severely comminuted fractures |
| | Osteomyelitis: More common in open fractures |
| | Respiratory distress: More common in multiple-trauma situations |
| | Amputation: Rare |
| | Compartment syndrome: Rare |
| | Neurological deficit to peripheral nerves: Rare |
| | Vascular complications: Rare |
| **Procedure code** | 27506 |
| **Pain score** | 9-10 (due to extensive open fracture) |

### PATIENT POPULATION CHARACTERISTICS

| | |
|---|---|
| **Age range** | Any age, but predominance of males < 30 yrs |
| **Male:Female** | 5:1 |
| **Incidence** | Common |
| **Etiology** | Motorcycle and motor vehicle accidents<br>Falls<br>Industrial injury |
| **Associated conditions** | Frequently associated with trauma to other organ systems, including head and neck, chest, abdomen, and extremities; these will often be treated simultaneously with the femur fracture. |

---

## ANESTHETIC CONSIDERATIONS

See "Anesthetic Considerations for Lower-Extremity Procedures" at the end of "Orthopedic Surgery for Lower Extremities" section.

**References**

1. Bucholz RW, Brumback RJ: Fractures of the shaft of the femur. In *Rockwood and Green's Fractures in Adults*, 3rd edition. Rockwood CA Jr, Green DP, Bucholz RW, eds. JB Lippincott, Philadelphia: 1991, 1653-1723.
2. Crenshaw AH: Delayed union and nonunion of fractures. In *Campbell's Operative Orthopaedics*. Crenshaw AH, ed. CV Mosby, St. Louis: 1987, Vol 3, 2053-2118.
3. Rankin EA, Baker GI: Complications of treatment of fractures of the femoral shaft. In *Complications in Orthopaedic Surgery*. Epps CH Jr, ed. JB Lippincott, Philadelphia: 1986, 513-36.
4. Russell TA: Malunited fractures. In *Campbell's Operative Orthopaedics*. Crenshaw AH, ed. CV Mosby, St. Louis: 1987, Vol 3, 2015-52.

# ARTHROPLASTY OF THE KNEE

## SURGICAL CONSIDERATIONS

**Description**: In this procedure, an arthrotomy of the knee joint is performed, and metallic and plastic components are used for replacement of the knee joint surfaces (**total knee replacement**). The femur, patella, and tibia are exposed; cartilage and minimal bone are excised with a saw. The new components may be cemented or uncemented. Alternatively, arthroplasty may be performed on only one compartment of the knee (i.e., medial/lateral **unicompartmental knee replacement**). In **revision procedures**, one or more components of the old joint are removed and new components are placed. In a **resection or excision arthroplasty** of the knee, normally done for infection of the prosthesis, the components are removed but not replaced.

**Usual preop diagnosis**: Arthritis of knee; arthrosis of knee; loose (or malpositioned) knee prosthesis; infected knee

### SUMMARY OF PROCEDURE

| | Knee Replacement | Revision | Resection/Excision |
|---|---|---|---|
| **Position** | Supine | ⇐ | ⇐ |
| **Incision** | Anterior or anteromedial over patella | ⇐ | ⇐ |
| **Special instrumentation** | Appropriate prostheses and instrumentation | Special instruments for excising cement | ⇐ |
| **Unique considerations** | ± Tourniquet; ± SCD | ⇐ | ⇐ |
| **Antibiotics** | Broad-spectrum cephalosporin (e.g., cefamandole 1 gm iv q 6 hrs x 48 hrs) | Broad spectrum cephalosporin after cultures taken | ⇐ |
| **Surgical time** | 2 - 3 hrs | 3 - 5 hrs or more | 3 - 4 hrs |
| **Closing considerations** | In infected or complex revision cases (rare), a local or free flap is required. | ⇐ | ⇐ |
| **EBL** | 300-500 cc | 500-1000 cc | ⇐ |
| **Postop care** | Bulky dressing or splint; or continuous passive motion is begun, using a machine. | ⇐ | Splint/cast |
| **Mortality** | Minimal | ⇐ | ⇐ |
| **Morbidity** | DVT, without prophylaxis: 50-75% | ⇐ | ⇐ |
| | DVT, with prophylaxis (e.g., Coumadin®, adjusted-dose heparin, SCD, anti-embolism stockings): 10-20% | ⇐ | ⇐ |
| | Postop subluxation/dislocation of patella: ≤ 35% | >35% | – |
| | Superficial wound necrosis: 10-15% | >10-15% | ≥10-15% |
| | Wound infection: | >5-10% | Rare |
| | Primary rheumatoid or psoriatic arthritis, diabetes: 5-10% | | |
| | Primary OA: 1% | | |
| | PE: 1-7% | ⇐ | ⇐ |
| | Postop subluxation/dislocation of knee joint: 1-6% | ≥1-6% | – |
| | Late aseptic loosening requiring revision (after ~10 yrs: 5% | – | – |

| | Knee Replacement | Revision | Resection/Excision |
|---|---|---|---|
| **Morbidity, continued** | Peroneal nerve injury: 1-5% | >1-5% (more common in difficult revisions) | 1-5% |
| | Urinary retention requiring catheterization: Common | – | – |
| | Hematoma: Rare - 1% | – | – |
| | Hypotension | – | – |
| | Knee stiffness | – | – |
| | Intraop fracture: Rare | ⇐ | ⇐ |
| | Wound dehiscence: Rare | – | – |
| | Fat embolism: Extremely rare | – | – |
| | Vascular injury to popliteal vessels: Extremely rare | – | – |
| **Procedure code** | 27447 | 27487 | 27488 |
| **Pain score** | 7 | 8 | 9 |

## PATIENT POPULATION CHARACTERISTICS

| | |
|---|---|
| **Age range** | Generally >60 yrs<br>Arthritis of the knee, e.g., rheumatoid arthritis or juvenile rheumatoid arthritis, hemophilia, 18 yrs or older |
| **Male:Female** | 1:1 |
| **Incidence** | Common; approximately 100,000/yr in U.S. |
| **Etiology** | Arthrosis of the knee (DJD or OA)<br>Sero-positive or sero-negative arthritis<br>Traumatic arthritis<br>Hemophiliac arthropathy of the knee |
| **Associated conditions** | Dependent on primary condition |

# ANESTHETIC CONSIDERATIONS

See "Anesthetic Considerations For Knee Procedures," following "Repair of Tendons – Knee and Leg" (below).


**References**

1. Fortune WP: Complications of total and partial arthroplasty in the knee. In *Complications in Orthopaedic Surgery*. Epps CH Jr, ed. Lippincott, Philadelphia: 1986, 1109-45.
2. Insall JN: Total knee replacement. In *Surgery of the Knee*. Insall JN, ed. Churchill Livingstone, New York: 1984, 587-695.
3. Tooms RE: Arthroplasty of the ankle and knee. In *Campbell's Operative Orthopaedics*. Crenshaw AH, ed. CV Mosby, St. Louis: 1987, Vol 2, 1145-1211.

# ARTHRODESIS OF THE KNEE

## SURGICAL CONSIDERATIONS

**Description**: In this procedure, the femur is fused to the tibia, obliterating the knee joint. Through a midline incision and anterior arthrotomy, the cartilage surface and a small amount of bone are excised. The cut ends are opposed and aligned in 0-20° of flexion and 5-10% of valgus. The bones are stabilized with plates, screws, an intramedullary rod or an external fixator.

**Usual preop diagnosis**: Arthritis or other arthrosis of the knee; previous septic arthritis of the knee, failed or infected knee arthroplasty

### SUMMARY OF PROCEDURE

| | |
|---|---|
| **Position** | Usually supine |
| **Incision** | Anterior midline over knee |
| **Special instrumentation** | External fixator; internal fixation with plates and screws or intramedullary nail |
| **Unique considerations** | Intraop radiographs or image intensifier; tourniquet |
| **Antibiotics** | Broad-spectrum antibiotic (e.g., cefamandole 1 gm iv q 6 hrs x 48 hrs |
| **Surgical time** | 3 hrs (+ 1 hr, if necessary, to excise total knee arthroplasty) |
| **Closing considerations** | Cast or splint while anesthetized |
| **EBL** | < 100 cc if tourniquet and local fixation used. 500-1000 cc, if no tourniquet used, or if intramedullary procedures are used. |
| **Mortality** | Rare, but depends primarily on age and medical condition of patient. |
| **Morbidity** | Thromboembolism — probably similar to, or greater than, %'s for total knee replacement:<br>DVT: 50-75% (without prophylaxis)<br>DVT: 10-20% (if prophylaxis used)<br>PE: 1-7% (if no prophylaxis; reduced if anti-coagulation or SCDs used)<br>Failure of fusion (nonunion), malunion: 10% (higher after failed knee replacement: 19-44%; with Charcot joint, as high as 50%)<br>Pin tract infection: 1-10% or more<br>Wound infection: 5%<br>Deep infection and osteomyelitis<br>Urinary retention requiring catheterization; UTI: Common<br>Breakage or failure of internal or external fixation: Rare<br>Fat embolism: Rare<br>GI bleed, MI: Rare |
| **Morbidity, continued** | Hematoma: Rare<br>Hypotension: Rare<br>Intraop femoral or tibial fracture: Rare<br>Neurological injury, usually popliteal nerve or peroneal nerve: Rare<br>Superficial wound necrosis and wound dehiscence: Rare<br>Vascular injury to popliteal vessels: Rare<br>Amputation: Extremely rare (usually due to acute arterial occlusion or uncontrollable local sepsis) |
| **Procedure code** | 27580 |
| **Pain score** | 9 |

### PATIENT POPULATION CHARACTERISTICS

| | |
|---|---|
| **Age range** | Any age |
| **Male:Female** | 1:1 |
| **Incidence** | Rare |
| **Etiology** | Failed or infected total knee replacement (probably most common etiology)<br>Trauma to knee: unreconstructable, intra-articular fractures<br>Total unstable knee or failed ligament repairs with severe DJD in a young patient |

## ANESTHETIC CONSIDERATIONS

See Anesthetic Considerations For Knee Procedures, following "Repair of Tendons – Knee and Leg" (below).


**References**

1. Carnesale PG, Stewart MJ: Complications of arthrodesis surgery. In *Complications in Orthopaedic Surgery.* Epps CH Jr, ed. JB Lippincott, Philadelphia: 1986, 1289-98.
2. Fortune WP: Complications of total and partial arthroplasty in the knee. In *Complications in Orthopaedic Surgery.* Epps CH Jr, ed. JB Lippincott, Philadelphia: 1986, 1109-45.
3. Hohl M, Larson RL: Complications of treatment of fractures and dislocations of the knee. In *Complications in Orthopaedic Surgery.* Epps CH Jr, ed. JB Lippincott, Philadelphia: 1986, 537-84.
4. Russell TA: Arthrodesis of the lower extremity and hip. In *Campbell's Operative Orthopaedics.* Crenshaw AH, ed. CV Mosby, St. Louis: 1987, Vol 2, 1091-1130.


# OPEN REDUCTION AND INTERNAL FIXATION (ORIF) OF PATELLAR FRACTURES

## SURGICAL CONSIDERATIONS

**Description**: In ORIF of patellar fractures, a short incision over the patella is used to perform a reduction by direct visualization of the fracture fragments of the patella. Since this is generally an intra-articular fracture, the fragments should be reduced precisely. The torn quadriceps retinaculum is also repaired. Part or all of the patella may be excised; pins, wires and/or screws are normally used to fix the patellar fragments together internally. Thereafter, the knee is casted or early motion of the knee is started.

**Usual preop diagnosis**: Fracture of patella; severe degenerative arthritis of patellofemoral joint

### SUMMARY OF PROCEDURE

| | |
|---|---|
| **Position** | Supine |
| **Incision** | Anterior over patella |
| **Special instrumentation** | Wire, pins, screws as necessary |
| **Unique considerations** | Intraop radiographs may be obtained; tourniquet |
| **Antibiotics** | Broad-spectrum cephalosporin (e.g., cefamandole 1 gm iv q 6 hrs x 48 hrs) |
| **Surgical time** | 1.5 - 2 hrs |
| **Closing considerations** | Splint or cast usually applied. |
| **EBL** | < 100 cc |
| **Mortality** | < 1% |
| **Morbidity** | Late degenerative arthritis of patellofemoral joint: ~50-60%<br>DVT: ~5%<br>Wound infection, septic arthritis, osteomyelitis: ~5%<br>Delayed union, nonunion, malunion: ~2-5%<br>Knee stiffness: Common<br>Weakness: Common<br>Avascular necrosis: Rare<br>Sympathetic dystrophy: Rare |

**Morbidity, continued** Following patellectomy:
Quadriceps strength: ~75% of normal
**Procedure code** 27524
**Pain score** 7

### PATIENT POPULATION CHARACTERISTICS

**Age range** Any age; frequently seen in young, active, healthy adults.
**Male:Female** 1:1
**Incidence** ~1% of all skeletal injuries
**Etiology** Trauma:
Falls: 60%
Motorcycle and motor vehicle accidents: 25-35%
Industrial injury: 6%
Degenerative arthritis of patellofemoral joint: Rare

## ANESTHETIC CONSIDERATIONS

See Anesthetic Considerations following "Repair of Tendons – Knee and Leg" (below).

**References**


1. Hohl M, Larson RL: Complications of treatment of fractures and dislocations of the knee. In *Complications in Orthopaedic Surgery*. Epps CH Jr, ed. JB Lippincott, Philadelphia: 1986, 537-84.
2. Hohl M, Johnson EE, Wiss DA. Fractures of the knee. In *Rockwood and Green's Fractures in Adults*, 3rd edition. Rockwood CA Jr, Green DP, Bucholz RW, eds. JB Lippincott, Philadelphia: 1991, 1725-97.
3. Russell TA: Malunited fractures. In *Campbell's Operative Orthopaedics*. Crenshaw AH, ed. CV Mosby, St. Louis: 1987, Vol 3, 2015-52.
4. Sisk TD: Fractures of lower extremity. In *Campbell's Operative Orthopaedics*. Crenshaw AH, ed. CV Mosby, St. Louis: 1987, Vol 3, 1607-1718.


# REPAIR OR RECONSTRUCTION OF KNEE LIGAMENTS

## SURGICAL CONSIDERATIONS

**Description**: Collateral ligaments are usually repaired by direct suture or by stapling the torn ligaments to bone. Cruciate tears are generally repaired only if bone is avulsed at one end of the ligament, again with direct suture, staples, or screws. For collateral ligament repair, a longitudinal incision is made directly over the ligament medially or laterally. The ligament is exposed by deep dissection and elevation of skin flaps. The torn ligament is repaired by direct suture or by fixing it to bone with a screw or staple. Following closure, the knee is immobilized with a long leg splint or cast. Cruciate ligaments are repaired in similar fashion except for the approaches: medial parapatellar (with anterior arthrotomy) for the anterior cruciate ligament (ACL) and posteromedial (with posterior arthrotomy) for the posterior cruciate lateral (PCL). Cruciate ligament reconstruction is performed for instability 2° intra-substance tears of these ligaments. Homografts, such as a portion of the patellar tendon or semitendinosus tendon, are usually used, but allografts or synthetics are also available. (The ligaments of the knee are illustrated in Fig 10.3-5, 10.3-6.)

**Usual preop diagnosis**: Trauma

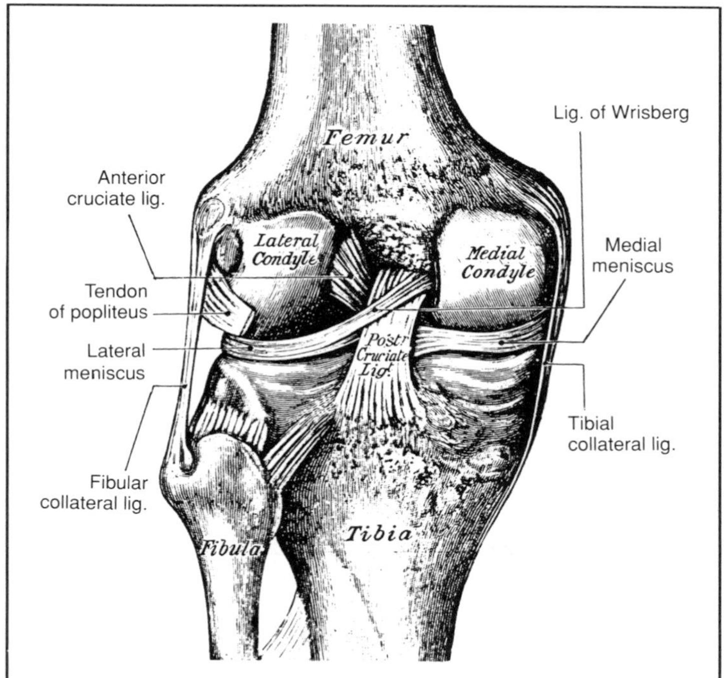


Figure 10.3-5. Left knee-joint (from behind), showing interior ligaments. (Reproduced from Goss CM, ed: *Gray's Anatomy of the Human Body, 27th edition.* Lea & Febiger: 1959.)

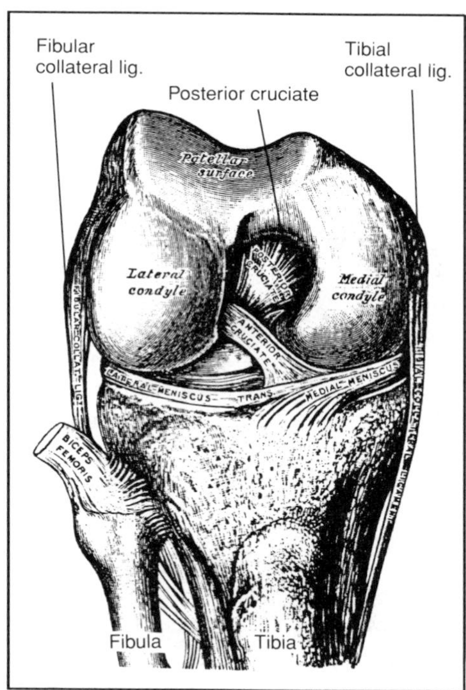


Figure 10.3-6. Right knee-joint, dissected from the front. (Reproduced from Goss CM, ed: *Gray's Anatomy of the Human Body, 27th edition.* Lea & Febiger: 1959.)

## SUMMARY OF PROCEDURE

| | Repair or Collateral Reconstruction | Repair or Cruciate Reconstruction |
|---|---|---|
| **Position** | Supine | ⇐ |
| **Incision** | Over collateral ligament | Anterior and lateral ACL or medial PCL |
| **Special instrumentation** | Staples | Drill guides, staples, screws |
| **Unique considerations** | Often arthroscopically assisted; tourniquet | ⇐ |
| **Antibiotics** | None | Cefazolin 1 gm iv preop |
| **Surgical time** | 2 hrs | ⇐ |
| **Closing considerations** | Splint or cast while anesthetized | ⇐ |
| **EBL** | 100 cc | ⇐ |
| **Postop care** | PACU → room or home | ⇐ |
| **Mortality** | Minimal | ⇐ |
| **Morbidity** | Infection: < 1% | ⇐ |
| | Thrombophlebitis: < 5% | ⇐ |
| **Procedure code** | 27405 (primary repair, ligament/capsule) | 27428 |
| | 27407 (cruciate ligament) | |
| | 27409 (collateral and cruciate ligaments) | |
| **Pain score** | 4 | 7 |

## PATIENT POPULATION CHARACTERISTICS

| | |
|---|---|
| **Age range** | Young adult |
| **Male:Female** | 2:1 |
| **Incidence** | Common |
| **Etiology** | Trauma: 100% |

## ANESTHETIC CONSIDERATIONS

See Anesthetic Considerations following "Repair of Tendons – Knee and Leg" (below).


**References**

1. Crenshaw AH, ed: *Campbell's Operative Orthopaedics*, 8th edition. Mosby-Year Book, St. Louis: 1992.


# PATELLAR REALIGNMENT

## SURGICAL CONSIDERATIONS

**Description**: The goal of this procedure is prevention of chronic subluxation or dislocation of the patella. Soft tissue components of the surgery include incision (release) of the lateral patellar retinaculum and reefing or tightening of the medial retinaculum (Fig 10.3-7). In cases of severe malalignment of the extensor mechanism, the insertion of the patellar tendon may be moved to a new, more medial location (tibial tubercle transfer). In this procedure, the tibial tubercle generally is detached with a saw or osteotomes, leaving a bone pedicle attached distally. The tubercle is then rotated medially on the pedicle and fixed in its new position with a screw. Many surgeons routinely perform an anterior compartment fasciotomy to prevent postop compartment syndrome.

**Usual preop diagnosis**: Chronic patellar subluxation or dislocation

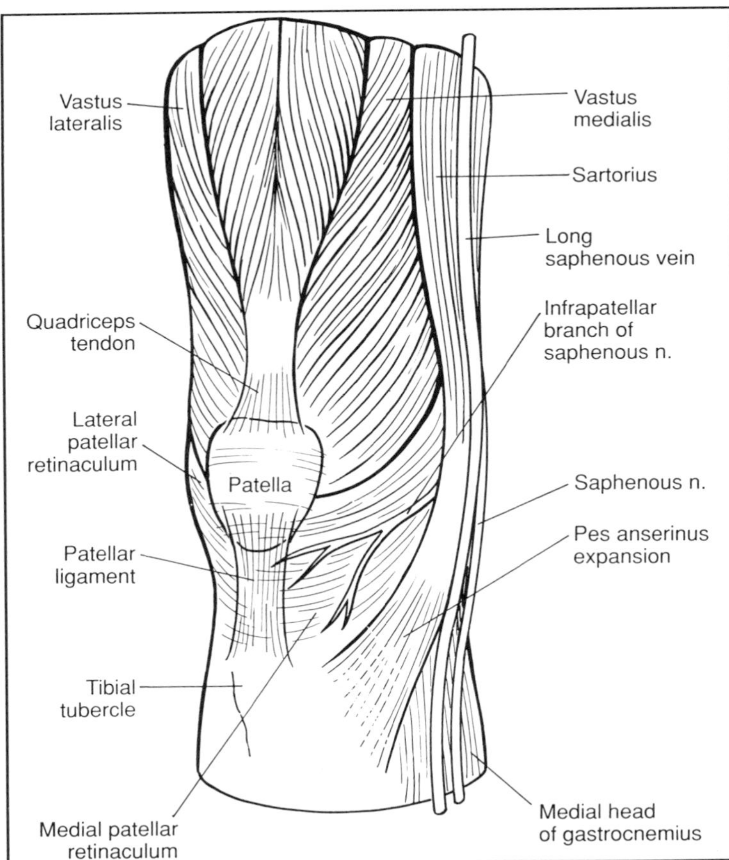


**Figure 10.3-7.** Anatomy of the patellar retinaculum. (Reproduced with permission from Hoppenfeld S, deBoer P: *Surgical Exposures in Orthopaedics: The Anatomic Approach.* JB Lippincott: 1984.)

## SUMMARY OF PROCEDURE

| | Patellar Realignment | Tibial Tubercle Transfer |
|---|---|---|
| **Position** | Supine | ⇐ |
| **Incision** | Anteromedial or anterolateral to knee | ⇐ |
| **Special instrumentation** | None | Screws or staples |
| **Unique considerations** | Tourniquet | ⇐ |
| **Antibiotics** | None | Cefazolin 1 gm iv preop |
| **Surgical time** | 1 hr | 1.5 hrs |
| **Closing considerations** | None | Splint or cast while anesthetized |
| **EBL** | 50 cc | 100 cc |
| **Postop care** | PACU → room or home | ⇐ |
| **Mortality** | Minimal | ⇐ |
| **Morbidity** | Hemarthrosis: 100% | 5% |
| | Re-dislocation: 20% | 25% |
| | Thrombophlebitis: 10-20% | ⇐ |
| | Compartment syndrome: < 1% | ⇐ |
| | Infection: < 1% | ⇐ |
| **Procedure code** | 27425 | 27420; 27422 (with soft tissue realignment) |
| **Pain score** | 6 | 7 |

## PATIENT POPULATION CHARACTERISTICS

| | |
|---|---|
| **Age range** | Usually young adult |
| **Male:Female** | 1:2 |
| **Etiology** | Trauma: 70% |
| | Congenital: 30% |
| **Associated conditions** | Patellofemoral dysphasia: 60-70% |

## ANESTHETIC CONSIDERATIONS

See Anesthetic Considerations following "Repair of Tendons – Knee and Leg" (below).

**References**

1. Epps CH Jr, ed: *Complications in Orthopaedic Surgery*, 2nd edition. JB Lippincott, Philadelphia: 1986.

# ARTHROSCOPY OF THE KNEE

## SURGICAL CONSIDERATIONS

**Description:** **Knee arthroscopy** is used to diagnose and treat intra-articular problems, most commonly torn meniscus, but the procedure is also used for ligament injuries (Fig 101.3-5, 10.3-6), osteochondral fractures, loose bodies, arthritis and infections. In knee arthroscopy, multiple portals or entry points for the arthroscope and instruments are generally used. The most common portals are anteromedial and anterolateral adjacent to the patellar ligament. Other portals may be suprapatellar, parapatellar and posterior. Portals are made by making a stab wound with a knife and then entering the joint with a combination of sharp and blunt trochars. A diagnostic inspection from one of the anterior portals is normally performed at the outset. A second portal is used with a nerve hook to manipulate intra-articular tissues. If resection or repair is performed, the appropriate instruments are inserted through one of the portals. Meniscus repair and cruciate reconstruction may require separate longitudinal incisions, which are usually posteromedial or posterolateral, for placement of sutures and/or drill holes.

**Meniscectomy** and/or **debridement** is often performed in conjunction with arthroscopy. **Cruciate ligament reconstruction** usually is performed with arthroscopic assistance. At the end of the procedure, the knee joint is copiously irrigated with NS or LR solution through one of the portals. Portals are closed with Steri-Strips® or a single suture; compression bandages are applied; and often a knee immobilizer is used.

**Usual preop diagnosis:** Torn meniscus; cruciate ligament tear; arthritis

### SUMMARY OF PROCEDURE

| | Arthroscopy | Meniscectomy/Debridement | Cruciate Reconstruction |
|---|---|---|---|
| **Position** | Supine | ⇐ | ⇐ |
| **Incision** | 3-4.5 cm portals | ⇐ | ⇐ + Anterior midline and lateral |
| **Special instrumentation** | Arthroscopic video system; small biters and graspers | ⇐ + Shaver | ⇐ + Drill guides and drills; fixation screws |
| **Unique considerations** | Thigh holder; foot of table 90°; ± tourniquet | ⇐ | ⇐ |
| **Antibiotics** | None | None | Cefazolin 1 gm iv preop |
| **Surgical time** | 0.5 hr | 1 - 2 hrs | 2 - 3 hrs |
| **Closing considerations** | No splint; local anesthetic injected | ⇐ | ⇐ |
| **EBL** | Minimal | ⇐ | 50 cc |
| **Postop care** | PACU → home | ⇐ | ⇐ Or overnight |
| **Mortality** | < 0.1% | ⇐ | ⇐ |
| **Morbidity** | Hemarthrosis: 5-20% | 5% | ⇐ |
| | Thrombophlebitis: < 2% | ⇐ | ⇐ |
| | Infection: 0.1% | ⇐ | ⇐ |
| | Stiffness: < 0.1% | < 1% | ⇐ |
| **Procedure code** | 29871 | 29880 (medial/lateral meniscectomy)<br>29881 (medial or lateral meniscectomy)<br>29877 (debridement) | 29888 (anterior cruciate)<br>29889 (posterior cruciate) |
| **Pain score** | 3 | 4 | 6 |

### PATIENT POPULATION CHARACTERISTICS

| | |
|---|---|
| **Age range** | 10-70 yrs (usually 20-40 yrs) |
| **Male:Female** | 2:1 |
| **Incidence** | The most common arthroscopic procedure (85% of total) |
| **Etiology** | Trauma: ~85%<br>Arthritis: ~10%<br>Infection: ~5% |

| | |
|---|---|
| **Associated conditions** | Usually healthy<br>Systemic arthritis: < 5% |

## ANESTHETIC CONSIDERATIONS

See Anesthetic Considerations following "Repair of Tendons – Knee and Leg" (below).


**References**

1. McGinty JB, ed: *Operative Arthroscopy.* Raven Press, New York: 1991.


# KNEE ARTHROTOMY

## SURGICAL CONSIDERATIONS

**Description**: **Arthrotomy** of the knee is the opening of the joint for drainage, excision of intra-articular tissue (synovium, meniscus, loose bodies), ligament repair/reconstruction, or fracture fixation. The knee is generally opened with a parapatellar incision, either medial or lateral, and the joint capsule is incised just adjacent to the patella. After the intra-articular pathology is addressed, a tight capsular closure is performed, followed by subcutaneous tissue and skin closure.

**Variant procedure or approaches**: **Arthrotomy with debridement** may be used for infection or arthropathy which produces debris. In both cases, **synovectomy** may be necessary.

**Usual preop diagnosis**: Infection; trauma (fracture, sprain, torn meniscus); arthritis

### SUMMARY OF PROCEDURE

| | Arthrotomy | Arthrotomy with Debridement | Arthrotomy with Synovectomy |
|---|---|---|---|
| **Position** | Supine | ⇐ | ⇐ |
| **Incision** | Medial or lateral parapatellar | ⇐ | ⇐ |
| **Special instrumentation** | Tourniquet | ⇐ | ⇐ |
| **Antibiotics** | Cefazolin 1 gm iv preop | ⇐ | ⇐ |
| **Surgical time** | 1 hr | 2 hrs | 2 - 3 hrs |
| **Closing considerations** | Compressive dressing; may be splinted; suction drain | ⇐ | ⇐ |
| **EBL** | 100 cc | ⇐ | ⇐ |
| **Postop care** | PACU → room | ⇐ | ⇐ |
| **Mortality** | Minimal | ⇐ | ⇐ |
| **Morbidity** | Hemarthrosis: 100% | ⇐ | ⇐ |
| | Degenerative arthritis: 5-20% | ⇐ | ⇐ |
| | Stiffness: 5% | ⇐ | ⇐ |
| | Thrombophlebitis: 5% | ⇐ | ⇐ |
| | Infection: 1% | 10% | 20% |
| **Procedure code** | 27310 | 27331 | 27334 (anterior or posterior)<br>27335 (anterior/posterior) |
| **Pain score** | 7 | 7 | 8 |

### PATIENT POPULATION CHARACTERISTICS

| | |
|---|---|
| **Age range** | Infant - elderly (usually young adult) |
| **Male:Female** | 1:1 |
| **Incidence** | Common |
| **Etiology** | Infection<br>Trauma<br>Arthritis |
| **Associated conditions** | Inflammatory arthritis: 20% |

## ANESTHETIC CONSIDERATIONS

See Anesthetic Considerations following "Repair of Tendons – Knee and Leg" (below).

**References**

1. Epps CH Jr, ed: *Complications in Orthopaedic Surgery*, 2nd edition. JB Lippincott, Philadelphia: 1986.

# REPAIR OF TENDONS – KNEE AND LEG

## SURGICAL CONSIDERATIONS

**Description**: Acute ruptures of tendons in the lower limb are repaired by **direct suture** and sometimes reinforced with part of another tendon. At the knee, patellar tendon ruptures are most common; at the ankle, Achilles tendon ruptures are most common. A longitudinal incision generally is made directly over the tendon. The tendon sheath is opened and tendon ends reapproximated with a nonabsorbable tendon stitch. If necessary, the repair may be augmented by synthetic tape or fascia or protected with a wire which takes tension off the repair. The tendon sheath is closed separately from the skin incision; and a cast or splint is applied. **Achilles tendon** and **posterior tibial tendon repair** require different positioning. The patient is placed prone, and a longitudinal incision is made just medial to the tendon, spanning the rupture. The tendon sheath is incised and carefully protected. Torn ends of the tendon are approximated with multiple tendon stitches and may be protected with a fascial flap developed from the gastrocnemius fascia. The tendon sheath is carefully closed, followed by skin wound closure. A splint or cast is applied with the foot in equinus.

**Usual preop diagnosis**: Tendon rupture

### SUMMARY OF PROCEDURE

| | Tendon Repair | Achilles Tendon Repair |
|---|---|---|
| **Position** | Supine | Prone |
| **Incision** | Over tendon | ⇐ |
| **Special instrumentation** | Wire or synthetic tape for augmentation | ⇐ |
| **Unique considerations** | Tourniquet | ⇐ |
| **Antibiotics** | If young, none; in elderly or infirm, cefazolin 1 gm iv preop | ⇐ |

| | Tendon Repair | Achilles Tendon Repair |
|---|---|---|
| **Surgical time** | 1 hr | ⇐ |
| **Closing considerations** | Splint or cast while anesthetized. | ⇐ |
| **EBL** | Minimal | ⇐ |
| **Postop care** | PACU → room or home | ⇐ |
| **Mortality** | Minimal | ⇐ |
| **Morbidity** | Weakness: ~ 10% | – |
| | Wound slough: 5% | ⇐ |
| | Adhesions: < 1% | ⇐ |
| | Infection: < 1% | ⇐ |
| | | Re-rupture: 5-10% |
| **Procedure code** | 27380 (primary suture of infrapatellar tendon)<br>27385 (primary suture of quadriceps or hamstring muscle rupture)<br>27658 (repair of flexor tendon)<br>27664 (repair of extensor tendon) | 27650 |
| **Pain score** | 3 | 3 |

### PATIENT POPULATION CHARACTERISTICS

| | |
|---|---|
| **Age range** | Any age |
| **Male:Female** | 1:1 |
| **Incidence** | Uncommon |
| **Etiology** | Trauma: 90%<br>Chronic tendinitis: 10% |
| **Associated conditions** | Obesity<br>Diabetes mellitus (DM)<br>Inflammatory arthritis |

---

## ANESTHETIC CONSIDERATIONS FOR KNEE PROCEDURES

**(Procedures covered: arthroplasty; arthrodesis; repair of ligaments; patellar realignment; arthroscopy; arthrotomy; tendon repair)**

### PREOPERATIVE

Trauma and osteoarthritis are the most common indications for these procedures. Trauma patients (e.g., those with sports injuries) are often young and healthy, whereas arthritic patients are often elderly and anesthetic management must be tailored to any concurrent disease. Patients with rheumatoid and other inflammatory arthritides form another group of candidates for these procedures – the special anesthetic considerations for these patients are described in "Arthroplasty of the Hip." A final group of patients undergoing these procedures are hemophiliacs, who develop arthritis from recurrent bleeding into their joints. The hematologic management of these patients is discussed below.

**Respiratory** These patients often have rheumatoid arthritis and associated pulmonary conditions. For example, pulmonary effusions are common. Limited respiratory reserve warrants farther evaluation. Pulmonary fibrosis (rare) often manifests as a cough and dyspnea. Rheumatoid arthritis involving the cricoarytenoid joints may manifest as hoarseness, glottic narrowing and difficult intubation. Arthritic involvement of the TMJ and cervical spine may further complicate airway management.
**Tests:** As indicated from H&P.

**Cardiovascular** The severity of the arthritis often limits exercise, and makes assessment of cardiovascular status difficult. ECHO and dipyridamole thallium imaging may be necessary for an adequate cardiac evaluation. Rheumatoid arthritis is associated with pericardial effusion, cardiac valve fibrosis, cardiac conduction abnormalities and aortic regurgitation.
**Tests:** ECG and others as indicated from H&P.

**Neurological** In arthritic patients, a thorough preop neurological exam often yields evidence of cervical nerve root compression. After the stability of the neck has been established, the full range of neck motion should be evaluated for evidence of nerve compression and cerebral ischemia (suggesting

| | |
|---|---|
| | vertebral artery compression). Consider preop lateral neck films to determine stability of atlanto-occipital joint. **Tests:** As indicated from H&P. |
| **Musculoskeletal** | Pain and decreased joint mobility may make positioning and regional anesthesia difficult in this patient population. |
| **Hematologic** | Hemophiliacs require restoration of clotting factors preop. Administer 1 U of factor concentrate/kg body weight for each 2% increase necessary to achieve clotting factor activity of 40% normal. FFP contains 1 U/cc and cryoprecipitate 20 U/cc. Hemophilia B, but not hemophilia A, can be treated with prothrombin complex concentrate; however, these products can activate clotting factors and → DIC. Approximately 10% of hemophiliacs develop antibodies to exogenous clotting factors, and the care of these patients should be guided by a consulting hematologist. **Tests:** Hct; other tests as indicated from H&P. |
| **Laboratory** | Other tests as indicated from H&P. |
| **Premedication** | Diazepam 5-10 mg po 1 hr preop. Preop patellar pain is effectively treated with a femoral nerve block at the inguinal ligament using 10 ml of lidocaine 1.5% epinephrine 1:200,000. |

## INTRAOPERATIVE

**Anesthetic technique:** For many of these patients, regional anesthesia may be the preferred technique, offering the advantages of ↓blood loss, ↓DVT, minimal respiratory impairment and effective postop analgesia. Patients with rheumatoid arthritis rarely have involvement of the lumbar spine. Since rheumatoid arthritis frequently affects the cervical spine, however, these patients may have limited range of neck motion, an unstable atlanto-occipital joint, and cricoarytenoid and TMJ arthritis. Careful airway evaluation, therefore, is important to determine the appropriateness of special intubation techniques (e.g., fiber optic, light wand).

**Regional anesthesia:** Either subarachnoid or epidural blocks are useful techniques, depending on the patient population (e.g., younger patients may be at ↑risk of spinal headache following SAB). Anesthesia extending from S2 to T12 (T8 if tourniquet is used) is adequate for knee surgery. Full motor blockade is essential for fixation of the patella, or placement of the joint prosthesis and assessment of the passive ROM of the prosthesis. Typical drugs and doses include: subarachnoid – 15 mg of 0.75% bupivacaine with morphine 0.2 mg; epidural – 15-20 cc 2% lidocaine with epinephrine 1:200,000 in divided doses.

**General anesthesia:**

| | |
|---|---|
| **Induction** | Standard induction (see Appendix) is appropriate for patients with normal airways. |
| **Maintenance** | Standard maintenance (see Appendix). Neuromuscular relaxation facilitates the placement of the prosthesis. Hemophiliacs will require infusion of clotting factors. For hemophilia A and von Willebrand's disease, 1.5 U/kg/hr and for hemophilia B, 0.75 U/kg/hr. |
| **Emergence** | The tourniquet is deflated around the time of emergence. In patients with moderate-to-severe lung disease, controlled ventilation should be continued until after the lactic acid that has accumulated in the leg has been metabolized (3-5 min), since these patients may be unable to increase ventilation to buffer this acid load. |

| | | |
|---|---|---|
| **Blood and fluid requirements** | IV: 14-16 ga x 1<br>NS/LR @ maintenance during the case and 5-10 cc/kg bolus prior to tourniquet deflation. | A tourniquet blocks intraop blood loss. When it is deflated, prepare for a 1-2 U blood loss over the ensuing hr; more, if the posterior tibial artery has been damaged in the dissection. |
| **Control of blood loss** | Tourniquet | Inflation pressure is typically 100 mmHg greater than systolic pressure. Maximum "safe" tourniquet time is 1.5-2 hr, followed by a 5-to-(preferably) 15-min reperfusion interval, if further tourniquet time is necessary. |
| **Monitoring** | Standard monitors (see Appendix).<br>± CVP line | A CVP line is indicated in the presence of significant cardiac or pulmonary disease. |
| **Positioning** | √ and pad pressure points.<br>√ eyes. | In rheumatoid arthritic patients, meticulous padding of the extremities is mandatory. |
| **Complications** | Posterior tibial artery trauma<br>Peroneal nerve palsy | A 20% fall in mean BP is common on tourniquet deflation. Additional crystalloid (5-10 cc/kg) may be necessary to replace edema fluid and blood loss to the leg. |

## POSTOPERATIVE

| | | |
|---|---|---|
| **Complications** | Hemorrhage from the posterior tibial artery | √ surgical drain output. |
| | Peroneal nerve palsy → foot drop<br>Tourniquet-related nerve injury | Examine patient for evidence of neurologic dysfunction and notify surgeons as necessary. |
| | Post-tourniquet syndrome (PTS) | PTS is a self-limiting condition in which the affected limb is edematous, pale and weak. |
| **Pain management** | Spinal opiates:<br>- Epidural anesthesia<br>- Spinal anesthesia | Epidural hydromorphone 50 μg/cc infused at 100-250 μg/hr provides excellent analgesia. Intrathecal morphine 0.2-0.3 mg provides analgesia for up to 24 hrs after administration. |
| **Tests** | Hct; other studies as indicated. | |

**References**

1. Epps CH Jr, ed: *Complications in Orthopaedic Surgery*, 2nd edition. JB Lippincott, Philadelphia: 1986.

# OPEN REDUCTION AND INTERNAL FIXATION (ORIF) OF THE TIBIAL PLATEAU FRACTURE

## SURGICAL CONSIDERATIONS

**Description**: ORIF of the tibial plateau or proximal tibia fracture involves making a longitudinal incision along the proximal leg lateral to the knee, obtaining a reduction by direct visualization of the fracture fragments, and applying plates and screws along the tibia for rigid internal fixation. An iliac crest bone graft may be necessary. A **proximal tibial osteotomy** involves correcting malalignment (valgus and varus) of the lower extremity by excising a wedge of bone from the tibia and correcting the mechanical axis.

**Usual preop diagnosis**: Tibial plateau or proximal tibial fracture; nonunion/malunion of the tibial plateau or proximal tibia; degenerative arthritis of the knee, with varus or valgus deformity

### SUMMARY OF PROCEDURE

| | Tibial Plateau Fracture | Proximal Tibial Osteotomy |
|---|---|---|
| **Position** | Supine | ⇐ |
| **Incision** | Lateral to knee, usually; medial, rarely | Transverse or lateral incision |
| **Special instrumentation** | Special plates, screws; reduction clamps; radiolucent table | ⇐ |
| **Unique considerations** | Intraop radiographs or image intensifier; tourniquet | ⇐ |
| **Antibiotics** | Broad-spectrum cephalosporin (e.g., cefamandole 1 gm iv q 6 hrs x 48 hrs) | ⇐ |
| **Surgical time** | Approximately 2.5 - 3 hrs; more, depending on difficulty | ⇐ |
| **Closing considerations** | Splint, cast while anesthetized | ⇐ |
| **EBL** | < 200 cc | ⇐ |
| **Postop care** | Multiple-trauma victim → ICU; others → PACU; ± continuous passive motion | None |
| **Mortality** | Rare, except in severe multiple trauma | ~2% |
| **Morbidity** | Wound infection: 7-15% | 2% |
| | DVT (symptomatic): 3-5% | 10-20% |
| | Peripheral nerve damage: 3% | 1-25% |
| | Compartment syndrome | Nonunion, malunion: < 5% |
| | Delayed union, nonunion, malunion | Intra-articular fracture: 2% |
| | Hypotension (multiple trauma) | |
| | Intra-articular fracture | |
| | Leg-length discrepancy | |
| | Osteomyelitis, septic arthritis | |
| | Respiratory distress and fat embolism | |
| | Vascular complications | |
| **Procedure code** | 27535; 27536 | 27705 |
| **Pain score** | 7 | 7 |

### PATIENT POPULATION CHARACTERISTICS

| | |
|---|---|
| **Age range** | Any age; fracture most common in younger trauma patients and elderly<br>Degenerative arthritis of knee, < 60 yrs |
| **Male:Female** | 1:1 |
| **Incidence** | Common |
| **Etiology** | Trauma: falls, motorcycle and motor vehicle accidents, industrial injuries<br>Degenerative: arthritis of knee |

## ANESTHETIC CONSIDERATIONS

See "Anesthetic Considerations for Lower-Extremity Procedures" at the end of "Orthopedic Surgery for Lower Extremities" section.

**References**

1. Crenshaw AH: Delayed union and nonunion of fractures. In *Campbell's Operative Orthopaedics.* Crenshaw AH, ed. CV Mosby, St. Louis: 1987, Vol 3, 2053-2118.
2. Hohl M, Larson RL: Complications of treatment of fractures and dislocations of the knee. In *Complications in Orthopaedic Surgery.* Epps CH Jr, ed. JB Lippincott, Philadelphia: 1986, 537-84.
3. Hohl M, Johnson EE, Wiss DA: Fractures of the knee. In *Rockwood and Green's Fractures in Adults*, 3rd edition. Rockwood CA Jr, Green DP, Bucholz, eds. JB Lippincott, Philadelphia: 1991, 1725-97.
4. Russell TA: Malunited fractures. In *Campbell's Operative Orthopaedics.* Crenshaw AH, ed. Mosby, St. Louis: 1987, 2015-52.
5. Aglietti P, Chambat P: Fractures of the knee. In *Surgery of the Knee.* Insall JN, ed. Churchill Livingstone, New York: 1984, 395-490.

# INTRAMEDULLARY NAILING, TIBIA

## SURGICAL CONSIDERATIONS

**Description**: In intramedullary nailing of the tibia, a metal nail is placed into the medullary canal of the tibia to stabilize (or prevent) a fracture. The affected leg generally is placed in traction, on a fracture table, via stirrup or calcaneal pin. Following the incision, an awl is used to make an entry hole in the proximal metaphysis of the tibia, through which a guide wire is introduced. The guide wire is placed across the aligned fracture, and the nail is introduced and driven over the guide wire. Prior to nail insertion, the medullary canal is often reamed to allow use of a larger nail. Most nails are interlocked both proximally and distally with screws which pass from the bone through holes in the nail.

**Usual preop diagnosis**: Fracture, nonunion or malunion of the tibia

### SUMMARY OF PROCEDURE

| | |
|---|---|
| **Position** | Supine, on fracture table. Consider inducing anesthesia before moving patient to the fracture table. |
| **Incision** | Proximal longitudinal incision over the patellar tendon; stab wound for screws |
| **Special instrumentation** | Nails, screws and insertion instruments; intramedullary reamers |
| **Unique considerations** | Image intensifier |
| **Antibiotics** | Cefazolin 1 gm iv preop |
| **Surgical time** | 2 hrs |
| **Closing considerations** | No splint or cast |
| **EBL** | 200 cc |
| **Postop care** | PACU → room |
| **Mortality** | Minimal |
| **Morbidity** | Compartment syndrome: < 5%<br>Infection: < 2%<br>Neuropraxia: < 1% |
| **Procedure code** | 27806 |
| **Pain score** | 5 |

### PATIENT POPULATION CHARACTERISTICS

| | |
|---|---|
| **Age range** | >16 yrs |
| **Male:Female** | 5:1 |
| **Etiology** | Trauma: 95%<br>Tumor: 5% |
| **Associated conditions** | Multiple trauma: 50%<br>Compartment syndrome: 5% |

## ANESTHETIC CONSIDERATIONS

See "Anesthetic Considerations for Lower-Extremity Procedures" at the end of "Orthopedic Surgery for Lower Extremities" section.

**References**

1. Rockwood CA Jr, Green DP, Bucholz RW, eds: *Rockwood and Green's Fractures in Adults*, 3rd edition. JB Lippincott, Philadelphia: 1991.

# EXTERNAL FIXATION, TIBIA

## SURGICAL CONSIDERATIONS

**Description**: Fractures of the tibia are fixed with percutaneous pins which are clamped to an external frame. Stainless steel pins are drilled into the proximal and distal fragments of the fracture through stab wounds in the skin and subcutaneous tissues. Usually 2-3 pins are placed on either side of the fracture. Pin clamps and an external frame are attached and the fracture aligned with the assistance of the image intensifier or under direct vision. Following fracture alignment, the pin clamps and frames are tightened to hold fracture alignment. External fixation is often used with open fractures. **Small-pin fixators** (e.g., Ilizarov) are used for fracture fixation, leg lengthening and treatment of bony defects. Wound irrigation and debridement often accompany application of the fixation frame.

**Usual preop diagnosis**: Tibia fracture; tibial nonunion or malunion; tibial shortening.

### SUMMARY OF PROCEDURE

| | |
|---|---|
| **Position** | Supine |
| **Incision** | Stab wounds. Small-pin fixator may require metaphyseal incision for osteotomy. |
| **Special instrumentation** | Pins; fixation frame |
| **Unique considerations** | Image intensifier |
| **Antibiotics** | Cefazolin 1 gm iv preop |
| **Surgical time** | 0.5 - 1 hr<br>Small-pin fixator: 3 - 5 hrs |
| **Closing considerations** | May be open fracture (usually left open) |
| **EBL** | 50 cc; small-pin fixator, 100 cc |
| **Postop care** | PACU → room |
| **Mortality** | Minimal |
| **Morbidity** | Infection: 15%<br>Compartment syndrome: < 2%<br>Neuropraxia: < 1% |
| **Procedure code** | 27806 |
| **Pain score** | 2-3 |

### PATIENT POPULATION CHARACTERISTICS

| | |
|---|---|
| **Age range** | All ages |
| **Male:Female** | 5:1 |
| **Incidence** | Common |
| **Etiology** | Trauma: 95%<br>Shortened limb: < 2%<br>Un-united or malunited fracture: < 2% |
| **Associated conditions** | Open fracture: 95%<br>Compartment syndrome: < 2%<br>Congenital anomaly: < 1% |

## ANESTHETIC CONSIDERATIONS

See "Anesthetic Considerations for Lower-Extremity Procedures" at the end of "Orthopedic Surgery for Lower Extremities" section.

**References**

1. Rockwood CA Jr, Green DP, Bucholz RW, eds: *Rockwood and Green's Fractures in Adults*, 3rd edition. JB Lippincott, Philadelphia: 1991.

# OPEN REDUCTION AND INTERNAL FIXATION (ORIF) OF DISTAL TIBIA, ANKLE, AND FOOT FRACTURES

## SURGICAL CONSIDERATIONS

**Description**: ORIF is nearly always required for displaced fractures involving the ankle or joints in the foot. A longitudinal incision is made over the fractured medial and/or lateral malleoli. Dissection is carried directly down to the bone and the fracture is identified and reduced under direct vision. Open fractures may require irrigation and debridement. The fractures are realigned under direct vision and fixed and stabilized with pins, plates and/or screws. An intraop radiograph is obtained to confirm reduction and placement of hardware. The incisions are closed and a splint or cast is applied.

**Usual preop diagnosis**: Fracture of the distal tibia, ankle or foot

### SUMMARY OF PROCEDURE

| | ORIF Ankle | With Irrigation and Debridement |
|---|---|---|
| **Position** | Supine | ⇐ |
| **Incision** | Longitudinal over fracture site | ⇐ + Extension of existing wound |
| **Special instrumentation** | Pins, plates and screws | ⇐ |
| **Unique considerations** | Tourniquet; x-ray or image intensifier | ⇐ |
| **Antibiotics** | Cefazolin 1 gm iv preop | ⇐ |
| **Surgical time** | 2 hrs | 2 - 3 hrs |
| **Closing considerations** | Splint or cast while anesthetized. | Splint or cast; may leave wound open. |
| **EBL** | 50 cc | 100 cc |

| | ORIF Ankle | With Irrigation and Debridement |
|---|---|---|
| **Postop care** | PACU → room | ⇐ |
| **Mortality** | Minimal | ⇐ |
| **Morbidity** | Wound dehiscence: 10% | ⇐ |
| | Loss of reduction: 7% | ⇐ |
| | Infection: 3% | 15% |
| **Procedure code** | 27766 (distal tibia); 27792 (distal fibula); 27814 (bimalleolar); 27822 (trimalleolar) | ⇐ |
| **Pain score** | 4 | 4 |

### PATIENT POPULATION CHARACTERISTICS

| | |
|---|---|
| **Age range** | Infant - elderly (usually >60 yrs) |
| **Male:Female** | 1:1 |
| **Incidence** | ~ 250,000 cases/yr in U.S. |
| **Etiology** | Trauma: 100% |
| **Associated conditions** | Alcohol abuse<br>Obesity<br>Diabetes mellitus (DM) |

## ANESTHETIC CONSIDERATIONS

See "Anesthetic Considerations for Lower-Extremity Procedures" at the end of "Orthopedic Surgery for Lower Extremities" section.

### References


1. Carragee EJ, Csongradi JJ, Bleck EE: Early complications in the operative treatment of ankle fractures. Influence of delay before operation. *J Bone Joint Surg* [Br] 1991; 73(1):79-82.
2. Epps CH Jr, ed: *Complications in Orthopaedic Surgery*, 2nd edition. JB Lippincott, Philadelphia: 1986.
3. Rockwood CA Jr, Green DP, Bucholz RW, eds: *Rockwood and Green's Fractures in Adults*, 3rd edition. JB Lippincott, Philadelphia: 1991.


# REPAIR NONUNION/MALUNION, TIBIA

## SURGICAL CONSIDERATIONS

**Description**: This procedure is used to treat a fracture which is not healed or which has healed misaligned. The fracture is mobilized, usually grafted with autogenous or allograft bone, and realigned. With an **anterior approach**, a longitudinal incision is made anteromedial or anterolateral to the shaft of the tibia. Dissection is carried directly down to the bone and the nonunion identified. If the tibia is approached with a **posterolateral** incision, the patient is turned prone and a longitudinal incision is made just posterior to the fibula. Dissection is carried down posteriorly to the interosseous membrane, to the tibia, and the procedure becomes identical to the anterior approach. Tissue interposed between the bone ends may or may not be debrided. The cortex of the bone adjacent to the nonunion is roughened with an osteotome. Autogenous or allograft bone is placed adjacent to or in the nonunion site. In the case of a malunion, the bone may be osteotomized with a saw or osteotomes to allow realignment. If skeletal fixation is used, a plate may be attached to the bone through the same incision. Alternatively, an intramedullary nail may be placed through an incision anterior to the tibial tubercle. If an intermedullary device is used, the canal may be reamed with intermedullary reamers prior to placement of the nail. A third type of skeletal fixation is the external fixator which stabilizes the non-union via percutaneous pins placed into the proximal and distal tibia, which are then spanned by a device with pin clamps at both ends. An intraop x-ray is often used to confirm fixation and placement of devices; alternatively, an image intensifier may be used.

**Variant procedure or approaches**: Autogenous **bone grafting from the iliac crest** is commonly used to stimulate healing. Stabilization is often achieved with internal or external **skeletal fixation**. An incision is made directly over the iliac crest and muscles are stripped from the crest and table of the ilium. Osteotomes and gouges are used to remove either the inner or outer table of the ilium and cancellous bone between the two tables. The wound is closed over a suction drain.

**Usual preop diagnosis**: Un-united or malunited fracture

**SUMMARY OF PROCEDURE**

| | Basic Repair | With Iliac Graft | With Skeletal Fixation |
|---|---|---|---|
| **Position** | Supine (prone with posterior lateral graft) | ⇐ | ⇐ |
| **Incision** | Anteromedial or posterolateral to shaft of tibia | Anteromedial, parallel to iliac crest | ⇐ |
| **Special instrumentation** | None | ⇐ | Pins, plates, screws, rods, external fixator |
| **Unique considerations** | Tourniquet; x-ray or image intensifier | ⇐ | ⇐ |
| **Antibiotics** | Cefazolin 1 gm iv preop. (If infected nonunion anticipated, antibiotics are withheld until cultures are obtained.) | ⇐ | ⇐ |
| **Surgical time** | 2 hrs | 2.5 hrs | 3 hrs |
| **Closing considerations** | Splint or cast applied while anesthetized. | ⇐ | No splint or cast |
| **EBL** | 100 cc | 200-300 cc | ⇐ |
| **Postop care** | PACU → room | ⇐ | ⇐ |
| **Mortality** | Minimal | ⇐ | ⇐ |
| **Morbidity** | Thrombophlebitis: 5% | ⇐ | ⇐ |
| | Compartment syndrome: 1% | ⇐ | ⇐ |
| | Infection: 1% | ⇐ | ⇐ |
| | Hematoma: < 1% | 5% | 1-3% |
| **Procedure code** | 27720 | 27724 | 27720 |
| **Pain score** | 5 | 8 | 5-8 |

**PATIENT POPULATION CHARACTERISTICS**

| | |
|---|---|
| **Age range** | 10-80 yrs (usually 20-40 yrs) |
| **Male:Female** | 5:1 |
| **Incidence** | 5-10% of tibia fractures; 50-75% of open fractures |
| **Etiology** | Trauma: 100% |
| **Associated conditions** | Poor nutrition: 50%<br>Infection: 10%<br>Metabolic disease: 10% |

## ANESTHETIC CONSIDERATIONS

See "Anesthetic Considerations for Lower-Extremity Procedures" at the end of "Orthopedic Surgery for Lower Extremities" section.

**References**

1. Epps CH Jr, ed: *Complications in Orthopaedic Surgery*, 2nd edition. JB Lippincott, Philadelphia: 1986.
2. Csongradi JJ, Maloney WJ: Ununited lower limb fractures. *West J Med* 1989; 150(6):675-80.

# ARTHROSCOPY OF THE ANKLE

## SURGICAL CONSIDERATIONS

**Description**: **Ankle arthroscopy** is usually a diagnostic procedure, although it may be used for debridement or removal of loose bodies. The ankle joint is generally inspected through anterolateral and anteromedial portals. Posterolateral and posteromedial portals also may be used. Each portal (entry wound) is made via a 5 mm stab wound in the skin (Fig 10.3-8); then instrumentation is placed, using trochars. If the ankle joint is tight, a mechanical distractor (external fixator distraction apparatus spanning the ankle joint) may be used. The distractor is attached to the bones via percutaneous pins, as in the case of the application of an external fixator. The portals are closed with sterile tape or a single suture. **Debridement** may be used to reduce local or generalized articular damage.

**Usual preop diagnosis**: Trauma; infection; arthritis

### SUMMARY OF PROCEDURE

| | Arthroscopy | Arthroscopy + Debridement |
|---|---|---|
| **Position** | Supine | ⇐ |
| **Incision** | 2 - 3.5 cm portals (incisions) | ⇐ |
| **Special instrumentation** | Arthroscopic video system; small biters and graspers | ⇐ + Shaver |
| **Unique considerations** | ± Tourniquet. May use distractor with pins through tibia and calcaneus. | ⇐ |
| **Antibiotics** | Cefazolin 1 gm iv preop (optional) | ⇐ |
| **Surgical time** | 1 hr | 1 - 2 hrs |
| **Closing considerations** | No splint; incisions injected with local anesthetic. | ⇐ |
| **EBL** | Minimal | 50 cc |
| **Postop care** | PACU → home | ⇐ |
| **Mortality** | < 0.01% | ⇐ |
| **Morbidity** | Hemarthrosis: 5% | ⇐ |
| | Thrombophlebitis < 2% | ⇐ |
| | Infection: < 1% | ⇐ |
| **Procedure code** | 29894 | 29887 (limited); 29898 (extensive) |
| **Pain score** | 2-3 | 3 |

### PATIENT POPULATION CHARACTERISTICS

| | |
|---|---|
| **Age range** | 12-70 yrs (usually 20-40 yrs) |
| **Male:Female** | 1:1 |
| **Incidence** | Uncommon |
| **Etiology** | Trauma: 70%<br>Arthritis: 20%<br>Infection: 5% |
| **Associated conditions** | Usually healthy<br>May have systemic arthritis |

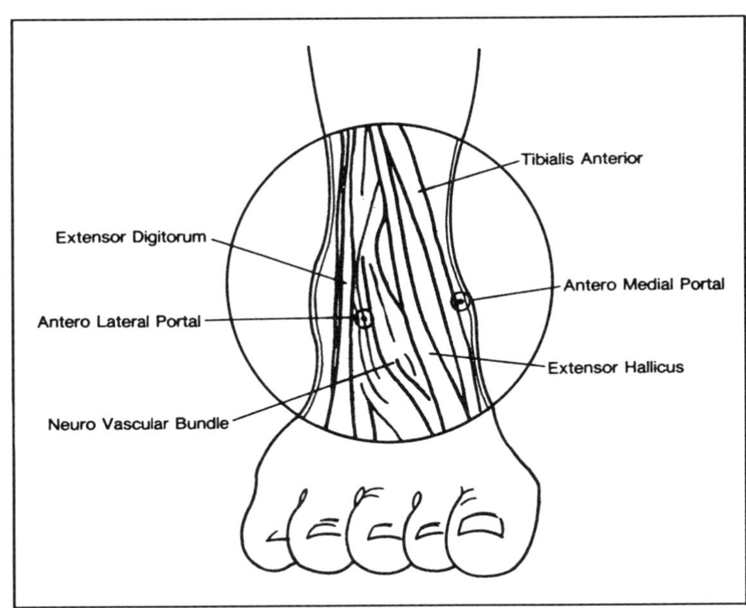


**Figure 10.3-8.** Portals for ankle arthroscopy. (Reproduced with permission from Chapman MW, ed: *Operative Orthopaedics*. JB Lippincott: 1988.)

## ANESTHETIC CONSIDERATIONS

See "Anesthetic Considerations for Lower-Extremity Procedures" at the end of "Orthpedic Surgery for Lower Extremities" section.

**References**

1. McGinty JB, ed: *Operative Arthroscopy*. Raven Press, New York: 1991.

# ANKLE ARTHROTOMY

## SURGICAL CONSIDERATIONS

**Description**: Arthrotomy of the ankle is the opening of the joint for drainage, debridement or fracture treatment. The joint is usually opened with an anterolateral, midline or an anteromedial longitudinal incision. Tendons and neurovascular structures are carefully retracted to expose the joint capsule, which is then opened in line with the skin incision. After intra-articular pathology is addressed, careful closure of the capsule is performed, taking care to obtain good hemostasis.

**Usual preop diagnosis**: Infection; trauma; arthritis

### SUMMARY OF PROCEDURE

| | |
|---|---|
| **Position** | Supine |
| **Incision** | Anterior midline or anteromedial longitudinal |
| **Special instrumentation** | Tourniquet |
| **Antibiotics** | Cefazolin 1 gm iv preop |
| **Surgical time** | 1 - 2 hrs |
| **Closing considerations** | ± Splint while anesthetized; may have suction drain. |
| **EBL** | Minimal |
| **Postop care** | PACU → room |
| **Mortality** | Minimal |
| **Morbidity** | Hemarthrosis: 20%<br>Thrombophlebitis: 5%<br>Infection: 1% |
| **Procedure code** | 27610 (for infection, with exploration, drainage or removal of foreign body); 27620 (with joint exploration, ± Bx, ± removal of loose or foreign body); 27625 (for synovectomy) |
| **Pain score** | 5 |

### PATIENT POPULATION CHARACTERISTICS

| | |
|---|---|
| **Age range** | Infant - elderly |
| **Male:Female** | 1:1 |
| **Incidence** | Rare |
| **Etiology** | Trauma: 70%<br>Arthritis: 20%<br>Infection: 10% |
| **Associated conditions** | Inflammatory arthritis<br>Multiple trauma<br>Immunosuppression |

## ANESTHETIC CONSIDERATIONS

See "Anesthetic Considerations for Lower-Extremity Procedures" at the end of "Orthpedic Surgery for Lower Extremities" section.

**References**

1. Crenshaw AH, ed: *Campbell's Operative Orthopaedics*, 8th edition. Mosby-Year Book, St. Louis: 1992.

# ANKLE ARTHRODESIS

## SURGICAL CONSIDERATIONS

**Description:** An **ankle fusion** may need to be performed for severe pain 2° arthritis of the ankle. In most cases, an anterior approach is made to the ankle joint. An alternative approach is through the medial malleolus. The ankle joint is exposed and the surfaces of the joint are debrided either with osteotomes or a burr. Cancellous bone is exposed on the distal tibia and talus and the joint is clamped together either with a simple external fixation device with pins going through the distal tibia and talus or with bone screws that go from the distal tibia into the talus. The wound is closed over a drain and a splint may be applied.

**Usual preop diagnosis:** Arthritis of the ankle

### SUMMARY OF PROCEDURE

| | |
|---|---|
| **Position** | Supine |
| **Incision** | Anterior midline over distal tibia |
| **Special instrumentation** | Tourniquet; external fixator or bone screws |
| **Unique considerations** | Intraop radiographs |
| **Antibiotics** | Cefazolin 1 gm iv preop |
| **Surgical time** | 2 hrs |
| **Closing considerations** | May be splinted; suction drain. |
| **EBL** | 100 cc |
| **Postop care** | PACU → room |
| **Mortality** | Minimal |
| **Morbidity** | Nonunion (late): 15%<br>Thrombophlebitis: 10%<br>Hematoma: 5%<br>Wound dehiscence: 5%<br>Infection: 1% |
| **Procedure code** | 27870 |
| **Pain score** | 8 |

### PATIENT POPULATION CHARACTERISTICS

| | |
|---|---|
| **Age range** | All adult |
| **Male:Female** | 1:1 |
| **Etiology** | Degenerative arthritis<br>Trauma<br>Avascular necrosis of talus<br>Septic arthritis |

| | |
|---|---|
| **Associated conditions** | Inflammatory arthritis<br>Any disease requiring steroids |

## ANESTHETIC CONSIDERATIONS

See "Anesthetic Considerations for Lower-Extremity Procedures" at the end of "Orthpedic Surgery for Lower Extremities" section.

**References**

1. Chapman MW, ed: *Operative Orthopaedics*. JB Lippincott, Philadelphia: 1988.
2. Crenshaw AH, ed: *Campbell's Operative Orthopaedics*, 8th edition. Mosby-Year Book, St. Louis: 1992.

# REPAIR/RECONSTRUCTION OF ANKLE LIGAMENTS

## SURGICAL CONSIDERATIONS

**Description:** Lateral ankle ligaments may be repaired acutely, but generally are reconstructed at a later date, if necessary, with the peroneus brevis used in most reconstructions. An incision is made posterior to the distal fibula, curving around the lateral malleolus and ending in the anterolateral foot. The peroneus brevis tendon is identified and detached from its musculotendinous junction in the leg, and the peroneus brevis muscle is sutured to the peroneus longus tendon. A hole is drilled from anterior to posterior in the distal lateral malleolus; then the detached end of the peroneus brevis tendon is threaded through the hole. It is then attached to either the calcaneus or the talus, anterior to the lateral malleolus, with a staple or by suturing into a hole in the bone. The skin and subcutaneous tissues are closed and a splint or cast is applied.

**Usual preop diagnosis:** Lateral instability of the ankle

### SUMMARY OF PROCEDURE

| | |
|---|---|
| **Position** | Supine or lateral decubitus |
| **Incision** | Posterolateral aspect of ankle |
| **Special instrumentation** | Bone staples |
| **Unique considerations** | Tourniquet |
| **Antibiotics** | Cefazolin, 1 gm iv preop |
| **Surgical time** | 2 hrs |
| **Closing considerations** | Splint or cast while still anesthetized. |
| **EBL** | Minimal |
| **Postop care** | PACU → room or home |
| **Mortality** | Minimal |
| **Morbidity** | Infection: < 1%<br>Re-rupture: < 1%<br>Wound dehiscence: < 0.1% |
| **Procedure code** | 27695 (suture, primary, torn, ruptured or severed ligament, ankle; collateral); 27696 (both collateral ligaments); 27698 (suture, secondary repair, torn, ruptured or severed ligament, ankle, collateral) |
| **Pain score** | 5 |

### PATIENT POPULATION CHARACTERISTICS

| | |
|---|---|
| **Age range** | Young adults |
| **Male:Female** | 2:1 |
| **Etiology** | Ankle sprain |
| **Associated conditions** | Alcohol abuse<br>Obesity<br>Diabetes mellitus (DM) |

## ANESTHETIC CONSIDERATIONS

See "Anesthetic Considerations for Lower-Extremity Procedures" at the end of "Orthpedic Surgery for Lower Extremities" section.


**References**

1. Epps CH Jr, ed: *Complications in Orthopaedic Surgery*, 2nd edition. JB Lippincott, Philadelphia: 1986.


# AMPUTATION THROUGH ANKLE (SYME)

## SURGICAL CONSIDERATIONS

**Description**: **Syme amputation** is ankle disarticulation with closure, using a posterior flap, including the heel pad (Fig 10.3-9). It is more functional than below-knee amputation because patients can bear weight on the end of the stump, but success is poor in patients with vascular disease or peripheral neuropathy. The posterior flap is dissected directly from the calcaneus, carefully preserving the tough heel pad and its blood supply. The heel pad is sutured directly to the distal tibia to prevent migration and to cover the bone end. The posterior flap is then sutured to the anterior flap with interrupted sutures and a compression dressing applied.

**Usual preop diagnosis**: Trauma; infection

### SUMMARY OF PROCEDURE

| | |
|---|---|
| **Position** | Supine |
| **Incision** | Anterior and posterior flaps |
| **Unique considerations** | Tourniquet |
| **Antibiotics** | Cefazolin 1 gm iv preop |
| **Surgical time** | 1.5 - 2 hrs |
| **Closing considerations** | Bulky dressing; if infection present, wound may be left open. |
| **EBL** | 100 cc |
| **Postop care** | PACU → room |
| **Mortality** | Minimal |
| **Morbidity** | Phantom pain: 90%<br>Infection: 10-15%<br>Wound breakdown: 10-15%<br>Pneumonia: 12%<br>MI: 7%<br>PE: 6%<br>Hematoma: 5%<br>Stroke: 5% |
| **Procedure code** | 27888 |
| **Pain score** | 5 |

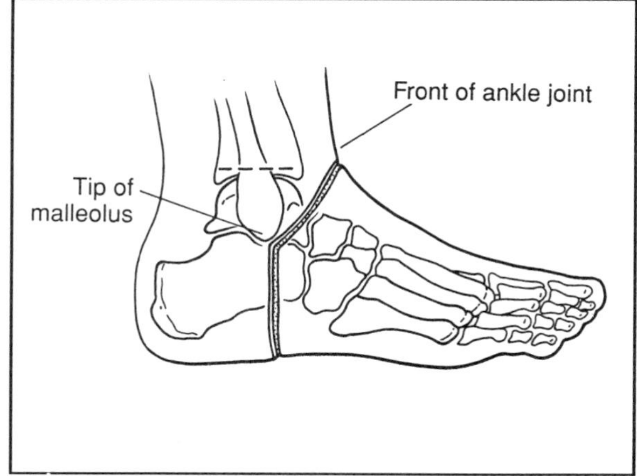


**Figure 10.3-9.** Incision for Syme amputation. (Reproduced with permission from Chapman MW, ed: *Operative Orthopaedics*. JB Lippincott: 1988. Redrawn from Wagner WF Jr: The Syme amputation. In *American Academy of Orthopaedic Surgeons: Atlas of limb prosthetics*. Mosby-Year Book: 1981.)

### PATIENT POPULATION CHARACTERISTICS

| | |
|---|---|
| **Age range** | Typically, >60 yrs |
| **Male:Female** | 3:1 |
| **Incidence** | 20,000-30,000/yr |
| **Etiology** | Trauma: 50%<br>Infection: 30%<br>Congenital anomaly: 5% |
| **Associated conditions** | Peripheral vascular disease: 30-40%<br>Diabetes: < 20% |

## ANESTHETIC CONSIDERATIONS

See "Anesthetic Considerations for Lower-Extremity Procedures" at the end of "Orthpedic Surgery for Lower Extremities" section.


**References**

1. Epps CH Jr, ed: *Complications in Orthopaedic Surgery*, 2nd edition. JB Lippincott, Philadelphia: 1986.


# AMPUTATION, TRANSMETATARSAL

## SURGICAL CONSIDERATIONS

**Description**: This amputation, usually for infection or ischemic necrosis of the toes, is performed at the mid-metatarsal level, leaving the patient able to walk without a prosthesis. A transverse dorsal incision is made at the transmetatarsal level, and a plantar incision is made beginning at the corners of the dorsal incision and extending distally to the metatarsal heads to create a long plantar flap. The plantar flap is reflected proximally to the mid-metatarsal level and tapered distally. The metatarsals are sectioned with a saw, and nerves and tendons are sectioned proximal to the osteotomies. The plantar flap is then brought over the ends of the bones and sutured with interrupted sutures to the dorsal flap. A compression dressing is applied.

**Variant procedure or approaches**: Other partial-foot amputations, such as **mid-tarsal** and **ray amputation**, are much less common. They are managed in a fashion similar to that of the transmetatarsal amputation.

**Usual preop diagnosis**: Gangrene of the toes; infection

### SUMMARY OF PROCEDURE

| | |
|---|---|
| **Position** | Supine |
| **Incision** | Dorsal and plantar flaps |
| **Unique considerations** | Tourniquet |
| **Antibiotics** | Cefazolin 1 gm iv preop |
| **Surgical time** | 1 - 2 hrs |
| **Closing considerations** | Bulky dressing |
| **EBL** | 50 cc |
| **Postop care** | PACU → room |
| **Mortality** | Minimal |

| | |
|---|---|
| **Morbidity** | Phantom pain: 90%<br>Infection: 10-15%<br>Wound breakdown: 10-15%<br>Hematoma: 5% |
| **Procedure code** | 28805 |
| **Pain score** | 5 |

**PATIENT POPULATION CHARACTERISTICS**

| | |
|---|---|
| **Age range** | >60 yrs |
| **Male:Female** | 3:1 |
| **Incidence** | 20,000-30,000 total amputations/yr |
| **Etiology** | Vascular disease: 70%<br>Infection: 25%<br>Trauma: < 5%<br>Congenital anomalies: < 1% |
| **Associated conditions** | Vascular disease: 70%<br>Diabetes mellitus: 30%<br>Pulmonary disease: 30% |

## ANESTHETIC CONSIDERATIONS

See "Anesthetic Considerations for Lower-Extremity Procedures" at the end of "Orthpedic Surgery for Lower Extremities" section.

**References**

1. Crenshaw AH, ed: *Campbell's Operative Orthopaedics*, 8th edition. Mosby-Year Book, St. Louis: 1992.
2. Epps CH Jr, ed: *Complications in Orthopaedic Surgery*, 2nd edition. JB Lippincott, Philadelphia: 1986.

# LENGTHENING OR TRANSFER OF TENDONS, ANKLE AND FOOT

## SURGICAL CONSIDERATIONS

**Description**: In cases of motor imbalance from neuromuscular disease or trauma, tendons are lengthened or transferred to a new insertion to partially restore balance or normalize joint motion. For **tendon lengthening**, a longitudinal incision generally is made directly over the tendon. Subcutaneous tissues and tendon sheath are incised to expose the tendon, which is transected with a Z-type incision. The tendon is placed in its lengthened position and the ends of the Z are closed with absorbable suture. If present, the tendon sheath is closed separately from the skin closure. In a **tendon transfer**, the tendon is usually cut close to its insertion, and transferred to a new bony insertion, which often requires a separate incision. The tendon is attached to the bone either with a metal staple or by suturing it into a drill hole in the bone.

**Variant procedure or approaches**: **Achilles' tendon lengthening** is used to bring the ankle out of equinus. A **posterior tibial tendon lengthening** and/or **posterior ankle capsulotomy** may accompany the procedure.

**Usual preop diagnosis**: Contracture of muscle

### SUMMARY OF PROCEDURE

| | Tendon Lengthening | Achilles Tendon Lengthening |
|---|---|---|
| **Position** | Supine | Prone |
| **Incision** | Over tendon; sometimes multiple incisions | Over tendon |
| **Unique considerations** | Tourniquet | ⇐ |
| **Antibiotics** | If young, none; in elderly or infirm, cefazolin 1 gm iv preop | ⇐ |
| **Surgical time** | 2 hrs | 1 hr |
| **Closing considerations** | Splint or cast while anesthetized | ⇐ |
| **EBL** | 10 cc | ⇐ |
| **Postop care** | PACU → room | PACU → room or home |
| **Mortality** | Minimal | ⇐ |
| **Morbidity** | Infection: < 1% | ⇐ |
| **Procedure code** | 27685 (single); 27690 (transfer or transplant of single tendon; superficial; 27691 (anterior or posterior tibial through interosseous space) | 27685 |
| **Pain score** | 4 | 3 |

### PATIENT POPULATION CHARACTERISTICS

| | |
|---|---|
| **Age range** | Any age |
| **Male:Female** | 1:1 |
| **Incidence** | Rare |
| **Etiology** | Neuromuscular disease: 80%<br>Trauma: 20% |
| **Associated conditions** | Static encephalopathy/cerebral palsy: 75%<br>Other neuromuscular disease: 25% |

## ANESTHETIC CONSIDERATIONS

See "Anesthetic Considerations for Lower-Extremity Procedures" at the end of "Orthpedic Surgery for Lower Extremities" section.

**References**

1. Crenshaw AH, ed: *Campbell's Operative Orthopaedics*, 8th edition. Mosby-Year Book, St. Louis: 1992.

# AMPUTATION ABOVE THE KNEE

## SURGICAL CONSIDERATIONS

**Description**: In above-the-knee amputations, the distal part of the lower extremity is excised, starting just above the knee at the level of the distal third of the femur (Fig 10.3-10). A stump is fashioned, and will require prosthetic fitting at a later time. The most commonly performed stumps incorporate anterior and posterior flaps of equal length. The underlying muscles (hamstrings and quadriceps) are either sewn to each other (**myoplasty**) or to bone (**myodesis**). In a **guillotine**, or **open amputation**, the stump is not fashioned (tissues are not closed) until later. This is a multi-stage procedure used for dirty, traumatic amputations, infection, or above-knee amputations with questionable survival, and is usually done as a life-saving procedure. Internal fixation of part of the remaining femur may be indicated in traumatic amputations. The patient returns to the OR every 1-3 days for re-debridement until closure of the clean stump can be performed.

**Usual preop diagnosis**: Peripheral vascular disease or gangrene of lower extremity; trauma to lower extremity; open-femur fracture with traumatic amputation; tumor of lower extremity

### SUMMARY OF PROCEDURE

| | |
|---|---|
| **Position** | Supine |
| **Incision** | Anterior and posterior on thigh |
| **Special instrumentation** | Amputation saw and rasp; drill for myodesis |
| **Unique considerations** | Patient often very ill from sepsis, chronic disease or trauma |
| **Antibiotics** | Broad-spectrum cephalosporin (e.g., cefamandole 1 gm iv q 6 hrs), ± gentamicin (80 mg iv q 8 hrs); adjust dosage for renal status, ± penicillin (1-2 million U iv q 4 hrs) |
| **Surgical time** | 1- 2 hrs |
| **Closing considerations** | Compressive dressing ± special stump sock |
| **EBL** | 250 cc or more; higher for traumatic amputations |
| **Postop care** | Generally PACU → room (if medically unstable → ICU) |
| **Mortality** | Approximately 10-20%; higher in PVD (10-39%) |
| **Morbidity** | Phantom limb: 85-95%; phantom pain: 2-15%<br>Wound infection ± deep infection: < 15% in PVD<br>Respiratory failure or pneumonia: 10-15%<br>MI: 7-10%<br>Thromboembolism: 6-10%<br>Cerebrovascular accident: 5-10%<br>Failure to heal ± wound dehiscence: Uncommon<br>Contractures – flexion and abduction contracture: Common<br>Urinary retention requiring catheterization: Common<br>Hematoma: Rare<br>Reamputation: Rare<br>Neuromas: Rare<br>UTI: Rare<br>Contralateral amputation, especially in diabetics and those with PVD<br>Postop depression |
| **Procedure code** | 27590 (above-knee amputations)<br>27592 (open above-knee amputation)<br>27596 (reamputation) |
| **Pain score** | 7-10 |

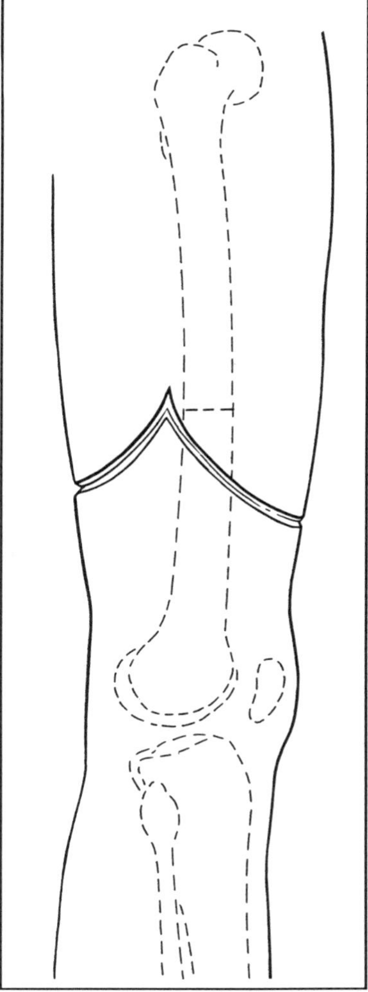

**Figure 10.3-10.** Amputation through middle third of thigh. (Reproduced with permission from Crenshaw AH: *Campbell's Operative Orthopaedics*, 7th edition. CV Mosby: 1987.)

### PATIENT POPULATION CHARACTERISTICS

| | |
|---|---|
| **Age range** | 70-90% >60 yrs: peripheral vascular disease, diabetic gangrene<br>18-35 yrs: multiple trauma with traumatic amputation; tumor of lower extremity |
| **Male:Female** | Overall 3-9:1<br>Elderly, predominance of males<br>Multiple trauma, 4-5:1<br>Tumor 1:1 |
| **Incidence** | Common for peripheral vascular disease patients<br>Rare for trauma or tumor |
| **Etiology** | Peripheral vascular disease and diabetic gangrene: 70-90%<br>Multiple trauma (younger patients): Rare – usually with severe Grade IIIC injuries with neurovascular severance<br>Tumor: Rare<br>Uncontrollable infection (e.g., gas gangrene): Rare |
| **Associated conditions** | Diabetes: 70-80% of patients presenting for this procedure<br>Numerous other serious medical conditions<br>Multiple trauma in younger patients |

## ANESTHETIC CONSIDERATIONS

See Anesthetic Considerations following "Amputation Below Knee" (below).

**References**

1. McCollough NC III: Complications of amputation surgery. In *Complications in Orthopaedic Surgery*. Epps CH Jr, ed. JB Lippincott, Philadelphia: 1986, 1335-67.
2. Tooms RE: Amputations of lower extremity. In *Campbell's Operative Orthopaedics*. Crenshaw AH, ed. CV Mosby, St. Louis: 1987, Vol 1, 607-27.

# AMPUTATION BELOW THE KNEE

## SURGICAL CONSIDERATIONS

**Description**: **Below-the-knee amputation** is ablation of the lower limb, usually at the level of the mid-leg. A long, posterior flap normally is used to cover the stump. The condition of the soft tissues may dictate the level and/or type of flaps used. The procedure begins with an anterior transverse incision made over the mid-tibia. A long posterior flap, which is 2-3 times the diameter of the leg in length, is then made. The bone is exposed anteriorly and the anterolateral neurovascular structures and muscles are transected and ligated as appropriate (Fig 10.3-11). The bone is then transected with a bone saw, and the posterior structures are transected and ligated as appropriate. The amputated leg and foot are then removed from the table and the posterior flap is tapered and shaped for closure. Deep sutures are placed to secure the posterior muscles to the anterior tibia. The skin opening and subcutaneous tissues are closed with interrupted sutures (Fig 10.3-12). Finally, a drain is placed (sometimes), and either a compression dressing or an immediate postop cast is applied.

**Variant procedure or approaches**: **Guillotine amputation** may be used as the first of a two-stage procedure in infected or contaminated cases. With a guillotine amputation, the bone and soft tissues are transected very quickly in guillotine fashion at the mid-tibial level. Neurovascular structures are ligated as appropriate. These wounds are usually left open and a compression dressing applied.

**Usual preop diagnosis**: Dysvascular limb; infection; trauma

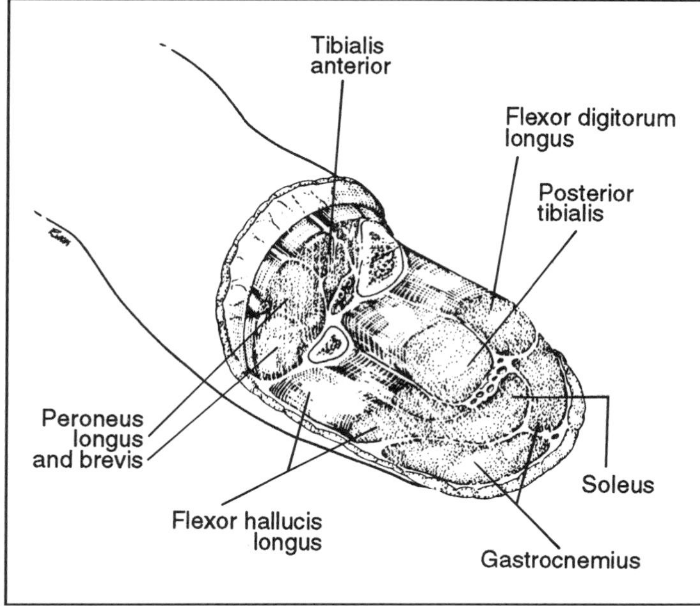


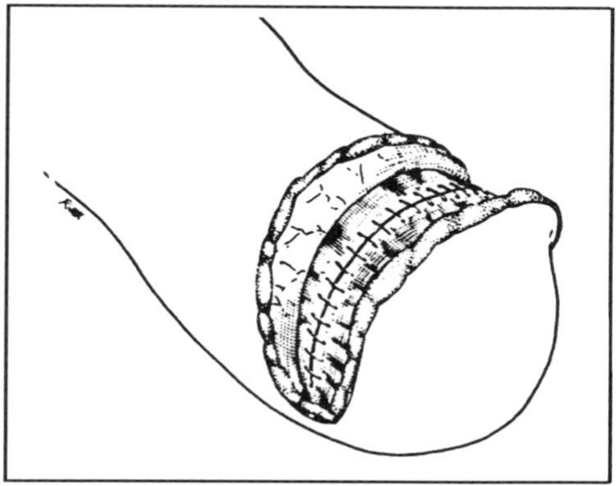

↑**Figure 10.3-12.** Suture of flap to deep fascia and periosteum anteriorly.

←**Figure 10.3-11.** Below-knee amputation prior to closure.

(Both figures reproduced with permission from Crenshaw AH: *Campbell's Operative Orthopaedics*, 8th edition. CV Mosby: 1992. Redrawn from Burgess EM and Zettl JH: Artif Limbs 1969; 13:1.)

## SUMMARY OF PROCEDURE

| | |
|---|---|
| **Position** | Supine |
| **Incision** | Anterior and posterior flaps; for guillotine amputation, circumferential incision |
| **Special instrumentation** | Bone saw |
| **Unique considerations** | Tourniquet, if traumatic (tourniquet contraindicated if infected or avascular) |
| **Antibiotics** | Cefazolin 1 gm iv preop |
| **Surgical time** | 1.5 hrs; for guillotine amputation, 0.5 hr |
| **Closing considerations** | May use cast; drain. Bulky dressing needed for guillotine amputation. |
| **EBL** | 200 cc |
| **Postop care** | PACU → room |
| **Mortality** | 10% |
| **Morbidity** | Phantom pain: 90%<br>Infection: 10-15%<br>Wound breakdown: 10-15%<br>Pneumonia: 12%<br>MI: 7%<br>PE: 6%<br>Hematoma: 5%<br>Stroke: 5% |
| **Procedure code** | 27880; 27881 (includes immediate prosthetic fitting) |
| **Pain score** | 5 |

## PATIENT POPULATION CHARACTERISTICS

| | |
|---|---|
| **Age range** | Usually >60 |
| **Male:Female** | 3:1 |
| **Incidence** | 20,000-30,000 total amputations/yr |
| **Etiology** | Dysvascular limb: 70%<br>Trauma: 20%<br>Infection : 5%<br>Tumor: 5%<br>Congenital anomaly: < 1% |

| | |
|---|---|
| **Associated conditions** | Vascular disease: 70-80%<br>Malnutrition: 50%<br>Diabetes mellitus: 30%<br>Pulmonary disease: 30% |

## ANESTHETIC CONSIDERATIONS FOR ABOVE- AND BELOW-KNEE AMPUTATION

### PREOPERATIVE

Vascular disease and tumors are the two most common indications for these surgeries. Patients presenting for amputations often have severe systemic vascular disease. Their inability to perform exercise limits the usefulness of preop history in evaluating cardiopulmonary reserve, and often necessitates invasive studies for full evaluation.

| | |
|---|---|
| **Respiratory** | Smoking is a risk factor common to both vascular and pulmonary diseases. Chronic bronchitis or COPD patients should have maximum medical therapy (e.g., inhaled bronchodilators, theophylline and steroids, when appropriate) prior to anesthesia. Regional anesthesia is an excellent choice for patients with severe pulmonary disease.<br>**Tests:** As indicated from H&P. |
| **Cardiovascular** | Significant cardiovascular disease is present in 30% of patients presenting for vascular surgery. Particularly in diabetics, CAD is often silent. Dipyridamole thallium imaging of the heart can reveal the preop myocardium at risk of ischemia, however, therapy of stenotic coronary arteries can usually be undertaken only after the amputation. Medical management, to include ß-blockers when tolerated, will reduce perioperative MIs.<br>**Tests:** ECG; others as indicated from H&P. |
| **Neurological** | Peripheral and autonomic neuropathies may be present in the diabetic patient. Hence, these patients may be more susceptible to injury from malpositioning and are less able to tolerate the hemodynamic changes associated with regional anesthesia. Pre-existing neurological deficits should be carefully documented. |
| **Musculoskeletal** | Rhabdomyolysis can occur in the presence of partial ischemia. (See Renal section, below.) |
| **Hematologic** | Often a trial of heparin, warfarin or thrombolytic therapy will have been undertaken prior to amputation. Coagulation studies, including PT, PTT and bleeding time are, therefore, often necessary to determine the appropriateness of epidural or intrathecal anesthesia. Warfarin-induced elevation of the PT can be reversed preop with FFP 5-10 ml/kg body weight. This therapy may induce fluid overload in patients with poor cardiac reserve. For these patients, diuretics should be administered to maintain normovolemia.<br>**Tests:** As indicated from H&P. |
| **Renal** | Limb ischemia can result in myoglobinemia from rhabdomyolysis. Evidence of progressive renal failure or rising CPK-MM fractions should be treated with hydration, forced alkaline diuresis and prompt amputation.<br>**Tests:** Creatinine; BUN; CPK enzymes, if creatinine is elevated. |
| **Laboratory** | Diabetic patients require control of blood glucose preop and perioperative glucose monitoring. |
| **Premedication** | Standard premedication (see Appendix). |

### INTRAOPERATIVE

**Anesthetic technique:** Either regional or GA may be appropriate.

**Regional anesthesia:** Both SAB and epidural blocks are useful techniques. Subarachnoid anesthesia has the advantage of limited spread of the block above the level of surgery, while obtaining adequate blockade of the sacral roots that are resistant to low-dose epidural techniques. Epidural anesthesia allows for extending the duration of anesthesia and for the administration of postop epidural analgesia. Anesthesia from T12 (T8 with tourniquet) is adequate. Full motor blockade is not necessary. Typical drugs and doses include: subarachnoid – 75 mg of 5% lidocaine in 5% dextrose with morphine 0.2 mg; epidural – 12-15 cc 2% lidocaine with epinephrine 1:200,000 in divided doses.

**General anesthesia:**

| | |
|---|---|
| **Induction** | Standard induction (see Appendix) is appropriate for patients with normal airways. Intubation is indicated for diabetic patients with gastroparesis. |
| **Maintenance** | Standard maintenance (see Appendix). |
| **Emergence** | No special considerations |

| | | |
|---|---|---|
| **Blood and fluid requirements** | Moderate blood loss<br>IV: 16 ga x 1<br>NS/LR @ 4-6 cc/kg/hr | Expect 100-200 cc blood loss, mostly during cleaning of wound made while developing a flap. |
| **Control of blood loss** | Tourniquet may be used. | Inflation pressure is typically 100 mmHg greater than systolic pressure. Maximum "safe" tourniquet time is 1.5-2 hr, followed by a 5-to-(preferably) 15-min reperfusion interval, if further tourniquet is necessary. |
| **Special considerations** | Tourniquet deflation and limb reperfusion | Mild hypotension is common. In patients with moderate-to-severe lung disease, continue controlled ventilation until after the lactic acid that has accumulated in the ischemic leg is metabolized (3-5 min) since these patients may be unable to increase ventilation adequately to buffer this acid load. |
| **Monitoring** | Standard monitors (see Appendix).<br>± CVP line<br>± Arterial line | Invasive monitoring is indicated in the presence of severe cardiac or pulmonary disease. Serial blood glucose determination should be made in the diabetic patient. |
| **Positioning** | √ and pad pressure points.<br>√ eyes. | Meticulous padding of the extremities is necessary to prevent ischemic skin ulceration in patients with vascular insufficiency. |

### POSTOPERATIVE

| | | |
|---|---|---|
| **Complications** | Hematoma<br>Bleeding | √ drains. |
| **Pain management** | Spinal opiates<br>Epidural analgesia | Epidural hydromorphone 50 $\mu$g/cc infused at 50-200 $\mu$g/hr provides excellent analgesia. |
| **Tests** | CXR if CVP was placed. | Other studies as indicated. |

**References**

1. Epps CH Jr, ed: *Complications in Orthopaedic Surgery*, 2nd edition. JB Lippincott, Philadelphia: 1986.

# FASCIOTOMY OF THE THIGH

## SURGICAL CONSIDERATIONS

**Description**: Increased intracompartmental pressure in the thigh requires surgical release of tight skin and fascial structures (Fig 10.3-13). This usually occurs after severe trauma to the thigh (e.g., crush injury, comminuted fracture, etc.) or, after prolonged vascular surgery, with ischemia to the thigh. Compartment syndrome is a true emergency and must be treated within minutes of recognition. Failure to do so may result in loss of limb or death. Conventional devices may be used to measure intracompartmental pressure, which usually is abnormal if >30-35 mmHg (normal = approximately < 30 mmHg). Fasciotomy of the thigh involves incising the skin and fascia over the thigh and debriding any necrotic tissue. The wound is left open for later re-debridement, delayed primary closure or skin grafting. Thus, the fasciotomy begins a multi-stage procedure of incision and debridement, with subsequent reconstruction.

**Usual preop diagnosis**: Compartment syndrome of thigh; crush injury to thigh

## SUMMARY OF PROCEDURE

| | |
|---|---|
| **Position** | Supine or lateral decubitus |
| **Incision** | Lateral thigh |
| **Unique considerations** | Patient may be very ill. If an ipsilateral femoral fracture is present with a compartment syndrome, the surgeon may want to perform ORIF, intramedullary nailing, or external fixation of the fracture. |
| **Antibiotics** | Broad-spectrum cephalosporin (e.g., cefamandole 1 gm iv q 6 hrs) |
| **Surgical time** | 1.5 - 2 hrs for fasciotomy alone |
| **Closing considerations** | Wound left open and covered by sterile dressings. |
| **EBL** | 250-500 cc |
| **Postop care** | If surgery is performed acutely, patient frequently will be a multiple-trauma victim with numerous injuries and extensive blood loss, and usually goes to ICU. |
| **Mortality** | Dependent on extent of multiple trauma |
| **Morbidity** | Hypotension and fluid loss: Common<br>Neurological deficit to peripheral nerves: Common, if decompression delayed<br>Respiratory distress and fat embolism: Not uncommon, if concomitant femur fracture<br>Vascular complications: Not uncommon<br>Amputation: Rare if decompression prompt<br>Systemic sepsis: Rare<br>Wound infection: Rare<br>New compartment syndrome; insufficient fasciotomy: Rare |
| **Procedure code** | 27025 |
| **Pain score** | 7-8 |

## PATIENT POPULATION CHARACTERISTICS

| | |
|---|---|
| **Age range** | Any age, but predominance of males < 30 yrs |
| **Male:Female** | 5:1 |
| **Incidence** | Extremely rare |
| **Etiology** | Trauma: motorcycle and motor vehicle accidents, falls, industrial injury, crush injuries<br>Post-surgery: local hematoma and swelling<br>Thrombosis or disruption of blood supply to thigh (e.g., failed proximal vascular bypass surgery, aortic dissection, etc.)<br>Massive infection of thigh compartment (e.g., gas gangrene) |
| **Associated conditions** | Burns<br>Drug and alcohol overdose<br>Frequently associated with trauma to other organ systems |

---

# ANESTHETIC CONSIDERATIONS

See Anesthetic Considerations following "Fasciotomy of the Leg" (below).

#### References


1. Mubarak SJ: Compartment syndromes. In *Operative Orthopaedics*. Chapman MW, ed. JB Lippincott, Philadelphia: 1988, 179-95.
2. Richardson EG: Miscellaneous nontraumatic disorders. In *Campbell's Operative Orthopaedics*. Crenshaw AH, ed. CV Mosby, St. Louis: 1987, Vol 2, 1014-15.

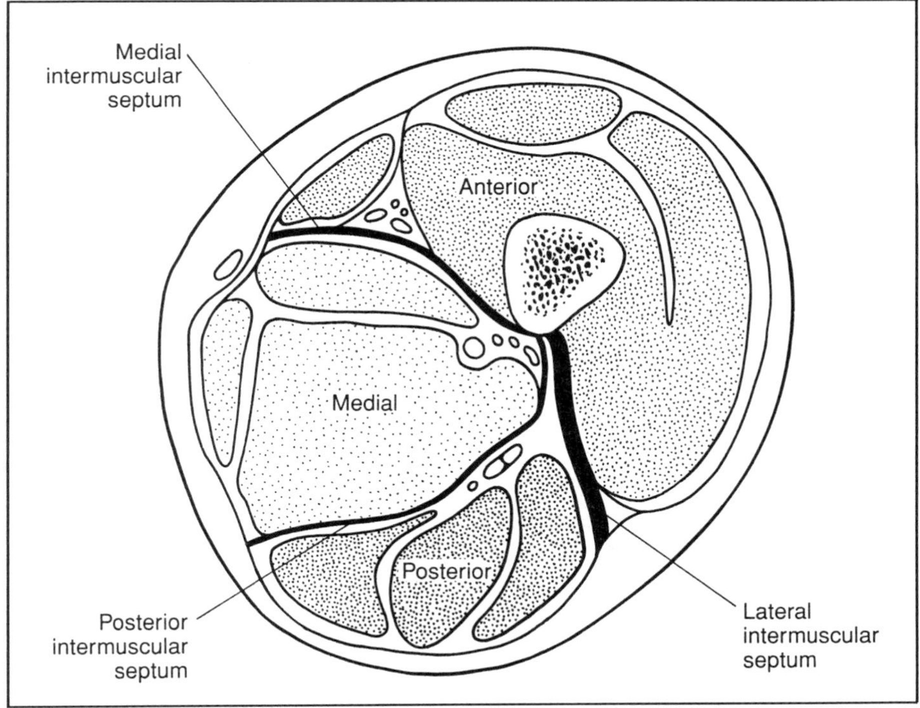


**Figure 10.3-13.** Cross-section of the thigh showing the 3 major compartments. (Reproduced with permission from Tarlow SD, Achterman C, Hayhurst J, Ovadin D: Acute compartment syndrome of the thigh. *J Bone Joint Surg* [Am] 1986; 68:1441.)

# FASCIOTOMY OF THE LEG

## SURGICAL CONSIDERATIONS

**Description**: This procedure is the surgical decompression of fascial compartments for treatment or prevention of compartment syndrome. Patients are often very ill and unstable with other injuries or disease. Compartment syndrome is a true emergency and must be treated within minutes of recognition. Failure to do so may result in loss of limb or death. There are four compartments in the leg: anterior, lateral, deep posterior and superficial posterior (Fig 10.3-14). Generally, all four compartments are released during the procedure. A four-compartment fascial decompression can be performed through two incisions – medial and lateral. A medial longitudinal incision is made just posterior to the tibia; through this incision, the superficial and deep posterior compartments are identified and the fascia incised in longitudinal fashion. A straight, lateral, longitudinal incision is made and the deep fascia overlying the anterior and lateral compartments is identified. The fascia of each compartment is then incised longitudinally. Skin incisions are rarely closed because of the swelling. A compression dressing is applied and splints may be used.

**Usual preop diagnosis**: Compartment syndrome; vascular trauma

### SUMMARY OF PROCEDURE

| | |
|---|---|
| **Position** | Supine |
| **Incision** | Medial and lateral parallel to tibia |
| **Unique considerations** | Often associated with fracture; may require fixation. |
| **Antibiotics** | Cefazolin 1 gm iv preop |
| **Surgical time** | 0.5+ hr |
| **Closing considerations** | Wounds left open; splint may be required. |

| | |
|---|---|
| **EBL** | 100 cc |
| **Postop care** | PACU → room; vascular monitoring is carried out clinically via a pulse oximeter on toes |
| **Mortality** | Minimal |
| **Morbidity** | Myonecrosis: 50%<br>Thrombophlebitis: 10-20%<br>Infection: 10-15% |
| **Procedure code** | 27602 |
| **Pain score** | 3 |

### PATIENT POPULATION CHARACTERISTICS

| | |
|---|---|
| **Age range** | All ages |
| **Male:Female** | 1:1 |
| **Incidence** | ~ 5% of tibia fractures |
| **Etiology** | Trauma – blunt fracture, vascular: 90%<br>Drug overdose: 10%<br>Burns: < 5%<br>Revascularization: < 5% |
| **Associated conditions** | Multiple trauma: 60%<br>Vascular disease: 15% |

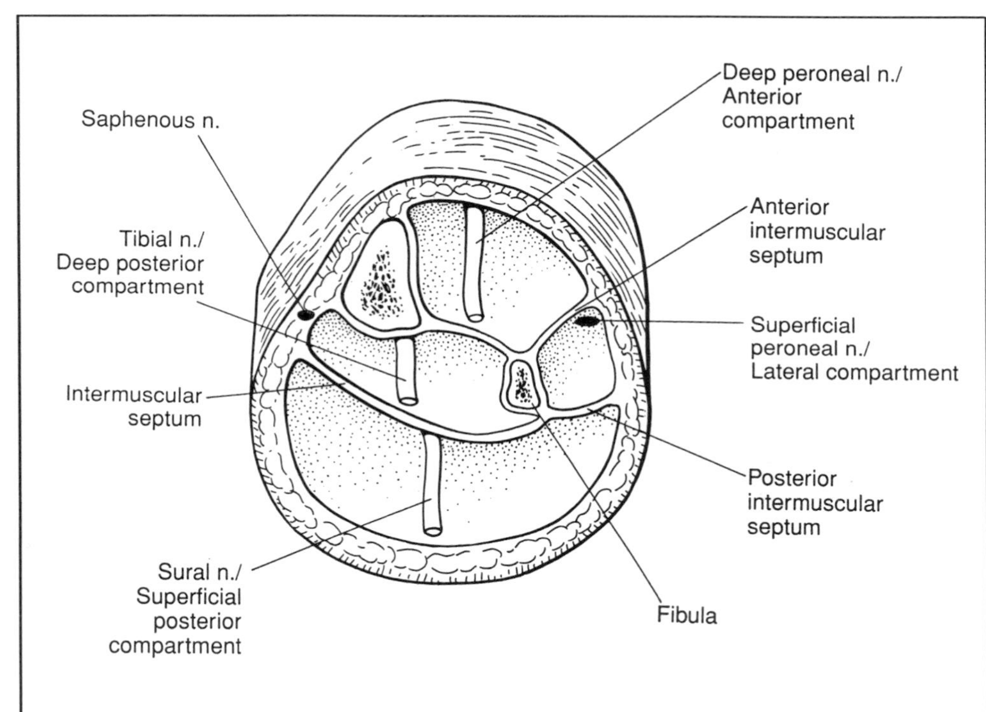


**Figure 10.3-14.** Cross-section of the left leg, middle lower third, showing the 4 compartments with associated peripheral nerves. (Reproduced with permission from Mubarak SJ, Owen CA: Double-incision fasciotomy of the leg for decompression in compartment syndromes. *J Bone Joint Surg* [Am] 1977; 59:184-87.)

---

## ANESTHETIC CONSIDERATIONS FOR FASCIOTOMY OF THIGH AND LEG

### PREOPERATIVE

Compartment syndromes and necrotizing fasciitis are the indications for these procedures. Patients with compartment syndrome often have no systemic disease, while patients with necrotizing fasciitis have a rapidly life-threatening infection that requires prompt surgical debridement, and often is complicated by rhabdomyolysis and DIC.

| | |
|---|---|
| **Respiratory** | Usually no special considerations, unless massive sepsis. |

| | |
|---|---|
| **Cardiovascular** | Sepsis is uniformly present in patients with necrotizing fasciitis. Management includes antibiotics and hemodynamic support with dopamine (5-15 $\mu$g/kg/min) or epinephrine (15-250 ng/kg/min) with therapy guided by invasive hemodynamic monitoring, which may include PA catheter. |
| **Neurological** | If fasciotomy is for compartment syndrome, there may be compromise of distal nerves and blood flow. Perform a thorough neurologic exam of the involved extremity to document preop deficits. |
| **Hematologic** | If infection is the indication for the fasciotomy, DIC is likely. Evaluate for pathologic bleeding. Administer factors necessary to correct coagulopathy during the procedure.<br>**Tests:** PT; PTT; fibrinogen; D-dimer; fibrin split products; platelet count |
| **Renal** | Both necrotizing fasciitis and compartment syndrome often cause myoglobinuria and rhabdomyolysis. Myoglobinuria can be inferred from urine that is dipstick-positive for occult blood but microscopically free of RBCs in the absence of hemolysis. |
| **Laboratory** | Hct; serial $K^+$ levels if there is an active diuresis; other studies as indicated from H&P. |
| **Premedication** | Diazepam 5-10 mg po 1 hr preop |

## INTRAOPERATIVE

**Anesthetic technique:** Regional techniques are appropriate for compartment syndrome decompression, unless there is evidence of DIC. These surgeries are usually of short duration (< 1 hr). Sepsis and hemodynamic instability usually mandate GETA for fasciotomy in patients with necrotizing fasciitis.

**Regional anesthesia:** Either subarachnoid or epidural blocks are useful in the absence of infection or severe coagulopathy. Subarachnoid anesthesia has the advantage of adequate blockade of the sacral roots that are resistant to low-dose epidural techniques. Anesthesia from T10-S2 is adequate. Typical drugs and dosages include: subarachnoid – 15 mg of 0.5% bupivacaine; epidural – 12-15 cc 2% lidocaine with epinephrine 1:200,000 in divided doses.

**General anesthesia:**

| | |
|---|---|
| **Induction** | Standard induction (see Appendix). |
| **Maintenance** | Standard maintenance (see Appendix). |
| **Emergence** | Consider postop ventilation for patients with impaired oxygenation or ongoing hemodynamic instability. Otherwise, no special considerations. |

| | | |
|---|---|---|
| **Blood and fluid requirements** | IV: 16 ga x 1 (compartment syndrome)<br>14-16 ga x 2 (necrotizing fasciitis) | To prevent renal damage, insure adequate circulatory volume; induce osmotic diuresis with mannitol 0.25 gm/kg iv. Furosemide 10-100 mg also may be necessary to maintain diuresis. Replace UO with half NS with 50 mEq bicarbonate/L, or as guided by invasive monitoring. |
| **Monitoring** | Standard monitors (see Appendix).<br>UO<br>± Arterial line<br>± CVP or PA catheter | Patients with necrotizing fasciitis require an arterial line and either a CVP or PA catheter to guide fluid and inotropic/pressor therapy. |
| **Positioning** | ✓ and pad pressure points.<br>✓ eyes. | |

## POSTOPERATIVE

| | | |
|---|---|---|
| **Complications** | DIC<br>Renal failure 2° rhabdomyolysis<br>Hypo/hyperkalemia<br>Sepsis syndrome including ARDS | |
| **Pain management** | PCA or epidural analgesia | See Appendix. |
| **Tests** | Hct<br>Electrolytes<br>UA (dipstick and microscopic) | For patients with sepsis, coagulation profile, including PT/PTT, D-dimer, fibrin split products and platelet count. |

References

1. Epps CH Jr, ed: *Complications in Orthopaedic Surgery*, 2nd edition. JB Lippincott, Philadelphia: 1986.
2. Rockwood CA Jr, Green DP, Bucholz RW, eds: *Rockwood and Green's Fractures in Adults*, 3rd edition. JB Lippincott, Philadelphia: 1991.

# BIOPSY, LEG AND FOOT

## SURGICAL CONSIDERATIONS

**Description**: Biopsy is performed to excise tissues for pathologic evaluation, usually through a small, longitudinal wound. For **incisional biopsy**, a longitudinal incision is made over the mass. Overlying soft tissues are incised with minimal undermining. The area in question is incised and the biopsy removed, with care being taken to prevent spillage into the adjacent tissues. The pathologist often is asked to perform a frozen section to determine whether diagnostic tissue is present. The wound is closed with interrupted sutures and a compression dressing applied. A splint or cast may be used if a significant amount of bone has been removed. If the lesion is small, x-ray control or image intensification may be necessary for localization. **Needle biopsy** may be used for distinct osseous lesions to obtain small amounts of tissue for culture or histology. **Excisional biopsy** may be used for benign lesions like exostoses or lipomas.

**Usual preop diagnosis**: Tumor; infection

### SUMMARY OF PROCEDURE

| | Incisional Biopsy | Needle Biopsy | Excisional Biopsy |
|---|---|---|---|
| **Position** | Supine | ⇐ | ⇐ |
| **Incision** | Short longitudinal | Stab wound | Over lesion |
| **Special instrumentation** | Bone-cutting instruments; x-ray or image intensifier | Trephine (e.g., Craig needle); x-ray or image intensifier | X-ray or image intensifier |
| **Unique considerations** | Tourniquet | ⇐ | ⇐ (Bone graft may be necessary. |
| **Antibiotics** | None (may be given postop) | ⇐ | ⇐ |
| **Surgical time** | 1 hr | 0.5 hr | 0.5 - 2 hrs |
| **Closing considerations** | May be splinted. | Usually no splint | May be splinted. |
| **EBL** | 50 cc | Minimal | 100-200 cc |
| **Postop care** | PACU → room or home | ⇐ | PACU → room |
| **Mortality** | Minimal | ⇐ | ⇐ |
| **Morbidity** | Hematoma: 5% | ⇐ | ⇐ |
| | Tumor spread: < 5% | ⇐ | ⇐ |
| | Infection: < 1% | ⇐ | ⇐ |
| **Procedure code** | 27607 (deep incision + opening of bone cortex)<br>27640 (partial excision [craterization, saucerization or diaphysectomy] of bone)<br>27641 (fibula)<br>28005 (deep incision + opening of bone cortex) | 20220 (bone biopsy, trocar or needle; superficial)<br>20225 (deep [vertebral body, femur]) | 20240 (excisional biopsy, superficial)<br>20245 (deep)<br>27635 (bone cyst or benign tumor, tibia or fibula)<br>28100 (bone cyst or benign tumor, talus or calcaneus)<br>28104 (bone cyst or benign tumor, other tarsal or metatarsal bones)<br>28108 (benign tumor, phalanges of foot) |
| **Pain score** | 3 | 2 | 3 |

### PATIENT POPULATION CHARACTERISTICS

| | |
|---|---|
| **Age range** | All ages |
| **Male:Female** | 1:1 |
| **Incidence** | Rare |
| **Etiology** | Tumor: 75%<br>Infection: 25% |
| **Associated conditions** | Metastatic disease<br>Immune compromise |

## ANESTHETIC CONSIDERATIONS

See Anesthetic Considerations following "Biopsy or Drainage of Abscess/Excision of Tumor" (below).

**References**

1. Enneking WF: *Musculoskeletal Tumor Surgery*. Churchill Livingstone, New York: 1983.

# BIOPSY OR DRAINAGE OF ABSCESS/EXCISION OF TUMOR

## SURGICAL CONSIDERATIONS

**Description**: This procedure involves obtaining a piece of tissue for histologic and/or bacteriologic diagnosis by closed, percutaneous means or by open biopsy. Subsequently, the area may be drained (abscess or infection) or an open excision of a tumor may follow (with or without internal fixation). For excision of tumors of the pelvis, acetabulum or femur, please consult the appropriate section describing fractures of the area. Each case must be individualized.

**Variant procedure or approaches**: Excision of infection or tumor of proximal or distal femur, femoral shaft, pelvis or acetabulum.

**Usual preop diagnosis**: Femur: biopsy of mass; infection; osteomyelitis. Pelvis or acetabulum: biopsy of pelvis or acetabulum; drainage of abscess or infection of pelvis or acetabulum; osteomyelitis of pelvis or acetabulum; septic arthritis of acetabulum

### SUMMARY OF PROCEDURE

| | |
|---|---|
| **Position** | Supine or lateral decubitus |
| **Incision** | Percutaneous, short or long; location depends on surgical approach. |
| **Special instrumentation** | Bx needles and instruments to take core Bx; bone cement may be used to plug Bx site. |
| **Unique considerations** | May require intraop frozen section and gram stain. Some surgeons use fracture table or radiolucent table with image intensifier. |
| **Antibiotics** | After tissue has been obtained, a broad-spectrum cephalosporin antibiotic (e.g., cefamandole 1 gm iv q 6 hrs x 48 hrs). A gram stain will help decide immediate antibiotic coverage, but cultures and sensitivities are ultimately necessary. |
| **Surgical time** | 1 hr for simple procedures; much longer (up to 12 hrs) for more extensive excisional procedures ± further reconstruction. |
| **EBL** | 100 cc - 1000 cc or more |
| **Postop care** | If procedure is extensive with much blood loss, or the patient is unstable or ill from chronic sepsis or invasive tumor, it is prudent to send patient to ICU. |
| **Mortality** | Dependent on extent of procedure. Bx or drainage of a small, localized abscess in soft tissue or bone is rarely life-threatening. Wide/radical excision of a malignant tumor in the pelvis or extremities is frequently life/limb-threatening. |
| | The following are dependent on site and procedure: |
| **Morbidity** | Intraop fracture<br>Nonunion<br>Chronic osteomyelitis<br>Hypotension 2° to blood loss<br>Respiratory distress<br>Neurological injury to peripheral nerves<br>Vascular injury<br>Compartment syndrome |

**Morbidity, continued**
Residual instability of pelvis or hip joint
Fracture of pelvis or acetabulum, nonunion
Chronic osteomyelitis or septic arthritis
Hypotension 2° to blood loss
Respiratory distress
Neurological injury to lumbosacral plexus, sciatic nerve or other peripheral nerves
Vascular injury to iliac or other vessels
Injury to GI, genitourinary or gynecological organs

**Procedure code** Multiple codes (e.g., 20000, 20005, 26990, 26991, 26992, 27040, 27041, 27047, 27048, 27049, 27070, 27071, 27075-9; 27301, 27303, 27323, 27324, 27327, 27328, 27329, 27360, 27365)

**Pain score** 2-10

### PATIENT POPULATION CHARACTERISTICS

**Age range** Any age; predominance of elderly patients with tumors

**Male:Female** 1:1

**Incidence** Rare

**Etiology**
Benign and malignant tumors: Common
Infection: Rare
Previous surgery: Rare
Previous trauma: Rare

**Associated conditions** Metastatic disease or other foci of infection

---

## ANESTHETIC CONSIDERATIONS FOR LOWER-EXTREMITY PROCEDURES

**(Procedures covered: ORIF femur; tibia; closed reduction and external fixation femur; tibia and intermedullary nailing of femur and tibia; distal tibial and ankle procedures; biopsy, leg and foot; biopsy or drainage of abbscess/excision of tumor)**

### PREOPERATIVE

Trauma victims comprise the largest group of patients for these procedures. Minimizing the time between fracture and surgery for open wounds significantly reduces the incidence of wound infection. Evaluations for other injury, adequacy of fluid resuscitation and pre-existing conditions need to be undertaken promptly and used as a guide for anesthetic management. Patients with bone cancer form another subset of patients and often have concurrent medical conditions and have undergone chemotherapy or radiation therapy preop.

**Respiratory** Pulmonary fat embolus occurs in 10-15% of patients following bone fracture. Sx include hypoxemia, ↑HR, tachypnea, respiratory alkalosis, mental status changes and conjunctival petechiae. Lab analysis may reveal fat in the urine. Preop therapy for this condition should include supplemental $O_2$ with mechanical ventilation, to correct hypoxemia, and meticulous fluid management to prevent worsening pulmonary capillary leak.

**Tests:** CXR; others as indicated from H&P.

**Cardiovascular** Cardiac contusion or tamponade are possible if blunt chest trauma has occurred during the injury. A large volume of blood can be hidden around a long bone fracture site. ↑HR, orthostasis or ↓BP indicate hypovolemia, and this should be corrected with crystalloid (10-40 ml/kg) or blood if Hct < 24%. In patients with a tibial or distal femur fracture, and who are presenting with hemodynamic instability and ongoing blood loss, consider applying a tourniquet to the thigh prior to induction.

**Tests:** ECG, CPK enzyme levels and ECHO will help evaluate the presence of cardiac injury.

**Neurological** Perform a thorough neurological evaluation, including mental status and peripheral sensory exams. A CT scan of the head is indicated for any patient with prolonged loss of consciousness prior to anesthesia. Drug abuse is common in trauma patients and they should be asked specifically about any drug use.

**Tests:** Patients with inappropriate behavior or a positive drug abuse Hx should undergo a urine and plasma drug screen.

| | |
|---|---|
| **Musculoskeletal** | Consider cervical instability and obtain spine films if mechanism of injury included rapid deceleration or trauma to the head or neck. Myoglobinemia and ↑$K^+$ may result from crush injury. |
| **Hematologic** | Patients with cancer who have undergone chemotherapy and multiple transfusions often develop sensitivities to blood products and may require specialized blood products such as leukocyte-poor PRBC or red cells negative for a particular antigen. The availability of these blood products should be confirmed prior to surgery.<br>**Tests:** Hct and others as indicated from H&P. |
| **Renal** | **Tests:** UA |
| **Laboratory** | Other tests as indicated from H&P. |
| **Premedication** | Due to the risk of gastric aspiration, minimal or no premedication is given to trauma victims. For other patients, diazepam 5-10 mg po 1 hr preop. Narcotic premedication (morphine 1-2 mg iv q 10 min titrated to effect) is appropriate for patients experiencing pain with movement. |

## INTRAOPERATIVE

**Anesthetic technique:** For trauma patients, regional anesthesia permits evaluation of mental status, provides intact airway reflexes and ↓blood loss. Combative patients, those requiring multiple concurrent surgical procedures or prolonged (>2 hr) procedures are often managed with GETA.

**Regional anesthesia:** Either subarachnoid or epidural blocks are useful techniques. Subarachnoid anesthesia has the advantage of adequate blockade of the sacral roots that are resistant to low-dose epidural techniques. Epidural anesthesia allows for the administration of postop epidural analgesia. Anesthesia from T12 (T8 with tourniquet) to S2 is adequate. Full motor blockade is desirable. Typical drugs and doses include: subarachnoid – 15 mg of 0.5% bupivacaine with morphine 0.2 mg (omit if outpatient); epidural – 12-15 cc 2% lidocaine with epinephrine 1:200,000 in divided doses (Na bicarbonate 0.1 mg/ml will speed onset of block).

**General anesthesia:**

| | |
|---|---|
| **Induction** | Standard induction (see Appendix) is appropriate for patients with normal airways. Trauma patients require a rapid-sequence induction and intubation with cricoid pressure to prevent gastric aspiration. |
| **Maintenance** | Standard maintenance (see Appendix). Trauma patients are often cold and require active warming if < 35°C (convection blanket and active humidifier). Warming the patient may unmask severe hypovolemia that should be corrected. |
| **Emergence** | Trauma patients should have full return of protective airway reflexes and, given the possibility of fat embolus, evidence of adequate oxygenation on 50% $O_2$ prior to extubation. |

| | | |
|---|---|---|
| **Blood and fluid requirements** | IV: 14-16 ga x 2<br>NS/LR @ 4-8 cc/kg/hr<br>Warm fluids.<br>Humidify gasses. | Some fractures can involve large (30 cc/kg) blood losses that are hidden in the leg or thigh. Clinical signs of hypovolemia and serial Hct determination should guide fluid therapy. |
| **Control of blood loss** | Tourniquet | Inflation pressure is typically 100 mmHg greater than systolic pressure. Maximum "safe" tourniquet time is 1.5-2 hr, followed by a 5-to-(preferably) 15-min reperfusion interval, if further tourniquet time is necessary. |
| **Monitoring** | Standard monitors (see Appendix).<br>± Arterial line<br>± CVP line | Arterial and CVP lines are indicated for patients with ↓BP not readily correctable with crystalloid infusion, massive blood loss (>1 blood volume) or the need for postop ventilation. |
| **Positioning** | ✓ and pad pressure points.<br>✓ eyes. | |
| **Special considerations** | Release of tourniquet | A 20% fall in mean BP is common on tourniquet deflation. Additional crystalloid (5-10 cc/kg) may be necessary to replace edema fluid and blood loss to the leg. |
| **Complications** | Fat embolism<br>Myoglobinemia | |

## POSTOPERATIVE

| | | |
|---|---|---|
| **Complications** | Hypoxemia | May be 2° fat embolism. |
| **Pain management** | Spinal opiates:<br>Epidural anesthesia<br>Spinal anesthesia | Epidural hydromorphone 50 μg/cc infused at 100-250 μg/hr provides excellent analgesia. Intrathecal morphine 0.2-0.3 mg provides analgesia for up to 24 hrs after administration. (Monitor for delayed respiratory depression.) |
| **Tests** | Hct<br>CXR, if CVP placed or oxygenation is impaired. | Other studies as indicated. |

### References


1. Wilkins RM, Winter WG: Complications of treatment of fractures and dislocations of the hip. In *Complications in Orthopaedic Surgery*. Epps CH Jr, ed. JB Lippincott, Philadelphia: 1986, 469-511.
2. Carnesale PG: Infections. In *Campbell's Operative Orthopaedics*. Crenshaw AH, ed. CV Mosby, St. Louis: 1987, Vol 1, 649-709.
3. Carnesale PG: General principles of tumors. In *Campbell's Operative Orthopaedics*. Crenshaw AH, ed. CV Mosby, St. Louis: 1987, Vol 2, 713-46.

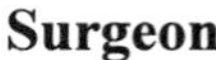

**Surgeon**

**Eugene J. Carragee, MD**

---

## 10.4 SPINE SURGERY

---

# ANTERIOR SPINAL RECONSTRUCTION AND FUSION - THORACIC AND THORACOLUMBAR SPINE

## SURGICAL CONSIDERATIONS

**Description**: Most spinal procedures have traditionally been approached posteriorly. The advent of surgical treatment for vertebral TB and post-polio spinal deformities during the 1960s saw the development of surgical approaches to the anterior spine.[1] Initially, these procedures were reserved for patients with significant deformities, especially kyphosis. More recently, the treatment of traumatic, neoplastic and degenerative conditions have been included in the anterior approach. Regardless of the condition under treatment, the approach is similar for a given level. There are several more or less distinct types of surgical exposures, depending on the level.

**Cervicothoracic approach:** Most cephalad and difficult is the approach to the upper thoracic spine (T1-T3). This generally includes a modified anterior cervical exposure with a caudal extension, including a resection of the clavicle, part of the manubrium and sometimes the rib at the thoracic outlet. Dangers in this exposure are to the great vessels at the thoracic outlet, trachea (rare) and esophagus (more common), lung parenchyma, sympathetic ganglia, lymphatic duct (on the left) and brachial plexus. Once the spine is exposed and the discs and/or vertebrae are removed, the spinal cord is at risk. This procedure involves entering the thoracic cavity, in which case it is usually done intrapleurally – that is, through the parietal pleura. The lung needs to be collapsed at least partially. Spinal cord monitoring is usually performed; wake-up tests are not.

**Transthoracic approach:** Further down the spine, the levels from T5-T10 are more easily reached via a transthoracic approach. This involves a typical thoracotomy with the resection of a rib. The level of the rib resection is usually 1-2 levels above the highest vertebral level being approached. The great vessels and lung parenchyma are at risk, as is the thoracic duct (on the left) (Fig 10.4-1). The patient is in the lateral decubitus position and the mediastinum and heart usually fall to the opposite side, out of harm's way. Risk to the spinal cord depends on the difficulty and extent of the vertebral disease and the reconstruction. Spinal cord monitoring usually is performed intraop. The need for the lung to be deflated varies with the extent of the exposure. In centers where this procedure is frequently performed and the surgeons are accustomed to the respiratory motion during operation, DLTs are not routinely used. Since there is no (intended) violation of the lung parenchyma, air leaks and parenchymal repairs are not common.

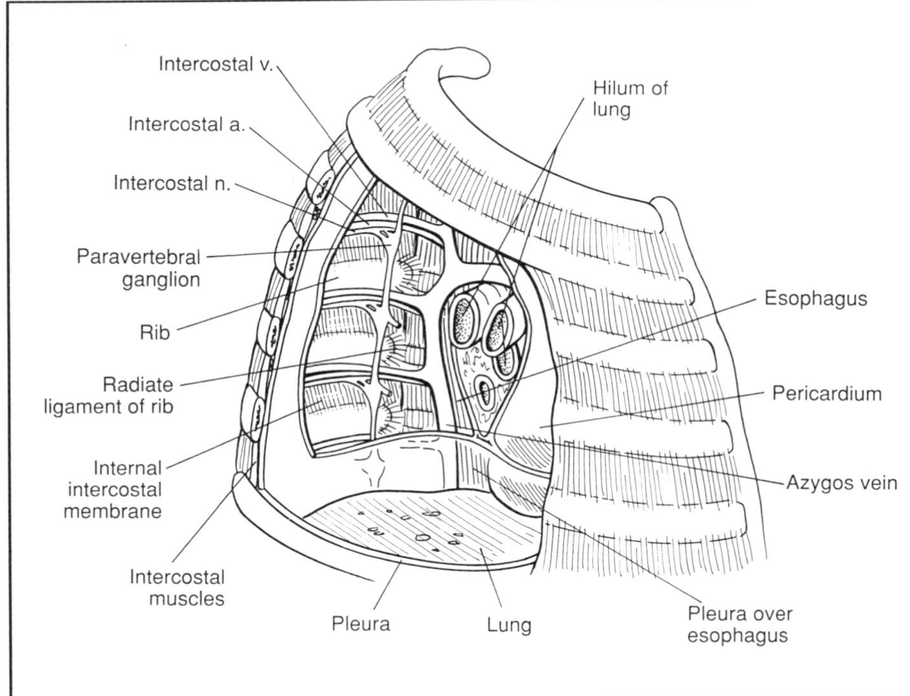


**Figure 10.4-1.** Surgical anatomy of the transthoracic approach. (Reproduced with permission from Hoppenfeld S, deBoer P: *Surgical Exposures in Orthopaedics*. JB Lippincott: 1984.)

**Transdiaphragmatic approach:** When the exposure must transverse the diaphragm, a combined retroperitoneal and transthoracic approach is used. This requires the diaphragm to be sectioned circumferentially from the chest wall and spine. If only the very low segments of the thoracic spine (T10-T12) are exposed, the required deflation of the involved lung is minimal. The risks are the same as those encountered with the transthoracic or retroperitoneal approaches alone. Regardless of the level of exposure, the operating table is normally used during the procedure to manipulate the spine for better exposure and to "lock in" implants, bone grafts, etc. Usually, the area of the spine to be exposed is centered above the "breaking" joint and kidney rests of the table (Fig 10.4-2). After the initial exposure, the table is angled in the center with the head and legs pointing down and kidney rests elevated to "open up" the section of spine facing the surgeon. After removal of the disk, abscess or tumor, a reconstruction – using bone graft, metal implants, bone cement, or a combination of these – is performed. The operating table is straightened and, with the spine in neutral alignment, the stability of the reconstruction is tested. This maneuver may need to be repeated several times.

The **morbidity** of these procedures depends primarily on the nature of the underlying disease. Obviously, bleeding and visceral injury is more likely when debriding a grapefruit-sized Potts abscess with several destroyed vertebrae than in removing a degenerated lumbar disk for fusion.

In some instances, the anterior procedure may be followed with a posterior fusion, either immediately or after 5-7 days' convalescence. If done immediately after, the patient needs to be repositioned prone, and the second procedure done through a midline exposure. Sometimes anterior and posterior surgery are performed simultaneously by two surgical teams. The most common reason for a staged anterior/posterior procedure (in the U. S.) is scoliosis; however, fracture at the thoracolumbar junction, after anterior decompression and reconstruction, are often instrumented and fused posteriorly.

**Usual preop diagnosis**: Fractures (usually at thoracic lumbar junction); idiopathic scoliosis; primary neoplasm or metastatic disease to the spine; pyogenic or TB osteomyelitis of the spine; Scheuermann's kyphosis

**SUMMARY OF PROCEDURE**

| | **Cervicothoracic Approach** | **Transthoracic Approach** | **Transdiaphragmatic Approach** |
|---|---|---|---|
| **Position** | Supine; towel roll placed between shoulder blades, head slightly extended and turned away from operated side | Lateral decubitus; intended segments over the table break and kidney rests; axillary roll (Fig 10.4-2) | ⇐ |
| **Incision** | Inverted "L" longitudinally along manubrium to sternal notch, then transversely above clavicle | Along a rib 2 levels above the highest segment to be exposed | ⇐ |
| **Special instrumentation** | Instrumentation rarely used. Strut grafts, using rib, fibula, clavicle or cement, may be used to replace excised vertebrae. | For thoracolumbar scoliosis, a Zielke-type rod and screws may be used; more rigid instrumentation sometimes used in fractures. | ⇐ More common to use instrumentation at the affected level than above. |
| **Unique considerations** | Difficulty and dangers of exposure to vessels and viscera (described above); postop respiratory distress well-described | In performing spinal reconstruction, manipulation of operating table is essential to "lock in" graft or implant (see above). | ⇐ |
| **Antibiotics** | Cefazolin 1 gm iv (+ gentamicin 80 mg iv, if indwelling bladder catheter) | ⇐ | ⇐ |
| **Surgical time** | 2 - 6 hrs | ⇐ | ⇐ |
| **Closing considerations** | Patient usually transferred to bed prior to being aroused; sudden jerking motions may dislodge graft or implant. | ⇐ | ⇐ |
| **EBL** | 200-5000 cc; blood loss is extremely variable; when bleeding occurs, it may be torrential from the aorta, vena cava or iliac vessels and branches. In non-tumor or infection cases, 200-400 cc is usual. | ⇐ | ⇐ |

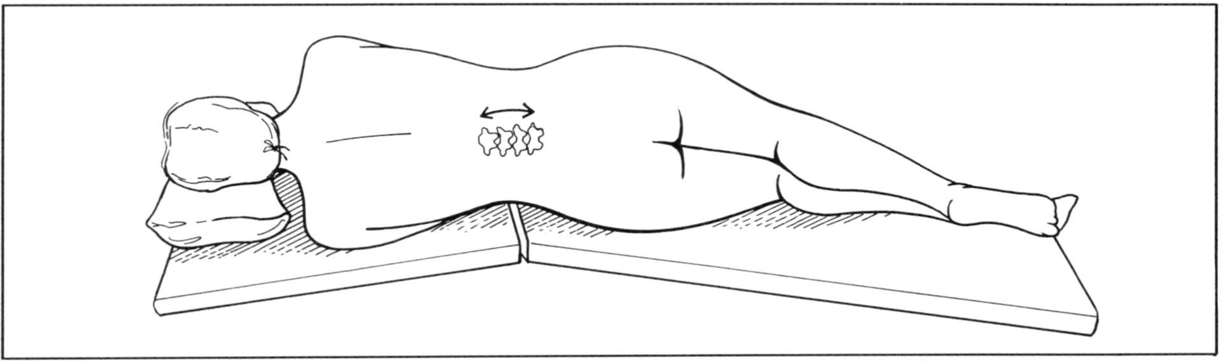

**Figure 10.4-2.** Patient position for transdiaphragmatic or retroperitoneal approach. (Reproduced with permission from Hoppenfeld S, deBoer P: *Surgical Exposures in Orthopaedics*. JB Lippincott: 1984.)

| | Cervicothoracic Approach | Transthoracic Approach | Transdiaphragmatic |
|---|---|---|---|
| **Postop care** | Chest drain, NG suction usually needed; short period of ICU observation is usual. | ⇐ | ⇐ |
| **Mortality** | < 0.1%, except in cases of malignancy or sepsis | ⇐ | ⇐ |
| **Morbidity** | For elective degenerative cases: 5-10% overall | ⇐ | ⇐ |
| | DVT: 6% | ⇐ | ⇐ |
| | Neurological: 3% | ⇐ | ⇐ |
| | Infection: 1% | ⇐ | ⇐ |
| | Sexual dysfunction | ⇐ | ⇐ |
| | For sepsis or tumor: 50-80% (overall) | ⇐ | ⇐ |
| | Cardiorespiratory failure | ⇐ | ⇐ |
| | Sepsis | ⇐ | ⇐ |
| **Procedure code** | 22141, 63085-22 | 22141, 63085 | 22141, 63087 |
| **Pain score** | 7-8 (if patient sensate at level of surgery) | ⇐ | ⇐ |

### PATIENT POPULATION CHARACTERISTICS

| | |
|---|---|
| **Age range** | 12-30 yr (scoliosis surgery); >40 (tumor and infection surgery) |
| **Male:Female** | 1:1, except more scoliosis surgery in females |
| **Incidence** | 20,000/yr |
| **Etiology** | Scoliosis, idiopathic: 50%<br>Trauma: 20%<br>Scoliosis, neuromuscular: 15%<br>Infections, tumors: 10%<br>Scoliosis, congenital: 5% |
| **Associated conditions** | Same as above |

## ANESTHETIC CONSIDERATIONS

See "Anesthetic Considerations for Spinal Reconstruction and Fusion" in "Pediatric Orthopedic Surgery."

## References


1. Hodgson AR, Stock FE, Fang HSY et al: Anterior spinal fusion: the operative approach and pathological finding in 412 patients with Potts disease of the spine. *Br J Surg* 1980; 48:172-86.
2. Emery SE, Chan DP, Woodward HR: Treatment of hematogenous pyogenic vertebral osteomyelitis with anterior debridement and primary bone grafting. *Spine* 1989; 14(3):284-91.
3. Hoppenfeld S, deBoer P: *Surgical Exposures in Orthopaedics*. JB Lippincott, Philadelphia:1984, 209-301.
4. Kostuik JP, Carl A, Ferron S: Anterior Zielke instrumentation for spinal deformity in adults. *J Bone Joint Surg* [Am] 1989; 71(6):898-906.
5. Kurz LT, Pursel SE, Herkowitz HN: Modified anterior approach to the cervicothoracic junction. *Spine* 1991; 16(10 Suppl):S542-47.
6. Sundaresan N, Shah J, Feghali JG: A transsternal approach to the upper thoracic vertebrae. *Am J Surg* 1984; 148(4):473-77.


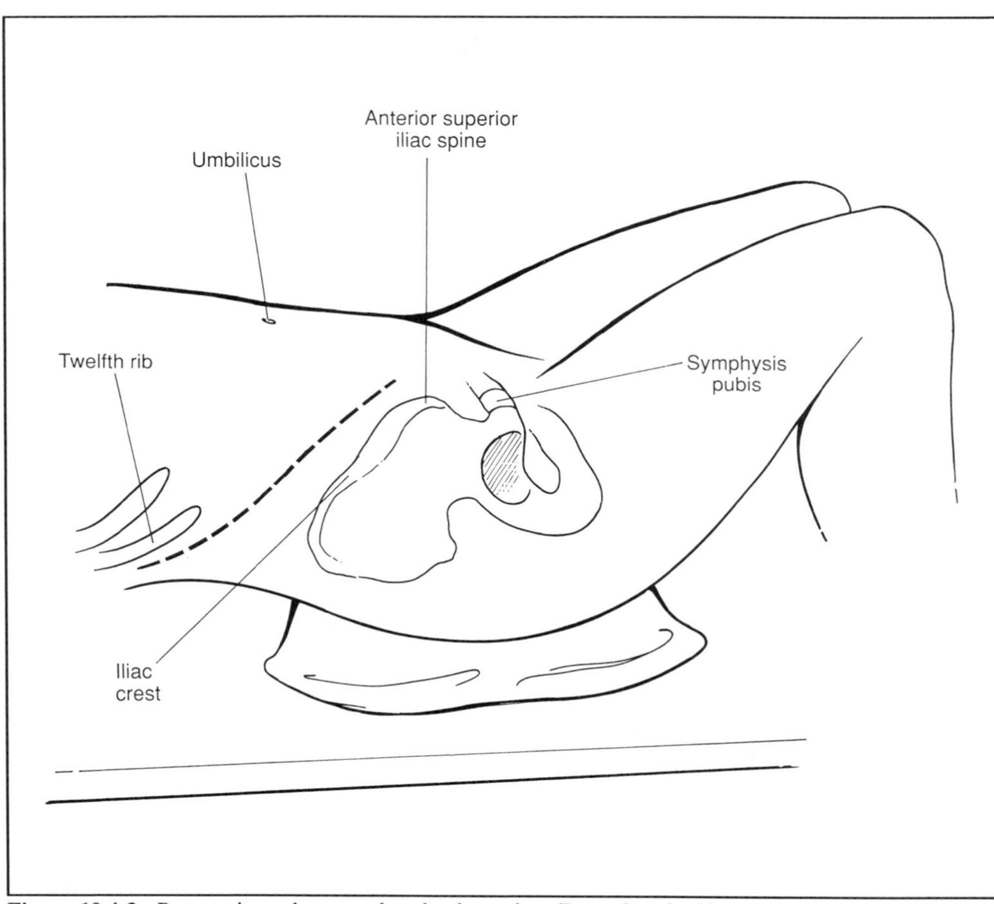


**Figure 10.4-3.** Retroperitoneal approach to lumbar spine. (Reproduced with permission from Hoppenfeld S, deBoer P: *Surgical Exposures in Orthopaedics*. JB Lippincott: 1984.)

# ANTERIOR SPINAL RECONSTRUCTION AND FUSION – LUMBOSACRAL SPINE

## SURGICAL CONSIDERATIONS

**Description**: The same general considerations apply here as in thoracolumbar reconstruction segments. The thoracic cavity is not entered, nor is the diaphragm sectioned. Careful preop assessment is needed, as these patients vary greatly in morbidity. The same operative procedure is performed for removal of a degenerative disk in a healthy patient as is carried out to decompress the caudae equina in a debilitated patient with metastatic breast carcinoma.

**Retroperitoneal approach**: Below the diaphragm, exposure of the lumbar spine L2-S1 can be performed through a retroperitoneal approach (Fig 10.4-3). This involves a flank incision, often with resection of the 11th or 12th rib. The patient lies in a decubitus or partial decubitus position. At risk here are the great vessels above and below the bifurcation of the aorta (L4-L5). The ureter crosses the operative field and must be identified and protected. The sympathetic chain may be damaged along the vertebra, but the consequences of this are minimal. The pre-sacral plexus further down may be injured and result in persistent retrograde ejaculation.

Regardless of the level of exposure, the operating table normally is used during the procedure to manipulate the spine for better exposure and to "lock in" implants, bone grafts, etc. Usually the area of the spine to be exposed is centered above the "breaking" joint and kidney rests of the table (Fig 10.4-2). After initial exposure, the table is angled in the center with the head and legs pointing down and the kidney rests elevated to "open up" the section of spine facing the surgeon. After the removal of the disk, abscess or tumor, a reconstruction – using bone graft, metal implants, bone cement, or a combination of these – is performed. The table is then straightened; and with the spine in neutral alignment, the stability of the reconstruction is tested by this maneuver, which may need to be repeated several times.

In some instances, the anterior reconstruction and fusion is followed with a **posterior fusion**, either immediately or after 5-7 days' convalescence. If done immediately after, the patient needs to be positioned prone on the operating table, and the second procedure done through a midline exposure. Sometimes anterior and posterior surgeries can be performed simultaneously by two surgical teams. The most common reason for a staged anterior/posterior procedure (in the U. S.) is scoliosis. Recent trends in degenerative lumbar disk surgery indicate that anterior and posterior fusions are becoming more common, with some evidence suggesting better results in fusion and pain relief.

**Variant procedure or approaches**: When the L5 vertebra and sacrum need to be widely exposed, a **transperitoneal approach** may be needed. This involves a laparotomy or Pfannenstiel's incision, displacement of the bowels out of the pelvis and exposure of the lumbosacral junction (Figs 10.4-4). The patient is supine for this procedure and the surgical risks are similar, as with other intra-abdominal approaches.[1]

**Usual preop diagnosis**: Degenerative disc disease; segmental instability,[2,3] vertebral fractures requiring decompression; vertebral osteomyelitis or tuberculosis,[4,5] neoplastic disease of the lumbar spine.[1]

### SUMMARY OF PROCEDURE

| | Retroperitoneal Approach | Transperitoneal Approach |
|---|---|---|
| **Position** | Lateral decubitus, affected side up. The up hip and knee are flexed to relax psoas muscle and allow its reflection to expose the lumbar vertebral bodies. | Supine |
| **Incision** | Flank incision curving anteriorly to the lateral margin of the rectus abdomenus (Fig 10.4-3) | Pfannenstiel above the pubis |
| **Special instrumentation** | Occasional use of anterior instrumentation to stabilize fractures or to reconstruct the spine when entire vertebrae are removed. | ⇐ |
| **Unique considerations** | In performing spinal reconstruction, manipulation of operating table is essential to "lock in" graft or implant (see above). | ⇐ + A general bowel prep usually is performed preop. |
| **Antibiotics** | Cefazolin 1 gm iv (+ gentamicin 80 mg iv, if indwelling bladder catheter already in place); exception is when infection is suspected and specific cultures are obtained intraop. | ⇐ |

| | Retroperitoneal Approach | Transperitoneal Approach |
|---|---|---|
| **Surgical time** | 3 - 6 hrs | ⇐ |
| **Closing considerations** | The spine may be more or less stable after reconstruction, and patient usually transferred to bed prior to being awakened. Sudden jerking motions, etc., may dislodge graft or implant. | ⇐ |
| **EBL** | 200-5000 cc. Blood loss is extremely variable. When bleeding occurs, it may be torrential from the aorta, vena cava or iliac vessels and branches. In non-tumor/infection cases, 200-400 cc is usual. | ⇐ |
| **Postop care** | Patients with degenerative conditions and elective surgeries normally recover in PAR and return to ward. Patients with infections, fractures and tumors are usually observed in ICU for 24 hrs postop. Ileus for 24-72 hrs is usual; NG suction usually continues until bowel sounds and passing flatus are present. Generally, mobilization depends on final stability. | ⇐ |
| **Mortality** | Malignancy or sepsis: 1-2% | ⇐ |
| | Elective: < 0.1% | ⇐ |
| **Morbidity** | In patients with malignancy, sepsis or fractures with caudae equinae compression, overall serious complications: 25-50% | ⇐ |
| | Cardiopulmonary failure | ⇐ |
| | Sepsis | ⇐ |
| **Procedure code** | 63090, 63091, 22142, 22148 | ⇐ |
| **Pain score** | 6 | 6 |

### PATIENT POPULATION CHARACTERISTICS

| | |
|---|---|
| **Age range** | Variable (infant-adult) |
| **Male:Female** | 1:1, except more scoliosis surgery in females |
| **Incidence** | Uncommon |
| **Etiology** | Infection |
| | Trauma |
| | Congenital neoplasia |

## ANESTHETIC CONSIDERATIONS

See "Anesthetic Considerations for Spinal Reconstruction and Fusion" in "Pediatric Orthopedic Surgery."

### References

1. Hoppenfeld S, deBoer P: *Surgical Exposures in Orthopaedics*. JB Lippincott, Philadelphia: 1984, 209-301.
2. Kozak JA and O'Brien JP: Simultaneous combined anterior and posterior fusion. An independent analysis of a treatment for the disabled low-back pain patient. *Spine* 1990; 15(4):322-28.
3. Leong JCY: Anterior interbody fusion. In *Lumbar Interbody Fusion*. Lin PM and Gill K, eds. Aspen Pub, Rockville: 1989, 133-47.
4. Emery SE, Chan DK, Woodward HR: Vertebral osteomyelitis. *Spine* 1989; 14:284-91.
5. Hodgson AR, Stock FE, Fang HSY et al: Anterior spinal fusion: the operative approach and pathological finding in 412 patients with Potts disease of the spine. *Br J Surg* 1980; 48:172-86.
6. Kostuik JP, Carl A, Ferron S: Anterior Zielke instrumentation for spinal deformity in adults. *J Bone Joint Surgery* [Am] 1989; 71(6):898-906.

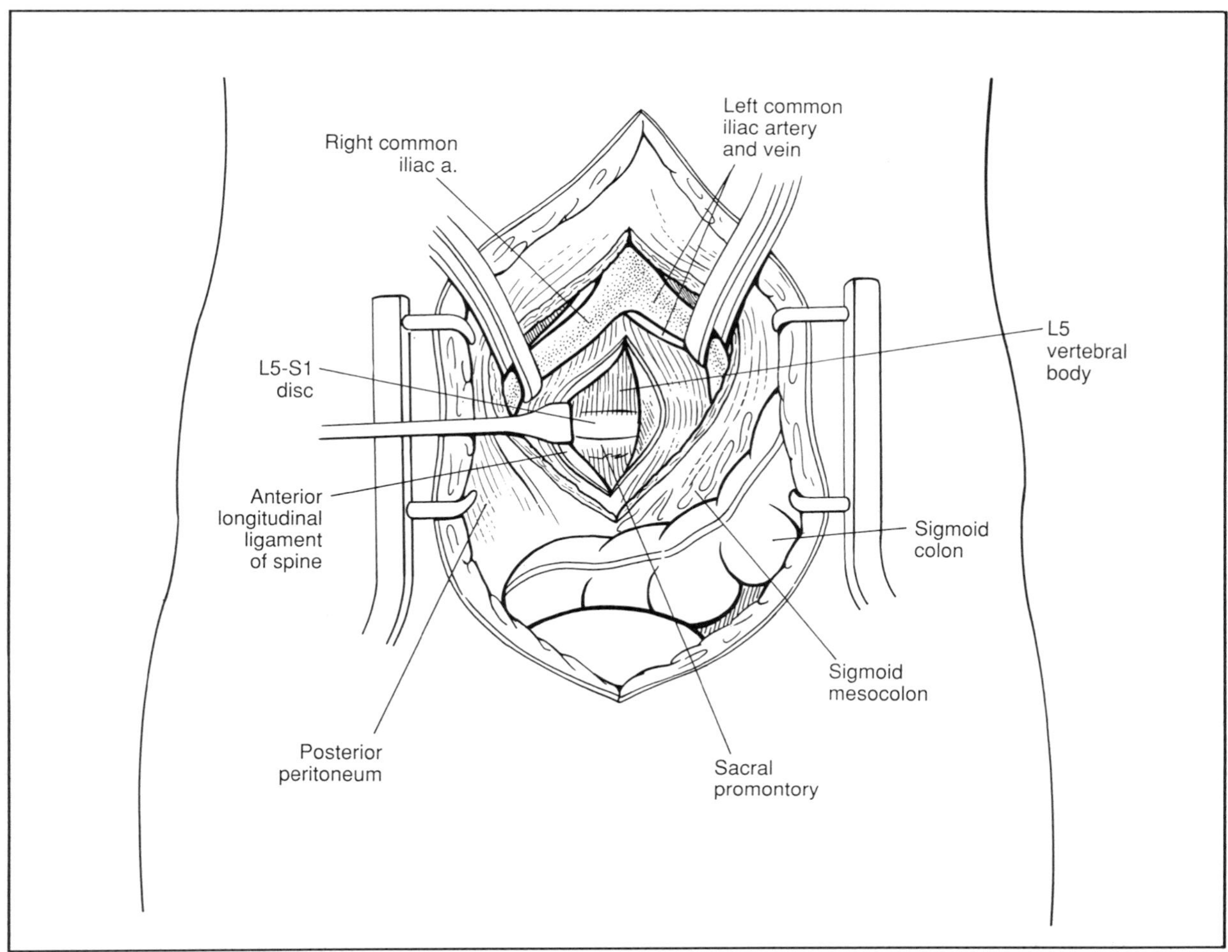


**Figure 10.4-4.** Transperitoneal approach to lumbosacral junction. (Reproduced with permission from Hoppenfeld S, deBoer P: *Surgical Exposures in Orthopaedics*. JB Lippincott: 1984.)

**Surgeons**

**Lars M. Vistnes, MD, FRCS(C)** *(Aesthetic Surgery)*
**Barry Press, MD, FACS** *(Burn Surgery)*
**Stephen A. Schendel, MD, DDS** *(Congenital Malformation, Restorative Surgery)*

---

# 11. RECONSTRUCTIVE SURGERY

---

**Anesthesiologists**

**Rona G. Giffard, MD, PhD** *(Aesthetic, Burn Surgery)*
**Yuan-Chi Lin, MD, MPH** *(Congenital Malformation Surgery)*
**Stanley I. Samuels, MB, BCh, FFARCS** *(Restorative Surgery)*
**Richard A. Jaffe, MD, PhD** (Restorative Surgery)

**Surgeon**

**Lars M. Vistnes, MD, FRCS(C)**

---

# 11.1 AESTHETIC SURGERY

---

**Anesthesiologist**

**Rona G. Giffard, MD, PhD**

# ABDOMINOPLASTY

## SURGICAL CONSIDERATIONS

**Description:** **Abdominoplasty** is most commonly performed for true abdominal skin and wall laxity. Such laxity is often found in conjunction with a diastasis of the recti muscles and a partial herniation of abdominal contents into the abdominal wall through this diastasis. The procedure is often performed in combination with abdominal **liposuction** to get rid of excess fat in the panniculus adiposis found in both men and women. Abdominoplasty is less commonly performed than it was prior to the advent of liposuction (approximately a decade ago).

It is performed through an incision made just above the pubic hairline, and extended bilaterally to the area of both anterior and superior iliac spines. The operation involves total undermining of the flap that is raised at the level of the abdominal wall musculature, extending as far up as the costal margin on both sides. Then the excess skin is pulled down and resected, which usually requires the placement of the umbilicus at a new site in the abdominal wall. In the case of morbidly obese persons undergoing abdominoplasty, the procedure is essentially as described above, but consists more of a **wedge resection** of skin and fat with minimal-to-no amount of undermining. The individual who has had liposuction is usually up and about with a girdle and quite comfortable within 24-48 hours, whereas the abdominoplasty patient who has suction drains and a very tight closure usually ambulates with some difficulty for the first 7-10 days after surgery.

**Usual preop diagnosis:** Abdominal laxity; rectus diastasis

### SUMMARY OF PROCEDURE

| | Abdominoplasty | Liposuction |
|---|---|---|
| **Position** | Supine | ⇐ |
| **Incision** | Extended Pfannenstiel; periumbilical | Periumbilical; suprapubic |
| **Special instrumentation** | Soft tissue | Suction device |
| **Unique considerations** | Must be able to flex table to facilitate closure. | ⇐ |
| **Antibiotics** | Cefazolin 1 gm iv intraop | ⇐ |
| **Surgical time** | 2.5 hrs | < 2.5 hrs |
| **Closing considerations** | Flex table | ⇐ |
| **EBL** | 200-600 cc; greater in morbidly obese | ⇐ |
| **Postop care** | Pillows under knees; head of bed raised to maintain flexed position. | ⇐ |
| **Mortality** | 0-1% | ⇐ |
| **Morbidity** | Ileus: 10% | ⇐ |
| | Infection: 2-3% | ⇐ |
| | Dehiscence: 1% | ⇐ |
| | Fat embolism: 1% | ⇐ |
| **Procedure code** | 15877 | ⇐ |
| **Pain score** | 4-6 | 2-4 |

### PATIENT POPULATION CHARACTERISTICS

| | |
|---|---|
| **Age range** | 30-55 yrs |
| **Male:Female** | 1:5 |
| **Incidence** | 10,000+/yr (This procedure is one of the most commonly performed of all plastic surgical operations.) |
| **Etiology** | Overeating |
| **Associated conditions** | Morbid obesity |

## ANESTHETIC CONSIDERATIONS

### PREOPERATIVE

Typically, there are two patient populations for abdominoplasty: the generally healthy, and the morbidly obese. Many have a history of amphetamine, cocaine or thyroid hormone abuse.[2] For the healthy patient, liposuction may be done on an outpatient basis; for the obese, however, it should be done only as an inpatient procedure. The following considerations focus on the morbidly obese patient (body weight [kg] ≥ 2 x ideal weight. Ideal body weight [kg] is estimated by subtracting 100 [male] or 105 [female] from height in cm).

**Respiratory** In the morbidly obese patient, findings include[3]: ↑$O_2$ consumption, ↑$CO_2$ production, restrictive lung disease, ↓FRC, ↓ERV, ↓VC, ↓IC, and ↓$PaO_2$. These changes are exacerbated by the supine position. Younger patients may show alveolar hyperventilation in response to hypoxemia; older patients may not and may retain $CO_2$. Patients may have obesity hypoventilation syndrome (Pickwickian syndrome): intermittent airway obstruction, hypoxemia and hypercarbia during sleep. Obese patients are at increased risk of pulmonary aspiration due to increased incidence of hiatal hernia and gastroesophageal reflux, and increased gastric volumes (>25 cc with pH < 2.5 in >75%). See Premedication (below) for aspiration prophylaxis.

**Tests:** CXR; room-air ABG and PFT (helpful, but generally do not predict postop complications, e.g., atelectasis, pneumonia).

**Cardiovascular** ↑CO and ↑blood volume → LVH. Chronic hypoxia and pulmonary compromise may produce right heart failure, severely decreased exercise tolerance, increased risk of CAD. Patient with LVH may have ↑dysrhythmias.

**Tests:** ECG (↑HR, conduction abnormalities, LVH); CXR (cardiomegaly)

**Metabolic** Increased incidence of diabetes, hypercholesterolemia, hypertriglyceridemia, liver abnormalities; ↓plasma folate, $B_{12}$; ↑incidence of cholelithiasis, nephrolithiasis. Determine whether electrolyte abnormalities are present in patient S/P ileojejunal bypass.

**Tests:** LFTs; electrolytes; glucose

**Hematologic** Polycythemia suggests chronic hypoxemia (see Respiratory, above).

**Tests:** Hb/Hct and coagulation studies.

**Laboratory** Other tests as indicated from H&P.

**Premedication** Sedative premedication is avoided in the morbidly obese due to their pulmonary compromise. Aspiration prophylaxis is essential: ranitidine 100 mg po or iv the evening before, and 60-90 min before surgery, plus non-particulate antacids (Na citrate 0.3 M, 30 cc po) pre-induction. Additionally, metoclopramide 10 mg iv may be given, although it has not been shown to be more effective in combination with an $H_2$-blocker than the $H_2$-blocker alone. For the healthy outpatient, midazolam 1-2 mg iv immediately preop may lessen anxiety.

### INTRAOPERATIVE

**Anesthetic technique:** GETA. Morbidly obese patients may not tolerate the supine position for an extended period of time.

**Induction** Standard induction (see Appendix) for healthy patients. Special considerations for the morbidly obese include prophylaxis for aspiration (see above), followed by rapid-sequence induction. If mandibular and cervical mobility are decreased by excessive soft tissue, plan awake fiber optic intubation; anticipate rapid $O_2$ desaturation during periods of hypoventilation, even with adequate preoxygenation.

**Maintenance** Standard maintenance (see Appendix). In the obese, increased plasma fluoride concentrations are found after anesthesia with halothane and enflurane; controlled ventilation with large TV and high inspired $O_2$ concentration is recommended. Since epinephrine infiltration is generally used to decrease blood loss, isoflurane is recommended as the least dysrhythmogenic of the inhalation agents in the presence of epinephrine. **NB:** Midazolam has a prolonged half-life in obese patients, but awakening times from inhalational or narcotic-based anesthetics are comparable to those of non-obese patients.

**Emergence** Smooth emergence with minimal bucking, coughing or retching to minimize tension on the suture line; give anti-emetics (metoclopramide 10 mg or droperidol 1 mg iv) 1 hr before conclusion of surgery. Maintenance of flexed position will minimize tension on suture line. Small additional doses of narcotic (e.g., meperidine 10 mg) may be titrated to RR if patient is allowed to resume spontaneous respiration before the end of the case.

| | | |
|---|---|---|
| **Blood and fluid requirements** | Moderate blood loss<br>IV: 16-18 ga x 1<br>NS/LR @ 6-10 cc/kg/hr | For liposuction, blood loss is generally estimated at 25-30% of the aspirate volume,[4] but the observed range is large. Aspirate volumes up to 1000-2000 cc are generally tolerated with no need of transfusion. Replace with crystalloid @ 1:3. Blood loss is decreased by local infiltration with dilute solutions of epinephrine prior to liposuction, and is also limited by staging the procedure. Patients may donate autologous blood. Prompt application of pressure garments to the area is recommended. |
| **Monitoring** | Standard monitors (see Appendix).<br>± Arterial line<br>± CVP line | Additional monitoring for the morbidly obese patient may include arterial and CVP lines. |
| **Positioning** | Flexed position<br>Pillows under knees<br>✓ and pad pressure points.<br>✓ eyes. | Flexed position minimizes tension on suture line. Morbidly obese may require 2 OR tables side-by-side. Supine position may be poorly tolerated; monitor ventilation closely. |
| **Complications** | Fat emboli | Micro fat emboli are common during liposuction. |

## POSTOPERATIVE

| | | |
|---|---|---|
| **Complications** | Patients may have postop ileus of 1-2 d duration. | The morbidly obese should not be outpatients; they have an increased incidence of wound infection, DVT, PE and postop pulmonary complications. They generally should receive supplemental $O_2$ for the first 2 d postop. Keep patient in semi-sitting or flexed position to avoid undue stress on wound. |
| **Pain management** | Depending on extent of surgery and whether or not it is inpatient, epidural narcotics or PCA may be used (see Appendix). | |
| **Tests** | Pulse oximetry | Maximum reduction of arterial saturation may occur on postop day 2-3.[5] |

**References**


1. Vistnes, LM: *Procedures in Plastic and Reconstructive Surgery: How They do it.* Little, Brown, Boston: 1991.
2. Klein JA: Anesthesia for liposuction in dermatologic surgery. *J Dermatol Surg Oncol* 1988; 14(10):1124-32.
3. Cooper JR, Brodsky JB: Anesthetic management of the morbidly obese patient. *Seminars in Anesthesia* 1987; Vol VI: 260-70.
4. Goodpasture JC, Bunkis J: Quantitative analysis of blood and fat in suction lipectomy aspirates. *Plast Reconstr Surg* 1986; 78(6):765-69.
5. Vaughan RW, Wise L: Postoperative arterial blood gas measurements in obese patients: effects of position on gas exchange. *Ann Surg* 1975; 182(6):705-9.

# MAMMOPLASTY

## SURGICAL CONSIDERATIONS

**Description:** There are at least four patient population categories for mammoplasty: those presenting for breast augmentation, breast lift or reduction mammoplasty and those presenting for reconstruction of breast, usually following cancer surgery.

**Augmentation mammoplasty**, by definition, is an operation in which the skin and mammary tissues are augmented by the placement of a prosthesis. The most commonly used prosthesis at the present time is a saline-filled silicone prosthesis. Placement of the prosthesis may be above or below the pectoralis muscle, depending on surgeon's choice and amount of tissue available. The operation can be done under local anesthesia or GA.

**Breast lift**: There is usually enough ptosis of the breast that it is necessary to replace the ptotic breast tissue at a higher level. This requires resection of the skin and placement of a nipple areolar complex at a higher level on the chest wall. It may be combined with a modest augmentation – i.e., placement of a prosthesis above or below the pectoralis major muscle – at the same time. This is a more extensive operation than augmentation mammoplasty and requires more time.

**Breast reduction**: Depending on the size of the breast to be reduced, the amount of tissue removed from each breast may be anywhere from 200-1000 gm. The nipple is usually transplanted to a higher site, based on an inferior pedicle of dermis and breast tissue. If the reduction is in the 1000-gm range, however, the nipple is usually transplanted as a free graft.

**Breast reconstruction**: Done in three basic ways: (1) Reconstruction using tissue expansion, with the eventual placement of a breast implant. (2) Use of a breast implant and augmentation by local flaps, such as a latissimus dorsi musculocutaneous flap, in order to make up for tissue lost at the time of the surgery. (3) Use of total autogenous tissue, usually with a transverse rectus abdominis muscle (TRAM) flap. In this procedure, a wedge of abdominal wall skin and subcutaneous tissue is moved on its blood supply of one or both of the recti muscles to the new site on the chest wall, fashioned in such a way as to construct a new breast. This is the longest and most complicated procedure. In some situations it can be done as a free (microsurgical) flap. All three procedures are discussed in more detail in "Breast/Chest Wall Reconstruction" in "Restorative Surgery" section.

**Usual preop diagnosis**: Hypomastia; hypermastia; breast ptosis; S/P mastectomy

**SUMMARY OF PROCEDURE**

| | Breast Augmentation | Breast Lift | Reduction Mammoplasty | Reconstruction Of Breast |
|---|---|---|---|---|
| **Position** | Supine | ⇐ | ⇐ | ⇐ |
| **Incision** | Inframammary, subareolar, or axillary incisions | ⇐ | ⇐ | ⇐ |
| **Unique considerations** | May put patient in sitting position during procedure. | ⇐ | ⇐ | May need to turn patient on side if reconstruction involves use of latissimus dorsi flap. |
| **Antibiotics** | Cefazolin 1 gm iv intraop | ⇐ | ⇐ | ⇐ |
| **Surgical time** | 1 hr | 1.5 hr | 2 - 3 hrs | ⇐ |
| **Closing considerations** | May need patient sitting up for application of dressing. | ⇐ | ⇐ | ⇐ |
| **EBL** | Minimal | Usually requires transfusion of 1 U autologous blood. | ⇐ | 1-2 U, particularly if combined immediately with breast resection. |
| **Postop care** | None | Suction drains | ⇐ | ⇐ |
| **Mortality** | Minimal | 0-0.1% | 0-0.5% | ⇐ |

| | Augmentation | Breast Lift | Reduction | Reconstruction |
|---|---|---|---|---|
| **Morbidity** | Prosthesis failure: 5% | ⇐ | N/A | 5% |
| | Infection: 1% | ⇐ | ⇐ | ⇐ |
| | Dehiscence: < 1% | ⇐ | 1% | ⇐ |
| | | | Graft failure: 2% | Flap failure: 2% |
| **Procedure code** | 19325 | 19316 | 19318 | 19360 |
| **Pain score** | 2-3 | 2-4 | 2-4 | 3-5 |

### PATIENT POPULATION CHARACTERISTICS

| | |
|---|---|
| **Age range** | 17-45 yrs |
| **Incidence** | 5000+/yr in U.S. |
| **Etiology** | Absence of development<br>Atrophy 2° childbearing |
| **Associated conditions** | None common |

**References**

1. Vistnes LM: *Procedures in Plastic Surgery: How They Do It.* Little, Brown, Boston: 1991.

## ANESTHETIC CONSIDERATIONS

### PREOPERATIVE

Typically, three patient populations present for mammoplasty: 1) healthy individuals, for reduction or augmentation mammoplasty; 2) morbidly obese, for reduction mammoplasty; 3) breast cancer patients, for reconstruction after mastectomy. (For preop considerations in the morbidly obese patient, see Anesthetic Considerations for "Abdominoplasty," above.) Breast cancer patients undergoing mastectomy with immediate reconstruction will not have had either chemotherapy or radiation. The following considerations are for breast cancer patients undergoing delayed reconstruction post-chemotherapy.

| | |
|---|---|
| **Respiratory** | Pulmonary fibrosis may complicate chemotherapy. Bleomycin (>200 mg/m[1]) has the greatest pulmonary toxicity, but alkylating agents, including cyclophosphamide and melphalan, used to treat breast cancer, have some pulmonary toxicity. Avoid high $FiO_2$ (>40%) with bleomycin. Consider pulmonary fibrosis in a patient reporting dyspnea, nonproductive cough and fever.<br>**Tests:** CXR; ABG and PFTs as indicated from H&P. |
| **Cardiovascular** | Cardiomyopathy and CHF may result from chemotherapy, especially doxorubicin (Adriamycin®) >550 mg/m[1].<br>**Tests:** ECG; ECHO, if indicated from H&P. |
| **Neurological** | Note any previous damage to long thoracic nerves, as evidenced by winged scapula deformity. |
| **Musculoskeletal** | Avoid ivs and BP cuff on mastectomy side. |
| **Hematologic** | Leukopenia, thrombocytopenia and anemia from chemotherapy can be present.<br>**Tests:** CBC; platelet count; coagulation profile; bleeding time; Hb/Hct |
| **Renal/Hepatic** | Methotrexate can produce some renal and hepatic dysfunction.<br>**Tests:** Electrolytes; BUN; creatinine; LFTs |
| **Laboratory** | Other tests as indicated from H&P, prior chemotherapy, obesity. |
| **Premedication** | Midazolam 1-2 mg iv immediately preop or valium 5-10 mg po 1 hr preop |

### INTRAOPERATIVE

**Anesthetic technique:** GETA

| | |
|---|---|
| **Induction** | Standard induction (see Appendix). Check with surgeons as to whether they will use a nerve stimulator during dissection. |

| | | |
|---|---|---|
| **Maintenance** | Standard maintenance (see Appendix). Surgeons may want patient sitting for part of the procedure. Pneumothorax should be considered with any change in lung inflation pressure, $O_2$ saturation, or BP. | |
| **Emergence** | During some of the procedure and for application of dressing, patient may be moved to sitting position, with consequent coughing, bucking, etc. (Rx: deeper anesthesia, e.g., propofol 0.5 mg/kg or lidocaine 1 mg/kg.) Watch BP carefully and treat orthostatic hypotension if it occurs, usually with a fluid bolus if the patient is not fluid sensitive (Hx of CHF or renal failure). | |
| **Blood and fluid requirements** | IV 16-18 ga x 1<br>NS/LR @ 4-8 ml/kg/hr | Minimal blood loss for simple reconstruction, augmentation or reduction; larger blood losses anticipated for combined procedures (mastectomy with immediate reconstruction or flap reconstruction). |
| **Monitoring** | Standard monitors (see Appendix).<br>Arterial line in the morbidly obese | |
| **Positioning** | Patient may need to be sitting for application of dressing. | Avoid HTN, bucking and straining; these may cause or exacerbate bleeding at reconstruction site. |

## POSTOPERATIVE

| | |
|---|---|
| **Complications** | Pneumothorax |
| **Pain management** | PCA (see Appendix). |

References

1. Cooper Jr, Brodsky JB: Anesthetic management of the morbidly obese patient. *Seminars in Anesthesia* 1987; Vol VI: 260-70.

**Surgeon**

**Barry Press, MD, FACS**

## 11.2 BURN SURGERY

**Anesthesiologist**

**Rona G. Giffard, MD, PhD**

# FREE SKIN GRAFT FOR BURN WOUND

## (WITH TANGENTIAL EXCISION, EXCISION TO FASCIA, OR DEBRIDEMENT)

## SURGICAL CONSIDERATIONS

**Description:** Until the mid-1970s, management of burn wounds involved daily debridement, hydrotherapy and spontaneous eschar separation, with subsequent skin grafting to the underlying granulation tissue. Recently, operative management has become much more aggressive with the description of **tangential excision** (TE) by Janzekovic[1]. This surgical approach to the burn wound involves operative excision of eschar (burned necrotic tissue), and it can be performed as TE. Thin slices of burned tissue are removed with either manual or power dermatomes, until a healthy wound bed is developed. Assessment of the wound bed is done with visualization of bleeding and/or the clinical appearance of the excised bed.

It has become apparent that early eschar excision is advantageous even if wounds are so extensive they cannot be closed with autografts. In this situation, TE or **excision to fascia** is performed, but the wounds are closed with the application of cadaver allograft (preferred), porcine xenograft or synthetic biologic dressings. The wound is maintained in this way, with further debridement and changing of the biologic dressings as necessary, until autograft becomes available from the patient. The recently developed ability to apply cultured keratinocytes to these wounds has added another option for definitive permanent coverage of excised burns.

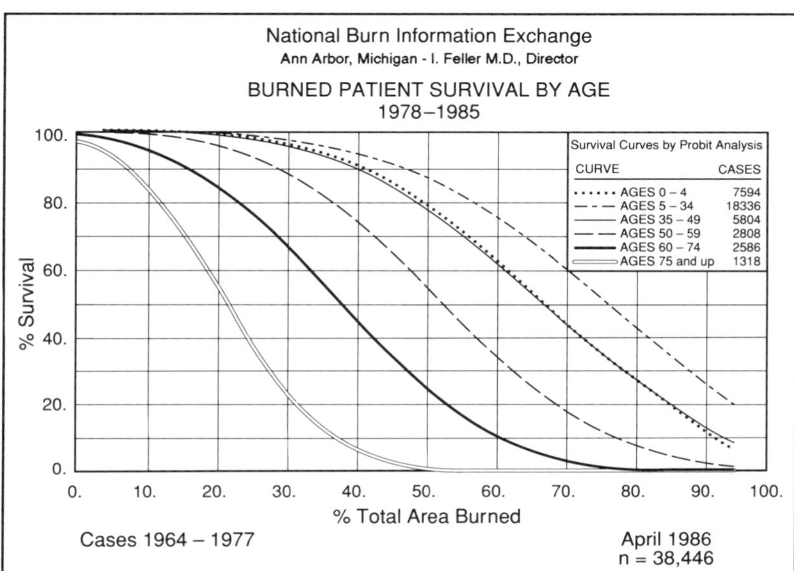


**Table 11.2-1.** Curves showing survival rates of different age groups according to percent of TBSA burned. (Reproduced with permission from Feller I, Jones CA: Use of a national burn registry to evaluate and address the burn problem. *Surg Clin N Am* 1987; 67(2):167-89.)

In patients with serious burns (>40% total body surface area [TBSA]), excision usually commences on the third hospital day, after completion of the fluid resuscitation phase. In general, repeated excisions and coverage as described above are performed every 2-3 days, as the patient's condition permits. If eschar excision can be completed before secondary sepsis supervenes, management of the patient is easier and the complications and morbidity are considerably lessened. For deep burns in high-risk patients, **excision to fascia** can be performed. This generally is done with a cutting electrocautery or cold knife, and involves removal of all burned and unburned tissue down to the deep muscle fascia. Generally, the fascia is viable and will support a skin graft. Fascial excision can be performed more rapidly and with less blood loss than TE. Its disadvantages, however, are the marked cosmetic deformities that occur because of the loss of all soft tissue overlying the musculature and, often, functional limitations for the same reason. TE is the more frequently performed procedure.

**Usual preop diagnosis**: Thermal burns; electrical or chemical burn

### SUMMARY OF PROCEDURE

| | |
|---|---|
| **Position** | Supine, prone or lateral. Prone generally is preferred for early excisions so that large areas, such as the back, buttocks and posterior thighs, can be excised initially for maximum reduction of eschar load. Patients tolerate the prone position better before secondary sepsis or pulmonary complications have supervened. Position changes may be necessary intraop if, for example, donor skin is to be harvested from the back for application to the anterior surface of the body. |
| **Incision** | Anywhere eschar is to be excised. |

| | |
|---|---|
| **Special instrumentation** | Dermatomes of surgeon's choice. Manual dermatomes include Weck, Humby, and Eschmann knives. Powered dermatomes (generally used in the U.S. for harvesting skin grafts) include Padgett, Zimmer and Brown. Because blood loss is generally diffuse and can be massive, several techniques are used to minimize it. TEs of extremities can be performed by experienced surgeons under pneumatic tourniquet control. |
| **Temperature considerations** | Due to loss of skin integrity and large exposed surfaces, these patients lose heat rapidly. Fluids, gasses, and the OR should be warm, although there is no demonstrable benefit to warming the OR past the point of isothermic neutrality (~82°F [28°C]).[2] |
| **Unique considerations** | In excising burn eschar or harvesting skin grafts, depending on location of recipient and donor sites, many surgeons use subcutaneous infiltration of NS to smooth out irregularities (e.g., underlying ribs) to physically improve the ease of taking skin grafts. Substantial amounts of NS can be infiltrated subcutaneously (e.g., up to 2-3 L). In a small child, this may be a significant fluid bolus and should be figured into the total fluids administered to patient by anesthesiologist. |
| **Antibiotics** | Cefazolin 1 gm iv on induction of anesthesia (unless receiving systemic antibiotics) |
| **Surgical time** | **NB**: The endpoints for surgical excision are: (1) a **time of 2-3 hrs**; (2) **core temperature of 35°C**; or (3) **blood loss of 10 U PRBC**. The violation of any of these parameters invites coagulopathy and increasing problems with hemostasis and vital sign stability. Adverse affects occurring after 3-4 hrs of operative time are more closely associated with massive transfusion or hypothermia than with time itself. |
| **Closing considerations** | After excision of wounds and attainment of hemostasis, wounds are closed, using either autograft, allograft, xenograft or synthetic biologic dressings (described above). Postop dressing, splinting and positioning can be quite time-consuming. Uncontrolled patient movement poses a problem for graft security; however, most of the time grafts are secured with circumferential dressings (to protect against this eventuality). Application of these dressings may be very time-consuming, and any uncontrolled patient movement is detrimental to graft positioning at that point. |
| **EBL** | Varies with magnitude of procedure, but the goal is to **keep it under 10 U PRBC**. Blood ordered varies with surgeon and procedure, and whether pneumatic tourniquet control is used. Bleeding is also controlled with the application of dilute solutions of epinephrine (e.g., 1:200,000). Substantial absorption occurs and very high plasma epinephrine levels have been measured in these patients. Complications from this, however, are minimal in patients with severe burns because of high endogenous catecholamine secretion. Other topical agents used for hemostasis include thrombin and microcrystalline collagen. These modalities are often combined with compressive wraps and elevation of excised extremities to promote hemostasis. Because blood loss may be massive and difficult to control, close communication between anesthesiologist and surgeon is essential. In large excisions, blood replacement often is begun prior to excision so that the anesthesiologist does not get behind in blood replacement. As a rule, replacement with blood and crystalloid is preferable to artificial plasma expanders such as hetastarch or dextran. |
| **Postop care** | Generally, patients can be extubated at the end of these procedures, recovered in the PACU and returned to the burn center. If patient remains intubated, generally he/she is transported directly back to the burn center, where body temperature can be more easily maintained. |
| **Mortality** | 18-40% (Mortality is a function of the burn size, plus other associated conditions [especially inhalation injury] as seen in Table 11.2-1.) |
| **Morbidity** | Massive blood loss<br>Sepsis<br>Infection 2° to catheters and lines |
| **Procedure code** | 15000, 15100, 15101 |
| **Pain score** | 2-5 (most patients are maintained on methadone for perioperative pain control) |

## PATIENT POPULATION CHARACTERISTICS

| | |
|---|---|
| **Age range** | All |
| **Male:Female** | More commonly male |
| **Incidence** | 2.5 - 3 million/year |
| **Etiology** | Scald<br>Flame burns<br>Chemicals |
| **Associated conditions** | Generally few |

## ANESTHETIC CONSIDERATIONS

### PREOPERATIVE

The extent of physiologic derangement depends on the percent of TBSA burned, time since burn was sustained, and treatment received in the interval. Patients are usually young and healthy; older patients generally have a poorer outcome. Generally, after major burns, the patient is fluid-resuscitated and stabilized, then brought to the OR on about the third day to begin tangential excision (TE) and coverage of the burned area with skin grafts. Blood loss and hypothermia are the predominant considerations during surgery on burn patients. Blood loss can be rapid and massive, as much as 8 U in 15 min, and can be difficult to estimate as it generally is not collected into the suction.

**Respiratory** — **Upper airway**: A patient with burns around the airway should be intubated on arrival at ER, as subsequent intubation may become more difficult, or even impossible. Careful assessment of airway, face, head and neck is essential to anticipate problems with subsequent airway management.

**Lower airway**: Patients may suffer from ARDS, and ventilator settings should be noted preop. High PIP and minute-volume requirements may necessitate the use of an ICU-type ventilator in OR. Patients with extensive burns can be severely hypermetabolic (patient with 40% TBSA burn may have twice the normal metabolic rate) with ↑$CO_2$ production. These patients may require high-minute ventilation (as much as 30 L/min), and high levels of PEEP to maintain normocarbia. Other possible effects of severe burns include: ↓lung and chest-wall compliance, ↓FRC, ↑A-a gradient, ↑carboxyhemoglobinemia and ↑methemoglobinemia.

**Tests:** ABG, depending on pulmonary status; CXR

**Cardiovascular** — The hypermetabolism associated with burns increases cardiac demand, and burn patients have greatly elevated circulating levels of catecholamines → ↑HR.

**Tests:** As indicated from H&P.

**Neurological** — Evaluate for burn encephalopathy. Characterize baseline mental status before anesthesia to allow evaluation of recovery postop.

**Musculoskeletal** — Damaged muscle ↑acetylcholine receptor density, resulting in ↓sensitivity to non-depolarizing muscle relaxants and potentially fatal elevations of potassium in response to succinylcholine. In burns >5% TBSA, avoid succinylcholine after the 4th day post-burn. Recovery of normal response to muscle relaxants does not occur until the burns have completely healed.

**Hematologic** — Coagulopathies may result directly from the burn injury, as well as from rapid replacement of blood loss during fluid resuscitation.

**Tests:** Hb/Hct; electrolytes; coagulation profile

**IV access** — May be difficult; assess preop. Consider central line placement.

**Laboratory** — Other tests as indicated from H&P.

**Premedication** — Adequate analgesia should be given (titrate dose to effect) to allow transport.

**Transport** — For patients with severe ARDS, transportation from burn unit to OR may pose formidable challenges with regard to ventilation. Cardiopulmonary monitoring must be continued during transport; the ventilation system used in transport must be capable of delivering high minute-volumes, PEEPs and PIPs. These requirements may not be satisfied by standard bag-valve systems.

### INTRAOPERATIVE

**Anesthetic technique:** GETA

**Induction** — Thiopental (3-5 mg/kg), if patient is already volume-resuscitated; otherwise, use etomidate 0.3 mg/kg or ketamine 1-3 mg/kg. Pancuronium (0.15 mg/kg) or vecuronium (0.3 mg/kg) for intubation. In patients with extensive burns, 1.5 times the usual intubation dose may be required. If the face is burned, mask induction or awake FOL may be necessary. The ETT should be sutured in place or wired to the teeth by the surgeon to avoid dislodging it, especially during procedures in the prone position. Alternatively, the tube may be secured with umbilical tape.

**Maintenance** — Standard maintenance (see Appendix). These patients may require minute-volumes >30 L/min, high inspiratory pressures and PEEP for adequate ventilation. For these cases a Siemens® or ICU-type ventilator is recommended. Surgeons may give epinephrine topically to decrease blood loss. Epinephrine is well-absorbed from the disrupted skin surface → ↑↑plasma catecholamine levels; thus, isoflurane is preferred over halothane to decrease the risk of dysrhythmias.

**Emergence** — Estimation of an adequate dose of narcotic to provide good postop analgesia may be difficult as these patients are often on high doses of narcotics preop.

| | | |
|---|---|---|
| **Blood and fluid requirements** | Extensive blood loss<br>IV: 14-16 ga x 2<br>NS/LR @ 8-10 ml/kg/hr<br>Keep UO 0.5-1 cc/kg/hr<br>Blood: ~200 cc/1% BSA excised and grafted.[6]<br>Fluid warmer<br>T&C 2-4 U PRBC (to keep ahead) | Blood must be in OR prior to induction. The major blood loss is generally associated with eschar excision, usually the first part of the procedure. For patients without contraindications to hemodilution, it is often better to delay PRBC transfusion until major blood loss is complete. IV hyperalimentation should be continued during surgery; or, replace the same volume with 10% dextrose infusion to avoid hypoglycemia. If sudden ↓BP occurs during very rapid infusion of blood (>150 ml/min), consider using calcium to counteract the chelating effect of citrate. Avoid fluid overload, especially if patient has ARDS, is a small child, or is elderly. As the surgical site is superficial, there is not much 3rd-space loss. It may be necessary to have an additional person available to help administer blood. |
| **Thermal considerations** | Room = 80-82°F<br>Warm all fluids.<br>Humidify gasses.<br>Warming blanket<br>Head cover | Temperature must be monitored throughout the case. The surgeon should be notified if patient's core temperature decreases to 35°. |
| **Monitoring** | Standard monitors (see Appendix).<br>± CVP line, PA catheter<br>Urinary catheter | ECG may require needle electrodes if there is no skin to apply adhesive electrodes. Patients who are hemodynamically unstable should be monitored with PA catheters. |
| **Positioning** | ✓ and pad pressure points.<br>✓ eyes. | The burn patient may be uniquely susceptible to laryngeal or upper airway edema in the prone position, so examination of the upper airway before extubation is recommended to avoid emergent reintubation. |
| **Complications** | Massive blood loss | |

**POSTOPERATIVE**

| | | |
|---|---|---|
| **Complications** | Hypothermia<br>Coagulopathy | May occur as the result of massive blood loss and replacement. |
| **Transport** | Continue cardiopulmonary monitoring.<br>High minute-ventilation requirements<br>↑PIP<br>↑PEEP | Verify adequacy of transport ventilation system before departing OR. |
| **Pain management** | Oral methadone<br>IV fentanyl | Titrate analgesia to effect. |
| **Tests** | Hct, ABG, electrolytes, PT, PTT, PLT, if massive transfusion given. | |


**References**

1. Janzekovic Z: A new concept in the early excision and immediate grafting of burns. *J Trauma* 1970; 10(2):1103-8.
2. Jankovich GH, Austin EN: Environmental Injuries. In *Surgery: Scientific Principles and Practice*. Greenfield LJ, et al, eds. JB Lippincott, Philadelphia: 1993, 359.
3. Burke JF, Quinby WC Jr, Bondoc CC: Primary excision and prompt grafting as routine therapy for the treatment of thermal burns in children. *Surg Clin North Am* 1976; 56(2):477-94.
4. Heimbach DM: Early burn excision and grafting. *Surg Clin North Am* 1987; 67(1):93-107.
5. Pavlin EG: *Surgical Management of the Burn Wound.* Heimbach DM, Engrav LH, eds. Raven Press. New York: 1985, Ch 9, 139-53.
6. Moran KT, O'Reilly TJ, Furman W, Munster AM: A new algorithm for calculation of blood loss in excisional burn surgery. *Am Surg* 1988; 54(4):207-8.

**Surgeon**

**Stephen A. Schendel, MD, DDS**

# 11.3 CONGENITAL MALFORMATION SURGERY

**Anesthesiologist**

**Yuan-Chi Lin, MD, MPH**

# CLEFT LIP REPAIR – UNILATERAL/BILATERAL

## SURGICAL CONSIDERATIONS

**Description**: Cleft lip may be either unilateral or bilateral, associated frequently with clefts of the alveolus and palate. Surgical repair involves the design and execution of geometric flaps on the medial and lateral sides of the cleft. The most common technique is the **rotation advancement flap of Millard** (Fig 11.3-1).

**Variant procedure or approaches**: Other approaches commonly performed are those of the **Davies** or **Tennison** type (Z-plasty) lip repairs (Fig 11.3-2). In large clefts, a lip adhesion may be performed as an initial stage several months prior to the actual definitive correction of the cleft lip. This procedure basically involves creating a wound on either side and suturing the muscles, mucosa and skin together. The procedure itself is very short – approximately a half hour or less of actual surgical time.

**Usual preop diagnosis**: Cleft lip/palate

### SUMMARY OF PROCEDURE

| | |
|---|---|
| **Position** | Supine; table rotated either 90° or 180° with oral RAE® or anode tube. |
| **Incision** | Medial and lateral cleft margins into the nose and in the maxillary vestibule on the left side. |
| **Special instrumentation** | Plastic surgery throat pack (**NB:** removal important); oral RAE® or anode tube |
| **Unique considerations** | Pediatric patients should wake up in an unagitated state, as undue crying may place excessive tension on repair. Elbow restraints for children. |
| **Antibiotics** | Cefazolin 1 gm iv |
| **Surgical time** | 0.75 - 1.5 hrs |
| **Closing considerations** | Smooth emergence |
| **EBL** | 5-10 cc |
| **Postop care** | Elbow restraints for 2 wks |
| **Mortality** | Minimal |
| **Morbidity** | Infection<br>Wound breakdown |
| **Procedure code** | 40701 (unilateral); 40702 (bilateral one-stage); 40700 (bilateral two-stage) |
| **Pain score** | 4 |

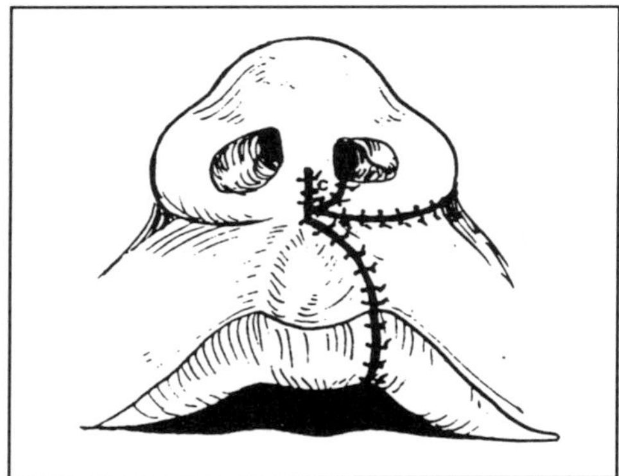

**Figure 11.3-1.** Completion of the rotation flap of Millard. (Reproduced with permission from McCarthy JG, ed: *Plastic Surgery*. WB Saunders: 1990).

### PATIENT POPULATION CHARACTERISTICS

| | |
|---|---|
| **Age range** | 1 wk - 6 mo |
| **Male:Female** | 2:1 – cleft lip and palate. Left cleft more common than right; both more common than bilateral, in the ratio of 6:3:1. |
| **Incidence** | 1/750 for Caucasians; more common in Asians; less in Blacks. |
| **Etiology** | Multi-factorial, including both genetic and environmental aspects |
| **Associated conditions** | Associated anomalies are seen in approximately 29% of cleft lip cases, and may include major chromosomal deletions and/or duplications, along with possible severe mental retardation.[1]<br>Pierre Robin syndrome<br>CHD<br>Treacher-Collins syndrome<br>Subglottic stenosis |

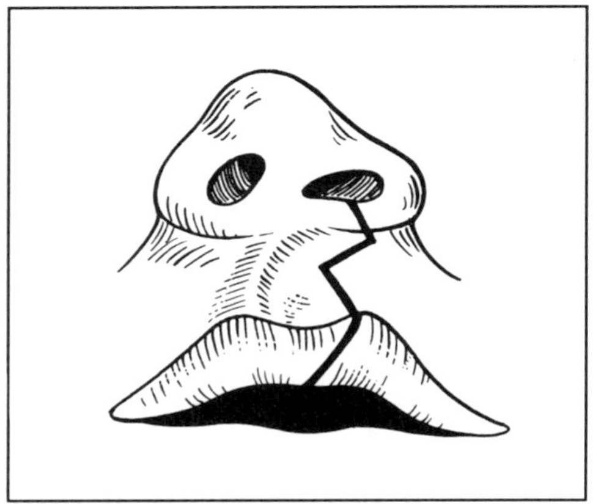

**Figure 11.3-2.** Z-plasty closure of lip. (Reproduced with permission from McCarthy JG, ed: *Plastic Surgery*. WB Saunders: 1990).

## ANESTHETIC CONSIDERATIONS

See "Anesthetic Considerations for Lip and Nose Surgery" following "Lip/Nose Revisions" (below).


**References**

1. Gorlin RJ, Cohen MM, Levin LS: *Syndromes of the Head and Neck*, 3rd edition. Oxford University Press, New York: 1990.


# ABBE-ESTLANDER REPAIR/CROSS LIP FLAP

## SURGICAL CONSIDERATIONS

**Description**: Occasionally, the individual born with a cleft lip and palate is severely deficient in tissue of the upper lip. This occurs most frequently in the bilateral condition. Correction involves switching tissue from the midline of the lower lip to the central portion of the upper lip, maintaining a pedicle of soft tissue between the lips, which usually contains the labial artery on one side. This pedicle normally is cut between 7-11 days. The redundant tissue in the mid-portion of the upper lip is transferred to the columellar portion of the nose at the same time, which elongates this section (Fig 11.3-3).

**Variant procedure or approaches**: Only minor technical variants

**Usual preop diagnosis**: Severely cleft lip/palate

### SUMMARY OF PROCEDURE

| | |
|---|---|
| **Position** | If nasal RAE® tube used, table is either rotated 90° or left in usual position. If oral RAE® tube is used, table is rotated either 90° or 180°. The nasal RAE® tube has the advantage of easier extubation of a patient with the central portion of his lips essentially sewn together. Nasal intubation, however, somewhat limits the surgeon's ability to visualize and reconstruct the nasal section of the surgery. The oral RAE® tube has the opposite advantages and disadvantages. |
| **Incision** | Midline upper and lower lips (Fig 11.3-3) |
| **Special instrumentation** | Nasal or oral RAE® tube (surgeon's preference); plastics setup |
| **Unique considerations** | Central portion of lips are attached by a thin, easily damaged soft-tissue pedicle. Patient should wake up unagitated. |
| **Antibiotics** | Cefazolin 1 gm iv |
| **Surgical time** | 1 - 2 hrs |
| **Closing considerations** | **NB:** Remove throat pack. |
| **EBL** | 25-50 cc |
| **Mortality** | Rare |
| **Morbidity** | Flap necrosis: < 1%<br>Suture line dehiscence: < 1% |
| **Procedure code** | 40761 |
| **Pain score** | 4 |

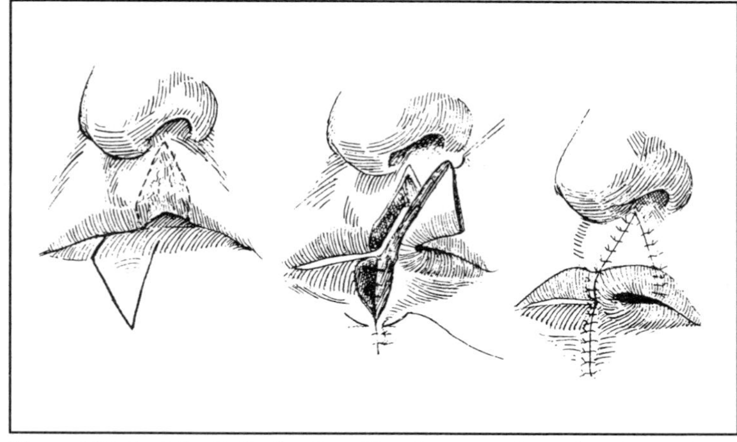

**Figure 11.3-3.** Abbe-Estlander flap. Note lips sutured together. (Reproduced with permission from Converse JM, ed: *Reconstructive Plastic Surgery*, Vol 3, 2nd edition. WB Saunders Co: 1977.)

### PATIENT POPULATION CHARACTERISTICS

| | |
|---|---|
| **Age range** | 3+ yrs |
| **Male:Female** | 2:1 |
| **Incidence** | 1/750 Caucasians (>Asians; < Blacks) |
| **Etiology** | Multi-factorial, including both genetic and environmental aspects |
| **Associated conditions** | Associated anomalies are seen in approximately 29% of the clefts and may include major chromosomal deletions or duplications, with a possibility of severe mental retardation.[1]<br>CHD<br>Pierre Robin syndrome<br>Treacher-Collins syndrome<br>Subglottic stenosis |

## ANESTHETIC CONSIDERATIONS

See "Anesthetic Considerations for Lip and Nose Surgery" following "Lip/Nose Revisions" (below).

**References**

1. Gorlin RJ, Cohen MM, Levin LS: *Syndromes of the Head and Neck*, 3rd edition. Oxford University Press, New York: 1990.

# PALATOPLASTY

## SURGICAL CONSIDERATIONS

**Description**: Cleft palate can be seen as either an isolated condition or in conjunction with clefting of the lip. The mildest form of cleft palate is the submucous, or occult cleft, in which there is no visible cleft but, rather, a nonunion of the soft-palate muscles. This is followed by the incomplete soft-palate cleft and, finally, the complete cleft, which includes soft and hard palates and may extend through the alveolar portion of the maxilla. Repair involves mobilizing the lateral soft tissue and moving it toward the midline to close the cleft and elongate the palate, if necessary. The most important goal of cleft-palate repair is the attainment of normal speech. Children with unrepaired or inadequately repaired clefts develop nasal-sounding speech patterns termed "rhinolalia." Cleft-palate repair, therefore, is usually done when the child is 12-18 months old, before consequential speech development. In addition to closing the cleft itself, an important goal of palate repair is approximation, in normal alignment, of the levator palati muscles, which are responsible for oronasal valving in speech and swallowing. The cleft palate is closed by loosening the palatal mucoperiosteum from the underlying bone and either approximating it in the midline (**Langenbeck technique**) or using a V-Y type of retrodisplacement and closure (**Wardill-Kilner technique**). In either method, the levator muscles are specifically dissected and the levator sling is reconstructed. A layered closure is usually done, including repositioning of the alveolar muscles.

There are several different approaches to the muscle reconstruction in the soft palate, which can generally be termed **intravelarveloplasties**. One of the newer techniques is a Z-plasty of the soft palate, also called a **Furlow procedure**. The other procedures are basically closures of the muscles and a push-back to lengthen the palate.

**Usual preop diagnosis**: Cleft palate

### SUMMARY OF PROCEDURE

| | |
|---|---|
| **Position** | Supine; table rotated 90°-180° with oral RAE® tube extending down the midline of the lower jaw and taped to the chin. |
| **Incision** | Edges of the cleft palate and possibly the alveolar and pterygomandibular raphe areas |
| **Special instrumentation** | Dingmann mouth gag and, usually, a headlight; oropharyngeal pack |

| | |
|---|---|
| **Unique considerations** | Minimal-to-moderate amount of blood in the oropharynx at end of procedure; should be carefully suctioned. Also, there may be some respiratory difficulties on emergence. Traction with a tongue suture often proves helpful in restoring patient's airway. Usually oral or nasopharyngeal airways should not be placed in children. |
| **Antibiotics** | Cefazolin 1 gm q 4-6 hrs x 5-7 d |
| **Surgical time** | 1 - 1.5 hr |
| **Closing considerations** | Child should not wake up crying and hypertensive. Tongue suture may be placed prior to extubation. |
| **EBL** | 50 cc |
| **Postop care** | Elbow restraints |
| **Mortality** | Rare |
| **Morbidity** | Recurrent bleeding<br>Hematoma under the palate<br>Dehiscence of the palate |
| **Procedure code** | 42200 |
| **Pain score** | 4 |

### PATIENT POPULATION CHARACTERISTICS

| | |
|---|---|
| **Age range** | 6-9 mo |
| **Male:Female** | 1:3 |
| **Incidence** | 1/1,000 |
| **Etiology** | Failure of fusion of the palatal shelves from anterior to posterior. (Can be due to a persistent high-tongue position *in utero*, increased facial width, reduced facial mesenchyme and/or drugs such as steroids, anticonvulsants and benzodiazepines, or infection.) |
| **Associated conditions** | Multiple associated conditions. Most common is the Pierre Robin anomaly, in which cleft palate is found in association with glossoptosis and a micrognathic retruded mandible. These children frequently have airway obstruction and, even at an older age, may have sleep apnea.[1] |

## ANESTHETIC CONSIDERATIONS

See "Anesthetic Considerations for Lip and Nose Surgery" following "Lip/Nose Revisions" (below).

**References**

1. Gorlin RJ, Cohen MM, Levin LS: *Syndromes of the Head and Neck*, 3rd edition. Oxford University Press, New York: 1990.

# PHARYNGOPLASTY

## SURGICAL CONSIDERATIONS

**Description**: Following the initial repair of palatal clefts, some children or young adults demonstrate continued hypernasal speech patterns, a condition called "velopharyngeal incompetence." This can be 2° a short, soft palate, a large nasopharynx, or a soft palate which has inadequate movement either 2° scarring or due to neurogenic problems. The typical repair would be a superiorly based **pharyngeal flap** to the soft palate.

**Variant procedure or approaches**: An **Orticochea flap**, using the posterior tonsillar pillars, which are repositioned along with the palatoglossus muscle to the posterior pharynx

**Usual preop diagnosis**: Velopharyngeal incompetence

### SUMMARY OF PROCEDURE

| | |
|---|---|
| **Position** | Supine, table rotated 90° or 180°; oral RAE® tube exited out the midline and taped in that position. |
| **Incision** | Involves incisions in soft and hard palates, and in the posterior pharyngeal wall. |
| **Special instrumentation** | Dingmann mouth gag; headlight |
| **Unique considerations** | Avoid oral or nasopharyngeal airways or nasal suctioning. |
| **Antibiotics** | Cefazolin 1 gm iv |
| **Surgical time** | 1 - 1.5 hr |
| **Closing considerations** | Pediatric patients should not become hypertensive (↑bleeding). There will be some nasopharyngeal drainage; thorough oral suctioning is important. |
| **EBL** | 50-100 cc |
| **Postop care** | Avoid postop oral or nasopharyngeal airways or nasal suctioning. Be aware of possible occlusion of nasopharynx with flap and bleeding. |
| **Mortality** | Rare |
| **Morbidity** | Recurrent bleeding<br>Hematoma under the palate<br>Dehiscence of the palate<br>Nasopharyngeal obstruction<br>Secondary sleep apnea |
| **Procedure code** | 42225 (pharyngeal flap); 42226 (pharyngeal flap with palatal lengthening) |
| **Pain score** | 4 |

### PATIENT POPULATION CHARACTERISTICS

| | |
|---|---|
| **Age range** | 3-11 yrs most common |
| **Male:Female** | 1:1 |
| **Incidence** | Approximately 1/3 of children undergoing cleft palate repair will need some type of secondary palatal lengthening procedure after 3 yrs. |
| **Etiology** | Short and scarred palate<br>Neurogenic palate<br>Palate-to-pharyngeal ratio which is too small |
| **Associated conditions** | Sleep apnea<br>Pierre Robin syndrome, glossoptosis and micrognathia<br>Treacher-Collins syndrome<br>Microtia with craniofacial malformation<br>Subglottic stenosis<br>CHD |

## ANESTHETIC CONSIDERATIONS

See "Anesthetic Considerations for Lip and Nose Surgery" following "Lip/Nose Revisions" (below).

# ALVEOLAR CLEFT REPAIR WITH BONE GRAFT

## SURGICAL CONSIDERATIONS

**Description:** Alveolar cleft occurs as both bony and soft-tissue defects in the alveolar portion of the maxilla in the position of the lateral incisor tooth; thus, an oral/nasal fistula exists with this deformity. The size of the cleft is variable; it may be unilateral or bilateral and it is most often associated with cleft lip and palate. The surgical procedure involves raising mucosal gingival flaps, advancing them, and performing a layered closure, starting with the nasal floor and working toward the oral cavity. A bone graft is placed in between these two layers to consolidate the upper arch. Cancellous bone is usually taken from the iliac crest or from the outer table of the skull.

**Variant procedure or approaches:** In young children, the procedure may be performed without the use of bone grafts.

**Usual preop diagnosis:** Congenital alveolar cleft

### SUMMARY OF PROCEDURE

| | |
|---|---|
| **Position** | Supine; table rotated 90°-180° |
| **Incision** | Oral, with the addition of iliac crest incision or scalp incision, either parasagittal or coronal |
| **Special instrumentation** | Throat pack; Dingmann mouth gag; headlight. Normally, 2 instrument setups used, with hip instruments kept separate from oral instruments. |
| **Unique considerations** | Important to assure that the hip from which iliac crest bone graft will be procured is on the opposite side from the anesthesiologist if the table is rotated only 90°. Midline oral RAE® tube. |
| **Antibiotics** | Cefazolin 1 gm iv |
| **Surgical time** | 1.5 - 2.5 hrs |
| **Closing considerations** | **NB:** Insure that throat pack has been removed. Pediatric patients should not wake up in agitated state. Oral mouth gag and gentle oral suctioning permissible; avoid nasal suctioning, especially from the cleft side. |
| **EBL** | 100-200 cc |
| **Mortality** | Rare |
| **Morbidity**[1] | Bone graft loss: 2-10%<br>Infection: 2-10%<br>Refistulization: 2-10%<br>Prolonged hip discomfort |
| **Procedure code** | 42210 |
| **Pain score** | 6 |

### PATIENT POPULATION CHARACTERISTICS

| | |
|---|---|
| **Age range** | 8-12 yrs |
| **Male:Female** | 2:1 |
| **Incidence** | Unknown |
| **Etiology** | Multi-factorial, including both genetic and environmental aspects |
| **Associated conditions** | Associated anomalies are seen in approximately 29% of cleft lip cases; and may include major chromosomal deletions and/or duplications, with the possibility of severe mental retardation.[2]<br>CHD<br>Pierre Robin syndrome<br>Treacher-Collins syndrome<br>Subglottic stenosis |

## ANESTHETIC CONSIDERATIONS

See "Anesthetic Considerations for Lip and Nose Surgery" following "Lip/Nose Revisions" (below).

**References**


1. Wolfe SA, Price GW, Stuzin JM, Berkowitz SI: Alveolar and anterior palatal clefts. In *Plastic Surgery*, Vol 4. McCarthy JG, ed. WB Saunders Co, Philadelphia: 1990, 2753-70.
2. Gorlin RJ, Cohen MM, Levin LS: *Syndromes of the Head and Neck*, 3rd edition. Oxford University Press, New York: 1990.

# LIP/NOSE REVISIONS

## SURGICAL CONSIDERATIONS

**Description**: Secondary deformities of the nose and lip develop following the initial repair of either bilateral or unilateral cleft lip deformities. These subsequent deformities depend on the extent of the initial congenital anomaly, the quality of the surgical repair and resulting oral facial function. Revision can consist of a minimal scar revision, to a complete opening and reconstruction of the lip and nose, with or without ancillary procedures such as **cartilage grafting** to the nose and **septorhinoplasty**.

**Usual preop diagnosis**: Secondary deformity

### SUMMARY OF PROCEDURE

| | |
|---|---|
| **Position** | Supine, rotated 90°-180°, with oral RAE® tube. |
| **Incision** | Variable, in lip or nasal areas |
| **Special instrumentation** | Throat pack; possibly rhinoplasty instruments; oral RAE® tube |
| **Unique considerations** | Procurement of a cartilage graft is usually from the nasal septum or ear; thus, the head may need to be turned to one side and this area also prepped. Elbow restraints for children. |
| **Antibiotics** | Cefazolin 1 gm iv |
| **Surgical time** | Variable, depending on the extent of revision: 0.5 - 3 hrs |
| **EBL** | Minimal - 75 cc |
| **Mortality** | Rare |
| **Morbidity** | Infection<br>Wound breakdown |
| **Procedure code** | 40720 |
| **Pain score** | 5 |

### PATIENT POPULATION CHARACTERISTICS

| | |
|---|---|
| **Age range** | 2-50 yrs |
| **Male:Female** | 1:1 |
| **Incidence** | 20-60% of patients with primary clefts |
| **Etiology** | Unsatisfactory outcome of previous lip/nose surgery |
| **Associated conditions** | Associated anomalies are seen in approximately 29% of the clefts and may include major chromosomal deletions or duplications, with a possibility of severe mental retardation.[1]<br>Pierre Robin syndrome<br>CHD<br>Treacher-Collins syndrome<br>Subglottic stenosis |

---

## ANESTHETIC CONSIDERATIONS FOR LIP AND NOSE SURGERY

**(Procedures covered: cleft lip repair; Abbe-Estlander repair/cross lip flap; palatoplasty; pharyngoplasty; alveolar cleft repair with bone graft; lip/nose revisions)**

### PREOPERATIVE

The anesthesiologist should be aware of the parent's feelings about their malformed child.[2] The whole family needs to be treated with sensitivity and compassion. Cleft lip closure may be carried out as early as the first week of life in the healthy neonate; however, many surgeons and anesthesiologists find the "rule of ten" helpful: the child should have an Hb >10 gm, be 10 weeks old, and weigh 10 kg. The hard palate is usually closed between the ages of 1-5 years; however, the soft palate should be closed prior to speech development (12-15 months). **Palatoplasty** and **pharyngoplasty** are usually carried out from 5-15 years. Patients with these midline facial defects are most likely to have other associated anomalies, including CHD, subglottic stenosis, and Pierre Robin or Treacher-Collins syndromes.

**Respiratory** Careful assessment is necessary as associated anomalies may affect airway or lungs. Chronic otitis 2° eustachian tube dysfunction is common. Treat with antibiotics before surgery. Postpone surgery (~2 wks) if Sx of acute upper RTI present (e.g., runny nose, fever, sore throat, cough). Palatoplasty patients may have sleep apnea and airway obstruction on induction.
**Tests:** as indicated from H&P.

**Airway** Be aware of other congenital anomalies affecting the airway, such as Apert's, Goldenhar's, Klippel-Feil, Pierre Robin, Turner's or Treacher-Collins syndromes or Crouzon's disease. Review any previous anesthetic records for insights into airway management. Consider elective tracheostomy under local anesthesia in patients with severe airway abnormalities. Patients with severe subglottic stenosis may require preop tracheostomy.

**Cardiovascular** CHD is frequently associated with cleft palate.[3] Preop evaluation of a patient with a known or suspected heart defect should include thorough H&P, ECG, Hct, baseline $O_2$ sat and CXR. For children with Sx of cardiac dysfunction or those requiring cardiac medication, it is advisable to consult with a pediatric cardiologist to optimize the patient's condition prior to surgery.
**Tests:** Preop ECG indicated for patients with CHD; others as indicated from H&P.

**Nutritional** Infants with cleft lip/palate may have problems with oral feeding. Assess nutritional status from physical exam and by comparison to expected growth for age.
**NB:** NPO after midnight for solids. Patients should continue to have clear liquids up until 2 hrs preop.

**Neurological** Delayed development of speech is common in the older child with cleft palate. Some of these children may be hearing-impaired. Preop preparation and discussion is important to minimize the impact of these communication problems.

**Psychological** Many patients with orofacial congenital malformations require multiple procedures; emotional support and psychological assessment of these patients are essential.

**Hematologic** High incidence of iron deficiency anemia; T&C for 1 U PRBC (cleft palate).
**Tests:** Hct

**Laboratory** Other tests as indicated from H&P.

**Premedication** < 1 yr old rarely needs premedication; >1 yr old, either oral midazolam (0.75 mg/kg) or oral ketamine (6 mg/kg) ~30 min preop is adequate.

## INTRAOPERATIVE

**Anesthetic technique:** GETA

**Induction** Typically, an inhalational induction (halothane ± $N_2O/O_2$) while patient is breathing spontaneously. Airway obstruction is best treated with an oral airway. Anticipate difficult laryngoscopy if large, pre-palatal cleft present. Intubate with oral RAE® tube and secure in midline of lower lip. In patients with difficult airways, FOL is the technique of choice. Avoid muscle relaxants for difficult intubations until ETT is placed.

**Maintenance** Standard pediatric maintenance (see Appendix) ± muscle relaxant. Airway is shared with the surgeons. The Dingmann mouth gag is used for surgical exposure and may inadvertently compress the ETT or cause an endobronchial intubation. Flexion of the neck may also cause endobronchial intubation. Extension of the neck may cause complete or partial extubation. Adequacy of ventilation should be checked after every position change. Bilateral breath sounds should be equal after final positioning. ETT should be sutured to the alveolar ridge.

**Emergence** Pharyngeal (throat) packs are usually placed to prevent aspiration of blood. **NB:** Packs must be removed before extubating the trachea. Consider laryngoscopy to inspect airway and remove blood and clots before extubation. A tongue stitch is useful postop following cleft palate surgery. It may be used to pull the tongue forward to relieve postop respiratory obstruction. Extubation in the lateral (tonsillar) position is useful in promoting drainage of blood and secretions.

**Blood and fluid requirements**
IV: 18-20 ga x 1
NS/LR @:
4 cc/kg/hr – 0-10 kg
+ 2 cc/kg/hr – 11-20 kg
+ 1 cc/kg/hr – >20 kg
(e.g., 25 kg = 65 cc/hr)

Blood loss replaced by 3:1 crystalloid or 1:1 colloid (e.g., 5% albumin or 6% hetastarch). Rarely, a blood transfusion may be indicated for hemorrhage.

**Monitoring** Standard monitors (see Appendix).

| | | |
|---|---|---|
| **Positioning** | √ and pad pressure points.<br>√ eyes. | |
| **Complications** | Obstructed ETT → ↑PIP | √ ETT to see that it is not partially or completely obstructed by mouth gag. |
| | Mucous plugging<br>Hemorrhage | √ bilateral breath sounds. |

**POSTOPERATIVE**

| | | |
|---|---|---|
| **Complications** | Retained throat pack | √ for retained throat pack if there are Sx of airway obstruction in immediate postop period. |
| | Airway edema → croup<br>Hemorrhage | Treatment of post-intubation croup consists of cool, humidified, 100% $O_2$ mask, or nebulization 2.25% racemic epinephrine (0.5 ml in 3 ml NS). Racemic epinephrine is given for its vasoconstrictor, rather than its bronchodilator, effect. |
| **Pain management** | Acetaminophen 20 mg/kg<br>Suppository narcotics<br>Morphine 0.05-0.1 mg/kg iv | |
| **Tests** | Hct | Others as indicated. |


**References**

1. Gorlin RJ, Cohen MM, Levin LS: *Syndromes of the Head and Neck*, 3rd edition. Oxford University Press, New York: 1990.
2. Jones RG: A short history of anaesthesia for hare-lip and cleft palate repair. *Br J Anaesth* 1971; 43(8):796-802.
3. Wallbank WA: Cardiac effects of halothane and adrenaline in hare-lip and cleft-palate surgery. *Br J Anaesth* 1970; 42(6):548-52.


# OTOPLASTY

## SURGICAL CONSIDERATIONS

**Description**: There are a number of congenital ear malformations which result in an ear of abnormal shape, frequently with a lack of the antihelical fold. Surgical reconstruction consists of creating an antihelical fold and decreasing the prominence of the ear, as measured by its projection from the mastoid process. This usually involves an elliptical skin incision in the posterior ear area, dissection over the mastoid, and/or cartilage scoring or resection.

**Variant procedure or approaches**: All procedures are similar, with minor differences in suturing and amount of resection tissue. In addition to the posterior incision, an anterior incision can be used in some approaches. **Microtia reconstruction** is a much larger procedure and, therefore, is staged.

**Usual preop diagnosis**: Ear malformation; ear trauma

### SUMMARY OF PROCEDURE

| | |
|---|---|
| **Position** | Supine; table rotated either 90° or 180°; oral intubation |
| **Incision** | Posterior ear; occasionally anterior ear |
| **Unique considerations** | Head turned from side-to-side during operation. |
| **Antibiotics** | Cefazolin 1 gm iv |
| **Surgical time** | 2 hrs |

| | |
|---|---|
| **Closing considerations** | Ear dressing requires 5-10 min at end of procedure. **NB:** Remove throat pack. |
| **EBL** | 10-20 cc |
| **Mortality** | Rare |
| **Morbidity** | Hematoma formation: < 1%<br>Infection: < 1%<br>Unsymmetrical ear reduction: < 1% |
| **Procedure code** | 69300 |
| **Pain score** | 4 |

#### PATIENT POPULATION CHARACTERISTICS

| | |
|---|---|
| **Age range** | 6+ yrs |
| **Male:Female** | Unknown |
| **Incidence** | Unknown |
| **Etiology** | Unknown |

### ANESTHETIC CONSIDERATIONS

See "Anesthetic Considerations for Ear Surgery" (in "Otolaryngology - Head and Neck Surgery" section).

## PRIMARY CORRECTION OF CRANIOSYNOSTOSIS, CRANIOFACIAL ANOMALIES

### SURGICAL CONSIDERATIONS

**Description**: Premature closure of cranial sutures causes various abnormal skull shapes, of which the most common are: **scaphocephaly**, involving the sagittal suture; **plagiocephaly**, involving a unilateral coronal suture or lambdoid suture; and **trigonocephaly**, involving the metopic suture. Surgical correction involves releasing or resecting the affected suture and simultaneously correcting the asymmetric skull by bone flap repositioning or advancement, usually a fronto-orbital advancement with supraorbital bar. Procedures are extradural.

**Variant procedure or approaches**: In older children (>2 yrs), split cranial bone grafts may be required to correct defects caused by bone-flap advancement. Excision of skull segments is commonly accompanied by **micro-plate fixation**.

**Usual preop diagnosis**: Premature closure of cranial sutures; syndromes such as Apert's, and Crouzon's disease; ↑ICP

#### SUMMARY OF PROCEDURE

| | |
|---|---|
| **Position** | Usually supine; prone for correction of lambdoidal suture synostosis |
| **Incision** | Usually coronal |
| **Special instrumentation** | Horseshoe headrest, usually pediatric; occasionally, Gardiner tongs |
| **Unique considerations** | Control of intracranial pressure – spinal drain may be placed. |
| **Antibiotics** | Pediatric: cefazolin 15-30 mg/kg q 8 hrs, or vancomycin 10-15 mg/kg q 6 hrs, and cefotaxime 25-50 mg/kg q 6 hrs for oropharyngeal contamination and following dural tears. |
| **Surgical time** | 2 - 6 hrs |
| **Closing considerations** | Full head-wrap dressing causes head/neck movement → bucking. |
| **EBL** | 200-800 cc; may be formidable. |

**Postop care** ICU: 1-2 d

**Mortality** 0.6-1.6%

**Morbidity** Major complications: 14.3%
Bone infection: 3-7%
CSF leak: 4.5%
Air embolus: < 1%
Blindness: < 1%[1]
Massive bleeding: < 1%

**Procedure code** 21175 and/or 61557 (craniotomy for craniosynostosis with correction)

**Pain score** 4

### PATIENT POPULATION CHARACTERISTICS

**Age range** 2-24 mo (primary correction)

**Male:Female** 1:1

**Incidence** 1/10,000 births

**Etiology** Idiopathic; however, some are associated with specific genetic conditions (e.g., Crouzon's disease and Apert's syndrome).

**Associated conditions** Hydrocephalus
↑ICP
Mental retardation
Airway problems
Ocular abnormalities
Exotropia (20% Crouzon's disease or Apert's syndrome)
Lagophthalmus
Exorbitism

---

## ANESTHETIC CONSIDERATIONS

**(Procedures covered: primary correction of craniosynostosis, craniofacial anomalies; plagiocephaly, scaphocephaly, trigonocephaly)**

### PREOPERATIVE

Patients may have craniofacial anomalies – particularly Apert's syndrome and Crouzon's disease – which are associated with maxillary hypoplasia and difficult intubation. Hence, detailed preop airway evaluation is necessary. Children with single-suture craniosynostosis are usually healthy. Surgery is often performed between 3-6 months of age, preferably when the infant weighs > 5 kg.

**Respiratory** Patients with long-standing upper airway obstruction due to choanal atresia, mandibular and maxillary hypoplasia or other causes, may have chronic hypoventilation and hypoxia, and may experience episodes of apnea. If the patient has Sx of acute RTI, delay elective surgery at least 2 wks. The presence of fever, cough and abnormal chest auscultation necessitates radiographic evaluation and pediatric consultation.
**Tests:** As indicated from H&P.

**Airway** Be aware of other congenital anomalies affecting the patient's airway, such as Apert's, Goldenhar's, Klippel-Feil, Pierre Robin, Turner's or Treacher-Collins syndromes or Crouzon's disease. Review any previous anesthetic records for patient to gain insights into appropriate airway management. Consider elective tracheostomy under local anesthesia in patients with severe airway abnormalities.

**Cardiovascular** Consider the coexistence of congenital cardiopulmonary anomalies, particularly in patients with Apert's syndrome (autosomal dominant trait, craniosynostosis, syndactyly of hands and feet). Preop evaluation of a patient with a known or suspected heart defect should include thorough H&P, ECG, Hct, baseline $O_2$ sat and CXR. For children with Sx of cardiac dysfunction or those requiring cardiac medication, it is advisable to consult with a pediatric cardiologist to optimize the patient's condition prior to surgery.
**Tests:** Preop ECG indicated for patients with CHD; others as indicated from H&P.

| | |
|---|---|
| **Neurological** | If only the sagittal suture is involved, the resulting deformity is primarily cosmetic, and ICP is usually normal. If more than one suture is involved, brain growth will be impaired, the patient will be developmentally retarded, and intracranial HTN may be present. |
| **Hematologic** | Surgery in early infancy (< 9 mo) is common; thus, allowable blood loss is small; blood transfusion is usually required.<br>**Tests:** Hct; PT; PTT; T&C blood. |
| **Laboratory** | Other tests as indicated from H&P. |
| **Premedication** | Patients < 12 mos old usually do not require premedication. Antibiotic prophylaxis for CHD (e.g., ampicillin 25 mg/kg + gentamicin 2.5 mg/kg iv). |

## INTRAOPERATIVE

**Anesthetic technique:** GETA. Anticipate possible difficult airway. Heat OR to 78-80°.

| | |
|---|---|
| **Induction** | Surgery for craniectomies is extradural. Either mask induction with $N_2O$ and inhalational agent or iv induction is suitable for the infant with a normal airway. For a difficult airway, intubation may be facilitated by using a FOL while patient is awake or lightly anesthetized and spontaneously ventilating. In rare situations, tracheostomy, under sedation and local anesthesia, may be necessary. Consider suturing ETT to prevent accidental extubation. |
| **Maintenance** | Maintenance anesthesia with inhalational agent, or balanced anesthesia and long-acting muscle relaxant, should be adequate. Surgery may be prolonged. Control of ICP may be necessary (see below). |
| **Emergence** | Prompt awakening to allow neurological evaluation is an important goal. |

| | | |
|---|---|---|
| **Blood and fluid requirements** | Anticipate large blood loss.<br>IV: 18 ga x 1-2<br>NS/LR @:<br>4 cc/kg/hr – 0-10 kg<br>+ 2 cc/kg/hr – 11-20 kg<br>+ 1 cc/kg/hr – >20 kg<br>(e.g., 25 kg = 65 cc/hr)<br>Warm all fluids.<br>Humidify gasses. | Have 1-2 U PRBC available. Use NS/LR for replacing deficit, maintenance and 3rd-space fluid loss. Replace blood loss with colloid and PRBC cc for cc. Significant blood loss begins with scalp incision; allowable blood loss is small, so that it is important to begin transfusion early before hypovolemia occurs.[2] EBV for an infant in this age group is 75 cc/kg. A good rule is to infuse a volume of blood equal to 10% of EBV prior to incision in the healthy infant. |
| **Control of ICP** | Hyperventilation<br>Osmotic diuretic<br>Loop diuretic | In some cases, it may be desirable to ↓ICP. This can be accomplished by ↑ventilation ($PaCO_2$ 25-30 mmHg), diuretics (furosemide 1 mg/kg iv). |
| **Monitoring** | Standard monitors (see Appendix).<br>± Arterial line<br>± CVP line<br>± Precordial Doppler[3]<br>± Urinary catheter | Arterial cannulation for continuous monitoring of ABG, Hct, electrolytes, etc. VAE has been reported during craniectomies in infants; hence, a precordial Doppler and CVP line will be helpful. |
| **Positioning** | ✓ and pad pressure points.<br>✓eyes. | Positioning depends on surgical approach; most are performed with patient prone; however, use of the head-up position is not uncommon. |
| **Complications** | Oculocardiac reflex (OCR) → ↓↓HR and ↓↓BP. | Notify surgeons and Rx with atropine 0.02 mg/kg. |
| | VAE | Be prepared to make prompt Dx of VAE (↓$ETCO_2$, change in Doppler sounds, ↑$ETN_2$ ↓$O_2$ sat, ↓BP, ↑HR) and Rx: notify surgeons, flood wound, ± head down, aspirate CVP, ± vasopressors. |

## POSTOPERATIVE

| | | |
|---|---|---|
| **Complications** | Hypovolemia with ↓BP<br>Hypothermia | Inadequate volume replacement may result in ↓BP. ✓ Hct to establish need for further fluid or blood therapy. |
| **Pain management** | Parenteral narcotics (see Appendix). | |
| **Tests** | Followup Hct postop | Transfuse to keep Hct ≥30%. |

**References**

1. McCarthy JG, Thorne CHM, Wood-Smith D: Principles of craniofacial surgery: Orbital hypertelorism. In *Plastic Surgery*, Vol 4. McCarthy JG, ed. WB Saunders Co, Philadelphia: 1990, 2974-3012.
2. Davies DW, Munro IR: The anesthetic management and intraoperative care of patients undergoing major facial osteotomies. *Plast Reconstr Surg* 1975; 55(1):50-5.
3. Harris MM, Yemen TA, Davidson A, Strafford MA, Rowe RW, Sanders SP, Rockoff MA: Venous embolism during craniectomy in supine infants. *Anesthesiology* 1987; 67(5):816-19.

# SECONDARY CORRECTION OF CRANIOFACIAL MALFORMATIONS

## SURGICAL CONSIDERATIONS

**Description**: These procedures usually are performed on children 5 years and older. There are two basic approaches. The first involves advancement of the upper face and frontal bone, frequently described as a **mono-block** or **frontofacial advancement**. The second variation, called **facial bipartition** or **periorbital osteotomies**, is for correction of telorbitism (wide-spaced eyes), usually accomplished by a combined extra- and intracranial approach, using both plastic and neurosurgical teams.

**Variant procedure or approaches**: Many different variations of the above-named procedures can be performed; but from an anesthetic standpoint, they are not significantly different. The use of cranial bone grafts and rigid fixation have shortened these somewhat lengthy procedures. Other bone grafts, however, from ribs and iliac crest, are occasionally required. These procedures frequently last six hours or longer and blood loss can be very heavy. Reconstruction of the forehead orbital area following a tumor excision, for example, uses a similar approach, but requires additional bone grafts.

**Usual preop diagnosis**: Craniofacial malformations

### SUMMARY OF PROCEDURE

| | Mono-block or Frontofacial Advancement | Facial Bipartition or Periorbital Osteotomies |
|---|---|---|
| **Position** | Prone | ⇐ |
| **Incision** | Coronal, oral | Coronal, infraorbital |
| **Special instrumentation** | Neurosurgical power tools; mini/micro plates | ⇐ |
| **Unique considerations** | ↑ICP; may require hyperventilation and spinal drain. | ⇐ |
| **Antibiotics** | Cefazolin 1 gm iv or vancomycin and cefotaxime | ⇐ |
| **Surgical time** | 4 - 10 hrs | ⇐ |
| **Closing considerations** | Head and neck movement with application of head-wrap dressing → bucking. | ⇐ |
| **EBL** | 400-800 cc | ⇐ |
| **Postop care** | ICU: 1 d | ⇐ |
| **Mortality** | 0.6-1.6% | ⇐ |
| **Morbidity** | Major complications: 14.3% | ⇐ |
| | Bone infection: 3-7% | ⇐ |
| | CSF leak: 4.5% | ⇐ |
| | Air embolus: < 1% | ⇐ |
| | Blindness: < 1% | ⇐ |
| | Massive bleeding: < 1% | ⇐ |
| **Procedure code** | 21159 | 21172, 21182, 21261, 21260 |
| **Pain score** | 6 | 6 |

### PATIENT POPULATION CHARACTERISTICS

| | |
|---|---|
| **Age range** | 3-20 yrs |
| **Male:Female** | 1:1 |
| **Incidence** | 1/100,000 |
| **Etiology** | Congenital: 80%<br>Occasionally trauma or tumor: 20% |
| **Associated conditions** | Depends greatly on the syndrome or disease (e.g., Apert's syndrome, Crouzon's disease, etc.). See "Primary Correction of Craniosynostosis, Craniofacial Anomalies.") |

---

## ANESTHETIC CONSIDERATIONS

### PREOPERATIVE

Craniofacial syndromes often are associated with maxillofacial deformities, mandibular abnormalities and challenging airway management.[1]

**Respiratory** Patients with long-standing upper airway obstruction due to choanal atresia, mandibular and maxillary hypoplasia, etc. may have chronic hypoventilation and hypoxia, and may have apnea episodes. If Sx of acute upper RTI, delay elective surgery at least 2 wks. The presence of fever, cough and abnormal chest auscultation necessitates radiographic evaluation and pediatric consultation.

**Tests:** As indicated from H&P.

**Airway** Be aware of other congenital anomalies affecting the airway, such as Apert's, Goldenhar's, Klippel-Feil, Pierre Robin, Turner's or Treacher-Collins syndromes or Crouzon's disease. Review any previous anesthetic records for insights into airway management. Consider elective tracheostomy under local anesthesia in patients with severe airway abnormalities.

**Cardiovascular** Frequency of CHD is increased in patients with craniofacial abnormalities. Preop evaluation of patient with known or suspected heart defect should include H&P, ECG, Hct, baseline $O_2$ sat and CXR. For children with Sx of cardiac dysfunction or those requiring cardiac medication, it is advisable to consult with a pediatric cardiologist to optimize patient's condition prior to surgery.

**Tests:** Preop ECG indicated for patients with CHD; others as indicated from H&P.

**Neurological** Neurologic deficits, if any, should be documented preop.

**Laboratory** Hb/Hct; therapeutic drug levels for patients taking anticonvulsants.

**Premedication** Premedication is helpful for patients > 1 yr – oral midazolam 0.5-0.75 mg/kg or oral ketamine 6 mg/kg about 30-60 min before induction.

### INTRAOPERATIVE

**Anesthetic technique:** GETA, with special consideration given to associated CHD, pulmonary and airway problems.

**Induction** In an otherwise healthy patient, inhalational induction with subsequent placement of iv lines is appropriate. Muscle relaxants facilitate intubation but should be used only when adequate mask ventilation can be assured. An oral RAE® ETT is useful for this procedure and should be secured carefully in place (often by suturing). Intubation in a patient with airway abnormalities may be facilitated by using a FOL with patient awake or lightly anesthetized and spontaneously ventilating. In rare situations, tracheostomy, under sedation and local anesthesia, may be necessary.[2,3]

**Maintenance** Standard pediatric maintenance (see Appendix).

**Emergence** Extubate trachea when patient is awake and protective airway reflexes have returned. Patients with reactive airway disease may require deep extubation.

**Blood and fluid requirements**

Anticipate large blood loss.
IV: 18 ga x 1-2
NS/LR @:
4 cc/kg/hr – 0-10 kg
+ 2 cc/kg/hr – 11-20 kg
+ 1 cc/kg/hr – >20 kg
(e.g., 25 kg = 65 cc/hr)

The goal of intraop fluid therapy is to replace preop deficits, intraop fluid, electrolyte and blood losses, while providing maintenance fluids. Half of the calculated deficit (hrs fasting x hourly maintenance fluid requirement) generally is replaced during the 1st hr of anesthesia and the balance over the next 1-2 hrs. Surgical manipulation of tissue will cause 3rd-space fluid loss pro-

| | | |
|---|---|---|
| | Warm fluids.<br>Humidify gasses. | portional to the degree of surgical trauma and tissue exposure. It may range from 0-10 ml/kg/hr. |
| **Control of blood loss** | Deliberate hypotension | Deliberate hypotension can be accomplished by use of SNP, esmolol or potent inhalational agents titrated to effect (MAP 50-60 mmHg). |
| **Monitoring** | Standard monitors (see Appendix).<br>Arterial line<br>± CVP line | Arterial line is essential for monitoring BP during deliberate hypotension and for ABGs and blood chemistries. |
| **Control of ICP** | Hyperventilation<br>Mannitol<br>Loop diuretics<br>CSF drainage (>1 yr old) | For some procedures, it is essential to reduce intracranial volume to facilitate surgical access. If prolonged brain retraction is required, postop cerebral edema may ensue. |
| **Positioning** | ✓ and pad pressure points.<br>✓eyes. | Positioning head above the heart facilitates venous drainage, but also increases the incidence of VAE. Do not hyperextend or hyperflex the head and neck. Flexion of the neck will move the ETT downward (mainstem intubation); extension will move the ETT upward (cuff leak). |
| **Complications** | Displacement of ETT<br>Oculocardiac reflex (OCR) → ↓↓HR, ↓BP<br>VAE<br>Major blood loss | Suture ETT to alveolar ridge.<br>Notify surgeon. RX: atropine 0.02 mg/kg.<br>VAE should be suspected if sudden ↑$ETN_2$, ↓$ETCO_2$, ↓$O_2$ sat, ↓BP, ↑HR. Notify surgeon, flood surgical field with NS, support patient hemodynamically and D/C $N_2O$. |

**POSTOPERATIVE**

| | | |
|---|---|---|
| **Complications** | ↑ADH secretion<br>DI<br>Cerebral edema<br>Pneumothorax<br>Bleeding | SIADH or DI may follow brain manipulation and may re-quire pharmacologic intervention for Rx. Cerebral edema may → ↑ICP (headache, N&V, ↓mental status, etc.)<br>Pneumothorax (Sx = ↑respirations, wheezing, ↓BP, ↓CO, ↓$O_2$ sat) may occur 2° rib resection for bone graft. ✓ CXR. |
| **Pain management** | PCA (see Appendix). | |
| **Tests** | Hct | |

**References**


1. Christianson L: Anesthesia for major craniofacial operations. *Int Anesthesiol Clin* 1985; 23(4):117-30.
2. MacLennan FM, Robertson GS: Ketamine for induction and intubation in Treacher-Collins Syndrome. *Anesthesia* 1981; 36(2):196-98.
3. Rasch DK, Browder F, Barr M, Greer D: Anaesthesia for Treacher-Collins and Pierre Robin syndromes: a report of three cases. *Can Anaesth Soc J* 1986; 33(3P+1):364-70.

**Surgeon**

**Stephen A. Schendel, MD, DDS**

---

## 11.4 RESTORATIVE SURGERY

---

**Anesthesiologists**

**Stanley I. Samuels, MB, BCh, FFARCS**
**Richard A. Jaffe, MD, PhD**

# REPAIR OF FACIAL FRACTURES

## SURGICAL CONSIDERATIONS

**Description:** Facial fractures are characterized by location. Fractures of the maxilla are classified either as **Le Fort I, II** or **III**, depending on the level of the fracture (Fig 11.4-1). **Le Fort III** is essentially a disassociation of the cranium and face. **Le Fort II** is a triangular fracture with a fracture line across the nose, through the infraorbital rims, and extending to the entire lower maxillary structures. **Le Fort I** is a horizontal fracture, separating the teeth and maxillary components from the upper facial structures. In these cases, the maxilla is usually mobile, or impacted posteriorly, occasionally closing off the posterior airway. Associated fractures in the maxillary region include fractures of the zygoma. Orbital fractures (most common is the orbital floor fracture), isolated nasal fractures, and nasal orbital ethmoid fractures (usually with severe comminution of the upper face and telecanthus, and possible intracranial fractures) have the potential for CSF rhinorrhea.

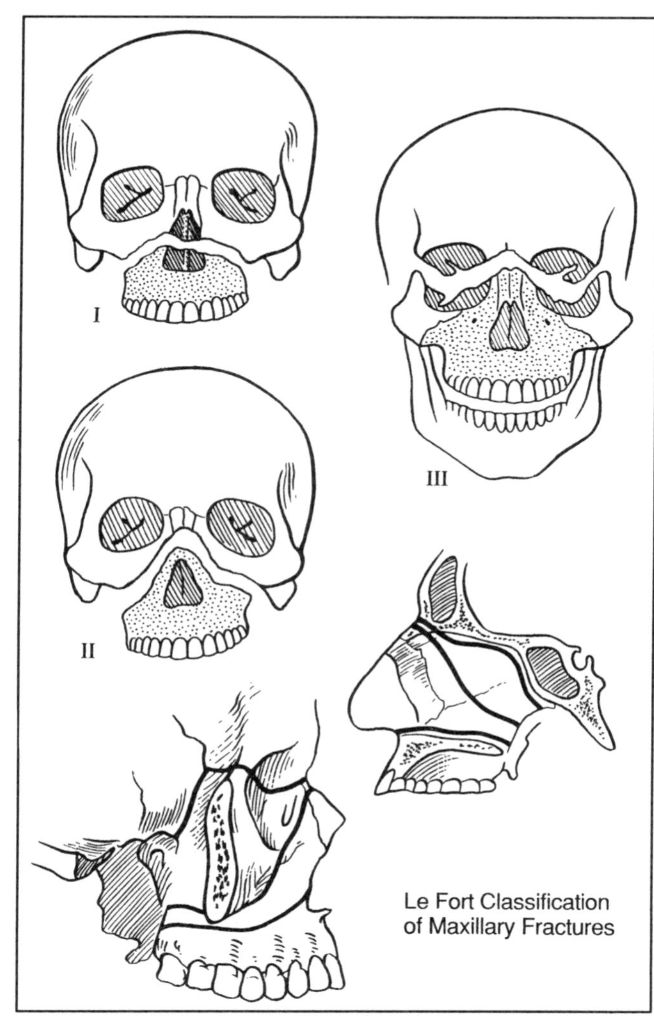


**Figure 11.4-1.** Le Fort I is a horizontal fracture involving mobilization of the dentition and maxilla. Le Fort II is a pyramid-shaped fracture including the dentition and nasal structures. Le Fort III fracture involves separation of the cranium from facial bone structure. (Reproduced with permission from Schultz RC: *Facial Injuries*. Yearbook Medical Pub: 1988.)

Fractures of the mandible are classified by the type of fracture and location (Fig 11.4-2), the most common being the subcondylar fracture. Fractures involving the mandibular body, such as the parasymphyseal fracture, may end up with a mobile mandible. In cases of bilateral mandibular body fractures associated with symphyseal fractures, the mandible can be flail and fall posteriorly in the supine position, blocking off the airway. All the fractures involving change in occlusion (Le Fort maxillary and all mandibular fractures), require reestablishment of a normal occlusion by intermaxillary wiring and the application of arch bars. This may be combined with rigid fixation, most commonly internal plates. Many approaches are possible, requiring, for example, external excisions under the eyelid, along the inferior border of the mandible, or, in extreme cases, a bicoronal incision, depending on the extent of the fracture and associated facial lacerations. Oral incisions may be associated with external incisions.

**Usual preop diagnosis**: Facial trauma

### SUMMARY OF PROCEDURE

| | Mandibular | Maxillary Orbital Zygomatic | Nasal |
|---|---|---|---|
| **Position** | Supine | ⇐ | ⇐ |
| **Incision** | Intraoral; lateral submandibular | Intraoral, ± subciliary incisions); possibly coronal | Closed reduction; possibly intranasal |
| **Special instrumentation** | Air power tools; plate fixation; headlight | ⇐ | ⇐ |

| | Mandibular | Orbital Zygomatic | Nasal |
|---|---|---|---|
| **Unique considerations** | Nasal RAE®; throat pack; ETT | Fractures not involving change in occlusion (e.g, orbital zygomatic, nasal fractures) can be handled by oral intubation. All fractures with a change in occlusion should undergo nasal intubation, with either RAE® or 60° curved connector. | ⇐ |
| **Antibiotics** | Cefazolin 1 gm iv q 4-6 hrs x 5-7 d | ⇐ | ⇐ |
| **Surgical time** | 1 - 3 hrs | 1 - 6 hrs | 1 hr |
| **EBL** | Minimal | 50-600 cc | Minimal |
| **Postop care** | PACU (uncomplicated fractures); ICU (large fractures ± intracranial trauma) | ⇐ + Patient may wake up with jaws wired together. | ⇐ |
| **Mortality** | Minimal | ⇐ | ⇐ |
| **Morbidity** | Pain | ⇐ | ⇐ |
| | Swelling | ⇐ | ⇐ |
| | Infection | ⇐ | ⇐ |
| | Bone loss | ⇐ | ⇐ |
| | Poor occlusal or cosmetic result | – | |
| | Visual problems | ⇐ | |
| **Procedure code** | 21440-21470 (mandibular fractures)<br>21480-21490 (TMJ fractures) | 21343-21344 (frontal sinus fractures)<br>21345-21348 (Le Fort II)<br>21355-21366 (malar zygomatic fractures)<br>21385-21408 (orbital fractures)<br>21421-21423 (Le Fort I)<br>21431-21436 (Le Fort III) | 21310-21337 (nasal/septal fractures)<br>21388-21340 (nasoethmoid fractures) |
| **Pain score** | 5 | 4 | 4 |

## PATIENT POPULATION CHARACTERISTICS

| | |
|---|---|
| **Age range** | >4 yrs |
| **Male:Female** | 1:1 |
| **Incidence** | The most common bones to be fractured are nasal bones, followed by the zygoma and arch, mandible and orbital floor; 2/3 of patients involved in motor vehicle accidents (MVAs).[1] |
| **Etiology** | MVAs: 54%<br>Home accidents: 17%<br>Athletic injuries: 11% |
| **Associated conditions** | Dental fractures<br>Intracranial injury<br>Cervical spine fractures: 10%<br>Shock<br>Globe injuries |

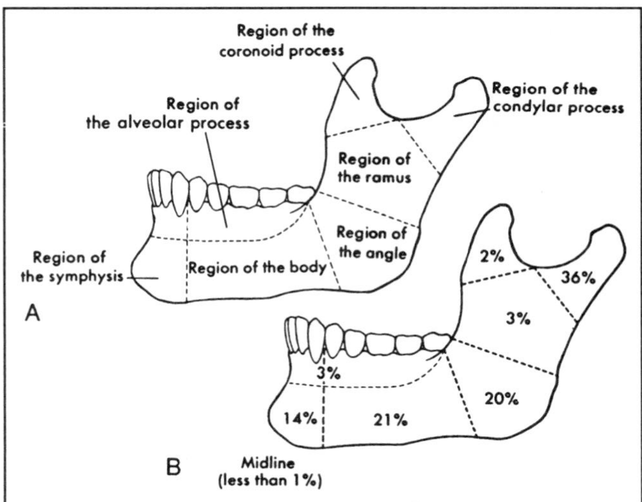


**Figure 11.4-2.** (A) Mandibular regions. (B) Percentage of fractures occurring in each region. (Reproduced with permission from Kruger GO: *Textbook of Oral and Maxillofacial Surgery*, 6th edition. CV Mosby Co: 1984.)

# ANESTHETIC CONSIDERATIONS

## PREOPERATIVE

Frequently, the anesthesiologist's first encounter with these patients is in the ER where prompt airway management decisions are essential, often before diagnostic imaging studies are complete. Several options exist: often the airway can be managed simply by inserting an oropharyngeal airway. Failing this, an emergency intubation will be necessary. Blind nasal intubation should be avoided in patients with CSF rhinorrhea or other evidence of nasopharyngeal trauma. The potential for creating false passages and additional trauma is significant. An awake oral intubation with topical anesthesia is often the safest approach. Emergency oral intubation may be complicated by an unstable C-spine and limited jaw opening, together with blood and debris in the oropharynx, making visualization difficult, if not impossible. Often the only recourse is tracheostomy under local anesthesia. As with any trauma victim, attention is first directed toward maintaining the airway and restoration of fluid volume. The repair of the facial fracture may be carried out incidentally to the primary trauma surgery or, more often, is deferred until the patient's condition is stabilized. This preop assessment will focus on the patient coming to the OR for semi-elective repair of facial fracture.

**Airway** — Usually facial swelling and intraoral bleeding will have resolved, although mouth opening may be limited 2° pain or mechanical factors. Airway management requires detailed knowledge of the fracture site(s). Patients with a Le Fort fracture may benefit from an oral intubation to allow inspection of the nasopharynx before nasal intubation and definitive repair. The possibility of an awake fiber optic intubation should be discussed with the patient. Patients with isolated orbital, zygomatic or nasal fracture do not usually present airway management problems. The surgeon should be consulted regarding the preferred intubation route.

**Respiratory** — Evaluate for associated trauma. ✓ that chest tubes are functioning properly.
**Tests:** CXR; others as indicated from H&P.

**Cardiovascular** — Blunt chest trauma may be associated with myocardial contusion and pericardial effusion/ tamponade. Typically, several days will have elapsed since the initial trauma and the patient will be hemodynamically stable.
**Tests:** ECG; others as indicated from H&P.

**Neurological** — Meningitis may occur in patients with persistent rhinorrhea or pneumocephalus. Document any neurological deficit.

**Musculoskeletal** — May be associated with other fractures and soft-tissue trauma which may affect patient positioning.

**Hematologic** — **Tests:** Hct; others as indicated from H&P.

**Laboratory** — Other tests as indicated from H&P.

**Premedication** — Standard premedication (see Appendix) is appropriate for neurologically intact patients.

## INTRAOPERATIVE

**Anesthetic technique:** GETA

**Induction** — If there is any doubt regarding the ease of intubation, an awake FOL should be performed (see "Anesthetic Considerations for Thoracolumbar Procedures" under "Neurosurgery"). Nasal intubation is preferred for patients with mandibular and maxillary (Le Fort) fractures involving a change in occlusion. Patients with orbital, zygomatic or nasal fractures are usually intubated orally. In patients with normal airways, a standard induction (see Appendix) is appropriate. Nasal or oral ETTs (RAE®), or anode ETTs are commonly used to minimize intrusion into the surgical field.

**Maintenance** — Standard maintenance (see Appendix); muscle relaxation is usually required. Administration of an anti-emetic (e.g., metoclopramide 10 mg iv or ondansetron 4 mg iv) is beneficial in patients who have their jaws wired or banded together.

**Emergence** — Patients with difficult airways or with jaws wired together should be extubated when fully awake. A wire cutter (or scissors for elastic bands) should be at the bedside at all times. Insure that all throat packing has been removed before extubation. Some patients with multiple trauma or extensive soft-tissue swelling may require continued postop intubation and mechanical ventilation.

| | | |
|---|---|---|
| **Blood and fluid requirements** | Moderate blood loss<br>IV: 16-18 ga x 1<br>NS/LR @ 6-8 cc/hr | Maxillary repairs may be associated with significant blood loss. |
| **Monitoring** | Standard monitors (see Appendix). | Invasive monitoring may be required in patients with intracranial or other trauma. |

| | | |
|---|---|---|
| **Positioning** | √ and pad pressure points.<br>√ eyes. | Some surgeons prefer that the OR table be rotated 90° or 180°. Be prepared with long hoses and appropriate connectors. Protect eyes with an ophthalmic ointment. |
| **Complications** | ETT damage | Nasal ETT may be inadvertently wired to the maxilla, making extubation difficult. |

**POSTOPERATIVE**

| | | |
|---|---|---|
| **Complications** | Airway obstruction | Wire cutters (or scissors) should be available at bedside to facilitate emergent re-intubation or other form of airway management. Consider retained throat pack. |
| | N&V | Vigorous treatment of nausea is important. |
| **Pain management** | Parenteral narcotics or PCA with anti-emetics (see Appendix). | |

**References**

1. Manson PN: Facial Injuries. In *Plastic Surgery*, Vol 2. McCarthy JG, ed. WB Saunders Co, Philadelphia: 1990, 867-1141.

# LE FORT OSTEOTOMIES

## SURGICAL CONSIDERATIONS

**Description:** Le Fort osteotomies are used to correct maxillary deformities. The most common is the **Le Fort I**, a transverse osteotomy above the apices of the teeth used to correct maxillary retrusion or maxillary vertical excess. Intraoral vestibular incision is used for this approach, followed by an osteotomy of the maxilla, using either a burr or a saw, and completed with osteotomes. The osteotomy goes through both sinuses and frequently into the nasal cavity. **Le Fort II** or, occasionally, **Le Fort III maxillary osteotomies** (Fig 11.4-1) may be used to correct severe mid-facial retrusion with an orbital component. In these cases, infraorbital incisions are used with either brow or coronal incisions. With maxillary advancements, iliac or cranial bone grafts are often necessary. Most of these patients have orthodontic appliances and will require maxillary fixation with either wire or elastics at the end of the procedure. The maxilla is usually rigidly fixed in the new position with small mini-plates.

**Usual preop diagnosis**: Facial deformities

**SUMMARY OF PROCEDURE**

| | Le Fort I | Le Fort II | Le Fort III |
|---|---|---|---|
| **Position** | Supine; table may be rotated 90° or 180° | ⇐ | ⇐ |
| **Incision** | Intraoral | Intraoral and facial or coronal | ⇐ |
| **Special instrumentation** | Mini-plates and screws for maxilla | ⇐ | ⇐ |
| **Unique considerations** | Jaw frequently closed, either by wires or elastics, at end of procedure; RAE® or armored tube used. | ⇐ | ⇐ |
| **Antibiotics** | Cefazolin 1 gm iv x 5 d | ⇐ | ⇐ |
| **Surgical time** | 3 - 6 hrs | ⇐ | ⇐ |
| **EBL** | 400-800 cc | ⇐ | ⇐ |
| **Postop care** | PACU → room | ICU x 1 d | ⇐ |

| | Le Fort I | Le Fort II | Le Fort III |
|---|---|---|---|
| **Mortality** | Minimal | ⇐ | ⇐ |
| **Morbidity** | Relapse | ⇐ | ⇐ |
| | Infection | ⇐ | ⇐ |
| | Bone/tooth loss: Uncommon | ⇐ | ⇐ |
| | Intraop bleeding: Uncommon | ⇐ | ⇐ |
| **Procedure code** | 21144 - 21147 (variable) | 21150 | 21154 |
| **Pain score** | 4 | 5 | 5 |

### PATIENT POPULATION CHARACTERISTICS

| | |
|---|---|
| **Age range** | 15 yrs - adulthood, usually < 20 yrs |
| **Male:Female** | 1:1 |
| **Incidence** | Up to 5% of population |
| **Etiology** | Usually developmental in nature |
| **Associated conditions** | None, unless part of a recognized condition (e.g., Apert's syndrome, Crouzon's disease). May be associated with congenital anomalies, such as cleft lip and palate. |

## ANESTHETIC CONSIDERATIONS

See Anesthetic Considerations following "Mandibular Osteotomies/Genioplasty" (below).

**References**

1. Lanigan DT, Hey JH, West RA: Major vascular complications of orthognathic surgery: hemorrhage associated with Le Fort I osteotomies. *J Oral Maxillofac Surg* 1990; 48(6):561-73.
2. Hilley MD, Ghali GE, Giesecke AU: Anesthesia for orthognathic surgery in modern practice. In *Orthognathic Reconstructive Surgery*, 2nd edition. Bell WH, ed. WB Saunders Co, Philadelphia: 1992, 128-53.

# MANDIBULAR OSTEOTOMIES/GENIOPLASTY

## SURGICAL CONSIDERATIONS

**Description:** Mandibular deformities include either a retruded mandible or a prognathic mandible involving a malocclusion (Class II or III) and may be combined with a small chin (microgenia). Surgical correction of the basic mandibular deformity involves either advancing or retruding the mandible. The most common procedure for this is the **sagittal ramus split osteotomy (Obwegesser)**. This may be combined with a **genioplasty** to correct the chin deformity. Genioplasty also may be performed as an isolated procedure, the most common type being one in which a horizontal osteotomy of the inferior mandible is performed and the chin segment repositioned. A variety of approaches for mandibular osteotomies often involve the ramus area of the mandible and are performed via an intraoral approach. In some very large deformities, an external incision (**Risdon** type) and bone graft placement may be necessary to complete the mandibular ramus reconstruction. Occasionally, deformities may be corrected by mandibular body osteotomies. **Rigid fixation** of mandibular osteotomies is often accomplished by the use of small mini-plates or screws. Fixation can also be accomplished with elastic traction (rarely, wire fixation) between mandible and maxilla, placed either at the time of surgery, or several days following, and held in position for 1-2 weeks. Microgenia may be corrected by placement of an implant without performing an osteotomy. This procedure can be done either via the oral route or the extraoral route by a small submental incision. Most frequently, this isolated procedure is performed with local anesthesia and sedation.

**Usual preop diagnosis**: Mandibular deformity

## SUMMARY OF PROCEDURE

| | |
|---|---|
| **Position** | Supine; table may be rotated 90° or 180° |
| **Incision** | Usually oral, but may be in the submental or posterior mandibular area externally. |
| **Special instrumentation** | Mini-plates and screws |
| **Unique considerations** | Postop, patient may have bimaxillary fixation with inability to open the mouth. |
| **Antibiotics** | Cefazolin 1 gm iv |
| **Surgical time** | Genioplasty: 0.5 - 1 hr<br>Mandibular osteotomy: 2 - 4 hrs |
| **EBL** | Genioplasty: 50 cc<br>Mandibular osteotomy: 100-200 cc |
| **Postop care** | PACU → room |
| **Mortality** | Rare |
| **Morbidity** | Mandibular relapse: ≤ 30%<br>Mental nerve paresthesia: 5-20% |
| **Procedure code** | 21121 (genioplasty sliding osteotomy); 21120 (genioplasty augmentation by prosthetic material); 21195 (mandibular ramus sagittal split osteotomy); 21196 (with rigid internal fixation); 21193, 21194 (mandibular ramus with bone graft); 21198 (segmental maxillary osteotomy) |
| **Pain score** | 4 |

**Figure 11.4-3.** Standard anesthesia and surgical setup for a maxillofacial surgical procedure and certain craniofacial surgical procedures. The table may be rotated 90°-180° with anesthesia equipment and personnel at the foot or off to one side. (Reproduced with permission from Bell WH, ed: *Modern Practice of Orthognathic Surgery*, Vol I. WB Saunders: 1990.)

### PATIENT POPULATION CHARACTERISTICS

| | |
|---|---|
| **Age range** | 8 yrs-adult |
| **Male:Female** | Unknown |
| **Incidence** | Unknown |
| **Etiology** | Developmental: 90%<br>Acquired: 10% |

## ANESTHETIC CONSIDERATIONS

**(Procedures covered: Le Fort osteotomies; mandibular osteotomies/genioplasty)**

### PREOPERATIVE

These surgeries are usually performed on patients with facial disproportion. In general, this patient population is young (< 8 yrs) and healthy; however, many of them will present with challenging airway management problems. In addition, facial disproportion will alter congenital anomalies (e.g., Crouzon's disease, Apert's syndrome). (For discussion of specific syndromes, see Anesthetic Considerations for "Pediatric Orthopedic Surgery for Extremities.")

| | |
|---|---|
| **Airway** | As usual, a careful airway evaluation is essential since many of these patients have abnormal airway anatomy. Visual inspection often reveals the reasons for the surgery and allows the anesthesiologist to determine the safest approach to intubation. When a difficult intubation is anticipated, the need for awake fiber optic intubation should be discussed with the patient. |
| **Respiratory** | Consider the anesthetic implications of associated congenital syndromes in this patient population.<br>**Tests:** As indicated from H&P. |
| **Cardiovascular** | Consider the anesthetic implications of associated congenital syndromes in this patient population.<br>**Tests:** As indicated from H&P. |
| **Hematologic** | Encourage autologous blood donation for maxillary procedures.<br>**Tests:** Hct |
| **Laboratory** | Other tests as indicated from H&P. |
| **Premedication** | Standard premedication (see Appendix) is usually appropriate. |

## INTRAOPERATIVE

**Anesthetic technique:** GETA

**Induction** If there is any doubt regarding the ease of intubation, an awake FOL should be performed (see description in "Anesthetic Considerations for Thoracolumbar Procedures" under "Neurosurgery"). Nasal intubation is preferred for patients with mandibular and maxillary (Le Fort) fractures involving a change in occlusion. Patients with orbital, zygomatic or nasal fractures are usually intubated orally. In patients with normal airways, a standard induction (see Appendix) is appropriate. Nasal or oral ETTs (RAE®), or anode ETTs, are commonly used to minimize intrusion into the surgical field.

**Maintenance** Standard maintenance (see Appendix); muscle relaxation is usually required. Administration of an anti-emetic (e.g., metoclopramide 10 mg iv or ondansetron 4 mg iv) is essential in patients who have their jaws wired or banded together.

**Emergence** Patients with difficult airways or with their jaws wired (or banded) together should be extubated when fully awake. A wire cutter (or scissors for elastic bands) should be at the bedside at all times. Insure that all throat packing has been removed before extubation. Some patients with multiple trauma or extensive soft-tissue swelling may require continued postop intubation and mechanical ventilation.

| | | |
|---|---|---|
| **Blood and fluid requirements** | Moderate blood loss<br>IV: 16 ga x 1<br>NS/LR @ 5-8 cc/kg/hr | Maxillary osteotomies may be associated with major blood loss (e.g., 2000 cc). Deliberate hypotension may be useful during maxillary surgery and blood should be readily available. |
| **Monitoring** | Standard monitors (see Appendix).<br>± Arterial line<br>± CVP line or 2nd iv | Direct arterial pressure measurements are useful for deliberate hypotension. Central venous access or a 2nd peripheral iv may be useful for vasodilator infusions. |
| **Positioning** | ✓ and pad pressure points.<br>✓ eyes. | Eyes should be protected with an ophthalmic ointment and possible tarsorrhaphy by the surgeons. Some surgeons prefer to have the OR table rotated 90° or 180°. Be prepared with long hoses and appropriate connectors. |
| **Complications** | ETT damage<br>Hemorrhage | ETT may be cut during maxillary osteotomy, necessitating rapid re-intubation. |

## POSTOPERATIVE

| | | |
|---|---|---|
| **Complications** | Airway obstruction<br>N&V | Wire cutters (or scissors) should be available at bedside to facilitate emergent re-induction or other form of airway management. Consider retained throat pack. Vigorous treatment of nausea is important. |
| **Pain management** | Parenteral narcotics or PCA with anti-emetics (see Appendix). | |

# MICROVASCULAR FREE-TISSUE/FLAP TRANSFER

## SURGICAL CONSIDERATIONS

**Description:** Soft-tissue or bony defects, not amenable to surgical treatment by local flaps, are corrected by the **transfer of appropriate tissue ("free-flap")**, using microvascular techniques. The location and extent of the defect determines which type of free-flap is most appropriate. Head and neck defects following tumor ablation are usually composite in nature and require transfer of bony tissue and overlying soft tissues. Typical donor sites are the radial forearm, scapula, iliac crest and fibula. Facial paralysis or soft-tissue defects are occasionally treated by insertion of a serratus flap through a face-lift incision.

Upper-extremity defects can be treated by a number of different **free-tissue transfers**. Lower-extremity defects are often traumatic in nature and occur most frequently in the distal two-thirds of the lower extremity. In this instance, **rectus abdominis** and **latissimus dorsi flaps** are frequently used. Bony defects can be treated by the transfer of a free fibula, usually from the other leg or iliac bone. The patient is usually in the supine position, although occasionally the prone position is used, depending on which flap is being procured. The extremity involved will always be isolated. If it is an upper extremity, a hand table or arm board may be needed. The incision is variable, depending on the flap. The most common upper extremity flaps are the radial forearm and lateral upper arm. The most common lower extremity flaps are lateral or medial leg flaps in the thigh, including tensor fascia lata and the lower leg gastrocnemius flap.

**Variant procedure or approaches**: Depending on site and size of wound, **skin grafting** and **pedicle flaps** are alternatives.

**Usual preop diagnosis:** Tissue defect

### SUMMARY OF PROCEDURE

| | Scapular Flap/ Latissimus | Serratus | Rectus | Extremity Flaps |
|---|---|---|---|---|
| **Position** | Prone (donor site); supine (graft) | Lateral decubitus (donor site); supine (graft) | Supine | Generally supine; occasionally prone |
| **Incision** | Lateral back | Mid-axillary line | Abdomen; hip–iliac; lateral leg–fibular; forearm–radial | Variable, depending on flap |
| **Special instrumentation** | Microscope, microvascular instruments; fluid warmer for irrigation | ⇐ | ⇐ | Hand table or arm board (upper extremity) |
| **Unique considerations** | Microvascular only: ASA, usually given as a suppository at beginning of procedure. Dextran (40 cc bolus) or heparin (5,000-7,000 U bolus, check PT, PTT) also may be used. | ⇐ | ⇐ | ⇐ |
| **Antibiotics** | Cefazolin 1 gm iv | ⇐ | ⇐ | ⇐ |
| **Surgical time** | 4 - 12 hrs | ⇐ | ⇐ | ⇐ |
| **Closing considerations** | Extensive dressing | ⇐ | ⇐ | ⇐ |
| **EBL** | 100-600 cc | ⇐ | ⇐ | ⇐ |
| **Postop care** | PACU → room; flap needs to be monitored by laser Doppler, direct vision. | ⇐ | ⇐ | ⇐ |
| **Mortality** | Minimal | ⇐ | ⇐ | ⇐ |

| | Scapular Flap | Serratus | Rectus | Extremity Flaps |
|---|---|---|---|---|
| **Morbidity** | Hematoma<br>Wound infection<br>Partial flap loss<br>Total flap loss: 2-5% | ⇐<br>⇐ | ⇐<br>⇐ | ⇐<br>⇐ |
| **Procedure code** | 15410 (free skin flap transplantation)<br>15755 (microvascular transfer free-flap) | ⇐ | ⇐ | 15732 (muscle, myocutaneous or fasciocutaneous flap, head and neck); 15734 (trunk); 15736 (upper); 15738 (lower) |
| **Pain score** | 4 | 4 | 4 | 4 |

### PATIENT POPULATION CHARACTERISTICS

| | |
|---|---|
| **Age range** | 15-45 yrs |
| **Male:Female** | 1:1 |
| **Incidence** | Unknown |
| **Etiology** | Trauma<br>Cancer<br>Congenital |
| **Associated conditions** | Depend on underlying disease. |

## ANESTHETIC CONSIDERATIONS

See Anesthetic Considerations following "Breast/Chest Wall Reconstruction" (below).

# PRESSURE-SORE AND WOUND RECONSTRUCTION

## SURGICAL CONSIDERATIONS

**Description:** Pressure sores are frequently seen in para/quadriplegics or other non-ambulatory patients. In the supine patient, pressure sores are commonly located in the sacral and trochanteric areas. Ischial ulcers are most commonly found in the wheelchair-bound patient. Surgical reconstruction of pressure sores in these patients involves debridement of the wound and transposition of adjacent tissue flaps. Other areas in which pressure sores are frequently found are the heel and knee. Closure of these involves rotation of flaps and, occasionally, skin grafting of the donor site or flap.

**Variant procedure or approaches**: Rotation or transposition myocutaneous flap, fasciocutaneous flap, or muscle flaps covered by split-thickness skin grafts

**Usual preop diagnosis:** Pressure sores

### SUMMARY OF PROCEDURE

| | Sacral | Ischial | Trochanteric |
|---|---|---|---|
| **Position** | Prone, flexed at waist; (occasionally lithotomy) | Prone, flexed at waist | Lateral decubitus |
| **Incision** | Back or gluteal | Back, gluteal or thigh | Posterior or lateral thigh |
| **Antibiotics** | Cefazolin 1 gm iv until drains removed, 7-14 d | ⇐ | ⇐ |
| **Surgical time** | 2 - 4 hrs | ⇐ | ⇐ |

| | Sacral | Ischial | Trochanteric |
|---|---|---|---|
| **Closing considerations** | No sheer forces or pressure to surgical area. Patient may be transferred to a non-pressure bed immediately postop. | ⇐ | ⇐ |
| **EBL** | 100-400 cc | ⇐ | ⇐ |
| **Postop care** | PACU → room; occasionally, spinal rehabilitation unit | ⇐ | ⇐ |
| **Mortality** | Rare | ⇐ | ⇐ |
| **Morbidity** | Infection<br>Wound breakdown<br>Late recurrence of ulcer | ⇐ | ⇐ |
| **Procedure code** | 15933-15937 | 15940-15946 | 15950-15958 |
| **Pain score** | 2 | 2 | 2 |

### PATIENT POPULATION CHARACTERISTICS

| | |
|---|---|
| **Age range** | 20-40 yrs |
| **Male:Female** | Predominantly male |
| **Incidence** | Typically in paraplegic or quadriplegic patients |
| **Etiology** | Prolonged bed rest with pressure in traumatized patients or those with altered sensation |
| **Associated conditions** | Infection<br>Paraplegia<br>Debilitation<br>Quadriplegia |

## ANESTHETIC CONSIDERATIONS

See Anesthetic Considerations following "Breast/Chest Wall Reconstruction" (below).

# BREAST/CHEST WALL RECONSTRUCTION

## SURGICAL CONSIDERATIONS

**Description:** Breast defects are usually the result of mastectomy for cancer. Congenital defects (e.g., Poland syndrome) are rare. Chest wall defects are occasionally seen following cardiovascular surgery or can be radiation-induced. There are three approaches to **breast reconstruction**: **tissue expansion** of the overlying skin by placement of an expander, followed by a permanent prosthesis; **transfer of a flap**, such as a latissimus dorsi myocutaneous flap, to the defect, followed by placement of a breast prosthesis; and complete **soft-tissue reconstruction**, most frequently using a pedicled rectus abdominis flap. Breast reconstruction following breast ablation can be accomplished using a latissimus dorsi myocutaneous flap as shown in Fig 11.4-4. The flap and skin pedicle are transferred from the ipsilateral back to the anterior chest where they are inserted into position. It is always necessary to use an implant with a latissimus dorsi reconstruction as the flap itself is not of adequate size to totally reconstruct an absent breast. Alternatively, the breast may be reconstructed by using the TRAM flap, which is a rectus abdominis muscle myocutaneous flap. This flap can be transferred with the superior epigastric vessels as a pedicled flap of either the contralateral or ipsilateral side, although the contralateral is preferred. The TRAM flap also may be transferred as a free-flap with microvascular anastomoses, as demonstrated in Fig 11.4-5. **Chest wall reconstruction** is frequently accomplished by rotation or transfer of the pectoralis muscles, followed by advancement of skin pedicles with split-thickness skin grafts. Occasional defects will need a pedicular or a free-rectus flap for adequate coverage.

**Usual preop diagnosis**: Carcinoma of the breast; radiation therapy; cardiovascular surgery; Poland syndrome

### SUMMARY OF PROCEDURE

| | Tissue Expander/Prothesis | Latissimus Flap | Rectus Flap |
|---|---|---|---|
| **Position** | Prone | Lateral decubitus; prone | Prone; table flexed |
| **Incision** | Breast | ⇐ | ⇐ |
| **Antibiotics** | Cefazolin 1 gm q 4-6 hrs iv x 5-7 d | ⇐ | ⇐ |
| **Surgical time** | 1 hr | 3 hrs | 4 - 6 hrs |
| **Closing considerations** | Extensive dressing required | ⇐ | ⇐ |
| **EBL** | Minimal-100 cc | 200-400 cc | 300-500 cc |
| **Postop care** | PACU → room | ⇐ | ⇐ |
| **Mortality** | Rare | ⇐ | ⇐ |
| **Morbidity** | Capsular contraction: ± 30% | – | – |
| | Decreased sensation: 15% | ⇐ | ⇐ |
| | Hematoma: 2.2% | ⇐ | ⇐ |
| | Fat/skin necrosis: 1.7-1.9% | ⇐ | ⇐ |
| | Nipple areola necrosis: 1.4% | ⇐ | ⇐ |
| | | Flap loss: Rare | ⇐ |
| | | Abdominal hernia: Rare | ⇐ |
| **Procedure code** | 19340 (immediate insertion of breast prosthesis)<br>19342 (delayed insertion of breast prosthesis) | 19360 (reconstruction with muscle and myocutaneous flap) | ⇐ |
| **Pain score** | 4-5 | 4-5 | 4-5 |

### PATIENT POPULATION CHARACTERISTICS

| | |
|---|---|
| **Age range** | 30-45 yrs |
| **Male:Female** | Breast reconstruction: mostly female |
| **Incidence** | Breast reconstruction is performed in 9% of female population; incidence of chest wall unknown |
| **Etiology** | Cancer<br>Trauma<br>Idiopathic<br>Radiation or post-cardiovascular surgery (chest wall reconstruction) |
| **Associated conditions** | Breast cancer<br>Cardiovascular disease<br>S/P chemotherapy<br>Pulmonary disease |

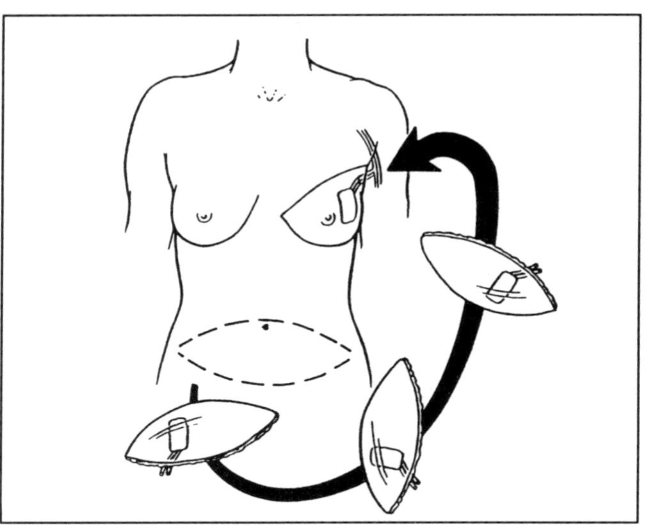

**Figure 11.4-4.** Breast reconstruction using free TRAM flap. (Reproduced with permission from Barton FE Jr: Breast cancer, preventive mastectomy, and breast reconstruction. *SRPS* 1991; 6(30):14.)

## ANESTHETIC CONSIDERATIONS

**(Procedures covered: microvascular free-tissue transfer/musculocutaneous flaps; pressure sore and wound reconstruction; breast/chest well reconstruction)**

### PREOPERATIVE

These surgeries are carried out on patients who have sustained major soft-tissue losses and require a flap procedure to

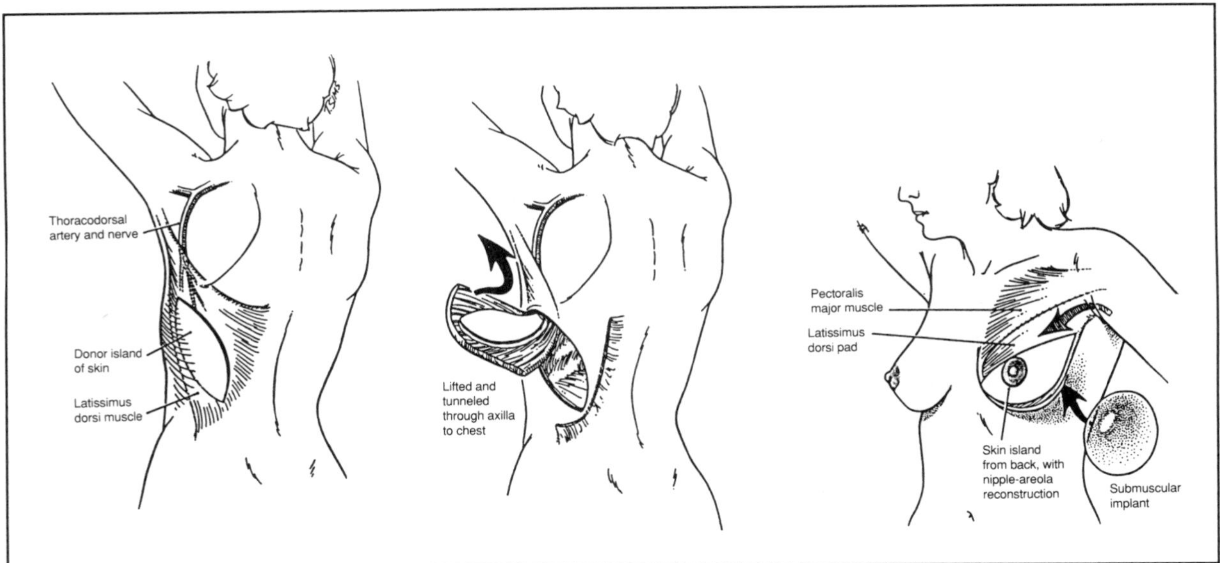


**Figure 11.4-5.** Breast reconstruction using latissimus dorsi myocutaneous flap. (Reproduced with permission from Barton FE Jr: Breast cancer, preventive mastectomy, and breast reconstruction. *SRPS* 1991; 6(30):14.)

cover the defect. There are typically four patient populations presenting for surgery: (1) Those presenting for reconstruction following cancer surgery, such as radical neck and breast reconstruction. (See Anesthetic Considerations for the primary procedure.) (2) Patients following trauma, usually upper or lower limb defects. (3) Patients with congenital defects. (4) Non-ambulatory, or quadriplegic/paraplegic patients who develop decubitus ulcer. In general, groups 1-3 should present few problems for the anesthesiologist. In a patient with a congenital lesion, however, it is prudent to look for evidence of CHD, musculoskeletal deformities and, of course, airway problems. The last group may well present several anesthetic challenges, as discussed below.

**Respiratory** Intercostal muscle weakness → atelectasis and ↓clearance of secretions → recurrent RTIs and V/Q mismatching + hypoxemia.
**Tests:** PFT; ABG; others as indicated from H&P.

**Cardiovascular** Autonomic hyperreflexia (AH) may occur in patients with a sensory level of T10 or above. Manifestations include ↑BP, ↓HR, dysrhythmia and vasodilatation in response to stimulation below the lesion. Seizures and cerebral hemorrhage also have been reported. Identify triggering stimuli (e.g., bowel or bladder distension, cutaneous stimulation).
**Tests:** ECG; others as indicated from H&P.

**Neurological** AH in patient with spinal cord injury (see Cardiovascular, above) may manifest as headaches, sweating, facial flushing or syncope.

**Musculoskeletal** Immobility → skeletal muscle atrophy, osteoporosis and decubitus ulcer formation.

**Renal** Chronic spinal cord injury → recurrent UTIs → renal failure.
**Tests:** UA; BUN; creatinine; others as indicated from H&P.

**Laboratory** Immobility → ↑$Ca^{++}$ → dysrhythmia and nausea.
**Tests:** Others as indicated from H&P.

**Premedication** Standard premedication (see Appendix) is usually appropriate. Patients with limited respiratory reserve should receive minimal sedation.

## INTRAOPERATIVE

**Anesthetic technique:** GETA. If flap donor and recipient sites are confined to the lower half of the body, regional anesthesia may be considered for short procedures. Spinal or epidural anesthesia will prevent AH, but may not be tolerated for prolonged surgery. Lighter levels of GA will not prevent AH.

**Induction** Standard induction (see Appendix) and intubation. Avoid succinylcholine in patients with muscle paralysis (2° ↑$K^+$).

**Maintenance** Standard maintenance (see Appendix). Muscle relaxation is usually appropriate. The patient should be kept warm and well-hydrated to minimize peripheral vasoconstriction, which might impair graft perfusion.

| | | |
|---|---|---|
| **Emergence** | AH 2° distended bladder or rectum may occur on emergence from anesthesia. | |
| **Blood and fluid requirements** | Moderate blood loss<br>IV: 16 ga x 1<br>NS/LR @ 4-6 cc/kg/hr<br>Warm fluids.<br>Humidify gasses. | Keep patient warm and maintain a positive fluid balance. |
| **Monitoring** | Standard monitors (see Appendix).<br>UO<br>± Arterial line | An arterial line may be useful in patients susceptible to AH and for prolonged procedures where regular ABGs and blood chemistries will be useful. |
| **Positioning** | ✓ and pad pressure points.<br>✓ eyes. | Many of these patients may be osteoporotic, so great care should be used in moving and positioning. |
| **Complications** | Hypothermia | Patients with spinal cord injury often have impaired thermoregulation. Maintain normal body temperature with warming blankets, fluid and airway warmers. |
| | AH | AH should be promptly controlled with SNP bolus and infusion while anesthesia is deepened. |
| | Decubitus ulcer | Pressure necrosis can occur in as little as 2 hrs. Carefully pad and repeatedly ✓ pressure points. |
| | Dextran reaction | Prophylactic use of very low molecular weight dextran (Promit®) usually prevents allergic reactions to higher molecular weight dextrans. |

## POSTOPERATIVE

| | | |
|---|---|---|
| **Complications** | Respiratory insufficiency | Quadriplegic patients may have ↓VC and ↓ERV and be uniquely susceptible to residual respiratory depressant effects. |
| | AH | AH may occur 2° distended bladder or rectum. Rx: SNP bolus/infusion; removal of stimulus. |
| **Pain management** | Parenteral opiates (see Appendix).<br>PCA (see Appendix). | Pain should be promptly treated to minimize reflex peripheral vasoconstriction and impaired graft perfusions. |

**Surgeons**

**Bruce A. Reitz, MD** *(Pediatric Cardiovascular Surgery)*
**Gary E. Hartman, MD** *(Pediatric General Surgery)*
**John A. Duncan III, MD, PhD** *(Pediatric Neurosurgery)*
**Lawrence M. Shuer, MD** *(Pediatric Neurosurgery)*
**Gary K. Steinberg, MD, PhD** *(Pediatric Neurosurgery)*
**Lawrence A. Rinsky, MD** *(Pediatric Orthopedic Surgery)*

---

# 12. PEDIATRIC SURGERY

---

**Anesthesiologists**

**Robert J. Moynihan, MD** *(Pediatric Cardiovascular Surgery)*
**George Lederhaas, MD** *(Pediatric General Surgery)*
**Alvin Hackel, MD** *(Pediatric General Surgery)*
**C. Philip Larson, Jr, MD, MS** *(Pediatric Neurosurgery)*
**Yuan-Chi Lin, MD, MPH** *(Congenital Malformation Surgery)*

**Surgeon**

**Bruce A. Reitz, MD**

## 12.1 PEDIATRIC CARDIOVASCULAR SURGERY

**Anesthesiologist**

**Robert J. Moynihan, MD**

# SURGERY FOR TETRALOGY OF FALLOT

## SURGICAL CONSIDERATIONS

**Description:** Tetralogy of Fallot (TOF) consists of underdevelopment of the RV infundibulum, with resulting RV-outflow (pulmonary) stenosis, a large malalignment (overriding aorta) type of VSD, RVH (Fig 12.1-1), and occasionally, ASD (pentalogy of Fallot). TOF, which causes reduced pulmonary flow, accounts for approximately 10% of all surgery performed to correct congenital heart defects (CHDs). The variation in presentation depends primarily on the type of RV-outflow tract obstruction (RVOTO). The operation to correct TOF consists of relieving the obstruction and closing the VSD with a patch.

Patients with TOF were first treated palliatively beginning in 1944, with the introduction of the **Blalock-Taussig procedure**, which produced a systemic artery-to-PA shunt. This procedure augments the amount of blood traversing the pulmonary bed and returning oxygenated to the left atrium, thus increasing the percent saturation in the systemic circulation. As modern cardiac surgery has developed, this palliative approach has given way to early, complete correction in most cases. Palliation is reserved for patients with severe pulmonary arterial hypoplasia and/or with an anomalous left-anterior, descending coronary artery originating from the right coronary artery. Total correction is now performed routinely, even in neonates. RVOTO is treated as necessary by infundibular muscle resection, pulmonary valvotomy or valvectomy, and augmentation of the main PA or PA branches with patching. Pericardium, Gortex® or other type of biologic membrane material can be used for patching at any level, from the RV to PA. The VSD is closed with a Dacron® patch using standard techniques, with care being taken to avoid injury to the bundle of His, which would produce heart block.

**Usual preop diagnosis:** TOF; cyanotic CHD; severe cyanotic spells; failure to thrive

### SUMMARY OF PROCEDURE

| | **Neonate Repair with Hypothermia And Circulatory Arrest** | **Infant & Adult Repair With Standard CPB** |
|---|---|---|
| **Position** | Supine | ⇐ |
| **Incision** | Standard median sternotomy | ⇐ |
| **Cannulation for CPB** | Ascending aortic cannula and single right-atrial cannula | Ascending aortic cannula and separate SVC and IVC cannula with chokers to exclude the heart and give total CPB, with access to the right atrium. |
| **Unique considerations** | Shunting R → L allows any gaseous or particulate emboli entering the iv to become systemic emboli by crossing the VSD to the systemic circulation. | ⇐ |
| **Antibiotics** | Cefazolin 15-30 mg/kg q 8 hrs | ⇐ |
| **Myocardial** | Blood or crystalloid cardioplegia, in addition to topical myocardial hypothermia | ⇐ |
| **Intraop sequence** | Right ventriculotomy<br>Resection of infundibular obstructing muscle bands<br>Patch closure of VSD<br>Closure of ASD<br>Reinstitution of CPB<br>Repair of RVOTO, with patch, as needed | Right ventriculotomy with excision of obstructing muscle<br>Patch closure of VSD<br>Augmentation of RV and PA, with patch, as needed<br>Right atriotomy with closure of ASD |
| **Surgical time** | Circulatory arrest: 30 - 45 min<br>Cross-clamp: 60 min<br>Total: 3 - 4 hrs | 45 - 75 min<br>60 - 90 min<br>3 - 4 hrs |
| **Closing considerations** | Chest tube in pericardial (and possibly pleural) space, if opened | ⇐ |
| | Temporary ventricular pacing wires applied to heart | ⇐ |
| | Possible right- or left-atrial line for monitoring, as necessary | |

| | | |
|---|---|---|
| **EBL** | Moderate | ⇐ |
| **Postop care** | Cardiac ICU x 2-3 d. 1-2 d assisted ventilation; inotropics for right heart dysfunction. | ⇐ |
| **Mortality** | 4-5% | 2-4% |
| **Morbidity** | Bleeding<br>Infection<br>Low CO<br>Stroke<br>Heart block<br>Residual VSD<br>Transient, right-side CHF | |
| **Procedure code** | 33692 | ⇐ |
| **Pain score** | 8-10 | 8-10 |

## PATIENT POPULATION CHARACTERISTICS

**Age range** 2 mo-65 yrs (usually < 5 yrs)

**Male:Female** 60:40

**Incidence** 0.5/1,000

**Etiology** No apparent correlation with any specific genetic disorder; higher than expected prevalence of older maternal age at time of conception of affected children.

**Associated conditions** Other CHDs, such as AV canal
PDA
Previous palliative shunt
Anomalous left coronary artery
Metabolic acidosis in cases of profound hypoxia
Right-side aortic arch

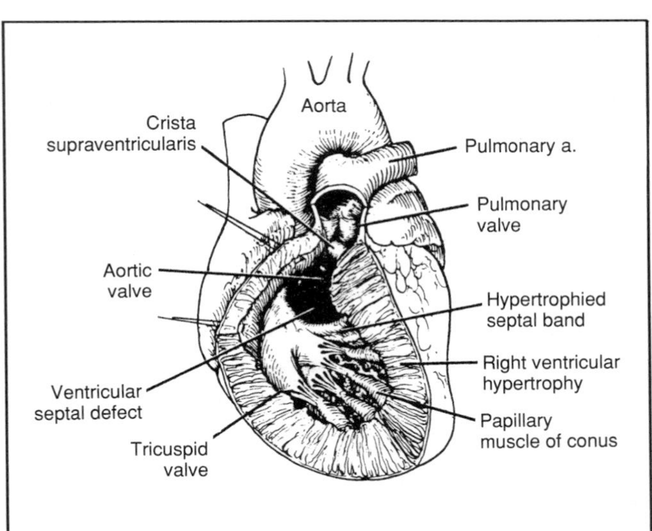


**Figure 12.1-1.** Tetralogy of Fallot. (Reproduced with permission from Dunphy JE, Way LW: *Current Surgical Diagnosis and Treatment.* Lange Medical Publications: 1973.)

---

# ANESTHETIC CONSIDERATIONS

## PREOPERATIVE

**Pathophysiology** **R → L shunting** via VSD → systemic desaturation (hypoxemia) → ↑R → L shunting by:
- ↑systemic venous return (tachypnea)
- ↑RV outflow tract obstruction (RVOTO) (infundibular spasm, volume depletion, ↑↑ in PVR)
- ↓SVR (acidosis, arteriolar dilation)

**"TET" spells** **Hypercyanotic ("TET") spells:** etiology uncertain. Probably initiated by ↑$O_2$ demand → ↓$PaO_2$, ↓pH and ↑$PaCO_2$ → ↑RR → ↑venous return, ↑R → L shunt. Infundibular spasm and ventricular dysfunction may also initiate an episode.

Rx: Rapid and vigorous treatment often essential to break a potentially malignant cycle. Specificity of Rx also essential, requiring considerable insight into state of pathophysiology:
- "Squatting" (knees-to-chest) → ↑SVR and ↓venous return.
- Phenylephrine → ↑SVR: bolus 10 μg/Kg; infusion 2-5 μg/Kg/min. Excessive ↑BP → ↑PVR.
- $NaHCO_3$ 1-2 mEq/kg → correction of acidosis → ↑SVR.
- Volume (NS/LR bolus 10-20 cc/kg) → ↑RV end-systolic volume [RVESV]) → ↓RVOTO.
- Propranolol (ß-blockade) → ↓HR and ↓inotropy → ↑RVESV and ↓RVOTO → ↓infundibular spasm.
- Halothane → similar effect to ß-blockade. It is the preferred volatile agent 2° minimal ↓SVR effect. Use with caution in cases associated with severe CHF.

- Morphine sedation/GA → ↓infundibular spasm, ↓$VO_2$.
- Hyperventilation → ↓$PaCO_2$ → ↓PVR. PVR seldom a major contributor to RVOTO, except in the presence of ↓↓pH, ↑↑$PaCO_2$, ↓↓$PaO_2$ or some form of reactive pulmonary HTN.
- Avoid low MAP → atelectasis → ↑PVR; 100% $O_2$ → ↓PVR.

**Respiratory** Any infectious/asthmatic pulmonary process will complicate pre- and postop cardiopulmonary function. Where possible, patient condition should be optimized preop.

**Tests:** CXR; AoE; ↓pulmonary vascular markings

**Cardiovascular** CHF is rare in young patients, except in those with large L → R shunts, i.e., PDA or bronchopulmonary collaterals. CHF is more common in older children/adults 2° RV cardiomyopathy, chronic hypoxia and functionally induced aortic insufficiency (AoI). Thorough knowledge of the patient's anatomic defects and their pathophysiology is essential (e.g., is RVOTO fixed or dynamic).

**Tests:** ABG; ECG – RVH; RAD ± complete or incomplete RBBB; CXR – normal heart size; "coeur en sabot" – elevation of apex 2° RVH, RAE; ECHO – general anatomic confirmation; cardiac cath with angiography – site and severity of RVOTO; source and quantity of pulmonary blood flow; AI, tricuspid regurgitation (TR), coronary artery anatomy; degree of CHF (LVEDP)

**Hematologic** Polycythemia (typical with chronic $O_2$ sat < 90%) → ↑blood viscosity (critical above Hct 70) and propensity to cerebral and PA thrombotic events. Coagulopathy associated with polycythemia and with postop coagulopathy thrombocytopenia, hypofibrinogenemia, and ↓factors V, VIII, ± fibrinolysis, ± low-grade DIC).

**Tests:** CBC; platelets; bleeding time; coagulation profile

**Laboratory** Other tests as indicated from H&P.

**Premedication** Premed desirable in patients >6 mo old. Midazolam 0.5-0.75 mg/kg po in 15-30 cc apple juice 30 min prior to induction.

## INTRAOPERATIVE

**Anesthetic technique:** GETA. Children are brought into prewarmed OR (80°F, isothermal for infants). If iv is placed preinduction (implying very fragile hemodynamics), it will be used for iv induction, thereby avoiding potent inhalational agents.

**Induction** Typically mask halothane, $O_2$ ± $N_2O$. If iv in place, fentanyl (10 $\mu$g/Kg) and pancuronium (0.2 mg/Kg) ± volatile agent. Intubation via nasal route is preferred for stability and patient comfort. The ETT is advanced gently until a mainstem intubation occurs. It is then withdrawn until bilateral breath sounds are once again heard (carinal position), then withdrawn an additional distance so that the tip of the ETT is approximately mid-trachea (taped position). Positive pressure leak between 30-40 cm $H_2O$ is desirable. Leaks < 30 cm result in volume loss and difficulty providing appropriate ventilation during critical phases intraop or postop. Conversely, leaks 40 cm $H_2O$ carry a higher risk of subglottic edema and/or stenosis.

**Maintenance** Fentanyl (100-200 $\mu$g/kg total, in divided doses), pancuronium (0.2 mg/kg prn), midazolam (0.1-0.2 mg/kg as hemodynamically tolerated) ± volatile agent. $FiO_2$ = 1. "TET" spells can occur 2° surgical manipulation. Rx as in preop spells.

**Emergence** Transport to ICU intubated and ventilated. Inotropic support usually required 24-48 hrs.

**Blood and fluid requirements**

IV: 22-24 ga x 2, taped securely
NS @ TKO
D5 ¼ NS @ 1-2 cc/min
Warm fluids.
Humidify and warm gasses.

Proximal CVP port: NS used for volume and drug administration as well as blood sampling, CVP transduction. Distal CVP port: D5 ¼ NS at ~1-2 cc/min, carrier solution for vasoactive infusion.

**Monitoring**

Standard monitors (see Appendix).
Urinary catheter
Arterial line (usually radial)
CVP line: 4 Fr double-lumen (usually right IJ)

Usually a 22-ga catheter is placed percutaneously in the radial artery (avoid Blalock-Taussig shunt side, usually right side). On infants, a fiber optic transilluminator may facilitate arterial cannulation. Dorsalis pedis and posterior tibial arteries are avoided, due to problems with spasm and clotting when coming off CPB. Femoral arteries are cannulated as a last resort, using a 2½ or 3 Fr 2-4 cm catheter. If all else fails, a surgical cut-down is performed. Older children (>20 kg) may receive adult-size central lines, as well as PA catheters, if medically indicated.

| | | |
|---|---|---|
| **Pre-CPB** | Heparinization (3 mg/kg)<br>ACT >400 sec<br>MAP ~70 mmHg<br>Cannulae placed<br>Drips off<br>√ pupils.<br>√ UO. | In the pre-CPB period, crystalloid and/or 5% albumin is administered as needed to compensate for bleeding and 3rd-space losses. Blood replacement is reserved for major blood loss situations associated with re-do's and/or surgical entry into major vessels/heart chambers. |
| **CPB** | Ventilation stopped.<br>Hypothermia: 22-26°C<br>Hct 20-25 typical during CPB<br>√ adequate flow/pressure.<br>√ anesthetic/NMB levels.<br>√ pupils.<br>√ peripleural perfusion, edema, venous congestion.<br>√ ABG, electrolytes, UO, Hct and ACT q 30-60 min. | Drugs are injected into the pump reservoir as appropriate. (For example, use phentolamine for HTN and/or slow/inadequate body cooling; methylprednisolone for deep hypothermic cardiac arrest [DHCA] situations; lasix for suboptimal UO; and heparin in accordance with ongoing ACT analysis). Perfusion pressure, CVP and flow rates are monitored in tandem with the perfusionists. Observation for venous congestion is ongoing during the procedure. Monitoring electrolytes and arterial/venous blood and formulation of appropriate therapeutic interventions is essential. |
| **Transition off CPB** | Rewarming<br>Vasoactive infusions started at 34°C.<br>Flush lines.<br>√ waveforms.<br>Suction ETT.<br>Resume ventilation.<br>√ bilateral breath sounds.<br>√ ABC, electrolytes, Hct (~30).<br>√ ACT (>400).<br>√ ECG: pacing may be necessary.<br>Supplement NMB and deepen anesthesia. | Aerosolized albuterol may be indicated if wheezing is present. Air emboli must be removed from the pulmonary veins, aorta and cardiac chambers. Full-flow CPB at normothermia is often allowed to rebuild myocardial ATP stores. The cross-clamp is removed and the empty heart (vented) is allowed to beat. The vent is discontinued and the heart is gradually allowed to work with progressively less "pump" support. |
| **Post-CPB** | Inotropic support (dopamine, dobutamine, epinephrine)<br>RV afterload reduction (↓PVR):<br>$FiO_2 = 1$<br>$PaCO_2$ ~30<br>NTG ± $PGE_1$<br>Minimize mean airway pressure.<br>AV sequential pacemaker (heart block not uncommon).<br>Surgical PA or LA line usually placed to monitor cardiac status.<br>Reverse anticoagulation.<br>Rx coagulopathy: (fresh (< 48° old), whole blood preferred.<br>FFP/platelets/cryo/EACA/DDAVP, as necessary. | ↓RV compliance is expected (↑RVEDP = RV failure). This RV "failure" is 2° to RVH, CPB, hypothermic arrest, infundibulotomy and pulmonary regurgitation, as well as general surgical manipulation of the RV. RV afterload reduction is essential, initially through ventilatory efforts: clear unobstructed ventilation, do not allow wheezing (albuterol prn), use gentle hyperventilation on 100% $O_2$. If these maneuvers are not sufficient, then NTG/PGE are used. Inotropic support of RV also typically is used – dopamine/dobutamine initially and epinephrine reserved for severe RV dysfunction. Inotropic support, especially dopamine and epinephrine, may ↑PVR, thus confounding overall resuscitation. R → L intra-atrial shunting possible even if PFO/ASD "closed." Large volume requirements may be 2° bleeding and capillary leak. |
| **Positioning** | √ and pad pressure points.<br>√ eyes. | |
| **Complications** | Cerebral/cardiac embolization<br>Aortic dissection<br>Unilateral carotid hypoperfusion<br>Pump/oxygenator failure<br>Massive blood transfusion | Massive blood transfusion with citrated blood products (>2 cc/kg/min) → coagulopathy, ↓$Ca^{++}$, ↑K. Rx: includes stopping transfusion (if possible), $CaCl_2$, hyperventilation. |

### POSTOPERATIVE

| | | |
|---|---|---|
| **Complications** | Persistent shunt R → L, usually at atrial level, L → R, at ventricular level<br>Hypothermia<br>Persistent bleeding<br>RV failure<br>Pneumo/hemothorax<br>Dysrhythmias<br>Cardiac tamponade | Sometimes a PFO will be left surgically open, especially if RV failure is severe, in order to allow RV decompression via a R → L intra-atrial shunt. This will often result in profound systemic $O_2$-Hb desaturation. Theory is that it is better to have systemic desaturation than uncompensated RV failure. ECHO will confirm the existence of intra-atrial shunting. |
| **Tests** | ABGs<br>Electrolytes<br>Coagulation profile<br>CXR – ✓ line placement, ETT placement<br>ECHO | TEE monitoring is emerging as an invaluable anatomical and physiological monitor. |


**References**

1. Strong MJ, Keats AS, Cooley DA: Anesthesia for cardiovascular surgery in infancy. *Anesthesiology* 1966; 27(3):257-65.
2. Engstrom R, Fitzgerald D: *Manual of Pediatric Cardiac Anesthesia.* Stanford University Hospital Medical Center, Stanford: 1988.
3. Lake CL: *Pediatric Cardiac Anesthesia.* Appleton & Lange, Norwalk, CT: 1988.
4. Kaplan JA: *Cardiac Anesthesia,* Volume 2. WB Saunders, Philadelphia: 1987.
5. Ryan JF, Todres ID, Coté CJ, Goudsouzian N: A practice of anesthesia for infants and children. In *Anesthesia for Children with Heart Disease.* Hickey PR, ed. Grune and Strattan, Orlando: 1986, ch 16.


# SURGERY FOR TOTAL ANOMALOUS PULMONARY VENOUS CONNECTION

## SURGICAL CONSIDERATIONS

**Description:** Total anomalous pulmonary venous connection (TAPVC) is a congenital cardiac malformation in which there is no direct connection between any pulmonary vein and the left atrium. Typically, all of the pulmonary veins connect to the right atrium or to one of its tributaries. A patent foramen ovale (PFO) or an atrial septal defect (ASD) must be present to insure survival after birth. The object of the repair is to enable the pulmonary vein to drain into the left atrium.

TAPVC was first successfully repaired in 1956 by Lewis and Varco at the University of Minnesota, with joining of the pulmonary venous sinus to the left atrium and closure of the ASD. Although mortality for this lesion was initially quite high, particularly in infants with obstruction of the pulmonary veins, recent improvements in intraop and postop management have allowed successful correction in the majority of neonates and infants. TAPVC is supercardiac in about 45% of cases, cardiac in about 25%, infracardiac in about 25%, and mixed in about 5%. The anomalous drainage in supercardiac TAPVC is usually by a left vertebral vein into the innominate vein. In cardiac TAPVC, drainage is usually to the coronary sinus and occasionally to the right atrium. In infracardiac TAPVC, drainage is usually into the portal vein. Usually, the right and left pulmonary veins drain into a common pulmonary venous sinus in each of these entities. This allows for anastomosis of the common venous sinus to the left atrium and, thus, definitive repair. When pulmonary venous drainage is obstructed, patients present with severe pulmonary edema, pulmonary HTN, and low cardiac output. Symptomatic TAPVC is repaired at any age, frequently with induced hypothermia and circulatory arrest (children < 5 kg), and success is often related to adequate control of elevated pulmonary vascular resistance (PVR) in the early postop period. The heart is exposed through a standard median sternotomy. The aorta and venous cannulae are placed (described below) and CPB with cooling is started. The aorta is cross-clamped and cardiac arrest is induced with cardioplegia. CPB is stopped and venous cannulae are removed. The cardiac apex is reflected and the pulmonary veins are dissected superiorly through the posterior pericardium. The left atrium is opened transversely with extension out on the left atrial appendage. Direct anastomosis of the pulmonary venous confluence to the left atrium is accomplished using continuous sutures. Through a right atriotomy, the ASD or PFO is closed, the atria are repaired and CPB with rewarming is started. (Alternative repair may be through the right atrium and across the atrial septum, constructing the anastomosis from inside the left atrium.)

**Usual preop diagnosis**: TAPVC; total anomalous venous return; total anomalous pulmonary venous drainage – all of these ± obstruction and either supracardiac, cardiac, or infracardiac types

### SUMMARY OF PROCEDURE

| | |
|---|---|
| **Position** | Supine |
| **Incision** | Standard median sternotomy |
| **Cannulation for CPB** | Ascending aorta for arterial return and single right atrial cannula (when hypothermia and circulatory arrest employed) or bicaval venous cannulation (children > 5 kg). |
| **Unique considerations** | Patients often require urgent or emergency surgery. Obligatory R→L shunting permits venous air bubbles or particulate emboli to become systemic emboli. Myocardial preservation using blood or crystalloid cardioplegia, in addition to topical myocardial hypothermia is used. |
| **Antibiotics** | Cefazolin 15-30 mg/kg q 8 hrs |
| **Surgical time** | Aortic cross-clamp: 40 min<br>Circulatory arrest: 30 - 35 min<br>Total: 2.5 - 3 hrs |
| **Closing considerations** | A fine polyvinyl catheter inserted through the free wall of the RV and advanced into the pulmonary trunk will permit drug infusions for pulmonary HTN. A chest tube is inserted in the pericardial space and temporary ventricular pacing wires are applied to the heart. |
| **EBL** | Moderate |
| **Postop care** | 2-4 d of assisted ventilation, sedation and hyperventilation, pulmonary vasodilators, including isoproterenol, $PGE_1$, SNP and inotropes, as needed for right heart dysfunction. |
| **Mortality** | 2-20%, depending on presence of preop pulmonary venous obstruction and preop acidosis. |
| **Morbidity** | Pulmonary vasospasm: 25-40%<br>Low CO: 10%<br>Bleeding: 2-3% |
| **Procedure code** | 33730 |
| **Pain score** | 8-10 |

### PATIENT POPULATION CHARACTERISTICS

| | |
|---|---|
| **Age range** | 1 d - 20 yrs (usually < 1 mo) |
| **Male:Female** | 4:1 in infradiaphragmatic type; equal distribution in other types |
| **Incidence** | 0.5%-2% of cases of CHD |
| **Etiology** | No apparent correlation |
| **Associated conditions** | PDA – present in nearly all infants within the first few wks of life and in about 15% of cases overall.<br>VSD – occasionally occur (may be associated with tetralogy of Fallot, double outlet RV, interrupted aortic arch and other lesions). |

---

## ANESTHETIC CONSIDERATIONS

### PREOPERATIVE

**Pathophysiology** R → L shunting (partial or total) must be balanced by R → L shunting via an ASD. This "balanced" situation results in systemic cyanosis and mild-to-moderate increase in volume load to the RV → mild CHF (↑RVEDP) and pulmonary HTN. Obstruction of anomalous pulmonary venous connection is common → pulmonary venous congestion, pulmonary edema and severe pulmonary HTN → ↑↑ cyanosis. As infant grows and demand for systemic output increases,

ASD may become relatively restrictive. Restrictive ASD → right heart volume overload → dilatation and right CHF → ↑↑ cyanosis. Those with significant pulmonary HTN, pulmonary venous obstruction and ↓pulmonary blood flow, are most likely to present in early infancy with severe cyanosis and CHF.

**Respiratory** Pulmonary edema, pulmonary HTN, ↓↓pulmonary compliance as described above.

**Tests:** CXR – pulmonary edema, conspicuous pulmonary vascularity, large cardiac silhouette

**Cardiovascular** The severity of the symptoms associated with this defect depends on several factors, including partial vs total shunt, size of ASD, existence of pulmonary venous obstruction and degree of CHF. Symptomatic infants usually severely cyanotic, often acidotic and subject to rapid cardiovascular deterioration associated with pharmacologically exacerbated myocardial dysfunction and/or ↑PVR. If restrictive ASD → balloon atrial septostomy, may improve R → L interatrial shunting. Obstructed pulmonary venous channel can also be dilated in this method. These present palliative measures only until definitive surgical therapy.

**Laboratory** Other tests as indicated from H&P.

**Premedication** Sedatives seldom used in these cases. Atropine (iv) useful in < 6-mo old to minimize bradycardiac reflexes.

## INTRAOPERATIVE

**Anesthetic technique:** GETA

**Induction** Typically via iv with titrated fentanyl (10 μg/kg) and pancuronium (0.2 mg/kg). ETT appropriately sized and placed nasally in small children and infants for ↑stability/comfort. The ETT is advanced gently until a mainstem intubation occurs. It is then withdrawn until bilateral breath sounds are once again heard (carinal position), then withdrawn an additional distance so that the tip of the ETT is approximately mid-trachea (taped position). Positive pressure leak between 30-40 cm $H_2O$ is desirable. Leaks < 30 cm result in volume loss and difficulty providing appropriate ventilation during critical phases intraop or postop. Conversely, leaks 40 cm $H_2O$ carry a higher risk of subglottic edema and/or stenosis. Volatile agents may be poorly tolerated in the severely ill infant. Inhalation induction OK for hemodynamically stable and vigorous children.

**Maintenance** Fentanyl (100-200 μg/kg in divided doses), pancuronium (0.2 mg/kg prn), midazolam (0.1-0.2 mg/kg as titrated) ± volatile agent, $FiO_2$ = 1.0.

**Emergence** Transport to ICU intubated and ventilated. Inotropic support usually required 24-48 hrs.

**Blood and fluid requirements**

IV: 22-24 ga x 2
NS/LR prn
5% albumin (20 cc/kg max)
Hetastarch (20 cc/kg max)
1 U PRBC

**Monitoring**

Standard monitors (see Appendix).
Urinary catheter
Arterial line (usually radial)
CVP line: 4 Fr double-lumen (usually right IJ)

Usually a 22-ga catheter is placed percutaneously in the radial artery. On infants, a fiber optic transilluminator may facilitate arterial cannulation. Dorsalis pedis and posterior tibial arteries are avoided, due to problems with spasm and clotting when coming off CPB. Femoral arteries are cannulated as a last resort, using a 2½ or 3 Fr 2-4 cm catheter. If all else fails, a surgical cut-down is performed. Older children (>20 kg) may receive adult-size central lines, as well as PA catheters if medically indicated.

Severely ill infants may present with invasive lines in place, full ventilatory support via an ETT and with inotropic support. In these patients, volatile agents are poorly tolerated. Fentanyl and pancuronium become the anesthetic. Increased $FiO_2$ is unlikely to significantly improve $PO_2$ since shunting is fixed. Deep GA will ↑venous $PO_2$ → ↓pulmonary HTN → improved general condition.

| | | |
|---|---|---|
| **Pre-CPB** | Heparinization (3 mg/kg)<br>ACT >400 sec<br>Cannulae placed<br>✓ pupils.<br>✓ UO. | In the pre-CPB period, crystalloid and/or 5% albumin is administered as needed to compensate for bleeding and 3rd-space losses. Blood replacement is reserved for major blood loss situations associated with re-do's and/or surgical entry into major vessels/heart chambers. |
| **CPB** | Hypothermia 18°C<br>Hct 20-25%<br>Adequate CPB flow ± pressure<br>Infusions off<br>Ventilation stopped | |

**CPB** Management of CPB is discussed in Intraoperative Considerations for "Tetralogy of Fallot." Differences in management will be discussed below.

**Post-CPB** Eccentric RV hypertrophy 2° chronic volume overload → characteristically dilated ventricle → net ↑compliance and ↓contractility. RV afterload reduction is essential, initially via ventilatory maneuver: clear unobstructed ventilation, no wheezing (albuterol prn), gentle hyperventilation on 100% $O_2$. If these maneuvers are not sufficient, then NTG/$PGE_1$ are used. Deep level of GA also is essential to keep PVR low. Inotropic support of RV typically used: dopamine/dobutamine initially and epinephrine reserved for severe RV dysfunction. Excessive inotropic support ↑PVR → ↑shunt. Adequate preload of this compliant ventricle is essential and must be determined by gentle volume challenge post-CPB.

| | | |
|---|---|---|
| **Complications** | Cerebral/cardiac embolization<br>Aortic dissection<br>Unilateral carotid hypoperfusion<br>Pump/oxygenator failure<br>Massive blood transfusion | Massive blood transfusion with citrated blood products (>2 cc/kg/min) → coagulopathy, ↓$Ca^{++}$, ↑K. Rx: includes stopping transfusion (if possible), $CaCl_2$, hyperventilation. |

## POSTOPERATIVE

| | | |
|---|---|---|
| **Complications** | Persistent R → L shunt, usually at atrial level; L → R, at ventricular level<br>Hypothermia<br>Persistent bleeding<br>RV failure<br>Pneumo/hemothorax<br>Dysrhythmias<br>Cardiac tamponade | Some degree of arterial desaturation is possible after repair if the coronary sinus continues to drain highly desaturated blood into the LA. Typically, $O_2$ sats would range from 92-96% due to this shunt. |
| **Tests** | ABGs<br>Electrolytes<br>Coagulation profile<br>CXR – ✓ line placement, ETT placement<br>ECHO | TEE monitoring is emerging as an invaluable anatomical and physiological monitor. |

**References**


1. Kirklin JW, Barrett-Boyes BG: Total anomalous pulmonary venous connection. In *Cardiac Surgery*, 2nd edition. Churchill-Livingstone, New York; 1993, 645-73.
2. Engstrom R, Fitzgerald D: *Manual of Pediatric Cardiac Anesthesia*. Stanford University Hospital Medical Center, Stanford: 1988.
3. Lake CL: *Pediatric Cardiac Anesthesia*. Appleton & Lange, Norwalk, CT: 1988.
4. Kaplan JA: *Cardiac Anesthesia*, Volume 2. WB Saunders, Philadelphia: 1987.
5. Ryan JF, Todres ID, Coté CJ, Goudsouzian N: A practice of anesthesia for infants and children. In *Anesthesia for Children with Heart Disease*. Hickey PR, ed. Grune and Strattan, Orlando: 1986, ch 16.

# SURGERY FOR COMPLETE TRANSPOSITION OF THE GREAT ARTERIES

## SURGICAL CONSIDERATIONS

**Description:** Complete transposition of the great arteries (TGA) is a congenital defect in which the aorta arises from the RV, and the PA from the LV (Fig 12.1-2). In this lesion, there is atrial-ventricular concordance and ventricular-arterial discordance. The earliest surgical treatment for TGA was described by **Blalock** and **Hanlon** in 1950, with a procedure in which an **atrial septectomy** was performed, improving the mixing of pulmonary and systemic blood at the atrial level. In the 1950s, a variety of partial physiologic corrections were developed in which the pulmonary veins or the vena cava were transposed to the alternate atria. Palliative treatment was advanced by **Rashkind's** description of a **balloon atrial septostomy** in 1966. More complete palliation was obtained by **atrial inversion** operations described by **Senning** in 1959 and **Mustard's procedure** introduced in 1963. These procedures were the standard in a strategy which combined balloon atrial septostomy and an atrial inversion operation 3-24 months later. TGA with other anomalies, such as VSD and LV outflow tract obstruction (LVOTO) was successfully repaired in 1969 by **Rastelli** and colleagues. The anatomic correction of transposition by **arterial switch and reimplantation** of coronary arteries had been suggested for many years, but was successfully advanced by the work of **Jantene, Yacoub** and others from the mid-1970s on. Widespread application of the arterial switch technique in neonates became the standard in about 1987.

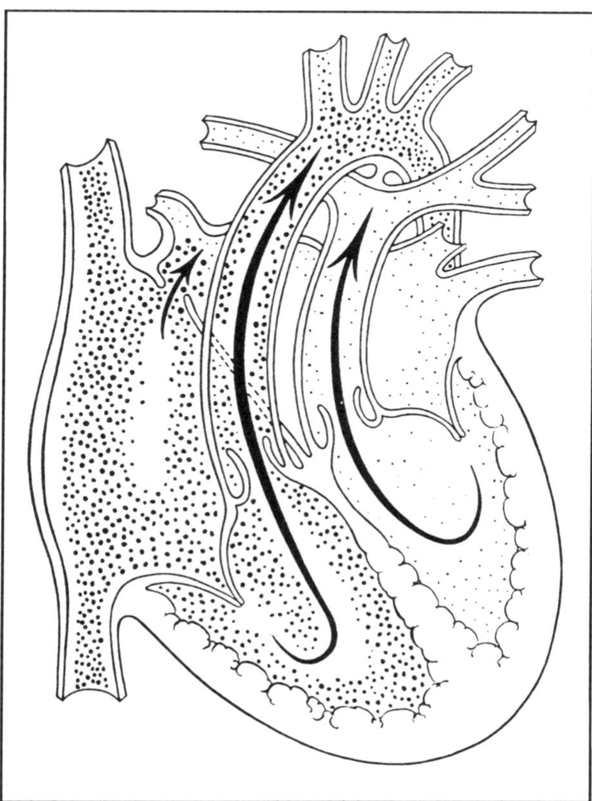

**Figure 12.1-2.** Transposition of the great arteries. (Reproduced with permission from Waldenhausen JA, Pierce WS: Transposition of the great arteries. In Hardy JD, ed: *Rhoads Textbook of Surgery, 5th ed.* JB Lippincott: 1977.)

Total correction is now performed routinely in the first three weeks of life. Following a standard median sternotomy, the heart is exposed and CPB is instituted. The aorta is cross-clamped, cardiac arrest is instituted with cardioplegia, and induced hypothermia is begun. Transection of the anterior great vessel and removal of the coronary arteries with an aortic button is carried out. The posterior great vessels are transected with the creation of a suitable-sized opening in the adjacent sinus of the posterior great vessel, and reanastomosis of the aortic button. The PA bifurcation is transposed anterior to the distal portion of the ascending aorta, pericardial patches are placed in the openings remaining after removal of the anterior coronary buttons, and associated atrial or VSDs are repaired. Then, reanastomosis of the great arteries is performed. If hypothermia has been induced, a brief period of circulatory arrest is sustained in order to repair the ASD and/or VSD, if present. Next, reperfusion and rewarming are begun. End-to-end suture of the PA outflow is performed. The aorta is unclamped and cardiac resuscitation and de-airing maneuvers are performed. CPB is discontinued, and closure is routine.

**Usual preop diagnosis**: Complete TGA; transposition of the great vessels; transposition ± VSD; ASD; PDA

### SUMMARY OF PROCEDURE

| | |
|---|---|
| **Position** | Supine |
| **Incision** | Standard median sternotomy |
| **Cannulation for CPB** | Ascending aortic cannula; right atrial appendage or direct bicaval cannulation |
| **Unique considerations** | Operation to be performed before LV pressure falls substantially by ↓PVR. If LV becomes deconditioned, failure may result, following arterial switch. Coronary artery anomalies are not uncommon; but the only significant anomaly is the intramural coronary artery, which complicates repair. |

| | |
|---|---|
| **Myocardial preservation** | Blood or crystalloid cardioplegia, in addition to topical myocardial hypothermia |
| **Antibiotics** | Cefazolin 15-30 mg/kg q 8 hrs |
| **Surgical time** | Cross-clamp: 45 - 70 min<br>Circulatory arrest: 10 - 15 min<br>Total: 3 hrs |
| **Closing considerations** | Routine closure with chest tube in the pericardial space; temporary ventricular pacing wire; possible right or left atrial line for monitoring, as necessary. |
| **EBL** | Minimal |
| **Postop care** | 24-48 hrs of assisted ventilation; pulmonary HTN protocol; hyperventilation and sedation; use of pulmonary vasodilators; use of inotropes for adequate CO. |
| **Mortality** | 5% |
| **Morbidity** | Bleeding<br>Coronary artery kinking and myocardial ischemia<br>Pulmonary vascular spasm |
| **Procedure code** | 33778 |
| **Pain score** | 8-10 |

### PATIENT POPULATION CHARACTERISTICS

| | |
|---|---|
| **Age range** | 1-21 d; up to 3-6 mo in patients with VSD |
| **Male:Female** | 2:1; 3.3:1 when no VSD present |
| **Incidence** | 7-8% of all CHD; 1/2100-1/4500 births |
| **Etiology** | Usually no associated syndromes or other non-cardiac abnormalities. |
| **Associated conditions** | ASD<br>VSD<br>PDA<br>LVOTO<br>Pulmonary atresia<br>Coarctation of the aorta |

---

## ANESTHETIC CONSIDERATIONS

### PREOPERATIVE

**Pathophysiology** Ventriculoarterial discordance disrupts the normal sequential relationship between the pulmonary and systemic circulations. Deoxygenated systemic venous blood is ejected via the RV into the aorta (systemic circulation), while oxygenated pulmonary venous blood is misdirected by the LV to the pulmonary circulation. This represents a parallel circulation, rather than the normal series circulation. Circuit communication (mixing) via intracardiac (VSD, ASD, PFO) or extracardiac (PDA, bronchopulmonary collaterals). Physiological mechanisms affecting the degree of intercirculatory mixing are complex and not well-understood, and ultimately are reflected in the degree of arterial saturation. ↓mixing can result from ↓ventricular compliance/↓CO, ↓pulmonary blood flow (↑PVR 2° hypoxia, hypercarbia, hypothermia, acidosis) and/or LVOT obstruction (subpulmonic fibromuscular ridge, dynamic subaortic stenosis or ↓number and size of anatomic communications.

**Respiratory** Frequent respiratory infections and dyspnea are common. $PGE_1$ therapy may induce apnea → mechanical ventilatory support. Pulmonary edema often correlates with existence of a VSD.

**Tests:** CXR – cardiomegaly, egg-shaped heart, ± pulmonary plethora

**Cardiovascular** Large volumes of blood recirculate in patients with this lesion, → CHF. Degree of mixing (Qp:Qs) directly proportional to systemic saturation. Pulmonary vascular disease common and often complicates approach and management.

**Tests:** ECG – right axis deviation, RV hypertrophy. ECHO – diagnostic. Cardiac cath – defines anatomy, especially presence of ASD, PFO, PDA, VSD, pulmonary collaterals, coronary artery anatomy and LV size and function estimation; also measures PVR, shunt fraction. Raskind Miller atrial septostomy and $PGE_1$ are palliative treatments used to improve mixing.

**Hematologic** Polycythemia typical in children > 6 mo (uncorrected) → induced pulmonary vascular disease. Also, polycythemia typical with chronic $O_2$ sat < 90% → ↑blood viscosity (critical if Hct > 70) and propensity to cerebral and PA thrombotic events. Coagulopathy associated with polycythemia (thrombocytopenia, hypofibrinogenemia and ↓factors V, VIII and ± fibrinolysis, low-grade DIC). **Tests:** Hct; PT; PTT; FSP; others as indicated from H&P.

**Laboratory** Other tests as indicated from H&P.

**Premedication** Sedatives seldom used, 2° very young patient population.

## INTRAOPERATIVE

**Anesthetic technique:** GETA

**Induction** Infants usually have ivs in place and often are mechanically ventilated. Atropine (iv) useful in < 6-mo-old children to minimize bradycardic reflexes. IV induction with fentanyl (10 μg/kg) and pancuronium (0.2 mg/kg). Inhalation induction OK for the older child, but must be done cautiously, as some patients may not tolerate the hemodynamic changes associated with volatile agents.

**Maintenance** Fentanyl 100-200 μg/kg, pancuronium 0.2 mg/kg, midazolam 0.1-0.2 mg/kg (redose during rewarming) ± volatile agent. $FiO_2$ = 1.0. ETT appropriately sized and placed nasally in small children and infants for ↑stability and comfort. Deep GA favorably affects "mixing" in these patients as long as ventricular function and, thus, CO are preserved. In addition to better mixing, deep GA will ↓$O_2$ consumption → ↑venous $PO_2$ → ↑arterial $PO_2$. Also, any pulmonary HTN will be decreased by an ↑venous $PO_2$ and ↑$FiO_2$ (1.0), thus improving mixing. Beware the newborn who presents critically ill with cyanosis, acidosis, variable ductal patency, uncertain intravascular volume status, etc. Hypoxia, acidosis and ventricular dysfunction can create highly labile hemodynamics during all phases of the pre-CPB period.

**Emergence** These patients are transported to ICU intubated and ventilated.

**Blood and fluid requirements**

Anticipate major blood loss.
IV: umbilical venous line or 22-24 ga peripheral line
NS/LR @ 4 cc/kg/hr
5% albumin (20 cc/kg max)
Hetastarch (20 cc/kg max)
PRBC: 1 U in OR

Intravascular volume depletion should be avoided perioperatively. Beware of complications 2° massive blood transfusion with citrated blood products (>2 cc/kg/min): ↓Ca++, ↑K. Rx: includes stopping transfusion, $CaCl_2$, hyperventilation.

**Monitoring**

Standard monitors (see Appendix).
Urinary catheter
Arterial line (umbilical or radial)
CVP line: 4 Fr double-lumen IJ
Umbilical venous line

Commonly, an infant presents to the OR with ivs and invasive lines (umbilical) in place, often mechanically ventilated due to $PGE_1$-induced apnea, or general hemodynamic/pulmonary instability.

**Pre-CPB**

Heparinization (3 mg/kg)
ACT >400 sec
✓ pupils.
✓ UO.

During the pre-CPB period, crystalloid and/or 5% albumin is administered as needed to compensate for bleeding and 3rd-space losses. Blood replacement is reserved for major blood loss situations associated with re-do's and/or surgical entry into major vessels/heart chambers.

**CPB**

Ventilation stopped
Hypothermia: 22-26°C
± Ice packs around head.
Hct 20-25 typical during CPB
✓ adequate flow/pressure.
✓ anesthetic/NMB adequacy.
✓ pupils.
✓ peripleural effusion, edema, venous congestion.
✓ ABG, electrolytes, UO, Hct, ACT q 30-60 min.

Drugs are injected into the pump reservoir as appropriate (i.e., phentolamine for HTN and/or slow/inadequate body cooling, methylprednisolone for deep hypothermic cardiac arrest [DHCA] situations, furosemide for suboptimal UO, and heparin in accordance with ongoing ACT analysis). Perfusion pressure, CVP and flow rates are monitored in tandem with perfusionists. Observation for venous congestion is ongoing. Monitoring electrolytes and arterial/venous blood and formulation of appropriate therapeutic interventions is essential.

**Transition off CPB**

Rewarming
Vasoactive infusions starting at 34°C.
Flush lines.
✓ waveforms.
Suction ETT.
Resume ventilating.
✓ bilateral breath sounds.
✓ ABC, electrolytes, Hct (~30).
✓ ACT (>400).
✓ ECG – pacing may be necessary.
Supplement NMB and deepen anesthesia.

Aerosolized albuterol may be indicated if wheezing present. Air emboli must be removed from the pulmonary veins, aorta and cardiac chambers. Full-flow CPB at normothermia is often allowed to rebuild myocardial ATP stores. The cross-clamp is removed and the empty heart (vented) is allowed to beat. The vent is removed and the heart is gradually allowed to work with progressively less "pump" support.

**Post-CPB**

Inotropic support (dopamine, dobutamine, epinephrine)
RV afterload reduction (↓PVR):
$FiO_2 = 1$
$PaCO_2$ ~30
NTG ± $PGE_1$
Minimize mean airway pressure.
AV sequential pacemaker (heart block not uncommon).
Surgical PA line or LA line are normally placed to monitor cardiac status.
Large volume requirements 2° bleeding and capillary leak.
Reverse anticoagulation.
Rx coagulopathy: (fresh (< 48° old), whole blood preferred.
FFP/platelets/cryo/EACA/DDAVP as necessary.

In patients without a VSD, the LV can become "deconditioned" when the PVR falls soon after birth. Reconditioning can be done by PA banding prior to the definitive switch procedure. Life-threatening LV failure can result if an inadequately "prepared" LV is forced to function as the sole systemic ventricle. Intense LV inotropic support and occasionally LV assist devices (LVADs) or ECMO may be necessary. Anatomic stenosis at the site of great vessel re-anastomosis may be hemodynamically significant.

**Positioning**

✓ and pad pressure points.
✓ eyes.

**Complications**

Cerebral/cardiac embolization
Aortic dissection
Unilateral carotid hypoperfusion
Pump/oxygenator failure

## POSTOPERATIVE

**Complications**

Hypothermia
Persistent surgical/medical bleeding
Pneumo/hemothorax
Dysrhythmias
Cardiac tamponade
Myocardial ischemia
LV failure
Residual structural defects: AI, supravalvular PS or AS

Ischemia 2° coronary artery stenosis, stretching, spasm, compression, etc., can badly damage myocardial tissues. Spasm can be treated with NTG and ↑aortic pressure. If the now-anterior PA dilates (↓$PaO_2$, ↑$PaCO_2$, ↓temp, ↓pH, excessive or too little PIP, or RV failure), then the coronary arteries may be compressed. Measures to decrease PA pressure are often essential.

**Tests**

ABGs
Electrolytes
Coagulation profile
CXR (✓ line placement, ptx, CT placement)
ECHO

TEE monitoring is emerging as an invaluable anatomical and physiological monitor.

**References**

1. Kirklin JW, Barrett-Boyes BG: Complete transposition of the great arteries. In *Cardiac Surgery*, 2nd edition. Churchill-Livingstone, New York: 1993, 1383-1467.
2. Strong MJ, Keats AS, Cooley DA: Anesthesia for cardiovascular surgery in infancy. *Anesthesiology* 1966; 27(3):257-65.
3. Engstrom R, Fitzgerald D: *Manual of Pediatric Cardiac Anesthesia.* Stanford University Hospital Medical Center, Stanford: 1988.
4. Lake CL: *Pediatric Cardiac Anesthesia.* Appleton & Lange, Norwalk, CT: 1988.
5. Kaplan JA: *Cardiac Anesthesia,* Volume 2. WB Saunders, Philadelphia: 1987.
6. Ryan JF, Todres ID, Coté CJ, Goudsouzian N: A practice of anesthesia for infants and children. In *Anesthesia for Children with Heart Disease.* Hickey PR, ed. Grune and Strattan, Orlando: 1986, ch 16.

# SURGERY FOR ATRIOVENTRICULAR CANAL DEFECT

## SURGICAL CONSIDERATIONS

**Description:** Atrioventricular (AV) canal defects occur as a result of deficiency of septal tissue immediately above and below the level of the AV valves and deficiency of the AV valves in continuity with the septal defects. When the defect involves the atrial septum and not the ventricular septum, it is called a partial AV canal defect or an ostium primum atrial septal defect (ASD).

Early palliative repair of AV canal defects consisted of PA banding to reduce excessive pulmonary flow. The first total corrections, which included repair of the septal defects and suture of valvular defects, took place in the mid-1950s with the availability of CPB techniques. As modern cardiac surgery has developed, this difficult lesion has become increasingly correctable at an earlier age and with greater safety and reliability. **Palliation** is rare and is reserved for very small infants with associated conditions, such as CHF and pneumonia. **Total correction** is now performed routinely, even in neonates. Repair consists of closure of ventricular defects and ASDs, with or without closure of the defect in the anterior leaflet of the mitral valve, and repair of associated defects, such as PDA or secundum ASD. These septal defects may be repaired with either a two-patch technique, consisting of a Dacron® patch on the ventricular septum and pericardial patch on the atrial septum, or a single Dacron® patch covering both atrial and ventricular defects. The ASD is frequently closed by placing the coronary sinus return on the left atrial side in order to avoid suturing in the area of the bundle of His.

The heart is exposed through a standard median sternotomy. For **ostium primum ASD** or **partial AV canal**: CPB is instituted and aorta cross-clamped. The heart is arrested with cardioplegia. Tapes are placed around the vena caval cannula and right atriotomy, and the mitral valve cleft is sutured. A pericardial patch is placed across the top of the ventricular septum, around the orifice of the coronary sinus, and along the free edge of the superior portion of the ASD. The atriotomy is closed and the aorta unclamped. Cardiac resuscitation and de-airing procedures are carried out and closure commenced.

For **complete AV canal defect**: Following median sternotomy, aortic and bicaval cannulation are carried out. The aorta is cross-clamped and the heart arrested with cardioplegia. Caval tapes are applied and right atriotomy is performed. It may be necessary to divide the common anterior and posterior bridging leaflets in the plane of the ventricular septum. VSD sutures are placed on the RV side of the septum and an appropriately sized half-moon shaped Dacron® patch is cut. The VSD sutures are placed through the circular margin of the patch and reapproximation of the mitral anterior leaflet to the top of the ventricular septal patch. Next, attention is paid to suturing of the mitral valve cleft and of a pericardial patch to the top of the ventricular septal patch, carrying the pericardial patch anastomosis around the coronary sinus and the superior margin of the ASD. The tricuspid valve is reattached to the level of the top of the ventricular patch. Closure of the right atrium, aortic unclamping, rewarming, and resuscitation of the heart are commenced and CPB discontinued.

**Usual preop diagnosis**: AV canal defect: common, complete and partial AV canal; ostium primum ASD

### SUMMARY OF PROCEDURE

| | Ostium Primum ASD Or Partial AV Canal | Complete AV Canal Defect |
|---|---|---|
| **Position** | Supine | ⇐ |
| **Incision** | Standard median sternotomy | ⇐ |
| **Cannulation for CPB** | Ascending aortic cannula, direct bicaval cannulation | ⇐ |
| **Unique considerations** | None | Repair performed through a right atrial incision, no ventriculotomies required. |
| **Myocardial preservation** | Blood or crystalloid cardioplegia, in addition to topical myocardial hypothermia | ⇐ |
| **Antibiotics** | Cefazolin 15-30 mg/kg q 8 hrs | ⇐ |
| **Surgical time** | Cross-clamp: 30 - 40 min<br>Total: 2 - 3 hrs | 60-80 min<br>3 - 4 hrs |
| **Closing considerations** | Chest tube in the pericardial space, temporary ventricular pacing wire, possible right or left atrial line for monitoring, as necessary | ⇐ |
| **EBL** | Moderate | ⇐ |
| **Postop care** | ICU x 1-2 d; 12-24 hrs assisted ventilation; minimal need for inotropes | 1-3 d assisted ventilation; pulmonary HTN protocol consisting of hyperventilation and sedation. Use of pulmonary vasodilators (e.g., Isoproterenol® or $PGE_1$). Use inotropes for adequate CO. Avoid excessive volume to prevent distention and mitral valve regurgitation. |
| **Mortality** | 0-1% | 2-4% |
| **Morbidity** | Bleeding<br>Infection<br>Transient heart block | Pulmonary vasospasm<br>Right heart dysfunction<br>Mitral valve regurgitation<br>Low CO<br>Bleeding<br>Heart block<br>Residual VSD |
| **Procedure code** | 33641 | 33670 |
| **Pain score** | 8-10 | 8-10 |

### PATIENT POPULATION CHARACTERISTICS

| | | |
|---|---|---|
| **Age range** | 1-20 yrs (usually 4-5 yrs) | 2 mo-1 yr |
| **Male:Female** | 1:1 | ⇐ |
| **Incidence** | 0.5-1% of CHD cases | ⇐ |
| **Etiology** | Down syndrome: Rare (in patients with partial AV canal defect) | Down syndrome: Common (~ 75% in patients with complete AV canal defect) |
| **Associated conditions** | Left AV valve incompetence | Pulmonary arterial HTN<br>Left AV valve incompetence<br>Minor associated cardiac anomalies (e.g., PDA or secundum ASD, tetralogy of Fallot) |

## ANESTHETIC CONSIDERATIONS

### PREOPERATIVE

**Pathophysiology** Mild-to-moderate L → R shunting via ASD (ostium primum) → RAE, eccentric EVH 2° chronic volume overload, pulmonary HTN. Commonly associated with cleft anterior leaflet of the mitral valve → MR → ↑↑L → R shunt, predisposing to pulmonary HTN and volume-overload-induced CHF. Complete AV canal defect: severe L → R shunting → early onset of pulmonary HTN and CHF. ↑SVR or ↓PVR may → ↑L → R shunt → exacerbation of CHF.

**Respiratory** Chronic pulmonary congestion → pulmonary edema, ↓pulmonary compliance, airway closure, ↓FRC, atelectasis, V/Q mismatch → intrapulmonary R → L shunt and ↓$PaO_2$. Pulmonary infections are common.

**Tests:** CXR – cardiomegaly, RAE, ↑pulmonary vascular markings.

**Cardiovascular** Ostium primum: RV volume overload → RV failure and pulmonary HTN associated with size of ASD and existence of MR. Complete AV canal defect: bi-ventricular failure and pulmonary HTN early and common.

**Tests:** ABG; ECG (RAE, RVE), ↑PR interval; cardiac cath – shows extent of AV valve dysfunction, size of VSD, shunt fraction, degree of pulmonary HTN; also ✓ for PDA, TOF.

**Down Syndrome** Commonly associated with complete AV canal defect. Mental retardation (100%), hearing loss (50%), small trachea (25%), frequent pulmonary infection, airway obstruction (intrathoracic and extrathoracic). Possibly difficult intubation in this patient population. All patients with Down syndrome should be considered at risk from atlanto-axial instability, and one should avoid excessive neck flexion or rotation.

**Neurological** Neck pain, torticollis, gait disturbance, hyperreflexia, limb weakness or paresthesias suggest atlanto-axial subluxation (neurology consultation prior to surgery).

**Laboratory** Other tests as indicated from H&P.

**Premedication** Usually midazolam 0.5-0.75 mg/kg po. Older children with Down syndrome occasionally may not cooperate for oral premed → ketamine (4-6 mg/kg im).

## INTRAOPERATIVE

**Anesthetic technique:** GETA

**Induction** Typically mask halothane ± $N_2O$. If iv in place, fentanyl (10 μg/kg) and pancuronium (0.2 mg/kg) ± volatile agent. Due to relative macroglossia, Down syndrome patients often present difficult mask airway management, necessitating the use of an oral airway. ETT appropriately sized and placed nasally in small children and infants for ↑stability/comfort. The ETT is advanced gently until a mainstem intubation occurs. It is then withdrawn until bilateral breath sounds are once again heard (carinal position), then withdrawn an additional distance so that the tip of the ETT is approximately mid-trachea (taped position). Positive pressure leak between 30-40 cm $H_2O$ is desirable. Leaks < 30 cm result in volume loss and difficulty providing appropriate ventilation during critical phases intraop or postop. Conversely, leaks 40 cm $H_2O$ carry a higher risk of subglottic edema and/or stenosis.

**Maintenance** Fentanyl 100-200 μg/kg, pancuronium 0.2 mg/kg, midazolam 0.1-0.2 mg/kg ± volatile agent. $FiO_2$ = 0.3 and $ETCO_2$ 35-40.

**Emergence** Children with uncomplicated ASD are usually extubated within 2 hrs in the ICU. Typically, in more complicated septal defects, patients are kept deeply anesthetized and paralyzed overnight. Measures to lower PVR and inotropically support the RV continue and are treated as clinically indicated.

**Blood and fluid requirements** NS/LR prn
5% albumin (20 cc/kg max)
1 U PRBC

**Monitoring** Standard monitors (see Appendix).
Urinary catheter
Arterial line (usually radial)
CVP line: 4 Fr double-lumen (usually right IJ)

Usually a 22-ga catheter is placed percutaneously in the radial artery (avoid Blalock-Taussig shunt side, usually right side). On infants, a fiber optic transilluminator may facilitate arterial cannulation. Dorsalis pedis and posterior tibial arteries are avoided, due to problems with spasm and clotting when coming off CPB. Femoral arteries are cannulated as a last resort, using a 2½ or 3 Fr 2-4 cm catheter. If all else fails, a surgical cut-down is performed. Older children (>20 kg) may receive adult-size central lines, as well as PA catheters, if medically indicated.

Percutaneous radial line placement is often difficult in Down syndrome patients due to tortuous radial arteries. This may necessitate femoral artery approaches and/or radial artery cutdowns.

**CPB** Management of CPB is discussed in Intraoperative Considerations for "Tetralogy of Fallot." Differences in management are discussed below.

**Pre-CPB** Pulmonary over-circulation is typical with these lesions. Degree and direction of shunting depends on relative compliance of the 2 ventricular chambers and the size/location of the defect. Small-to-moderate pulmonary blood flow (QP/QS $\leq$ 1.5) is well-tolerated and usually associated with ASD. With the addition of a VSD component, QP/QS ratios can easily exceed 3.0, resulting in pulmonary HTN and over-circulation-induced CHF. If pulmonary blood flow large enough, for long enough, shunt can reverse (↑↑PVR → Eisenmengers syndrome). Goal during anesthesia (pre-correction) is to not ↑SVR or ↓PVR, which could exacerbate L → R shunt and CHF. Therefore, $FiO_2$ = 0.21-0.25, $ETCO_2$ = 35-40 and deep GA so that SVR is not excessive. Due to pulmonary congestion, these patients tend to have excessive pulmonary secretions and are prone to bronchospasm, necessitating vigorous pulmonary toilet and bronchodilator treatment.

**Post-CPB** ↓RV compliance is expected (↑RVEDP – RV failure) and therapeutic maneuvers are focused on improvement of RV function. RV afterload reduction is essential (see discussion in "Tetralogy of Fallot").

## POSTOPERATIVE

**Complications**

- Residual structural defects – AV valve regurgitation, VSD, ASD
- Systemic $O_2$ desaturation (92-96%) if coronary sinus drainage → LA after repair.

Other structural residual defects can affect hemodynamics, e.g., MR, requiring systemic vasodilation. Analysis of post-repair function is best-performed by TEE.

**Tests**

ABGs
Electrolytes
Coagulation profile
CXR (✓ line placement, ETT placement)
ECHO

TEE monitoring is emerging as an invaluable anatomical and physiological monitor.

**References**

1. Kirklin JW, Barrett-Boyes BG: Atrioventricular canal defect. In *Surgery*, 2nd edition. Churchill-Livingstone, New York: 1993, 693-74.
2. Strong MJ, Keats AS, Cooley DA: Anesthesia for cardiovascular surgery in infancy. *Anesthesiology* 1966; 27(3):257-65.
3. Engstrom R, Fitzgerald D: *Manual of Pediatric Cardiac Anesthesia*. Stanford University Hospital Medical Center, Stanford: 1988.
4. Lake CL: *Pediatric Cardiac Anesthesia*. Appleton & Lange, Norwalk, CT: 1988.
5. Kaplan JA: *Cardiac Anesthesia*, Volume 2. WB Saunders, Philadelphia: 1987.
6. Ryan JF, Todres ID, Coté CJ, Goudsouzian N: A practice of anesthesia for infants and children. In *Anesthesia for Children with Heart Disease*. Hickey PR, ed. Grune and Strattan, Orlando: 1986, ch 16.

**Surgeon**

**Gary E. Hartman, MD**

## 12.2 PEDIATRIC GENERAL SURGERY

**Anesthesiologists**

**George Lederhaas, MD**
**Alvin Hackel, MD**

# REPAIR OF ESOPHAGEAL ATRESIA/TRACHEOESOPHAGEAL FISTULA

## SURGICAL CONSIDERATIONS

**Description**: The vast majority (86%) of infants with esophageal atresia (EA) have an associated distal tracheo-esophageal fistula (TEF) (Fig 12.2-1). Aspiration of gastric contents or GI distension via the distal fistula generally mandates urgent operative intervention. Many surgeons continue to advocate **gastrostomy**, either as part of the primary repair or as a preliminary procedure in complicated cases. Primary repair with or without gastrostomy is possible in large infants with no associated anomalies or aspiration pneumonitis. **Staged procedures** – initial gastrostomy, followed within days or weeks by **right thoracotomy** for esophageal repair – are used in premature infants with associated anomalies or aspiration, or by surgeons' preference.

Debate continues regarding the choice of retropleural vs transpleural repair. Transpleural repair is quicker, but it exposes the pleural space to anastomotic leak and is potentially more disruptive to respiratory physiology. Preop identification of right aortic arch (5%) will allow for consideration of a **left thoracotomy** for the esophageal repair. A **lateral thoracotomy** is used on the side opposite the aortic arch. Initial attention is directed at identification and division of the distal fistula, if present, with the trachea open during the division. The proximal pouch generally requires significant dissection and also may require a circular **myotomy** to gain enough length for a primary anastomosis, which is almost always possible and is done in a single layer.

**Variant procedure or approaches**: EA without fistula (8%) is treated with initial **gastrostomy**, followed by attempted primary repair, at 6-8 weeks, after dilation of the proximal or both pouches. A less desirable alternative is **proximal esophagostomy** with delayed interposition of colon or gastric tube. TEF without atresia (4%) is usually diagnosed later in the first few years of life, due to recurrent aspiration, and is usually approached through a cervical incision.

**Usual preop diagnosis**: Esophageal atresia; TEF

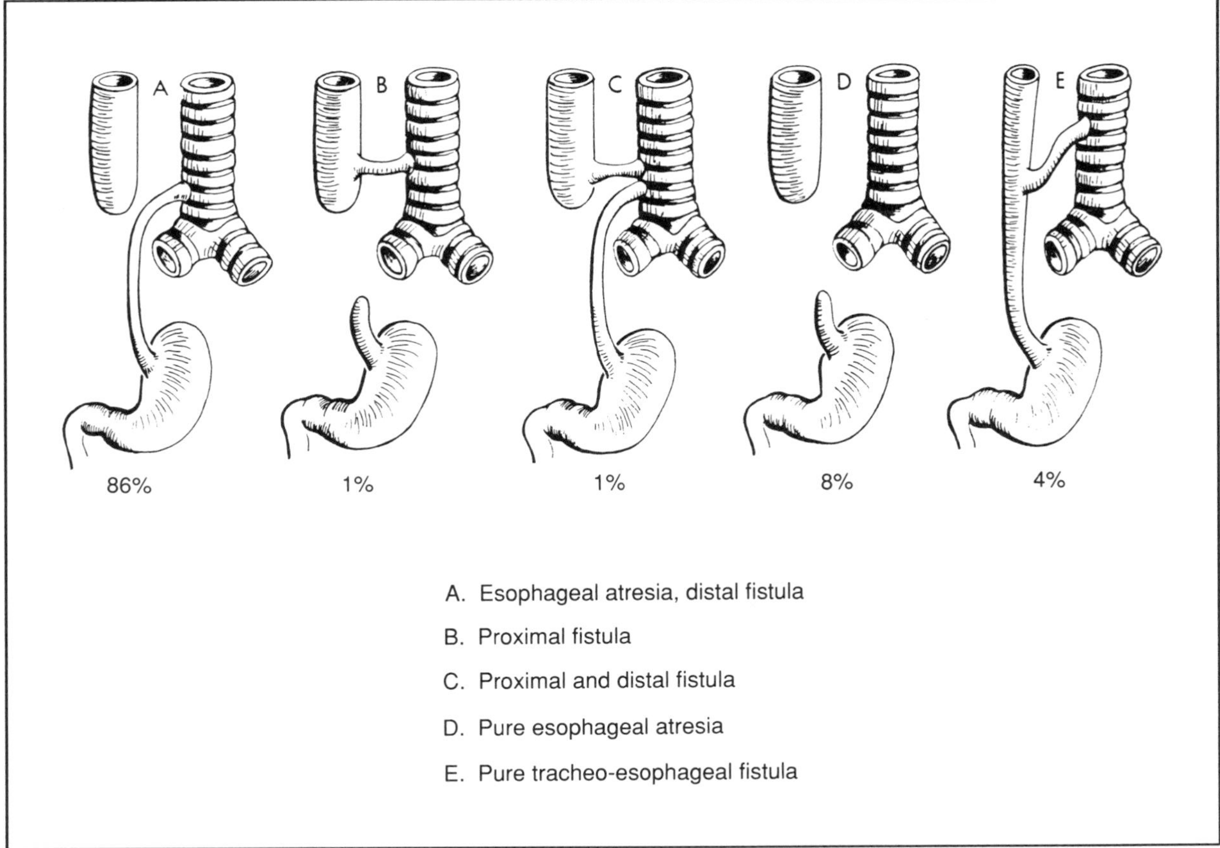


**Figure 12.2-1.** Types of esophageal atresia. (Reproduced with permission from Ravitch MM, et al eds: *Pediatric Surgery*, Vol 1, 3rd edition. Year Book Medical Pub: 1979.)

### SUMMARY OF PROCEDURE

| | Primary Repair | Gastrostomy |
|---|---|---|
| **Position** | Lateral | Supine |
| **Incision** | Posterolateral thoracotomy (side opposite aortic arch) | Paramedian, midline |
| **Special instrumentation** | Bougie in upper pouch | Whiskey nipple |
| **Unique considerations** | Loss of ventilation via fistula | May be done under local anesthesia. |
| **Antibiotics** | Preop: ampicillin 25 mg/kg iv + gentamicin 2.5 mg/kg iv; intraop: cephalosporin irrigation (1 gm/500 cc NS) | ⇐ ⇐ |
| **Surgical time** | 2 - 4 hrs | 1 hr |
| **Closing considerations** | Extubation favored | Local anesthetic; wound infiltration |
| **EBL** | 10 cc/kg | 5 cc/kg |
| **Postop care** | NICU; humidified mist; avoid CPAP and neck hyperextension | ⇐ |
| **Mortality** | 1-20%, depending on associated anomalies | 5% |
| **Morbidity** | Stricture: 20-40%<br>Leak: 10-20%<br>Atelectasis<br>Aspiration<br>Stridor | Aspiration |
| **Procedure code** | 43312 | 48331 |
| **Pain score** | 7-8 | 3-4 |

### PATIENT POPULATION CHARACTERISTICS

| | |
|---|---|
| **Age range** | Days-weeks |
| **Male:Female** | 1:1 |
| **Incidence** | 1/4000 births |
| **Etiology** | Unknown |
| **Associated conditions** | Imperforate anus<br>Cardiac anomalies (VATER association)<br>Renal anomalies (VATER association)<br>Vertebral anomalies, rectal anomalies, cardiac, TEF, renal, limb (VACTERL association)<br>Trisomy 13, 18<br>Hydrocephalus |

## ANESTHETIC CONSIDERATIONS

### PREOPERATIVE

Esophageal atresia (EA) and tracheoesophageal fistula (TEF) are usually detected in the first day of life, although TEF without atresia may be difficult to diagnose until the patient experiences recurrent pneumonia, cyanosis associated with feeding, or abdominal distention. The fistula is usually at the distal trachea near the carina. Because of the risk of pulmonary aspiration, gastrostomy is performed within hours of detection. In some premature infants or those with respiratory complications, the gastrostomy is done under local anesthesia prior to thoracotomy. These abnormalities are frequently associated with prematurity (30-40%) and other congenital anomalies, particularly cardiac (20-35%). The VATER association includes the following defects: vertebral (or VSD), anal, TEF, esophageal atresia and radial (or renal) anomalies. Routine neonatal preop evaluation includes H&P, serum electrolytes, blood sugar and Hct. Evidence of UO is needed before surgery.

**Respiratory** The upper esophageal pouch is continuously suctioned to minimize aspiration. Premature infants are at risk for respiratory distress syndrome (RDS). These patients frequently have respiratory insufficiency 2° meconium aspiration or RDS, and may be intubated and on mechanical ventilation with supplemental $O_2$ prior to surgery.
**Tests:** CXR; ABG

**Cardiovascular** Associated cardiac abnormalities include (in approximate order): VSD, PDA, tetralogy of Fallot, ASD and coarctation. At risk for pulmonary HTN with R → L shunt (e.g., PFO).
**Tests:** ECG; ECHO; catheterization, as indicated from H&P in consultation with pediatric cardiologist.

**Gastrointestinal** Multiple associated GI anomalies (e.g., VATER association, pyloric stenosis, duodenal atresia) in 20% of patients.

**Musculoskeletal** Musculoskeletal anomalies (e.g., VATER association) occur in ~30% of these patients, but are usually of little anesthetic significance, except cervical spine.
**Tests:** C-spine flexion, extension

**Hematologic** For the first 2-3 mo of life, the $O_2$-carrying capacity of blood is increased because of the presence of fetal Hb with its decreased sensitivity to 2,3-DPG. A shift to the right of the $O_2$ saturation curve results in ↑$O_2$-Hb affinity. As a result, tissue oxygenation may be reduced, especially with anemia (Hb < 12 gm/dl @ < 2-3 mos).
**Tests:** Hct; T&C; others as indicated from H&P.

**Laboratory** Serum electrolytes, UA, ABG, blood glucose, to determine metabolic state.

**Premedication** Usually none

## INTRAOPERATIVE

**Anesthetic technique:** GETA, using a pediatric circle or Bain circuit with humidified and warmed gasses. Maintain body temperature as close to 37°C as possible. Warm room to at least 78-80°F. If child is otherwise healthy and extubation is planned at end of the case, consider placing a caudal anesthetic (e.g., bupivacaine 0.25% with epinephrine 1:200,000 1 cc/kg + NS 0.5 cc/kg for a total volume of 1.5 cc/kg) after airway is secured and the child is anesthetized.

**Induction** Atropine (0.02 mg/kg iv) is given before induction to ablate vagal response to laryngoscopy. Awake intubation is preferred. Advance ETT to right mainstem and withdraw until bilateral breath sounds are present. Have flexible pediatric bronchoscope available to verify placement of ETT and site of TEF. Keep air leak around ETT to a minimum (~20 cm $H_2O$) to minimize alterations in ventilation 2° changes in chest and pulmonary compliance.

**Maintenance** Avoid high $FiO_2$; use air/$O_2$ mixture for ventilation to maintain $O_2$ sat between 95-100%. Use low PIPs to avoid gastric distention by gasses passing through fistula. Careful adjustment of ventilation may be necessary during surgical retraction of lung. Concurrent manual ventilation provides direct monitoring of pulmonary compliance. Air/$O_2$/opiate (e.g., fentanyl 5-10 μg/kg/hr) and low-dose volatile technique preferred because of better hemodynamic stability. Muscle relaxation (pancuronium or vecuronium 0.1 mg/kg iv) is usually necessary. If combined caudal anesthetic is used, GA drug requirements will be reduced. Frequent tracheal suctioning may be needed.

**Emergence** Extubation in OR is preferable, but not always possible. Supplemental $O_2$ is usually necessary to keep $PaO_2$ = 60-80 mmHg ($SpO_2$ = 95-100%). Cardiac or pulmonary complications, or any question regarding adequacy of ventilation, mandate continued intubation and ventilation.

**Blood and fluid requirements** Blood loss usually minimal
IV: 22-24 ga x 1-2
NS/LR @ (maintenance):
4 cc/kg/hr – 0-10 kg

Continue dextrose-containing solution from ICN. Replace 3rd space losses (6-8 cc/kg/hr) with NS/LR. Replace blood loss with 5% albumin cc for cc blood loss; maintain Hct >35%.

**Monitoring** Standard monitors (see Appendix).
Left axillary precordial stethoscope
Arterial line (24 ga)

ABG, Hct and glucose q 60 min

**Positioning** ✓ and pad pressure points.
✓ eyes.
Axillary roll
Arms should be positioned to be visible and easily available to anesthesiologist.

The patient is turned to the left lateral decubitus position for a right thoracotomy. Monitor breath sounds in dependent lung.

| | | |
|---|---|---|
| **Complications** | Hypothermia<br>Metabolic acidosis<br>Hypo- or hyperventilation<br>Aspiration<br>Pneumothorax<br>Atelectasis<br>Mucus plug | ETT placement may interfere with TEF closure. |

**POSTOPERATIVE**

| | | |
|---|---|---|
| **Complications** | Apnea<br>Pneumothorax<br>Hypoventilation<br>Tracheal leak<br>Inadequate neuromuscular reversal<br>Recurrent laryngeal nerve injury<br>Pneumonia | Maintenance of normothermia lessens incidence of apnea, hypoventilation and metabolic acidosis.<br><br>Spontaneous hip flexion is the most reliable indication of adequate neuromuscular function. |
| **Pain management** | Acetaminophen 10-20 mg/kg pr q 4 hr prn<br>Fentanyl 0.5-1.0 $\mu$g/kg iv q 60 min prn | |
| **Tests** | ABG, Hct | |


**References**

1. Chittmittrapap S, Spitz L, Kiely EM, Brereton RJ: Anastomotic leakage following surgery for esophageal atresia. *J Pediatr Surg* 1992; 27(1):29-32.
2. Goh DW, Brereton RJ: Success and failure with neonatal tracheo-oesophageal anomalies. *Br J Surg* 1991; 78(7):834-37.
3. Randolph JG: Esophageal Atresia and Congenital Stenosis. In *Pediatric Surgery*, 4th edition. Ravitch MM, et al, eds. Year Book Medical Publishers, Inc, Chicago: 1986, 682-93.
4. Gregory GA, ed: *Pediatric Anesthesia*, 2nd edition. Churchill Livingstone, New York: 1989, 920-27.
5. Motoyama EK, Davis PC, eds: *Smith's Anesthesia for Infants and Children*, 5th edition. CV Mosby, St. Louis: 1990, 450-53.
6. Holzki J: Bronchoscopic findings and treatment in congenital tracheo-oesophageal fistula. *Paediatric Anaesthesia* 1992; 2:297-303.


# ABDOMINAL TUMOR: RESECTION OF NEUROBLASTOMA, WILMS' TUMOR, HEPATOBLASTOMA

## SURGICAL CONSIDERATIONS

**Description**: Neuroblastoma and Wilms' tumor (50% of retroperitoneal masses) are the most common abdominal tumors in childhood. Hepatic tumors or malformations (hemangioma) are less common, but challenging lesions. These tumors usually occur in young (< 5 yrs) children, and are generally explored with the intent of complete resection. Limited explorations with biopsy only are uncommon. The principles of the operative approach are similar for these tumors and include a generous transperitoneal exposure, followed by careful exploration. If the lesion appears resectable, mobilization of the tumor from the posterior body wall and adjacent viscera usually should precede attempts to control the vascular pedicle. Not infrequently the tumor must be divided to preserve major vessels (Fig 12.2-2). If the tumor is fully mobilized prior to major vessel dissection, then hemorrhage can be controlled by application of vascular clamps and rapid tumor excision. The large size of these tumors frequently precludes the strategy of early vascular pedicle control, which frequently needs to wait for full mobilization of the mass. Surgeon and anesthesiologist need to be prepared for thoracic extension of the procedure and major vessel control. **Neuroblastoma** arises from sympathetic tissue in the adrenal or other retroperitoneal ganglia. While urinary catecholamine levels are frequently elevated, these tumors rarely produce cardiovascular symptoms. **Wilms' tumor** frequently has direct tumor extension

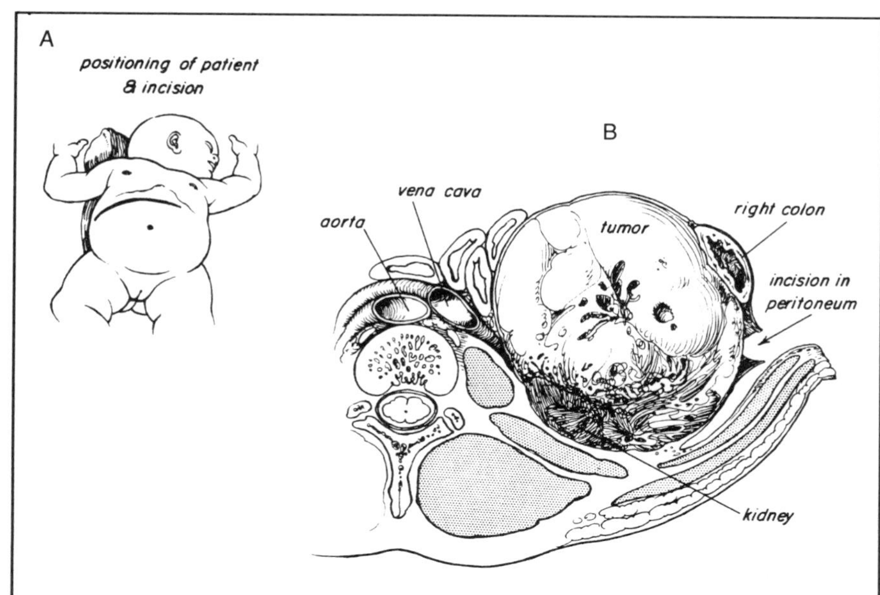


**Figure 12.2-2.** (A) Patient elevated, with transverse incision that can be extended into the flank. (B) Anatomic relationship of retroperitoneal tumor (Wilms') to major vascular structures. (Reproduced with permission from Ravitch MM, et al, eds: *Pediatric Surgery*. Year Book Medical Pub: 1986.)

into the IVC or right atrium, particularly with right-side tumors. Preop preparation should include ultrasound imaging and prepping for CPB if major venous extension is suspected. Major **hepatic resections** may be required for tumors or hemangiomas producing CHF or thrombocytopenia not responsive to steroids, hepatic artery embolization or ligation.

**Usual preop diagnosis**: Neuroblastoma; Wilms' tumor; hepatoblastoma

**SUMMARY OF PROCEDURE**

| | Neuroblastoma | Wilms' Tumor | Hepatic Resections |
|---|---|---|---|
| **Position** | Supine, 15° lift (see Fig 12.2-2, inset) | ⇐ | ⇐ |
| **Incision** | Transverse, possible thoracic extension (see Fig 12.2-2, inset) | ⇐ | ⇐ |
| **Special instrumentation** | None | Bypass instruments | CUSA; laser |
| **Unique considerations** | None | Atrial tumor; IVC may be obstructed →↓↓CO | Possible CHF, platelets |
| **Antibiotics** | Preop: ampicillin 25 mg/kg iv + gentamicin 2.5 mg/kg | ⇐ | ⇐ |
| | iv; intraop: cephalosporin irrigation (1 gm/500 cc NS) | ⇐ | ⇐ |
| **Surgical time** | 3 - 6 hrs | ⇐ | ⇐ |
| **Closing considerations** | None | None | Hypoglycemia |
| **EBL** | 20-50 cc/kg | ⇐ | 20-100 cc/kg |
| **Postop care** | PICU | ⇐ | ⇐ |
| **Mortality** | < 5% | ⇐ | ⇐ |
| **Morbidity** | Intestinal obstruction: 10% | ⇐ | – |
| | Postop respiratory atelectasis | ⇐ | ⇐ |
| | | | Hypoglycemia: 10% |
| | | | Bile leak: 5-10% |
| **Procedure code** | 60545 | 50230 | 47120, 47122, 47125, 47130 |
| **Pain score** | 7-8 | 7-8 | 7-8 |

### PATIENT POPULATION CHARACTERISTICS

| | | | |
|---|---|---|---|
| **Age range** | Few months–school age | ⇐ | ⇐ |
| **Male:Female** | 1:1 | ⇐ | ⇐ |
| **Incidence** | 1/10,000 | < 1/10,000 | ⇐ |
| **Etiology** | Unknown | ⇐ | ⇐ |
| **Associated conditions** | Beckwith-Wiedemann syndrome<br>Aniridia<br>Hemi-hypertrophy<br>HTN: Rare | None | ⇐ |

---

## ANESTHETIC CONSIDERATIONS

### PREOPERATIVE

Neuroblastoma, Wilms' tumor (nephroblastoma) and hepatoblastoma commonly present as abdominal masses in infants and children < 4 yrs old. Abdominal pain, fever and ↑BP (2° ↑catecholamines or renal ischemia) are often associated findings. These patients may have received chemotherapy or XRT preop, and the timing of surgery may be based on multiple factors.

**Respiratory** There may be respiratory compromise (as a result of a large abdominal mass pushing up on the diaphragm) which may worsen in the supine position. Wilms' tumor commonly metastasizes to the lungs.
**Tests:** CXR, if indicated from H&P.

**Cardiovascular** ↑BP is associated with both Wilms' tumor and neuroblastoma, and volume status should be assessed carefully. Tumor bulk may impede venous return by occluding the IVC. Wilms' tumor may extend through the IVC into the right atrium. These patients may have received doxorubicin, which is associated with cardiomyopathy and CHF (most commonly at doses >200 mg/m$^2$). Consultation with a pediatric cardiologist may be appropriate.

**Renal** Wilms' tumor may present with hematuria and other GU anomalies. Renal function is usually normal.
**Tests:** BUN; creatinine

**Endocrine** Neuroblastomas are associated with ↑catecholamine production. Preop adrenergic blockade (as would be required for a pheochromocytoma) is not necessary.
**Tests:** Urine VMA and HVA

**Gastrointestinal** Persistent, watery diarrhea (→ hypovolemia, ↓$K^+$) is associated with neuroblastoma 2° VIP secretion. Intestinal compression from tumor may ↑risk of gastric aspiration. A surgical bowel prep may cause additional fluid and electrolyte disturbances.
**Tests:** Electrolytes

**Hematologic** Severe anemia and thrombocytopenia may be present. Blood should be available because of possible massive intraop blood loss.
**Tests:** CBC; T&C. ✓ availability of parental/directed donor blood, if requested.

**Laboratory** Other tests as indicated from H&P.

**Premedication** In patients at risk for gastric aspiration, prophylaxis with metoclopramide (0.1 mg/kg iv) and ranitidine (0.8 mg/kg iv) should be considered. Patients >12 mos may benefit from midazolam (0.5-0.75 mg/kg po) 30 min before surgery.

### INTRAOPERATIVE

**Anesthetic technique:** GETA, using a pediatric circle or Bain circuit with humidified and warmed gasses. Warm OR to 75°-80°F; use warming pad on OR table. Warming all IV fluids is mandatory in order to maintain body temperature at 37°C.

**Induction** IV catheter insertion prior to induction may be preferable An upper extremity or EJ site is preferred due to potential for obstruction of IVC during surgery. A modified rapid-sequence induction is recommended in those patients with a large intra-abdominal mass compressing the GI tract. Otherwise, standard pediatric induction (see Appendix) is appropriate. Children < 12

| | | |
|---|---|---|
| **Induction, continued** | months may benefit from a preinduction dose of atropine (0.2 mg/kg iv) to ablate vagal response to laryngoscopy. In children < 8 yrs of age, an uncuffed ETT should be used. The appropriate size for the ETT is one that will allow a small leak around the tube when positive pressure is applied (20-30 cm $H_2O$). | |
| **Maintenance** | Standard maintenance (see Appendix). Muscle relaxation is appropriate. Hypertension associated with tumor manipulation can be treated with SNP (0.5-2.0 $\mu$g/kg/min) or labetalol (0.1 mg/kg iv) boluses. | |
| **Emergence** | In most instances, patient can be extubated at the end of surgery. Suction NG tube prior to extubation. | |
| **Blood and fluid requirements** | Potential for large blood loss/moderate 3rd-space loss<br>IV: 18-20 ga x 1-2<br>NS/LR @ (maintenance):<br>4 cc/kg/hr - 0-10 kg<br>+ 2 cc/kg/hr - 11-20 kg<br>+ 1 cc/kg/hr - >20 kg<br>(e.g., 25 kg = 65 cc/hr) | Tumor resection may be associated with massive blood loss, especially with IVC or renal vein involvement. Avoid placement of iv catheter in lower extremities. 5% albumin may be useful to replace third-space losses (8-10 cc/kg/hr). Transfuse to maintain Hct >23. Over 12 mos of age, dextrose-containing solutions are not required. |
| **Monitoring** | Standard monitors (see Appendix).<br>Arterial line: 22 ga<br>CVP line: 4 Fr (subclavian or IJ)<br>Urinary catheter | ABG, Hct, blood glucose should be measured hourly. CVP measurement may useful to evaluate fluid status. UO monitored and kept at 1 cc/kg/hr. |
| **Positioning** | ✓ and pad pressure points.<br>✓ eyes. | |
| **Complications** | Hypotension<br>HTN<br>PE<br>Hypothermia<br>Hypoventilation | ↓BP 2° blood loss or IVC obstruction or PE<br>↑BP 2° tumor or adrenal manipulation<br>2° tumor embolization usually from IVC →↓BP.<br>Abdominal retractors and packing will interfere with ventilation. |

## POSTOPERATIVE

| | | |
|---|---|---|
| **Complications** | Atelectasis<br>Hypoventilation | If supplemental $O_2$ required, pulse oximetry useful for weaning from $O_2$. |
| **Pain management** | Morphine 0.05-0.1 mg/kg iv q 2-4 hrs prn, or<br>Ketorolac 0.9 mg/kg iv q 6 x 2 d | |
| **Tests** | Hct<br>ABG<br>CXR | <br><br>If CVP placed. |

**References**


1. Grosfeld JL: Neuroblastoma. In *Pediatric Surgery*, 4th edition. Ravitch MM, et al, eds. Year Book Medical Publishers, Chicago: 1986, 283-93.
2. Othersen HB Jr: Wilms' Tumor. In *Pediatric Surgery*, 4th edition. Ravitch MM, et al, eds. Year Book Medical Publishers, Chicago: 1986, 293-302.
3. Randolph JG, Guzzetta PC: Tumors of the Liver. In *Pediatric Surgery*, 4th edition. Ravitch MM, et al, eds. Year Book Medical Publishers, Chicago: 1986, 302-11.
4. Gregory GA, ed: *Pediatric Anesthesia*, 2nd edition. Churchill Livingstone, New York: 1989, 920-27.
5. Motoyama EK, Davis PC, eds: *Smith's Anesthesia for Infants and Children*, 5th edition. CV Mosby, St. Louis: 1990, 450-53.
6. Creagh-Barry P, et al: Neuroblastoma and anaesthesia. *Paed Anaesth* 1992; 2:147-52.
7. Charlton GA, Sedgwick J, Sutton DN: Anaesthetic management of renin-secreting nephroblastoma. *Br J Anaesth* 1992; 69(2):206-09.

# REPAIR OF CONGENITAL DIAPHRAGMATIC HERNIA

## SURGICAL CONSIDERATIONS

**Description**: Congenital diaphragmatic hernia remains a highly lethal anomaly, due to associated pulmonary vascular HTN and pulmonary hypoplasia. Once considered a surgical emergency, it is now common to treat newborns with a period of stabilization or **ECMO support** (see "ECMO") prior to repair of the diaphragmatic defect. Most surgeons prefer an abdominal approach to allow for treatment of associated intestinal anomalies, to close skin only, or to place a Silastic® pouch, if replacing the intestine in the abdominal cavity is associated with undue tension. *In utero* diagnosis allows for maternal transport to a tertiary center, preferably one with ECMO capability. **Laparotomy** by subcostal or upper transverse incision is followed by reduction of viscera from thorax. Diaphragm may be repaired by primary suture if adequate tissue remains. Otherwise it is closed with a patch of Silastic® or Gortex®. Use of a chest tube is optional. If significant adhesions or obstruction related to intestinal malrotation are identified, they are corrected. Replacement of the bowel into the abdomen may be impossible or may produce excessive tension, in which case a Silastic® silo may be used or the skin closed without closing the abdominal wall muscles.

**Variant procedure or approaches**: **Thoracotomy** is preferred by a few surgeons for primary repair, usually of right-sided lesions, and is the approach of choice for recurrent hernias. Hernias initially requiring ECMO support may be repaired prior to or following decannulation. Because the risk of postop hemorrhage is increased if anticoagulation is prolonged, most centers repair the hernia at the completion of the ECMO run. Once the patient has been shown to tolerate weaning from ECMO, the circuit flow is increased to 100 cc/kg/min to allow operating during reduced anticoagulation; patients are then weaned fairly rapidly after repair (12-24 hrs). **Lateral** or **anterolateral thoracotomy**, using the 6th or 7th interspace, provides adequate exposure for closing the defect in the diaphragm, which is done as from the abdomen. The ability to deal with intestinal abnormalities or abdominal tension, however, is limited by this approach.

**Usual preop diagnosis**: Diaphragmatic hernia; Bochdalek's hernia (posterolateral diaphragm)

### SUMMARY OF PROCEDURE

| | |
|---|---|
| **Position** | Supine (lateral for thoracic approach) |
| **Incision** | Subcostal (posterolateral for thoracic approach) |
| **Special instrumentation** | Pre- and post-ductal arterial catheters, soft-tissue patch, Gortex® |
| **Unique considerations** | Reactive pulmonary vasculature |
| **Antibiotics** | Preop: ampicillin 25 mg/kg iv + gentamicin 2.5 mg/kg iv; intraop: cephalosporin irrigation (1 gm/500 cc NS) |
| **Surgical time** | 1 - 2 hrs |
| **Closing considerations** | Assess for changes in ventilation (e.g., PIP, pre- and post-ductal ABG). |
| **EBL** | 5-10 cc/kg |
| **Postop care** | Paralysis maintained; hyperventilation, fentanyl infusion @ 2-5 μg/kg/min |
| **Mortality** | 50% without ECMO<br>25-30% with ECMO |
| **Morbidity** | Pulmonary HTN<br>Respiratory failure<br>Sepsis<br>Intestinal obstruction/dysfunction |
| **Procedure code** | 39540 |
| **Pain score** | 6-7 (7-8 for thoracic approach) |

### PATIENT POPULATION CHARACTERISTICS

| | |
|---|---|
| **Age range** | Newborn–weeks or months |
| **Male:Female** | 1-2:1 |
| **Incidence** | 1/4000 |
| **Etiology** | Unknown |

**Associated conditions** Malrotation: 40-100%
Congenital heart disease: 15%
Renal anomalies: Rare
Esophageal atresia: Rare
CNS abnormalities: Rare

## ANESTHETIC CONSIDERATIONS

### PREOPERATIVE

These infants present with varying degrees of respiratory distress. The majority are already mechanically ventilated, sedated and paralyzed in the ICN prior to anesthesia consultation. Associated defects are myelomeningocele, hydrocephalus, PDA and esophageal atresia (EA). Some infants may be on ECMO.

**Respiratory** The lung on affected side is usually hypoplastic or aplastic. The prognosis is correlated with magnitude of pulmonary hypoplasia and pulmonary muscular abnormalities present on the contralateral side. There is decreased compliance, with resultant risk for hypoventilation. ↑PIP → ↑risk for pneumothorax. Persistent pulmonary HTN and progressive hypoxemia may be present.
**Tests:** CXR; ABG

**Cardiovascular** R → L shunting may occur at level of PDA or preductally (e.g., PFO). The degree of R → L shunting may be dramatically increased by ↑pulmonary vasoconstriction (2° ↓$PO_2$, ↑$PCO_2$, ↓pH, ↑sympathetic tone) → severe systemic hypoxemia. ↓cardiac output 2° persistent pulmonary HTN and hypoxemia will lead to metabolic acidosis.
**Tests:** CXR; ECHO; ABG

**Neurological** Myelomeningocele and/or hydrocephalus may be present. Repeated bouts of hypoxemia predispose to intraventricular hemorrhage (IVH) in preterm infant. These areas of hemorrhage have loss of cerebral autoregulation and BP increases are directly transmitted to the microvasculature, with ↑risk of recurrent hemorrhage and edema.
**Tests:** Head ultrasound

**Hematologic** Hct should be maintained at 36%. HbF has ↑affinity for $O_2$ and ↓sensitivity to 2,3-DPG. This will aggravate cellular hypoxia in the patient with compromised circulatory status. Confirm that vitamin K was administered at birth.
**Tests:** CBC; T&C; PT; PTT

**Metabolic** Negligible glycogen stores in neonate; therefore, dextrose hyperalimentation should be initiated early. In patients with CHF, diuretic administration leads to ↓$K^+$.
**Tests:** Electrolytes; glucose; BUN; creatinine

**Gastrointestinal** Constant NG/OG suction. Gastric distention will worsen ventilation.

**Laboratory** Other tests as indicated from H&P.

**Premedication** None

### INTRAOPERATIVE

**Anesthetic technique:** GETA, using a pediatric circle or Bain circuit with humidified and warmed gasses. Use pressure-limited ventilation (PIP < 30 cm $H_2O$). Maintain body temperature as close to 37°C as possible. Warm room to at least 75-80°F. Warming blanket on OR table. Consider use of ICN ventilator (e.g., Baby Bird®) particularly if high RR (>30/min) is required.

**Induction** Transported from ICN to OR by anesthesia team. If infant is already intubated tracheally, confirm paralysis prior to transport. This is to lessen the risk of patient movement and self-extubation. Transport with full monitoring (ECG, pulse oximetry, arterial pressure tracing). Have airway equipment available (Miller 1 laryngoscope blade, ET 3.0-3.5 with stylets, neonatal mask). Resuscitation drugs (e.g., epinephrine 10 μg/cc) should be drawn up. Syringe with NS/LR flush. Prior to any further anesthetic administration, re-establish all monitoring in OR. Atropine (0.02 mg/kg iv) given prior to opiates to counteract bradycardia. For non-intubated patients, standard pediatric induction (see Appendix) is appropriate. Avoid $N_2O$ and maintain PIPs as low as possible.

| | | |
|---|---|---|
| **Maintenance** | Opiate-based anesthetic (fentanyl 10-25 μg/kg iv total) with isoflurane supplementation. Ventilate with air/$O_2$ to maintain $O_2$ saturation 95-100%, as measured by preductal ABGs/pulse oximetry. Continue neuromuscular blockade with pancuronium or vecuronium (0.05 mg/kg/hr). | |
| **Emergence** | Patient will remain intubated. Transport back to ICN with full monitoring, airway equipment and drugs. | |
| **Blood and fluid requirements** | Blood loss minimal<br>IV: 22-24 ga x 2<br>D5 NS/LR @ 4 cc/kg/hr maintenance | These infants are fluid-restricted in ICN. If not in overt CHF, albumin 5% (5-10 cc/kg) slow bolus prior to opiates. Continue dextrose-containing solution (dextrose 4-6 mg/kg/min) from ICN. If umbilical venous line not present, dopamine may be infused via peripheral iv with dextrose solution serving as the carrier fluid. In emergency, NS/LR, albumin 5%, PRBCs (Hct < 50%) may be given via umbilical artery line. |
| **Monitoring** | Standard monitors (see Appendix).<br>Right-side precordial stethoscope<br>Arterial line (umbilical artery or radial – 24-ga)<br>± umbilical vein line<br>Preductal and postductal pulse oximetry | ABG, Hct, glucose q 30-60 min. Contralateral pneumothorax is detected using a right axillary precordial stethoscope.<br><br>Changes in pre- and postductal pulse oximetry provide early warning of R → L shunt/pulmonary HTN. |
| **Positioning** | ✓ and pad pressure points.<br>✓ eyes. | Arms/iv access sites should be positioned to be visible and easily available. |
| **Complications** | Pneumothorax<br>Hypoventilation<br>Hypothermia<br>Metabolic acidosis<br>R → L shunting<br>CHF | With acute deterioration in $O_2$ saturation, pneumothorax on unaffected side is likely. With removal of abdominal contents from thorax, do not attempt to expand lungs vigorously. Hypoplasia, not atelectasis, is the primary problem. Keep PIP < 30 cm $H_2O$, if possible. |

## POSTOPERATIVE

| | | |
|---|---|---|
| **Complications** | Same as Intraoperative Complications, above. | Those infants whose oxygenation continues to worsen are possible candidates for ECMO. Discuss with ICN team their criteria for initiation of ECMO. |
| **Pain management** | Fentanyl (0.5-2.0 μg/kg/hr iv) | Tachyphylaxis can develop in 24-48 hrs. |
| **Tests** | CXR; ABG; Hct; glucose; electrolytes | |


**References**

1. Anderson KD: Congenital diaphragmatic hernia. In *Pediatric Surgery*, 4th edition. Ravitch MM, et al, eds. Year Book Medical Publishers, Chicago: 1986, 589-601.
2. Falconer AR, Brown RA, Helms P, Gordon I, Baron JA: Pulmonary sequelae in survivors of congenital diaphragmatic hernia. *Thorax* 1990; 45(2):126-29.
3. Wilson JM, Lund DP, Lillehei CW, Vacanti JP: Congenital diaphragmatic hernia: predictors of severity in the ECMO era. *J Pediatr Surg* 1991; 26(9):1028-33.
4. Cook DR, Marcy JH, eds: *Neonatal Anesthesia*, 1st edition. Appleton Davies Inc, Pasadena: 1988.
5. Stehling L, ed: *Common Problems in Pediatric Anesthesia*, 2nd edition. Mosby-Year Book, St. Louis: 1992, 7-11.
6. Goldsmith JP, Karokin EH, eds: *Assisted Ventilation of the Neonate*, 2nd edition. WB Saunders Co, Philadelphia: 1988.

# LAPAROTOMY FOR INTESTINAL PERFORATION, NECROTIZING ENTEROCOLITIS

## SURGICAL CONSIDERATIONS

**Description**: Necrotizing enterocolitis (NEC) is an ischemic/inflammatory condition of the GI tract (1° terminal ileum and splenic flexure of the colon) occurring primarily in stressed prematures. It may progress to full-thickness necrosis and perforation, which have traditionally been treated by **resection** with **enterostomy** or **primary anastomosis** in selected cases. These infants are usually bacteremic with thrombocytopenia, complex respiratory distress and severe prematurity. Blood loss may be significant. Volume replacement and temperature regulation, therefore, must be precise. Laparotomy via an upper abdominal, transverse incision allows inspection of the entire GI tract for areas of perforation or full-thickness necrosis. Areas of irreversible injury are resected and any questionable areas are retained. Occasionally, primary anastomosis may be suitable, but most often proximal enterostomy and mucous fistula at the lateral margins of the incision are safe and expeditious.

**Variant procedure or approaches**: In extremely small infants (< 1500 gm) a few centers have utilized **peritoneal drainage** under local anesthesia as a temporizing or definitive management. This procedure consists of a small, RLQ incision with evacuation of intestinal contents or purulent material from the peritoneal cavity and placement of Penrose drain(s) through the incision. It is performed in the NICU, with minimal physiologic disturbance.

**Usual preop diagnosis**: Perforated NEC

### SUMMARY OF PROCEDURE

| | Resection | Drainage |
|---|---|---|
| **Position** | Supine | ⇐ |
| **Incision** | Transverse | RLQ |
| **Special instrumentation** | None | Penrose drains |
| **Unique considerations** | Temperature support | ⇐ |
| **Surgical time** | 1 - 2.5 hrs | 0.5 hrs |
| **EBL** | 10-100 cc/kg | 1-2 cc/kg |
| **Postop care** | NICU | ⇐ |
| **Mortality** | 20-25% | 16-20% |
| **Morbidity** | Respiratory failure<br>Sepsis<br>Stricture<br>Intracranial hemorrhage | ⇐ |
| **Procedure code** | 44120 (enterectomy with anastomosis)<br>44125 (enterectomy with stoma) | 49020 |
| **Pain score** | 6-7 | 3-4 |

### PATIENT POPULATION CHARACTERISTICS

| | |
|---|---|
| **Age range** | Newborn–wks |
| **Male:Female** | >1:1 |
| **Incidence** | 5-8% NICU admissions |
| **Etiology** | Multifactorial including:<br>Intestinal ischemia<br>Bacterial colonization<br>Perinatal stress<br>Immaturity<br>Hypoxia<br>Hyperosmolar feeding<br>Splanchnic ischemia |
| **Associated conditions** | Prematurity: 80-90%<br>Respiratory distress, PDA |

# ANESTHETIC CONSIDERATIONS

## PREOPERATIVE

Most (80-90%) of these patients are premature infants (< 36 weeks gestational age) presenting with sepsis and pulmonary insufficiency. In addition to sepsis, significant 3rd-space losses contribute to hypovolemia and metabolic acidosis.

**Respiratory** — Premature infants are at risk for RDS. These infants are usually on mechanical ventilation with ↑$FiO_2$ prior to surgery. They also are at increased risk for pneumonia, pneumothorax and pulmonary edema 2° to sepsis and/or CHF. ✓ ventilator settings and recent ABG in preparation for OR mechanical ventilation.
**Tests:** CXR; ABG

**Cardiovascular** — Intrinsically labile BP. Inotropes (e.g., dopamine 5-10 μg/kg/min) may be required to maintain adequate CO. Associated cardiac anomalies (e.g., VSD, PDA) can lead to CHF, further complicating fluid management. Pulmonary over-circulation and intrinsic pulmonary disease contribute to pulmonary HTN.
**Tests:** CXR; ABG; ECG; ± ECHO

**Neurological** — Intraventricular hemorrhage (IVH) may be 2° to prematurity or birth asphyxia. These hemorrhagic regions have impaired autoregulation, and wide variations in BP (20-30 mmHg) can aggravate ischemia/hemorrhage. In addition, these patients may have a seizure disorder. Should this be the case, ✓ medication list for appropriate anticonvulsant therapy.
**Tests:** Head ultrasound, if indicated from H&P.

**Renal** — Presence of PDA and prior Rx with NSAID (e.g., indomethacin) can lead to impaired renal perfusion and clearance. Aggravating factors are aminoglycoside antibiotics, sepsis and CHF.
**Tests:** BUN; creatinine

**Metabolic** — Metabolic acidosis 2° to sepsis/CHF will further worsen myocardial function. Neonate has minimal glycogen stores and impaired ability to mobilize calcium.
**Tests:** ABG; $Ca^{++}$; glucose; electrolytes

**Hematologic** — DIC, thrombocytopenia, hemolysis and T-antigen activation on RBCs are present with overwhelming sepsis, particularly clostridial infections.
**Tests:** CBC; PT; PTT; fibrinogen; T-antigen; availability of washed RBCs and platelets (plasma can contain antibody against T-antigen that causes hemolysis)

**Antibiotics** — Triple antibiotic therapy (ampicillin 50 mg/kg iv, gentamicin 2.5 mg/kg, clindamycin 10 mg/kg iv). ✓ nursing records for time of administration of antibiotics.
**Tests:** Cultures

**Laboratory** — Others as indicated from H&P.

**Premedication** — None

## INTRAOPERATIVE

**Anesthetic technique:** GETA, using a pediatric circle or Bain circuit with warmed, humidified gasses. Use air/$O_2$ mixture for ventilation that maintains $SpO_2$ between 95-100%. Avoid high concentrations of $O_2$. Consider use of ICN ventilator (e.g., Baby Bird®) if patient requires ↑RR or ↑PIPs.

**Induction** — These patients are usually intubated. If not, awake intubation is favored. Give atropine 0.02 mg/kg iv (0.1 mg minimum dose) prior to laryngoscopy. Pre-oxygenate for 2 min. Miller 0/1 blade with $O_2$ side port, if available. Suction NG. Apply cricoid pressure until airway secured. ETT should have leak at 20-30 cm $H_2O$ pressure.

**Maintenance** — Narcotic technique (fentanyl 20-30 μg/kg iv total) – avoid myocardial depression from volatile agents. Avoid $N_2O$ (↑bowel size). Muscle relaxation required.

**Emergence** — Postop ventilation is required. Transport to ICN with full monitoring (ECG, arterial line, pulse oximetry). Have laryngoscope and appropriately sized mask and ETT available. Extra volume (albumin 5% in 20 cc syringes) may be needed during transport.

**Blood and fluid requirements** — Anticipate moderate-to-large blood and fluid losses.
IV: 22-24 ga x 2
Continue dextrose-containing solution from ICN (dextrose requirements 4-6 mg/kg/min)
Warm fluids.

Neonates are usually fluid-restricted in ICN to lessen incidence of PDA. 3rd-space losses are usually significant. Rx: ↓BP with volume before increasing dopamine. Maintain Hct >35%. Albumin 5% (10 cc/kg iv) boluses as needed. Crystalloid/colloid >100 cc/kg total

| | | |
|---|---|---|
| **Blood, continued** | | not uncommon. Hct, glucose, $Ca^{++}$, ABG, platelet count, PT/PTT, electrolytes q 30-60 min. |
| **Monitoring** | Standard monitors (see Appendix).<br>Arterial line 24 ga – preferably preductal<br>± CVP line (subclavian, IJ, femoral) 3 Fr | Central line not as important as arterial line for intraop care. Catheters that can be antibiotic-coated are preferred to lessen risk of subsequent line infection. |
| **Positioning** | √ and pad pressure points.<br>√ eyes. | |
| **Complications** | Hypothermia<br>Metabolic acidosis<br>Hypovolemia | Aggressive volume repletion and maintaining normothermia will prevent or ameliorate metabolic acidosis. Bicarbonate replacement = base deficit x wt (kg) x 0.3 → ↓SVR. |
| | Hemolysis 2° blood products (rare) | Minimized by use of washed PRBCs. |
| | Pneumothorax | ↓$O_2$ sats, ↑PIPs. √ for mucus plugging or mainstem intubation. |
| | Hypocalcemia | Frequent blood sampling is necessary. Rx: $CaCl_2$ (10 mg/kg iv) via central line or Ca gluconate (30 mg/kg iv) via peripheral line. |
| | Hypoglycemia | Continue 10% dextrose infusion from ICN. |

## POSTOPERATIVE

| | | |
|---|---|---|
| **Complications** | Retrolental fibroplasia<br>Hypovolemia from continued 3rd-spacing<br>Metabolic acidosis/sepsis<br>Pulmonary edema with fluid remobilization | Maintain $PaO_2 < 70$ mmHg to lessen incidence of retrolental fibroplasia. |
| **Pain management** | Morphine (0.05-0.10 mg/kg iv) q 1-2 hrs prn or via continuous infusion for initial 24-48 hrs | |
| **Tests** | CBC; electrolytes; $Ca^{++}$; glucose; ABG | CXR, if central line placed. |

**References**


1. Ein SH, Shandling B, Wesson D, Filler RM: A 13-year experience with peritoneal drainage under local anesthesia for necrotizing enterocolitis perforation. *J Pediatr Surg* 1990; 25(10):1034-37.
2. Harberg FJ, McGill CW, Saleem MM, Halbert R, Anastassiou P: Resection with primary anastomosis for necrotizing enterocolitis. *J Pediatr Surg* 1983; 18(6):743-46.
3. Kleigman RM: Neonatal necrotizing enterocolitis: implication for an infectious disease. *Pediatr Clin North Am* 1979; 26:327-42.
4. Santulli TV, Schullinger JN, Heird WC, Gongaware RD, Wiggens J, Barlow B, Blanc WA, Berdon WE: Acute necrotizing enterocolitis in infancy: a review of 64 cases. *Pediatrics* 1975; 55(3):376-87.
5. Cook DR, Marcy JH, eds: *Neonatal Anesthesia*, 1st edition. Appleton Davies, Pasadena: 1988.
6. Diaz JH, ed: *Perinatal Anesthesia and Critical Care*, 1st edition. WB Saunders Co, Philadelphia: 1991.

# REPAIR OF PECTUS EXCAVATUM/CARINATUM

## SURGICAL CONSIDERATIONS

**Description**: Pectus excavatum (funnel chest) is a deformity of the sternum and costal cartilages occurring primarily in boys. It is 8-10 times more common than the carinatum (pigeon breast) deformity. While some surgeons believe excavatum deformities are purely cosmetic, recent studies confirm cardiopulmonary deficits in moderate and severe cases. Many children have an antecedent or coincidental respiratory problem, usually in the form of reactive airway disease. The operative procedure consists of **resection** of the costal cartilages of ribs 3-7 bilaterally, **excision** of the xiphoid, and **transverse osteotomy** of the sternum. A transverse incision is used to elevate skin flaps. Pectoralis muscles are elevated from the chest wall and costal cartilages 3-7 are excised, leaving posterior perichondrium intact. The xiphoid is excised and the sternum is fractured at the 2nd interspace. The pectoralis muscles are reattached to the sternum and drains are placed in the mediastinum. If entry into the pleura occurs, the pleura space is evacuated and repaired. In older children and adolescents, the sternum may be reinforced with a metal strut or pin. Operative correction of the excavatum and carinatum deformities is essentially identical, although the timing of operation is frequently different. Excavatum deformities are best repaired at 5-6 yrs to allow improved thoracic volume during growth. Carinatum or minor excavatum deformities are usually repaired following the pubertal growth spurt.

**Usual preop diagnosis**: Pectus excavatum; carinatum

### SUMMARY OF PROCEDURE

| | |
|---|---|
| **Position** | Supine |
| **Incision** | Transverse |
| **Special instrumentation** | Air drill; sternal strut; K-wire |
| **Unique considerations** | Possible pleural entry |
| **Antibiotics** | Preop: ampicillin 25 mg/kg iv + gentamicin 2.5 mg/kg iv; intraop: cephalosporin irrigation (1 gm/500 cc NS) |
| **Surgical time** | 3 - 5 hrs |
| **EBL** | 5-20 cc/kg; greater in older patients |
| **Postop care** | PICU, ICU; aggressive respiratory support; analgesia (epidural catheter, PCA–see Appendix.) |
| **Mortality** | 0.2% |
| **Morbidity** | Pneumothorax<br>Fluid accumulation |
| **Procedure code** | 21740 |
| **Pain score** | 7-8 |

### PATIENT POPULATION CHARACTERISTICS

| | |
|---|---|
| **Age range** | 5 yrs - adolescent |
| **Male:Female** | 5-9:1 |
| **Incidence** | Uncertain |
| **Etiology** | Relationship with reactive airway disease |
| **Associated conditions** | Marfan syndrome: 5%<br>Mitral valve prolapse: 5% |

## ANESTHETIC CONSIDERATIONS

### PREOPERATIVE

**Pectus excavatum** (a condition in which there is concave depression of the lower sternum) may be associated with CHD and restrictive lung disease. If the deformity is present without cardiac or pulmonary disease, the patient is asymptomatic and the procedure is cosmetic. Surgery usually occurs between 5-10 years of age. **Pectus carinatum**

(a convex lower sternum) is usually repaired for cosmetic reasons only. Surgery usually occurs in the teenage years. Cardiac abnormalities (VSD, PDA, mitral valve anomalies) may be associated with the pectus disorder.

| | |
|---|---|
| **Respiratory** | Restrictive lung disease 2° chest wall deformity may be present. If a longstanding condition, patient may have chronic hypoxemia, with resultant pulmonary HTN and polycythemia. If patient has exercise limitations, there is a need to differentiate between cardiac and pulmonary components.<br>**Tests:** CXR: AP, lateral; PFTs; ABG, if symptomatic |
| **Cardiovascular** | In both conditions, CHD should be investigated if present. Pulmonary HTN may be 2° pulmonary over-circulation (e.g., VSD).<br>**Tests:** ECG; ECHO |
| **Laboratory** | Hct; T&C; electrolytes |
| **Premedication** | If patient is asymptomatic, midazolam (0.75 mg/kg po up to 20 mg) or diazepam (0.1-0.2 mg/kg po up to 5 mg) or a combination of the two can be given. |

## INTRAOPERATIVE

**Anesthetic technique:** GETA, using a pediatric circle or Bain's circuit with warmed, humidified gasses. Heating pad on OR table. Maintain body temperature close to 37°C.

| | |
|---|---|
| **Induction** | IV preferable but, if asymptomatic, may proceed with mask induction. With restrictive lung disease, there is ↓FRC, which will shorten the time to alveolar equilibration for the volatile anesthetics. Hypercarbia will aggravate pulmonary HTN. Tracheal intubation, facilitated by neuromuscular blockade (pancuronium 0.1 mg/kg, vecuronium 0.1 mg/kg). Use cuffed ETT for patient >8 yrs old. With uncuffed ETT, keep air leak to minimum (20-30 cm $H_2O$) to avoid alterations in chest and pulmonary compliance. |
| **Maintenance** | Primarily narcotic-based with air/$O_2$ low-percent volatile agent. In older age group, insertion of lumbar epidural catheter is possible for treatment of postop pain relief. When locating epidural space, use loss of resistance with NS. This avoids hemodynamic risk from air embolus. Use morphine (preservative-free) 0.06-0.08 mg/kg. Avoid local anesthetics since surgical incision extends to C3 dermatome. |
| **Emergence** | Plan for extubation in OR. Ensure adequate reversal of neuromuscular blockade with neostigmine (0.07 mg/kg iv) and glycopyrrolate (0.014 mg/kg iv). |

| | | |
|---|---|---|
| **Blood and fluid requirements** | Usually minimal blood and 3rd-space losses<br>IV: 18 or 20 ga x 1<br>NS/LR @ 3-5 kg/hr | With chronic hypoxemia or right-side heart disease, maintain Hct >30. If otherwise healthy, maintain Hct >22. |
| **Monitoring** | Standard monitors (see Appendix). | |
| **Positioning** | ✓ and pad pressure points.<br>✓ eyes. | Elbow padding to avoid ulnar nerve compression |
| **Complications** | Pneumothorax<br>Atelectasis<br>Subglottic edema | |

## POSTOPERATIVE

| | | |
|---|---|---|
| **Complications** | Respiratory insufficiency 2° splinting, pre-existing restrictive pulmonary disease<br>Pneumothorax | |
| **Pain management** | Epidural (lumbar) or PCA (see Appendix). | Epidural – morphine (0.03 mg/kg-0.05 mg/kg) q 12-24 hrs x 48 hrs<br>Ketorolac (0.9 mg/kg iv q 6 hrs x 48 hrs), in addition to the above measures |

**References**


1. Arn PH, Scherer LR, Haller JA Jr, Pyeritz RE: Outcome of pectus excavatum in patients with Marfan syndrome and in the general population. *J Pediatr* 1989; 115(6):954-58.
2. Derveaux L, Ivanoff I, Rochette F, Demedts M: Mechanism of pulmonary function changes after surgical correction for funnel chest. *Eur Respir J* 1988; 1(9):823-25.
3. Ravitch MM: The chest wall. In *Pediatric Surgery*, 4th edition. Ravitch MM, et al, eds. Year Book Medical Publishers, Chicago: 1986, 563-89.
4. Chidambaram B, Mehta AV: Currarino-Silverman syndrome (pectus carinatum type 2 deformity) and mitral valve disease. *Chest* 1992; 102(3):780-82.
5. Gregory GA, ed: *Pediatric Anesthesia*, 2nd edition. Churchill Livingstone, New York: 1989, 934-35.
6. Motoyama EK, Davis PJ, eds: *Smith's Anesthesia for Infants and Children*, 5th edition. CV Mosby, St. Louis: 1990, 464-5.


# PYLOROMYOTOMY

## SURGICAL CONSIDERATIONS

**Description**: Pyloric stenosis due to idiopathic hypertrophy of the muscular layers of the antrum and pylorus occurs in infants, producing projectile vomiting with subsequent dehydration and metabolic alkalosis. Surgical division of the hypertrophied muscle fibers — **pyloromyotomy** — has been the treatment of choice for this condition since the early 20th century. The operative procedure is quite straightforward, with mucosal entry, usually on the duodenal side, being the only significant technical problem. Preop hydration, replacement of electrolytes, and prevention of aspiration are crucial to a successful outcome. The operation is performed through a short, right-upper-quadrant incision. After delivering the antrum and pylorus, a superficial incision through the serosa of the hypertrophied muscle is carried through an avascular region. Blunt division of the muscle fibers can be done with the back of a scalpel handle or the specialized Benson pyloric spreader. Careful inspection for entry into the lumen may be facilitated by injecting air through a NG tube. Mucosal injury is usually at the duodenal end of the myotomy and can be treated either by simple repair or by closing the myotomy and performing another myotomy at an alternate site.

**Variant procedure or approaches**: **Laparoscopic myotomy** and **balloon dilation** of the pylorus have been done, but cannot match the simplicity, reliability and low complication rate of open myotomy.

**Usual preop diagnosis**: Pyloric stenosis

### SUMMARY OF PROCEDURE

| | |
|---|---|
| **Position** | Supine |
| **Incision** | Transverse |
| **Special instrumentation** | Benson pyloric spreader |
| **Intraop antibiotics** | Cephalosporin irrigation (1 gm/500 cc NS) |
| **Surgical time** | 0.5 - 1 hr |
| **EBL** | < 5 cc/kg |
| **Postop care** | Cardiac/apnea monitoring |
| **Mortality** | 0.3% |
| **Morbidity** | Duodenal perforation<br>Incomplete myotomy<br>Dehiscence |
| **Procedure code** | 43520 |
| **Pain score** | 4-5 |

### PATIENT POPULATION CHARACTERISTICS

| | |
|---|---|
| **Age range** | 1-12 wks |
| **Male:Female** | 4:1 |
| **Incidence** | 3/1000 births |
| **Etiology** | Unknown |
| **Associated conditions** | Has occurred following repair of other congenital anomalies, such as esophageal atresia, omphalocele. |

---

## ANESTHETIC CONSIDERATIONS

### PREOPERATIVE

Patients with pyloric stenosis are usually term infants that present in the first month of life with mild-to-moderate dehydration 2° intractable vomiting. Correction of volume deficit and metabolic abnormalities is the first line of treatment. Surgery should proceed only after patients are medically stabilized.

| | |
|---|---|
| **Cardiovascular** | Mild-to-moderate dehydration (50-100 cc/kg) is common and this defect should be replaced with NS over approximately 12 hrs.<br>**Tests:** Urinary $Cl^-$ >20 mEq/L or plasma Cl >100 meq/L, when fluid volume restored. |
| **Metabolic** | Protracted vomiting → dehydration with hypochloremic hypokalemic metabolic alkalosis. $\downarrow K^+$ should be treated once alkalemia is resolved and urine output is confirmed.<br>**Tests:** ABGs; electrolytes; $Ca^{++}$; glucose |
| **Gastrointestinal** | Full-stomach precautions. |
| **Laboratory** | Hct; other tests as indicated from H&P. |
| **Premedication** | None |

### INTRAOPERATIVE

**Anesthetic technique:** GETA, using a pediatric circle or Bain circuit with warmed, humidified gasses. Warm OR to 75-80° F. Use air/$O_2$ or $N_2O/O_2$ mixture to maintain $O_2$ sat @ 95-100%. Maintain body temperature close to 37°C.

| | |
|---|---|
| **Induction** | An iv catheter usually will be in place prior to induction. Decompress stomach with NG or OG tube. Atropine (0.02 mg/kg iv, 0.1 mg minimum) prior to induction. Preoxygenate 2-3 min. Rapid-sequence induction with cricoid pressure should be performed, using STP (4 mg/kg iv) and succinylcholine (1-2 mg/kg iv). Use awake laryngoscopy if difficulty with intubation is anticipated. Intubate trachea with a 3.5 uncuffed ETT. Should have air leak at 20-30 cm $H_2O$ pressure. Do not wait for return of muscle function before administering vecuronium (0.1 mg/kg iv) or atracurium (0.4 mg/kg iv). |
| **Maintenance** | Volatile agent (isoflurane) and air/$O_2$ or $N_2O/O_2$. Avoid opiates to lessen risk of postop apnea. Maintain muscle relaxation. Surgeon can infiltrate wound site with bupivacaine 0.25% (with epinephrine 1:200,000) – not to exceed 2.5 mg/kg (1.0 cc/kg), for postop pain relief. |
| **Emergence** | Reverse with neostigmine (70 $\mu$g/kg iv) and atropine (0.02 mg/kg iv). Prior to extubation, suction stomach contents via NG/OG tube. Extubate only when fully awake. |

| | | |
|---|---|---|
| **Blood and fluid requirements** | Minimal blood loss<br>IV - 22 ga x 1<br>D5 NS/LR @ (maintenance):<br>4 cc/kg/hr – 0-10 kg | Minimal blood loss or 3rd-space loss. Continue maintenance fluid to provide dextrose at 4-6 mg/kg/min. After D5 NS/LR 10 cc/kg iv bolus, D5 NS/LR is continued for duration of case. |
| **Monitoring** | Standard monitors (see Appendix). | |
| **Positioning** | ✓ and pad pressure points.<br>✓ eyes. | |
| **Complications** | Aspiration | ETT in trachea does not prevent aspiration absolutely. Active inspiration and vomiting may permit vomitus to pass around ETT. |

### POSTOPERATIVE

| | | |
|---|---|---|
| **Complications** | Apnea | Should be on pulse oximetry/apnea monitor on ward x 12 hrs. Continue dextrose solution until tolerating po. Differential diagnosis of apnea includes hypoglycemia and hypothermia. |
| | Hypoglycemia | Rx of hypoglycemia: dextrose 0.5 gm/kg iv |
| **Pain management** | Acetaminophen (10-15 mg po/pr q 4 hrs prn) | |
| **Tests** | None routinely indicated. | |

**References**

1. Benson CD: Infantile hypertrophic pyloric stenosis. In *Pediatric Surgery*, 4th edition. Ravitch MM, et al, eds. Year Book Medical Publishers, Chicago: 1986, 811-15.
2. Eriksen CA, Anders CJ: Audit of results of operations for infantile pyloric stenosis in a district general hospital. *Arch Dis Child* 1991; 66(1):130-33.
3. Goh DW, Hall SK, Gornall P, Buick RG, Green A, Conkery JJ: Plasma chloride and alkalemia in pyloric stenosis. *Br J Surg* 1990; 77(8):922-23.
4. Bissonnette B, Sullivan PJ: Pyloric stenosis. *Can J Anaesth* 1991; 38(5):668-76.

# ESOPHAGEAL REPLACEMENT, COLON INTERPOSITION, WATERSTON PROCEDURE, GASTRIC TUBE PLACEMENT

## SURGICAL CONSIDERATIONS

**Description**: Esophageal replacement in children is usually performed for complicated caustic stricture or esophageal atresia (EA). Patients with failed repair of EA usually have a proximal esophagostomy and may have pulmonary dysfunction or other congenital anomalies. Caustic stricture of the esophagus occurs primarily in children 1-3 years old, and may require esophageal replacement after failed attempts at dilation. The ideal long-term esophageal substitute does not exist, but segments of colon or a tube fashioned from the greater curvature of the stomach are the most suitable. Pulling the stomach up into the bed of the esophagus is also an option. The **proximal anastomosis** is usually performed in the neck at the site of a previous esophagostomy or in the chest, well above the level of stricture. The interposed segment may be brought through the bed of the resected esophagus or transpleural behind the root of the lung. Substernal routes are not favored in children. Depending on the level of the anastomosis, the operation may be accomplished by thoracoabdominal, thoracic or abdominal, or thoracic, abdominal and cervical incisions. Consequently, the operation may be performed in a single position or may require position and drape changing.

**Usual preop diagnosis**: EA; caustic stricture

### SUMMARY OF PROCEDURE

| | |
|---|---|
| **Position** | Supine, tilted; or supine, then lateral |
| **Incision** | Thoracoabdominal ± cervical; or transverse abdominal, posterolateral thoracic |
| **Special instrumentation** | Bougie (upper esophagus) |
| **Antibiotics** | Preop: ampicillin 25 mg/kg iv + gentamicin 2.5 mg/kg iv; intraop: cephalosporin irrigation (1 gm/500 cc NS) |
| **Surgical time** | 3 - 5 hrs (4 - 6 hrs with position change) |
| **EBL** | 20-40 cc/kg |
| **Postop care** | PICU |
| **Mortality** | 5% |

| | |
|---|---|
| **Morbidity** | Respiratory failure<br>Anastomotic leak<br>Sepsis<br>Stricture |
| **Procedure code** | 43110, 43499 |
| **Pain score** | 7-8 |

### PATIENT POPULATION CHARACTERISTICS

| | |
|---|---|
| **Age range** | 1-5 yrs |
| **Male:Female** | 2:1 |
| **Incidence** | ~200/yr in U.S. |
| **Etiology** | Caustic ingestion; esophageal atresia |
| **Associated conditions** | Caustic stricture<br>Imperforate anus<br>VACTERL association |

## ANESTHETIC CONSIDERATIONS

### PREOPERATIVE

These patients usually are children presenting with a Hx of caustic substance ingestion and subsequent development of esophageal stricture. They have undergone multiple esophageal dilations under GA. Previous anesthesia records should be obtained. Preop, these patients are admitted for bowel prep and, consequently, may be hypovolemic.

| | |
|---|---|
| **Gastrointestinal** | Varying degrees of esophageal reflux may be present. Preop $H_2$-blocker administration is appropriate (e.g., ranitidine 0.8 mg/kg iv) the night before and morning of surgery. A gastrostomy may be present in some patients.<br>**Tests:** Review prior barium swallow studies and upper GI endoscopy reports; electrolytes |
| **Hematologic** | Anemia due to poor nutrition.<br>**Tests:** CBC; T&C |
| **Laboratory** | Other tests as indicated from H&P. (✓ parental/directed donor blood availability.) |
| **Premedication** | IV may already be in place and midazolam (0.05-0.1 mg/kg iv) can be administered in holding area. Alternatively, midazolam usually can be given po (0.5-0.75 mg/kg) 30 min before surgery. |

### INTRAOPERATIVE

**Anesthetic technique:** GETA, using a pediatric circle or Bain circuit with humidified and warmed gasses. Heating pad on OR table. Warm room to 78-80°F. An epidural catheter (for postop pain management) may be placed once child is anesthetized and airway is secured.

| | |
|---|---|
| **Induction** | IV induction preferred. If reflux concerns present, preoxygenate for 2-3 min and perform rapid-sequence induction with cricoid pressure (see Appendix). Children > 2 yrs of age do not require pretreatment with atropine. Intubate trachea with uncuffed ETT that has air leak at ~20 cm $H_2O$. Continue neuromuscular blockade with vecuronium or pancuronium (0.1 mg/kg iv). |
| **Maintenance** | Use air/$O_2$/isoflurane. Local anesthetic is not administered. Avoid $N_2O$ to minimize increase in size of possible pneumothorax during mediastinal dissection. Appropriate use of non-depolarizing muscle relaxant with train-of-four monitoring. Epidural catheter is used for opiate administration (preservative-free morphine 0.05-0.07 mg/kg). |
| **Emergence** | Plan for extubation in OR. |

| | | |
|---|---|---|
| **Blood and fluid requirements** | Blood loss mild to moderate<br>IV: 22 ga x 2<br>NS/LR @ ~10 cc/kg/hr | Replace 3rd-space losses with NS/LR (~10 cc/kg/hr). Replace blood loss cc for cc with albumin 5%. Transfuse to maintain Hct >22. |
| **Monitoring** | Standard monitors (see Appendix).<br>CVP 4 Fr double-lumen<br>± Arterial line (22-ga)<br>Foley catheter<br>Axillary stethoscope | CVP line used for postop TPN (maintain 1 lumen for that purpose); also enables blood draws.<br>Marked arterial waveform variation with ventilation is a sensitive indicator of hypovolemia. ABG/Hct prn. |

| | | |
|---|---|---|
| **Positioning** | Shoulder roll<br>✓ and pad pressure points.<br>✓ eyes. | Beware of tracheal extubation with head extension. Confirm ETT position with laryngoscopy. |
| **Complications** | Hypoventilation<br>Hypothermia<br>Pneumothorax<br>Dysrhythmias<br>Aspiration | Suprasternal dissection involves traction on trachea and recurrent laryngeal nerve. Mediastinal pullthrough may damage great vessels, and lead to pneumothorax, manipulation-induced dysrhythmias and impaired chest-wall compliance. |

**POSTOPERATIVE**

| | | |
|---|---|---|
| **Complications** | Subglottic edema<br>Hypoventilation<br>Pneumothorax<br>Recurrent laryngeal nerve injury<br>Mediastinitis | Inadequately treated pain → hypoventilation. |
| **Pain management** | Epidural morphine (0.03-0.05 mg/kg bolus q 8-16 hrs x 2-3 d)<br>Acetaminophen (10-20 mg/kg pr q 4 hrs prn)<br>Ketorolac (0.5-0.9 mg/kg iv up to 30 mg q 6 hrs x 2 d) | Ketorolac's opiate-sparing effect is of particular benefit, but no study comparing acetaminophen to ketorolac has been performed to date. |
| **Tests** | CXR; Hct | |

**References**

1. Anderson KD: *Esophageal Substitution in Pediatric Surgery*. Holder TM, Ashcraft KW, eds. WB Saunders Co, Philadelphia: 1980, 284-91.
2. Cywes S, et al. Corrosive strictures of the oesophagus in children. *Ped Surg Int* 1993; 8:8-13.
3. Schecter NL, Berde CB, Yaster M, eds: *Pain in Infants, Children, and Adolescents*, 1st edition. Williams and Wilkins, Baltimore: 1993, 357-83.

# HEPATIC PORTOENTEROSTOMY (KASAI PROCEDURE)

## SURGICAL CONSIDERATIONS

**Description**: Biliary atresia is a misnomer, since the pathology is that of an obliterative inflammation of the extrahepatic biliary tree. The obstruction develops postnatally and is progressive, eventually involving the intrahepatic biliary radicles and producing obstructive hepatopathy. Biliary atresia was uniformly fatal (mean survival 13 months) prior to the introduction of the **Kasai procedure (hepatic portoenterostomy)**. The success of this procedure is highly dependent upon operative technique and the age of the infant, with less than 10% achieving bile drainage if operated at 12 wks or more. The operation consists of an initial limited exploration with cholangiogram. If patency of the biliary tree is established, a liver biopsy is done and the procedure terminated. If biliary atresia is confirmed, the gallbladder and biliary tree remnants are excised with extensive dissection of the porta hepatis. The biliary tree is then reconstructed, usually employing a Roux-en-Y of jejunum anastomosed directly to the liver capsule at the porta. A variety of procedures have been described, based on the use of different areas of the GI tract (jejunum, appendix) as the biliary substitute, or based on the use or non-use of a cutaneous stoma or intussuscepted valve in the conduit. All successful procedures include extensive dissection of the extrahepatic biliary tree to the surface of the liver with portoenterostomy. If operating for choledochal cyst, the procedure is similar. **Hepatic transplantation** is indicated for patients with a poor response to portoenterostomy or delay in initial diagnosis (age >3 months).

**Usual preop diagnosis**: Biliary atresia; choledochal cyst; obstructive jaundice

### SUMMARY OF PROCEDURE

| | |
|---|---|
| **Position** | Supine |
| **Incision** | Upper transverse-chevron; right transverse for cholangiogram |
| **Special instrumentation** | Cholangiography equipment |
| **Unique considerations** | Cholangiogram, if gall bladder patent; increased glucose requirement (4-8 mg/kg/min) |
| **Antibiotics** | Preop: ampicillin 25 mg/kg iv + gentamicin 2.5 mg/kg iv; intraop: cephalosporin irrigation (1 gm/500 cc NS) |
| **Surgical time** | 4 - 6 hrs (1-2 hrs if cholangiography/Bx only) |
| **EBL** | 10-20 cc/kg (5-100 cc/kg for cholangiogram) |
| **Postop care** | PICU |
| **Mortality** | < 5% |
| **Morbidity** | Bile leak: 10-15%<br>Obstruction: 10%<br>Sepsis: 5-10%<br>Respiratory failure: 5% |
| **Procedure code** | 47701 (Kasai); 47700 (with cholangiogram) |
| **Pain score** | 7-8 (4-5 for cholangiogram) |

### PATIENT POPULATION CHARACTERISTICS

| | |
|---|---|
| **Age range** | 6-12 wks |
| **Male:Female** | >1:1 |
| **Incidence** | 1/15,000 births |
| **Etiology** | Viral, autoimmune |
| **Associated conditions** | **NB:** Asplenia syndrome: 5-10%<br>Polysplenia: 5-10% |

---

## ANESTHETIC CONSIDERATIONS

### PREOPERATIVE

Biliary atresia is a postnatal inflammatory disorder of the hepatobiliary tree involving the intrahepatic biliary radicles → obstructive jaundice. Progressive symptomatology in the first year of life necessitates exploratory laparotomy and cholangiography, with consequent hepatic portoenterostomy, should the diagnosis be biliary atresia. Infants presenting at 3-6 months of age with diagnosis of biliary atresia usually have undergone extensive workup to rule out viral hepatitis. These infants tend to have normal growth and development, unlike those with an infectious etiology for liver disease.

| | |
|---|---|
| **Gastrointestinal** | Hepatic function preserved initially (i.e., normal albumin synthesis). Cholestatic jaundice usually present. There may be impaired elimination of drugs, particularly non-depolarizing muscle relaxants. Glucose homeostasis is usually normal. |
| **Hematologic** | Anemia 2° hepatic disease. Impaired vitamin K absorption 2° lack of bile salts. Elevated PT will correct with vitamin K administration (phytonadione 1 mg im/iv). Have FFP available if PT not corrected after vitamin K.<br>**Tests:** PT; PTT; CBC; T&C |
| **Laboratory** | Electrolytes; BUN; creatinine; LFTs; albumin; bilirubin, direct and indirect glucose; others as indicated from H&P. Confirm availability of blood products (PRBCs, FFP). (✓ parental/directed donor blood availability.) |
| **Premedication** | None |

### INTRAOPERATIVE

**Anesthetic technique:** GETA, using a pediatric circle with warmed and humidified gasses. Warm OR to 75°-80°F; use warming pad on OR table. (Remember: majority of heat loss is radiant).

| | | |
|---|---|---|
| **Induction** | Mask induction is preferred. IV placed once child anesthetized. Pancuronium (0.1 mg/kg iv) to facilitate tracheal intubation, using an uncuffed 3.5-4.0 ETT (with leak at 20-30 cm $H_2O$). | |
| **Maintenance** | Isoflurane/air/$O_2$. No $N_2O$ to avoid bowel distension. Administer fentanyl (10-25 $\mu$g/kg iv total), with pancuronium continued to facilitate abdominal closure. | |
| **Emergence** | Patient remains intubated and is transported to ICU. For transport, ventilate with 100% $O_2$, have laryngoscope and additional ETT available. Assure adequate neuromuscular blockade to minimize patient movement and possibility of self-extubation. | |
| **Blood and fluid requirements** | Moderate blood loss<br>IV: 22 ga x 1-2 (in upper extremities)<br>NS/LR @ 10 cc/kg/hr<br>Albumin 5% | Potential for large 3rd-space losses. Plan 10 cc/kg/hr of NS/LR for replacement, and be prepared for sudden blood loss. Use albumin 5%, replacing cc for cc blood loss; transfuse to maintain Hct >22%. If dextrose infusion required, give 4-6 mg/kg/min. |
| **Monitoring** | Standard monitors (see Appendix).<br>Urinary catheter<br>NG tube<br>Arterial line (22-24 ga) | ABG, Hct, blood glucose q 60 min and prn. Maintain UO @ 1 cc/kg/hr. Arterial line helpful for lab draws. The presence of ↑↑BP variations with respiration is a useful indicator of hypovolemia. |
| **Positioning** | ✓ padding – heels, elbows, occiput.<br>✓ eyes. | |
| **Complications** | Hypothermia<br>Hypovolemia<br>Hypoventilation<br>Metabolic acidosis | In upper abdominal surgery, the retractors and abdominal packing may limit diaphragmatic excursion, thus requiring higher PIP to adequately ventilate the patient. ETT leak (PIP) > 20 cm $H_2O$ to insure adequate ventilation. |

## POSTOPERATIVE

| | | |
|---|---|---|
| **Complications** | Hypovolemia<br>Transfusion-associated disease<br>Atelectasis<br>Cholangitis | 3rd-space losses continue in the immediate postop period. Postop mechanical ventilation with TV 10-12 cc/kg and PEEP 3-5 cm $H_2O$ to minimize atelectasis. |
| **Pain management** | Fentanyl (1-2 mg/kg/iv q 1 hr prn)<br>MS (0.05-0.1 mg/kg iv q 2-4 hrs prn) | Regional anesthesia avoided because of concerns over perioperative coagulopathy. |
| **Tests** | Hct, ABG | |

### References


1. Engelskirchen R, Holschneider AM, Gharib M, Vente C: Biliary atresia – a 25-year survey. *Eur J Pediatr Surg* 1991; 1(3):154-60.
2. Karrer FM, Hall RJ, Stewart BA, Lilly JR: Congenital biliary tract disease. *Surg Clin North Am* 1990; 70(6):1403-18.
3. Kasai M, Suzuki H, Ohashi E, Ohi R, Chiba T, Okamoto A: Technique and results of operative management of biliary atresia. *World J Surg* 1978; 2(5):571-79.
4. Katz J, Steward DJ, eds: *Anesthesia and Uncommon Pediatric Diseases*, 2nd edition. WB Saunders Co, Philadelphia: 1993.

# RESECTION OF CYSTIC HYGROMA, BRANCHIAL CLEFT CYST, THYROGLOSSAL DUCT CYST, OR OTHER CERVICAL MASS

## SURGICAL CONSIDERATIONS

**Description:** Lesions requiring extensive dissection in the neck and parotid region that occur during the patient's childhood are generally due to malformations of the lymphatic system (cystic hygroma, lymphangioma), branchial cleft or thyroglossal duct remnants, or infection of the lymph nodes and salivary glands with atypical mycobacteria. Cystic hygromas are usually large lesions centered about the IJ vein. Careful, tedious dissection of the cervical vessels, brachial plexus and the facial, vagus, phrenic, spinal accessory and hypoglossal nerves is common. Extension into the mediastinum occurs in 10-15% of cervical hygromas and should be evaluated preop by x-ray. Branchial cleft anomalies usually require much less extensive dissection. Thyroglossal duct remnants are excised with the central portion of the hyoid bone. Atypical mycobacterial adenitis frequently involves the high jugulodigastric nodes and the submaxillary or parotid gland, with the facial nerve and its marginal mandibular branch being the most vulnerable structures. This midline lesion connects to the pharynx at the foramen cecum and resection must include this tract and the mid portion of the hyoid bone to prevent recurrence. Other lesions in this location are dermoid cysts or ectopic thyroid, which may represent all of the functioning thyroid tissue and, thus, should be preserved.

**Usual preop diagnosis:** Cystic hygroma; branchial cleft cyst/fistula; thyroglossal duct cyst; atypical mycobacterial adenitis

### SUMMARY OF PROCEDURE

| | Lateral Lesions/Hygroma/ Branchial Mycobacterial | Midline Lesions/ Thyroglossal Duct |
|---|---|---|
| **Position** | Neck extended, head rotated | Neck extended, head midline |
| **Incision** | Oblique | Transverse |
| **Special instrumentation** | Facial nerve monitor; nerve stimulator | None |
| **Unique considerations** | Nerve testing | None |
| **Antibiotics** | Preop: ampicillin 25 mg/kg iv + gentamicin 2.5 mg/kg iv; intraop: cephalosporin irrigation (1 gm/500 cc NS) | ⇐ |
| **Surgical time** | 2 - 6 hrs | 1 hr |
| **EBL** | 5-20 cc/kg | $<$ 5 cc/kg |
| **Postop care** | PICU; airway monitoring | None |
| **Mortality** | 2-5% | $<$ 1% |
| **Morbidity** | Airway compromise | ⇐ |
| | Fluid accumulation | ⇐ |
| | Infection | ⇐ |
| **Procedure code** | 38555 (excision cystic hygroma)<br>42410 (excision parotid tumor)<br>42815 (branchial cleft excision) | 60280 |
| **Pain score** | 3-4 | 3-4 |

### PATIENT POPULATION CHARACTERISTICS

| | |
|---|---|
| **Age range** | Newborn - school age |
| **Male:Female** | 1:1 |
| **Incidence** | Common |
| **Etiology** | Developmental anomaly<br>Mycobacteria |
| **Associated conditions** | Hygroma-mediastinal airway involvement<br>Branchial cleft: 10% (bilateral) |

## ANESTHETIC CONSIDERATIONS

### PREOPERATIVE

These patients generally are otherwise healthy children. A cystic hygroma (cystic lymphangioma), as with other neck masses, may cause airway obstruction and difficult intubation.

**Respiratory** — The size and extent of the neck mass should be defined carefully in an effort to detect the potential for airway compromise and to avoid soft-tissue trauma during intubation, with consequent acute airway obstruction. Inspiratory stridor suggests supraglottic obstruction, while expiratory stridor is associated with subglottic/intrathoracic obstruction. These patients should have had prior CT/MRI imaging; anesthesia records for these studies should be reviewed.
**Tests:** CXR ± CT/MRI scans

**Cardiovascular** — Cervical masses may be adherent to and/or cause compression of the great vessels.
**Tests:** CT/MRI scans

**Hematologic** — T&C for cystic hygroma, or if a cervical mass involves great vessels or extends into the mediastinum (~3%).
**Tests:** Hct

**Laboratory** — Other tests as indicated from H&P.

**Premedication** — If 1-10 yrs old and asymptomatic, midazolam (0.5-0.75 mg po) 30 min prior to arrival in OR. Avoid all premedication in patients with potential airway compromise.

### INTRAOPERATIVE

**Anesthetic technique:** GETA with pediatric circle, and warm, humidified gasses. OR temperature 75-80°; warming pad on OR table.

**Induction** — Standard pediatric induction (see Appendix) in patients without airway compromise. IV should be secured prior to induction when airway obstruction is present. Mask induction with halothane in 100% $O_2$. As plane of anesthesia deepens, gently assist ventilation. (Keep PIP < 20 cm $H_2O$). Give atropine (0.02 mg/kg iv) prior to laryngoscopy. If partial airway obstruction exists, maintain spontaneous ventilation and perform laryngoscopy at ~3 MAC of volatile agent. FOB should be available. Have full range of ETT sizes available, since airway narrowing may be present. Once airway is secured, proceed with neuromuscular blockade (vecuronium 0.1 mg/kg iv or atracurium 0.4 mg/kg iv).

**Maintenance** — Standard pediatric maintenance (see Appendix). Surgeon may infiltrate incision with local anesthetic. Limit bupivacaine to 2.5 mg/kg.

**Emergence** — Reverse neuromuscular blockade with neostigmine (0.07 mg/kg iv) and atropine (0.02 mg/kg iv). Extubate when fully awake.

| | | |
|---|---|---|
| **Blood and fluid requirements** | Minimal blood loss<br>IV: 20-22 ga x 1<br>Great vessel involvement: IV: 20 ga x 2<br>NS/LR @ 3 cc/kg/hr | Minimal 3rd-space losses. Each cc blood loss can be replaced with 3 cc NS/LR. When great vessels involved, place at least one iv in lower extremity. Blood loss can be quite sudden; have blood available in OR. |
| **Monitoring** | Standard monitors (see Appendix).<br>± Arterial line - 22 ga | An arterial line is used when there is risk of large blood loss or perioperative airway compromise. |
| **Positioning** | ✓ and pad pressure points.<br>✓ eyes. | |
| **Complications** | ETT dislodged/loss of airway<br>Laryngospasm<br>Bronchospasm<br>Hemorrhage | ETT must be carefully secured. Liberal use of benzoin.<br>Avoid tension on ETT by circuit hoses.<br>Hold ETT during surgeon's intraoral examination. |

### POSTOPERATIVE

| | | |
|---|---|---|
| **Complications** | Subglottic edema<br>Upper airway obstruction from edema related to tumor resection<br>Recurrent laryngeal nerve injury | Dexamethasone (0.5-1 mg/kg iv) and nebulized racemic epinephrine (1.25%) with mist $O_2$ to treat subglottic edema. |

| | | |
|---|---|---|
| **Pain management** | Morphine (0.05-0.1 mg/kg iv q 2-4 hrs)<br>Acetaminophen (10-15 mg/kg po/pr q 4 hrs) | The majority of these procedures are performed on outpatient basis (except cystic hygroma). |
| **Tests** | None | |

**References**

1. Filston, HC: Head and Neck-sinuses and Masses. In *Pediatric Surgery*, Holder TM, Ashcraft KW, eds. WB Saunders Co, Philadelphia: 1980, 1062-79.
2. Ravitch MM, Rush BF Jr: Cystic Hygroma. In *Pediatric Surgery*, 4th edition. Ravitch MM, et al, eds. Year Book Medical Publishers, Chicago: 1986, 533-39.
3. Soper RT, Pringle KC: Cysts and Sinuses of the Neck. In *Pediatric Surgery*, 4th edition. Ravitch MM, et al, eds. Year Book Medical Publishers, Chicago: 1986, 539-52.
4. Gregory GA (ed): *Pediatric Anesthesia*, 2nd ed. Churchill Livingstone, New York: 1989.
5. Motoyama EK, Davis PC, eds: *Smith's Anesthesia for Infants and Children*, 5th ed. CV Mosby, St. Louis: 1990.

# REPAIR OF OMPHALOCELE/GASTROSCHISIS

## SURGICAL CONSIDERATIONS

**Description**: The goals of treatment for the abdominal wall defects (gastroschisis/omphalocele) are the safe return of the herniated viscera to the abdominal cavity and closure of the abdominal wall muscles and skin. Gastroschisis, with no covering membrane and few associated anomalies, generally requires urgent operative treatment. Omphalocele, with an intact membrane, may be managed non-operatively if associated anomalies require more urgent diagnosis or treatment. While primary closure is ideal, many patients have inadequate abdominal domain, which produces unacceptable respiratory or cardiovascular compromise if primary repair is attempted. Elevation of skin flaps and removal of umbilical cord may require extending the incision in the midline. In omphalocele, the membrane is left intact if possible and the wound closed or Silastic® sheeting attached. In gastroschisis, the defect is usually extended and a gastrostomy is placed. If reduction of the viscera is not possible, or if it produces unacceptable respiration or cardiovascular compromise, then a **staged procedure** is performed. This consists of suturing Silastic® sheeting to the full-thickness abdominal wall, creating a silo or pouch to contain the abdominal viscera. This pouch is reduced in size day-by-day until the viscera are returned to the abdominal cavity. The reductions may be done in the nursery or the OR and usually will allow definite closure of the abdominal wall in 7-10 d. Omphalocele, under unusual circumstances, can be treated by skin coverage only or by topical application of iodine or mercurochrome to the membrane.

**Usual preop diagnosis**: Omphalocele; gastroschisis; pentalogy of Cantrell; exstrophy cloaca

### SUMMARY OF PROCEDURE

| | |
|---|---|
| **Position** | Supine |
| **Incision** | Midline |
| **Special instrumentation** | None; for staged repair, nylon-reinforced Silastic® sheeting |
| **Antibiotics** | Preop: ampicillin 25 mg/kg iv + gentamicin 2.5 mg/kg iv; intraop: cephalosporin irrigation (1 gm/500 cc NS) |
| **Surgical time** | 2 hrs |
| **Closing considerations** | Assess respiratory and cardiovascular function after muscle closure by PIP, ABG, MAP. Impaired ventilation and venous return will result from over-aggressive attempts at closure. |
| **EBL** | 5-10 cc/kg |

| | |
|---|---|
| **Postop care** | Assisted ventilation; volume support (gastroschisis) |
| **Mortality** | Omphalocele: 28%<br>Gastroschisis: 15-23% |
| **Morbidity** | Respiratory failure<br>Intestinal ischemia/obstruction<br>Infection |
| **Procedure code** | 49600-05(primary); 49611 (staged repair) |
| **Pain score** | 5-6 (primary); 4-5 (staged repair) |

### PATIENT POPULATION CHARACTERISTICS

| | |
|---|---|
| **Age range** | Newborn |
| **Male:Female** | 1:1 |
| **Incidence** | 1/3000 - 1/10,000 live births |
| **Etiology** | Unknown |
| **Associated conditions** | Gastroschisis - malrotation, intestinal atresia<br>Omphalocele - cardiac, renal anomalies<br>Trisomy 13, 18<br>Beckwith-Wiedemann syndrome (hypoglycemia, macroglossia)<br>Pentalogy of Cantrell - omphalocele, sternal, diaphragmatic, pericardial, cardiac anomalies<br>Exstrophy cloaca - omphalocele, exstrophy bladder, imperforate anus |

---

## ANESTHETIC CONSIDERATIONS

### PREOPERATIVE

Newborns with omphalocele/gastroschisis present for urgent surgery. The large exposed surface area of abdominal contents allows substantial evaporative heat and fluid losses. Omphalocele is associated with other congenital anomalies (e.g., VSD, Beckwith-Wiedemann syndrome [infantile gigantism, macroglossia]). The majority of these patients should be medically stabilized in the nursery prior to coming to the OR.

| | |
|---|---|
| **Respiratory** | If premature (< 36 wks gestational age), is at increased risk for RDS. Respiratory insufficiency may be present.<br>**Tests:** CXR; ABG |
| **Cardiovascular** | With omphalocele, there is a 20% incidence of cardiac anomalies (VSD, PDA). Presence of murmur.<br>**Tests:** ECHO, if indicated |
| **Gastrointestinal** | Intestinal atresia may be present. Hypovolemia from evaporative loss also may be present. Use full-stomach precautions. ✓ administration of antibiotics to prevent peritonitis. |
| **Endocrine** | Beckwith-Wiedemann associated with hypoglycemia (term infant glucose – normal >36 mg/dL).<br>**Tests:** Glucose; electrolytes |
| **Laboratory** | CBC; T&C; PT; PTT; UA |

### INTRAOPERATIVE

**Anesthetic technique:** GETA, using a pediatric circle or Bain circuit with humidified and warmed gasses. Maintain body temperature close to 37°C. Warm room to 78-80°F. (Remember majority of heat loss is radiant.)

**Induction** Atropine (0.02 mg/kg iv, minimum dose 0.1 mg) is given before induction to ablate vagal response to laryngoscopy. Pass an OG tube to decompress stomach. Assure adequate intravascular volume status (capillary refill < 2 sec; warm, pink extremities). Preoxygenate with 100% $O_2$ for 2-3 min. Consider awake intubation if hypovolemic; otherwise, apply cricoid pressure. STP (4-6 mg/kg iv) and succinylcholine (1-2 mg/kg iv) administered to facilitate tracheal intubation. 3.5 ETT is most appropriate for this age group. Once airway is secured, administer vecuronium or pancuronium (0.1 mg/kg iv). Keep air leak around ETT at approximately 30-40 cm $H_2O$. Lower pressure air leak may make ventilation difficult if primary closure of abdomen is accompanied by significant rise in intra-abdominal pressure.

| | | |
|---|---|---|
| **Maintenance** | Avoid high $FiO_2$. Use air/$O_2$ mixture for ventilation to maintain $O_2$ sat 95-100% and $PaO_2 < 100$. Primarily narcotic-based technique with fentanyl (10-25 μg/kg iv total), low-dose isoflurane as needed. Note initial PIP prior to abdominal closure. Maintain neuromuscular blockade with vecuronium or pancuronium to facilitate abdominal closure. | |
| **Emergence** | Remain intubated postop. Transport to ICN on 100% $O_2$ to increase margin of safety in case of accidental extubation. | |
| **Blood and fluid requirements** | Marked 3rd-space fluid loss<br>Minimal-moderate blood loss<br>IV: 22-24 ga x 1-2, upper extremities | Continue dextrose-containing solution from ICN (4-6 mg/kg/min). Replace 3rd-space losses (10-15+ cc/kg/hr). Replace blood loss with albumin 5% and/or blood cc for cc. Maintain Hct >35%. All lines in upper extremities. Lower extremities usually edematous due to abdominal venous and lymphatic compression. |
| **Monitoring** | Standard monitors (see Appendix).<br>Arterial line (24-ga radial)<br>± CVP – 3 Fr subclavian or 4 Fr IJ<br>Urinary catheter | ABG pre- and post-abdominal closure. Hct, glucose, electrolytes q 60 min. CVP – maintain 1 lumen sterile, if possible, for postop TPN. Respiratory variation on arterial waveform is sensitive indicator of hypovolemia. |
| **Positioning** | Arms positioned to have ready access to arterial line.<br>✓ and pad pressure points.<br>✓ eyes. | |
| **Complications** | Hypothermia<br>Hypovolemia<br>Respiratory insufficiency/hypoventilation<br>Atelectasis<br>Volume overload/pulmonary edema | Some institutions monitor intra-abdominal pressure. If intragastric pressure is >20 mmHg and CVP increases by 4 mmHg with initial primary closure, it should be converted to a staged repair. Raised abdominal pressure will cause an acute restrictive ventilatory defect and promote abdominal visceral ischemia. |

**POSTOPERATIVE**

| | | |
|---|---|---|
| **Complications** | Respiratory failure<br>Bowel ischemia/necrosis<br>Renal failure<br>Peritonitis<br>Sepsis/metabolic acidosis<br>Pneumothorax<br>RDS<br>Hypothermia | Abdominal 3rd spacing will persist in immediate postop period → ↑intra-abdominal pressure → bowel ischemia + ↓renal perfusion. Persistent metabolic and/or respiratory acidosis mandates staged repair. |
| **Pain management** | Fentanyl (1-3 μg/kg/hr) continuous infusion if delayed closure<br>Fentanyl (1-2 μg/kg iv q 30 min prn) | |
| **Tests** | ABG; Hct; glucose; electrolytes, $Ca^{++}$<br>UO maintained at >0.5 cc/kg/hr | |

**References**


1. Sauter ER, Falterman KW, Arensman RM: Is primary repair of gastroschisis and omphalocele always the best operation? *Am Surg* 1991; 57(3):142-44.
2. Schier F, Schier C, Stute MP, Wurtenberger H: 193 cases of gastroschisis and omphalocele – postoperative results. *Zentralbl Chir* 1988; 113(4):225-34.
3. Schuster S: Omphalocele and gastroschisis. In *Pediatric Surgery*, 4th edition. Ravitch MM, et al, eds. Year Book Medical Publishing, Chicago: 1986, 740-63.
4. Yaster M, et al: Hemodynamic effects of primary closure of omphalocele/gastroschisis in human newborns. *Anesthesiology* 1988; 69:84-8.
5. Gregory GA, ed: *Pediatric Anesthesia*, 2nd edition. Churchill Livingstone, New York: 1989.
6. Motoyama EK, Davis PC, eds: *Smith's Anesthesia for Infants and Children*, 5th edition. CV Mosby, St. Louis: 1990.

# HERNIA REPAIR

## SURGICAL CONSIDERATIONS

**Description:** Repair of inguinal hernia is the most common operation performed in children. Inguinal hernias in children are almost always indirect type due to failure of the processus vaginalis to obliterate. They are more common and more likely to incarcerate in premature infants. Bilateral hernias are common at < 2 years of age. Hydroceles are identical to inguinal hernia in origin and treatment. Complications of hernia repair are uncommon and are most commonly related to the effects of GA on an immature CNS and respiratory system. Umbilical hernias are more common in Blacks and will usually undergo spontaneous closure if given enough time; 75-80% will close by 2 years of age and 95-98% by 5 years. Inguinal hernia repair is performed via an inguinal skin crease incision. The sac is separated from the spermatic cord structures, dissected to the level of the internal ring, and ligated. The distal sac and floor of the inguinal canal are not disturbed. Bilateral procedures are usually done in children < 2 years of age. Umbilical repair is performed through a transverse incision with excision of the sac after detaching it from the undersurface of the skin. The fascia is repaired transversely and little, if any, intraperitoneal exploration done.

**Usual preop diagnosis**: Inguinal hernia; hydrocele; umbilical hernia

### SUMMARY OF PROCEDURE

| | Inguinal | Umbilical |
|---|---|---|
| **Position** | Supine | ⇐ |
| **Incision** | Inguinal, bilateral | Infraumbilical |
| **Unique considerations** | Prematurity | Abdominal compression if hernia large |
| **Antibiotics** | Intraop: cefazolin irrigation 1 gm/500 cc NS | None |
| **Surgical time** | 1 hr | ⇐ |
| **Closing considerations** | Nerve block, caudal | None |
| **EBL** | 5 cc/kg | ⇐ |
| **Postop care** | Apnea monitor; hospitalization for prematures | None |
| **Mortality** | < 1% | ⇐ |
| **Morbidity** | Apnea<br>Recurrence | None |
| **Procedure code** | 49500 | 49580 |
| **Pain score** | 3-5 | 3-5 |

### PATIENT POPULATION CHARACTERISTICS

| | | |
|---|---|---|
| **Age range** | Premature - adolescent | > 2 yrs |
| **Male:Female** | 5:1 | N/A |
| **Incidence** | 1-2% | 1% |
| **Etiology** | Patent processes vaginalis | Persistent umbilical defect |
| **Associated conditions** | Gonadal dysgenesis | None |

## ANESTHETIC CONSIDERATIONS

### PREOPERATIVE

Hernia repair is most commonly performed in otherwise healthy infants in the first two years of life, often on an outpatient basis. It is also performed on premature infants (< 36 weeks gestational age at birth) and other neonates requiring intensive care. Premature infants are particularly prone to inguinal hernias. Postop apnea can occur in infants of 50-60 weeks gestational age, particularly if the infant was premature, has neurologic disease and/or Sx, or required intensive care in the early neonatal period.

**Respiratory** Bronchopulmonary dysplasia (BPD), tracheomalacia and subglottic stenosis are consequences of prolonged mechanical ventilation and immature lungs at birth. ✓ prior ICN Hx. ↓FRC and ↑PVR makes infants with this disease more susceptible to hypoxia. They may require supplemental nasal $O_2$ on a chronic basis.
**Tests:** CXR

**Cardiovascular** Prior PDA ligation is possible. These patients may be on diuretic therapy for intrinsic lung disease (e.g., BPD) with resultant decreased intravascular volume.
**Tests:** CXR; electrolytes

**Neurological** Premature infants may be prone to seizure disorders. Premature infants have immature respiratory centers and may exhibit paradoxical apneic/bradycardic episodes in response to hypoxemia.
**Tests:** Anticonvulsant levels

**Hematologic** Anemia is common at ~3 mos of age and increases risk of postop apnea.
**Tests:** Hct; PT; PTT; platelets, as indicated from H&P.

**Laboratory** Other tests as indicated from H&P.

**Premedication** If >1 yr of age, midazolam (0.5-0.75 mg po) 30 min prior to arrival in OR.

## INTRAOPERATIVE

**Anesthetic technique:** Typically, GETA or mask GA (± caudal block), using a pediatric circle or Bain circuit with warm, humidified gasses. Warm OR to 75°-80°F; use warming pad on OR table.

**Induction** Mask induction with halothane/$N_2O/O_2$. Secure iv. If appropriate, position child for placement of caudal anesthetic: bupivacaine 0.25% with epinephrine 1:200,000 @ 1 cc/kg. If child otherwise healthy and >1 yr old, may proceed with mask anesthetic; otherwise, tracheal intubation with uncuffed ETT is preferred (air leak should = 20-30 cm $H_2O$). Atropine (0.02 mg/kg iv) given prior to laryngoscopy. Intubation facilitated with vecuronium (0.1 mg/kg) or atracurium (0.4 mg/kg iv).

**Maintenance** Standard pediatric maintenance (see Appendix) is appropriate. With caudal anesthetic, decrease amount of volatile anesthetic and avoid opiates. 2 MAC of inhalational agents at incision is required to avoid laryngospasm in this patient population. Caudal bupivacaine onset time ~15 min.

**Emergence** Reverse neuromuscular blockade with neostigmine (0.07 mg/kg iv) and atropine (0.02 mg/kg iv). Extubate only when fully awake.

| | | |
|---|---|---|
| **Blood and fluid requirements** | Negligible blood loss<br>IV: 22 ga x 1<br>NS/LR @ (maintenance):<br>4 cc/kg/hr – 0-10 kg<br>+ 2 cc/kg/hr – 11-20 kg | Infants receiving diuretics will require 10-20 cc/kg iv of NS/LR to avoid hypotension 2° volatile anesthetics. In children < 1 mo old, use dextrose-containing iv solution. |
| **Monitoring** | Standard monitors (see Appendix). | Premature infants may become hypoglycemic. ✓ blood glucose during surgery. |
| **Positioning** | ✓ and pad pressure points.<br>✓ eyes. | With too-large mask, beware ocular compression/corneal abrasion. |
| **Complications** | Laryngospasm | |
| | Bronchospasm | Rx bronchospasm: albuterol inhaler. Mist $O_2$ after extubation. |
| | Hypothermia | |
| | Pulmonary hypertensive episode | |
| | Local anesthetic toxicity | |
| | Hypoglycemia | Avoid hyperglycemia → diuresis and dehydration. |

## POSTOPERATIVE

| | | |
|---|---|---|
| **Complications** | Apnea/bradycardia<br>Subglottic edema | Can lessen incidence of apnea/bradycardia by administering caffeine (10 mg/kg iv) intraop or in PACU. |
| **Pain management** | Field block<br>Acetaminophen (10-20 mg po q 4-6 hrs prn) | If no caudal used, a field block (bupivacaine 0.25% 2-3 cc) at end of surgery reduces pain in the immediate postop period. It is usually performed by the surgeon. |

| | | |
|---|---|---|
| **Tests/monitoring** | Apnea monitor and pulse oximeter for 12-18 hrs for premature infants < 60 wks gestational age | Caffeine is no substitute for monitoring and attentive parents/nurses. |

**References**

1. Grosfeld JL: Current concepts in inguinal hernia in infants and children. *World J Surg* 1989; 13(5):506-15.
2. Kurth CD, Spitzer AR, Broennle AM, Downes JJ: Postoperative apnea in preterm infants. *Anesthesiology* 1987; 66(4):483-88.
3. Welborn LG, Hannallah RS, Fink R, Ruttimann VE, Hick JM: High-dose caffeine suppresses postoperative apnea in former preterm infants. *Anesthesiology* 1989; 71(3):347-49.
4. Stehling L, ed. *Common Problems in Pediatric Anesthesia*, 2nd edition. Mosby Year Book, St. Louis: 1992, 69-85.
5. Beckerman RC, Brouillette RT, Hunt CE, eds: *Respiratory Control Disorders in Infants and Children*, 1st edition. Williams and Wilkins, Baltimore: 1991, 161-77.

# ORCHIOPEXY, CIRCUMCISION, HYPOSPADIAS REPAIR

## SURGICAL CONSIDERATIONS

**Description:** Operations to repair undescended testis or hypospadias are among the most common procedures performed in childhood. Most of these procedures are performed on an outpatient basis and the anesthetic considerations are similar. The majority of patients are young (< 2 years) and in good health.

**Orchiopexy**, a procedure to correct undescended testis, is now being recommended at earlier ages. The operative approach is identical to that of inguinal hernia (which frequently accompanies the undescended testis), with the addition of a scrotal incision. Occasionally, **intraperitoneal dissection** or **laparoscopy** are part of the exploration. On rare occasions, inadequate length of spermatic vessels requires **microvascular anastomosis** to the inferior epigastric vessels. Complicated orchiopexy generally requires postop hospitalization for closer observation of associated ileus.

**Circumcision** is performed upon parental request and can be done with metal (Gomco®) or disposable (Plastibel®) devices. Alternatively, resection of the prepuce with scissors and suturing of the two skin layers is termed "free-hand" circumcision.

**Hypospadias repair** consists of releasing the fibrous tissue to produce curvature of the shaft (chordee) and advancement of the abnormal meatus to a position on the tip of the glans. Since most hypospadic meati are distal (glans or coronal), the advancement is usually straightforward, with use of available tissue, such as prepuce or the glans tissue. More proximal lesions require more extensive tissue replacement, which may include bladder mucosa or full-thickness skin as a free graft.

**Variant procedure or approaches**: The number of reported variations in repair of hypospadias is extremely large. The magnitude of the procedure is best assessed by the distance the meatus needs to be advanced and the techniques favored by the surgeon.

**Usual preop diagnosis**: Undescended testis; hypospadias

### SUMMARY OF PROCEDURE

| | Orchiopexy | Hypospadias | Circumcision |
|---|---|---|---|
| **Position** | Supine/frog leg | Supine | ⇐ |
| **Incision** | Inguinal skin crease; scrotal | Shaft | Preputial |
| **Special instrumentation** | Possible laparoscopy or microvascular equipment | Urethral sounds; cystourethroscopy | None |
| **Unique considerations** | Prematurity | None | ⇐ |

| | Orchiopexy | Hypospadias | Circumcision |
|---|---|---|---|
| **Antibiotics** | Preop: ampicillin 25 mg/kg iv + gentamicin 2.5 mg/kg iv; intraop: cephalosporin irrigation (1 gm/500 cc NS) | ⇐ | None |
| **Surgical time** | 1 - 2 hrs | 2 - 3 hrs | 30 min |
| **Closing considerations** | None | Dressing application | None |
| **EBL** | 5-10 cc/kg | ⇐ | < 5 cc/kg |
| **Postop care** | Possible apnea monitoring in prematures | Analgesia | Apnea monitor, if premature |
| **Mortality** | < 1% | ⇐ | ⇐ |
| **Morbidity** | Apnea<br>Recurrence<br>Urinary retention | Fistula: 10%<br>Stenosis: 5% | Infection<br>Bleeding |
| **Procedure code** | 54640 | 54300 | 54152 |
| **Pain score** | 3-5 | 5-6 | 2-3 |

### PATIENT POPULATION CHARACTERISTICS

| | | | |
|---|---|---|---|
| **Age range** | Premature - several yrs | 6 mo - several yrs | ⇐ |
| **Incidence** | Hernia: 1-4%<br>Undescended testis: 0.8% | 0.8% | Common |
| **Etiology** | Patent processus vaginalis | Unknown | N/A |
| **Associated conditions** | Undescended testis, renal anomalies: 9%<br>Hernia, gonadal dysgenesis: 2% | Undescended testis: 10% | N/A |

---

## ANESTHETIC CONSIDERATIONS

### PREOPERATIVE

Orchiopexy, circumcision and hypospadias repair are most commonly performed in the first 2 years of life in otherwise healthy children. Vaginoscopy and cystoscopy, however, may be done on any age group, usually prepubertal. Occasionally, there may be concerns of sexual abuse.

**Renal** — With phimosis, there may be Hx of UTIs. Possible pyelonephritis. Hematuria requires GU workup.
**Tests:** UA; renal function (BUN, creatinine), as clinically indicated.

**Laboratory** — Hct; others as indicated from H&P.

**Premedication** — If >1 yr of age, consider midazolam (0.5-0.75 mg/kg po) or diazepam (0.1-0.2 mg/kg po up to 10 mg) induction. If >10 yrs old: standard premedication (see Appendix).

### INTRAOPERATIVE

**Anesthetic technique:** GETA or mask anesthetic, using a pediatric circle or Bain circuit with humidified and warmed gasses. A combined technique with caudal anesthesia or regional nerve block is often used for non-endoscopic procedures. For small children, warm OR to 70-75°F. Use warming pad on OR table.

**Induction** — In younger patients, mask induction is customary before iv placement. Mask GA is preferred for circumcision to minimize coughing/bucking at end of case, thereby decreasing bleeding. If the surgical procedure will be >30 min, tracheal intubation is preferred. Vecuronium (0.08 mg/kg iv) or atracurium (0.4 mg/kg iv) is administered to facilitate tracheal intubation. If appropriate, caudal anesthesia can be obtained using bupivacaine 0.25% with epinephrine 1:200,000; for circumcision and hypospadias repair, 0.5 cc/kg; for orchiopexy, 0.75 cc/kg.

| | | |
|---|---|---|
| **Maintenance** | Standard pediatric maintenance (see Appendix). At least 2 MAC analgesia is required prior to skin incision to prevent laryngospasm. Caudal anesthesia can be used to provide the majority of analgesia in non-endoscopic procedures. | |
| **Emergence** | If neuromuscular blockade is used, reverse with neostigmine (0.07 mg/kg iv) and atropine (0.02 mg/kg iv). Extubate when patient is fully awake. | |
| **Blood and fluid requirements** | Negligible blood loss<br>IV: 20-22 ga x 1<br>NS/LR @ maintenance | Pediatric maintenance:<br>4 cc/kg/hr – 0-10 kg<br>+ 2 cc/kg/hr – 11-20 kg<br>+ 1 cc/kg/hr – >20 kg |
| **Monitoring** | Standard monitors (see Appendix). | |
| **Positioning** | ✓ and pad pressure points.<br>✓ eyes. | Ocular compression/corneal abrasion may occur with oversize mask. |
| **Complications** | Laryngospasm | Rx: 100% $O_2$, jaw thrust, positive pressure. If necessary, administer succinylcholine (1-2 mg/kg iv). |
| | Intravascular local anesthetic administration | Epinephrine in caudal anesthetic (to detect intravascular administration) does not significantly prolong analgesia. |

### POSTOPERATIVE

| | | |
|---|---|---|
| **Complications** | Bleeding | |
| **Pain management** | Caudal or regional block<br>Acetaminophen (10-20 mg po/pr q 6 hrs prn) | Optimal analgesia and presence of parents in PAR will minimize child's agitation/movement/crying. |

**References**


1. Belman AB: Hypospadias. In *Pediatric Surgery*, 4th edition. Ravitch MM, et al, eds. Year Book Medical Publishers, Chicago: 1986, 1286-1302.
2. Duckett JW, Snyder HM: Meatal advancement and glanuloplasty hypospadias repair after 1,000 cases: avoidance of meatal stenosis and regression. *J of Urol* 1992; 147(3):665-69.
3. Ellis GF, Patil U: Urologists' perspectives of single-stage hypospadias repair in the 1980s. Experience of 100 patients. *Urology* 1989; 34(5):262-64.
4. Fonkalsrud EW: Undescended Testes. In *Pediatric Surgery*, 4th edition. Ravitch MM, et al, eds. Year Book Medical Publishers, Chicago: 1986, 793-807.
5. Gregory GA, ed: *Pediatric Anesthesia*, 2nd edition. Churchill Livingstone, New York: 1989.
6. Motoyama EK, Davis PC, eds: *Smith's Anesthesia for Infants and Children*, 5th edition. CV Mosby, St. Louis: 1990.


# ESOPHAGOSCOPY, FOREIGN BODY REMOVAL, ESOPHAGEAL DILATION

## SURGICAL CONSIDERATIONS

**Description**: Flexible, diagnostic **esophagogastroduodenoscopy**, a common procedure in pediatrics, is usually performed under heavy sedation in an endoscopy suite or special procedure area. **Rigid esophagoscopy** is usually performed for therapeutic indications, such as removal of a foreign body, dilation of an esophageal stricture or injection of varices. The procedure is similar for each diagnosis and generally is performed with ET intubation. Foreign body removal is normally a very short procedure, while dilation and variceal injection can be prolonged and may require multiple insertions/removals of the endoscope. Compression of the trachea, distal to the ETT by the rigid esophagoscope, is not an uncommon occurrence.

**Usual preop diagnosis**: Esophageal foreign body; stricture; esophageal varices

### SUMMARY OF PROCEDURE

| | |
|---|---|
| **Position** | Supine |
| **Special instrumentation** | Rigid esophagoscopes; forceps; dilators |
| **Unique considerations** | Esophagoscope may obstruct airway; dilation may perforate esophagus. |
| **Surgical time** | 5 min - 2 hrs |
| **Closing considerations** | Abrupt ending |
| **EBL** | < 5 cc/kg |
| **Postop care** | Airway support |
| **Mortality** | < 5% |
| **Morbidity** | Esophageal perforation: 2-5% |
| **Procedure code** | 43200 |
| **Pain score** | 2-3 |

### PATIENT POPULATION CHARACTERISTICS

| | |
|---|---|
| **Age range** | Newborn - school age |
| **Male:Female** | 1:1 |
| **Incidence** | 1/1000 |
| **Etiology** | Varices - portal HTN<br>Foreign body - possible stricture |
| **Associated conditions** | Esophageal atresia - stricture<br>Portal HTN - varices |

## ANESTHETIC CONSIDERATIONS

### PREOPERATIVE

Esophagoscopy for foreign body removal is usually performed in healthy infants and children, although esophageal lodging of a foreign body can occur in any age group. All of these patients should be treated with full-stomach precautions. Esophageal dilation usually performed in 2 distinct patient populations: (1) those with prior tracheoesophageal fistula (TEF) repair, and (2) those with prior ingestion of a caustic substance.

| | |
|---|---|
| **Respiratory** | Patients with prior caustic ingestion may have Hx of pulmonary aspiration, with resultant chemical pneumonitis and/or fibrosis. Prolonged intubation after TEF repair may → subglottic stenosis. √any recent anesthesia records for ETT size required.<br>**Tests:** CXR, if clinically indicated. |
| **Cardiovascular** | There may be persistent congenital cardiac anomalies in the TEF patient.<br>**Tests:** Cardiology consultation, as needed. |
| **Laboratory** | No routine lab analyses are required if patient has no underlying chronic illnesses. |
| **Premedication** | For esophageal dilation, patient preference is extremely important since some patients have undergone this procedure several times. For foreign body removal, iv access may be necessary before induction. No premedication if < 1 yr old. |

### INTRAOPERATIVE

**Anesthetic technique:** GETA, using a pediatric circle or Bain circuit. Room temperature can be maintained at 65-70°F, as long as patient is covered.

| | |
|---|---|
| **Induction** | A rapid-sequence induction is usually appropriate for this patient population, unless patient is presenting for dilation alone and has no evidence to suggest reflux. Atropine (0.02 mg/kg iv) administered to attenuate bradycardia from succinylcholine. Preoxygenate for 2-3 min. Apply cricoid pressure. STP (4-6 mg/kg iv), followed by succinylcholine (1-2 mg/kg iv). Confirm absence of train-of-four prior to laryngoscopy. Intubate trachea with age-appropriate ETT ([16 + age] ÷ 4). Once airway is secured, administer atracurium (0.04 mg/kg iv) or vecuronium (0.1 mg/kg iv). |

| | | |
|---|---|---|
| **Maintenance** | Maintain anesthesia with volatile agent/$N_2O/O_2$. No need for opiates since there is negligible post-procedural pain. Maintain neuromuscular blockade. Movement must be avoided, particularly with rigid esophagoscopy. | |
| **Emergence** | Extubate when fully awake. Neostigmine (0.07 mg/kg iv) and atropine (0.02 mg/kg iv) to reverse neuromuscular blockade. Do not attempt reversal of neuromuscular blockade until first twitch of train-of-four has returned. | |
| **Blood and fluid requirements** | IV: 20-22 ga x 1<br>NS/LR @ 4-6 cc/kg/hr | |
| **Monitoring** | Standard monitors (see Appendix).<br>Peripheral nerve stimulator | |
| **Positioning** | ✓ and pad pressure points.<br>✓ eyes.<br>✓ radial pulse of dependent arm. | Axillary roll as needed; avoid brachial plexus compression. |
| **Complications** | Pneumothorax<br>Aspiration<br>Accidental extubation<br>Stridor 2° subglottic edema | Esophageal perforation, more common with rigid esophagoscopy, will lead to pneumothorax (right > left). |

### POSTOPERATIVE

| | | |
|---|---|---|
| **Complications** | Residual neuromuscular blockade<br>Pneumothorax | |
| **Pain management** | Negligible postop pain | If patient reports marked substernal discomfort, suspect esophageal perforation. |
| **Tests** | None | |

**References**

1. Gans SL, ed: Esophagoscopy. In *Pediatric Endoscopy*. Grune and Stratton, New York: 1983, 55-66.
2. Johnson DG: Esophagoscopy. In *Pediatric Surgery*, 4th edition. Ravitch MM, et al, eds. Year Book Medical Publishers, Chicago: 1986, 677-81.

# LARYNGOSCOPY, BRONCHOSCOPY

## SURGICAL CONSIDERATIONS

**Description:** Congenital or acquired lesions of the upper airway are common problems in pediatric surgery. Management of the airway, while allowing operative manipulation, can be challenging, and it requires the cooperation of an experienced anesthesiologist and endoscopist. The options for airway management depend on the level of the lesion and presence or absence of a tracheostomy. Laryngeal and subglottic lesions require **suspension laryngoscopy** and generally preclude the use of an ETT, although occasionally a small ETT can be positioned so as not to interfere with the operative procedure (Fig 12.2-3). Normally, ventilation is accomplished with a venturi or a nasopharyngeal system. For lower lesions, where the procedure is performed via **rigid bronchoscopy**, ventilation can be performed through the side arm of the bronchoscope; however, it requires high pressure. Currently, many of these lesions are being treated with $CO_2$ or KTP lasers. Consequently, all standard laser precautions, including those for airway ignition, must be observed. The procedure for airway foreign body is similar to other pediatric bronchoscopy, but it includes the need to manipulate loose objects in the airway with the ever-present risk of total airway obstruction. The bronchoscope and foreign body are generally removed as a unit, resulting in temporary, and frequently recurrent, loss of control of the airway.

**Usual preop diagnosis:** Airway foreign body; subglottic stenosis; hemangioma; papillomatosis

## SUMMARY OF PROCEDURE

| | Suspension Laryngoscopy | Bronchoscopy |
|---|---|---|
| **Position** | Supine | ⇐ |
| **Special instrumentation** | Suspension laryngoscope; venturi ventilation equipment; ± laser | ⇐ + Rigid bronchoscope |
| **Unique considerations** | Non-intubated ventilation | Embolectomy catheter; loss of airway |
| **Surgical time** | 1 - 2 hrs | 1 hr |
| **Closing considerations** | Abrupt end of procedure | ⇐ |
| **EBL** | < 5 cc/kg | ⇐ |
| **Postop care** | Airway support | ⇐ |
| **Mortality** | < 5% | Minimal |
| **Morbidity** | Loss of airway<br>Pneumothorax<br>Tracheobronchial rupture: Rare | ⇐ |
| **Procedure code** | 31571 | 31622 |
| **Pain score** | 2-3 | ⇐ |

## PATIENT POPULATION CHARACTERISTICS

| | |
|---|---|
| **Age range** | Newborn-school age |
| **Male:Female** | 1:1 |
| **Incidence** | Subglottic stenosis: 1/1000<br>Papillomatosis: 1/100,000 |
| **Etiology** | Prolonged intubation |
| **Associated conditions** | Prematurity |

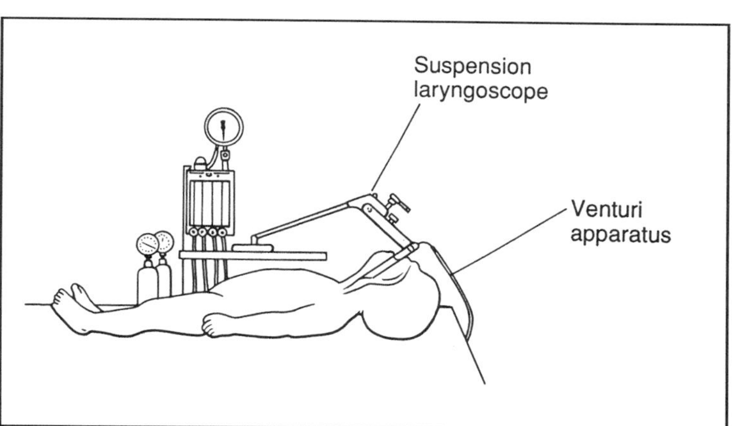


**Figure 12.2-3.** Suspension laryngoscopy with venturi ventilation. (Redrawn with permission from Gans SL, ed: *Pediatric Endoscopy*. Grune and Stratton, New York: 1983.)

# ANESTHETIC CONSIDERATIONS

See Anesthetic Considerations for "Laryngoscopy/Bronchoscopy/Esophagoscopy" in "Otolaryngology" section.

**References**

1. Benjamin B: Laryngoscopy. In *Pediatric Endoscopy*, Gans SL, ed. Grune and Stratton, New York: 1983, 17-36.

# PULLTHROUGH FOR HIRSCHSPRUNG'S DISEASE; SOAVE, DUHAMEL, SWENSON PULLTHROUGH

## SURGICAL CONSIDERATIONS

**Description:** Congenital aganglionosis (Hirschsprung's disease) produces functional obstruction of the colon with symptoms related to the length of bowel involved. The absence of ganglion cells is continuous in retrograde fashion from the anus with most (75%) cases having the transition to ganglionic bowel in the sigmoid colon. Symptoms range from constipation to complete colonic obstruction, with some patients developing a toxic enterocolitis requiring **emergency colostomy** after initial resuscitation. Most medical centers perform correction of this anomaly in two stages — **initial colostomy** in the transition zone, followed by **definitive pullthrough**. Definitive procedures are generally performed at 10 kg or 12-18 months of age. Some centers are performing definitive pullthrough in the first month, without a preliminary colostomy.

The three popular types of pullthrough procedures include resection of most of the aganglionic bowel and delivery of ganglionic bowel to the distal anal canal. They vary in the method of intrapelvic dissection and the type of coloanal anastomosis. All procedures include an initial intraperitoneal dissection, followed by a transanal anastomosis. Some surgeons prefer total lower-body prep, with legs included; others use a modified lithotomy position, with abdominal and perineal prep. After mobilization of the aganglionic colon, the rectum is either transected (**Duhamel**) or dissected to the level of the levator muscle. In the **Swenson procedure (abdominal-perineal pullthrough)**, the rectal dissection is done on the external surface of the muscular layer, whereas in the **Soave (mucosal stripping and pullthrough** of the resulting muscular tunnel) it is done between the submucosal and inner muscular layers. In the **Duhamel (double-barrelled pullthrough)**, the proximal rectum is closed and the ganglionic bowel is delivered behind the rectum to allow an end-to-side anastomosis just above the levator. The Swenson procedure consists of an end-to-end anastomosis of ganglionic bowel to full-thickness rectal stump. In the Soave procedure, the bowel is delivered within the muscular remnant of rectum and sutured to the remnant of mucosa and submucosa 1 cm above the dentate line.

Some surgeons perform the initial colostomy in the right colon, regardless of the location of the transition zone. In this circumstance, biopsies with frozen sections are required during the definitive pullthrough and a subsequent colostomy closure will follow after adequate healing of the coloanal anastomosis is confirmed.

**Usual preop diagnosis:** Hirschsprung's disease; congenital aganglionosis; congenital megacolon

### SUMMARY OF PROCEDURE

| | Preliminary Colostomy | Pullthrough |
|---|---|---|
| **Position** | Supine | Supine → lithotomy |
| **Incision** | Left lower-quadrant transverse | Low transverse |
| **Special instrumentation** | None | Staplers |
| **Unique considerations** | Frozen section to confirm ganglion cells | No monitors or iv lower extremity |
| **Antibiotics** | Preop: ampicillin 25 mg/kg iv + gentamicin 2.5 mg/kg iv; intraop: cephalosporin irrigation (1 gm/500 cc NS) | ⇐<br>⇐ |
| **Surgical time** | 1 - 1.5 hrs | 4 - 5 hrs (Soave)<br>3 - 4 hrs (Duhamel) |
| **Closing considerations** | None | Re-prep/drape |
| **EBL** | < 5 cc/kg | 5-10 cc/kg |
| **Postop care** | Cardiac/apnea monitor | PICU |
| **Mortality** | With enterocolitis: 10%<br>Without enterocolitis: 0-2% | < 5% |
| **Morbidity** | Prolapse<br>Stricture<br>Hernia | Anastomotic leak: 5%<br>Wound infection: 4%<br>Pelvic abscess: 3% |
| **Procedure code** | 44320 | 45120 |
| **Pain score** | 4 | 6-7 |

## PATIENT POPULATION CHARACTERISTICS

| | | |
|---|---|---|
| **Age range** | Newborn - 18 mo (normally) | 1 yr |
| **Male:Female** | 4:1 | ⇐ |
| **Incidence** | 1/5000 | ⇐ |
| **Etiology** | Unknown | ⇐ |
| **Associated conditions** | Trisomy 21: 5%<br>Genitourinary anomalies: < 5%<br>Neurofibromatoses | ⇐ |

---

# ANESTHETIC CONSIDERATIONS

## PREOPERATIVE

Infants (~12 months of age) with Hirschsprung's disease (congenital aganglionosis) have had prior colostomies and now present for colorectal reanastomosis. They may be mildly malnourished, but otherwise healthy.

**GI** Diarrhea may be present with associated malabsorption state.
**Tests:** Electrolytes

**Laboratory** Hct; T&C

**Premedication** Midazolam 0.5-0.75 mg/kg po administered 30 min before induction for child >12 mo.

## INTRAOPERATIVE

**Anesthetic technique:** GETA, using a pediatric circle with humidified and warmed gasses. A combined technique with caudal anesthesia is preferred. Warm OR to 75-80°F; use warming pad on OR table.

**Induction** Mask induction is preferable, unless iv is already in place. Uncuffed ETT used in this age group, with usual size being 4.0-4.5 mm ID. Keep air leak around ETT to a minimum (~20 cm $H_2O$) to minimize alterations in ventilation 2° changes in chest and pulmonary compliance. The patient is placed in a lateral decubitus position for caudal anesthesia (bupivacaine 0.25% with epinephrine 1:200,000 @ 1 cc/kg with preservative-free morphine 30-50 $\mu$g/kg).

**Maintenance** Low-dose volatile agent and air/$O_2$ with muscle relaxation for majority of cases. During last 30 min, $N_2O$ can be substituted for air. Caudal anesthesia will provide the majority of analgesia, but not the degree of muscle relaxation that will be necessary. Supplemental muscle relaxants (e.g., vecuronium 0.1 mg/kg), therefore, are required. High lesions may require turning the patient from prone to supine following mobilization of the colon.

**Emergence** The goal is to extubate at end of case. Reverse neuromuscular blockade with neostigmine (0.07 mg/kg iv) and atropine (0.02 mg/kg iv.) Often admitted to ICU for continued fluid and analgesic management.

| | | |
|---|---|---|
| **Blood and fluid requirements** | Mild blood loss<br>IV: 20-22 ga x 1-2 in upper extremities<br>NS/LR @ (maintenance):<br>4 cc/kg/hr – 0-10 kg<br>+ 2 cc/kg/hr – 11-20 kg<br>+ 1 cc/kg/hr – >20 kg<br>(e.g., 25 kg = 65 cc/hr) | Potential for large 3rd-space losses; plan 10 cc/kg/hr of crystalloid for replacement. Attempt to limit crystalloid to 50 cc/kg for case. Use 5% albumin for rapid volume expansion; transfuse to maintain Hct >23%. As a result of bowel prep, patient may require 10-20 cc/kg iv of NS/LR to offset volume deficit.<br>For children >1 mo of age, dextrose-containing solutions not required. |
| **Monitoring** | Standard monitors (see Appendix).<br>Urinary catheter<br>± Arterial line (22 ga) | ABG, Hct, blood glucose prn. Maintain UO @ 1 cc/kg/hr. Arterial line helpful for monitoring BP, lab draws and presence of respiratory variations as indicator of volume status. |
| **Positioning** | ✓ padding, particularly over lateral fibular head (common peroneal nerve).<br>✓ eyes. | |

| | | |
|---|---|---|
| **Complications** | Hypothermia<br>Hypovolemia | Majority of heat loss is radiant (skin), but potential for large volume shifts mandates warming fluids. |

**POSTOPERATIVE**

| | | |
|---|---|---|
| **Complications** | Hypothermia<br>Hypovolemia<br>Respiratory depression 2° opiates | |
| **Pain management** | Caudal block | Bupivacaine with epinephrine and morphine (as described above) will provide analgesia for 8-16 hrs. |
| **Tests** | Hct | |

**References**

1. Sieber WK: Hirschsprung's disease. In *Pediatric Surgery*, 4th edition. Ravitch MM, et al, eds. Year Book Medical Publishers, Chicago: 1986, 995-1016.
2. Swenson O, Sherman JO, Fisher JH, Cohen E: The treatment and postoperative complications of congenital megacolon: A 25-year followup. *Ann Surg* 1975; 182(3):266-73.
3. Raffensperger JG, ed. *Swenson's Pediatric Surgery*, 5th edition. Appleton & Lange, Norwalk: 1990, 555-78.

# PULLTHROUGH FOR IMPERFORATE ANUS, SACRO-PERINEAL PULLTHROUGH (PERINEAL ANOPLASTY), ABDOMINO-SACRO-PERINEAL PULLTHROUGH

## SURGICAL CONSIDERATIONS

**Description:** Imperforate anus anomalies are classified as high or low, depending on whether the distal end of the rectum ends above or below the levator ani muscle complex. **Low lesions** are repaired from a perineal approach (**perineal anoplasty**), without a preliminary colostomy. **High lesions** are treated with a preliminary **colostomy**, usually right transverse colon, followed by definitive repair at 10 kg, or 12-18 months of age. High lesions are initially approached from the sacrum to identify the end of the bowel and deliver it to the perineal location, either through a tunnel created anterior to the levator muscle, or by dividing the levator and external sphincter and reconstructing them around the rectum. If the rectum ends high and cannot be adequately mobilized from behind, the path to the perineum is established and the patient is turned to allow intraperitoneal mobilization of an adequate length of colon. After adequate mobilization, the neoanus is constructed either by passing the colon through the previously identified tunnel or by turning the patient again to perform the perineal anastomosis and reconstruct the muscle complex. The varieties of sacro-perineal pullthrough and posterior sagittal anorectoplasty vary in the manner of handling the levator muscle, but the level of the rectal atresia will determine whether the procedure is accomplished entirely from the posterior approach or whether an abdominal procedure will be required.

**Usual preop diagnosis:** Imperforate anus

**SUMMARY OF PROCEDURE**

| | Low Lesions | High Lesions |
|---|---|---|
| **Position** | Supine, lithotomy | Prone, possible turn to spine or lithotomy |
| **Incision** | Midline perineal | Midline sacral, transverse abdominal |
| **Special instrumentation** | Muscle stimulator | ⇐ + Urethral sound; vaginal pack |

| | Low Lesions | High Lesions |
|---|---|---|
| **Unique considerations** | None | Pressure points; prone position |
| **Antibiotics** | Preop: ampicillin 25 mg/kg iv + gentamicin 2.5 mg/kg iv; intraop: cephalosporin irrigation (1 gm/500 cc NS) | ⇐<br>⇐ |
| **Surgical time** | 1 - 1.5 hrs | 3 - 6 hrs |
| **EBL** | < 5 cc/kg | 5-20 cc/kg |
| **Postop care** | Apnea monitor if neonate | PICU |
| **Mortality** | ≤ 20%, due to associated anomalies | ≤ 40%, due to associated anomalies |
| **Morbidity** | Anal stenosis: 5-10%<br>Mucosal prolapse: 5% | ⇐<br>Intestinal obstruction: 5-10%<br>Neurogenic bladder: < 5%<br>Urethral stricture: 1-3% |
| **Procedure code** | 46715 (cutback anoplasty)<br>46716 (transplant anoplasty) | 46730 (sacrococcygeal approach)<br>46735 (abdominal and perineal approach) |
| **Pain score** | 3-4 | 5-6 |

**PATIENT POPULATION CHARACTERISTICS**

| | | |
|---|---|---|
| **Age range** | Newborn - 6 mo | 12-18 mo |
| **Male:Female** | 1.5:1 | ⇐ |
| **Incidence** | 1/5000 | ⇐ |
| **Etiology** | Unknown | ⇐ |
| **Associated conditions** | CHD: Common<br>Esophageal atresia: 15%<br>Genitourinary anomalies<br>Sacral/spinal cord anomalies | ⇐ |

## ANESTHETIC CONSIDERATIONS

### PREOPERATIVE

Definitive repair is performed via the sacral and/or perineal route at ~12 months of age. Children with rectal or anal agenesis without fistula will have had colostomies in newborn period. Other anomalies (e.g., VATER association, VSDs, vertebral anomalies, anal agenesis, tracheoesophageal fistula [TEF]), esophageal atresia (EA), renal or radial bone abnormalities may be present.

| | |
|---|---|
| **Respiratory** | If VATER association present, ✓ cervical spine film and neck ROM. Avoid extreme head flexion. If prior TEF repair, concerns as previously noted in Anesthetic Considerations for "Repair of Esophageal Atresia/Tracheoesophageal Fistula," above.<br>**Tests:** CXR; cervical spine film |
| **Cardiovascular** | Patients with VATER syndrome have a 20% incidence of CHD (e.g., VSD). Prior cardiology consultation. |
| **Gastrointestinal** | Colostomy may be present; thus, anesthesia records may be available for review. |
| **Renal** | If renal abnormalities exist, obtain prior urological studies.<br>**Tests:** BUN; creatinine; electrolytes |
| **Musculoskeletal** | Radial bone deformities may be present. There is no evidence to suggest that these patients are at increased risk for malignant hyperthermia (MH). |
| **Laboratory** | Hct; T&C (✓ parental/directed donor blood availability.) |
| **Premedication** | Midazolam (0.5 mg/kg po) or ketamine (6 mg/kg po) 30 min prior to arrival in OR. If < 1 yr old, no premedication is given. |

### INTRAOPERATIVE

**Anesthetic technique:** GETA, using a pediatric circle or Bain circuit with humidified and warmed gasses. Warm OR to 75°-80°F; heating pad on OR table.

| | | |
|---|---|---|
| **Induction** | Awake intubation if airway management problems anticipated; otherwise, inhalational (mask) induction with halothane/$N_2O/O_2$. Secure iv access and administer vecuronium or pancuronium (0.1 mg/kg) to facilitate ET intubation. This age group usually requires 4.0-4.5 uncuffed ETT. Maintain air leak at ~20 cm $H_2O$. | |
| **Maintenance** | Volatile agent/$N_2O/O_2$ with morphine (0.1-0.25 mg/kg iv total) or fentanyl (5-10 $\mu$g/kg iv total). Maintain neuromuscular blockade as surgically indicated. | |
| **Emergence** | Usually extubated at end of case. Confirm air leak around ETT. Reverse neuromuscular blockade with neostigmine (0.07 mg/kg iv) and atropine (0.02 mg/kg iv). Ability to flex hips is a sign of adequate reversal. | |
| **Blood and fluid requirements** | Moderate blood/3rd-space losses<br>IV: 20-22 ga x 2<br>NS/LR @ (maintenance):<br>4 cc/kg/hr – 0-10 kg<br>+ 2 cc/kg/hr - 10-20 kg | Place iv's in upper extremities, since positioning of legs may impede venous flow. Maintain Hct >22. This age group does not require dextrose infusions.<br>3rd-space losses ~5 cc/kg/hr. |
| **Monitoring** | Standard monitors (see Appendix).<br>Urinary catheter<br>± 24-ga radial arterial line | Maintain UO @ 0.5-1.0 cc/kg/hr. Marked arterial waveform variation with ventilation is a sensitive indicator of hypovolemia. ABG/Hct/glucose prn. |
| **Positioning** | √ and pad pressure points.<br>√ eyes. | Patient may be turned during procedure. |
| **Complications** | Hypovolemia → ↓BP<br>Hypothermia<br>Metabolic acidosis | Mild metabolic acidosis may occur with significant bleeding, or when 3rd-space losses are replaced with bicarbonate-deficient fluids (NS, albumin 5%, PRBCs). |

## POSTOPERATIVE

| | | |
|---|---|---|
| **Complications** | Subglottic edema<br>Respiratory depression 2° to opiates | |
| **Pain management** | Fentanyl (1-2 mg/kg iv q 1 hr prn) or morphine (0.05-0.10 mg/kg iv q 1-4 hr) | Aggressive pain management warranted. |
| **Tests** | Hct, ABG, electrolytes | |

**References**


1. deVries PA, Pena A: Posterior sagittal anorectoplasty. *J Pediatr Surg* 1982; 17(5):638-45.
2. Templeton JM, O'Neill JA Jr: Anorectal malformations. In *Pediatric Surgery*, 4th edition. Ravitch MM, et al, eds. Year Book Medical Publishers, Chicago: 1986, 1022-35.
3. Smith EI, Tunell WP, Williams GR; A clinical evaluation of the surgical treatment of anorectal malformations (imperforate anus). *Ann Surg* 1978; 187(6):583-92.
4. Schecter NL, Berde CB, Yaster M, eds: *Pain in Infants, Children, and Adolescents*, 1st edition. Williams and Wilkins, Baltimore: 1993, 357-83.

# MEDIASTINAL MASS — BIOPSY OR RESECTION

## SURGICAL CONSIDERATIONS

**Description:** Mass lesions in the mediastinum may occur at any age, although congenital cystic lesions tend to occur in younger children, with malignant lesions occurring more often in pre-school and school-age children. Preop diagnosis is usually quite accurate and is assisted by considering patient age and anatomic location within the mediastinum (anterior, middle or posterior compartments) (Fig 12.2-4). Neurogenic tumors, most often neuroblastoma, and cystic duplications of the esophagus are the common lesions in the posterior compartment. Many of these lesions present with unusual symptoms (e.g., Horner's syndrome, opsoclonus). Minimal extension of neuroblastomas into the neural foramina are common and rarely require direct surgical approach (e.g., **laminectomy**). Although neuroblastomas may reach an impressive size, they are usually resectable. Middle mediastinal masses in older children are commonly lymphoproliferative disorders and may present with respiratory symptoms or SVC compression. They have been associated with cardiorespiratory collapse with GA; hence, obtaining diagnostic tissue safely may be problematic. In younger children (< 2 years average), middle mediastinal lesions frequently represent hemangioma or lymphangioma, which may extend to other compartments. Anterior mediastinal masses generally represent lesions of the thymus or malignant germ cell tumors or teratomas. The operative approach for most mediastinal tumors is via **posterolateral thoracotomy**, with occasional need for **median sternotomy**. With the availability of current diagnostic techniques, including CT-guided biopsy, the need for exploratory thoracotomy is unusual.

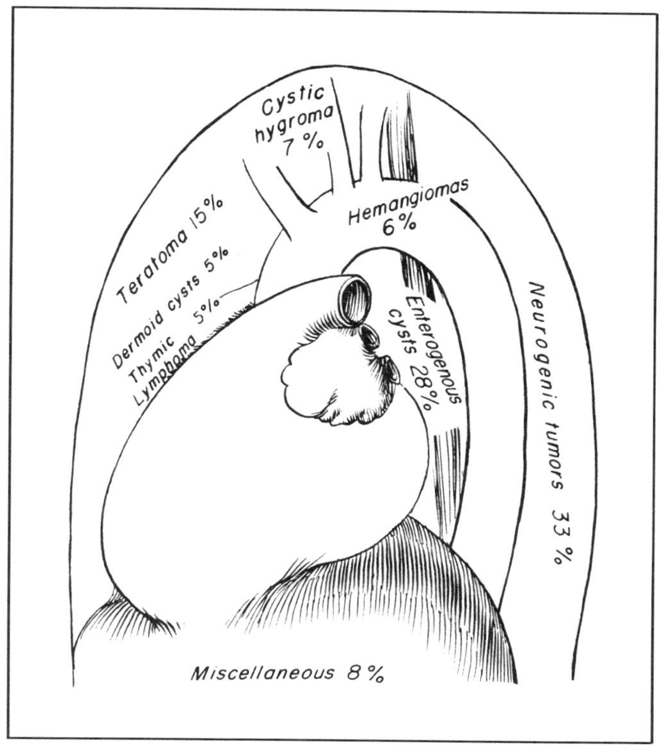


**Figure 12.2-4.** Distribution of mediastinal cysts and tumor. (Reprinted with permission from Ravitch MM, et al: *Pediatric Surgery*. Year Book Medical Publishers, Chicago: 1986.)

Most lesions can be approached through a right or left posterolateral thoracotomy. Neurogenic tumors are most common and can usually be completely excised, although blood loss may be significant if the chest wall is involved. Extension through a neural foramen usually can be delivered with the tumor. Middle and anterior lesions will require careful dissection around the pulmonary hilum and tracheobronchial tree. Median sternotomy may be required for anterior lesions, including the rare intrapericardial teratoma.

**Usual preop diagnosis:** Neuroblastoma; teratoma; duplication cyst of foregut; mediastinal mass (lymphoma)

### SUMMARY OF PROCEDURE

| | Lateral Thoracotomy | Median Sternotomy |
|---|---|---|
| **Position** | Lateral | Supine |
| **Incision** | Posterolateral | Median, parasternal |
| **Special instrumentation** | None | Bronchoscope; CPB |
| **Unique considerations** | Airway or cardiovascular collapse after induction in anterior mediastinal masses | ⇐ |
| **Antibiotics** | Preop: ampicillin 25 mg/kg iv + gentamicin 2.5 mg/kg iv; intraop: cephalosporin irrigation (1 gm/500 cc NS) | ⇐ |

| | Lateral Thoracotomy | Median Sternotomy |
|---|---|---|
| **Surgical time** | 2 - 4 hrs | 1 - 4 hrs |
| **Closing considerations** | Lung inflation; intercostal block; epidural catheter | ⇐ |
| **EBL** | 10-30 cc/kg | 10-50 cc/kg |
| **Postop care** | Aggressive respiratory therapy; analgesia | ⇐ |
| **Mortality** | < 5%, except symptomatic anterior masses | ⇐ |
| **Morbidity** | Atelectasis/respiratory | ⇐ |
| | Cardiovascular collapse with anterior masses | ⇐ |
| **Procedure code** | 39220 | ⇐ |
| **Pain score** | 7-8 | 6-7 |

### PATIENT POPULATION CHARACTERISTICS

| | |
|---|---|
| **Age range** | Newborn-teen yrs |
| **Male:Female** | 1:1 |
| **Incidence** | 1/5000 |
| **Etiology** | Unknown |
| **Associated conditions** | Cervical or axillary cystic hygroma<br>Hemangioma<br>SVC syndrome |

## ANESTHETIC CONSIDERATIONS

### PREOPERATIVE

The clinical presentation of a mediastinal mass is often non-specific in an otherwise healthy child. Often, a routine CXR (for some incidental Sx) will show the presence of an anterior mediastinal mass. These patients may suffer acute cardiorespiratory compromise on induction of anesthesia. Hence, a careful preop workup is essential.

**Respiratory** Respiratory Sx (e.g., dyspnea, cough, stridor, wheezing) are extremely important in guiding additional studies. The ability to lie supine without respiratory embarrassment should be determined. Tracheal and bronchial compression from the tumor may be positional. Preop chemotherapy may ↓tumor mass and relieve airway obstruction.

**Tests:** CXR; supine-sitting flow/volume loops (useful for evaluating location and extent of airway obstruction); ABG (or pulse oximetry), if symptomatic; chest CT/MRI

**Cardiovascular** Sx of a mediastinal mass may include SVC syndrome (e.g., venous engorgement of head and neck, edema of upper body). Other Sx may include syncope and headaches (↑ICP) made worse in the supine position. Papilledema should be sought.

**Tests:** ECHO; ECG, if symptomatic

**Musculoskeletal** If thymoma present, ✓ for Sx of myasthenia gravis.

**Tests:** Presence of acetylcholine-receptor antibodies

**Laboratory** Electrolytes; CBC; T&C for 2-4 U, depending on body weight and tumor size; other tests as indicated from H&P.

**Premedication** Avoid premedication in symptomatic patients.

### INTRAOPERATIVE

**Anesthetic technique:** GETA, with the ability to warm and humidify gasses. OR temperature 70-75°. Heating pad on OR table.

**Induction** An iv is mandatory before induction. If SVC syndrome is present, it is important to have iv access in the lower extremity. Atropine (0.02 mg/kg iv) is given to dry secretions and prevent bradycardia from deep halothane induction and laryngoscopy. An awake FOB and intubation in the sitting position may be necessary. Alternatively, a mask induction with halothane/$O_2$ in the semi-Fowler's (reclining) position may be appropriate. Intubation should be performed with preservation of spontaneous ventilation. Have small ETTs available, in light of possible tracheal

**Induction, continued** compression. Fiber optic bronchoscopy is useful to confirm ETT placement and to evaluate trachea/bronchi. Avoid muscle relaxants until the ETT is in place. Surgeon must be present with rigid bronchoscope immediately available in the event of acute airway obstruction on induction. **NB:** A simple positional change (e.g., supine to lateral or sitting) may relieve cardiorespiratory collapse.

**Maintenance** Spontaneous ventilation/assisted ventilation with volatile agent and 100% $O_2$ may be appropriate. Have surgeon infiltrate wound with bupivacaine 0.25% to reduce volatile anesthetic and opiate requirements.

**Emergence** Have all emergency airway equipment available and surgeon present. Patient should be fully awake before extubation.

| | | |
|---|---|---|
| **Blood and fluid requirements** | Usually minimal blood loss.<br>IV: 18-24 ga x 2, depending on age<br>NS/LR @ 10-20 cc/kg iv | If mediastinoscopy is performed, sudden blood loss from torn great vessel may occur. Volume-loading with NS/LR prior to induction may be appropriate because of myocardial depression and venodilation from deep inhalational induction. |
| **Monitoring** | Standard monitors (see Appendix).<br>Arterial line, if postop ventilation is planned. | Pulse oximeter on ear lobe detects desaturation sooner than probes on extremities. Precordial stethoscope earliest monitor of airway obstruction. |
| **Positioning** | ✓ and pad pressure points.<br>✓ eyes. | If obstruction worsens acutely, be prepared to change to lateral decubitus position, which may alleviate tracheal, bronchial compression and cardiovascular collapse. |
| **Complications** | Respiratory failure<br>Loss of airway<br>Bronchospasm<br>Laryngospasm<br>Hypotension | Careful attention to ABCs (airway, breathing, circulation). Have all resuscitation drugs (e.g., epinephrine 10 $\mu$g/kg iv) drawn up. |

## POSTOPERATIVE

| | | |
|---|---|---|
| **Complications** | Respiratory failure<br>Pneumothorax | Anesthesiologist must be readily available in the PACU to manage acute airway problems. |
| **Pain management** | Ketorolac 0.9 mg/kg (up to 30 mg) iv q 6° x 24 hrs | Cervical biopsy/mediastinoscopy have minimal postop pain and can be effectively treated with NSAID and local anesthetic infiltration. |
| **Tests** | Hct, ABG, CXR, as clinically indicated. | |

**References**


1. Ferrari LR, Bedford RF: General anesthesia prior to treatment of anterior mediastinal masses in pediatric cancer patients. *Anesthesiology* 1990; 72(6):991-95.
2. Mogul M, Hartman GE, Donaldson S, et al: Langerhans' Cell Histiocytosis presenting with superior vena cava syndrome: a case report. *Journal of Medical and Pediatric Oncology* (In Press).
3. Ravitch MM: Mediastinal cysts and tumors. In *Pediatric Surgery*, 4th edition. Ravitch MM, et al, eds. Year Book Medical Publishers, Chicago: 1986, 602-18.
4. Neuman GB, Weingarten AE, Abramowitz RM, Kushins LG, Abramson AL, Ladner W: The anesthetic management of the patient with an anterior mediastinal mass. *Anesthesiology* 1984; 60(2):144-47.
5. Watcha MF, et al: Comparison of ketorolac and morphine as adjuvants during pediatric surgery. *Anesthesiology* 1991; 76(3):368-72.

# EXTRACORPOREAL MEMBRANE OXYGENATION (ECMO)

## SURGICAL CONSIDERATIONS

**Description**: **Extracorporeal membrane oxygenation (ECMO)** for prolonged periods (3-21 days) has been perfected to allow cardiopulmonary support for newborns and children with reversible respiratory failure. The most common indications are meconium aspiration and pulmonary HTN associated with congenital diaphragmatic hernia. The procedure is performed in the NICU with OR technique. Patients are given anticoagulants prior to cannulation. Subsequently, repair of the diaphragmatic hernia also is performed in the NICU on ECMO support prior to decannulation. (Fig 12.2-5 shows ECMO schematic.)

The potential detrimental effects of the diaphragmatic repair on respiratory function can be managed with increased circuit flow in this setting. ECMO also has been helpful in some newborns with cardiopulmonary failure following correction of congenital cardiac defects. Vascular access is accomplished with one (veno venous) or two (veno arterial) cannulas. The IJ vein is cannulated in both methods with the tip of the cannula in the right atrium. In veno arterial ECMO, the common carotid artery is used with the tip of the cannula at the aortic arch. The wound is closed around the cannulas, which are secured to the infant's scalp.

**Usual preop diagnosis**: Meconium aspiration; diaphragmatic hernia; Bochdalek hernia

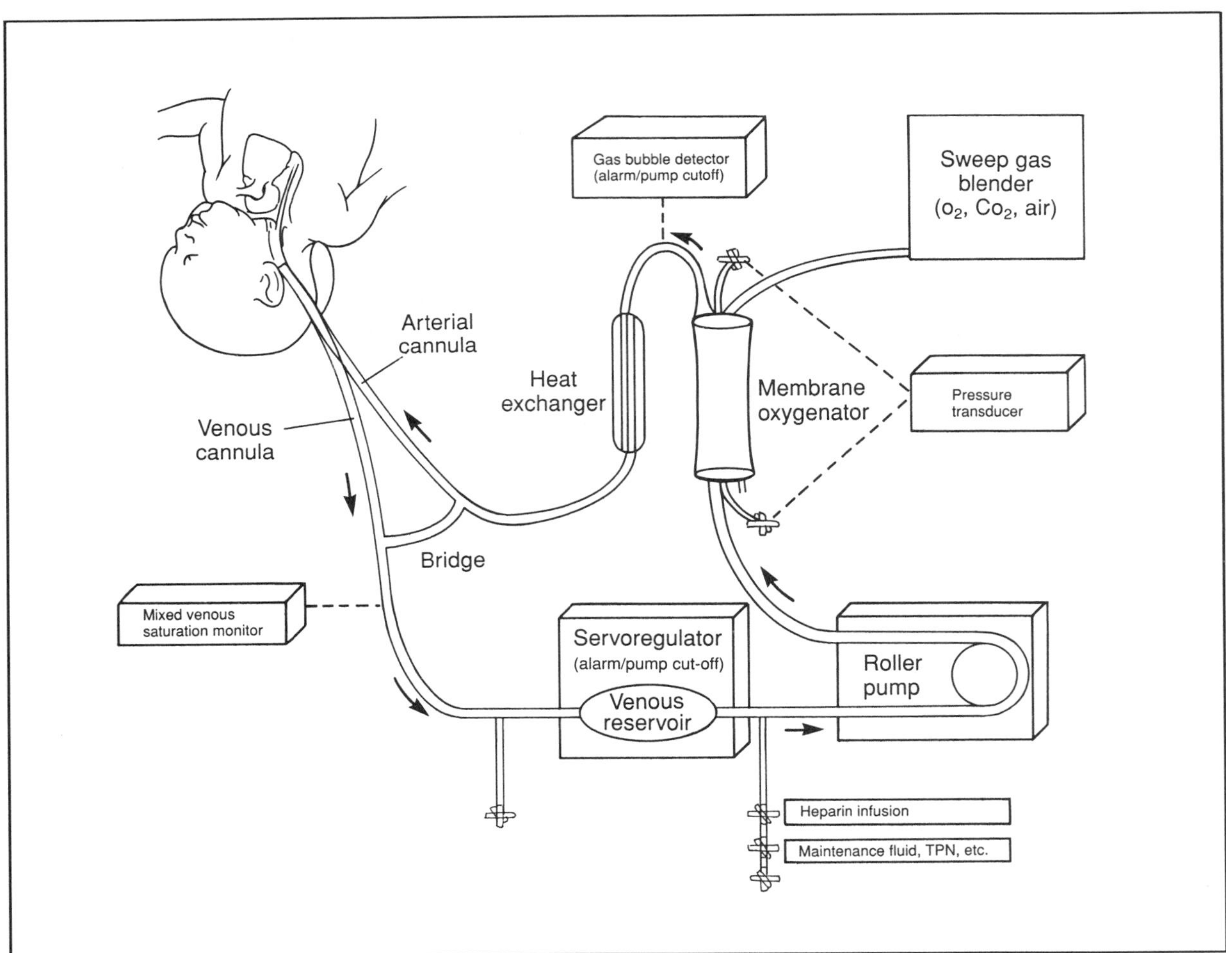


**Figure 12.2-5.** ECMO circuit. Venous blood is withdrawn by gravity through a servo regulator to prevent pump from actively siphoning venous return. Roller pump delivers blood back to the arterial cannula after it passes through the membrane oxygenator and heat exchanger. Venous return is from the right atrium, arterial infusion is into the aortic arch in double cannula (veno arterial) or right atrium (veno venous) techniques. (Reproduced with permission from Rhine W, Van Meurs K: Extracorporeal membrane and oxygenation. In *Nelson's Textbook of Pediatrics*, Update #8. WB Saunders Co: 1990.)

## SUMMARY OF PROCEDURE

| | |
|---|---|
| **Position** | Supine |
| **Incision** | Subcostal, right neck incision |
| **Special instrumentation** | ECMO circuit (Fig 12.2-3) |
| **Unique considerations** | Anticoagulation |
| **Antibiotics** | Preop: ampicillin 25 mg/kg iv + gentamicin 2.5 mg/kg iv; intraop: cephalosporin irrigation (1 gm/500 cc NS) |
| **Surgical time** | 1 - 2 hrs |
| **Closing considerations** | Assess for changes in ventilation (e.g., PIP, pre- and post-ductal ABG). |
| **EBL** | >5-10 cc/kg |
| **Postop care** | Paralysis maintained; hyperventilation; fentanyl infusion @ 2-5 $\mu$g/kg/min |
| **Mortality** | 25-30% |
| **Morbidity** | Respiratory failure<br>Sepsis |
| **Procedure code** | 36822 |
| **Pain score** | 6-7 |

## PATIENT POPULATION CHARACTERISTICS

| | |
|---|---|
| **Age range** | Newborn-weeks or months |
| **Male:Female** | 1-2:1 |
| **Incidence** | 1/4000 |
| **Etiology** | Unknown |
| **Associated conditions** | For diaphragmatic hernia:<br>Malrotation: 40-100%<br>Congenital heart disease: 15%<br>Renal anomalies<br>Esophageal atresia<br>CNS abnormalities |

**References**

1. Anderson KD: Congenital diaphragmatic hernia. In *Pediatric Surgery*, 4th edition. Ravitch MM, et al, eds. Year Book Medical Publishers, Chicago: 1986, 589-601.
2. Falconer AR, Brown RA, Helms P, Gordon I, Baron JA: Pulmonary sequelae in survivors of congenital diaphragmatic hernia. *Thorax* 1990; 45(2):126-29.
3. Wilson JM, Lund DP, Lillehei CW, Vacanti JP: Congenital diaphragmatic hernia: predictors of severity in the ECMO era. *J Pediatr Surg* 1991; 26(9):1028-33.

**Surgeons**

**John A. Duncan III, MD, PhD**
**Lawrence M. Shuer, MD**
**Gary K. Steinberg, MD, PhD**

## 12.3 PEDIATRIC NEUROSURGERY

**Anesthesiologist**

**C. Philip Larson, Jr, MD, MS**

# CRANIOFACIAL SURGERY

## SURGICAL CONSIDERATIONS

**Description**: Craniofacial surgery is a broad term which refers to both cranial and/or facial surgery for the correction of cranial dysostosis or craniofacial dysmorphism. Cranial dysostosis is the maldevelopment of the cranial base and/or vault, 2° to premature fusion of cranial sutures. This is commonly referred to as **craniosynostosis** and the surgical procedure involves removal of the affected suture(s). Craniosynostosis may involve one or more suture, and resulting deformities are characteristic and well-recognized. For example, scaphocephaly, the most common form of craniosynostosis, is caused by premature fusion of the sagittal suture. This results in an increase in the AP diameter of the head. The most common surgical procedure for correction of this condition is a **linear craniectomy**. Common cranial dysostoses and their corrective procedures include: scaphocephaly – linear craniectomy (sagittal); trigonocephaly – linear craniectomy (metopic); posterior plagiocephaly – linear craniectomy (lambdoid); anterior plagiocephaly – lateral canthal advancement; brachycephaly – bilateral canthal advancement (coronal).

Head growth to adult size occurs by 2-3 years of age; by this time, normal sutures have developed a fibrous union, which ossifies at 6-8 years. Craniosynostosis, therefore, is a developmental abnormality which presents within the first year of life. Early recognition and surgical correction are well-correlated with improved cosmetic outcome.[1-2] Most elective procedures are scheduled prior to 6 months of age; but many centers prefer surgical correction at approximately 3 months. Patient weight, blood volume and expected blood loss must be considered when surgery is scheduled. Most craniosynostoses (single and multiple) are sporadic, although a predisposition has been reported. In addition, several inheritable conditions exist, the most common being Crouzon's disease and Apert's syndrome, in which craniosynostosis is one of multiple genetic defects. Because of abnormalities in development of the cranial base, facial dysmorphism occurs, resulting in shallow, misplaced orbits and midface hypoplasia. Surgical correction today follows the guidelines established by **Tessier** and colleagues.[3,4,5] Surgical repair is often staged with correction of the cranial vault and base within the first year of life and advancement of the midface after primary dentition is complete. Multiple procedures are often required.

Positioning of patient, type of headrest and incision all vary, depending on location of the suture abnormality. Most commonly, the child is supine and a padded horseshoe headrest is used. A bicoronal, biparietal or Meisterschnitt incision is used. This provides good access to the anterior skull base, the pterion, the anterior fontanel and the coronal sutures. When the occipital region is involved (i.e., sagittal and/or lambdoidal craniosynostosis), the child may be placed prone and a biparietal or midsagittal incision used. Occasionally, the entire cranial vault needs to be exposed (multiple suture craniosynostosis), and a special headrest applied to the cheeks and suboccipital region is used. Pin fixation cannot be safely used in children < 2 yrs old.

Once the skin incision is made, blood loss should be minimized by the use of Raney clips along the skin edge. The craniectomy is performed, preferably with a high-speed craniotome such as the Midas Rex®. The extent of bone removal varies by the degree and number of sutures involved. Blood loss may be excessive, which is unacceptable; it should be controlled with bone wax. If a **sagittal linear craniectomy** is performed, injury to the superior sagittal sinus may occur. This is rare, but should be anticipated. The procedure is extradural and any defects in the dura should be repaired to prevent CSF leak. Increased intracranial pressure may result if reduction of the cranial vault is excessive and must be corrected prior to closure. Skin closure is routine.

**Usual preop diagnosis**: Craniosynostosis (sagittal, coronal, metopic, lambdoidal); craniofacial dysmorphism; Apert's syndrome; Crouzon's disease

### SUMMARY OF PROCEDURE

| | |
|---|---|
| **Position** | Supine or prone (less common); or table 180° |
| **Incision** | Bicoronal, biparietal, Meisterschnitt, midsagittal |
| **Special instrumentation** | Midas Rex® craniotome; mini- or micro-plates/screws |
| **Unique considerations** | ↑ICP and/or hydrocephalus may coexist. ↑ICP is usually seen with multiple-suture synostosis; it also occurs in single-suture craniosynostosis,[6] but is rare (< 5-10%). Hydrocephalus is typically seen in monogenic conditions (e.g., Apert's syndrome, Crouzon's disease). Most neurosurgeons shunt the hydrocephalus and treat the ↑ICP prior to craniosynostosis surgery. |
| **Antibiotics** | Vancomycin (13-15 mg/kg) or cloxacillin (25-50 mg/kg) for cranial surgery. Vancomycin or cloxacillin and cefotaxime (25-30 mg/kg) for craniofacial surgery involving nasal sinuses. |

**Closing considerations** Watch for increased blood loss from the scalp after hemostatic skin clips are removed. To prevent excessive blood loss, reapproximate only one portion of the scalp at a time.

**EBL** Highly variable; must be minimalized. Amount depends on the number of sutures involved and the magnitude of the repair. Operative injury to the superior sagittal sinus may be catastrophic if hemostasis cannot be achieved or volume loss is excessive.

**Postop care** ICU. Postop Hct and Hb levels required. Blood transfusion often necessary in infants (< 10 kg)

**Mortality** < 1-2%

**Morbidity** Meningitis
CSF rhinorrhea
↑ICP (2° skull reshaping)
Venous thrombosis
Neurological injury: Rare

**Procedure code** 61550 (single); 61552 (multiple sutures)

**Pain score** 1-3

### PATIENT POPULATION CHARACTERISTICS

**Age range** Newborn-young adult

**Male:Female** 1.2:1

**Incidence** 1/2,000/yr

**Etiology** Sporadic
Heritable (monogenic and chromosomal syndromes)
Environmentally induced (amniotic bands, iatrogenic)

**Associated conditions** Congenital defects (limbs, heart, brain, kidneys)
Hydrocephalus
Encephalocele (sincipital/basal)
Fibrous dysplasia
Craniometaphyseal dysplasia
Holoprosencephaly

---

## ANESTHETIC CONSIDERATIONS

### PREOPERATIVE

Craniofacial surgery encompasses a wide variety of procedures, with the two most common being linear craniectomy for craniosynostosis (or premature closure of the cranial sutures) and reconstructive (cosmetic surgery) for congenital deformities of the forehead, orbit ridges and nose. Craniosynostosis usually manifests itself in the first year of life, while surgery for other congenital deformities of the face and skull is usually performed from ages 1-6 years.

**Respiratory** As a result of their craniofacial deformities, some children may present difficult intubations. Their airways should be carefully evaluated preop.

**Neurological** Presenting Sx in infants with craniosynostosis include: progressively increasing irritability, crying, failure to eat and failure to grow in head circumference. These Sx may be due in part to ↑ICP. On physical examination, one or more of the cranial sutures are fused. Infants with other types of craniofacial deformity usually have no Sx related to their abnormalities.

**Laboratory** Tests as indicated from H&P.

**Premedication** For children, midazolam 0.5 mg/kg po generally provides satisfactory preop sedation after ~30 min. For young children (< 5 yrs) refusing po meds, instillation of midazolam 0.3 mg/kg intranasally provides rapid amnesia, sedation and easy separation from the parents.[7]

### INTRAOPERATIVE

**Anesthetic technique:** GETA.

**Induction** Standard pediatric induction (see Appendix). Orotracheal tubes are preferred over nasotracheal tubes because the surgery may involve reflection of the scalp down over the eyes and nose, in which case a nasal tube would be in the way. Following orotracheal intubation, make certain that the tube is endotracheal, not endobronchial. If in doubt, and the tube is uncuffed, advance tube until it is clearly endobronchial. Then, while listening with a stethoscope over the non-ventilated lung, remove it gradually until breath sounds are heard clearly. If the tube is cuffed, palpate cuff in the sternal notch. Tape the tube firmly in place at one side of the mouth using benzoin adherent. Ventilation is controlled to $PETCO_2$=35-40 mmHg with a mechanical ventilator, from the start of anesthesia until the surgical wound is closed. When craniofacial surgery is performed, the surgeon usually places plastic corneal shields in the eyes and sutures the lids shut to protect eyes from injury.

**Maintenance** Standard maintenance (see Appendix). Muscle relaxation is usually provided. Maintain a near normal BP. Maintain normal temperature by keeping the OR warm (78° F) and using warming lights as needed.

**Emergence** No specific considerations. The ETT is removed at the conclusion of the anesthetic. Patient usually goes to ICU.

| | | |
|---|---|---|
| **Blood and fluid requirements** | Large blood loss<br>IV: 18-20 ga x 1-2<br>D5 1/4 NS @ 4 cc/kg/hr<br>Fluid warmer | Administer crystalloid, usually D5 1/4 NS via a measured volume system (Volutrol®, continuous infusion pump, etc.). Blood is usually necessary. It is advisable to begin transfusion at the start of surgery, to avoid getting behind. Generally, it is better to administer warmed blood by syringe, in 10 ml increments. Serial Hct determinations are useful. |
| **Monitoring** | Standard monitors (see Appendix).<br>± Foley catheter<br>± Doppler<br>± Arterial line<br>± CVP line | If operation is anticipated to last several hrs, a Foley catheter should be inserted. If patient is semi-sitting, a Doppler ultrasound probe should be placed on the chest to monitor for air embolism. |
| **Positioning** | OR table rotated 180°<br>✓ and pad pressure points.<br>✓ eyes. | |

## POSTOPERATIVE CONSIDERATIONS

| | | |
|---|---|---|
| **Complications** | Bleeding<br>Hypovolemia | Major complications from this operation are uncommon. |
| **Pain management** | Parenteral opioids (see Appendix).<br>Avoid over-sedation. | Fentanyl 1-2 μg/kg q 60 min |
| **Tests** | Hct | Hct determinations are necessary to determine adequacy of blood replacement. |


**References**

1. Hoffman HJ, Hendrick EB: Early neurosurgical repair in craniofacial dysmorphism. *J Neurosurg* 1979; 51(6):796-803.
2. Hoffman HJ: Congenital malformations of the spine and skull. In *Practice of Surgery*. Goldsmith HS, ed. Harper & Row, New York; 1980.
3. Tessier P, Guiot G, Rougerie J, Delbet JP, Pastoriza J: Cranio-naso-orbito-facial osteotomies. Hypertelorism. *Ann Chir Plast* 1967; 12(2):103-18.
4. Tessier P: Total facial osteotomy. Crouzon's syndrome, Apert's syndrome: oxycephaly, scaphocephaly, turricephaly. *Ann Chir Plast* 1967; 12(4):273-86.
5. Tessier P: Relationship of craniostenoses to craniofacial dysostoses and to faciostenoses: a study with therapeutic implications. *Plast Reconstr Surg* 1971; 48(3):224-37.
6. Shillito J Jr, Matson DD: Craniosynostoses: a review of 519 surgical patients. *Pediatrics* 1968; 41(4):829-53.
7. Karl HW., Keifer AT, Rosenberger JL, Larach MG, Ruffle JM: Comparison of the safety and efficacy of intranasal midazolam or sufentanil for preinduction of anesthesia in pediatric patients. *Anesthesiology* 1992: 76(2):209-15.

# EPILEPSY SURGERY

## SURGICAL CONSIDERATIONS

**Description**: In the U.S., the prevalence of epilepsy is approximately 5-20/1,000 (0.5-2%), meaning that at least 1.5 million people have epilepsy.[1,2] In childhood, the incidence and prevalence is higher, with 90% of all new cases occurring before the age of 20.[3] Intractable epilepsy is defined as persistent seizure activity of such frequency or severity that prevents normal function and/or development. This diagnosis is made only after an adequate trial of anticonvulsant medication(s), with therapeutic levels, has been documented.[4] Of all those with epilepsy, 10-20% prove to be intractable; and it is estimated that approximately 20-30% of patients with intractable epilepsy may benefit from a surgical procedure.[5]

The causes of epilepsy are varied, ranging from idiopathic to neoplastic. Epilepsy surgery is most beneficial in patients with partial epilepsy 2° a structural lesion. Most commonly, this lesion is located in the temporal lobe; and, therefore, the most common operation is a **temporal lobectomy** in both children and adults. Cerebral dominance and, hence, the location of speech, must be determined using a preop Wada test (intracarotid amobarbital injection to localize language function).[6] Temporal lobe surgery may involve removal of only the structural lesion and associated epileptogenic cortex, cortical resection alone, excision of the amygdala and hippocampus or removal of the entire anterior temporal lobe, with the extent of posterior resection dependent on dominance. Depending on the center, intraop electrocorticography may be employed, requiring neuroleptic anesthesia. In addition, the speech center may need to be identified intraop, necessitating an awake procedure. These differing options will significantly alter the choice of anesthesia and must be established prior to surgery.

A standard **temporal lobectomy** is detailed as follows: The patient is placed supine on the operating table with the head turned 90° and held with pin fixation. A "question mark" temporal incision is often used, and hemostasis is achieved with skin clips. A flap – either a free temporal bone flap or an osteoplastic flap, based on the temporalis muscle – is elevated with a high-speed craniotome. A **subtemporal craniectomy** allows visualization of the entire anterior temporal lobe. The dura is opened, widely exposing the anterior 6-6.5 cm of the temporal lobe. The vein of Labbe must be preserved. At this point, surface and/or depth electrocorticography may be employed and **inhalation anesthetics must not be used**. After mapping the lesion, amygdala and hippocampus or anterior temporal lobe is removed. Temporal lobectomy involves resection of both the lateral and medial temporal structures, and is commonly performed in two steps. Often an operating microscope will be used to completely resect medial structures, including the uncus and hippocampal formation. Injury to the brain stem, 3rd and 4th cranial nerves, and either the middle cerebral or posterior cerebral arteries, can occur; these are known complications of this surgery. Closure of the dura, bone flap and scalp is routine.

**Variant procedure or approaches**: There are three common alternate procedures. The first is sectioning of the corpus callosum, known as a **corpus callosotomy**. This is usually employed for patients with atonic seizures or partial seizures with secondary generalization. Either the anterior two-thirds or the entire corpus callosum is divided in the midline. The approach is the same as any transcallosal, intraventricular procedure, and uses a bifrontal, paramedian scalp incision and elevation of free-bone flap adjacent to the midline in the region of the coronal suture. Injury to the sagittal sinus is possible and must be avoided. In addition, numerous bridging veins across the interhemispheric fissure must be preserved to avoid venous congestion and possible infarction. The right cerebral hemisphere is gently retracted from the falx, exposing the paired anterior cerebral arteries and underlying corpus callosum. If an anterior two-thirds transection is performed, an intraop x-ray is required to determine the posterior border.

The second alternate procedure is either a **frontal**, **temporal** or **occipital craniotomy** for resection of a structural, epileptogenic focus such as a tumor or AVM. This procedure may employ **stereotaxic localization** and the resultant craniotomy may be performed in the stereotaxic head frame, which alters the method of intubation. The subsequent craniotomy is similar to the excision of any structural lesion, with the exception of intraop electrocorticography of surrounding cortex, if used. Such monitoring alters the choice of anesthetic.

The third alternate procedure is diagnostic and involves placement of **surface and/or depth electrodes**. This may be performed with or without stereotaxic localization. Often only burr holes, outlining the future craniotomy flap, are used.

**Usual preop diagnosis**: Temporal lobe epilepsy; partial epilepsy; intractable epilepsy

### SUMMARY OF PROCEDURE

| | |
|---|---|
| **Position** | Supine, rarely prone for occipital lesions; or table 180° |
| **Incision** | Temporal question mark, reverse question mark, paramedian, frontal or occipital |
| **Special instrumentation** | Operating microscope; Cavitron®; bipolar cautery; surface electrode grids and strips; depth electrode |
| **Unique considerations** | Electrocorticography requiring neuroleptic anesthesia; awake procedures for mapping of temporal and/or frontal speech areas; stereotaxic craniotomy and lesionectomy |
| **Antibiotics** | Vancomycin (13-15 mg/kg) or cloxacillin (25-50 mg/kg) |
| **EBL** | Minimal for diagnostic procedures; 250-500 cc with craniotomy (adults) |
| **Postop care** | After craniotomy, ICU for 12-24 hrs |
| **Mortality** | < 1% |
| **Morbidity** | Hemiplegia<br>Dysphasia<br>Ophthalmoplegia<br>Brain stem surgery |
| **Procedure code** | 61538 (temporal lobectomy) |
| **Pain score** | 1-3 |

### PATIENT POPULATION CHARACTERISTICS

| | |
|---|---|
| **Age range** | 2-50 yrs |
| **Male:Female** | 1:1 |
| **Incidence** | 150,000/yr (new cases of epilepsy) |
| **Etiology** | Idiopathic (mesial temporal sclerosis)<br>Infectious (brain abscess, encephalitis)<br>Traumatic (glial scar)<br>Vascular (AVM, infarct)<br>Neoplastic (glioma, hamartoma, ganglioglioma)<br>Congenital (cortical dysplasia) |
| **Associated conditions** | Tuberous sclerosis<br>Sturge Weber<br>Infantile hemiplegia<br>Encephalitis<br>Hemimegalencephaly |

## ANESTHETIC CONSIDERATIONS

### PREOPERATIVE

Epilepsy is a common disorder among young adults. Anti-epileptic medication such as phenytoin will abolish seizure disorders in most patients, but some develop intolerable side effects to such medications, and others are refractory to medical therapy. Surgical ablation of the seizure focus may be the only effective therapy for some patients if they are to become self-sufficient and be able to operate a motor vehicle. Several operations may be done, the most common being placement of surface or depth electrodes to determine the focus of the seizure, and then subsequent temporal lobectomy for removal of the focus. In some cases, the lesion may be very focal and amenable to stereotactic localization and removal.

| | |
|---|---|
| **Neurological** | Usually the only neurological findings are a Hx of uncontrollable seizures, either focal or generalized. Obtain a description of seizure and prodromal Sx.<br>**Tests:** A Wada test or intracarotid injection of a barbiturate is usually performed to determine whether the area of proposed surgery has any cerebral dominance or speech function. |
| **Laboratory** | Tests as indicated from H&P. |
| **Premedication** | Standard premedication (see Appendix) is usually appropriate. |

## INTRAOPERATIVE

**Anesthetic technique:** Local anesthesia and GETA. The placement of surface or depth electrodes is done under GETA, as is a temporal lobectomy in the non-dominant hemisphere. If the seizure focus is in the dominant hemisphere, if there is any question about possible neurological injury by temporal lobectomy, the procedure is performed under local anesthesia, with intraop localization of the seizure focus. In this case, the patient should be told that the operation will be performed under local anesthesia, that every effort will be made to control discomfort, and that he/she will be expected to respond to some pictures and questions once the head is opened and the seizure area is identified. The patient should also be told that he/she probably will be amnesic for the operative events.

| | |
|---|---|
| **Induction** | Standard induction (see Appendix). If a difficult intubation is anticipated (e.g., stereotactic frame), orotracheal intubation is best accomplished before induction of GA. An awake fiber optic intubation is the best technique (see Anesthetic Considerations for "Thoracolumbar Neurosurgery Procedures" in the "Neurosurgery" section for a description of this technique). Once anesthesia is induced, a non-depolarizing neuromuscular relaxant is administered. |
| **Maintenance** | Standard maintenance (see Appendix). Generally, no further neuromuscular-blocking drugs are administered beyond that used for tracheal intubation. With adequate anesthesia, and the head fixed in the Mayfield-Kees skeletal fixation, patient movement of any consequence is highly unlikely. Furthermore, it is useful to see movement of an extremity as an indicator of inadequate depth of anesthesia. |
| **Emergence** | No special considerations. |

**Local anesthesia:** Initial sedation may be achieved with a combination of midazolam (0.07 mg/kg) and meperidine (1-1.5 mg/kg) or fentanyl (2-3 $\mu$g/kg). Nasal prongs should be placed on the patient and supplemental $O_2$ administered. If local anesthesia is used, continuous pump infusions of propofol (50-150 $\mu$g/kg/min) and an opiate (e.g., alfentanil 0.1-3 $\mu$g/kg/min) are extremely effective in providing amnesia and analgesia, while allowing the anesthesiologist to awaken the patient for about 30-60 min of testing, once the temporal lobe has been exposed surgically. A unique method of titrating infusion drugs is by monitoring ABG values continuously (see Monitoring, below).

| | | |
|---|---|---|
| **Blood and fluid requirements** | Moderate blood loss<br>IV: 18 ga x 2<br>NS/LR @ 4-6 cc/kg/hr | If local anesthesia used, 2 iv cannulae are needed – one for fluid administration, another for infusion of anesthetic drugs. If GA used, 1 peripheral iv and a CVP cannula are inserted. Blood transfusions seldom are needed for this operation since blood loss is usually < 500 ml. |
| **Monitoring** | Standard monitors (see Appendix).<br>Arterial line<br>CVP line (if GA)<br>UO | If the operation is to be performed under local anesthesia, continuous ABG monitoring[7] is useful for following the respiratory effects of the drugs being administered. These effects cannot always be followed accurately using $O_2$ sat and $ETCO_2$ monitoring, since frequent patient movement decreases the reliability of the former, and mouth breathing decreases the accuracy of the latter. |
| **Positioning** | Table rotated 180°<br>✓ and pad pressure points.<br>✓ eyes. | Semi-sitting position with head held in Mayfield-Kees skeletal fixation and rotated laterally with a roll under the shoulder on the operative side. Anesthetic hoses and intravascular lines must be long enough to be accessible. |
| **Complications** | Anxiety<br>Agitation<br>Seizure | Local anesthetic toxicity may produce agitation and seizures. |

## POSTOPERATIVE

| | | |
|---|---|---|
| **Complications** | Seizure<br>Bleeding<br>Cerebral edema | Monitor carefully for altered mental status. |
| **Pain management** | Codeine 30-60 mg 1 M q 4 hrs | Avoid over-sedation. |
| **Tests** | CT scan | If a patient exhibits any delay in emergence from anesthesia and surgery, or any new neurologic deficits appear, a CT scan is invariably obtained. |

**References**


1. Hauser WA, Kurland LT: The epidemiology of epilepsy in Rochester, Minnesota, 1935 through 1967. *Epilepsia* 1975; 16(1):1-66.
2. Hauser WA: *Epilepsy: frequency, causes, and consequences*. Demos, New York: 1990, 21-48.
3. O'Donohoe NV: *Epilepsies of Childhood.* Butterworths, Boston: 1985, 4.
4. Morrison G, Duchowny M, Resnick T, Alvarez L, Jayakan P, Prats AR, Dean P, Penate M: Epilepsy surgery in childhood. A report of 79 patients. *Pediatr Neurosurg* 1992, 18(5-6):291-7.
5. *Surgery for Epilepsy*. NIH Consensus Development Conference. Consensus Statement, 1990, Mar 19-21; 8(2) 2, and *JAMA* 1990; 264:729-33.
6. Blume WT, Grabow JD, Darley FL, Aronson AE: Intracarotid amobarbital test of language and memory before temporal lobectomy for seizure control. *Neurology* 1973, 23(8):812-19.
7. Larson CP, Vender J, Seiver A: Multi-site evaluation of a continuous intra-arterial blood gas monitoring system. Submitted to *Anesthesiology*.


# REPAIR OF MYELOMENINGOCELE OR MENINGOCELE

## SURGICAL CONSIDERATIONS

**Description:** Myelomeningocele and meningocele are birth defects which require early repair. Both of these conditions represent the failure of closure of the spinal canal in embryological development which may be detected before birth, using ultrasound and serum alpha-fetoprotein protein determinations. A myelomeningocele contains neural elements within the expanded dural sac, whereas the meningocele is an out-pouching of the dural sac. The timing of the repair of the defect depends on the integrity of the skin which is overlying the defect. Most myelomeningoceles have a very thin epithelium over the neural elements and some leak CSF. These situations constitute a relative emergency for risk of infection in the CNS. Most neurosurgeons prefer to repair these defects within the child's first 24 hours of life. Lumbar defects are most common, although some are quite large and may extend to the thoracic or, very rarely, to the cervical spine.

During the procedure, the child should be in the prone position. The defect is dissected such that the various anatomic layers can be separated. The neural elements are then freed and repair is begun with a dural closure. An attempt is then made to close the fascial layer. Sometimes it is necessary to free up some tissue from around the defect to close this layer; at other times this may be impossible. The subcutaneous layer and skin are closed last. Frequently, the surgeon has to rotate skin flaps in order to close the defect; occasionally, a plastic surgeon may be involved in complex skin closure.

**Variant procedure or approaches:** Occasionally, the defect is so well-covered that it can be repaired electively at a later stage in life. The exploration of a lumbar dermal sinus in an infant is an example of this to this procedure; however, instead of repairing a herniation of neural contents, the surgeon explores the sinus tract and frees it from neural structures, if attached.

**Usual preop diagnosis:** Myelomeningocele; meningocele; myelodysplasia; spina bifida

### SUMMARY OF PROCEDURE

| | |
|---|---|
| **Position** | Prone |
| **Incision** | Surrounding the defect, preserving skin which can be utilized in the closure |
| **Special instrumentation** | Loupes or operating microscope (optional) |
| **Unique considerations** | Child may have concomitant hydrocephalus, need for blood replacement. |
| **Antibiotics** | Cefotaxime (25-30 mg/kg iv), vancomycin (13-15 mg/kg iv, slowly) |

| | |
|---|---|
| **Surgical time** | 1.5 - 3 hrs |
| **Closing considerations** | Skin closure may be complex and require rotation of flaps or aid of plastic surgeon. |
| **EBL** | Negligible-25 cc |
| **Postop care** | Neonatal nursery. Postop, child often nursed on stomach or side. Head size is monitored for development of hydrocephalus, which may require shunting at a later date. |
| **Mortality** | Minimal-3% |
| **Morbidity** | The following occur in < 5% of cases:<br>Infection<br>Neurological problems<br>Aseptic meningitis<br>CSF leak<br>Massive blood loss |
| **Procedure code** | 63700-63706 (meningocele and myelomeningocele repairs); 61712 (microscopic procedure) |
| **Pain score** | 3-5 |

### PATIENT POPULATION CHARACTERISTICS

| | |
|---|---|
| **Age range** | Newborn-1 yr (usually within first 24 hrs) |
| **Male:Female** | ~1:1 |
| **Incidence** | 2/1000 live births |
| **Etiology** | Congenital |
| **Associated conditions** | Hydrocephalus<br>Neurologic impairment<br>Scoliosis<br>Vertebral abnormalities<br>Arnold Chiari malformation |

---

## ANESTHETIC CONSIDERATIONS

### PREOPERATIVE

Myelomeningoceles are congenital abnormalities of the spinal cord which result in a saccular protrusion near the base of the spine. The sac, containing neural elements and fluid (most often CSF), can vary in size from very small to occupying the whole lower spinal region. The diagnosis may be suspected by fetal ultrasound, and is confirmed at birth. It is generally believed that immediate removal of the sac and covering of the defect with skin is desirable to avoid rupture of the sac and contamination of the spinal cord. Hence, these newborns are usually brought to surgery within 24 hours of birth. Usually they do not have other important neurological deficits.

| | |
|---|---|
| **Neurological** | Although difficult to assess at this age, newborns may have motor and/or sensory deficits in the anal region or involving the lower extremities. |
| **Laboratory** | None except for routine preop studies. |
| **Premedication** | None necessary. |

### INTRAOPERATIVE

**Anesthetic technique:** GETA.

**Induction** The two most common induction techniques are: (1) Awake intubation of the trachea, followed by induction of GA with halothane, $N_2O$, $O_2$. (2) Induction of anesthesia with halothane, $N_2O$, $O_2$, followed by establishment of iv access, and then ET intubation (3.0-4.0 ETT) with the use of a muscle relaxant (e.g., vecuronium 0.15 mg/kg). Before intubation, administer atropine (0.1-0.2 mg to decrease secretions and prevent reflex bradycardia during manipulation of the airway. Halothane is preferred because it causes less airway irritability, thus allowing for a smoother induction. Verify that tube is endotracheal and not endobronchial. If in doubt, advance tube until it is clearly endobronchial; then, while listening with a stethoscope over the non-ventilated lung, remove it gradually until breath sounds are clearly heard. Tape tube firmly in place at one side of the mouth using benzoin adherent.

**Maintenance** Halothane 1% or less with $N_2O$ or air/$O_2$ mixture to maintain arterial $O_2$ sat at 95-96%. Depending on the duration of operation, additional doses of vecuronium (0.1 mg/kg) may be needed. Maintain a near-normal BP. Maintain normal temperature by keeping OR warm (78°F) and using warming lights as needed. Ventilation is controlled to maintain $PETCO_2$=35-40 mmHg with a mechanical ventilator, or manually from the start of anesthesia until surgical wound is closed.

**Emergence** The ETT is removed at the conclusion of the anesthetic. The newborn is nursed in the prone or lateral positions for the first few days postop.

| | | |
|---|---|---|
| **Blood and fluid requirements** | IV: 22-24 ga x 1<br>D5 1/4 NS @ 4 cc/kg/hr<br>Warm fluids. | Administer crystalloid, usually D5 1/4 NS via a measured volume system (Volutrol®, continuous infusion pump, etc.). Blood is rarely, if ever, necessary. |
| **Monitoring** | Standard monitors (see Appendix). | |
| **Positioning** | ✓ and pad pressure points.<br>✓ eyes. | Prone with shoulders and hips on bolsters to elevate abdomen off operating table. Head turned to the side which results in the tube being furthest from the bed. ✓ tube placement by listening to breath sounds after positioning. |

### POSTOPERATIVE

**Complications** CSF leak
Hydrocephalus

**Pain management** Parenteral opiates (see Appendix).

**References**

1. Reigel DH: Spinal bifida. In *Pediatric Neurosurgery: Surgery of the Developing Nervous System.* McLaurin R, Epstein F, eds. Grune & Stratton, New York; 1982, 23-48.

# SURGICAL CORRECTION OF SPINAL DYSRAPHISM

## SURGICAL CONSIDERATIONS

**Description:** Various congenital deformities of the spine classified as spinal dysraphism include: lipoma of the filum, lipomyelomeningocele, tethered spinal cord, diastematomyelia. Each of these conditions involve some sort of tethering of the spinal cord that can cause progressive neurologic dysfunction and/or pain over time. Often a prophylactic operation is advisable, even if the condition is diagnosed in an asymptomatic patient. The procedure involves a **laminectomy** type of approach (see "Lumbar Laminectomy"), exposing the defect, which has been imaged preop by appropriate radiologic studies. The cord is untethered by careful dissection of the neural structure from the offending structure. In the case of lipoma of the filum or simple tethering of the cord 2° a thick or fat filum terminale, it may only be necessary to incise the filum. In the case of lipomyelomeningocele, there is a bone or cartilaginous spicule within the spinal canal which usually splits the spinal cord into two hemi-cords. The spicule is resected and the cords are untethered in the process. In the case of the lipomyelomeningocele, the surgeon debulks the mass of fat which usually is contiguous from the subcutaneous tissues through the fascial planes, through a defect in the spinal canal (spina bifida) and dura, attaching itself to the spinal cord. The cord is freed through careful dissection of the fat mass. The surgeon must be careful not to sacrifice any of the nerve roots which traverse the most dependent portion of the lipoma toward the exiting root sleeves. The operating microscope and a $CO_2$ laser are often useful. A dural graft is required to close the defect created by the lipoma.

**Usual preop diagnosis:** Tethered spinal cord; fat filum terminale; lipomyelomeningocele; lipoma of the filum; diastematomyelia; spinal dysraphism

### SUMMARY OF PROCEDURE

| | |
|---|---|
| **Position** | Prone |
| **Incision** | Posterior midline centered over abnormality |
| **Special instrumentation** | Operating microscope; laser |
| **Unique considerations** | Blood replacement with loss of significant amount of blood in the infant |
| **Antibiotics** | Cefotetan (25-30 mg/kg iv) and vancomycin (13-15 mg/kg iv slowly), appropriate for weight |
| **Surgical time** | 1.5 - 5 hrs (longer for diastematomyelia and lipomyelomeningocele) |
| **Closing considerations** | Surgeon often wants to test integrity of dural closure with Valsalva maneuver: sustained (10-20 sec) inspiratory pressure at 20-40 cm $H_2O$. |
| **EBL** | 5-100 cc |
| **Postop care** | Patient often kept flat postop to protect dural closure. |
| **Mortality** | < 3% |
| **Morbidity** | Infection<br>Neurological<br>Aseptic meningitis<br>CSF leak<br>Massive blood loss |
| **Procedure code** | 61712 (microscopic); 63200 (untethering of cord); 63265-63273 (excision of lesion other than neoplasm) |
| **Pain score** | 3-5 |

### PATIENT POPULATION CHARACTERISTICS

| | |
|---|---|
| **Age range** | 3 mo - 15 yrs |
| **Male:Female** | ~1:1 |
| **Incidence** | Uncommon |
| **Etiology** | Congenital |
| **Associated conditions** | Ankle/foot deformity (size discrepancy)<br>Neurologic impairment<br>Scoliosis<br>Vertebral abnormalities<br>VACTERL association<br>Cutaneous anomaly over spine |

## ANESTHETIC CONSIDERATIONS

### PREOPERATIVE

A variety of spinal abnormalities fall under the category of spinal dysraphism, the most common being a tethered cord or a lipoma of the spinal cord. In the case of the tethered cord, there is usually a history of myelomeningocele repair at birth. Most patients range from 3-16 years of age.

| | |
|---|---|
| **Neurological** | Presenting Sx are usually those of pain in the lower back radiating into the legs and/or progressively worsening motor or sensory deficits in the anal region or involving the lower extremities (document carefully). |
| **Musculoskeletal** | Lower extremity sensory or motor deficits may be present and should be carefully documented. |
| **Renal** | Renal function may be impaired in patients with Hx of recurrent UTIs.<br>**Tests:** UA; BUN; Cr; others as indicated from H&P. |
| **Laboratory** | Other tests as indicated from H&P. |
| **Premedication** | For children, midazolam 0.5 mg/kg po generally provides satisfactory preop sedation after ~30 min. For young children (< 5 yrs) refusing po meds, instillation of midazolam 0.3 mg/kg intranasally provides rapid amnesia, sedation and easy separation from the parents. |

## INTRAOPERATIVE

**Anesthetic technique:** GETA.

**Induction** The two most common induction techniques are: (1) Standard induction (see Appendix). (2) Inhalation induction with halothane, $N_2O$, $O_2$, followed by establishment of iv access, and then ET intubation (3.0-4.0 ETT) with the use of a muscle relaxant (e.g., vecuronium 0.15 mg/kg). Before intubation, administer atropine (0.1-0.2 mg) to decrease secretions and prevent reflex bradycardia during manipulation of the airway. Halothane is preferred because it causes less airway irritability, thus allowing for a smoother induction. Following orotracheal intubation, make certain that the tube is endotracheal and not endobronchial. If in doubt, and the ETT is uncuffed, advance the tube until it is clearly endobronchial; then, while listening with a stethoscope over the non-ventilated lung, remove it gradually until breath sounds are clearly heard. If the ETT is cuffed, palpate the cuff in the sternal notch. Tape the tube firmly in place at one side of the mouth using benzoin adherent.

**Maintenance** Standard maintenance (see Appendix). Depending on the duration of operation, additional doses of vecuronium (0.1 mg/kg) may be needed. Ventilation is controlled to maintain $ETCO_2$=35-40 mmHg with a mechanical ventilator or manually from the start of anesthesia until the surgical wound is closed. Upon completion of placement of the dural graft, and before closure of the wound, the surgeon will want to check the integrity of the graft to eliminate any CSF leaks. The surgeon will ask that positive pressure be applied to the airway to at least 20 cm $H_2O$ for 10-20 sec. If graft leaks are detected, they will be repaired and the test repeated.

**Emergence** The ETT is removed at the conclusion of the anesthetic. The patient is nursed flat in the prone or lateral position for the first few days postop to lessen the chance of a CSF leak developing.

| | | |
|---|---|---|
| **Blood and fluid requirements** | IV: 18-20 ga x 1<br>NS/LR @ 4-6 cc/kg/hr | In children, administer fluids via a measured volume system (Volutrol®, continuous infusion pump, etc.) Blood is rarely, if ever, necessary. |
| **Monitoring** | Standard monitors (see Appendix).<br>± UO<br>± Foley catheter | If the operation is anticipated to last several hours, a Foley catheter should be inserted. |
| **Positioning** | ✓ and pad pressure points.<br>✓ eyes. | Prone with the shoulders and hips on bolsters to elevate the abdomen off the operating table. Head turned to the side, resulting in the tube being furthest from bed. ✓ tube placement by listening to breath sounds after positioning. |
| **Complications** | Severe bradycardia | Manipulation of the spinal cord may produce ↓↓HR reflexly. |

## POSTOPERATIVE

| | | |
|---|---|---|
| **Complications** | Possible neurological deficits<br>Infection<br>CSF leak | Major complications from this operation are uncommon, but include new neurological deficits from irritation of the spinal cord during surgery, localized infection and CSF leak from the wound site. |
| **Pain management** | Parental opiates or PCA (see Appendix). | |

**References**


1. Reigel DH: Sacral agenesis and diastematomyelia. In *Pediatric Neurosurgery: Surgery of the Developing Nervous System.* McLaurin R, Epstein F, eds. Grune & Stratton, New York: 1982, 79-90.
2. Pang D: Tethered cord syndrome: newer concepts. In *Neurosurgery Update II.* Wilkins RH, Rengachary SS, eds. McGraw-Hill, New York: 1991, 336-44.
3. Oakes WJ: Management of spinal cord lipomas and lipomyelomeningoceles. In *Neurosurgery Update II.* Wilkins RH, Rengachary S, eds. McGraw-Hill, New York: 1991, 345-52.

# CRANIOTOMY FOR VEIN OF GALEN ANEURYSM

## SURGICAL CONSIDERATIONS

**Description:** A vein of Galen aneurysm is a large, arteriovenous fistula between arteries of the posterior cerebral circulation and a massively enlarged vein of Galen (deep venous drainage of the brain). Patients can present with CHF (infants), hydrocephalus (infants, children, adults) or intracranial hemorrhage (adults).

Treatment is directed at staged occlusion of the arterial feeders to the arteriovenous fistula and thrombosis of the fistula itself from the venous side, using open microsurgical techniques, endovascular methods, or both. With reduction of aneurysmal flow, CO will decrease with ↑SVR and ↓mixed venous $PO_2$. **Subtemporal, midline occipital** or **bilateral occipital craniotomies** can be used to isolate and occlude arterial feeders to the vein of Galen aneurysm. Sometimes a **burr hole** is placed over the torcula (confluence of venous sinuses) for direct retrograde placement of thrombogenic coils into the arteriovenous fistula.

**Usual preop diagnosis:** Vein of Galen aneurysm, intracranial hemorrhage, hydrocephalus, progressive neurologic deficits

### SUMMARY OF PROCEDURE

| | |
|---|---|
| **Position** | Lateral decubitus, Concorde (modified prone), or semi-sitting; for burr-hole, lateral |
| **Incision** | Temporal or occipital; for burr-hole, occipital |
| **Special instrumentation** | Operating microscope, microscopic instruments; intraop angiography; for burr-hole, endovascular catheters and equipment |
| **Unique considerations** | Careful attention to blood loss in infants |
| **Antibiotics** | Vancomycin (1 gm iv slowly q 12 hrs for adults; 10-15 mg/kg iv slowly q 6 hrs for children); cefotaxime (1 gm iv q 6 hrs for adults; 40 mg/kg iv q 6 hrs for children) |
| **Surgical time** | 3 - 5 hrs |
| **Closing considerations** | Meticulous hemostasis; avoid hypotension or HTN (MAP 80-90 adults, 70-80 children). |
| **EBL** | < 250 cc |
| **Postop care** | Monitor for ↑ICP (using ventricular or subdural catheters) as a result of venous HTN 2° with rapid occlusion of arteriovenous fistula. ICU: 1-3 d. |
| **Mortality** | Approaches 100% if in CHF |
| **Morbidity** | Deep venous infarct: 5-10%<br>Hydrocephalus<br>Stroke<br>Subdural hygroma<br>Infection: Rare |
| **Procedure code** | 61686 (infratentorial, complex craniotomy); 61712 (microdissection); 61710 (intra-arterial embolization) |
| **Pain score** | 3-4 |

### PATIENT POPULATION CHARACTERISTICS

| | |
|---|---|
| **Age range** | 1 mo-3 yrs (typically) |
| **Male:Female** | 1:1 |
| **Incidence** | Rare |
| **Etiology** | Congenital |
| **Associated conditions** | Other intracranial vascular malformations<br>High-output CHF |

# ANESTHETIC CONSIDERATIONS

## PREOPERATIVE

Vein of Galen aneurysms are rare congenital abnormalities representing less than 1% of all aneurysms.[5] They are usually diagnosed in infants because they cause an abnormal increase in head size due to the aneurysmal dilatation and obstruction of the dural sinus. The abnormal vasculature constitutes a high-flow shunt, much like an arteriovenous malformation (AVM). If left untreated, the morbidity and mortality are high; however, treatment with radiologic embolization and/or surgical excision is also associated with high morbidity and mortality rates.

**Cardiovascular** Because these lesions constitute high-flow shunts through the brain, the infants are prone to develop CHF, which is fatal in more than 40% of patients.

**Neurological** Infants usually present with an abnormal head size, seizure disorder or bizarre neurological signs such as high-pitched crying, posturing, failure to eat or thrive, etc.

**Laboratory** CT; MRI; cerebral angiography. The infant may need sedation and anesthetic management to obtain adequate diagnostic studies.

**Premedication** None

## INTRAOPERATIVE

**Anesthetic technique:** GETA. The goals are the same as those for intracranial vascular malformations.

**Induction** Whenever possible, an intravenous induction is preferred. Thiopental 2-3 mg/kg, fentanyl 2-3 μg/kg, and vecuronium or atracurium, 0.1 mg/kg, are satisfactory induction agents.

**Maintenance** Thiopental ≤ 5 mg/kg, fentanyl ≤ 5 μg/kg, isoflurane ≤ 1% with $N_2O$ or air 60-70% to keep $O_2$ sat of 95-98%. Additional doses or non-depolarizing neuromuscular blocking drug may be administered as needed to maintain a single twitch response to nerve stimulation.

**Emergence** Plan to leave ETT in place for at least 24 hrs postop; infant should receive controlled ventilation and sedation during that interval. If infant does not show evidence of serious neurological injury postop, the ETT may be removed within 1-2 d.

| | | |
|---|---|---|
| **Blood and fluid requirements** | IV: 20-22 ga x 1-2<br>20-ga CVP, either IJ or subclavian | Replace blood as it is lost. Limit crystalloid fluid therapy to no more than 10 ml/kg above UO. |
| **Control of brain volume** | Same as for intracranial vascular malformations | |
| **Monitoring** | Same as for intracranial vascular malformations | |
| **Control of BP** | Goal = normal range for age<br>Neonate: 55-70/40 (HR 180)<br>1 yr: 70-100/60 (HR 140) | BP should be kept in the normal range for the infant with close monitoring from an arterial catheter. If HR becomes excessive, esmolol infusion is useful. |
| **Positioning** | Same as for intracranial vascular malformations | |
| **Complications** | Coagulopathy | If large volumes of blood are needed, a coagulopathy may ensue. Monitoring of coagulation status during surgery may be necessary. |
| | Hypothermia | Once the aneurysm is surgically corrected, immediate efforts must be made to return infant to a normal body temperature by the conclusion of the operation. |

## POSTOPERATIVE

| | |
|---|---|
| **Complications** | Neurological deficits<br>Intracranial hemorrhage<br>Heart failure |
| **Pain management** | Codeine 1-1.5 mg/kg im |
| **Tests** | Same as for intracranial vascular malformations |

**References**

1. Schmidek HH, Sweet WH, eds: *Operative Neurosurgical Techniques, Indications, Methods, Results*, Vol I - II. Grune & Stratton, Orlando: 1988.
2. Youmans JR, ed: *Neurological Surgery*, Vol 1-6. WB Saunders Co, Philadelphia: 1990.
3. Wilkins RL, Rengachary SS, eds: *Neurosurgery*, Vol 1-3. McGraw-Hill, New York: 1985.
4. Ojemann RG, Heros RC, Crowell RM: *Surgical Management of Cerebrovascular Disease*. Williams & Wilkins, Baltimore: 1988.
5. Lasjaunias P, Rodesch G, Pruvost P, Laroche FG, Landrieu P: Treatment of vein of Galen aneurysmal malformation. *J Neurosurg* 1989; 70(5):746-50.

**Surgeon**

**Lawrence A. Rinsky, MD**

## 12.4 PEDIATRIC ORTHOPEDIC SURGERY

**Anesthesiologist**

**Yuan-Chi Lin, MD, MPH**

# POSTERIOR SPINAL INSTRUMENTATION AND FUSION

## SURGICAL CONSIDERATIONS

**Description:** Posterior spinal instrumentation refers to implanted metal rods affixed to the spine to correct and internally splint the deformed spine. Originally designed for scoliosis, posterior spinal instrumentation is commonly performed simultaneously with spinal fusion for a variety of diagnoses including fracture, tumor, degenerative changes and developmental spinal deformity. The original **Harrington rod** is the simplest, and still considered by many to be "the gold standard."[1,3,4,6,7,10] The spine is approached by an extensive midline posterior incision in which a subperiosteal exposure (typically T2-5 down to L1-4) is used to elevate all the paraspinous muscles as far laterally as the tips of the transverse processes. One hook is placed at each end of the curve on the concave side and anchored by slipping the hook foot into the spinal canal (Fig 12.4-1). A ratcheted single rod is attached to the two hooks, and jacked into distraction, thus straightening out the concavity.

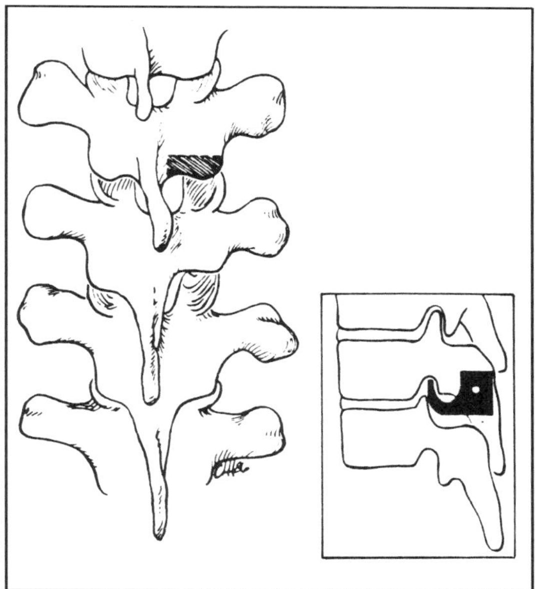

**Figure 12.4-1.** Placement of Harrington upper hook. (Reproduced with permission from Chapman MW, ed: *Operative Orthopaedics*, 2nd edition. JB Lippincott: 1993.)

Although excellent correction of moderate curves with Harrington instrumentation is possible, the ratchets are a weak point, and the presence of only two fixation points (the hooks) on the spine leaves a risk of hook dislodgement or fracturing of the laminae; thus, usually an extensive postop body case is required. To improve the fixation, many have added sublaminar wire loops[4,9-13] (Fig 12.4-2) at multiple levels (the **"Harri-Luque"**), or switched to two non-ratcheted, L-shaped rods with multiple sublaminar wires at each spinal level (**Luque rods**) (Fig 12.4-3). Others, fearful of the neurologic risks[14] caused by the sublaminar wires, have used supplemental wires passed through the base of the spinous processes.[5] This additional fixation eliminates the need for a cast, but a postop brace still is often used. The Luque rod system is most commonly used in scoliosis of neuromuscular etiology.

A more recent addition to posterior spinal instrumentation is the **Cotrel-Dubousset**[1,28] **system** in which multiple hooks are placed along bilateral rods. Hooks in this system can affix to the pedicles, laminae, or even transverse processes. Typically, 4-8 hooks are placed on each rod, with each hook affixed to some posterior element. By compressing along the convex surfaces, and distracting along the concave surfaces, some degree of even rotational correction is possible. This system is by far the most complex, but offers theoretic advantages in the possibility of a three-dimensional correction.

**Usual preop diagnosis**: Scoliosis (lateral deviation of the spine, usually idiopathic or neuromuscular); kyphosis (increased round back); reconstruction for tumor, trauma, etc.

### SUMMARY OF PROCEDURE

| | Harrington Rod | Luque Procedure or "Harri-Luque" | Cotrel-Dubousset |
|---|---|---|---|
| **Position** | Prone (on spinal frame or bolsters); avoid abdominal compression. | ⇐ | ⇐ |
| **Incision** | Posterior midline; optional separate iliac crest bone graft | ⇐ | ⇐ |
| **Special instrumentation** | Rods and hooks | Rods, wires and hooks | Rods, multiple hooks, hook connectors, transverse bars |
| **Unique considerations** | "Wake up" test and/or SSEPs. Frequently induced hypotension is requested. | ⇐ | ⇐ |
| **Antibiotics** | Cefazolin 1-2 gm iv | ⇐ | ⇐ |

| | Harrington Rod | Luque Procedure | Cotrel-Dubousset |
|---|---|---|---|
| **Surgical time** | 2 - 6 hrs | 3 - 7 hrs | ⇐ |
| **Closing considerations** | Greatest blood loss typically toward the end of procedure. | ⇐ | ⇐ |
| | Avoid hypotension after instrumentation is implanted. | ⇐ | ⇐ |
| **EBL** | 800-1500 cc | 1200-4000 cc | 1200-3000 cc |
| **Postop care** | ICU: 1-3 d | ⇐ | ⇐ |
| **Mortality**[1-7] | 0-0.5% | ⇐ | ⇐ |
| **Morbidity**[3-7,11-13] | Acute ileus: Very common | ⇐ | ⇐ |
| | Hook dislodgement requiring re-operation: 0-2% | 0-0.1% | 1% |
| | Wound infection: 0-2% | ⇐ | ⇐ |
| | Genitourinary infection: 5-7% | ⇐ | ⇐ |
| | Hematoma, massive bleeding: 1-5% | ⇐ | ⇐ |
| | Pneumothorax, pneumonia, atelectasis, etc: 1-5% | ⇐ | ⇐ |
| | Spinal cord injury: 0.23% | 0.86% | 0.6% |
| | Superior mesenteric syndrome: 0-1% | ⇐ | ⇐ |
| | Thromboembolism: < 1% | ⇐ | ⇐ |
| | Delayed: | | |
| | Pseudarthrosis: 0-5% | ⇐ | ⇐ |
| | Late rod fracture: 0-5% | ⇐ | ⇐ |
| | Decompensation: 0-2% | < 1% | Coronal decompensation: 0-5% |
| **Procedure code** | 22840 | 22842 | 22[illegible]42 |
| **Pain score** | 7-9 | 7-9 | 7-9 |

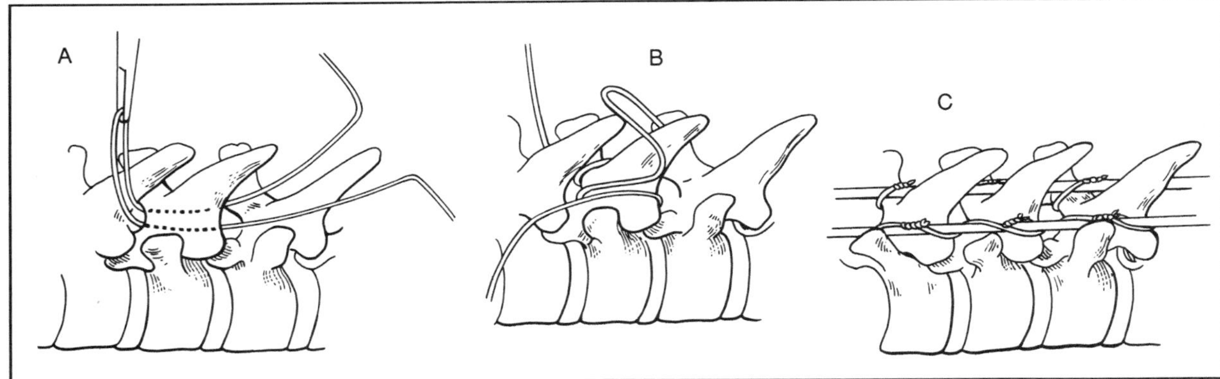


**Figure 12.4-2.** An example of passing and attaching sublaminar wires. (Reproduced with permission from Chapman MW, ed: *Operative Orthopaedics*, 2nd edition. JB Lippincott: 1993.)

## PATIENT POPULATION CHARACTERISTICS

| | |
|---|---|
| **Age range** | Usually 8-40 yrs |
| **Male:Female** | 1:5 |
| **Incidence** | 1:2/10,000 |
| **Etiology** | Idiopathic: 50-75% |
| | Neuromuscular: 20-30% |
| | Associated with syndromes such as osteocondyle dystrophies, osteogenesis imperfecta, etc: 5% |
| | Congenital scoliosis: 2-5% |

**Associated conditions**

Neuromuscular:
- Freidrich's ataxia (myocarditis and other cardiovascular anomalies; sudden death)
- Myelomeningocele
- Muscular dystrophy (muscle weakness, cardiomyopathy, dysrhythmias, succinylcholine → prolonged muscle contraction, ↑ sensitivity to respiratory depressant effect of barbiturates, opiates and benzodiazepines)
- Cerebral palsy
- GE reflux, ↓airway protective reflexes, ↑postop pulmonary complications
- Spina bifida
- Abnormalities of the spinal cord, e.g., tethered spinal cord, syringomyelia

Connective tissue disease:
- Ehlers-Danlos and Marfan syndrome – avoid ↑BP → aortic dissection; ↑risk of pneumothorax
- Osteogenesis imperfecta – position and intubate with great care.
- Congenital osteochondral dystrophies
- Dwarfing syndromes

CHD: 1-4%
- Coarctation: 0.5%
- Cyanotic CHD: 14%

MVP: 25% (avoid ↑LV emptying; consider antibiotics preop) cerebral palsy

Malignant hyperthermia (MH) risk

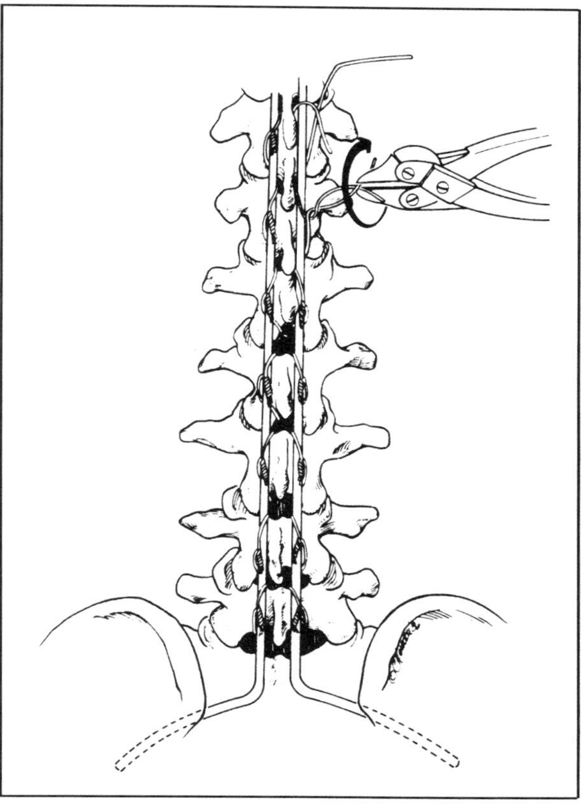

**Figure 12.4-3.** Positioning rods in pelvis; sublaminar wires being tightened. (Reproduced with permission from Chapman MW, ed: *Operative Orthopaedics*, 2nd edition. JB Lippincott: 1993.)

## ANESTHETIC CONSIDERATIONS

See "Anesthetic Considerations for Spinal Reconstruction and Fusion" following "Anterior Spinal Fusion for Scoliosis with Instrumentation" (below).

**References**


1. Akbarnia BA: Selection of methodology in surgical treatment of adolescent idiopathic scoliosis. *Orthop Clin North Am* 1988; 19(2):319-29.
2. Denis F: Cotrel-Dubousset instrumentation in the treatment of idiopathic scoliosis. *Orthop Clin North Am* 1988; 19(2):291-311.
3. Dickson JH, Harrington PR: The evolution of the Harrington instrumentation technique in scoliosis. *J Bone Joint Surg* [Am] 1973; 55(5):993-1002.
4. Dickson RA, Archer IA: Surgical treatment of late-onset idiopathic thoracic scoliosis. The Leeds procedure. *J Bone Joint Surg* [Br] 1987; 69(5):709-14.
5. Drummond DS, Guadagni J, Keene JS, Breed A, Narechania R: Interspinous process segmental spinal instrumentation. *J Pediatr Orthop* 1984; 4(4):397-404.
6. Dickson JH: An eleven-year clinical investigation of Harrington instrumentation. A preliminary report on 578 cases. *Clin Orthop* 1973; 93:113-30.
7. Lovallo JL, Banta JV, Renshaw TS: Adolescent idiopathic scoliosis treated by Harrington-rod distraction and fusion. *J Bone Joint Surg* [Am] 1986; 68(9):1326-30.
8. Lenke LG, Bridwell KH, Baldus C, Blanke K, Schoenecker PL: Cotrel-Dubousset instrumentation for adolescent idiopathic scoliosis. *J Bone Joint Surg* [Am] 1992; 74(7):1056-67.

9. Luque ER: *Segmental Spinal Instrumentation.* Slack Thorofare, NJ: 1984; 31-165.
10. Morrissy RT: *Atlas of Pediatric Orthopaedic Surgery.* JB Lippincott, Philadelphia: 1992; 1-57.
11. Rinsky LA, Gamble JG: personal series.
12. Silverman BJ, Greenberg PE: Idiopathic scoliosis posterior spine fusion with Harrington rod and sublaminar wiring. *Orthop Clin North Am* 1988; 19(2):269-79.
13. Sullivan JA, Conner SB: Comparison of Harrington instrumentation and segmental spinal instrumentation in the management of neuromuscular spine deformity. *Spine* 1982; 7(3):299-301.
14. Wilber RG, Thompson GH, Shaffer JW, Brown RH, Nash CL Jr: Postoperative neurological deficits in segmental spinal instrumentation. A study using spinal cord monitoring. *J Bone Joint Surg* [Am] 1984; 66(8):1178-87.


# ANTERIOR SPINAL FUSION FOR SCOLIOSIS, WITH INSTRUMENTATION

## SURGICAL CONSIDERATIONS

**Description**: Anterior spinal fusion is performed through a transthoracic and/or retroperitoneal approach to the vertebral bodies in which the intervertebral discs are removed and a bone graft placed between the vertebral bodies.[1-8] The disc removal ("release") loosens the spine and allows greater deformity correction than posterior-only procedures. It is often performed as a first stage to a "front-and-back" fusion, but may be performed alone, especially in cases of idiopathic lumbar scoliosis. **Dwyer** originated the technique[2] (1969) using a braided titanium cable through the screw heads, which are then crimped onto the cable (Fig 12.4-4). Although the correction is usually dramatic, the cable is not rigid and may decrease normal lumbar lordosis. **Zielke** (1976) exchanged the cable for a threaded rod with nuts holding the rod into slots in the screw head (Fig 12.4-5). The use of nuts allows a gradual controlled correction and a better lordosis control with at least some rigidity from the rod, but a slight increase in the "fiddle factor."[1,7] The procedure also may be performed without anterior instrumentation as a simple anterior release, normally followed by a posterior spinal fusion and instrumentation.[2-4]

The **Zielke procedure** is generally favored, especially if posterior spinal instrumentation is not otherwise needed. The approach is through a flank incision, then through a rib bed on the convex side (usually the 10th rib). The retroperitoneal plane is entered and developed by blunt dissection behind the transversus abdominis muscle. The pleural cavity is then entered, and the diaphragm usually must be divided circumferentially near its costal origin and around posteriorly to the spine. The prevertebral areolar plane is then entered and the segmental vessels to each vertebral body are clipped or cauterized in the midline. The psoas muscle is elevated off the lateral aspects of the vertebral bodies. Each disc in the fusion area (usually 3-5 discs) is then excised back to the posterior

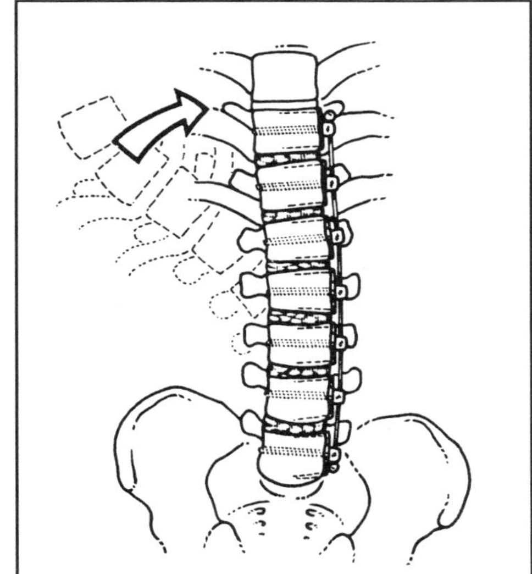

Figure 12.4-4. Dwyer instrumentation used to make spinal correction. (Reproduced with permission from Crenshaw AH, ed: *Campbell's Operative Orthopaedics*, 8th edition. Mosby-Year Book: 1992.)

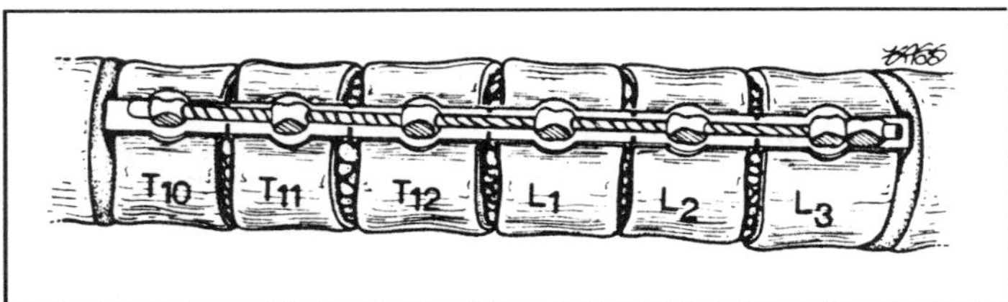


**Figure 12.4-5.** Instrumentation from T10-L3. (Reproduced with permission from Chapman MW, ed: *Operative Orthopaedics*, 2nd edition. JB Lippincott: 1993.)

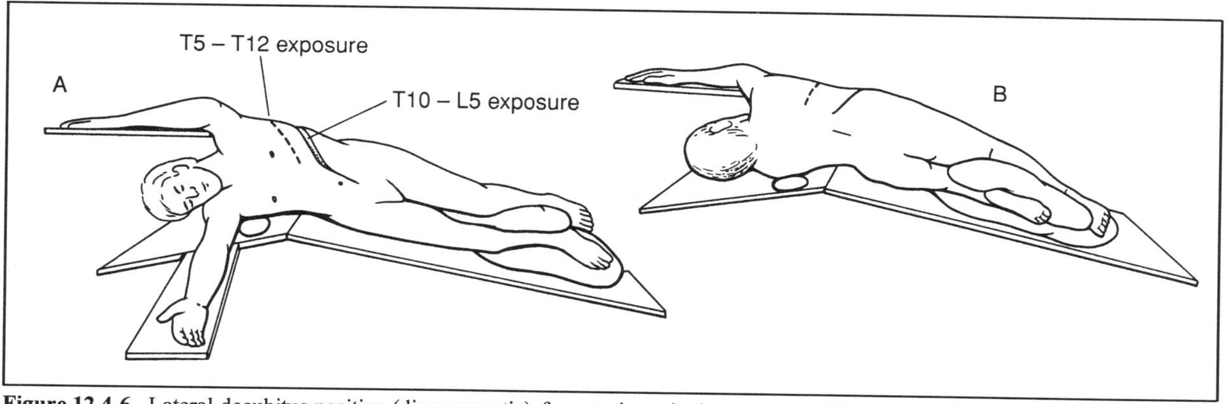


**Figure 12.4-6.** Lateral decubitus position (diagrammatic) for anterior spinal procedures: (A) anterior view; (B) posterior view. Roll is placed under axilla to minimize axillary artery compression. Skin incision for exposure of T5-T12 is shown with the dotted line. (Reproduced with permission from Chapman MW, ed: *Operative Orthopaedics*, 2nd edition. JB Lippincott: 1993.)

longitudinal ligament. Next, vertebral screws are inserted transversely across the appropriate bodies and joined at their heads by the Dwyer cable or Zielke rod. Compression is applied through the cable or rod, while the previously flexed OR table is slowly and gradually straightened. It is critical that the anesthesiologist straighten the table with great care to avoid excessive stress on the implants. Prior to closure of the disc spaces, bone graft is placed anteriorly to maintain lordosis.

**Usual preop diagnosis**: Scoliosis >45°; idiopathic or neuromuscular

**SUMMARY OF PROCEDURE**

| | Dwyer | Zielke | Release (No Instrumentation) |
|---|---|---|---|
| **Position** | Full lateral decubitus (Fig 12.4-6) | ⇐ | ⇐ |
| **Incision** | Flank: over rib at top vertebra in the curve (usually T9-T11) | ⇐ | ⇐ |
| **Special instrumentation** | Screws, staples, cable, crimper; DLT | Screws, staples, threaded rod, nuts; DLT | DLT |
| **Unique considerations** | OR table must be "broken" into flexed mode at start, then straightened after discs are removed to aid in reduction. Procedure often followed by posterior spinal fusion, sometimes on same day.[8] Proximity of great vessels, major bleeding a potential problem, although not common.[2,4-8] Patients with neuromuscular scoliosis often have poor generalized nutrition. Opening and closing sometimes performed by a separate team of general surgeons. Evoked cortical potentials often used to monitor spinal cord function. | ⇐ | ⇐ Uninstrumented release is always followed by posterior spinal fusion and usually instrumentation.[2,4] |
| **Antibiotics** | Cefazolin 25 mg/kg iv always used. | ⇐ | ⇐ |

| | Dwyer | Zielke | Release |
|---|---|---|---|
| **Surgical time** | 4 - 7 hrs | ⇐ | 3 - 6 hrs |
| **Closing considerations** | Chest tube always used; hypotension, if used electively, must be reversed before closure. | ⇐ | ⇐ |
| **EBL** | 500-3000 cc | ⇐ | 250-2000 cc |
| **Postop care** | ICU 2-4 d | ⇐ | ⇐ |
| **Mortality** | 0-2%, depending on underlying conditions[4,8] | ⇐ | ⇐ |
| **Morbidity** | Overall: 30% (significant problem or complication, depending on underlying condition[1-8] | ⇐ | 20% |
| | Ileus and atelectasis: ~ 50% | ⇐ | ⇐ |
| | Urinary tract infection: 10-25% (common in spina bifida) | ⇐ | ⇐ |
| | Minor transient root weakness, or paraesthesia: 10-20% | ⇐ | 1-5% |
| | Late kyphosis above instrumentation: 5-10% | ⇐ | ⇐ |
| | Nonunion and hardware failure: 5% | ⇐ | ⇐ |
| | Massive blood loss: 2-5% | ⇐ | ⇐ |
| | Respiratory failure: 1-2% | ⇐ | ⇐ |
| | Pneumonia: 1% | ⇐ | ⇐ |
| | Paraplegia (acute anterior spinal artery syndrome): < 1% | ⇐ | ⇐ |
| | Thromboembolism: Rare (< 5% in children) | ⇐ | ⇐ |
| **Procedure code** | 22845, 22810 | ⇐ | 22810 |
| **Pain score** | 5-8 | 5-8 | 4-7 |

## PATIENT POPULATION CHARACTERISTICS

| | |
|---|---|
| **Age range** | 5-35 yrs |
| **Male:Female** | Idiopathic: 1:10<br>Neuromuscular: 1:1 |
| **Incidence** | < 0.1/1000 |
| **Etiology** | Idiopathic scoliosis<br>Neuromuscular disease (especially cerebral palsy, spina bifida, polio, myopathies, muscular dystrophies)<br>Other genetic dysplasias of bone<br>Marfan syndrome (occasionally) |
| **Associated conditions** | Idiopathic: generally healthy<br>Cerebral palsy patients often retarded, often with poor general health<br>Spina bifida: usually with hydrocephalus and chronic urinary tract infection<br>Myopathy: malignant hyperthermia susceptible<br>Chronic restrictive lung disease in severe cases<br>Extremity contractures may make positioning difficult<br>Muscular dystrophy patients may have cardiomyopathy |

# ANESTHETIC CONSIDERATIONS FOR SPINAL RECONSTRUCTION AND FUSION

**(Procedures covered: anterior and posterior spinal reconstruction and fusion: thoracic, thorocolumbar and lumbar [Zielke, Dwyer, Harrington, Luque or Cotrel-Dubousset instrumentation])**

## PREOPERATIVE

Patients presenting for spinal reconstruction most commonly will have either idiopathic or acquired scoliosis. Scoliosis is a complex deformity involving both lateral curvature and rotation of the spine, as well as an associated deformity of the rib cage. Types of scoliosis include: idiopathic, congenital, neuromuscular, myopathic, trauma, tumor-related and mesenchenchymal disorders. The majority of cases are idiopathic, and the male:female ratio is 1:4. Normally, the cervical spine and lumbar spine are lordotic, while the thoracic spine is kyphotic. Surgery is indicated when the curvature is severe (angulation beyond 40° in the thoracic or lumbar spine[10]) or progressing rapidly. Non-scoliotic patients presenting for this surgery may have spinal instability as a result of trauma, metastatic carcinoma or infection (e.g., TB). These patients are usually healthy apart from their underlying pathology. The patients with disseminated lung or breast cancer may need a careful workup with regard to respiratory, nutritional and chemotherapeutic status. (See Anesthetic Considerations for "Lobectomy, Pneumonectomy" or "Mastectomy.")

**Respiratory** Respiratory impairment proportional to angle of lateral curvature (Fig 12.4-2)[11]

| Cobb Angle | 30° - 60° | 60° - 90° | >90° |
|---|---|---|---|
| VC | ↓25% | ↓50% | ↓70% |
| TLC | ↓27% | ↓37% | ↓50% |

Restrictive pattern: ↓TLC + ↓↓VC
-If VC >70% predicted, respiratory reserve is adequate.
-If VC < 40% predicted, postop ventilation usually is required.
Expect further significant (~40%) ↓VC immediately postop requiring 7-10 d to resolve.
↑RR + ↓TV → ↑dead space + ↓alveolar ventilation → V/Q mismatch → hypoxemia.[12]
**Tests:** CXR; ABG; PFT; assess exercise tolerance by Hx.

**Cardiovascular** ↑PVR (**NB**: independent of severity of scoliosis). High incidence of CHD and mitral valve prolapse.
**Tests:** ECG; ECHO – consult cardiologist if apical systolic murmur or other evidence of cardiovascular impairment is present.[13]

**Neurological** Some surgeons may request that the patient be awakened intraop to test anterior (motion) cord function. Practice wakeup testing preop to reveal any baseline deficits and reassure the patient that no pain will be felt during intraop testing. Tuberculous spondylitis (Pott's disease) frequently presents with focal neurological lesions ranging from loss of bowel and bladder control to paraplegia. Careful preop documentation of the neurological status is essential as surgery may worsen these symptoms.

**Musculoskeletal** When the angle of lateral curvature (Cobb angle) of the spine >25°, then the degree of respiratory impairment will be significant and the need for postop ventilatory support becomes more likely. Patients with muscular dystrophy may be more sensitive to myocardial depression from anesthetic agents and also may require postop ventilation 2° muscle weakness. Succinylcholine may cause severe rhabdomyolysis with hyperkalemia. These patients may also be at risk for MH.

**Hematologic** Avoid use of platelet inhibitors for 2-3 wks before surgery. Encourage autologous blood donation. (If Hb >11 gm/dL, may repeat donation q 3-7 d up to 14 d before surgery). Consider use of intraop hemodilution, controlled hypotension and cell-saver devices. Be aware that patients with previously placed spinal support (e.g., Milwaukee brace) for correction of scoliosis may have more blood loss than would otherwise occur.

**Laboratory** Hb/Hct; clotting profile: investigate all abnormalities before surgery. Other tests as indicated from H&P.

**Premedication** Standard premedication (see Appendix) if appropriate.

## INTRAOPERATIVE

**Anesthetic technique** GETA. For pediatric cases, preheat room to 78° F.

**Induction** Standard induction (see Appendix). A DLT may facilitate surgical access in the patient undergoing an anterior correction. The smallest available DLT is size 28 Fr (OD = 8.9 mm) typically suitable for a child aged 12-14 yrs.

| | | |
|---|---|---|
| **Maintenance** | Standard maintenance (see Appendix). It is important to use low concentrations and minimize changes of potent inhalational agents during measurement of SSEPs. Continue muscle relaxation. Droperidol is avoided as its α-blocking effect reduces the effectiveness of the epinephrine injected at the beginning of surgery to reduce incisional bleeding. | |
| **Emergence** | Patients are usually extubated; however, some may require continued intubation and admission to ICU (e.g., preop medical condition or massive intraop blood loss). Careful handling of the patient is necessary during transfer from OR table to bed. | |
| **Blood and fluid requirements** | Anticipate large blood loss.<br>IV: 14-16 ga x 2<br>NS/LR @ 8-10 cc/kg/hr<br>Warm all fluids.<br>Humidify gasses.<br>T&C 2-4 U PRBC. | Blood loss is a major consideration during scoliosis surgery. Profuse bleeding may occur when the erector spinal muscles are stripped and when large areas of cancellous bone are exposed. It may vary from 25%->100% of the patient's blood volume, although blood loss is usually less with the anterior approach (Dwyer's). Consider use of albumin or hetastarch – severe intravascular fluid deficit can be corrected more rapidly with a colloid solution. |
| **Control of blood loss** | Position to prevent venous engorgement.<br>↓MAP to 60-70 mmHg.<br>↓Hct to 25-28%. | Controlled hypotension to MAP = 60-70 mmHg in the fit patient has been shown to dramatically reduce blood loss, although there may be some ↑risk of spinal cord ischemia. In addition, deliberate hemodilution to Hct = 25-28% may prove useful. Maintain UO at 0.5-1.0 cc/kg/hr during controlled hypotension.[14] |
| **Monitoring** | Standard monitors (see Appendix).<br>Arterial line<br>CVP line<br>Urinary catheter<br>± SSEP[15] | Trends in CVP may be more reliable than measurement of UO to assess volume status in patients in the prone or lateral positions. |
| **Positioning** | ✓ eyes, neck.<br>✓and pad pressure points. | Pressure points must be carefully padded and checked frequently, especially during controlled hypotension. |
| **Wakeup test** | 40-60 min advance warning from surgeons is needed.<br>-Decrease inhalational agents.<br>-Reverse muscle relaxants (and narcotics, if necessary).<br>-Monitor train of four.<br>-Request hand squeeze; if present, elicit bilateral foot movement.<br>-Reinduce anesthesia with STP (1 mg/kg).<br>**Dangers:**<br>Air embolus<br>Dislodgement of spinal instrumentation<br>Accidental extubation[16] | Uncontrolled patient movement during wakeup test can result in accidental extubation or dislodgement of the spinal instrumentation. Unrestrained inspiratory efforts may provoke venous air embolism. The anesthesiologist must be prepared to rapidly re-anesthetize patient. |
| **SSEP monitoring** | Dorsal cord function only<br>SSEPs very sensitive to changes in volatile anesthetic in a dose-dependent manner.<br>Use $N_2O$/narcotic anesthetic. | The wakeup test assesses the integrity of motor pathways in the ventral cord. SSEPs are required to test sensory pathways in the dorsal cord. In some centers, SSEPs are followed throughout surgery. The SSEP technician should be informed of changes in the level of anesthesia. |
| **Complications** | Spinal cord ischemia<br>Massive blood loss<br>Fat embolism | SSEP indications of spinal cord ischemia should be treated by restoring normal BP and by decreased cord traction. Prompt transfusion may be necessary and blood should be available in the room (2-4 U PRBC). |

## POSTOPERATIVE

| | | |
|---|---|---|
| **Complications** | Pulmonary insufficiency<br>Hypothermia<br>Pneumothorax<br>Dislodgement of internal fixation | Postop ventilation may be required in patients with severe respiratory impairment (see "Preoperative Considerations," above). In addition, thoracotomy, surgical trauma to the diaphragm and fat embolism may further ↑ the risk of postop pulmonary insufficiency. Careful handling of patient in transfer is mandatory. |
| | Neurologic sequelae | Neurologic sequelae probably remain the most feared complication, and it is important to document postop neurologic exam. |
| **Pain management** | Intrathecal morphine 0.1-0.25 mg by surgeon intraop, dependent on age of child.<br>PCA (see Appendix). | Pain is a significant problem for postop scoliosis patients. Most need analgesia x 3-4 d. Preop consultation with patient (and parents) about different pain management techniques is important. |
| **Tests** | CXR; ABG; Hct | ✓ for pneumothorax and line placement. |

**References**

1. Brown JC, Swank S, Specht L: Combined anterior and posterior spine fusion in cerebral palsy. *Spine* 1982; 7(6):570-3.
2. Chapman MW: *Operative Orthopaedics*, 2nd edition. JB Lippincott, Philadelphia: 1993, 2899-2913.
3. Dwyer AF, Schafer MF: Anterior approach to scoliosis. Results of treatment in fifty-one cases. *J Bone Joint Surg* [Br] 1974; 56(2):218-24.
4. Ferguson RL, Allen BL Jr: Staged correction of neuromuscular scoliosis. *J Pediatr Orthop* 1983; 3:555-62.
5. Floman Y, Penny JN, Micheli LJ, Riseborough EJ, Hall JE: Combined anterior and posterior fusion in seventy-three spinally deformed patients: indications, results and complications. *Clin Orthop* 1982; 164:110-22.
6. McMaster MJ: Anterior and posterior instrumentation and fusion of thoracolumbar scoliosis due to myelomeningocele. *J Bone Joint Surg* [Br] 1987; 69(1):20-5.
7. Morrissy RT: *Atlas of Pediatric Orthopaedic Surgery*. JB Lippincott, Philadelphia: 1992, 75-97.
8. O'Brien JP, Yau AC, Gertzbein S, Hodgson AR: Combined staged anterior and posterior correction and fusion of the spine in scoliosis following poliomyelitis. *Clin Orthop* 1975; 110:81-9.
9. O'Brien T, Akmakjian J, Ogin G, Eilert R: Comparison of one-stage versus two-stage anterior/posterior spinal fusion for neuromuscular scoliosis. *J Pediatr Orthop* 1992; 12(5):610-15.
10. Goldstein LA, Waugh TR: Classification and terminology of scoliosis. *Clin Orthop* 1973; 93:10-22.
11. Smyth RJ, Chapman KR, Wright TA, Crawford JS, Rebuck AS: Pulmonary function in adolescents with mild idiopathic scoliosis. *Thorax* 1984; 39(12):901-4.
12. Smyth RJ, Chapman KR, Wright TA, Crawford JS, Rebuck AS: Ventilatory patterns during hypoxia, hypercapnia, and exercise in adolescents with mild scoliosis. *Pediatrics* 1986; 77(5):692-97.
13. Kafer ER: Respiratory and cardiovascular functions in scoliosis and the principles of anesthetic management. *Anesthesiology* 1980; 52(4):339-51.
14. Phillips WA, Hensinger RN: Control of blood loss during scoliosis surgery. *Clin Orthop* 1988; 229:88-93.
15. Grundy BL: Intraoperative monitoring of sensory-evoked potentials. *Anesthesiology* 1983; 58(1):72-87.
16. Sudhir KG, Smith RM, Hall J, Hall JE, Hansen DD: Intraoperative awakening for early recognition of possible neurologic sequelae during Harrington-rod spinal fusion. *Anesth Analg* 1976; 55(4):526-28.

# PELVIC OSTEOTOMY

## SURGICAL CONSIDERATIONS

**Description**: Pelvic osteotomy is used to improve hip instability in cases of congenital or developmental hip dysplasia and dislocation by "deepening" the shallow acetabulum.[1,2,5] It is frequently performed in conjunction with open reduction, and occasionally with femoral osteotomy. The surgical approach is made along the iliac crest, always exposing the external (gluteal) surface of the pelvis, and sometimes the internal (iliac) surface. The pelvis is osteotomized closely above the acetabulum, and sometimes through the pubis and ischium as well, depending on the direction of rotation and reorientation desired. Pelvic osteotomies either reorient an intact acetabular hyaline cartilage surface, or are designed as salvage procedures to enlarge the acetabulum by fibrocartilage metaplasia (see "Acetabular Augmentation, Chiari"). **Salter's innominate osteotomy** is the classic reorientation osteotomy, in which a complete cut of the supra-acetabular iliac bone allows rotation through the symphysis pubis.[4,7] **Pemberton's operation** is a slightly more difficult incomplete iliac osteotomy, rotating on the triradius cartilage (Fig 12.4-7), which is at the center of the acetabulum in young children.[3] The **Steel**,[6] **"Dial"** or **Eppright osteotomies** are the most difficult reorientation procedures. In each, the acetabulum is freed totally from any bony contact with the remainder of the pelvis, and rotated into better position.[5]

**Usual preop diagnosis**: Acetabular dysplasia due to congenital or developmental hip dislocation

### SUMMARY OF PROCEDURE

| | Salter | Pemberton | Steel, Dial |
|---|---|---|---|
| **Position** | Supine | ⇐ | ⇐ |
| **Incision** | Oblique or longitudinal anterior hip | ⇐ | ⇐ |
| **Special instrumentation** | Steinmann pins | Special curved, custom osteotomes | Steinmann pins |
| **Unique considerations** | Frequently follows previous unsuccessful open-hip surgery | ⇐ | ⇐ + Additional ischial incision |
| **Antibiotics** | Usually, cefazolin 25 mg/kg iv | ⇐ | ⇐ |
| **Surgical time** | 1.5 - 2 hrs | 2 - 3 hrs | 2 - 4 hrs |
| **Closing considerations** | 1.5 hip spica | ⇐ | ⇐ |
| **EBL** | 100-300 cc | ⇐ | 200-600 cc |
| **Postop care** | PACU → room; care as needed for spica cast. | ⇐ | ⇐ |
| **Mortality** | Minimal | ⇐ | ⇐ |
| **Morbidity** | Avascular necrosis of the hip: 5-6% | – | – |
| | Persistent hip subluxation: ~5% | ⇐ | ⇐ |
| | Infection: < 1% | ⇐ | ⇐ |
| | Sciatic or perineal palsy: < 0.1% | – | – |
| | Excess bleeding from superior gluteal artery: Rare | ⇐ | Occasional |
| | Ileus: Rare | ⇐ | Occasional |
| **Procedure code** | 27146; 27147 (with open Rx); 27151 (with femoral osteotomy); 27156 (with open Rx and femoral osteotomy) | ⇐ | ⇐ |
| **Pain score** | 2-5 | 2-5 | 3-6 |

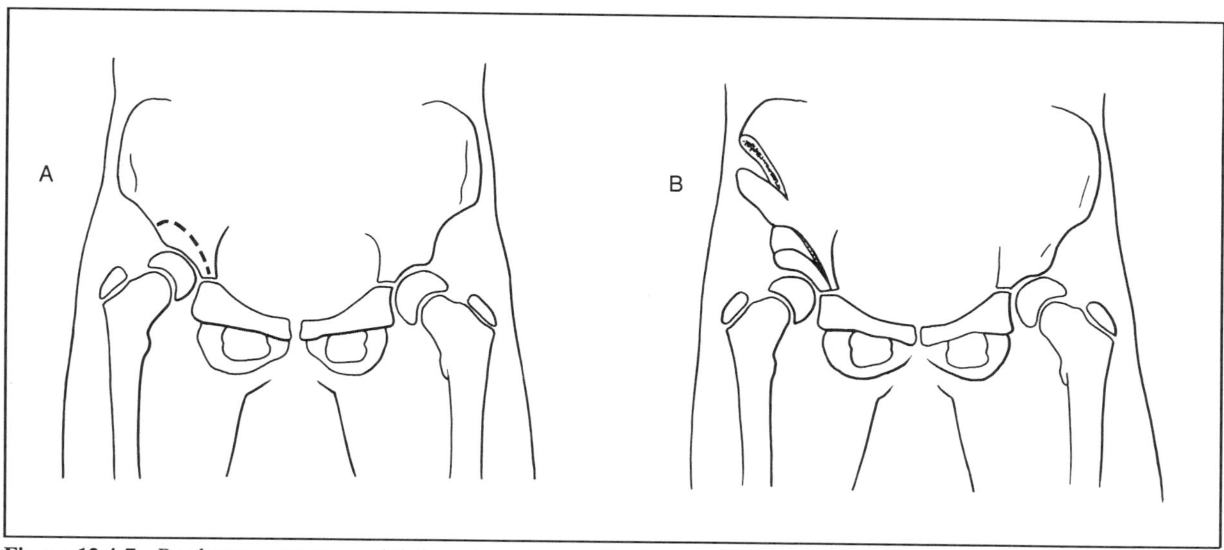


**Figure 12.4-7.** Pemberton osteotomy: (A) Osteotomy begins slightly superior to iliac spine, curves into triradiate cartilage. (B) Osteotomy completed with acetabular roof in corrected position. Wedge of bone is impacted into osteotomy site. (Reproduced with permission from Crenshaw AH, ed: *Campbell's Operative Orthopaedics*, 8th edition. Mosby-Year Book: 1992.)

## PATIENT POPULATION CHARACTERISTICS

| | Salter | Pemberton | Steel, Dial |
|---|---|---|---|
| **Age range** | 18 mo-6 yrs, if dislocated<br>18 mo-10 yrs, if only subluxated | 18 mo-7 yrs | >12 yrs |
| **Male:Female** | 1:2 | ⇐ | ⇐ |
| **Incidence** | 0.1/1000 | < 0.1/1000 | < 0.01/1000 |
| **Etiology** | Congenital and/or developmental hip dysplasia: 98%<br>Perthes disease: 1% | ⇐ | ⇐ |
| **Associated conditions** | Torticollis: < 1% | ⇐ | ⇐ |
| | Other joint contractures in cases of neuromuscular dislocation: < 1% | ⇐ | ⇐ |

## ANESTHETIC CONSIDERATIONS

See "Anesthetic Considerations for Pediatric Orthopedic Surgery for Extremities" at the end of this section.

**References**

1. Coleman SS: *Congenital Dysplasia and Dislocation of the Hip*. Mosby Year Book Inc, St. Louis: 1978.
2. MacEwen GD: Treatment of congenital dislocation of the hip in older children. *Clin Orthop* 1987; 225:86-92.
3. Pemberton PA: Pericapsular osteotomy of the ilium for the treatment of congenitally dislocated hips. *Clin Orthop* 1974; 98:41-54.
4. Salter RB, Duboi JP: The first fifteen years' personal experience with innominate osteotomy in the treatment of congenital dislocation and subluxation of the hip. *Clin Orthop* 1974; 98:72-103.
5. Staheli LT: Surgical management of acetabular dysplasia. *Clin Orthop* 1991; 264:111-21.
6. Steel HH: Triple osteotomy of the innominate bone. *J Bone Joint Surg* [Am] 1973; 55(2):343-50.
7. Waters P, Kurica K, Hall J, Micheli LJ: Salter innominate osteotomies in congenital dislocation of the hip. *J Pediatr Orthop* 1988; 8(6):650-55.

# ACETABULAR AUGMENTATION (SHELF) & CHIARI OSTEOTOMY

## SURGICAL CONSIDERATIONS

**Description:** Acetabular augmentation is a "salvage" procedure used to deepen the hip socket when a realignment osteotomy of the pelvis and/or femur would not adequately cover the femoral head.[5,8] This is accomplished by securing strips of cortical cancellous bone graft onto the proximal surface of the hip capsule. The surgical approach is anterior to the hip, elevating the gluteal muscles subperiosteally from the outer surface of the ilium. The reflected head of the rectus femoris tendon is elevated, and a domed-shaped slot is created just above the capsular attachment to the ilium. Abundant cortical cancellous strips of bone graft are then harvested from the upper two-thirds of the outer wall of the ilium. These bone grafts have a natural curve, and lie on the convexity of the hip capsule. No internal fixation, other than suture repair, is used to hold the bone graft in place. This creates a large bony augmentation (shelf) over the uncovered femoral capsule.

**Variant procedure or approaches:** The bone graft may be taken as a large, sculpted, solitary, cortical cancellous strut or wedge, or more commonly, as curved "shavings" anchored in a dome-shaped slot just above the hip capsule. In the **Chiari procedure,**[1-4] a complete dome-shaped osteotomy allows lateral displacement of the ilium just above the proximal hip capsule (Fig 12.4-8). The line of the osteotomy corresponds more or less with the slot of the shelf procedure. In either case, the result is abundant bony coverage over the hip capsule, which undergoes metaplasia into fibrocartilage.

**Usual preop diagnosis:** Acetabular dysplasia (shallow socket) due to congenital hip dislocation or developmental neurologic subluxation

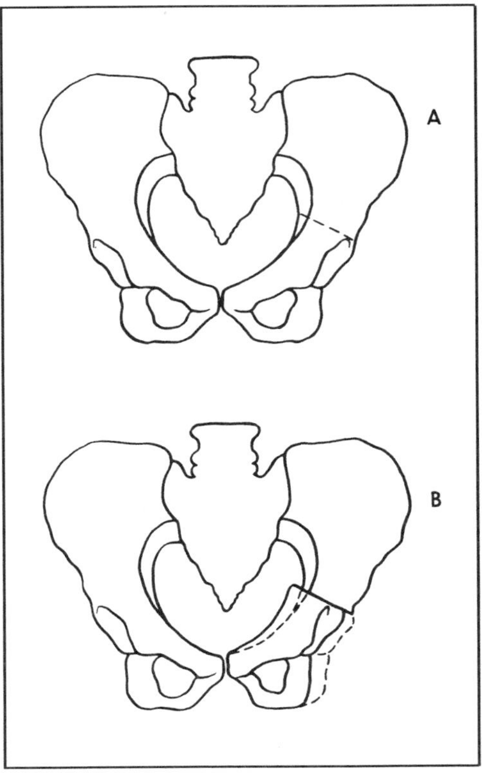


**Figure 12.4-8.** Chiari osteotomy: (A) Line of osteotomy. (B) Completed osteotomy. (Reproduced with permission from Crenshaw AH, ed: *Campbell's Operative Orthopaedics*, 8th edition. Mosby-Year Book: 1992.)

### SUMMARY OF PROCEDURE

| | Acetabular Augmentation | Chiari Osteotomy |
|---|---|---|
| **Position** | Supine or slightly tilted up (reverse Trendelenburg) | ⇐ or lateral decubitus |
| **Incision** | Oblique or longitudinal; anterior hip region | ⇐ |
| **Special instrumentation** | Usually no internal fixation | Two large screws or pins |
| **Unique considerations** | Image intensification or intraop x-ray | ⇐ |
| **Antibiotics** | Cefazolin 25 mg/kg iv | ⇐ |
| **Surgical time** | 1.5 - 3 hrs | ⇐ |
| **Closing considerations** | Single or 1.5 spica cast mandatory | Spica cast optional |
| **EBL** | 100-500 cc | 200-800 cc |
| **Postop care** | PACU → room. Care as necessary for cast. | ⇐ |
| **Mortality** | Minimal | ⇐ |
| **Morbidity** | Lateral femoral cutaneous nerve dysfunction: 30-50%[5-8]<br>Infection: 1% | Possible need[1-4] for later C-section: Rare<br>Sciatic or peroneal palsy: 2% |
| **Procedure code** | 27146 | ⇐ |
| **Pain score** | 4-6 | 4-6 |

### PATIENT POPULATION CHARACTERISTICS

| | |
|---|---|
| **Age range** | 6-35 yrs |
| **Male:female** | 1:1.5 |
| **Incidence** | < 0.1/1000 in general population; in neuromuscular population (e.g., cerebral palsy, poliomyelitis residuals): ≤ 5-10% |
| **Etiology** | Neuromuscular hip subluxation with shallow acetabulum<br>Residual shallow acetabulum (poor coverage from congenitally dislocated hip) |
| **Associated conditions** | Cerebral palsy<br>Polio<br>Spina bifida<br>Myopathy<br>Congenital atrophies<br>Charcot-Marie Tooth |

## ANESTHETIC CONSIDERATIONS

See "Anesthetic Considerations for Pediatric Orthopedic Surgery for Extremities" at the end of this section.

**References**

1. Betz RR, Kumar SJ, Palmer CT, MacEwen GD: Chiari pelvic osteotomy in children and young adults. *J Bone Joint Surg* [Am] 1988; 70(2):182-91.
2. Calvert PT, Augaust AC, Albert JS: The Chiari pelvic osteotomy. A review of the long-term results. *J Bone Joint Surg* [Br] 1987; 69(4):551-55.
3. Chiari K: Medial displacement osteotomy of the pelvis. *Clin Orthop* 1974; 98:55-69.
4. Morrissy RT: *Atlas of Pediatric Orthopaedic Surgery*. JB Lippincott, Philadelphia: 1992, 201-10.
5. Staheli LT: Slotted acetabular augmentation. *J Pediatr Orthop* 1981; 1(3):321-27.
6. Summers BN, Turner A, Wynn-Jones CH: The shelf operation in the management of late presentation of congenital hip dysplasia. *J Bone Joint Surg* [Br] 1988; 70(1):63-8.
7. White RE Jr, Sherman FC: The hip shelf procedure. A long-term evaluation. *J Bone Joint Surg* [Am] 1980; 62(6):928-32.
8. Zuckerman JD, Staheli LT, McLaughlin JF: Acetabular augmentation for progressive hip subluxation in cerebral palsy. *J Pediatr Orthop* 1984; 4(4):436-42.

# OBER FASCIOTOMY, YOUNT-OBER RELEASE

## SURGICAL CONSIDERATIONS

**Description**: **Ober's fasciotomy** is performed to release flexion, abduction and external rotation contracture at the hip.[1-4] This contracture usually occurs as a result of profound flaccid paralysis → prolonged positioning in a so-called "frog" position of 90° flexion, abduction, and lateral rotation at the hips. This results in tightening of the iliotibial (IT) band (the greatly thickened lateral aspect of the fascia lata) and related structures. The operation is performed through an anterolateral incision just distal to the iliac crest. All of the fascial investments of the tensor, sartorius, and at times the rectus femoris and gluteus medias and minimus, are divided while preserving any normal-appearing muscle fibers. The limb is stretched into progressively more adduction and extension, until a neutral position can be obtained. The **Yount procedure** is added when the knee is also contracted in a flexed mode due to tightness of the IT band. The Yount procedure consists of further resection of a segment of the IT band and a lateral intermuscular septum through a separate distal mid-lateral longitudinal incision just above the knee. An oblique segment of the IT band and septum are removed and not repaired.

**Usual preop diagnosis**: Flaccid paralysis and "frog" type contracture due to poliomyelitis, myelomeningocele or myopathy

## SUMMARY OF PROCEDURE

| | Ober Fasciotomy | Yount-Ober Release |
|---|---|---|
| **Position** | Supine; both legs must be prepped and draped to well above the iliac crest area for intraop stretching. | ⇐ |
| **Incision** | Oblique iliac crest | Mid-lateral longitudinal above knee joint, approximately 10 cm |
| **Unique considerations** | Patients with sensory and motor loss have a tendency to get pressure sores. | ⇐ |
| **Antibiotics** | Usually none | ⇐ |
| **Surgical time** | 1 hr/side | 30 min/side |
| **Closing considerations** | Bilateral above-knee casts | ⇐ |
| **EBL** | < 150 cc | < 50 cc |
| **Postop care** | PACU → room; extensive physical therapy program of stretching exercises. Myopathic patients will be at risk for postop respiratory compromise. | ⇐ |
| **Mortality** | Minimal | ⇐ |
| **Morbidity** | Hematoma: ~1% | ⇐ |
| | Fracture of atrophied bone postop: < 1% | ⇐ |
| | Infection: < 1% | ⇐ |
| | Pressure sores from positioning or casts: < 1% | ⇐ |
| **Procedure code** | 27025 | ⇐ |
| **Pain score** | 3-4 | 3-4 |

## PATIENT POPULATION CHARACTERISTICS

| | |
|---|---|
| **Age range** | 2-15 yrs |
| **Male:Female** | 1:1 |
| **Incidence** | Extremely rare in America-born children; however, polio is seen commonly in southeast Asian and Latin American immigrants. |
| **Etiology** | Polio<br>Myelomeningocele<br>Myopathy or dystrophy |
| **Associated conditions** | Other contractures<br>Incontinence<br>Pressure sores in myelomeningocele |

# ANESTHETIC CONSIDERATIONS

See "Anesthetic Considerations for Pediatric Orthopedic Surgery for Extremities" at the end of this section.

**References**

1. Beaty JH: Paralytic disorders. In *Campbell's Operative Orthopaedics*, 8th edition. Crenshaw AH, ed. Mosby Year Book, St. Louis: 1992, 2412-16.
2. Irwin CE: The iliotibial band, its role in producing deformity in poliomyelitis. *J Bone Joint Surg* [Am] 1949; 31:141-52.
3. Ober FR: The role of the iliotibial band and fascia lata as a factor in the causation of low-back disabilities and sciatica. *J Bone Joint Surg* [Am] 1936; 18:105-19.
4. Yount CC: The role of the tensor fasciae femoris in certain deformities of the lower extremities. *J Bone Joint Surg* [Am] 1926; 8:171-82.

# HIP, OPEN REDUCTION, ± FEMORAL SHORTENING

## SURGICAL CONSIDERATIONS

**Description:** Open reduction of the hip replaces a congenitally or developmentally dislocated femoral head into the anatomic acetabulum, usually after an unsuccessful attempt to reduce the hip by closed means.[1-6] It is often preceded by traction, and always followed by spica cast. A developmental dislocation presents with a more normal acetabulum and occurs around birth or later. Teratologic congenital dislocation of the hip occurs early *in utero*; and, as a result, is a high-riding dislocation with a poorly developed acetabulum, presenting much more difficulty in obtaining and maintaining reduction. The most common surgical approach is through an anterior groin incision. The hip capsule is exposed circumferentially, after division and tagging of the origins of the rectus, femoris and sartorius muscles, and retraction of the tensor and gluteal muscles. The capsule is opened in an oblique fashion, the ligamentum teres is excised, and any obstacle to reduction is removed. The iliopsoas tendon is lengthened; then the capsule is repaired in a "vest-over-pants" imbrication, with the hip reduced under direct visualization (Fig 12.4-9). A medial approach through the adductor region can be used in very young children (< 18 mo), but does not allow a capsular repair.[3] If femoral shortening is necessary, the surgical excision is either extended anterolateral, or a separate lateral incision is made longitudinally over the proximal femur.

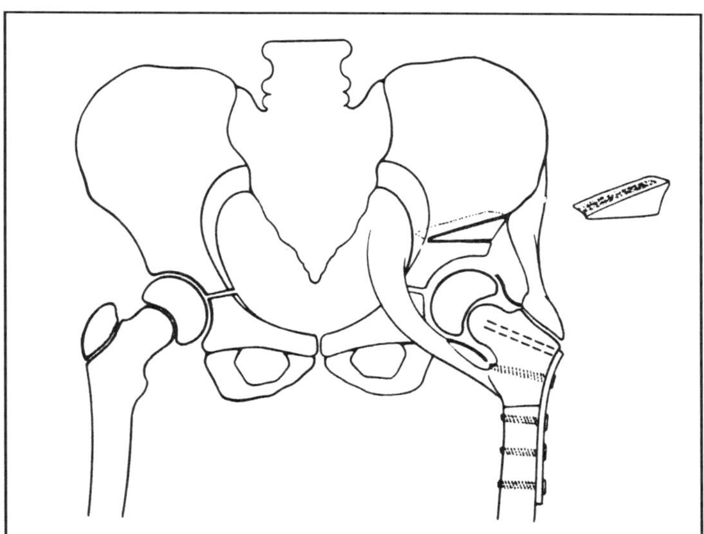

**Figure 12.4-9.** Open reduction with femoral shortening. (Reproduced with permission from Crenshaw AH, ed: *Campbell's Operative Orthopaedics*, 8th edition. Mosby-Year Book: 1992.)

**Variant procedure or approaches:** Most children < 2 yrs old can simply have the hip repositioned – closed or open – and subsequently have normal hip development. In older children, especially with a high dislocation, a segment of the femur is removed subtrochanterically to allow reduction without pressure (thus allowing "descent" of the femoral head). If the acetabulum is very shallow, a pelvic osteotomy may be added.

**Usual preop diagnosis:** Developmental dislocation of hip; teratologic congenital dislocation of hip

### SUMMARY OF PROCEDURE

| | Open Reduction | Open Reduction + Femoral Shortening |
|---|---|---|
| **Position** | Supine | ⇐ |
| **Incision** | Oblique groin ("bikini") or medial longitudinal over joint | ⇐ + Anterolateral thigh over joint |
| **Special instrumentation** | None | Plates and screws |
| **Unique considerations** | Preliminary arthrogram and, often, attempted closed reduction. Image intensifier is used. | ⇐ |
| **Antibiotics** | Usually cefazolin 25 mg/kg iv | ⇐ |
| **Surgical time** | 1.5 - 3 hrs | 2 - 4 hrs |
| **Closing considerations** | Hip spica cast applied on child's spica frame. **NB**: Do not wake patient until last radiograph is taken in case cast has to be reapplied. | ⇐ |
| **EBL** | < 100 cc | 100-400 cc |
| **Postop care** | PACU → room; care as necessary for spica cast. | ⇐ |
| **Mortality** | Minimal | ⇐ |

| | Open Reduction | Open Reduction + Femoral Shortening |
|---|---|---|
| **Morbidity** | Avascular necrosis of femoral head | ⇐ |
| | Stiffness and late arthritis | ⇐ |
| | Limb-length discrepancy | ⇐ |
| | Marked scrotal or labial swelling: Temporary | ⇐ |
| | Redislocation | ⇐ |
| | Infection | ⇐ |
| **Procedure code** | 27258, 27257 | 27259, 27151, 27156 |
| **Pain score** | 2-4 | 3-5 |

### PATIENT POPULATION CHARACTERISTICS

| | |
|---|---|
| **Age range** | Closed reduction: 3 mo-3 yrs<br>Open reduction: 6 mo-10 yrs<br>Open reduction femoral shortening: 2-14 yrs |
| **Male:female** | 1:5 (approximate) |
| **Incidence** | 1:10,000 |
| **Etiology** | Genetic background<br>Breech presentation<br>First-born girl |
| **Associated conditions** | Arthrogryposis<br>Larsen's disease<br>Myelomeningocele<br>Chromosomal anomalies<br>Congenital torticollis<br>Cerebral palsy |

## ANESTHETIC CONSIDERATIONS

See "Anesthetic Considerations for Pediatric Orthopedic Surgery for Extremities" at the end of this section.


**References**

1. Chapman MW: *Operative Orthopaedics*, 2nd edition. JB Lippincott, Philadelphia: 1993, 3101-62.
2. Coleman SS: *Congenital Dysplasia and Dislocation of the Hip*. Mosby Year Book Inc, St. Louis: 1978.
3. Galpin RD, Roach JW, Wenger DR, Herring JA, Birch JG: One-stage treatment of congenital dislocation of the hip in older children, including femoral shortening. *J Bone Joint Surg* [Am] 1989; 71(5):734-41.
4. Ferguson AB: Primary open reduction of congenital dislocation of the hip using a median adductor approach. *J Bone Joint Surg* [Am] 1973; 55:67189.
5. Morrissy RT: *Atlas of Pediatric Orthopaedic Surgery*. JB Lippincott, Philadelphia: 1992, 137-54.
6. Schoenecker PL, Strecker WB: Congenital dislocation of the hip in children. Comparison of the effects of femoral shortening and of skeletal traction in treatment. *J Bone Joint Surg* [Am] 1984; 66(1):21-7.

# ADDUCTOR RELEASE OR TRANSFER, PSOAS RELEASE

## SURGICAL CONSIDERATIONS

**Description**: The adductor tendon origins and/or the iliopsoas insertion are frequently released in spastic and other neurologic conditions (especially cerebral palsy) which cause crossing of the legs ("scissoring").[1-6] The goal is to allow greater abduction by decreasing the strength of the adductors and flexors. The releases are also performed for other causes of hip contracture due to developmental hip dislocation, juvenile arthritis, etc. The procedure is always performed on a supine patient through a groin incision in which the tendons (usually the adductor longus, brevis and gracilis) are isolated by blunt section and divided by electrocautery. In the classic procedure popularized by **Banks** and **Green**, the anterior branch of the obturator nerve is divided on the surface of the adductor brevis to effect more permanent adductor weakness. **Neurectomy** is now less popular because of the fear that the denervated muscle will fibrose into a worse scar.[6] The iliopsoas tendon may be released at its insertion on the lesser trochanter, in the base of the adductor incision; or, just the tendinous portion of the combined iliopsoas may be released at the pelvic rim, which produces a more modest degree of the flexor lengthening. Some surgeons transfer the adductor longus and gracilis muscles proximally and laterally, suturing them to the ischium to convert the adductors to hip extensors by changing their mechanics.[4,5] Theoretically, this is desirable; but it has not proven to be more effective overall than simple adductor release, and is a more complicated procedure.

**Usual preop diagnosis**: Adduction and flexion contracture of the hip with subluxation due to cerebral palsy, acquired encephalopathy or progressive neurologic disorder

### SUMMARY OF PROCEDURE

| | Adductor Release | Adductor Transfer | Psoas Release |
|---|---|---|---|
| **Position** | Supine | Supine or lithotomy | ⇐ |
| **Incision** | Medial proximal groin, longitudinal or transverse | Transverse medial groin | Anterior groin |
| **Unique considerations** | Frequently bilateral; often poor hygiene, especially if severe contracture; proximity to perineum | ⇐ | ⇐ |
| **Antibiotics** | Optional, cefazolin 25 mg/kg iv | ⇐ | ⇐ |
| **Surgical time** | 1 hr | 1.5 hrs | 1 hr |
| **Closing considerations** | Bilateral leg casts or double spica cast | ⇐ | ⇐ |
| **EBL** | < 100 cc | ⇐ | ⇐ |
| **Postop care** | PACU → room; care as necessary for spica cast. | ⇐ | ⇐ |
| **Mortality** | Minimal | ⇐ | ⇐ |
| **Morbidity** | Hematoma, drainage<br>Infection: < 1%<br>Recurrence of adduction deformity | ⇐ | ⇐ |
| **Procedure code** | 27001; 27003 (with obturator neurectomy) | 27098 | 27005 (release); 27111 (iliopsoas recession) |
| **Pain score** | 2-4 | 2-4 | 2-4 |

### PATIENT POPULATION CHARACTERISTICS

| | |
|---|---|
| **Age range** | 2-20 yrs |
| **Male:Female** | 1:1 |
| **Incidence** | 0 in general population; ≤ 30% of cerebral palsy patients (0.6-5.9/1,000)[6] |
| **Etiology** | Cerebral palsy: 90%<br>Slowly progressive degenerative neurologic conditions: 8-10%<br>Head injury and drowning: 1-2% |

**Associated conditions** Multiple other contractures
Gastroesophageal reflux
Poor general nutrition
Mental retardation

## ANESTHETIC CONSIDERATIONS

See "Anesthetic Considerations for Pediatric Orthopedic Surgery for Extremities" at the end of this section.


**References**

1. Banks HH, Green WT: Adductor myotomy and obturator neurectomy for the correction of adduction contracture of the hip in cerebral palsy. *J Bone Joint Surg* [Am] 1960; 42:111-26.
2. Bleck EE: *Orthopaedic Management in Cerebral Palsy.* JB Lippincott, Philadelphia: 1987, 282-319.
3. Bleck EE: The hip in cerebral palsy. *Orthop Clin North Am* 1980; 11(1):79-104.
4. Reimers J, Poulsen S: Adductor transfer versus tenotomy for stability of the hip in spastic cerebral palsy. *J Pediatr Orthop* 1984; 4(1):52-4.
5. Root L, Spero CR: Hip adductor transfer compared with adductor tenotomy in cerebral palsy. *J Bone Joint Surg* [Am] 1981; 63(5):767-72.
6. Tachdjian MD: *Pediatric Orthopaedics.* WB Saunders, Philadelphia: 1990, 1613-45.


# PINNING OF SLIPPED CAPITAL FEMORAL EPIPHYSIS (SCFE)

## SURGICAL CONSIDERATIONS

**Description**: During the rapid growth period of adolescence, the shearing stress of the body weight on the proximal femoral growth plate may cause the femoral head (capital epiphysis) to gradually move relative to the femoral neck physis (growth plate). The displacement occurs over weeks-to-months, with the head appearing to move posteriorly and inferiorly on the neck. ***In situ* pinning** (no reduction) is the most common treatment.[2-7] The goal is to prevent further slipping and subsequent arthritis by causing closure of the growth plate. The procedure must be performed under radiographic control (usually image intensifier), using a variety of threaded pins or screws which are passed through the neck into the femoral head. Currently, the favored technique uses 1 stout cannulated screw, which is passed percutaneously over a guide wire from the anterolateral aspect of the proximal femur. Traditionally, a small lateral incision was used at the base of the trochanter, with 2-4 pins placed; however, screws now in use are strong enough so that 1 is adequate for most chronic slips. More importantly, 1 screw can be placed "dead center" in the femoral head, avoiding the frequent complication of having a pin penetrate the joint.

**Variant procedure or approaches**: Although most slips are chronic, occasionally following mild trauma, an acute slip will supervene. Following severe trauma, a previous normal hip with an open physis (growth plate) may suffer an acute displacement, but this is rare. In such acute slips, some degree of reduction may be possible, and two pins are usually necessary.[3,7] Because pin-related complications are common, some surgeons prefer to close the growth plate by open drilling and curettement, with bone grafting across the cartilaginous plates.[1,8] This is performed through an anterior incision, opening the hip capsule widely from an oblique groin incision. No pins are used, but an iliac bone graft is placed across the physis. A body spica cast is frequently needed. Once the physis is closed, if there is severe residual deformity, a corrective osteotomy is performed in the trochanteric region (see "Femoral Osteotomy," Southwick procedure).

**Usual preop diagnosis**: Acute or chronic SCFE

## SUMMARY OF PROCEDURE

| | Pinning of SCFE | Variant Open Epiphysiodesis |
|---|---|---|
| **Position** | Supine | ⇐ |
| **Incision** | Short, proximal thigh or stab incision | Anterolateral groin |
| **Special instrumentation** | Guide wires; cannulated screws; image intensifier; ± fracture table | Image intensifier (recommended) |
| **Unique considerations** | Frequently bilateral (≤ 20%); often obese | ⇐ |
| **Antibiotics** | Cefazolin 1 gm iv | ⇐ |
| **Surgical time** | 0.5 - 2 hrs | 1 - 3 hrs |
| **Closing considerations** | None | Frequently needs spica cast |
| **EBL** | Negligible | 200-500 cc |
| **Postop care** | PACU → room | ⇐ + Body spica cast, occasionally |
| **Mortality** | Minimal | ⇐ |
| **Morbidity** | Unsuspected pin penetration: ≤ 37%[4,7] | ⇐ |
| | Avascular necrosis: ≤ 33% (in acute slip cases) | ⇐ |
| | Chondrolysis, hip stiffness: 1-28% | ⇐ |
| | Fracture after pin removal: < 1% | ⇐ |
| | Infection: < 1% | ⇐ |
| **Procedure code** | 27177 | ⇐ |
| **Pain score** | 2-3 | 2-3 |

## PATIENT POPULATION CHARACTERISTICS

| | |
|---|---|
| **Age range** | 10-16 yrs |
| **Male:Female** | 2-3:1 |
| **Incidence** | 1-3/100,000 (higher in African Americans) |
| **Etiology** | Excessive loading of the growth plate (obesity or increased angle of inclination of the physis)<br>Insufficient tensile strength of collagen and proteoglycans around the femoral neck<br>Increased thickness of the physis as from excessive growth hormone, hypogonadism, hypothyroidism, hyperparathyroidism, renal osteodystrophy, almost any other significant endocrinopathy<br>Radiation therapy |
| **Associated conditions** | Obesity<br>Endocrinopathies<br>Renal osteodystrophy |

## ANESTHETIC CONSIDERATIONS

See "Anesthetic Considerations for Pediatric Orthopedic Surgery for Extremities" at the end of this section.


**References**

1. Aadalen RJ, Weiner DS, Hoyt W, Herndon CH: Acute slipped capital femoral epiphysis. *J Bone Joint Surg* [Am] 1974; 56(7):1473-87.
2. Asnis SE: The guided screw system in slipped capital femoral epiphysis. *Contemp Orthop* 1985: 11:27-31.
3. Carlioz H, Vogt JC, Barba L, Doursounian L: Treatment of slipped upper femoral epiphysis: 80 cases operated on over 10 years (1968-1978). *J Pediatr Orthop* 1984; 4(2):153-61.
4. Lehman WB, Menche D, Grant A, Norman A, Pugh J: The problem of evaluating in situ pinning of slipped capital femoral epiphysis: an experimental model and a review of 63 consecutive cases. *J Pediatr Orthop* 1984; 4(3):297-303.
5. Morrissy RT: *Atlas of Pediatric Orthopaedic Surgery.* JB Lippincott, Philadelphia: 1992, 212-44.
6. O'Brien ET, Fahey JJ: Remodeling of the femoral neck after in situ pinning for slipped capital femoral epiphysis. *J Bone Joint Surg* [Am] 1977; 59(1):62-8.
7. Tachdjian MO: *Pediatric Orthopaedics.* WB Saunders, Philadelphia: 1990, 1016-81.
8. Weiner DS, Weiner S, Melby A, Hoyt WA Jr: A 30-year experience with bone graft epiphysiodesis in the treatment of slipped capital femoral epiphysis. *J Pediatr Orthop* 1984; 4(2):145-52.

# PROXIMAL FEMORAL OSTEOTOMY

## SURGICAL CONSIDERATIONS

**Description**: Femoral osteotomy is performed in the inter- or subtrochanteric area in order to redirect the proximal femur more superiorly (valgus), or inferiorly (varus), and/or for rotational correction of excessive medial/femoral torsion (anteversion). A plate and screws are commonly used, but an external fixator and/or spica cast may be placed instead. The usual surgical approach is directly and laterally over the proximal shaft of the femur, beginning at the greater trochanter. The deep fascia is split and the underlying vastus muscle is elevated subperiosteally to expose the femoral shaft. Normally, a power saw is used to make the osteotomy; and, depending on the correction desired, there are a variety of internal fixation devices which can be used.

**Variant procedure or approaches**: Different named plates (e.g., AO blade, Coventry screw, Richards screw, Wagner, etc.) may be used to affix the proximal to the distal femoral segments.[1,2,5,6] A 1-4 cm segment of femur may be removed in cases of superior hip dislocation to allow soft-tissue relaxation and descent of the femoral head into the socket.[3] An **external fixator** and/or spica cast may be used instead of a plate. Most proximal femoral osteotomies are performed in the subtrochanteric area, but some are performed in the intertrochanteric or base of the neck (**Kramer compensating**).[4] The **Southwick osteotomy** is a more complicated example of a subtrochanteric osteotomy, which corrects for three directions (varus, lateral rotation and extension).[6]

**Usual preop diagnosis**: Developmental hip subluxation; excessive hip anteversion; residual deformity from Perthes disease; coxa vara; slipped capital femoral epiphysis; residual deformity

### SUMMARY OF PROCEDURE

| | Varus Derotation Osteotomy with Plate and Screws | External Fixator | Southwick or Kramer |
|---|---|---|---|
| **Position** | Supine | ⇐ | ⇐ |
| **Incision** | Lateral thigh or, occasionally, long anterior thigh | ⇐ | ⇐ |
| **Special instrumentation** | Plate and screws; power drill and saw; image intensifier | External fixator; multiple pins; image intensifier | Plate and screws; power drill and saw; image intensifier |
| **Unique considerations** | Fracture or radiolucent table | ⇐ | ⇐ |
| **Antibiotics** | Usually cefazolin 25 mg/kg iv | ⇐ | ⇐ |
| **Surgical time** | 1.5 - 2.5 hrs | ⇐ | 2 - 4 hrs |
| **Closing considerations** | Spica cast, frequently | ± Spica cast | Spica cast, occasionally |
| **EBL** | 250-750 cc | ⇐ | 500-1000 cc |
| **Postop care** | PACU → room. Spica cast; non-weight-bearing ~6 wks; no full weight-bearing, 3 mo. | ⇐ | ⇐ |
| **Mortality** | Minimal | ⇐ | ⇐ |
| **Morbidity** | Persistent hip dysplasia: 5-20% (depending on etiology) | ⇐ | ⇐ |
| | Excess blood loss from a perforating branch of the profunda femoris: < 1% | ⇐ | ⇐ |
| | Infection: < 1% | ⇐ | ⇐ |
| | Loss of fixation, instrument failure: < 1% | ⇐ | ⇐ |
| | Nonunion: < 1% | ⇐ | ⇐ |
| | Persistent hip stiffness: < 1% | ⇐ | ⇐ |
| | Avascular necrosis: Rare | ⇐ | ⇐ |
| **Procedure code** | 27167 | ⇐ | 27181 |
| **Pain score** | 6-8 | 6-8 | 6-8 |

### PATIENT POPULATION CHARACTERISTICS

| | |
|---|---|
| **Age range** | 2-21 yrs |
| **Male:Female** | 1:1 |
| **Incidence** | Depending on diagnosis |
| **Etiology** | Coxa varum, coxa valgum due to muscle imbalance<br>Hip dislocation<br>Excessive medial femoral torsion (anteversion)<br>Osteochondrodystrophies (dwarfing syndromes)<br>Perthes disease, slipped capital femoral epiphysis |
| **Associated conditions** | Cerebral palsy<br>Myelomeningocele, neuromyopathies<br>Congenital hip dislocation<br>Occasionally, hypothyroidism as a cause of slipped capital femoral epiphysis |

## ANESTHETIC CONSIDERATIONS

See "Anesthetic Considerations for Pediatric Orthopedic Surgery for Extremities" at the end of this section.

**References**


1. Alonso JE, Lovell WW, Lovejoy JF: The Altdorf hip clamp. *J Pediatr Orthop* 1986; 6(4):399-402.
2. Canale ST, Holand RW: Coventry screw fixation of osteotomies about the pediatric hip. *J Pediatr Orthop* 1983; 3(5):592-600.
3. Coleman SS: *Congenital Dysplasia and Dislocation of the Hip*. Mosby, St. Louis: 1978.
4. Kramer WG, Craig WA, Noel S: Compensating osteotomy at the base of the femoral neck for slipped capital femoral epiphysis. *J Bone Joint Surg* [Am] 1976; 58(6):796-800.
5. Morrissy RT: *Atlas of Pediatric Orthopaedic Surgery*. JB Lippincott, Philadelphia: 1992, 264-304.
6. Southwick WO: Osteotomy through the lesser trochanter for slipped capital femoral epiphysis. *J Bone Joint Surg* [Am] 1967; 49(5):807-35.


# EPIPHYSIODESIS

## SURGICAL CONSIDERATIONS

**Description**: Epiphysiodesis[1-7] is performed in skeletally immature adolescents to eliminate or retard growth of the longer limb in cases of leg-length discrepancy (anisomelia). The timing of the procedure[1,5,7] is critical, based on the child's bone age and discrepancy, which are plotted on a graph or computer program. The procedure is most commonly performed through small incisions (1") about the knee, centered on the growth plate (physis) of the distal femur or proximal tibia. The original **Phemister technique**[6] is an approach in which a 3/4"-1¼" square or rectangular block of bone is removed using a box chisel centered on the physis, which is visualized directly. The bone block is rotated 90° or 180° and re-inserted, causing a bony bridge across the physis. **Blount**[2] subsequently used stout, reinforced staples to bracket the physis and "lock it." This provides theoretical advantage of reversibility (i.e., if staples are removed, growth may resume should the procedure have been performed at too early an age). More recently, a **percutaneous technique** of simply drilling directly across the cartilaginous physeal growth plate, causing a bony bridge. This is accomplished through small stab incisions, under image intensifier control.[3]

**Usual preop diagnosis**: Limb-length discrepancies of 2-5 cm in adolescents (willing to accept a slight diminution in adult stature)

## SUMMARY OF PROCEDURE

| | Open Epiphysiodesis | Percutaneous Epiphysiodesis | Epiphyseal Stapling |
|---|---|---|---|
| **Position** | Supine, with tourniquet | Supine | Supine, with tourniquet |
| **Incision** | 3-4 cm longitudinal incision, medial and laterally centered incisions over distal femoral and/or proximal tibial epiphysis | 1 cm, same area as open epiphysiodesis | 4-5 cm, same area as open epiphysiodesis |
| **Special instrumentation** | Box chisel | Drill point and sleeve | Heavy, reinforced staples |
| **Unique considerations** | Tourniquet used | Image intensifier control mandatory; no tourniquet | ⇐ |
| **Antibiotics** | Optional cefazolin 25 mg/kg iv | ⇐ | ⇐ |
| **Surgical time** | 1 hr | ⇐ | ⇐ |
| **Closing considerations** | Cylinder cast or knee immobilizer | ⇐ | ⇐ |
| **EBL** | < 50 cc | ⇐ | ⇐ |
| **Postop care** | PACU → room; crutches for comfort | ⇐ | ⇐ |
| **Mortality** | Minimal | ⇐ | ⇐ |
| **Morbidity** | Under- or overcorrection with regard to length: 5-10% | ⇐ | ⇐ |
| | Wound problems: < 5% | ⇐ | ⇐ |
| | Asymmetric growth arrest → valgus or varus deformity: 2-5% | ⇐ | ⇐ |
| | Anterior or lateral compartment syndrome: 1% | – | – |
| | Fracture: 1% | – | – |
| | Peroneal palsy: < 1% | – | – |
| **Procedure code** | 27475 (distal femur); 27477 (tibia and fibula); 27479 (combined femur and tibia) | ⇐ | ⇐ |
| **Pain score** | 3-5 | 2-3 | 3-5 |

## PATIENT POPULATION CHARACTERISTICS

| | |
|---|---|
| **Age range** | 9-14 yrs (adolescents, usually healthy with limb-length discrepancy 2-6 cm) |
| **Male:Female** | 1:1 |
| **Incidence** | < 1/1000 |
| **Etiology** | Idiopathic hemihypertrophy<br>Neurologic (e.g., polio, hemiplegia)<br>Congenital deformities of the lower extremities (e.g., congenitally short femur, fibular hemimelia)<br>Osteomyelitis; development of tumorous conditions (e.g., enchondromatosis)<br>Traumatic growth plate injuries occurring near puberty<br>Epiphyseal problems related to hip (slipped epiphysis, sequelae of Perthes disease)<br>Klippel-Trenaunay-Weber syndrome |
| **Associated conditions** | Other contractures in neurologic conditions (e.g., polio)<br>Neurofibromatosis, AV fistulae<br>Wilms' tumor: Rare |

## ANESTHETIC CONSIDERATIONS

See "Anesthetic Considerations for Pediatric Orthopedic Surgery for Extremities" at the end of this section.


**References**

1. Blair VP III, Walker SJ, Sheridan JJ, Schoenecker PL: Epiphysiodesis: a problem of timing. *J Pediatr Orthop* 1982; 2(3):281-4.
2. Blount WP, Clarke GR: Control of bone growth by epiphyseal stapling. *J Bone Joint Surg* [Am] 1949; 31:464-78.
3. Liotta FJ, Ambrose TA II, Eilert RE: Fluoroscopic technique vs Phemister technique for epiphysiodesis. *J Pediatr Orthop* 1992; 12(2):248-51.
4. Mayhall WST: Leg length discrepancy treated by epiphysiodesis. *Orthopaedics Rev* 1978; 7:441-4.
5. Moseley CF: A straight line graft for leg length discrepancies. *Clin Orthop* 1978; 136:33-40.
6. Phemister DB: Operative arrestment of longitudinal growth of bones in the treatment of deformities. *J Bone Joint Surg* 1933; [Am] 15:1-15.
7. Stephens DC, Herrick W, MacEwen GD: Epiphysiodesis for limb length inequality: results and indication. *Clin Orthop* 1978; 136:41-8.


# SOFIELD PROCEDURE

## SURGICAL CONSIDERATIONS

**Description**: The **Sofield procedure**, or **"fragmentation rodding,"** is most commonly performed for deformity of the long bones, and to prevent recurrent fracture, usually a result of osteogenesis imperfecta.[1-3,5,6] The procedure involves exposure of at least one end, and a varying amount of the bony shaft. If the deformity is severe, the entire shaft is exposed via a longitudinal incision, usually laterally. The bone is divided (osteotomized) into the minimum number of segments that will allow a straight intramedullary rod to traverse the segments (usually 2-4 osteotomies). The construct is justly referred to as a "shish-ka-bab." It is needed less frequently in the upper extremities.

**Variant procedure or approaches**: Because a growing bone will elongate beyond the end of a simple intramedullary rod after 1-2 years, the resulting unsupported portion of the bone will be liable to fracture or new deformity. To obviate this problem, **Bailey** and **Dubow** developed an **elongating rod system**,[1] which consists of an outer tubular rod sleeve (the female portion) and an inner obturator portion (male). Both ends of the telescoping rod are anchored in the ends of the bones. The system elongates much like a car radio antenna, and decreases the need for frequent revisions. The surgical technique is, however, identical to any fragmentation rodding, except that both ends of the bone must be exposed.

**Usual preop diagnosis**: Osteogenesis imperfecta; fibrous dysplasia (occasionally); rickets; congenital pseudarthrosis of the tibia

### SUMMARY OF PROCEDURE

| | |
|---|---|
| **Position** | Supine |
| **Incision** | Lateral for femur; anterolateral for tibia |
| **Special instrumentation** | ± Image intensifier table |
| **Unique considerations** | Tendency to hyperthermia; other bones may fracture in more severe cases, even as a result of a BP cuff. If dentinogenesis imperfecta is present, extreme care should be taken during intubation to prevent tooth trauma. In these patients, neck motion is often limited. |
| **Antibiotics** | Cefazolin 25 mg/kg iv |
| **Surgical time** | 1 - 1.5 hrs/tibia; 1.5 - 2.5 hrs/femur (often done sequentially on the same day) |
| **Closing considerations** | Double spica cast if femur is rodded. |

**EBL** Depending on age and size, as well as use of a tourniquet for the femur, 50-250 cc; for the tibia, 50-100 cc.

**Postop care** PACU → room; avoid trauma to teeth, mouth or other bones in PACU.

**Mortality** < 1% (usually related to severe restrictive lung disease, in the most severely involved cases[1-3,5])

**Morbidity** Intraop hyperthermia: Common
Intraop fracture of other bones or teeth
Late rod migration: Common
Late refracture: Common
Nonunion: Rare
Exuberant callus simulating osteosarcoma: Rare
Infection: < 1% of rodding
Radial nerve palsy (in cases of humerus or radius rodding)

**Procedure code** 27454 (femur); 27712 (tibia)

**Pain score** 2-3 (It is surprising how little discomfort these children have, especially the 2nd or 3rd time a bone is rodded.)

### PATIENT POPULATION CHARACTERISTICS

**Age range** 2-25 yrs

**Male:Female** 1:1

**Incidence** 1/20,000 (osteogenesis imperfecta); other etiologies much less common

**Etiology** Congenital (hereditary deficit in collagen synthesis) most commonly as autosomal dominant or spontaneous mutation): All cases

**Associated conditions** Dentinogenesis imperfecta
Diminished vital capacity due to associated kyphoscoliosis
Decreased hearing due to otosclerosis and impingement of the 8th cranial nerve
Pelvic distortion causing chronic constipation
Basilar impression and other C-spine abnormalities[4] causing brainstem compression or even hydrocephalus: Rare

---

## ANESTHETIC CONSIDERATIONS

See "Anesthetic Considerations for Pediatric Orthopedic Surgery for Extremities" at the end of this section.

---

**References**

1. Bailey RW, Dubow HI: Evolution of the concept of an extensible nail accommodating to normal longitudinal bone growth: clinical considerations and implications. *Clin Orthop* 1981, 159:157-70.
2. Gamble JG, Strudwick WJ, Rinsky LA, Bleck EE: Complications of intramedullary rods in osteogenesis imperfecta: Bailey-Dubow rods versus non-elongating rods. *J Pediatr Orthop* 1988; 8(6):645-49.
3. Marafioti RL, Westin GW: Elongating intramedullary rods in the treatment of osteogenesis imperfecta. *J Bone Joint Surg* [Am] 1977; 59(4):467-72.
4. Pozo JL, Crockard HA, Ransford AO: Basilar impression in osteogenesis imperfecta. A report of three cases in one family. *J Bone Joint Surg* [Br] 1984; 66(2):233-38.
5. Rodriquez RP, Bailey RW: Internal fixation of the femur in patients with osteogenesis imperfecta. *Clin Orthop* 1988; 159:126-33.
6. Sofield HA, Millar EA: Fragmentation, realignment and intramedullary rod fixation of deformities of the long bones in children. A ten-year appraisal. *J Bone Joint Surg* [Am] 1959; 41:1371-91.

# LIMB LENGTHENING

## SURGICAL CONSIDERATIONS

**Description**: Limb lengthening usually is performed in the lower extremity for congenital or acquired leg-length discrepancies of at least 5 cm.[1-8] Lesser discrepancies are dealt with by bone shortening or epiphysiodesis of the long side. The basic principles include: (1) application of an adjustable, external fixator; (2) "low-energy," transverse bone cut (osteotomy without use of a power saw) through a small, longitudinal incision over the involved bone; (3) preservation of the periosteal sleeve; (4) gradual lengthening, usually 1 mm/day in fractional adjustments; and (5) when desired limb length is obtained, either use bone graft and plate acutely, or leave until the bone gap fills in and stabilizes (average 38 days/cm gained).[5]

Limb lengthening dates back to the early 1900s; but it fell into disfavor because of the high rate of major complications.[1-2] **Wagner** improved the technique by introducing a simplified, unilateral, large-pin fixator, but performed the osteotomy in the mid-shaft, and began lengthening immediately[3-7] (Fig 12.4-10). This technique usually requires a bone graft and later plating as a second operation, to obtain healing. **DeBastiani** uses a similar large-pin fixator (**Orthofix**), but performs the osteotomy more toward the end of the bone (metaphysis), and waits a week before beginning the lengthening.[5] Spontaneous healing is usual. **Ilizarov** introduced a more complex, but more adaptable, small-pin transfixation system with a circular fixator.[4] In a similar fashion, the Ilizarov method stretches the healing callus[4] (callostasis). Typically, 4-10 cm/bone are gained with any of the above techniques.

**Usual preop diagnosis**: Congenital or acquired anisomelia (limb-length discrepancy) due to overgrowth or growth retardation >5 cm

### SUMMARY OF PROCEDURE

| | Wagner | Orthofix | Ilizarov |
|---|---|---|---|
| **Position** | Supine | ⇐ | ⇐ |
| **Incision** | Longitudinal mid-shaft | Longitudinal proximal shaft (metaphyseal) | ⇐ |
| **Special instrumentation** | Image intensifier; Wagner device (Fig 12.4-10); large bone pins | Image intensifier; Orthofix device; large bone pins | Ilizarov frame ("Erector set"); multiple 1.5-1.8 mm small-diameter wires |
| **Unique considerations** | Acute lengthening may cause ↑BP. | – | Frame should be prepped prior to surgery because of "fiddle factor." |
| **Antibiotics** | Cefazolin 25 mg/kg iv | ⇐ | ⇐ |
| **Surgical time** | 1 - 2 hrs | ⇐ | 2 - 4 hrs |
| **EBL** | < 100 cc | ⇐ | ⇐ |
| **Postop care** | PACU → room; early initiation of physical therapy and/or continuous passive motion (CPM) machine | ⇐ | ⇐ |
| **Mortality** | Minimal | ⇐ | ⇐ |
| **Morbidity** | While device remains in place at least one of the following complications is usual; frequently several occur before healing is complete.[3,6] | ⇐ | ⇐ |
| | Joint stiffness or localized infection: Very common - 50% (temporary) | ⇐ | ⇐ |
| | Edema, swelling, pressure sores: Common | ⇐ | ⇐ |
| | Joint subluxation: Common | ⇐ | ⇐ |
| | Psychological decompensation due to pain: Common | ⇐ | ⇐ |

| | Wagner | Orthofix | Ilizarov |
|---|---|---|---|
| **Morbidity, continued** | Premature consolidation: Common | ⇐ | ⇐ |
| | Skin necrosis: Common | ⇐ | ⇐ |
| | Wound infection: Common | ⇐ | ⇐ |
| | Localized osteomyelitis: Common | ⇐ | ⇐ |
| | Axial deviation of the bone: Common | ⇐ | ⇐ |
| | Delayed union, nonunion, late fracture: Common | ⇐ | ⇐ |
| | Pin penetration of a vessel or nerve: Rare | ⇐ | ⇐ |
| | Compartment syndrome: Rare | ⇐ | ⇐ |
| | Sudeck's atrophy: Rare | ⇐ | ⇐ |
| **Procedure code** | 27466 (femur); 27715 (tibia) | ⇐ | ⇐ |
| **Pain score** | 7-8 | 7-8 | 7-8 |

## PATIENT POPULATION CHARACTERISTICS

| | |
|---|---|
| **Age range** | 10-30 yrs |
| **Male:Female** | 1:1 |
| **Incidence** | Dependent on underlying diagnosis (common in polio) |
| **Etiology** | Congenital deficiencies of the lower extremities (e.g., proximal focal femoral deficiency, congenitally short femur, fibular hemimelia, etc.)<br>Osteomyelitis, traumatic growth plate injury, fracture<br>Asymmetric neurologic conditions (e.g., polio or cerebral palsy)<br>Congenital hemihypertrophy |
| **Associated conditions** | Hip and knee contractures<br>In cases of polio, other deformities and weaknesses<br>Arteriovenous malformations (AVMs)<br>Congenital or developmental hip dislocation |

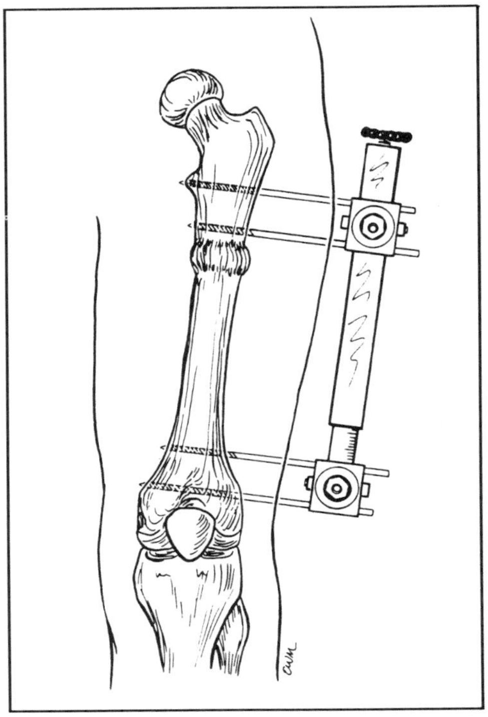

**Figure 12.4-10.** Wagner apparatus for leg lengthening. (Reproduced with permission from Chapman MW, ed: *Operative Orthopaedics*, 2nd edition. JB Lippincott: 1993.)

## ANESTHETIC CONSIDERATIONS

See "Anesthetic Considerations for Pediatric Orthopedic Surgery for Extremities" at end of this section.


**References**

1. Abbott LC: The operative lengthening of the tibia and fibula. *J Bone Joint Surg* [Am] 1927; 9:128-52.
2. Anderson WV: Leg lengthening. *J Bone Joint Surg* [Br] 1952; 34:150.
3. Coleman SS, Stevens PM: Tibial lengthening. *Clin Orthop* 1978; 136:92-104.
4. Dal Monte A, Donzelli O: Tibial lengthening according to Ilizarov in congenital hypoplasia of the leg. *J Pediatr Orthop* 1987; 7(2):135-38.

5. DeBastiani G, Aldegheai R, Renzi-Briviol, Trivella G: Limb lengthening by callus distraction (callotasis). *J Pediatr Orthop* 1987; 7(2):129-34.
6. Tachdjian MO: *Pediatric Orthopaedics*. WB Saunders, Philadelphia: 1990, 2895-3012.
7. Wagner H: Operative lengthening of the femur. *Clin Orthop* 1978; 136:125-42.

# PATELLAR REALIGNMENT

## SURGICAL CONSIDERATIONS

**Description**: Patellar realignment encompasses over 100 procedures designed to prevent lateral subluxation and dislocation of the patella.[1-10] These disorders include a spectrum of malalignments of the patella, ranging from simple excess lateral tilt, recurrent partial subluxation, and recurrent episodic dislocation, to irreducible chronic dislocation.[9] As such, the surgical procedures also encompass a spectrum of complexities, depending on the degree of instability. Nowadays, an arthroscopic inspection often is performed first. The basic principles of the repair include both proximal and distal realignment.[2-9] **Proximal realignment** includes: (1) lateral release, which is the division of the contracted lateral patellar retinacular joint capsule and other tight lateral tissue – the first step in all surgical repair – (2) medial tightening, including reefing and/or advancement of the medial capsule and vastus medialis muscle insertion; and (3) **distal realignment**, consisting of redirection of the patellar tendon more medially (and sometimes more anteriorly).

**Variant procedure or approaches**: Arthroscopic or open lateral release is the simplest, and first-step procedure. It may be sufficient when there is only subluxation and not true dislocation; and it has the advantage of being an outpatient procedure. For frank dislocation, an open "proximal realignment" also includes the medial tautening. If this is not sufficient to hold the patella centralized, and if the patient has open epiphyses (< 16 yrs), the lateral one-half of the patellar tendon may be released (distal realignment) and re-attached medially (**Roux-Goldthwait**); or the patella may be held medially by tenodesing the semitendinosis tendon to it.[1,8] In skeletally mature patients, the bony insertion of the patellar tendon is osteotomized and transferred medially (**Trillat**)[4], or anteriomedially (**Macquet**)[7]. The **Hauser procedure** of distal and medial transfer of the tibial tubercle has had a very poor, long-term outcome, and is seldom performed.

**Usual preop diagnosis**: Lateral patellar subluxation; recurrent dislocation; congenital or chronic lateral patellar dislocation

### SUMMARY OF PROCEDURE

| | Proximal Realignment | Trillat | Macquet |
|---|---|---|---|
| **Position** | Supine, with tourniquet | ⇐ | ⇐ |
| **Incision** | Anterior transverse or longitudinal or oblique, about the knee or arthroscopic | Anterior longitudinal | Transverse or oblique |
| **Special instrumentation** | None | Single bone screw | ⇐ |
| **Unique considerations** | Tourniquet | ⇐ | May use iliac or bank bone graft |
| **Antibiotics** | Optional, cefazolin 25 mg/kg iv | Usually, cefazolin 25 mg/kg iv | ⇐ |
| **Surgical time** | 1.5 hrs | 1 - 2 hrs | ⇐ |
| **Closing considerations** | Cylinder cast | ⇐ | Skin closure may be difficult, depending on elevation of tibial tubercle. |
| **Postop care** | PACU → home, if arthroscopic | PACU → room | ⇐ |
| **EBL** | < 100 cc | ⇐ | ⇐ |

| | Proximal realignment | Trillat | Macquet |
|---|---|---|---|
| **Mortality** | Minimal | ⇐ | ⇐ |
| **Morbidity** | Recurrence: 5-10% | ⇐ | ⇐ |
| | Late stiffness or increased knee pain: 5% | ⇐ | ⇐ |
| | Superficial wound dehiscence or infection: ≤ 5% | >5% | ≤ 5% |
| | Anterior compartment syndrome of the leg (Hauser procedure): 1-5% | ⇐ | ⇐ |
| | Deep infection: 1-2% | ⇐ | ⇐ |
| | Peroneal palsy: < 1% | ⇐ | ⇐ |
| **Procedure code** | 27422, 27425 (lateral release only | 27420, 27422 | 27418 |
| **Pain score** | 4-6 | 4-6 | 4-6 |

## PATIENT POPULATION CHARACTERISTICS

| | |
|---|---|
| **Age range** | 2-20 yrs (most commonly, 13-20 yrs) |
| **Male:Female** | 1:3[2] |
| **Incidence** | Subluxation: Very common<br>Recurrent dislocation: Rare<br>Congenital dislocation: Very rare[9] |
| **Etiology** | Generalized ligamentous laxity<br>Familial tendency, congenital hypoplasia at a lateral femoral condyle<br>Abnormal attachment or contracture of the IT band<br>Medial femoral torsion or genu valgum<br>Trauma |
| **Associated conditions** | Diffuse hyperlaxity syndromes (Ehlers-Danlos, Marfan, etc.)<br>Nail patella syndrome (hypoplastic nails and dislocated radial heads, as well as hypoplastic patellae) |

## ANESTHETIC CONSIDERATIONS

See "Anesthetic Considerations for Pediatric Orthopedic Surgery for Extremities" at the end of this section.

### References


1. Baker RH, Carroll N, Dewar FP, Hall JE: The Semitendinosus Tenodesis for recurrent dislocation of the patella. *J Bone Joint Surg* [Br] 1972; 54(1):103-9.
2. Bowker JH, Thompson EB: Surgical treatment of recurrent dislocation of the patella. A study of forty-eight cases. *J Bone Joint Surg* [Am] 1964; 46:1451-61.
3. Chrisman OD, Snook GA, Wilson TC: A long-term perspective study of the Hauser and Roux-Goldthwait procedures for recurrent patellar dislocation. *Clin Orthop* 1979; 144:27-30.
4. Cox JS: Evaluation of the Roux-Elmslie-Trillat procedure for knee extensor realignment. *Am J Sports* Med 1982; 10(5):303-10.
5. Fondren FB, Goldner JL, Bassett FH III: Recurrent dislocation of the patella treated by the modified Roux-Goldthwait procedure. A prospective study of forty-seven knees. *J Bone Joint Surg* [Am] 1985; 67(7):993-1005.
6. Hughston JC, Walsh WM: Proximal and distal reconstruction of the extensor mechanism for patellar subluxation. *Clin Orthop* 1979; 144:36-42.
7. Maquet P: Mechanics and osteoarthritis of the patellofemoral joint. *Clin Orthop* 1979; 144:70-3.
8. Morrissy RT: *Atlas of Pediatric Orthopaedic Surgery*. JB Lippincott, Philadelphia: 1992, 425-38.
9. Tachdjian MO: *Pediatric Orthopaedics*. WB Saunders, Philadelphia: 1990, 1551-95.
10. Trillat A, DeJour H, Louette A: Diagnostic et traitement des subluxations récidiventes de la rotule. *Rev Chir Orthop* 1964; 50:813-24.
11. Wall JJ: Compartment syndrome as a complication of the Hauser procedure. *J Bone Joint Surg* [Am] 1979; 61(2):185-91.

# TENDON TRANSFER, LENGTHENING (POSTERIOR TIBIAL)

## SURGICAL CONSIDERATIONS

**Description:** Extremity tendons may be lengthened (for contracture) or transferred to change the muscle force vector and compensate for paralysis or paresis of other muscle groups.[1,6] Originally used for the treatment of poliomyelitis sequelae, such lengthenings and transfers are now used for a variety of deformities 2° more common neuromuscular disorders such as cerebral palsy, muscular dystrophies, Charcot-Marie-Tooth disease, traumatic nerve palsies, etc. Basic principles are that the muscles to be transferred should be at least grade 4/5 strength, and that the loss of normal function should be well-compensated. The posterior tibial muscle (PTM) is a representative example, but many extremity muscles have one or more described lengthenings or transfers. Such procedures frequently are combined with other transfers or fusions.

For moderate spastic ankle varus, the simplest procedure, **PTM lengthening**, is accomplished by an intramuscular myotendinous "slide." This refers to simply cutting the tendinous fibers well within the distal muscle belly, and leaving a small gap in the tendon, while the surrounding muscle fibers remain intact.[6] An alternative for spastic varus is the **split posterior tibial transfer** of the PTM.[1,4] Four short, 2-3 cm incisions are used to expose and dissect ½ of the posterior tibia tendon at its insertion on the navicular. Then, ½ of the tendon is passed proximally up its sheath to a second incision just posterior to the distal tibial shaft medially. The freed ½ tendon is passed laterally to the peroneal tendon sheath just distal to the lateral malleolus, where, through a final incision, the tendon is anastomosed to the peroneus brevis.

For complete flaccid foot drop (e.g., peroneal nerve palsy), the entire posterior tibial tendon is transferred.[4,5] First, it is detached at its medial insertion, delivered proximally at the distal tibial posteriorly, passed **anteriorly** through a window in the interosseous membrane, and then subcutaneously passed to the mid-dorsal surface of the foot, where it is fixed into the middle cuneiform by a pull-out stitch.

**Usual preop diagnosis**: Flaccid or spastic developmental deformity such as varus or valgus foot neuromuscular disease.

### SUMMARY OF PROCEDURE

| | Lengthening | Split Transfer | Anterior Transfer |
|---|---|---|---|
| **Position** | Supine | ⇐ | ⇐ |
| **Incision** | Longitudinal posteromedial calf | Medial foot; posteromedial calf; lateral ankle; lateral foot | Medial foot; posteromedial calf; anterior ankle; dorsal foot |
| **Special instrumentation** | None | Tendon passers | Pull-out suture; buttons |
| **Unique considerations** | Underlying neurologic disease. Usually added to other procedures (e.g., Achilles tendon lengthenings.) | ⇐ | ⇐ |
| **Antibiotics** | Usually none | ⇐ | ⇐ |
| **Surgical time** | 30 min | 1 hr | ⇐ |
| **Closing considerations** | Below-knee cast | ⇐ | ⇐ |
| **EBL** | < 20 cc | < 50 cc | ⇐ |
| **Postop care** | PACU or room | ⇐ | ⇐ |
| **Mortality** | Rare | ⇐ | ⇐ |
| **Morbidity** | Over- or under-correction | ⇐ | ⇐ |
| | Hematoma | ⇐ | ⇐ |
| | Drainage: < 1% | ⇐ | ⇐ |
| **Procedure code** | 27685 | 27690 | 27691 |
| **Pain score** | 1-3 | 3-4 | 3-4 |

### PATIENT POPULATION CHARACTERISTICS

| | |
|---|---|
| **Age range** | 3-30 yrs |
| **Male:Female** | 1:1 |

| | |
|---|---|
| **Incidence** | Dependent on diagnosis |
| **Etiology** | Poliomyelitis<br>Cerebral palsy, spina bifida<br>Traumatic peroneal nerve injury<br>Neuropathies, myopathies (e.g., Charcot-Marie-Tooth disease) |
| **Associated conditions** | Multiple other contractures |

## ANESTHETIC CONSIDERATIONS

See "Anesthetic Considerations for Pediatric Orthopedic Surgery for Extremities" at the end of this section.


**References**

1. Green NE, Griffin PP, Shiavi R: Split posterior tibial-tendon transfers in spastic cerebral palsy. *J Bone Joint Surg* [Am] 1983; 65(6):748-54.
2. Hoffer MD, Barakat G, Koffman M: 10-year follow-up of split anterior tibial tendon transfer in cerebral palsied patients with spastic equinovarus deformity. *J Pediatr Orthop* 1985; 5(4):432-34.
3. Miller GM, Hsu JD, Hoffer MM, Rentfro R: Posterior tibial tendon transfer: a review of the literature and analysis of 74 procedures. *J Pediatri Orthop* 1982; 2(4):363-70.
4. Morrissy RT: *Atlas of Pediatric Orthopaedic Surgery*. JB Lippincott, Philadelphia: 1992, 645-68.
5. Richards BM: Interosseous transfer of tibialis posterior for common peroneal nerve palsy. *J Bone Joint Surg* [Br] 1989; 71(5):834-37.
6. Ruda R, Frost HM: Cerebral palsy. Spastic varus and forefoot adductus, treated by intramuscular posterior tibial tendon lengthening. *Clin Orthop* 1971; 79:61-70.


# TRIPLE ARTHRODESIS AND GRICE PROCEDURE (EXTRA-ARTICULAR SUBTALAR ARTHRODESIS)

## SURGICAL CONSIDERATIONS

**Description: Triple arthrodesis** is used to realign the hind foot of skeletally mature patients with significant fixed or flexible deformities of multiple etiologies. The technique involves denuding the cartilaginous surfaces of the talonavicular, talocalcaneal (subtalar) and calcaneocuboid joints and fusing them.[1-5] The approach is always through an oblique lateral sinus tarsi incision, and often an additional short medial incision over the talonavicular joint. For supple (passively correctable) deformities, the fusion is performed easily *in situ*. Fixed deformities are more difficult; but, basically, any deformity (valgus, varus, planus, cavus, etc.) can be corrected by resecting appropriate wedges of bone. Fixation is usually internal with pins, screws or staples, in addition to an external cast.

**Variant procedure or approaches**: Because the triple arthrodesis removes growth cartilage, it is unsuitable in growing children (< 12-14 years). **Grice** developed an **extra-articular subtalar fusion** which can be performed as early as age 3. It is basically a block of autologous bone graft placed between the talus and the calcaneus to stabilize a valgus heel. Tibial, fibular or, preferably, iliac autologous graft is used through the same lateral sinus tarsi incision as for a triple.

**Usual preop diagnosis**: Varus or cavo-varus foot deformities; severe valgus or equinovalgus

## SUMMARY OF PROCEDURE

| | Triple Arthrodesis | Grice Procedure |
|---|---|---|
| **Position** | Supine, slightly tilted up on the operative side | ⇐ |
| **Incision** | 2" oblique over the sinus tarsi; optional medial incision | ⇐ |
| **Special instrumentation** | Pins, screws or rods | Pin or screw |
| **Unique considerations** | Intraop x-ray to confirm pin position | Iliac or tibial autologous graft |
| **Antibiotics** | Usually - cefazolin 1 gm iv | Cefazolin 25 mg/kg iv |
| **Surgical time** | 1 - 2 hrs | 1.5 hrs |
| **Closing considerations** | Above-the-knee cast | ⇐ |
| **EBL** | < 100 cc | < 50 cc |
| **Postop care** | PACU → room | ⇐ |
| **Mortality** | Rare | ⇐ |
| **Morbidity** | Superficial skin slough | ⇐ |
| | Superficial infection | ⇐ |
| | Nonunion of at least one arthrodesis site (usually talonavicular) | ⇐ |
| | Aseptic necrosis of the talus: Rare | ⇐ |
| **Procedure code** | 28715 | 28725 |
| **Pain score** | 6-8 | 4-5 |

## PATIENT POPULATION CHARACTERISTICS

| | | |
|---|---|---|
| **Age range** | > 12 yrs | 3-10 yrs |
| **Male:Female** | 1:1 | ⇐ |
| **Incidence** | < 1% (depends on diagnosis and severity of deformity) | ⇐ |
| **Etiology** | Neuromuscular imbalance: Most cases | ⇐ |
| | Congenital malformations (e.g., coalitions, severe pes planus) | ⇐ |
| | Incomplete-treated or overcorrected clubfoot | ⇐ |
| | Post-fracture of calcaneus or talus | ⇐ |
| **Associated conditions** | Poliomyelitis | ⇐ |
| | Cerebral palsy – ↑GE reflux, ↓airway protective reflexes, ↑postop pulmonary complications | ⇐ |
| | Myelomeningocele | ⇐ |
| | Charcot-Marie-Tooth disease – ↑sensitivity to muscle relaxants | ⇐ |
| | Congenital tarsal coalition | ⇐ |

# ANESTHETIC CONSIDERATIONS

See "Anesthetic Considerations for Pediatric Orthopedic Surgery for Extremities" at the end of this section.

**References**

1. Chapman MW: *Operative Orthopaedics*, 2nd edition. JB Lippincott, Philadelphia: 1993, 2272-74.
2. Duncan JW, Lovell WW: Hoke triple arthrodesis. *J Bone Joint Surg* [AM] 1978; 60(6):795-98.
3. Dennyson WG, Fulford GE: Subtalar arthrodesis by cancellous grafts and metallic internal fixation. *J Bone Joint Surg* [Br] 1976; 58(4):507-10.

4. Grice DS: An extra-articular arthrodesis of the subastragalar joint for correction of paralytic flat feet in children. *J Bone Joint Surg* [Am] 1952; 34:927-40.
5. Morrissy RT: *Atlas of Pediatric Orthopaedic Surgery*. JB Lippincott, Philadelphia: 1992, 589-99.

# TURCO, SURGICAL CORRECTION OF CLUBFOOT

## SURGICAL CONSIDERATIONS

**Description:** Turco popularized the one-stage surgical correction of resistant (uncorrected by casting) clubfoot in 1971. The orthopedic literature, however, is replete with reports of varying techniques for surgical correction of clubfoot (talipes equino-varus). The three components of the deformity are: (1) hindfoot equinus (back of the heel is up); (2) varus (rolled inwardly); and (3) forefoot adductus (medial deviation). Beyond this, however, there exists considerable disagreement as to the pathologic anatomy, ideal skin incision, position, and which structures to release. Most surgeons vary the degree of release in proportion to the degree of deformity, often performing release of the same deep structures through totally different skin incisions. The most important structures release include: the entire posterior capsule of the ankle and subtalar joint; capsule of the subtalar, talonavicular and calcaneal cuboid joints; tendo-Achilles, posterior tibial tendon, and usually the toe flexors; and origin of the abductor, hallucis, and the plantar fascia. The navicular is repositioned on the talus and usually held with a small pin.

**Variant procedure or approaches**: **Turco's procedure**[10,11] is essentially a posteromedial procedure only and is performed through one incision on the medial aspect of the foot. **Crawford**[3] described a much more extensile approach through an incision that runs from anteromedial, around the back of the tendo-Achilles, and then anterolateral to the calcaneal cuboid joint. This approach is also used by **McKay**[5], **Simons**[7,8] and others for a more complete release. If there is severe equinus deformity, however, the incision is difficult to close posteriorly when the foot is brought up. **Carroll**[2] accomplishes much the same correction using a separate medial and posterolateral incision.

**Usual preop diagnosis**: Resistant idiopathic clubfoot (talipes equinovarus); secondary clubfoot due to paralysis

**SUMMARY OF PROCEDURE**

| | Turco | Cincinnati/McKay/Simon | Carroll |
|---|---|---|---|
| **Position** | Supine | Prone or supine | Supine |
| **Incision** | Straight medial foot | Transverse from the navicular bone medially-posteriorly across the heel cord, then laterally to the cuboid | Medial zigzag and posterolateral longitudinal |
| **Special instrumentation** | Usually loupe magnification; small K wires to hold reduction | ⇐ | ⇐ |
| **Unique considerations** | Tourniquet mandatory and often bilateral | ⇐ | ⇐ |
| **Antibiotics** | Cefazolin 25 mg/kg iv | ⇐ | ⇐ |
| **Surgical time** | 1 - 2 hrs/foot | ⇐ | ⇐ |
| **Closing considerations** | Well-padded, loose-fitting, above-the-knee cast x 10-14 d | ⇐ | ⇐ |
| **EBL** | < 30 cc | ⇐ | ⇐ |
| **Postop care** | PACU → room | ⇐ | ⇐ |
| **Mortality** | Rare | ⇐ | ⇐ |

| | Turco | Cincinnati/McKay/Simon | Carroll |
|---|---|---|---|
| **Morbidity**[5-11] | Mild, persistent deformity: Very common<br>Hematoma: 2%<br>Superficial infection: 1-2%<br>Avascular necrosis<br>Overcorrection valgus, planus<br>Pressure changes of the navicular<br>Wound dehiscence or necrosis<br>Transection of posterior tibial nerve or artery branch (rare, except in previously multiple-operated patient) | ⇐ | ⇐ |
| **Procedure code** | 28262 | ⇐ | ⇐ |
| **Pain score** | 2-5 | ⇐ | ⇐ |

### PATIENT POPULATION CHARACTERISTICS

| | |
|---|---|
| **Age range** | 3 mo-6 yrs |
| **Male:Female** | 2:1 (idiopathic type) |
| **Incidence** | 1.2/1000 live births (idiopathic type[9]) |
| **Etiology** | Genetic, or hereditary effects<br>Neuromuscular defects of the calf muscles<br>Primary defect of formation of the talus and/or other tarsal bones<br>Shortened ligaments and muscles |
| **Associated conditions** | Arthrogryposis (difficult intubation; ± VSD, other CHD)<br>Larsen's syndrome (difficult intubation; ± ↑ICP)<br>Freeman-Sheldon syndrome (difficult intubation)<br>Osteochondral dystrophies (e.g., diastrophic dwarfism)<br>Spinal dysraphism<br>Tethered spinal cord<br>Congenital constricting bands<br>Poliomyelitis |

## ANESTHETIC CONSIDERATIONS

See "Anesthetic Considerations for Pediatric Orthopedic Surgery for Extremities," below.

**References**

1. Beat JH: Congenital anomalies of the lower extremity. In *Campbell's Operative Orthopaedics*, 8th edition. Crenshaw AH, ed. Mosby Year Book, St. Louis: 1992, 2075-91.
2. Carroll NC: Congenital clubfoot: pathoanatomy and treatment. *AAOS Instr Course Lect* 1987; 36:117-21.
3. Crawford AH, Marxen JL, Osterfeld DL: The Cincinnati incision: a comprehensive approach for surgical procedures of the foot and ankle in childhood. *J Bone Joint Surg* [Am] 1982; 64(9):1355-58.
4. Lichtblau S: A medial and lateral release operation for clubfoot. *J Bone Joint Surg* [Am] 1973; 55(7):1377-84.
5. McKay DW: New concept of and approach to club foot treatment: Section II – correction of the club foot. *J Pediatr Orthop* 1983; 3(1):10-21.
6. Morrissy RT: *Atlas of Pediatric Orthopaedic Surgery*. JB Lippincott, Philadelphia: 1992, 523-28.
7. Simons GW: Complete subtalar release in clubfeet: Part I – a preliminary report. *J Bone Joint Surg* [Am] 1985 67(7):1044-55.
8. Simons GW: Complete subtalar release in clubfeet: Part II – comparison with less extensive procedures. *J Bone Joint Surg* [Am] 1985; 67(7):1056-65.
9. Tachdjian MO: *Pediatric Orthopaedics*. WB Saunders Co, Philadelphia: 1990, 2428-57.
10. Turco VJ: Surgical correction of the resistant club foot. One-stage posteromedial release with internal fixation: a preliminary report. *J Bone Joint Surg* [Am] 1971; 53(3):477-97.
11. Turco VJ: Resistant congenital club foot - one-stage posteromedial release with internal fixation. A follow-up report of a fifteen-year experience. *J Bone Joint Surg* [Am] 1979; 61(6A):805-14.

## ANESTHETIC CONSIDERATIONS

## FOR PEDIATRIC ORTHOPEDIC SURGERY FOR EXTREMITIES

**(Procedures covered: adductor release and/or transfer; psoas release; epiphysiodesis; Grice procedure; acetabular augmentation; Chiari osteotomy; proximal tibia; femoral osteotomy; limb lengthening; Ober fasciotomy; Yount Ober release; patellar realignment; syndactyly release; tendon lengthening or transfer; Turco procedure; triple arthrodesis; pollicization of finger; pinning of SCFE; pelvic osteotomy; hip open reduction)**

### PREOPERATIVE

Children undergoing orthopedic procedures of the extremities typically fall into two groups: (1) post-trauma but otherwise healthy and (2) those with a variety of chronic medical problems, including cerebral palsy, congenital hip dislocation, limb deformities, osteogenesis imperfecta, juvenile rheumatoid arthritis, epidermolysis bullosa, various myopathies and muscular dystrophies. The anesthesiologist should review the anesthetic implications of these various syndromes or diseases (see Table 12.4-1). Many of these patients will have cardiac, respiratory, endocrine and metabolic derangements, as well as airway abnormalities which may affect anesthetic management. In addition, the surgical procedures may run the gamut from a simple syndactyly repair of the fingers with little blood loss to pelvic osteotomies in small children with blood loss approaching patient blood volume.

**Respiratory** Patient's preop activity level is a good indication for baseline respiratory function. Careful assessment is necessary as associated anomalies may affect airway or lungs. Chronic otitis 2° eustachian tube dysfunction is common. Treat with antibiotics before surgery. Postpone surgery (~2 wks) if Sx of acute URTI (e.g., runny nose, fever, sore throat, cough) are present.

**Tests:** As indicated from H&P.

**Cardiovascular** Some pediatric patients with congenital musculoskeletal anomalies presenting for orthopedic procedures have coexisting cardiovascular anomalies. Although this is not common, preop review of patient's H&P is essential. A patient should not be accepted for orthopedic surgery and anesthesia until they are in the best possible physical and emotional condition. For children with CHD or who require cardiac medication, it is advisable to consult with a pediatric cardiologist before surgery.

**NB:** The consequences of VAE may be disastrous (e.g., cerebral or myocardial embolization) in patients with R → L shunt lesions. All iv lines, injection ports and syringes should be air-free.

**Tests:** ECG; Hct; baseline $O_2$ saturation; chest radiograph, as necessary

**Table 12.4-1. Preop anesthesia considerations for pediatric orthopedic diseases.**

| Disease | Anesthesia Considerations |
|---|---|
| Klippel-Feil | Limited cervical spine mobility; CHD |
| Septic arthritis | Systemic infection |
| Apert's syndrome | Hypoplastic maxilla → difficult airway management, ↑ICP, CHD |
| Marfan syndrome | Aortic dilation → aortic insufficiency; aortic dissection and aneurysm. Avoid ↑BP. Anticipate difficult intubation 2° narrow palate; lung cysts → pneumothorax. |
| Osteogenesis imperfecta | Bones fracture easily (e.g., with BP cuff): use extreme care in positioning and intubation. Hypermetabolic fever during anesthesia; platelet dysfunction; CHD; difficult airway. |
| Achondroplasia | Restrictive lung disease; poor cervical mobility. Anticipate difficult intubation. |
| Muscular dystrophy | ↑sensitivity to muscle relaxant; ↑MH susceptibility. Avoid succinylcholine. May have MVR and cardiac conduction abnormalities. May require postop ventilation. ✓ECG, ↓gastric emptying and weak laryngeal reflexes. |
| Myopathies | Avoid all muscle relaxants and respiratory depressants. Postop ventilation may be necessary. |
| Juvenile rheumatoid arthritis | Poor cervical mobility; TMJ ankylosis; carditis; possibility of difficult intubation. |
| Arthrogryposis | Poor cervical mobility; TMJ ankylosis; CHD; possible airway problems. |
| Cerebral palsy | Gastroesophageal reflux and pulmonary problems; ↑sensitivity to muscle relaxants. |

**Neurological** For patients with cerebral palsy presenting for orthopedic surgery, preop understanding of their intellectual functional capacity is necessary. Information about patient's behavioral or intellectual abilities is usually best obtained from parents or guardian. If patient is on seizure-control medication, it is recommended that the medication be continued until surgery. ✓ levels.

All patients who require Ober fasciotomy or Yount release will have profound weakness of lower extremities, if not of the entire body. Must be careful in choice of muscle relaxant (generally avoid depolarizing agents).

**Laboratory** Tests as indicated from H&P.

**Premedication** Premedication for separation anxiety (e.g., midazolam) and facilitating induction (e.g., atropine). Dosage must be individualized (see Appendix). Children with valvular disease, prosthetic valves, and/or most forms of CHD, as well as post-cardiac-correction patients, should receive antibiotics for bacterial endocarditis prophylaxis preop.[15]

## INTRAOPERATIVE

**Anesthetic technique:** As indicated in the preop considerations, these patient populations cover a vast spectrum, from fit and healthy children, to those suffering from a variety of clinical syndromes with airway and cardio-respiratory problems. Hence, anesthesia needs to be tailored to the individual patient. Some older children may benefit from regional anesthesia with sedation. Others may do well with a combined regional/GA technique, while still others with difficult airways may require awake FOL. The following sections address some (not all) of these concerns.

**Induction** **Normal:** standard pediatric (< 12 yrs) or adult induction (see Appendix).

**Difficult airway:** a mask induction and FOL during spontaneous respiration should be considered. Alternatives include use of an anterior commissure scope, blind oral or nasal intubation, use of FOL or light wand stylet, retrograde wire intubation and tracheostomy.

**Muscle abnormalities**: these patients may be very sensitive to muscle relaxants, have gastric hypomotility, and may be predisposed to MH. Induction should be accomplished by "non-triggering" agents (e.g., thiopental 1-3 mg/kg and atracurium or vecuronium if necessary for intubation). Succinylcholine is usually contraindicated in these patients. Dantrolene must be available, but it need not be administered prophylactically. A study of MH patients showed that 32 out of 89 had pre-existing musculoskeletal abnormalities.[13]

**Cardiorespiratory compromise**: inhalational induction, when administered cautiously, may be used safely in this group of patients. IV (e.g., etomidate 0.1-0.4 mg/kg iv) and intra-muscular (e.g., ketamine 4-8 mg/kg im) inductions are usually safe and effective in neonates and infants with severe cardiac disease.

**Maintenance** **Normal**: standard maintenance (see Appendix).

**Muscle abnormalities**: maintenance of anesthesia with a non-triggering agent (e.g., $N_2O$, opiates), and short-acting, non-depolarizing muscle relaxants is prudent. A peripheral nerve stimulator should be used to monitor muscle relaxation as the effects of muscle relaxants may be unexpectedly prolonged.

**Cardiorespiratory compromise**: the maintenance of anesthesia in this group is most commonly accomplished by use of inhalational agents, additional narcotics or other iv agents, depending on patient tolerance and postop plans for ventilatory management.

**Emergence** **Normal:** if muscle relaxant used, reverse with neostigmine (0.07 mg/kg) and glycopyrrolate (0.01 mg/kg iv) or edrophonium (0.5 mg/kg) and atropine (0.015 mg/kg iv). Make sure patient is awake and able to protect airway. A vital capacity of >15 ml/kg is considered an adequate sign of recovery of respiratory reserve.[16]

**Muscle abnormalities:** Anticipate postop respiratory impairment. Suction airway carefully. The response to neostigmine is unpredictable and may precipitate myotonia. Continued postop mechanical ventilation may be required.

**Cardiorespiratory compromise:** Tourniquet release may cause significant ↓CO and ↓BP, requiring temporary inotropic support. Otherwise, emergence as in normal patients.

**Regional anesthesia:** Used in patients undergoing lower extremity surgery.

**Caudal epidural** Use bupivacaine 0.25% or lidocaine 1%, ± epinephrine 1:200,000. Volume = 0.05 ml/kg/dermatome to be blocked.[18]

**Continuous epidural infusion** Use bupivacaine 0.1-0.125% ar rate of 0.1 ml/kg/hr in patients < 5 yrs; thereafter, patients may require 0.05-0.15 ml/kg/hr.

| | | |
|---|---|---|
| **Blood and fluid requirements** | IV: 22 ga or greater x 1-2<br>NS/LR @:<br>4 cc/kg/hr – 0-10 kg<br>+ 2 cc/kg/hr – 11-20 kg<br>+ 1 cc/kg/hr – >20 kg<br>(e.g., 25 kg = 65 cc/hr)<br>Warm fluids; humidify gasses. | There may be rapid fluid shifts in pediatric patients undergoing orthopedic procedures. Close monitoring and adequate fluid replacement will ensure hemodynamic stability. In hip or pelvis surgery, blood loss may be substantial, and adequate iv access is important as blood transfusion may be required. |
| **Control of blood loss** | Tourniquet – 120 min limit | Use of pneumatic tourniquets has become common practice in peripheral orthopedic procedures. They reduce intraop blood loss; however, they cause pain and, upon removal, release products of anaerobic metabolism.[17] |
| **Monitoring** | Standard monitors (see Appendix).<br>± Arterial line<br>± CVP line | Most pediatric patients presenting for extremity surgery do not require invasive monitoring. An arterial or CVP line may be helpful, depending on patient's medical condition, length of surgery and anticipated blood loss. |
| **Positioning** | ✓ and pad pressure points.<br>✓ eyes. | Patients with osteogenesis imperfecta or osteoporosis are at risk for fractures and joint dislocations and require special care in positioning. |
| **Complications** | MH | Early Sx of MH include: tachycardia, tachypnea, unstable BP, dysrhythmias, cyanotic mottling of skin, rapid rise in temperature (1°/15 min), discolored urine, metabolic acidosis, respiratory acidosis, hyperkalemia, myoglobinuria. Rx: stop surgery and anesthesia immediately; hyperventilate with 100% $O_2$; administer dantrolene sodium iv (starting dose = 1-2 mg/kg q 5-10 min; maximum cumulative dose = 10 mg/kg) by rapid infusion. Procainamide (15 mg/kg) over 15 min may be required for dysrhythmias. Initiate cooling, correct acidosis and hyperkalemia. Maintain UO of at least 2 ml/kg/hr. Monitor patient in ICU until danger of subsequent episodes is over (24 hrs). |

## POSTOPERATIVE

| | | |
|---|---|---|
| **Complications** | MH<br>Respiratory insufficiency | For MH considerations, see above. |
| **Pain management** | PCA (see Appendix).<br>Parenteral opiates<br>Spinal opiates | Caudal morphine (0.05 mg/kg) provides 8-24 hrs postop analgesia. Epidural fentanyl (0.3-1.0 $\mu$/kg/hr) may be administered by continuous infusion, ± low doses of bupivacaine. Patients with distal realignment are at risk for compartment syndrome postop and should not have a pain-relieving technique which could mask a compartment syndrome (e.g., epidural, etc.). |

**References**


1. Tait AR, Knight PR: The effects of general anesthesia on upper respiratory tract infections in children. *Anesthesiology* 1987; 67(6):930-35.
2. Britt BA, Kalow W: Malignant hyperthermia: a statistical review. *Can Anaesth Soc J* 1970; 17(4):293-315.
3. Brownell AK, Paasuke RT, Elash A, Fowlow SB, Seagram CG, Diewold RJ, Friesen C: Malignant hyperthermia in Duchenne muscular dystrophy. *Anesthesiology* 1983; 58(2):180-82.
4. Prevention of bacterial endocarditis. American Heart Assoc, Committee on Rheumatic Fever, Endocarditis and Kawasaki Disease of the Council on Cardiovascular Disease in the Young of the American Heart Association. *JAMA* 1990; 264(22):2919-22.
5. Shimada Y, Yoshiya I, Tanaka K, Yamazaki T, Kumon K: Crying vital capacity and maximal inspiratory pressure as clinical indicators of readiness for weaning of infants less than a year of age. *Anesthesiology* 1979; 51(5):456-59.
6. Brustowicz RM, et al: Metabolic responses to tourniquet release in children. *Anesthesiology* 1987; 67(5):792-94.
7. Takasaki M, Dohi S, Kawabata Y, Takahashi T: Dosage of lidocaine for caudal anesthesia in infants and children. *Anesthesiology* 1977; 47(6):527-29.

**Authors**

**Sarah S. Donaldson, MD, FACR** *(Pediatric Radiation Therapy)*
**Carol A. Shostak, RN, RTT, CMD** *(Pediatric Radiation Therapy)*

# 13. OUT-OF-OR PROCEDURES

**Anesthesiologists**

**Richard A. Jaffe, MD, PhD**
**Stanley I. Samuels, MB, BCh, FFARCS**

# PEDIATRIC RADIATION THERAPY

## SURGICAL CONSIDERATIONS

**Description:** Modern pediatric radiotherapy requires that the patient be in a stable and reproducible position for daily treatment. Sharply defined beams with secondary collimation are used to irradiate the tumor volume and to spare normal tissue. Patient movement may undermine techniques for sparing normal tissue and, while movement cannot be completely prevented, it must be minimized. In very young children, it is often impossible to prevent movement and achieve adequate cooperation for radiotherapy. In such cases, daily anesthesia is required. Close cooperation of the radiotherapy and anesthesia teams allows for safe and reproducible daily treatment.[1] In general, children older than 3 or 4 years can be induced to lie still for radiation therapy. Children from 2-1/2 to 4 years may cooperate during the treatment (which is usually less than 15 minutes), but not for the setup, in which an immobilization-stabilization device is made (often requiring 1 - 1.5 hours). In most infants and young children (< 2.5 years), anesthesia is essential.

The optimal position for radiotherapy must be one which is also optimal for the anesthesiologist. A series of radiographs are taken at the **setup**, which typically lasts 1-2 hours and requires GA. It is essential that there be no patient movement between exposures; if the patient moves, the entire procedure must be repeated. From the radiographs, individual beam-shaping devices are made. One or two days following setup, the patient has a simulation appointment, which usually is of shorter duration – often requiring only 30-60 minutes of anesthesia. Another series of radiographs is taken using the beam-shaping devices, which simulate the treatment to be given. When the setup and simulation procedures are successfully completed, the anesthetized patient is moved to the treatment room. He or she is put in the identical position achieved during the setup/simulation procedures, and treatment is administered. The first day or two, and weekly thereafter, a verification x-ray (called a "port film") is taken to confirm the accuracy of the treatment field. The treatment itself is of only a few minutes' duration for each field; ideally, the entire procedure is completed within 15-30 minutes. A course of treatment may be only a few days, or may last for 5-6 weeks, generally with the treatment given 5 times per week. Occasionally, multiple (2-3) treatments per day are given at 4- to 8- (usually 6-) hour intervals. At the initial appointment, the patient's optimal position is decided upon, an immobilization device constructed, and measurements taken. Initially, temporary marks or band-aids are used; however, when the final positioning has been determined, a more permanent mark, such as a tattoo, is applied. Often the use of a head holder with tape or velcro and/or a belt or mask is applied to ensure the position for radiotherapy.[3]

In managing certain brain tumors (e.g., medulloblastoma, high-grade intratentorial ependymoma, germ cell tumors and CNS leukemia), cranial spinal irradiation (CSI) is used. This procedure requires that the patient be placed in the prone position with the head flexed as much as possible to minimize a cervical lordosis. This positioning, however, creates special difficulties for the anesthesiologist. If the child is intubated for the setup, the radiation stabilization device must allow space for the ETT. If the child is not intubated, there must be adequate access to the airway.[5]

**Fractionation:** Pediatric protocols are currently testing the efficacy of giving multiple fractions (treatments) of radiation 2-3 times per day, usually at 6-hour intervals, to allow higher total radiation doses to be administered with possible less normal-tissue morbidity. These schemes have been, or are being evaluated for children with: brainstem gliomas; supratentorial glial tumors; medulloblastoma and other posterior fossa tumors; soft-tissue sarcomas, including rhabdomyosarcoma; some bone tumors, including Ewing's sarcoma; and total body irradiation in preparation for bone marrow transplantation. Until proven to be of increased efficacy, such schemes should remain part of large protocol studies. The timing of radiotherapy may be at 4-, 6-, or 8-hour intervals 2-3 times per day, depending on the protocol. These studies provide several challenges for anesthesiologists, radiotherapists and parents. Radiotherapy under anesthesia, however, has been successfully administered to infants undergoing multiple fractions per day.[9] Attention must be given to potential malnutrition and/or dehydration from prolonged periods of npo status.

**Total body irradiation (TBI):** Although most TBI techniques are administered with the patient standing, infants and small children must lie prone and supine for the treatment. This positioning requires sedation and/or anesthesia. Retching and vomiting, sometimes provoked by the radiation, present an additional challenge for proper radiotherapy technique, as well as for anesthetic management. Anesthesia for high-dose TBI has been accomplished with inhalation anesthetics and mechanical ventilation,[10] and with ketamine anesthesia.[11]

**Radiosurgery:** The technique of utilizing stereotactically localized radiosurgery with a highly collimated radiotherapy photon beam, as generated from a linear accelerator, is currently being employed for select patients with small CNS or base-of-skull tumors. There is increasing enthusiasm for this technique for infants and children with recurrent posterior fossa and cerebral tumors, craniopharyngiomas, optic nerve and chiasmal gliomas, and arteriovenous malformations (AVMs). Radiosurgery requires 6-8 hours of continuous anesthesia while a patient undergoes application of the metal halo frame, computed tomographic localization, and multiport radiotherapy treatment. This approach requires close coordination between the anesthesiologist, neurosurgeon and radiotherapist.

**Usual preop diagnosis:** Leukemia; retinoblastoma; most of the solid tumors of childhood

### SUMMARY OF PROCEDURE

| | Standard XRT | TBI | Radiosurgery |
|---|---|---|---|
| **Position** | Supine or prone | Supine and prone | Supine or prone |
| **Unique considerations** | If prone: head flexed for maximal straightening of the cervical spine. | May be repeated 2-3 times/ d at 4- to 6-hr intervals. | Halo frame placement at CT |
| **Anesthesia time** | Setup: 30 - 120 min<br>Treatment: < 15 min | < 20 min | 6 - 8 hrs |
| **Postop care** | PACU → home | PACU → room | PACU → room or home |

### PATIENT POPULATION CHARACTERISTICS

| | |
|---|---|
| **Age range** | Usually ≤ 4 yrs |
| **Male:Female** | 1:1 |
| **Incidence** | NA |
| **Associated conditions** | Brain tumors: Elevated ICP is of concern in these patients. Post-radiation edema following the first few treatments may further ↑ICP, with potential for brainstem herniation.[2] Some children with brainstem tumors are particularly difficult to anesthetize, perhaps because of disruption of nerve pathways in those areas of the brainstem which are affected by anesthetics.[1]<br>Diabetes insipidus (DI): It is often impossible to withhold fluids for 4-6 hrs prior to radiotherapy in an infant with symptomatic polydipsia from DI.<br>Neuroblastoma: Neuroblastomas are capable of secreting catecholamines and related substances; hence, there is a potential for paroxysmal HTN during anesthesia induction. In these children, the principles of anesthetic management are similar to those for pheochromocytoma.[13]<br>Retinoblastoma[14-17]: It is imperative that the patient be properly immobilized with no movement, as even a mm of change, as occurs with a sigh, may cause unnecessary radiation to the radiosensitive lens and anterior chamber. Optimal anesthesia prevents nystagmus and motion of the head. Even minimal lateral or rotary nystagmus may increase the risk of cataract induction.[6] A course of radiotherapy for retinoblastoma may involve 25-30 GA procedures in 5-6 wks. |

---

## ANESTHETIC CONSIDERATIONS

### PREOPERATIVE

A detailed pre-anesthesia visit is essential as this is the prime opportunity to gain the confidence of both child and parents. The importance of npo status needs to be stressed repeatedly to the parents, discussing the potential danger of vomiting during treatment. Breast milk may be given to infants < 6 mo of age, 4-6 hrs pre-treatment. Clear fluids are withheld for 2 hrs pre-treatment, while milk and solids should be withheld 6-8 hrs pre-treatment. Written instructions regarding preop protocol are extremely helpful in this context. In general, these patients are previously healthy children who have developed some life-threatening condition. Some of these children will have Sx of ↑ICP, which must be taken into account when designing an anesthetic plan.

**Respiratory** Patients with Sx of an URTI (runny nose, cough, fever) are commonly seen during XRT treatment and may pose problems for the anesthesia team. If the infection is acute, XRT should probably be delayed for a few d or until symptoms abate. Fortunately, most of the children can be managed without the use of an ETT, which might otherwise cause excessive secretions and postop laryngospasm. As always, the benefit of Rx must be balanced against the risks of anesthesia (induction laryngospasm, retained secretions, atelectasis/bronchospasm and postop laryngospasm).
**Tests:** As indicated from H&P.

**Neurological** Patients with intracranial tumors may have ↑ICP. Sx include irritability, headache, N&V and papilledema. Suspicion of ↑ICP probably mandates ET intubation and controlled ventilation to induce hypocarbia.

**Laboratory** Other tests as indicated from H&P.

**Premedication** Usually unnecessary in this patient group. Reliance on sedation or restraints is ill-advised and will lead to frustration on the part of the child, parents, technologists and physicians. Inappropriate sedation may cause respiratory and cardiovascular depression, and lead to a prolonged period of recovery.

## INTRAOPERATIVE

There is increasing enthusiasm for this technique for infants and children with recurrent posterior fossa and cerebral tumors, craniopharyngiomas, optic nerve and chiasmal gliomas, and arteriovenous malformations (AVM).

**Anesthetic technique:** Anesthesia for radiotherapy should be of brief duration, with rapid recovery and minimal cardiopulmonary depression, have good patient acceptance, allow maintenance of nutrition, and permit delivery of precise treatment by assuming immobility.[2] Inhalation, iv and intramuscular techniques have all been used successfully.

**Induction** IV: Propofol (1.5-2 mg/kg) iv slowly, followed by heparinized saline flush. Intubation is usually unnecessary, except for patients with ↑ICP or patients with potential for airway obstruction.

Inhalation: Mask induction with halothane is appropriate in children without iv access, and may be preferred by some children. Again, intubation is usually unnecessary. The airway may be maintained by extension of the neck and use of a head holder.[4] It is essential that this same degree of head flexion/extension be maintained for each daily treatment. An immobilization device may be molded, with the requirements for anesthesia kept in mind. If extreme neck flexion is required, ET intubation may be necessary.

**Maintenance** IV: Propofol (50-100 μg/kg/min) by continuous infusion. The airway can usually be well-maintained by careful positioning and the use of a head strap. Supplemental $O_2$ should be administered via nasal prongs or mask.

Inhalation: Maintain anesthesia with halothane in $O_2$, usually delivered by mask or insufflation.

**Emergence** IV: Flush iv with heparinized saline to prevent clotting. Patients will awaken rapidly following cessation of propofol infusion or inhaled agents. Extubation should be accomplished when the patient is fully awake, unless there is the possibility of ↑ICP, in which case a deep extubation is appropriate. This is important as there is frequently a long journey between the XRT department and PACU. Anti-emetics are usually unnecessary.

| | | |
|---|---|---|
| **Blood and fluid requirements** | IV: usually permanent access<br>NS/LR: infusion not usually required. | Many children receiving radiotherapy have a central venous access line, placed for long-term administration of chemotherapy. A planned course of anesthesia for radiotherapy, by itself, is an acceptable indication for placement of a central venous access line, even in the absence of plans for chemotherapy. Alternatively, an indwelling iv catheter with a heparin-lock for repeated iv injections has been effective in outpatient anesthesia for pediatric radiotherapy.[6] |
| **Monitoring** | Standard monitors (see Appendix). | A critical problem is the lack of access to the patient and monitors during XRT. A TV camera can focus on the visual displays of the monitors. Respiration may also be observed by direct visualization through a leaded-glass viewing port or a camera directed at the child. A small marker may be placed on the chest so that the rise and fall of chest motion is easily seen.[1] |
| **Positioning** | ✓ and pad pressure points.<br>✓ eyes. | |
| **Complications** | Airway obstruction | Respiratory obstruction occasionally occurs and responds to either nasopharyngeal or oropharyngeal airways. In rare instances, ET intubation may be required for persistent airway obstruction. |
| | Patient movements | Deepen anesthesia. |

## POSTOPERATIVE

| | | |
|---|---|---|
| **Complications** | Cerebral edema | In patients with ↑ICP, XRT can provoke an acute ↑ICP with consequent ↑headache, ↑N&V, ↓consciousness → cardiac arrest. These patients should be monitored x 24 hrs post-Rx. |
| **Pain management** | Standard approaches | Radiation treatments are not associated with pain, but may be useful in relieving pain associated with neoplastic disease. |


**References**

1. Murray WJ: Anesthesia for external beam radiotherapy. In *Pediatric Radiation Oncology,* Halperin EC, Kun LE, Constine LS, Tarbell NJ, eds. Raven Press, New York: 1989, 399-407.
2. Amberg HL, Gordon G: Low-dose intramuscular ketamine for pediatric radiotherapy: a case report. *Anesth Analg* 1976; 55(1):92-4.
3. Donaldson SS, Shostak CA, Samuels SI: Technical and practical considerations in the radiotherapy of children. *Front Radiat Ther* 1987; 21(1):256-69.
4. Browne CH, Boulton TB, Crichton TC: Anaesthesia for radiotherapy. A frame for maintaining the airway. *Anaesthesia* 1969; 24(3):428-30.
5. Maltby JR, Watkins DM: Repeat ketamine anaesthesia of a child for radiotherapy in the prone position. *Can Anaesth Soc J* 1983; 30(5):526-30.
6. Rodarte A: Heparin-lock for repeated anesthesia in pediatric radiation therapy. *Anesthesiology* 1982; 56(4):316-17.
7. Casey WF, Price V, Smith HS: Anaesthesia and monitoring for paediatric radiotherapy. *J R Soc Med* 1986; 79(8):454-56.
8. Davies DJ: Anesthesia and monitoring for pediatric radiation therapy. [LETTER] *Anesthesiology* 1986; 64(3):406-7.
9. Menache L, Eifel PJ, Kennamer DL, Belli JA: Twice-daily anesthesia in infants receiving hyper-fractionated irradiation. *Int J Radiat Oncol Biol Phys* 1990; 18(3):625-29.
10. Whitwan JG, Morgan M, Owen JR, Goolden AW, Spiers AS, Goldman JM, Gordan-Smith EC: General anaesthesia for high-dose total-body irradiation. *Lancet* 1978; 1(8056):128-29
11. Lo JN, Buckley JJ, Kim TH, Lopez R: Anesthesia for high-dose total body irradiation in children. *Anesthesiology* 1984; 61(1):101-3.
12. Greenberger JS, Cassady JR, Jaffe N, Vawter G, Crocker AC: Radiation therapy in patients with histiocytosis: Management of diabetes insipidus and bone lesions. *Int J Radiat Oncol Biol Phys* 1979: 5(10):1749-55.
13. Farman JV: Neuroblastomas and anaesthesia. *Br J Anaesth* 1965; 37(11):866-70.
14. Donaldson SS, Egbert PR: Retinoblastoma. In *Principles and Practice of Pediatric Oncology.* Pizzo PA, Poplack DG, eds, JB Lippincott, Philadelphia: 1989, 555-68.
15. Schipper J: An accurate and simple method for megavoltage radiation therapy of retinoblastoma. *Radiother Oncol* 1983; 1(1):31-41.
16. Harnett AN, Hungerford JL, Lambert GD, Hirst A, Darlison R, Hart BL, Trodd TC, Plowman PN: Improved external beam radiotherapy for the treatment of retinoblastoma. *Br J Radiol* 1987; 60(716):753-60.
17. Bagshaw MA, Kaplan HS: Supervoltage linear accelerator radiation therapy 8. Retinoblastoma. *Radiology* 1966; 86(2):242-46.

# APPENDIX

A. Standard Anesthetic Protocols

B. Table of Drug Interactions

C. Drugs Commonly Used in Anesthetic Management

D. Abbreviations and Acronyms

## STANDARD MONITORS (NON-INVASIVE)

Blood pressure

Capnometry or mass spectrometer: measurement of $ETCO_2$ and other respired gasses and anesthetics

Electrocardiogram (ECG): 5-lead preferred

Esophageal or precordial stethoscope: breath and heart sounds monitored; dysrhythmias and ↓BP detected

Nerve stimulator: monitor status of neuromuscular blockade

Oxygen analyzer: measurement of $FiO_2$

Pulse oximetry: measurement of $O_2$ saturation

Temperature: nasal or esophageal

Visual observation of patient: skin color, pupils, temperature, edema, sweating, movement

Ventilator function monitors

**NB:** The following sections are guidelines only. Specific drugs and drug dosages should be individualized based on the physiological and pharmacological status of the patient, including factors such as age, weight, medication and concurrent diseases.

## STANDARD ANESTHETIC MANAGEMENT (ADULT ASA 1 & 2)

### PREMEDICATION

| | | |
|---|---|---|
| **Light** | Diazepam 5-10 mg<br>Lorazepam 1-2 mg<br>Hydroxyzine 25-100 mg | po 1 hr preop<br>po 1 hr preop<br>po 1 hr preop |
| **Moderate** | Midazolam 1-2 mg iv<br>± Fentanyl 25-100 $\mu$g iv | Prior to induction (in patient holding area or OR) |
| **Heavy** | Diazepam 10 mg<br>+ Morphine 0.1 mg/kg<br>+ Scopolamine 0.2-0.4 mg | po 1-2 hrs preop<br>} im 30-60 min preop |

### INDUCTION TECHNIQUES

**Pre-induction**

1. ✓ anesthesia machine, suction, airway equipment, drugs.
2. Attach monitors and verify function.
3. Administer 100% $O_2$ by mask x 1-3 min.
4. Administer supplemental sedation/analgesia (as appropriate).
   e.g.: Fentanyl 1-3 $\mu$g/kg iv
   ± Midazolam 0.03-0.1 mg/kg iv

**Induction agents**

Thiopental 3-5 mg/kg iv
Propofol 1.5-2.5 mg/kg iv (in increments) **NB:** Pain on injection
Etomidate 0.2-0.4 mg/kg iv **NB:** Pain on injection; myoclonus

| | Drugs | Doses | Onset | Duration |
|---|---|---|---|---|
| **Muscle relaxants for intubation** | Succinylcholine: | 1.0 mg/kg | 30-60 sec | 4-6 min |
| | If given after 3 mg dTC for defasciculation: | 1.5 mg/kg | 30-60 sec | 4-6 min |
| | Infusion (titrated to effect): | 1 gm/250-500 NS | ~60 sec | While infusing (phase II block possible) |
| | Vecuronium: | 0.1 mg/kg | 2-3 min | 24-30 min |
| | | 0.2 mg/kg (rapid onset) | < 2 min | 45-90 min |
| | Pancuronium: | 0.1 mg/kg | 3-4 min | 40-65 min |
| | Mivacurium: | 0.1-0.2 mg/kg | 1-2 min | 6-10 min |
| | Atracurium: | 0.3-0.5 mg/kg | 2-3 min | 25-30 min |
| | d-tubocurarine (dTC): | 0.5 mg/kg | 3-5 min | 30 min |
| | Pipecuronium | 0.07-0.09 mg/kg | 2-3 min | 45-120 min |

## MAINTENANCE TECHNIQUES

| | | | |
|---|---|---|---|
| **Inhalational anesthesia** | 30-100% $O_2$<br>+ 0-70% $N_2O$<br>+ Isoflurane (MAC = 1.15%) titrated to effect | | |
| **Balanced anesthesia** | 30-100% $O_2$ in $H_2O$<br>+ 0-70% $N_2O$<br>+ Meperidine 0.5-1.5 mg/kg/3-4 hrs<br>or fentanyl 1-10 μg/kg/hr<br>+ Isoflurane ~0.5%<br>or propofol 50-200 μg/kg/min | | |
| **Total intravenous anesthesia** | 30-100% $O_2$ in $N_2O$<br>0-70% Air | | |
| | + Ketamine infusion<br>(infusion off 15-30 min<br>before end of surgery) | First hour<br>Hour 1-Hour 4<br>Hour 4 on | @ 1 mg/min/60-80 kg<br>@ 0.6 mg/min/60-80 kg<br>@ 0.4 mg/min/60-80 kg |
| | + Propofol infusion<br>(infusion off 5-10 min<br>before end of surgery) | First 10 min<br>10 min-2 hrs<br>After 2 hrs | @ 140-200 μg/kg/min<br>@ 100-140 μg/kg/min<br>@ 80-120 μg/kg/min |

If **continued muscle relaxation** is required during the above maintenance techniques, several options are available. Always use a nerve stimulator to assess block before redosing.

| | | |
|---|---|---|
| **Short-acting** | Mivacurium: | 0.1 mg/kg/10-20 min |
| **Intermediate** | Vecuronium: | 0.015 mg/kg/30 min |
| **Long** | Pancuronium:<br>Pipecuronium: | 0.02 mg/kg/60-90 min<br>0.015 mg/kg/60-90 min |

## EMERGENCE

| | |
|---|---|
| **1. Reversal of muscle relaxant** | As surgical conditions permit, reverse residual muscle relaxant (when at least 1 twitch is present in train-of-four) with one of the following:<br>Neostigmine 0.05-0.07 (maximum dose) mg/kg iv + glycopyrrolate 0.01 mg/kg iv, or<br>Edrophonium 0.5-1.0 (maximum dose) mg/kg iv + atropine 0.015 mg/kg iv. |
| **2. Nausea prophylaxis** | Metoclopramide 10 mg iv<br>Droperidol 0.625 mg iv<br>Ondansetron 4 mg iv |
| **3. $O_2$** | Discontinue $N_2O$/volatile agents and administer 100% $O_2$. |
| **4. Suction** | Suction oropharynx thoroughly. |
| **5. Extubation** | Extubate after protective air reflexes have returned, the patient is breathing spontaneously and is able to follow commands. |

**NB:** The following sections are guidelines only. Specific drugs and drug dosages should be individualized based on the physiological and pharmacological status of the patient, including factors such as age, weight, medication and concurrent diseases.

# STANDARD ANESTHETIC MANAGEMENT (PEDIATRIC)

## PREMEDICATION

In general, patients < 18 months of age do not need premedication – only atropine 0.02 mg/kg iv or im prior to intubation. Older children (18 months-10 yrs) can be successfully premedicated using oral midazolam (0.5-0.75 mg) in apple juice or grape Kool-Aid® 20-30 min prior to surgery.

## INDUCTION TECHNIQUES

**Pre-induction**

1. ✓ anesthesia machine, suction, airway equipment, drugs.
2. Attach monitors and verify function.
3. ± Premedication [< 18 mo: atropine only (0.02 mg/kg iv or im)].

**Induction**

Routes of administration:

1. Rectal – methohexital (5%) 30 mg/kg
2. Intramuscular – ketamine hydrochloride 3-5 mg/kg (with atropine 0.02 mg/kg)
3. IV – thiopental 2-5 mg/kg
   – methohexital 0.5-1 mg/kg
   – propofol 1-2.5 mg/kg
4. Inhalational-halothane (MAC = 0.87% [neonatal], 1-2% [infants], and 0.75% [adults]) initially diluted with $N_2O$ (up to 70%). Increase the inspired concentration of halothane incrementally every few breaths up to 2.5-3%. Monitor BP and HR closely.

**Muscle relaxation**

1. Succinylcholine: 1-2 mg/kg or 2-4 mg/kg im
2. Vecuronium or pancuronium: 0.1 mg/kg
3. Pipecuronium: 0.07-0.085 mg/kg
4. Atracurium: 0.3-0.5 mg/kg
5. Deep halothane and $O_2$

**Laryngoscope**

| Blade | Age |
|---|---|
| Miller 0 | Neonate |
| Miller 1 | 6-9 mo |
| Wis-Hipple 1.5 | 9 mo - 2 yrs |
| Miller 2 or Macintosh 2 | 2-5 yrs |
| Macintosh 2 | > 5 yrs |

**ETT**

| Age | Wt | ETT Size |
|---|---|---|
| Newborn | 3 kg | 3.0 |
| 6 mo | 6 kg | 3.5 |
| 1 yr | 10 kg | 4.0 |
| 3 yrs | 15 kg | Thereafter use formula: |
| 6 yrs | 20 kg | 4 + (age/4) = ETT size (to |
| 9 yrs | 30 kg | allow for a slight leak when |
| 12 yrs | 40 kg | positive pressure is applied. |

**NB:** This is a guide only; prepare an ETT one size larger and one size smaller than the ETT size selected. ✓✓ endotracheal placement of tube.

## MAINTENANCE TECHNIQUES

**Inhalational anesthesia**

30-100% $0_2$
+ 0-70% $N_2O$. In premies and infants, air may be used to lower $FiO_2$.
+ Isoflurane (MAC=1.15%) titrated to effect

**NB:** Warm and humidify all gasses in pediatric patients. Warm room to 75-80° F.

**Balanced anesthesia**

30-100% $O_2$
+ 0-70% $N_2O$

+ ~0.5% isoflurane
or propofol (50-200 μg/kg/min)

+ Meperidine (0.5-1.5 mg/kg/3-4 hrs)
or fentanyl (2-10 μg/kg/hr)

If **continued muscle relaxation** is required during the above maintenance techniques, several options are available. Always use a nerve stimulator to assess block before redosing.

| | | |
|---|---|---|
| **Short-acting** | Mivacurium: | 0.1 mg/kg → 6-10 min |
| **Intermediate** | Vecuronium: | 0.01 mg/kg → 25-30 min |
| **Long** | Pancuronium: | 0.1 mg/kg → 40-65 min |
| | Pipecuronium: | 0.08 mg/kg → 45-120 min |

## EMERGENCE

**1. Reversal of muscle relaxant**

As surgical conditions permit, reverse residual muscle relaxant (when at least 1 twitch is present in train-of-four) with one of the following:
Neostigmine 0.05-0.07 (maximum dose) mg/kg iv + glycopyrrolate 0.01 mg/kg iv, or
Edrophonium 0.5-1.0 (maximum dose) mg/kg iv + atropine 0.015 mg/kg iv.

**2. Nausea prophylaxis**

Metoclopramide 0.1 mg/kg iv (~1 hr before emergence)
Droperidol 0.1 mg/kg (single dose only)

**3. $O_2$**

Discontinue $N_2O$/volatile agents and administer 100% $O_2$.

**4. Suction**

Suction oropharynx thoroughly.

**5. Extubation**

Laryngeal spasm is common in children. It is, therefore, usual to extubate children when they are awake, moving all limbs, and breathing adequately. Infants and children with full stomachs or difficult airways must be extubated when they are fully awake. The pharynx should be suctioned thoroughly prior to extubation. Should laryngeal spasm occur, Rx with 100% $O_2$, and positive pressure ventilation. If spasm fails to resolve, then reintubate.

## RAPID-SEQUENCE INDUCTION OF ANESTHESIA (FULL-STOMACH PRECAUTIONS)

| | |
|---|---|
| **1. ↓gastric volume/acidity** | Ranitidine 50 mg iv at least 30-60 min before induction<br>Metoclopramide 5-10 mg iv 30-60 min before induction<br>0.3 M sodium citrate 30 ml po immediately before induction<br>Defasciculate: dTC 3 mg 3-5 min before succinylcholine |
| **2. Induction** | Pre-oxygenation > 3 min<br>Cricoid pressure (Sellick maneuver) by assistant<br>Etomidate 0.1-0.4 mg/kg or STP 3-5 mg/kg or ketamine 1 mg/kg iv<br>+ Succinylcholine 1.5 mg/kg for intubation (stylet ETT) |
| **3. Intubation** | Intubate when patient is fully relaxed.<br>Watch chest movement and auscultate for equal BBS.<br>✓ expired $CO_2$ on monitor.<br>Listen over stomach.<br>Secure ETT and stop cricoid pressure.<br>Pass NG tube and aspirate stomach. |
| **4. Failed intubation protocol** | See Anesthetic Considerations for "Cesarean Section" in "Obstetrics Surgery." |
| **5. Maintenance** | As indicated by patient's condition and type of surgery. |
| **6. Extubation** | Extubate when patient is awake and with active laryngeal protective reflexes. Remember, some may require postop ICU care until safe extubation can be assured. |

## SPECIAL PEDIATRIC CONSIDERATIONS

1. The same principles apply in children requiring surgery, and in those who may have full stomachs. Remember to empty the stomach with an OG tube prior to induction. If iv is placed, continue as indicated above. If iv access is difficult, $O_2$/halothane induction with cricoid pressure, succinylcholine (2-4 mg/kg) will permit intubation and minimize risks of gastric aspiration.

2. Awake intubation in neonates and sick infants may be the safest method.

# MONITORED ANESTHESIA CARE (MAC)

1. Standard monitoring with regular verbal contact.

2. Nasal $O_2$ (qualitative measurement of $ETCO_2$ can be accomplished by attaching a sampling catheter to the nasal cannula)

3. If the initial local anesthetic injection will be painful (e.g., retrobulbar block), then a brief period of analgesia, sedation and amnesia can be induced with:

| | Advantages: | Disadvantages: |
|---|---|---|
| A. Midazolam (0.5-2 mg)<br>3-5 min before injection<br>+ Ketamine (10-20 mg)<br>3 min before injection<br>+ Alfentanil 250-500 μg<br>2 min before injection | Profound amnesia<br>Excellent analgesia<br>No apnea<br>Airway reflexes maintained<br>Patient cooperation | Patient not "asleep"<br>Timing important<br>Possible ↑BP and HR |

or

| | Advantages: | Disadvantages: |
|---|---|---|
| B. STP (1-3 mg/kg)<br>± fentanyl (25-50 μg) | Patient "asleep" | Possible apnea<br>Possible loss of airway<br>↓BP<br>Patient unresponsive |

4. Light-to-moderate levels of sedation (± analgesia) can be maintained using a propofol infusion (25-100 μg/kg/min), or with intermittent bolus injections of midazolam (0.25-1 mg) ± fentanyl (10-25 μg), titrated to effect. Avoid respiratory depression.

## STANDARD ADULT POSTOP ANALGESICS AND ANTIEMETICS

| | | |
|---|---|---|
| **Analgesics** | Morphine | 2 mg/10 min, up to 6 mg iv |
| | Meperidine | 10 mg/10 min, up to 50-70 mg iv |
| | Fentanyl | 12.5-25 μg/5 min up to 100 μg iv |
| **Antiemetics** | Metoclopramide | 5-10 mg iv |
| | Droperidol | 0.625 mg iv |
| | Ondansetron | 4 mg iv – repeat if necessary after 30 min. |

## STANDARD PEDIATRIC POSTOP ANALGESICS AND ANTIEMETICS

| | | |
|---|---|---|
| **Analgesics** | Acetaminophen | 20 mg/kg po/pr prn q 4 hrs |
| | Morphine | 0.02 mg/kg iv q 5-10 min prn pain, may repeat up to 1.5 mg (for a 10-kg child) |
| | Meperidine | 0.5-1.0 mg/kg iv q 5-10 min prn pain, up to 1 mg/kg |
| **Antiemetics** | Droperidol | 0.02 mg/kg iv |
| | Metoclopramide | 0.1 mg/kg, may repeat up to 2 mg (for a 10 kg child) |
| | **NB:** Increased incidence of extrapyramidal reactions with both agents. | |

# EPIDURAL ANALGESIA

| Loading Dose | Morphine | Hydromorphone |
|---|---|---|
| Lower extremities | 2-3 mg | 0.3-0.5 mg |
| Pelvis | 3-4 mg | 0.5 mg |
| Abdomen | 5-7 mg | 0.5-1 mg |
| Thorax | 7-10 mg | 1-1.5 mg |

| Infusion | Morphine (0.15 mg/cc) | Hydromorphone (0.05 mg/cc) |
|---|---|---|
| Lower extremities | 2-3 cc/hr | 2-3 cc/hr |
| Pelvis | 2-4 cc/hr | 2-4 cc/hr |
| Abdomen | 3-5 cc/hr | 3-5 cc/hr |
| Thorax | 5-8 cc/hr | 5-8 cc/hr |

**Typical Orders for Postop Epidural/Spinal Analgesia**

1. Do not administer any opiates, antiemetics or sedatives unless ordered by anesthesiologist. If ordered by another service, notify anesthesiologist.
2. Label bed and Kardex "Epidural or Spinal Narcotic," as appropriate.
3. Put bed in 20- to 30-degree head-up position.
4. Resuscitation equipment at bedside or on medication cart: Ambu bag, oral airway, naloxone and syringe.
5. Maintain patent iv or heparin lock.
6. Check and record patient's sedation status q 1 hr for 12 hrs: awake, drowsy, asleep but easily arousable, unresponsive.
7. Respiratory monitoring: Select option A_____ or A and B _____ (pulse oximeter for _____ hrs).
   A. Check and record respiratory rate q 1 hr. (Appropriate for patients at low risk for respiratory depression.)
   B. Pulse oximeter. (Recommended if patient is obese, has had general anesthesia, sedatives or systemic opiates, or if there is any suggestion of respiratory compromise (e.g., low intra- or postop $O_2$ sat, sleep apnea). Mandatory if patient receiving depressant drugs other than as per this protocol.)
8. Treatment of respiratory depression:
   A. If RR < 10, or $O_2$ sat < 94% on 2 separate occasions less than 5 min apart, call anesthesiologist.
   B. If RR < 8, $O_2$ sat < 90%, or patient in obvious respiratory distress, call anesthesiologist STAT and encourage patient to breathe. If no immediate improvement, administer naloxone 0.2 mg iv STAT. Dose may be repeated up to 0.6 mg. Keep patient awake, administer $O_2$ at 10 L/min by non-rebreathing mask and assist ventilation if necessary. Apply pulse oximeter if not already in place.
9. Treatment of sedation:
   If patient complains of or exhibits excessive drowsiness (check for pinpoint pupils) call anesthesiologist and apply pulse oximeter. If patient is unarousable, immediately treat with naloxone as above (Step 8B).
10. Treatment of pruritus:
    Nalbuphine (Nubain®) 2.5-5 mg iv q 15 min (up to 10 mg). May be repeated every 2-4 hrs prn.
11. Treatment of nausea/vomiting:
    Nalbuphine (administer as in Step 10) or metoclopramide 10 mg iv every 3 hrs prn (up to 4 doses).
12. Treatment of pain:
    Nalbuphine 5-10 mg iv q 2-4 hrs prn, or oral analgesics after 6 hrs, as tolerated (see surgeon's orders for chosen oral analgesic).
13. Call anesthesiologist if:
    A. Sx of respiratory depression
    B. Patient very drowsy or has pinpoint pupils
    C. Pain relief inadequate
    D. Side effects are unresponsive to above therapy
14. Resume postop pain orders when epidural opioid orders end.

## PATIENT-CONTROLLED ANALGESIA (PCA)

| | | |
|---|---|---|
| **Loading dose** | Morphine<br>Meperidine | Titrate to comfort<br>Titrate to comfort |
| **PCA dose** | Morphine<br>Meperidine | 0.015 mg/kg/dose<br>0.15 mg/kg/dose* |
| **Lock-out dose** | 10-20 min | |
| **Basal rate** | Morphine<br>Meperidine | 1 mg/hr/70 kg<br>10 mg/hr/70 kg |
| **4-hr limit** | Morphine<br>Meperidine | 0.3 mg/kg<br>3 mg/kg |

***NB:** Toxic effect of normeperidine may become evident (e.g., seizures).

**Typical Orders**

1. Resume routine pain med orders after PCA discontinued.
2. Call anesthesiologist with any questions about PCA.
3. Check respiratory rate q 1 hr while PCA in use.
4. Call anesthesiologist if respiratory rate < 10/min. If rate < 8/min, treat with naloxone 0.4 mg iv push and assist ventilation while waiting for anesthesiologist.
5. Encourage patient to ambulate 4-6° after surgery unless contraindicated.

# TABLE OF DRUG INTERACTIONS

This table is intended only as an advisory overview of potential drug interactions between various drug classes that patients may be taking preoperatively with drugs used in anesthesia practice. In view of the constant flow of new drug information, the reader is strongly urged to check the primary literature of each drug and tailor drug usage to the specific clinical situation.

| Preop Drug Or Drug Class | Anesthetic Drug Or Drug Class | Interaction | Clinical Management |
|---|---|---|---|
| Amiodarone | fentanyl | ↓↓HR, ↓BP, sinus arrest | Monitor hemodynamic function.<br>Administer inotropic, chronotropic and pressor agents as indicated.<br>Large doses of vasopressors may be required.<br>Bradycardia is usually not responsive to atropine. |
| Aminoglycosides | enflurane | ↑potential for nephrotoxicity 2° fluoride | Monitor renal function postop. |
| | non-depolarizing muscle relaxants (NMR) | ↑NMR; possible protracted respiratory depression | Administer combination only when necessary.<br>Titrate NMR dose.<br>Antidotal use of Ca salts and anticholinesterases is unreliable.<br>Support respiration. |
| | succinylcholine | ↑depolarizing block | Delay administration of aminoglycosides as long as possible after recovery from block.<br>Support respiration. |
| Amphetamines | narcotic analgesics | ↑analgesia | Titrate dosage of narcotic. |
| Antacids | oral medication | Delayed drug absorption 2° delayed gastric emptying | Avoid administration within 2 hrs of each other. |
| Antibiotics, polypeptide (bacitracin, colismethate, polymyxin B) | non-depolarizing muscle relaxants (NMR) | ↑NMR | Monitor neuromuscular blockade.<br>Titrate dosage of NMR.<br>Support respiration. |
| Anticholinesterases (including ophthalmics) | non-depolarizing neuromuscular relaxants (NMR) | ↓NMR | Titrate dosage of NMR to therapeutic effectiveness. |
| Anticholinesterases | succinylcholine | ↑depolarizing block | Titrate succinylcholine.<br>Support respiration. |
| Asparaginase | physostigmine | Possible Parkinsonian effects | **Avoid combination.** |
| | droperidol | Possible Parkinsonian effects | **Avoid combination.** |

| Preop Drug Or Drug Class | Anesthetic Drug Or Drug Class | Interaction | Clinical Management |
|---|---|---|---|
| Azathioprine | non-depolarizing muscle relaxants (NMR) | ↓↓NMR | Monitor and support neuromuscular blockade.<br>Titrate NMR dosage. |
| Barbiturates | inhalation anesthetics, ketamine, narcotic analgesics | ↑respiratory depression | Monitor and support respiration. |
| Benzodiazepines | narcotic analgesics | ↓BP | Monitor and support BP. |
| | non-depolarizing muscle relaxants (NMR) | May ↑ or ↓NMR. | Monitor and support respiration. |
| | barbiturates | Drug actions may be additive. | Titrate dosage of barbiturate. |
| | bupivacaine | Reduces potential for CNS toxicity, but not for cardiovascular toxicity. | Seizure threshold raised; monitor and support cardiovascular status. |
| Benztropine | ketamine | ↑HR | Use ß-blocker if necessary. |
| ß-blockers | non-depolarizing muscle relaxants (NMR) | ↑ or ↓NMR | Monitor and support respiration. |
| | bupivacaine, lidocaine | ↓clearance of bupivacaine, lidocaine | Infuse slowly to prevent high peak levels. |
| ß-blockers, non-selective | epinephrine | ↑BP → ↓HR | **Avoid combination.**<br>Consider discontinuation of non-selective ß-blocker 3 d preop. |
| ß-blockers | droperidol | ↓BP | Monitor and support BP. |
| | neostigmine | ↓HR + ↓BP | Monitor and support cardiovascular status.<br>Use atropine. |
| | inhalation anesthetics | ↓HR, ↓BP; asystole | Monitor and support cardiovascular status. |
| Bretylium | inhalation anesthetics | Increased potential for ↓BP due to blunting of compensatory cardiovascular reflexes | Monitor and support cardiovascular status. |
| | d-tubocurarine | ↑NMR | Monitor and support neuromuscular blockade.<br>Monitor and support respiration. |
| Calcium channel blockers | inhalation anesthetics | Increased potential for cardiovascular depression, resulting in ↓BP, ↓HR, asystole | Monitor and support cardiovascular status. |

| Preop Drug Or Drug Class | Anesthetic Drug Or Drug Class | Interaction | Clinical Management |
|---|---|---|---|
| Carbamazepine | non-depolarizing muscle relaxants (NMR) | ↓NMR | Monitor neuromuscular blockade. Titrate dosage. |
| | diltiazem; verapamil | ↑carbamazepine levels → CNS toxicity | Monitor for neuromuscular disorders. |
| Chlorpropamide | barbiturates | ↑barbiturate activity | Monitor for CNS depression. |
| Cimetidine | lidocaine | ↑lidocaine toxicity | Use alternative $H_2$-antagonist. |
| | narcotic analgesics | ↑narcotic effects | Monitor for CNS depression. |
| | succinylcholine | ↑neuromuscular blockade (NMR) | Monitor neuromuscular blockade. Titrate succinylcholine. |
| Clindamycin & lincomycin | non-depolarizing muscle relaxants (NMR) | ↑↑NMR | **Avoid combination, if possible.** Monitor and support respiration. Anticholinesterases or $Ca^{++}$ may be of benefit. |
| Clonidine | inhalation anesthetics | ↓inhalation anesthetic requirements | Titrate inhalation anesthetic. |
| Corticosteroids | non-depolarizing muscle relaxants (NMR) | ↓, ↑ or no effect on NMR, depending on chronicity of dosing. | Carefully titrate NMR. |
| Cyclophosphamide | succinylcholine | ↓ metabolism → ↑block duration | ↓succinylcholine dosage. |
| Cyclosporine | non-depolarizing muscle relaxants (NMR) | ↑NMR | Monitor neuromuscular blockade and titrate dose. Support respiration. |
| Dantrolene | calcium channel blockers | Can precipitate hyperkalemia and cardiovascular collapse. | **Avoid combination.** |
| Digoxin | pancuronium | Precipitate new dysrhythmias or potentiate existing rhythm disturbances. | Monitor cardiac status. |
| | succinylcholine | Possible precipitation of new dysrhythmias or potentiate existing rhythm disturbances | Monitor cardiac status. |
| Disopyramide | neuromuscular relaxants (NMR) | ↑NMR | Monitor neuromuscular blockade. Consider use of a shorter-acting NMR. |
| Disulfiram | barbiturates | ↑barbiturate activity | Monitor for CNS depression. Titrate dose of barbiturates. |

| Preop Drug Or Drug Class | Anesthetic Drug Or Drug Class | Interaction | Clinical Management |
|---|---|---|---|
| Echothiophate, ophthalmic | succinylcholine | Systemic absorption → ↑↑NMR | **Use with extreme caution.** Titrate NMR dose. |
| Edetate (disodium EDTA) | barbiturates; inhalation anesthetics | Possible potentiation of cardio-depressant effects | Rx ↓BP with $CaCl_2$. |
| | NMR; succinylcholine | Potentiation of neuromuscular blockade ↑NMR; ↑depolarizing block | Titrate dose. Support respiration. |
| Ergotamine | ß-blocker | Severe peripheral vasospasm | **Avoid combination in patients with peripheral vascular disease.** |
| Erythromycin | alfentanil | ↑effect of alfentanil | Consider ↓dose of alfentanil. Monitor and support respiration. |
| | midazolam | ↑CNS depression | Titrate dose of midazolam. |
| Esmolol | succinylcholine | ↑NMR | Monitor neuromuscular blockade. Consider ↓dosage of esmolol. |
| | morphine | ↑ß-blockade | Monitor cardiovascular function. Consider ↓dose of esmolol. |
| Estrogens | succinylcholine | ↑NMR | Monitor neuromuscular blockade. Titrate succinylcholine. |
| Ethanol | alfentanil | Chronic alcohol consumption → pharmacodynamic tolerance to alfentanil. | May need to increase dose of alfentanil. |
| Glycopyrrolate | ketamine | ↑HR | Monitor HR. |
| | non-depolarizing muscle relaxants (NMR) | High doses may ↑NMR. | Monitor neuromuscular blockade. |
| Guanethidine | sympathomimetics | ↑direct-acting sympathomimetics (epinephrine, phenylephrine). ↓indirect-acting sympathomimetics (ephedrine, dopamine). | Use combination with caution. Titrate dosages. |
| Halothane | doxapram | ↑dysrhythmogenicity of halogenated hydrocarbons | Delay administration of doxapram for at least 10 min after discontinuing halothane. |
| Isoniazid | meperidine | ↓BP; ↑CNS depression | **Use combination with caution.** Monitor BP |
| | enflurane | Fast acetylators of INH facilitate defluorination of enflurane → high-output renal failure. | Monitor renal function postop. |

| Preop Drug Or Drug Class | Anesthetic Drug Or Drug Class | Interaction | Clinical Management |
|---|---|---|---|
| Ketamine | halothane | ↓BP + ↓CO | **Use combination with caution.** Monitor BP. |
| | succinylcholine | ↑NMR | Monitor neuromuscular blockade. Titrate dosage of succinylcholine. |
| Labetalol | inhalation anesthetics | ↓↓BP | **Use combination** (especially halothane) **with caution.** Monitor BP. |
| Levodopa | benzodiazepines | Possible antagonism of levodopa | **Avoid combination, if possible.** |
| | droperidol | Dopamine antagonist | **Avoid combination, if possible.** |
| Lidocaine | succinylcholine | ± ↑neuromuscular blockade | Monitor neuromuscular blockade. Titrate dosage of succinylcholine. |
| Lithium | neuromuscular relaxants (NMR) | ↑↑NMR | Titrate dosage of NMR. Monitor neuromuscular blockade. Support respiration. |
| Loop diuretics | non-depolarizing muscle relaxants (NMR) | ↑ or ↓NMR, possibly dosage dependent; $\downarrow K^+ \rightarrow$ ↑NMR | Monitor neuromuscular blockade. Titrate dose of NMR. Support respiration. |
| Magnesium salts, parenteral | non-depolarizing muscle relaxants (NMR) | ↑NMR | Monitor neuromuscular blockade. Titrate dosage of NMR. |
| Mercaptopurine | non-depolarizing muscle relaxants (NMR) | ↓NMR | Monitor neuromuscular blockade. Titrate dose of NMR. |
| Methocarbamol | anticholinesterases | Possible severe muscle weakness | Monitor neuromuscular blockade. Titrate dosage of anticholinesterase. |
| Methyldopa | naloxone | Naloxone may precipitate a mild ↑BP. | Monitor BP. |
| | ephedrine | ↓ephedrine effect | Use alternative pressor agents. |
| Metoclopramide | succinylcholine | ↑NMR | Monitor neuromuscular blockade. Titrate dosage of succinylcholine. |
| Monoamine oxidase inhibitors (MAO) | meperidine | Agitation, seizures, diaphoresis, fever, coma, apnea | **Avoid combination.** |
| Monoamine oxidase inhibitors (MAO) | sympathomimetics (including local anesthetic/epinephrine combinations) | Indirect- or mixed-acting sympathomimetic may cause severe headache, hyperpyrexia, or hypertensive crisis. (Direct-acting sympathomimetics appear to interact minimally.) | **Avoid combination.** Rx ↑BP with phentolamine. |

| Preop Drug Or Drug Class | Anesthetic Drug Or Drug Class | Interaction | Clinical Management |
|---|---|---|---|
| Narcotic analgesics | barbiturate anesthetics | Drug actions may be additive. | Monitor for CNS depression. |
| | propofol | ↓BP | Titrate dosage of propofol. |
| Nifedipine | fentanyl | ↓BP with high doses of fentanyl | Monitor BP.<br>Titrate fentanyl dosage. |
| Nitroglycerin (NTG) | pancuronium | ↑NMR | Monitor and support respiration. |
| Non-depolarizing muscle relaxants (NMR) | inhalation anesthetics | ↑NMR | Titrate dose of NMR.<br>Monitor neuromuscular blockade. |
| | ketamine | ↑NMR | Titrate dose of NMR.<br>Monitor neuromuscular blockade. |
| Oxytocic drugs (oxytocin, ergotamine, methylergonovine) | sympathomimetics | ↑BP 2° synergistic and additive vasoconstrictive effect | Monitor BP.<br>Titrate dosage. |
| Papaverine | droperidol, physostigmine | Possible development of Parkinsonian syndrome | **Avoid combination.** |
| Phenothiazines | narcotic analgesics | ↓analgesic effects | Titrate narcotic to analgesic effect. |
| | phenylephrine | ↓α-adrenergic effects | Use an alternative pressor agent. |
| Phenoxybenzamine | local anesthetics | ↑absorption of local anesthetics | Add epinephrine or other vasoconstrictor to local anesthetic. |
| Phenytoin | dopamine | ↓↓BP; cardiac arrest | **Use combination with extreme caution.**<br>Discontinue phenytoin infusion if ↓BP develops. |
| | inhalation anesthetics | Potentiation of inhalation anesthetics | Titrate dosage of inhalation anesthetics. |
| | non-depolarizing muscle relaxants (NMR) | Antagonism of NMR. Phenytoin alters pancuronium metabolism by enzyme induction, and has prejunctional effects similar to NMR. Atracurium not affected by phenytoin. | Increased dosage of NMR may be required.<br>Monitor neuromuscular function. |
| Probenecid | thiopental | ↑CNS depression | Titrate dosage of thiopental. |
| Procaine, procainamide | succinylcholine | ↑neuromuscular blockade 2° competition for pseudocholinesterases | Monitor neuromuscular blockade. |

| Preop Drug Or Drug Class | Anesthetic Drug Or Drug Class | Interaction | Clinical Management |
|---|---|---|---|
| Propofol | sedative/hypnotics inhalation anesthetics | ↑NMR | Titrate dose of NMR. Monitor neuromuscular blockade. |
| | succinylcholine | ↓↓HR | Consider atropine premed when propofol precedes succinylcholine. |
| Quinine, quinidine | non-depolarizing muscle relaxants (NMR) | ↑NMR | Titrate dosage of NMR. Monitor neuromuscular blockade. |
| | succinylcholine | ↑neuromuscular blockade 2° metabolism of succinylcholine | **Use this combination with caution.** |
| Ranitidine | non-depolarizing muscle relaxants (NMR) | Possible resistance to NMR | ↑dosage of NMR; if unsuccessful, use different NMR. |
| Rauwolfia alkaloids | sympathomimetics | ↑direct-acting sympathomimetics; ↓indirect-acting agents | Monitor BP. Titrate dosage. |
| | inhalation anesthetics | ↓inhalation anesthetic requirements; ↑CNS depressant effects; ↓BP. | Monitor CNS status. Monitor cardiovascular status. |
| Scopolamine | neuromuscular relaxants (NMR) | High doses of scopolamine may ↑NMR. | Monitor neuromuscular blockade. |
| | ketamine | ↑HR | Monitor HR. |
| Succinylcholine | anticholinesterases | ↑NMR | **Use combination with caution.** Monitor neuromuscular blockade. |
| Sympathomimetic amines | doxapram | Potentiation of sympathomimetic amines | Monitor cardiovascular and CNS status. |
| Theophylline | halothane | ↑catecholamine-induced dysrhythmias | Use an alternative inhalation agent. |
| | ketamine | Seizures | **Use combination with caution.** |
| | non-depolarizing muscle relaxants (NMR) | ↓NMR | May need ↑dosage of NMR. |
| | narcotic analgesic | ↑narcotic effects | Titrate narcotic. |
| Thiazide diuretics | non-depolarizing muscle relaxants (NMR) | ↑NMR (may be 2° ↓$K^+$) | Correct hypokalemia. Titrate NMR. |

| Preop Drug Or Drug Class | Anesthetic Drug Or Drug Class | Interaction | Clinical Management |
|---|---|---|---|
| Thiotepa | pancuronium | ↑NMR | Monitor neuromuscular block. |
| Tricyclic antidepressants (TCA) | sympathomimetics | ↑direct-acting sympathomimetics; ↓indirect-acting agents | Monitor for ↑BP and dysrhythmias. Titrate dosage. |
| | anticholinesterases | Anticholinergic effects of TCA may ↓anticholinesterase effect. | Titrate dose of anticholinesterase. |
| | halothane, pancuronium | ↑dysrhythmia | Monitor cardiac status. |
| Trimethaphan | non-depolarizing muscle relaxants (NMR) | ↑NMR | Monitor neuromuscular blockade. Titrate dosage of NMR. |
| Vancomycin | non-depolarizing muscle relaxants (NMR) | ↑NMR | Monitor neuromuscular blockade. Titrate dose of NMR. |
| Verapamil | etomidate | ↑respiratory depression; apnea | Monitor and support respiratory function. |
| | non-depolarizing muscle relaxants (NMR) | ↑NMR | ↓dosage of NMR. |

# DRUGS COMMONLY USED IN ANESTHETIC MANAGEMENT

| Usage | Generic Name | Commonly Used Brand Names |
|---|---|---|
| Premedication | diazepam<br>hydroxyzine<br>lorazepam<br>fentanyl citrate<br>midazolam hydrochloride<br>morphine sulfate<br>scopolamine<br>atropine sulfate | Valium®<br>Atarax®; Vistaril®<br>Ativan®<br>Sublimaze®<br>Versed®<br>Hyoscine; Transderm Scop® |
| Induction | propofol<br>etomidate<br>thiopental sodium<br>methohexital sodium<br>halothane | Diprivan®<br>Amidate®<br>Pentothal® sodium<br>Brevital® sodium<br>Fluothane® |
| Muscle relaxants | atracurium besylate<br>mivacurium<br>pancuronium bromide<br>pipecuronium<br>succinylcholine chloride<br>*d*-tubocurarine chloride<br>vecuronium bromide | Tracrium®<br>Mivacron®<br>Pavulon®<br>Arduan®<br>Anectine®<br><br>Norcuron® |
| Anesthetic maintenance | isoflurane<br>desflurane | Forane®<br>Suprane® |
| Intravenous agents | sufentanil citrate<br>fentanyl citrate<br>meperidine hydrochloride<br>propofol<br>ketamine hydrochloride | Sufenta®<br>Sublimaze®<br>Demerol®<br>Diprivan®<br>Ketaject®; Ketalar® |
| Muscle relaxant reversal agents | edrophonium chloride<br>neostigmine<br>glycopyrrolate | Enlon®, Reversol®, Tensilon®<br>Prostigmin®<br>Robinul® |
| Nausea prophylaxis | droperidol<br>metoclopramide hydrochloride<br>ondansetron | Inapsine®<br>Reglan®<br>Zofran® |
| Drugs for full-stomach precautions | ranitidine<br>metoclopramide<br>sodium citrate | Zantac®<br>Reglan®<br>Bicitra® |
| Local anesthetics - epidural | bupivacaine<br>lidocaine<br>chloroprocaine | Marcaine®; Sensorcaine®<br>Xylocaine®<br>Nesacaine® |
| Local anesthetics - spinal | bupivacaine<br>lidocaine<br>tetracaine | Marcaine® Spinal<br>Xylocaine®<br>Pontocaine® |
| Local anesthetics - regional | lidocaine<br>bupivacaine hydrochloride<br>etidocaine<br>mepivAcaine | Xylocaine®<br>Marcaine®<br>Duranest®<br>Carbocaine® |

# ABBREVIATIONS AND ACRONYMS

**hr(s):** hour(s)
**min:** minute(s)
**mo:** month(s)
**sec:** second(s)
**yr(s):** year(s)

**Bx:** biopsy
**D/C:** discontinue
**Dx:** diagnosis
**Hx:** history
**im:** intramuscular
**iv:** intravenous
**IV:** intravenous

**npo:** nothing by mouth
**po:** by mouth
**pr:** per rectum
**prn:** as needed
**qd:** every day
**qs:** every shift
**R/O:** rule out
**Rx:** treatment
**S/P:** status post
**Sx:** signs and symptoms
**TKO:** to keep open
**Tx:** transplant
**2°:** secondary to

**cc:** cubic centimeters
**dL:** deciliter
**ga:** gauge
**gm:** gram(s)
**kg:** kilogram(s)
**m:** meter(s)
**M:** molar
**mg:** milligram(s)
**ml:** milliliter(s)
**mm:** millimeter(s)
**U:** unit(s)

---

**A-a:** alveolar-arterial
**AAA:** abdominal aortic aneurysm
**ABG:** arterial blood gas
**AC:** anterior cruciate
**ACT:** activated clotting time
**ACTH:** adrenocorticotropic hormone
**ADH:** antidiuretic hormone (vasopressin)
**AF:** atrial fibrillation
**AH:** autonomic hyperreflexia
**A-I:** anterior-inferior
**AICD:** automatic implantable cardiac defibrillator
**ALT:** Alanine amino transferase
**AoE:** aortic enlargement
**AOVM:** angiography occult vascular malformations
**A-P:** anterior-posterior
**AR:** aortic regurgitation
**ARDS:** adult respiratory distress syndrome
**AS:** aortic stenosis
**ASA:** aspirin
**ASD:** atrial septal defect
**AST:** aspirated amino transferase
**AV:** atrioventricular
**AVM:** arteriovenous malformation
**AVR:** aortic valve replacement
**BAEP:** brainstem auditory evoked potential
**BAER:** brainstem auditory evoked response
**BB:** bronchial block
**BMR:** basal metabolic rate
**BP:** blood pressure
**BPD:** bronchopulmonary dysplasia
**BPF:** bronchopleural fistula
**bpm:** beats per minute
**BSA:** body surface area
**BSO:** bilateral salpingo-oophorectomy
**BUN:** blood urea nitrogen
**C-section:** cesarean section
**CABG:** coronary artery bypass graft(ing)
**CAD:** coronary artery disease
**CAJ:** cricoarytenoid joint
**CBC:** complete blood count
**CBF:** cerebral blood flow
**CCU:** coronary care unit
**CEA:** carotid endarterectomy
**CHD:** congestive heart disease
**CHF:** congestive heart failure
**CI:** cardiac index
**CMC:** carpometacarpal (joint)
**$CMRO_2$:** cerebral $O_2$ consumption
**CNS:** central nervous system
**CO:** cardiac output
**CoA:** coarctation of aorta
**COPD:** chronic obstructive pulmonary disease
**CPAP:** continuous positive airway pressure
**CPB:** cardiopulmonary bypass
**CPD:** citrate-phosphate-dextrose
**CPK:** creatinine phosphokinase
**CPM:** continuous passive motion
**CPP:** cerebral perfusion pressure
**CPR:** cardiopulmonary resuscitation
**CSF:** cerebrospinal fluid
**CSI:** cranial spinal irradiation
**CT:** computed tomography
**CTS:** carpal tunnel syndrome
**CUSA:** Cavitron ultrasonic aspirator
**CVA:** cerebrovascular accident
**CVP:** central venous pressure
**CXR:** chest x-ray
**D&C:** dilation & curettage
**DBP:** diastolic blood pressure
**DCR:** dacryocystorhinostomy
**DDAVP:** desmopressin acetate
**DHCA:** deep hypothermic cardiac arrest
**DI:** diabetes insipidus
**DIC:** disseminated intravascular coagulation
**DIP:** distal interphalangeal
**DJD:** degenerative joint disease
**DLT:** double lumen tube
**DM:** diabetes mellitus
**DOE:** dyspnea on exertion
**DORV:** double outlet right ventricle
**DPG:** diphosphoglycerate
**DSA:** digital subtraction angiography
**dTC:** d-tubocurarine
**DVT:** deep venous thrombosis
**EA:** esophageal atresia
**EACA:** aminocaprioic acid
**EBL:** estimated blood loss
**EBV:** estimated blood volume
**EC-IC:** extracranial-intracranial
**ECG:** electrocardiogram
**ECMO:** extracorporeal membrane oxygenation
**EDAS:** encephalo-duro-arteriosynangiosis
**EEA:** end-to-end anastomosis
**EF:** ejection fraction
**EJ:** external jugular
**EMG:** electromyogram

**ER:** emergency room
**ERCP:** endoscopic retrograde colangiopancreatography
**ERV:** expiratory reserve volume
**ET:** endotracheal
**$ETCO_2$:** end tidal $CO_2$
**$ETN_2$:** end tidal $N_2$
**ETOH:** alcohol
**ETT:** endotracheal tube
**FAP:** familial adenomatous polyposis
**FDP:** flexor digitorum profundus (tendon)
**FDS:** flexor digitorum superficialis (tendon)
**FDT:** forced duction test
**$FEV_1$:** forced expiratory volume (in 1 sec)
**FFP:** fresh frozen plasma
**FHR:** fetal heart rate
**FIGO:** International Federation of Gynecologists & Obstetrics
**$FiO_2$:** fraction of inspired oxygen
**FOB:** fiber optic bronchoscopy
**FOL:** fiber optic laryngoscopy
**FRC:** functional residual capacity
**FSP:** fibrin-split products
**FTSG:** full-thickness skin graft
**FVC:** forced vital capacity
**GA:** general anesthesia
**GCS:** Glasgow coma scale
**GETA:** general endotracheal anesthesia
**GFR:** glomerular filtration rate
**GI:** gastrointestinal
**GIA:** gastrointestinal anastomosis
**GNRH:** gonadotropin-releasing hormone
**GU:** genitourinary
**H&P:** history and physical examination
**Hb:** hemoglobin
**Hb/Hct:** hemoglobin/hematocrit
**HbA:** adult hemoglobin
**HbF:** fetal hemoglobin
**HCG:** human chorionic gonadotropin
**Hct:** hematocrit
**HELLP:** hemolysis, elevated liver enzymes and low-platelet count
**HFV:** high-frequency ventilation
**Hg:** mercury
**HIV:** human immune deficiency (virus)
**HLHS:** hypoplastic left heart (syndrome)
**HPV:** hypoxic pulmonary vasoconstrictive (reflex)
**HR:** heart rate
**HSV:** highly selective vagotomy
**HTN:** hypertension
**HVA:** homovanillic acid
**IABP:** intra-aortic balloon pump
**IC:** inspiratory capacity
**ICN:** intensive care nursery
**ICP:** intracranial pressure
**ICU:** intensive care unit
**IHSS:** idiopathic hypertrophic subaortic stenosis
**IJ:** internal jugular (vein)
**IMA:** internal mammary artery
**IMF:** intermaxillary fixation
**IOP:** intraocular pressure
**IORT:** intraoperative radiation therapy
**IPPV:** intermittent positive pressure ventilation
**ISS:** injury severity score
**IT:** iliotibial
**IVC:** inferior vena cava
**IVH:** intraventricular hemorrhage
**JVD:** jugular venous distention
**K:** potassium
**KTP:** potassium, titanium, phosphate
**LA:** left atrium
**LAD:** left anterior descending
**LEEP:** loop electrosurgical excision procedure
**LFT:** liver function test
**LH-RH:** luteinizing hormone-releasing hormone
**LHSV:** laparoscopic highly selective vagotomy
**LIMA:** left internal mammary artery
**LLETZ:** large loop excision of transitional zone
**LMP:** last menstrual period
**LR:** lactated Ringer's
**LRD:** living-related donor
**LTA:** lidocaine topical spray
**LV:** left ventricle (ventricular)
**LVAD:** left ventricular assist device
**LVEDP:** left ventricular end diastolic pressure
**LVH:** left ventricular hypertrophy
**LVOT:** left ventricular outflow tract
**LVOTO:** left ventricular outflow tract obstruction
**MAC:** maintained anesthesia care
**MAP:** mean arterial pressure
**MCA:** middle cerebral artery
**MEA:** multiple endocrine adenopathy
**mEq:** milliequivalent
**MH:** malignant hypothermia
**MI:** myocardial infarction
**MIF:** maximum inspiratory force
**MMEF:** maximum mid-expiratory force
**MS:** mitral stenosis
**MUGA:** multi-unit gated acquisition (scan)
**MV:** minute ventilation
**MVD:** microvascular decompression
**$MVO_2$:** mixed venous oxygen content
**N&V:** nausea & vomiting
**NB:** note well
**NEC:** necrotizing enterocolitis
**NG:** nasogastric tube
**NIBP:** non-invasive blood pressure
**NICU:** neonatal intensive care unit
**NLD:** nasolacrimal duct
**NO:** nitrous oxide
**NS:** normal saline (solution)
**NSAID:** non-steroid anti-inflammatory drug(s)
**NS/LR:** normal saline/lactated Ringer's solution
**NSR:** normal sinus rhythm
**NTG:** nitroglycerine
**NTP:** nitroprusside
**$N_2O$:** nitrous oxide
**OA:** osteoarthritis
**OCR:** oculocardiac reflex
**OG:** orogastric (tube)
**OLT:** orthotopic liver transplant
**OLV:** one-lung ventilation
**OPLL:** ossification of the posterior longitudinal ligament
**OR:** operating room
**ORIF:** open reduction and internal fixation
**OSA:** obstructive sleep apnea
**$O_2$:** oxygen
**PA:** pulmonary artery
**PACU:** post-anesthesia care unit
**$PaCO_2$:** partial pressure of $CO_2$ (arterials)
**PAD:** pulmonary artery diastolic
**PADP:** pulmonary artery diastolic pressure
**$PaO_2$:** partial pressure of oxygen (arterials)
**PAR:** post-anesthesia room
**PAWP:** pulmonary artery wedge pressure
**PCA:** patient controlled analgesia
**PCL:** posterior cruciate lateral
**PCWP:** pulmonary capillary wedge pressure
**PDA:** patent ductus arteriosus
**PDPH:** post-dural puncture headache

**PE:** pulmonary embolus
**PEEP:** positive end-expiratory pressure breathing
**PETCO$_2$:** end-tidal $CO_2$ partial pressure
**PFO:** patent foramen ovale
**PFTs:** pulmonary function test(s)
**PGE:** prostaglandin E
**PICU:** pediatric intensive care unit
**PID:** pelvic inflammatory disease
**PIH:** pregnancy-induced hypertension
**PIP:** peak inspiratory pressure
**PND:** paroxysmal nocturnal dyspnea
**POC:** product of conception
**PPV:** positive pressure ventilation
**PRBC:** packed red blood cells
**PT:** prothrombin time
**PTCA:** percutaneous transluminal coronary angioplasty
**PTM:** posterior tibial lengthening
**PTT:** partial thromboplastin time
**PVD:** peripheral vascular disease
**PVR:** pulmonary vascular resistance
**QRS:** QRS complex of ECG
**RA:** radial artery
**RBBB:** right bundle branch block
**RBC:** red blood cell
**RCA:** right coronary artery
**RDS:** respiratory distress syndrome
**RF:** regurgitant factor
**RFT:** renal function test
**RIND:** reversible ischemic neurological deficit
**RLQ:** right lower quadrant
**ROM:** range of motion
**ROP:** retinopathy of prematurity
**RR:** respiratory rate
**RSD:** reflux sympathetic dystrophy
**RTI:** respiratory tract infection
**RV:** right ventricle
**RVEDP:** right ventricular end diastolic pressure
**RVESV:** right ventricular end systolic volume
**RVH:** right ventricular hypertrophy
**RVOT:** right ventricular outflow tract
**RVOTO:** right ventricular outflow tract obstruction
**SA:** sinoatrial (node)
**SAB:** spontaneous abortion
**SAM:** systolic anterior motion
**SBP:** systolic blood pressure
**SCD:** sequential compression device
**SGOT:** liver enzyme
**SGPT:** liver enzyme
**SI:** sacroiliac
**SIADH:** syndrome of inappropriate antidiuretic hormone
**SMV:** superior mesenteric vein
**SNP:** sodium nitroprusside
**SOB:** short of breath
**SpO$_2$:** oxygen saturation measured by pulse oximetry
**SSEP:** somatosensory evoked potential
**SSS:** sick sinus syndrome
**STA:** superficial temporal artery
**STP:** sodium thiopental
**STSG:** split-thickness skin graft
**SVC:** superior vena cava
**SVR:** systemic vascular resistance
**SVT:** supraventricular tachycardia
**T/A:** tonsillectomy/adenoidectomy
**TAH:** total abdominal hysterectomy
**T&C:** type and cross-match
**TAPVC:** total anomalous pulmonary venous connection
**TB:** tuberculosis
**TBSA:** total body surface area
**TE:** tangential excision
**TEA:** thromboendarterectomy
**TEC:** (Larson)
**TEE:** transesophageal echocardiogram(graphy)
**TEF:** tracheoesophageal fistula
**TEG:** thromboelestograph
**TGA:** transposition of great arteries
**TIA:** transient ischemic attack
**TMJ:** temporomandibular joint
**TMJD:** temporomandibular joint dysfunction
**TOF:** Tetralogy of Fallot
**TPN:** total parenteral nutrition
**TR:** tricuspid regurgitation
**TSH:** thyroid-stimulating hormone
**TUR:** transurethral resection
**TURP:** transurethral resection of the prostate
**TV:** tidal volume
**TWR:** total wrist replacement
**UA:** urinalysis
**U/O:** urine output
**URTI:** upper respiratory tract infection
**UTI:** urinary tract infection
**VA:** ventriculoatrial
**VAE:** venous air embolism
**VC:** vital capacity
**VF:** ventricular fibrillation
**VO$_2$:** oxygen consumption
**VP:** ventriculoperitoneal
**V/Q:** ventilation-perfusion
**VSD:** ventricular septal defect
**VT:** ventricular tachycardia
**WBC:** white blood cell
**XRT:** x-ray therapy

# SUBJECT INDEX

Note: Page numbers appearing in bold refer to figures.